Thomson's

Special Veterinary Pathology

EDITION 3

Thomson's

Special Veterinary Pathology

M. Donald McGavin, MVSc, PhD, FACVSc
Diplomate, American College of Veterinary Pathologists;
Professor, Department of Pathology, College of Veterinary Medicine,
University of Tennessee, Knoxville, Tennessee

William W. Carlton, DVM, PhD, DSc (Hon)
Diplomate, American College of Veterinary Pathologists; Leslie Morton
Hutchings Distinguished Professor Emeritus of Veterinary Pathology,
Department of Veterinary Pathobiology, School of Veterinary Medicine,
Purdue University, West Lafayette, Indiana

James F. Zachary, DVM, PhD
Diplomate, American College of Veterinary Pathologists;
Professor of Veterinary Pathology, Department of Veterinary Pathobiology,
College of Veterinary Medicine, University of Illinois,
Urbana, Illinois

Mosby
A Harcourt Health Sciences Company
St. Louis London Philadelphia Sydney Toronto

Mosby
A Harcourt Health Sciences Company

Editor-in-Chief John A. Schrefer
Editorial Manager Linda L. Duncan
Developmental Editor Teri Merchant
Project Manager Carol Sullivan Weis
Production Editor Florence Achenbach
Designer Mark A. Oberkrom
Cover Art Photographs courtesy M. Donald McGavin, Mark Kuhlenschmidt, Joanne Messick, Howard Gelberg, James Zachary

THIRD EDITION

Mosby, Inc.
A Harcourt Health Sciences Company
11830 Westline Industrial Drive
St. Louis, Missouri 63146

Printed in the United States of America

Library of Congress Cataloging-in-Publication Data

Thomson, R. G. (Reginald G.)
Thomson's special veterinary pathology / [edited by] M. Donald McGavin, William W. Carlton, James F. Zachary.—3rd ed.
p. cm.
Includes bibliographical references (p.)
ISBN 0-323-00560-8 (hc.)
1. Veterinary pathology. I. Title: Special veterinary pathology. II. McGavin, M. Donald. III. Carlton, William W. IV. Zachary, James F. V. Title.
SF769.T464 2000
636.089'607—dc21

00-056224

01 02 03 04 05 GW/MV 9 8 7 6 5 4 3 2

Contributors

Helen M. Acland, BVSc
Diplomate, American College of Veterinary Pathologists; Veterinary Pathologist, Pennsylvania Veterinary Laboratory, Harrisburg, Pennsylvania

Charles C. Capen, DVM, MSc, PhD
Diplomate, American College of Veterinary Pathologists; Professor and Chairman, Department of Veterinary Biosciences, College of Veterinary Medicine; Professor of Endocrinology, Department of Internal Medicine, College of Medicine and Public Health,The Ohio State University, Columbus, Ohio

William W. Carlton, DVM, PhD, DSc (Hon)
Diplomate, American College of Veterinary Pathologists; Leslie Morton Hutchings Distinguished Professor Emeritus of Veterinary Pathology, Department of Veterinary Pathobiology, School of Veterinary Medicine, Purdue University, West Lafayette, Indiana

Anthony W. Confer, DVM, MS, PhD
Diplomate, American College of Veterinary Pathologists; Associate Dean for Research and Graduate Education, Endowed Chair for Food Animal Research, and Professor of Pathology, Department of Veterinary Pathobiology, College of Veterinary Medicine, Oklahoma State University, Stillwater, Oklahoma

John M. Cullen, VMD, PhD
Diplomate, American College of Veterinary Pathologists; Professor of Pathology, Department of Microbiology, Pathology, and Parasitology, College of Veterinary Medicine, North Carolina State University, Raleigh, North Carolina

†Cecil E. Doige, DVM, PhD
Western College of Veterinary Medicine, University of Saskatchewan, Saskatoon, Saskatchewan

Victor J. Ferrans, MD, PhD
Diplomate, American College of Veterinary Pathologists; Senior Research Scientist, Pathology Branch, National Heart, Lung, and Blood Institute, National Institutes of Health, Bethesda, Maryland

Howard B. Gelberg, DVM, PhD
Diplomate, American College of Veterinary Pathologists; Associate Dean for Research and Professor of Pathology, College of Veterinary Medicine, University of Illinois, Urbana, Illinois

Pamela E. Ginn, DVM
Diplomate, American College of Veterinary Pathologists; Associate Professor and Chief of Surgical Pathology, College of Veterinary Medicine, University of Florida, Gainesville, Florida

Ann M. Hargis, DVM, MS
Diplomate, American College of Veterinary Pathologists; Owner, DermatoDiagnostics, Edmonds, Washington; Affiliate Associate Professor, Department of Comparative Medicine, University of Washington School of Medicine, Seattle, Washington; Consultant, Phoenix Central Laboratory, Everett, Washington

Alfonso López, MVZ, MSc, PhD
Professor, Department of Pathology and Microbiology, Atlantic Veterinary College, University of Prince Edward Island, Charlottetown, Prince Edward Island

N. James MacLachlan, BVSc, MS, PhD
Diplomate, American College of Veterinary Pathologists; Professor and Chair, Department of Pathology, Microbiology, and Immunology, School of Veterinary Medicine, University of California, Davis, California

M. Donald McGavin, MVSc, PhD, FACVSc
Diplomate, American College of Veterinary Pathologists; Professor, Department of Pathology, College of Veterinary Medicine, University of Tennessee, Knoxville, Tennessee

Donald L. Montgomery, DVM, PhD
Diplomate, American College of Veterinary Pathologists; Head, Diagnostic Pathology, Texas Veterinary Medical Diagnostic Laboratory, Amarillo, Texas

Roger J. Panciera, DVM, MS, PhD
Diplomate, American College of Veterinary Pathologists; Professor, Department of Pathobiology, College of Veterinary Medicine, Oklahoma State University, Stillwater, Oklahoma

†Deceased.

James A. Render, DVM, PhD
Diplomate, American College of Veterinary Pathologists; Senior Pathologist, Pfizer Global Research and Development, Groton Laboratories, Groton, Connecticut

Gene P. Searcy, DVM, MSc, PhD
Diplomate, American College of Veterinary Pathologists; Professor, Department of Pathology, Western College of Veterinary Medicine, University of Saskatchewan, Saskatoon, Saskatchewan

Ralph W. Storts, DVM, PhD
Diplomate, American College of Veterinary Pathologists; Professor of Veterinary Pathology, Department of Veterinary Pathobiology, College of Veterinary Medicine, Texas A&M University, College Station, Texas

Beth A. Valentine, DVM, PhD
Diplomate, American College of Veterinary Pathologists; Assistant Professor, Department of Biomedical Sciences, College of Veterinary Medicine, Oregon State University, Corvallis, Oregon

John F. Van Vleet, DVM, PhD
Diplomate, American College of Veterinary Pathologists; Associate Dean for Academic Affairs and Professor of Veterinary Pathology, School of Veterinary Medicine, Purdue University, West Lafayette, Indiana

Steven E. Weisbrode, VMD, PhD
Diplomate, American College of Veterinary Pathologists; Professor, Department of Veterinary Biosciences, College of Veterinary Medicine, The Ohio State University, Columbus, Ohio

Preface

The third edition of *Thomson's Special Veterinary Pathology* has been revised with the same goals in mind that guided the first two editions: to provide the undergraduate student with a textbook comprehensive enough to meet every need in veterinary pathology. All chapters have been thoroughly updated, but the alimentary, endocrine, nervous, reproductive, and eye and ear chapters have been completely rewritten and the muscle chapter extensively revised. Well over 100 new illustrations have been added to augment text discussions and to achieve greater quality throughout.

In addition to the inclusion of new discussions and illustrations, another goal of this revision was to increase the lucidity of the text. Although all chapters do not have a standardized style, we have attempted to accentuate the role of pathogenesis and to use it as a basis of understanding of the sequence for the development of gross and microscopic changes. Also, we have attempted to continue to use standardized nomenclatures: Nomina Anatomica Veterinaria (NAV) for anatomical structures and the most current bacteriological terminology. The names of some bacteria have changed several times in the last decade; we have used the most recent name and placed the better known older term in parentheses on the initial use of the name of the organism. However, since these chapters went to press, the name change of *Pasteurella haemolytica* to *Mannheimia haemolytica* has been approved.

The editors have many persons to thank for help and support. First, we thank our contributing authors for their considerable efforts to achieve comprehensive and logical text suitable for veterinary students and to include information valuable to veterinary practitioners. Appreciation also goes to the secretarial staffs in our respective universities—Colleen Smith at the University of Tennessee and Carolyn Arnold and Jennifer Frazier at Purdue University. We appreciate the efforts and support of Linda Duncan, Editorial Manager, Harcourt, in helping to produce a quality product. Again we would extend our appreciation to our wives, Beverley McGavin and Jeanne Carlton, for their support and patience.

Although every effort is made to avoid errors, inevitably some occur, and we have been grateful to our colleagues who have alerted us to them in the past. We hope that readers will continue to refer any errors to us either by mail or by e-mail at mmcgavin@utk.edu or zacharyj@staff.uiuc.edu.

M. Donald McGavin
William W. Carlton
James F. Zachary

Contents

CHAPTER 7

The Hemopoietic System 325

GENE P. SEARCY

CHAPTER 8

The Nervous System 381

RALPH W. STORTS AND DONALD L. MONTGOMERY

CHAPTER 9

Muscle 461

M. DONALD MCGAVIN AND BETH A. VALENTINE

CHAPTER 10

Bone and Joints 499

STEVEN E. WEISBRODE AND CECIL E. DOIGE†

†Deceased.

CHAPTER 11

Integumentary System 537

ANN M. HARGIS AND PAMELA E. GINN

CHAPTER 12

Reproductive System: Female 601

HELEN M. ACLAND

CHAPTER 13

Reproductive System: Male 635

HELEN M. ACLAND

CHAPTER 14

The Eye and Ear 653

JAMES A. RENDER AND WILLIAM W. CARLTON

CHAPTER 1

Alimentary System

Howard B. Gelberg

The alimentary system is a long and complex tube that varies anatomically and functionally among animal species. For example, herbivores need fermentation chambers (either a rumen or expanded cecum) for the digestion of cellulose, a feature not present in carnivores. Although a large variety of gastrointestinal disturbances are clinically important in all species of animals, the predominant form of disease varies by species. Pet carnivores, partly because of their long life span, effective vaccines, and a lifestyle and diet similar to that of human beings, develop alimentary neoplasia far more often than herbivores. Meat, milk, and fiber-producing animals (ruminants and pigs) are host to a variety of infectious diseases that are largely resistant to vaccines. These pathogens may have evolved as a result of the herding instinct of these animals and the opportunity for pathogens to mutate within a large proximate host population. Equids are most prone to displacements of alimentary viscera.

A large part of the practice of veterinary medicine is devoted to the diagnosis and treatment of alimentary disorders. Many of the newer molecular and imaging tools have been designed specifically to increase the clinician's ability to make accurate diagnoses of the varied conditions of the alimentary system. Additionally, every physical examination includes the opportunity for a fecal analysis that allows the clinician a window into the functioning of the alimentary system as a whole.

Newer tools such as the polymerase chain reaction (PCR) allow the clinician to rapidly diagnose an infectious cause of enteritis without having to culture the organism in the traditional manner. Diagnosis of an infectious cause of disease of the alimentary system can also be made after biopsy from paraffin-embedded tissues by immunohistochemical staining or by in situ hybridization that allows visualization of the pathogen within target cells.

With the advent of fiberoptic endoscopes combined with laparoscopy, a thorough knowledge of normal and abnormal anatomy of the entire alimentary system is of clinical importance in disease diagnosis. This knowledge is now a necessity in clinical practice because gastrointestinal lumens, from the oral mucosa through the esophagus, stomach and duodenum, as well as the large colon, can be directly viewed in the live animal. With a small abdominal incision and insertion of a fiberoptic laparoscope, the entire serosal surface of the abdominal viscera can be viewed and sampled.

The most important point to keep in mind when making these examinations is that normal mucosal and serosal surfaces should be smooth and shiny. When they are not, animals should be examined thoroughly to determine why they deviate from normal.

ORAL CAVITY

Examination and evaluation of the oral cavity is one of the many places where the practice of pathology and clinical medicine meet. That is because the oral cavity can be examined by the clinician or pathologist using the same criteria for abnormality. The same can be said of the rectal mucosa.

The physiologically normal oral mucosa is smooth, shiny, and pink. In animals in which the oral mucosa is heavily pigmented, assessment of circulatory function (capillary refill time) and color as an indicator of red blood cell concentration can be difficult. In these cases, examination of conjunctiva, rectal, and urogenital mucosa can be substituted.

Developmental Anomalies

A variety of developmental abnormalities occur in the oral cavity. Some are incompatible with life unless surgically corrected. Of these congenital lesions, only a few have a proven hereditary component. Most are idiopathic. Thorough physical examination of neonates must include examination of the oral cavity for these defects.

Palatoschisis or cleft palate and **cheiloschisis** or cleft lip are among the most common developmental abnormalities of the oral cavity. Palatoschisis can be genetic or toxic in origin. It results from a failure of fusion of the lateral palatine processes and can be caused by steroid administration during pregnancy in primates, including human beings. Depending on the size of the defect, which can involve only the soft palate or both the soft and hard palates, the lesion can be surgically correctable. Important sequelae to the host are starvation due to an inability to create a negative pressure in the mouth and hence failure to suckle and aspiration

Table 1-1 Vesicular Stomatitides

Disease	Etiology	Ruminant	Pigs	Horses
Foot-and-mouth disease	Picornavirus	+	+	−
Vesicular stomatitis	Rhabdovirus	+	+	+
Vesicular exanthema of swine	Calicivirus	−	+	−
Swine vesicular disease	Enterovirus	−	+	−

+ = Species in which disease occurs.
− = Species in which disease does not occur.

pneumonia, since no effective separation is present between the oral and nasal cavities.

Cheiloschisis is sometimes referred to as "hare lip," since this is a normal feature of the rabbit. It is a failure of fusion of the upper lip along the midline or philtrum.

Stomatitis and Gingivitis

Stomatitis and gingivitis refer to inflammation of the mucous membranes of the oral cavity and gingiva, respectively. Because the oral cavity is constantly bombarded with ingested substances that are moved around by the tongue, the final result of a variety of insults to the lining of the oral cavity is a loss of mucosa—erosions, ulcerations, and necrosis. Thus, although inflammation is apparent, oftentimes clues as to the initiating process are absent. Lesions are classified as macules, papules, vesicles, erosions, and ulcers. These lesions can be caused by infectious agents, particularly viruses, chemical injury, trauma, intoxicants, autoimmune disease, and by systemic diseases. They often result in anorexia due to painful mastication. Hypersalivation (ptyalism) is also apparent. In the cat, gingivitis is the first and most consistent sign of feline immunodeficiency virus infection due to a reduction in CD4 lymphocytes, thymic atrophy, and lymph node atrophy.

Vesicular Stomatitides

The vesicular stomatitides are listed in Table 1-1. They are all viral induced, and all have identical appearances at gross and histopathologic examination. They are characterized in their early stages by vesicles or blisters of the oral mucosa. None are fatal. They produce great economic loss in the affected animals because of poor weight gain and sometimes abortions in gravid females. The exact cause of abortions is unknown but is probably related to the stress induced by the painful oral, cutaneous, and pedal lesions. Secondary bacterial invaders of these lesions can result in endotoxemia. Several diseases, such as foot-and-mouth disease and vesicular exanthema, affect the coronary bands of the digits resulting in lameness. Some of these diseases (foot-and-mouth disease, vesicular exanthema, swine vesicular disease) are exotic to the United States and thus are reportable to state or federal authorities, or both, if suspected by the examining clinician or pathologist. This requirement is due to the great expense involved in eradicating these diseases from the United States. Nontariff export barriers often arise from the presence of infectious agents in livestock that are foreign to countries with which we trade. These restrictions are designed to prevent introduction of highly contagious agents, such as foot-and-mouth disease, into resident animal populations.

The gross lesions begin as small, clear, fluid-filled vesicles of the lips, the buccal mucosa, and the surface and margins of the tongue. These lesions enlarge and coalesce to create bullae, which subsequently break and cause ulcers, exposing irregular patches of red, denuded submucosa. The epithelium covering large bullae can be readily pulled away with forceps or rubbed away with a gloved hand. Similar lesions occur in the nasal mucosa, particularly in pigs with vesicular exanthema, and in the esophagus and rumen of cattle with foot-and-mouth disease. Some animals have conjunctivitis and vesicular dermatitis of the interdigital cleft, coronary band, teats, and vulva. Microscopically, the lesions of these four diseases (foot-and-mouth disease, vesicular stomatitis, vesicular exanthema, and swine vesicular disease) are similar. Each lesion begins as intracellular edema affecting the epithelium, which results in ballooning degeneration of the cells of the stratum spinosum. These swollen cells have eosinophilic or clear, watery cytoplasm and pyknotic nuclei. Cell lysis and intercellular edema also occur. The overlying epithelium serves as a roof for the vesicle, which contains variable amounts of blood and sometimes neutrophils. Vesicles coalesce, producing bullae. Ulceration occurs when the epithelium is abraded or eroded. The denuded surface is coated initially by fibrin or fibrinopurulent exudate and later is covered by granulation tissue that proliferates from subjacent tissues. The hydropic ballooning of epithelial cells of the stratum spinosum is characteristic of the disease.

Clinical signs of the vesicular stomatitides include vesicles, bullae, detached epithelium, raw ulcerated areas on the tongue and lips, salivation, lameness, fever, and anorexia. This sequence of lesions develops as a result of rupture of initially infected cells and centripetal spread of virus to adjacent susceptible epithelium and multiple repeats of this infectious-lytic cycle. The diagnosis is based on characteristic gross and microscopic lesions, species affected, susceptibility of laboratory animal species to experimental inoculation, serology, and virus isolation.

Foot-and-mouth disease is an extremely important disease worldwide but has not appeared in U.S. livestock since 1929, when it was eradicated after an outbreak in California. It is characterized in its early stages by vesicles in the planum nasale, in the oral cavity, and tongue

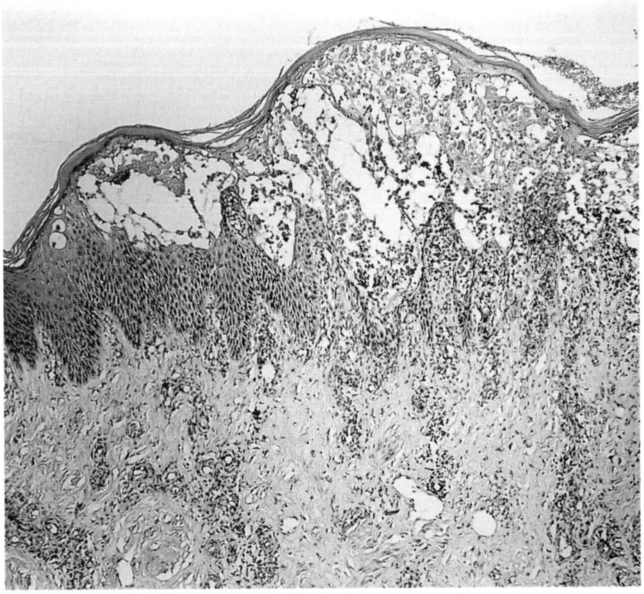

Figure 1-1 Oral mucosa; cow. Foot-and-mouth disease. Vesicles have formed from multiple coalescing foci of hydropic degeneration in the acanthotic epidermis. Hematoxylin-eosin (H & E) stain. *Courtesy Dr. D. Gregg.*

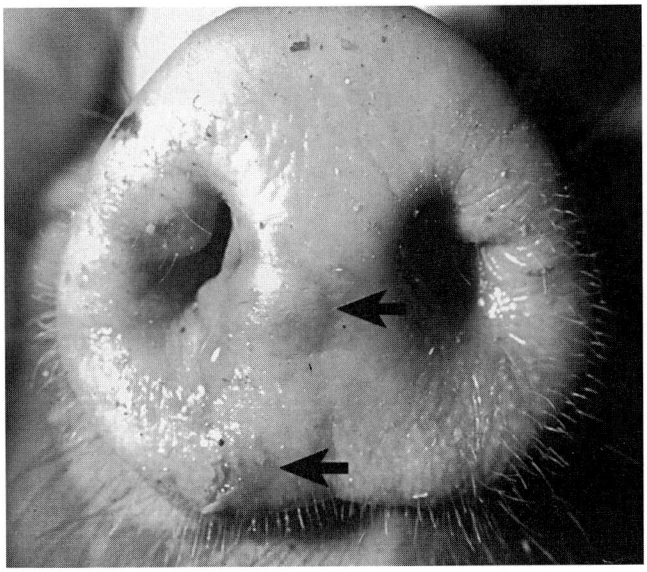

Figure 1-2 Snout; pig. Vesicular exanthema. Vesicles, both intact and ruptured *(arrows)*, are present on the planum nasale. *Gelberg H, Lewis RM. Vet Pathol 1982; 19:424-443.*

(Fig. 1-1). Fluid from ruptured vesicles spreads to areas of abraded skin, for example that of mammary gland. The coronary bands of the hooves can also be affected, which eventually can lead to sloughing of the hoof. Although this is not fatal, the pain and accompanying inappetence lead to weight loss. If allowed to heal, the hoof will regrow into a

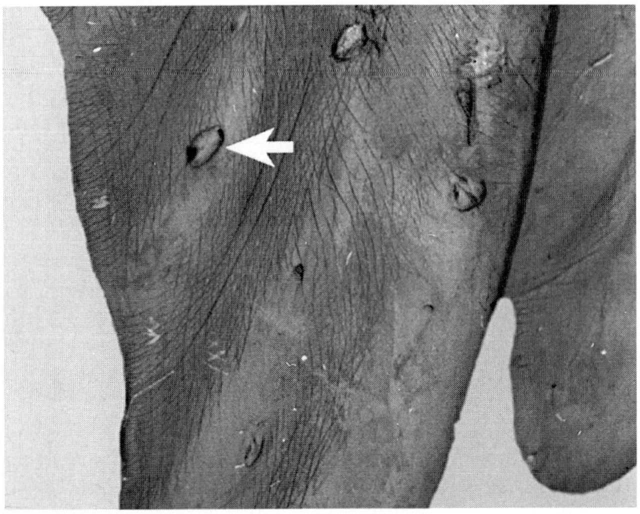

Figure 1-3 Flipper; northern fur seal. San Miguel sea lion virus infection. Vesicles, both intact *(arrow)* and ruptured are present on the non-haired portion of the foreflipper. *Gelberg HB, Dieterich RA, Lewis RM. Vet Pathol 1982; 19:413-423.*

ball-like structure. Young animals with foot-and-mouth disease frequently have a viral myocarditis.

Vesicular stomatitis is common in calves but does not occur in sheep or goats. In northern latitudes, it is generally a warm weather disease suggesting that insects act as vectors. As the name implies, vesicles in the oral cavity characterize the disease. Clinically, the disease is often recognized by inappetence in the affected animal, accompanied by hypersalivation.

Vesicular exanthema is a specific disease of pigs, which is indistinguishable clinically and pathologically from foot-and-mouth disease (Fig. 1-2). This disease was uniquely American and was believed eradicated from pigs in 1956 through enactment of federal laws requiring the cooking of garbage fed to pigs. More recent evidence indicates that vesicular exanthema of swine serovars are variants of San Miguel sea lion virus. This latter marine calicivirus occurs in coastal sea lion and fur seal populations from California to Alaska (Fig. 1-3).

Swine vesicular disease is indistinguishable from the other vesicular diseases and is exotic to the United States.

Erosive and Ulcerative Stomatitides

Erosive and ulcerative stomatitis can have a variety of causes. Erosions are defined by a loss of part of the surface epithelium, whereas ulcers are full-thickness epithelial loss exposing the basement membrane. Agents responsible include the viruses of bovine viral diarrhea, rinderpest, malignant catarrhal fever, feline calicivirus, equine viral rhinotracheitis, and bluetongue. Other causes include

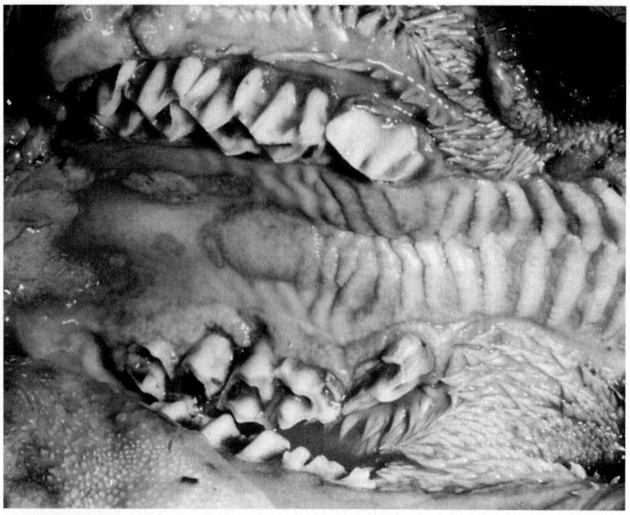

Figure 1-4 Palate; cow. Bovine papular stomatitis. Multiple, oval, plaquelike, depressed macules with hyperemic margins are in the soft and hard palates. *Courtesy Dr. M.D. McGavin.*

uremia and the feline eosinophilic granuloma complex. Oftentimes the oral lesions must be evaluated in the context of the clinical signs, together with histopathologic findings and ancillary testing, to arrive at a definitive diagnosis. Additionally, the vesicular stomatitides can progress, secondary to abrasion, to the point that they cannot be distinguished from the ulcerative stomatitides.

Papular Stomatitides

Parapox viruses cause the papular stomatitides. The two major diseases in this category are zoonotic. **Bovine papular stomatitis** is recognized by papules on the nares, muzzle, gingiva, buccal cavity, palate, and tongue (Fig. 1-4). Lesions also occur in the esophagus (Fig. 1-5), rumen, and omasum. Occasionally, eosinophilic cytoplasmic inclusion bodies are visible microscopically. In human beings, the disease is called milkers' nodules and is characterized by papules of the hands and arms.

Contagious ecthyma, or sore mouth, is a condition of sheep and goats characterized by macules, papules, vesicles, pustules scabs, scars and nodules in areas of skin abrasions including the corners of the mouth (fauces), mouth, udder, teats, coronary bands, and anus (Fig. 1-6). Occasionally, the mucosa of the esophagus and rumen also can be affected. Eosinophilic cytoplasmic inclusion bodies are visible at microscopic examination of lesions early in the course of disease. The condition in human beings is called orf.

Necrotizing Stomatitides

Necrotizing stomatitis occurs in cattle, sheep, and pigs. In cattle, it is sometimes referred to as **calf diphtheria.** Necrotizing stomatitis is characterized by yellow-gray

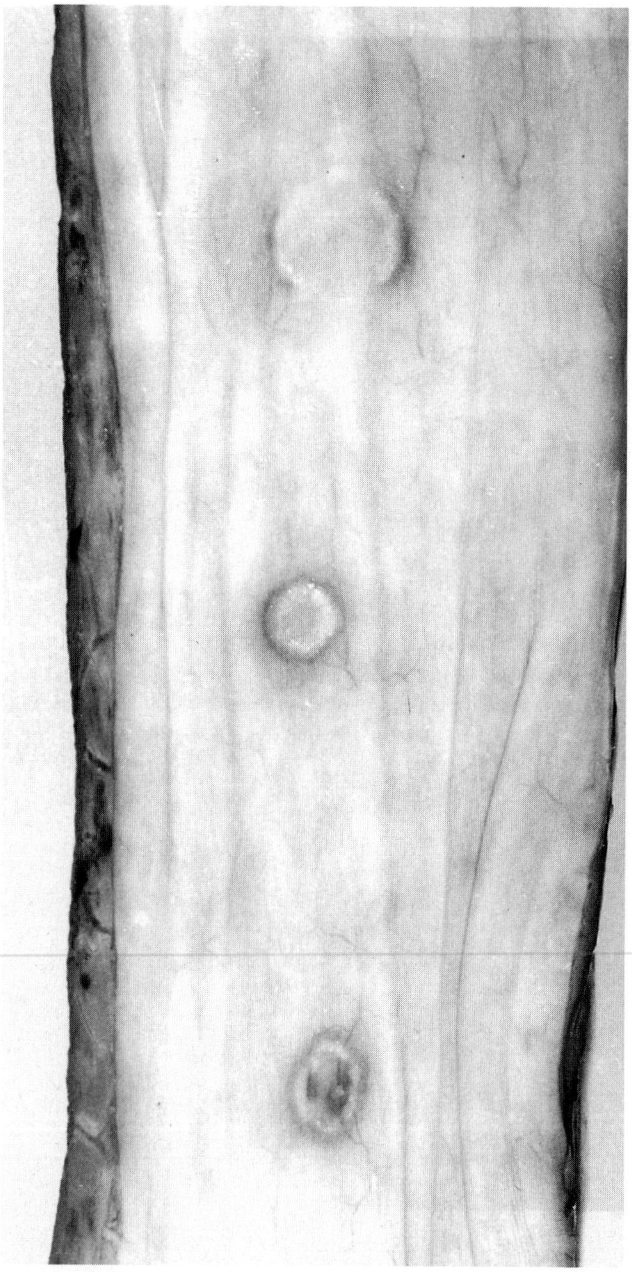

Figure 1-5 Esophagus; cow. Bovine papular stomatitis. Slightly raised and depressed oval lesions with hyperemic margins are in the esophagus. *Courtesy Dr. R.G. Thomson.*

round foci surrounded by a rim of hyperemic tissue in the oral cavity, larynx or pharynx or both. Necrotizing stomatitis is the end stage of all other forms of stomatitis when they are complicated by infection with *Fusobacterium necrophorum,* a gram-negative anaerobe. This organism appears as long, thin filaments, sometimes as rods or cocci, and is very difficult to demonstrate in tissue sections. Animals with oral necrobacillosis have swollen cheeks, anorexia, fever, and a characteristic fetid breath. The gross lesion consists of a raised core of tan-to-gray

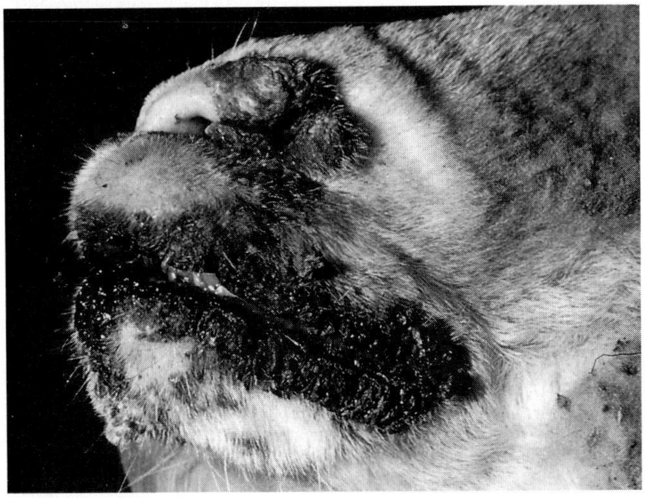

Figure 1-6 Muzzle; lamb. Ovine contagious ecthyma. Lips and external nares are covered with coalesced, blackened crusts. *Courtesy Dr. M.D. McGavin.*

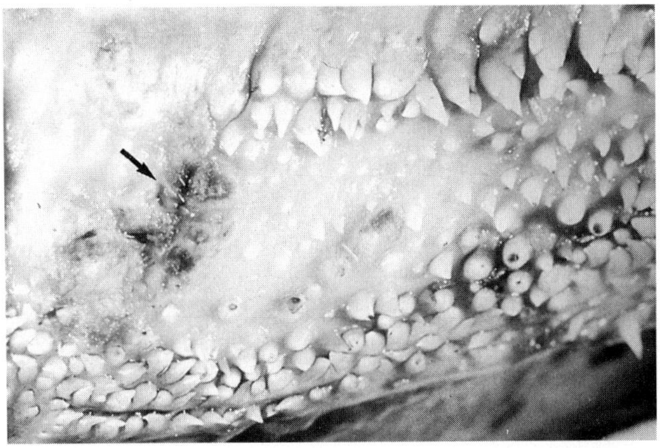

Figure 1-7 Buccal mucosa; calf. Oral necrobacillosis. An irregular, blackened erosion *(arrow)* is in the buccal mucosa. *Courtesy Dr. R.G. Thomson.*

necrotic material, which is readily separated from the adjacent viable crater (Fig. 1-7). Microscopically, the lesion is characterized by coagulation necrosis surrounded by a zone of granulation tissue and hyperemia.

Ulcerative gingivitis, also known as Vincent's gingivitis and trench mouth, is a fusospirochetal disease that affects human beings, chimpanzees, and some other species of nonhuman primates and rarely puppies. The acute inflammation and necrosis characteristic of this infection induce painful gums, a fetid mouth odor,

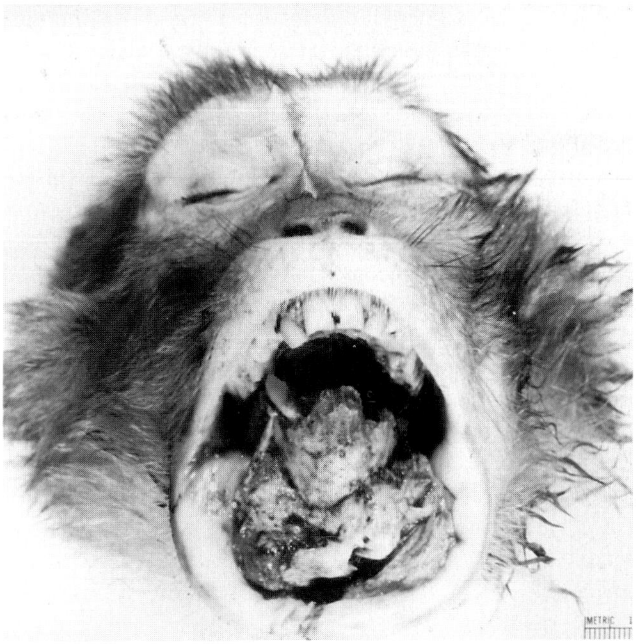

Figure 1-8 Oral mucosa; rhesus monkey. Noma. The mouth contains a mass of necrotic and inflammatory tissue. There has been a loss of lower incisors. *Adams RJ, Bishop JL. Lab Anim Sci 1980; 30:85-91.*

hemorrhages that occur with slight trauma, and increased salivation. Two anaerobes, *Borrelia vincentii,* a spirochete, and *Fusobacterium* spp. cause the disease. These organisms induce disease because of underlying nutritional deficiencies, debilitating conditions, or psychogenic factors. The lesion is an acute, necrotizing inflammation of the gingiva. Punched-out, craterlike ulcers occur in the interdental gingiva and the gingival margin, and are sometimes covered by a gray pseudomembrane. Large numbers of spirochetes and fusiform bacteria are present in smears of the lesions or are recovered by bacteriologic culture.

Noma, or cancrum oris, is an acute gangrenous stomatitis that has been recognized in human beings, rhesus monkeys, cynomolgus monkeys, and dogs. Spirochetes and fusiform bacteria cause this disease, perhaps with participation by other organisms of the mouth. It is similar to necrobacillosis, except the lesions are more severe, progressing to gangrenous perforation of the cheeks, lysis of bone, and death (Fig. 1-8). Spirochetes can be demonstrated in the lesions with a silver stain such as Warthin-Starry.

Eosinophilic Stomatitides

A focal granuloma or ulcer ("rodent ulcer") of oral tissues has been described infrequently in young dogs and more commonly in cats as **oral eosinophilic granuloma.** The cause is not known, but the lesions are suggestive of an immune-mediated mechanism, and similar lesions can be induced in experimental animals by injection of immune complexes. Antiepithelial autoantibodies also can be demonstrated in cats with eosinophilic granulomas. In both dogs and cats, a peripheral eosinophilia occurs in about half to two thirds of cases.

Gross lesions in the cat occur most frequently on the upper lips, particularly the commissure of the lips, but also can develop in the gingiva, palate, pharynx, tongue, or regional lymph nodes. In the Siberian husky, the ventral and lateral surfaces of the tongue and the palatine mucosa have been the sites of lesions (Fig. 1-9). The granuloma also occurs as an irregularly shaped ulcer, 8 to 15 mm in diameter, with a firm, indurated base. Alternatively, the mucosa can be intact and the lesion presents as a firm, granulomatous plaque, whose cut surface is off-white or yellow-white. Microscopically, the base of the ulcer and the granulomatous plaque consist of multiple granulomas. The center of the lesion has foci of collagenolysis. In these lesions, the collagen appears as amorphous or granular eosinophilic material with radiating projections. Eosinophils, mast cells, macrophages, epithelioid cells, and a few multinucleated giant cells surround these lesions. Lesions grouped as the eosinophilic granuloma complex of cats include **linear granulomas** and **eosinophilic plaques.** These lesions are strictly dermatologic lesions and do not affect the oral cavity. No proven etiologic link has been established between these cutaneous conditions and oral eosinophilic granulomas.

Lymphoplasmacytic Stomatitis

Lymphoplasmacytic stomatitis is an idiopathic condition of the cat named on the basis of the histologic appearance of the lesions (Fig. 1-10). It is an idiopathic, chronic condition characterized by red inflamed gums, fetid breath, and inappetence. The oral mucosa can be hyperplastic and ulcerated. The presence of plasma cells in the submucosa suggests an immune-mediated etiology.

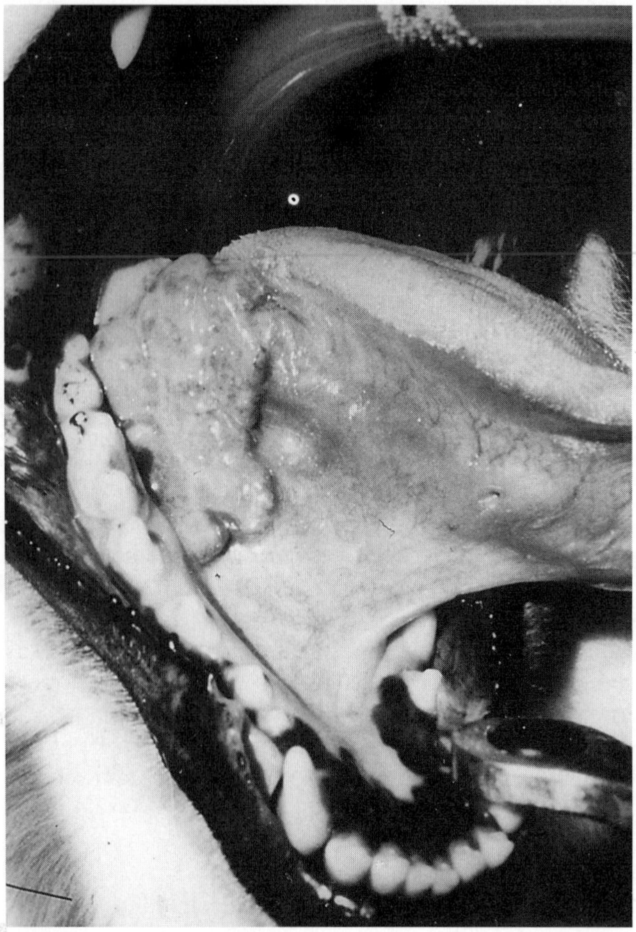

Figure 1-9 Lingual mucosa; dog. Eosinophilic granuloma. An irregular, raised, firm mass protrudes from the mucosa along the lateral margin of the tongue. *Potter, KA, Tucker RD, Carpenter JL. J Am Anim Hosp Assoc 1980; 6:595-600.*

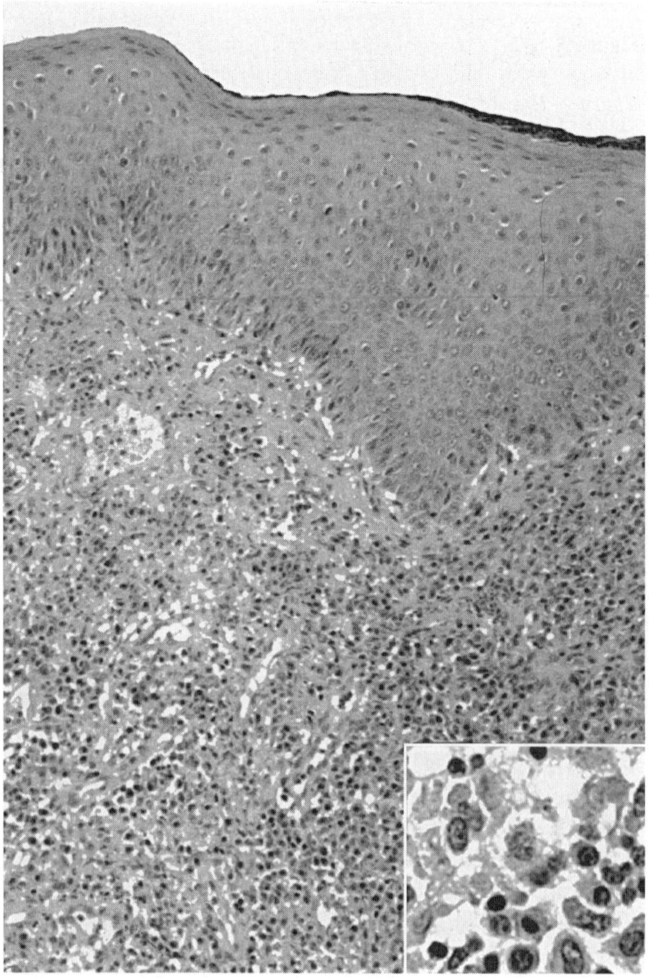

Figure 1-10 Gingiva; cat. Lymphoplasmacytic stomatitis. There is a florid infiltrate of inflammatory cells beneath the epithelium. *Inset:* The inflammatory cells are principally lymphocytes and plasmacytes. H & E stain.

Hyperplasia and Neoplasia

In the dog, 70% of tumors of the alimentary system are in the oral cavity. These tumors run the gamut of biologic behavior from simple epithelial hyperplasia to malignant neoplasms with metastases to distant sites.

Hyperplastic Diseases

Gingival hyperplasia is a simple overgrowth of gum tissues. The hyperplasia can become so severe as to bury incisor teeth (Fig. 1-11). Gingival hyperplasia is most common in brachycephalic dog breeds and is present in 30% of boxer dogs older than 5 years.

Grossly, gingival hyperplasia can be indistinguishable from an **epulis.** Epulis is a nonspecific term that designates a growth of the gingiva. The several kinds of epulides can only be distinguished by histopathologic examination. This distinction is not just an academic exercise because, although all epulides are considered benign, one form, acanthomatous epulis, invades bone and can be quite destructive (Fig. 1-12). Fortunately, this type of epulis can be managed therapeutically. Whether the epulides represent fibrous and epithelial hyperplasia or benign neoplasms of tooth germ is controversial.

Neoplasia

Squamous cell carcinomas occur in the oral cavity, particularly in the aged cat where they account for 60% of oral neoplasia. They generally occur on the ventrolateral surface of the tongue and tonsils (Fig. 1-13). Lingual squamous cell carcinomas are more common in cats, and

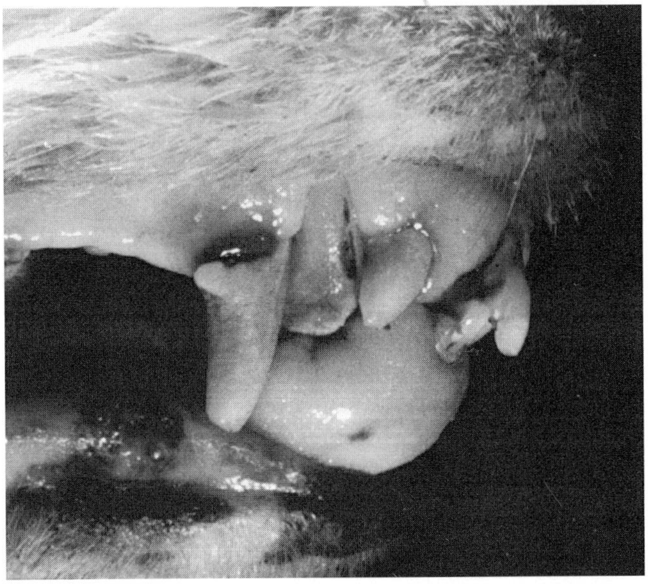

Figure 1-11 Gingiva; dog. Gingival hyperplasia. Hyperplastic gingiva buries some incisor teeth. Dental calculus (tartar) is also present.

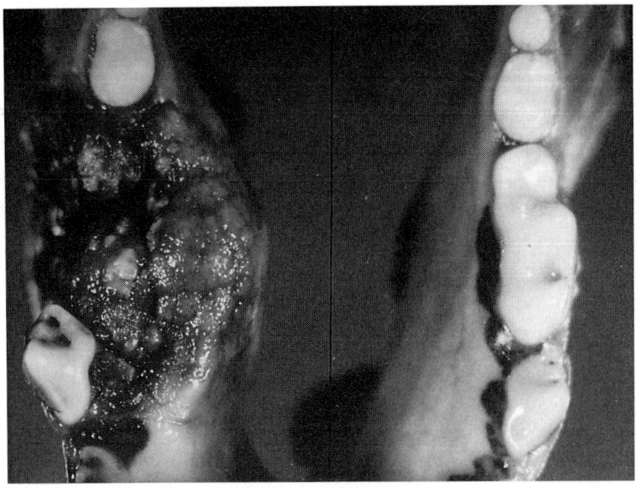

Figure 1-12 Mandible; dog. Acanthomatous epulis. This type of epulis can invade bone.

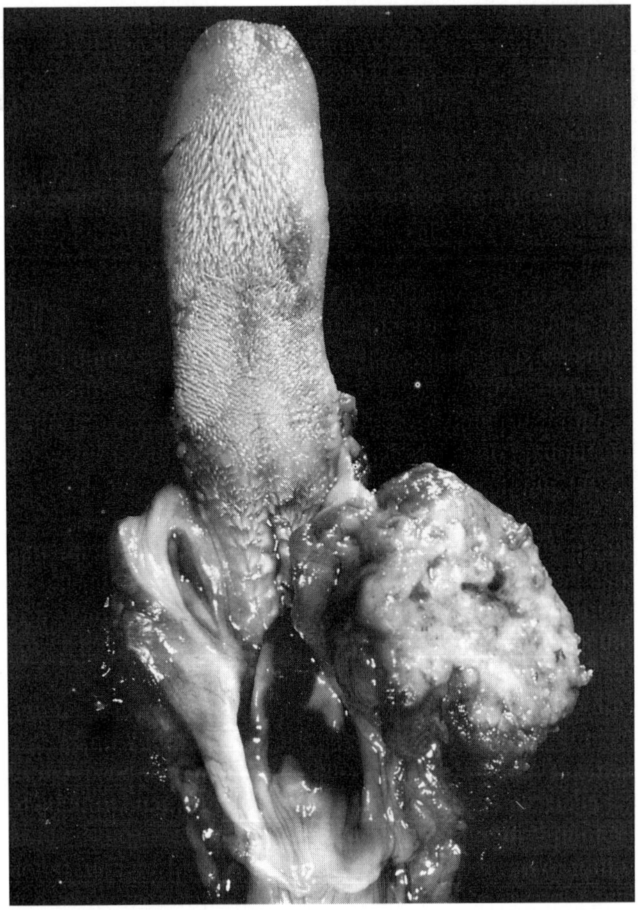

Figure 1-13 Tonsil; cat. Squamous cell carcinoma. The right tonsil has been replaced by a large, exophytic neoplasm. *Courtesy of Dr. R.W. Storts.*

tonsillar squamous cell carcinomas are more common in dogs.

About 5% to 10% of gingival squamous cell carcinomas metastasize to regional lymph nodes, and about 3% metastasize to distant sites. Squamous cell carcinomas of the tonsils metastasize to regional lymph nodes with much greater frequency, up to 98% of cases, and about 63% have metastasized to distant sites.

Squamous cell carcinomas, when small, are granular lesions and, with increased size, become beaded, cauliflower-like masses. Microscopically, irregular masses and cords of stratified squamous epithelial cells invade the submucosa or even subjacent muscle. The amount of keratin present depends on the degree of maturation of the neoplastic cells. Well-differentiated neoplasms have numerous keratin pearls, but poorly differentiated neoplasms have only a few keratinized cells and numerous mitotic figures. A characteristic feature is the presence of intercellular bridges (desmosomes) between adjacent epithelial cells. The amount of fibrous stroma varies considerably; some carcinomas induce a scirrhous response, whereas others have areas of necrosis caused by rapid tumor growth, collision necrosis, and loss of contiguity with the blood supply.

Ninety percent of **melanomas** of the oral cavity of dogs are malignant. A breed predilection exists for Scottish terriers, airedales, cocker spaniels, and Bedlington terriers. Some melanomas without pigment, termed amelanotic melanomas, present a greater diagnostic challenge to both the clinician and pathologist. Melanomas are composed of melanocytes and are of neural crest origin. The melanoma begins as a black macule and develops into a rapidly growing, firm mass. It can be dome shaped and smooth or have an ulcerated, red, and bleeding surface. Depending on the amount of pigment present, the interior of the mass is gray-white, dark brown, or black. Microscopically, the neoplasms consist of epithelioid or spindle-shaped melanocytes. Some neoplasms consist almost exclusively of epithelioid cells, whereas others are composed of spindle-shaped cells and resemble fibrosarcomas.

Canine oral papillomatosis is a papovavirus-induced transmissible condition and usually occurs in animals younger than 1 year (Fig. 1-14). The lesions are papilliform or cauliflower-like and can become quite florid. They are generally white and friable and occur on the mouth, tongue, palate, larynx, and epiglottis. The lesions usually regress spontaneously. Immunity is long lasting.

Grossly, these multiple tumors appear white or gray, are flat or smooth early, and, later, are gray, raised, and pedunculated with a keratinized surface. Microscopically, papillomas consist of an acanthotic, hyperplastic, stratified squamous epithelium and a proliferated connective tissue stroma, creating folds and fronds. Cells of the stratum spinosum enlarge greatly and have vesicular cytoplasm, so-called ballooning degeneration. At some stages, intranuclear inclusion bodies that contain virus particles are present.

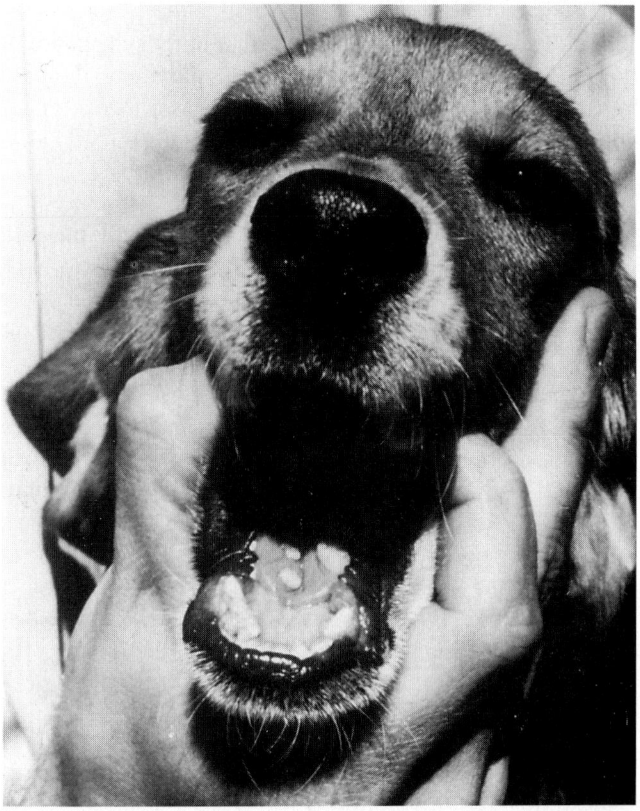

Figure 1-14 Tongue and gingiva; dog. Oral papillomas. Multiple, raised, gray nodules protrude from the tip of the tongue and gingiva. *Sundberg JP. Contr Oncol 1987;24:11-14.*

Fibrosarcomas arise from the collagen-producing cells (fibroblasts) of the oral cavity. Fibrosarcomas are most common in the cat, accounting for 20% of oral neoplasia in that species.

TEETH

The function of teeth is to provide mechanical advantage for mastication. Diseases that disrupt normal development and positioning of the teeth can adversely affect dental function. Acquired disease can result in the loss of integrity of the teeth or loss of rigid attachment of the teeth to the jawbones.

Proliferative, cystic or neoplastic diseases of the dental arcade can originate from cell rests that form from the dental lamina or the enamel organ (the cell rests of Malassez). In simple-toothed animals, such as carnivores, the tooth root is not covered by enamel. Receding gumlines therefore expose the dentin, resulting in pain and invasion by bacteria.

Malocclusions

Malocclusion refers to a failure of the upper and lower incisors to interdigitate properly. This feature is "normal" for some dogs, particularly the brachycephalic breeds. In the extreme, malocclusions can lead to difficulty in the prehension and mastication of food. Malocclusions are named according to the position of the mandible. Protrusion of the lower jaw is termed **prognathia,** whereas a short lower jaw with resultant protrusion of the upper jaw is termed **brachygnathia.** Sometimes these terms are incorrectly used, referring to brachygnathia as superior prognathia and prognathia as superior brachygnathia.

Malocclusions result from poor jaw conformation or, more rarely, from abnormal tooth eruption patterns. In some animals, such as rodents and rabbits, the teeth continue to grow throughout the animal's lifetime. If these animals are not provided with sufficient roughage in their diets, the teeth (both incisors and cheek teeth) overgrow and either "lock" the jaw or, because of a lack of occlusal grinding surfaces, prevent the animal from receiving proper nutrition.

Anomalies of Tooth Development

Tooth agenesis is fairly common and of little clinical significance in animals with simple teeth. Supernumerary tooth development is a rare curiosity. Abnormalities of tooth development can result from either primary dysplasias of the enamel organ or secondary consequences of trauma, infection, toxicosis, or metabolic abnormalities affecting tooth development. Primary dysplasias of the enamel organ usually result in failure of tooth development or severe malocclusion.

Dentigerous cysts are a result of abnormal tooth development's giving rise to epithelium-lined, cystic structures in the bone or soft tissues of the jaw. This lesion is rare, can remain asymptomatic or lead to painful or destructive diseases of the jaw, and occasionally can be the site of neoplasms. Usually, the cysts are lined by stratified squamous epithelium and often become filled with keratin. Infrequently, fragments of poorly developed teeth form within the cyst. In horses, a dentigerous cyst can result in a painful fistulous lesion. These draining tracts are seen most often in the temporal region, rostral and ventral to the ear (ear tooth). Infrequently, dentigerous cysts develop in mature animals with otherwise normal dentition. In these cases, the cysts arise as a result of the proliferation of epithelial cell rests remaining from the enamel organ (the cell rests of Malassez).

Segmental enamel hypoplasia occurs in the permanent teeth of dogs infected with the canine distemper virus during odontogenesis. Enamel is fully formed when the teeth are erupted; therefore virus infection of ameloblasts must occur during enamel formation, before 6 months of age, if enamel hypoplasia is to occur. The epithelium of the enamel organ during virus infection has typical viral lesions, including necrosis, disorganization, and lack of function of ameloblasts. After recovery from canine distemper virus infection, return of function and organization of the enamel organ is followed by reestablishment of normal enamel formation. Segmental enamel hypoplasia, corresponding to the zones with a lack of enamel formation during the time of distemper infection, is noted upon eruption of the permanent teeth (Fig. 1-15).

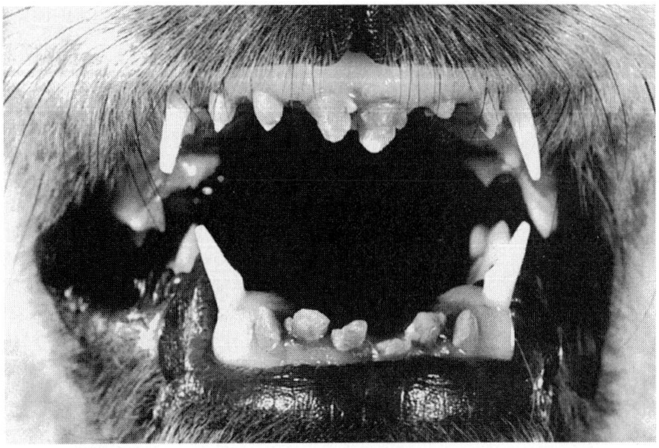

Figure 1-15 Teeth; dog. Enamel hypoplasia. There is a lack of enamel formation of the incisor teeth due to infection of ameloblasts with canine distemper virus during enamel formation.

Abnormal coloration of teeth can result from the incorporation of chemical agents, most typically tetracyclines, during mineralization. This result frequently occurs with the use of pediatric medications during permanent tooth development. Incorporation of porphyrins into the dentin in animals with congenital porphyria can cause pink discoloration of the teeth. Both tetracycline and porphyrins fluoresce under ultraviolet light, dramatically demonstrating these lesions.

Excessive fluoride incorporation into the enamel and dentin occurs in **fluoride toxicosis,** seen particularly in cattle and sheep. Toxic dietary concentrations of fluorine ingested during odontogenesis (from 6 to 36 months of age) can result in incorporation of the fluoride in the enamel and dentin of the permanent teeth, causing soft, chalky enamel. The discolored enamel is commonly yellow, dark brown, or black (Fig. 1-16). Clinical disease results from the loss of dental function through rapid dental attrition. Lesions of deciduous teeth have not been seen in experimentally induced fluorosis.

Lesions Caused by Attrition and Abnormal Wear

Alterations in dental appearance and function can be caused by normal or abnormal wear as a result of grinding forces. Loss of dental function due to normal dental attrition is an age-associated factor in domestic ruminants. Abnormal or irregular wear as a result of poor masticatory function, defective enamel, or abnormal oral cavity conformation can lead to serious dental malformation in horses. Aggressive dental maintenance is necessary to control irregular wear. In simple-toothed animals, the enamel cap is not usually exposed to abnormally harsh

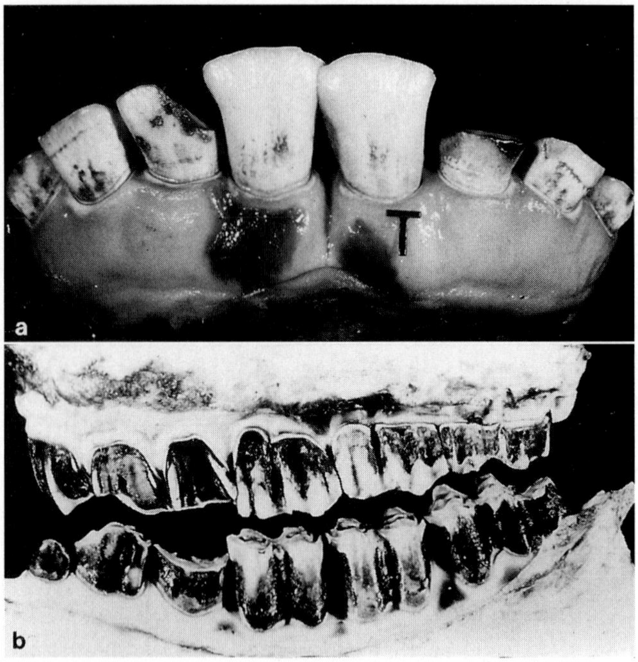

Figure 1-16 **A,** Incisor tooth; cow. Cow was fed a nonconstant toxic fluoride diet. There is abnormal pigmentation and an unusual wear pattern. **B,** Molar and premolar teeth; cow. The abnormal wear pattern seen here can cause problems with mastication. *Courtesy J.W. Suttie.*

grinding pressures. Habitual rock chewing in dogs or abnormal mastication can lead to erosion of the crown enamel and disfiguration of the tooth. Exposure of dentin or the pulp canal can lead to dental infection.

Feline External Resorptive Neck Lesions

External neck resorption of the teeth of cats can cause clinical signs referable to pain during mastication such as failure to eat or abnormal masticatory movements. Many cats with these tooth lesions have no history of prior dental disease. The disease is characterized by odontoclastic resorption of dental tissues. The resorption can occur in the root but most commonly occurs in the neck area of the tooth. Either a cementum or osteoid ingrowth subsequently lines the resorptive cavity, either partially or completely. This space can fill with a bacterial plaque that results in intense inflammation and osteoclastic resorption of dental tissues. Whether resorption is caused by inflammatory gum disease is unknown.

Infundibular Impaction

Impaction of the infundibulum is a cause of serious dental disease in ruminants and also occurs in horses. It is comparable in pathogenic mechanism to dental caries in simple-toothed animals. This disease has also been called infundibular necrosis and infundibular caries. Incomplete cementum formation in the infundibulum before the tooth erupts probably predisposes to infundibular impaction. Feed material is ground into the infundibulum (Fig. 1-17) where bacteria metabolize it to form acid, which causes demineralization. Also, bacterial enzymes digest the organic matrix of enamel and dentin. As a result of this matrix destruction, the pulp cavity is penetrated, resulting in pulpitis and periodontitis. Dental abscesses and formation of fistulous tracks lead to serious dental disease. The inflamed infundibular cavities often continue to become impacted with feed, increasing the likelihood that the lesion will develop further.

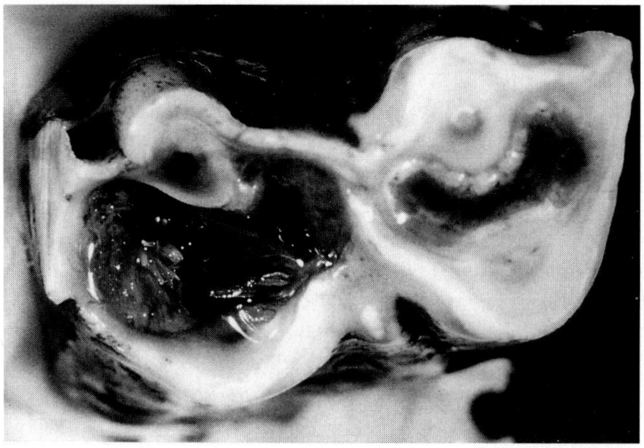

Figure 1-17 Molar teeth; cow. The infundibulum of the tooth on the left is impacted with feed.

Periodontal Disease

In addition to its destructive effect on mineralized dental matrices, the accumulation of a bacterial mass adherent to the tooth surface (dental plaque) has a destructive effect on the supporting soft tissues of the gingiva and periodontal ligament. Bacterial toxins and, possibly, the mechanical irritation of mineralized plaque (tartar or dental calculi) lead to atrophy and inflammation of the gingival epithelium and supporting stroma. The initial site for destructive inflammation is in the gingival crevice, that portion of the gingival epithelium that folds inward adjacent to the crown and attaches at the cementum-enamel junction of the tooth. After atrophy and destruction of the gingival stroma adjacent to the gingival crevice, the attachment of the epithelium moves lower on the tooth. Eventually, gingival-epithelial attachment occurs only on the root of the tooth, deep in the alveolar socket. As inflammation invades the connective tissues of the periodontal ligament, the suspensory apparatus is destroyed, and the tooth loosens. Additionally, alveolar osteomyelitis and pulpitis can result in abscesses, bacteremia, pain, reluctance to masticate, and a noxious odor to the breath. Periodontal disease is common in dogs, cats, and human beings. Diets that fail to provide an opportunity for forceful grinding in mastication predispose to periodontal disease.

Dental Neoplasia

Neoplasms of the enamel organ are named according to the extent of differentiation and the extent of odontogenesis seen in the neoplasms. The histologic appearance of these neoplasms is complex; persons with considerable experience in differentiating these uncommon neoplasms should be consulted when a precise diagnosis is indicated.

Odontogenic neoplasms can arise from the original dental lamina or from epithelial cell rests of Malassez that remain in the periodontal ligament. Dental neoplasms can also arise from dental epithelium in the superficial gingiva, in either the gingival crest or the surface epithelium. Odontogenic neoplasms also can arise from the cystic remnants of dysplastic odontogenesis. Poorly differentiated, strictly epithelial neoplasms usually occur in mature animals, presumably from the cell rests of Malassez. More fully differentiated neoplasms, displaying inductive formation of dentin or well-differentiated enamel matrix, arise in young animals, probably from dysplastic remnants of the original dental lamina. Dental neoplasms can either arise deeply in the jaw or originate on the surface epithelium. They usually occur near the teeth.

Odontomas are hamartomas of enamel organ origin and contain fully differentiated dentin and enamel. Ameloblasts, odontoblasts, and dental pulp also are present in some odontomas. Odontomas are nearly always found in young animals, most commonly in dogs and horses.

Ameloblastoma is the preferred generic name used for purely epithelial neoplasms of enamel organ origin. Several subtypes can be distinguished histologically. They are ameloblastic fibroma, ameloblastic odontoma, calcifying epithelial odontogenic tumor, peripheral odontogenic fibroma, and other rare tooth neoplasms.

Ameloblastoma occurs anywhere in the dental arcade, usually in adult dogs, and can be either superficial or deep. Ameloblastomas usually are locally invasive, resulting in lysis of alveolar bone. The histologic features characteristic of canine ameloblastomas include interbranching sheets and ribbons of epithelial cells with basal palisading and a central stellate reticulum. There is abrupt and intense keratinization, often with large, round, heavily keratinized cells and sometimes extracellular hyalin bodies between epithelial cells. These hyalin bodies often stain for amyloid. Ameloblastoma is differentiated from acanthomatous epulis by the absence of the characteristic stroma of the latter, absence of keratinization, and the presence of unique intercellular hyalin bodies. Ameloblastoma can be differentiated from squamous cell carcinoma by the nature and extent of the keratinization, the presence of intercellular hyalin bodies, and the formation of stellate, reticulum-like, epithelial sheets.

TONSILS

The palatine tonsils are pharyngeal lymphoid structures covered by stratified squamous epithelium. They do not possess afferent lymphatics and do not serve as lymph filters. Primary bacterial infections occur (tonsillitis), as well as primary neoplasms of either the lymphoid (lymphosarcoma) or epithelial (squamous cell carcinoma) components.

SALIVARY GLANDS

Inflammatory Diseases

Sialoadenitis or inflammation of a salivary gland is relatively rare in veterinary medicine. Although diagnosis of systemic diseases is not made by examining the salivary gland, rabies and canine distemper are two very important diseases that cause inflammation of the salivary glands. Saliva is a particularly important means of spread of the rhabdovirus that causes rabies. In the rat, a coronavirus termed sialodacryoadenitis virus is responsible for inflammation of the salivary gland and some adnexal ocular glands. *Salmonella typhisuis* has caused parotid sialoadenitis in pigs. Gross lesions of sialoadenitis are subtle, but can be accompanied by pain on palpation. Abscesses occasionally occur and are especially noticeable when they occur in the retrobulbar zygomatic gland.

Miscellaneous Diseases or Conditions

Changes in the salivary glands are uncommon in domestic animal species. A **ranula** is a cystic distension of the duct of the sublingual or submaxillary salivary gland that occurs on the floor of the mouth alongside the tongue. The cause is generally unknown, although some cases are due to sialoliths. A **salivary mucocoele,** in contrast, is a pseudocyst not lined by epithelium and filled with saliva. The cause of this lesion is also unknown, but they can occur secondary to traumatic rupture of the duct of a sublingual salivary gland with resultant leakage and encapsulation of saliva by reactive connective tissue.

Sialoliths are rare in domestic animal species. When they do occur, they are considered to be due to inflammation of the salivary gland with sloughed cells or inflammatory exudate forming a nidus for mineral accretion. Thus they are a cause of ranula formation.

Neoplasia

Salivary gland neoplasms, both benign and malignant, are uncommon but occur in all species (Fig. 1-18). They are composed of glandular or ductular elements or a combination of epithelial and mesenchymal components similar to those in mixed mammary neoplasms. A grossly similar condition, **salivary gland infarction** occurs infrequently in cats and rarely in dogs. The gross appearance of firmness and swelling of an infarcted gland must be distinguished microscopically from neoplasia

Necrotizing sialometaplasia

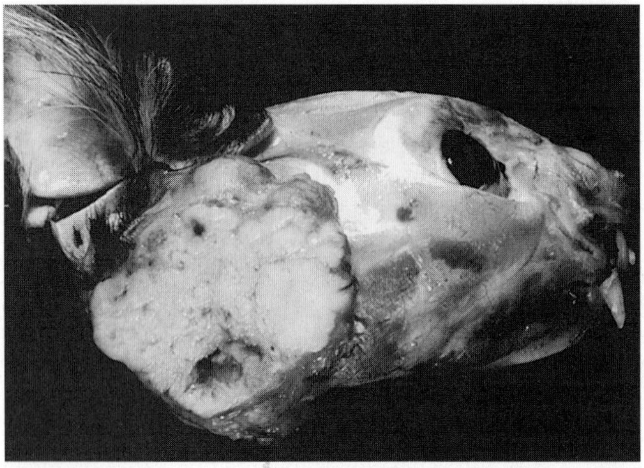

Figure 1-18 Head; cat. Salivary gland carcinoma. A large exophytic neoplasm of the parotid salivary gland replaces normal tissues.

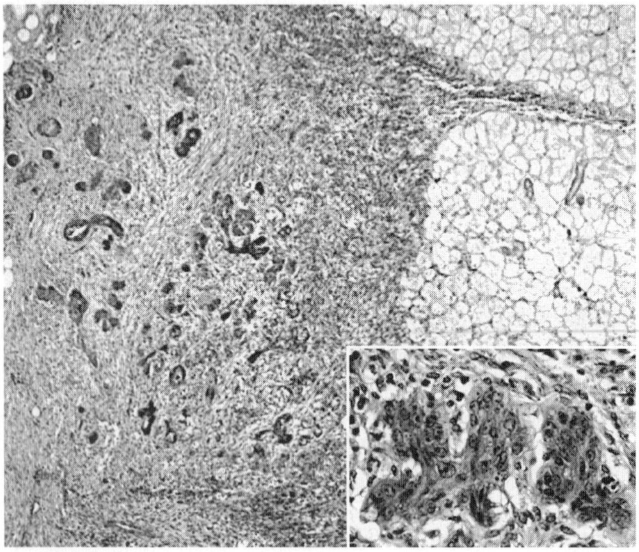

Figure 1-19 Salivary gland; cat. Salivary gland infarction. Note the areas of the gland that lack cell definition (necrosis) in the upper right of the photomicrograph. *Inset:* Hyperplasia of surviving salivary duct epithelial cells.

(Fig. 1-19). In salivary gland infarction, there are discrete foci of parenchymal necrosis with peripheral hemorrhage and inflammatory cells. Regeneration of the gland can be mistaken for neoplasia unless one is familiar with the former condition.

TONGUE

Developmental Anomalies

Congenital diseases of the tongue include epithelial defects such as fissures, epitheliogenesis imperfecta, or hair growing from the tongue. **Lethal glossopharyngeal**

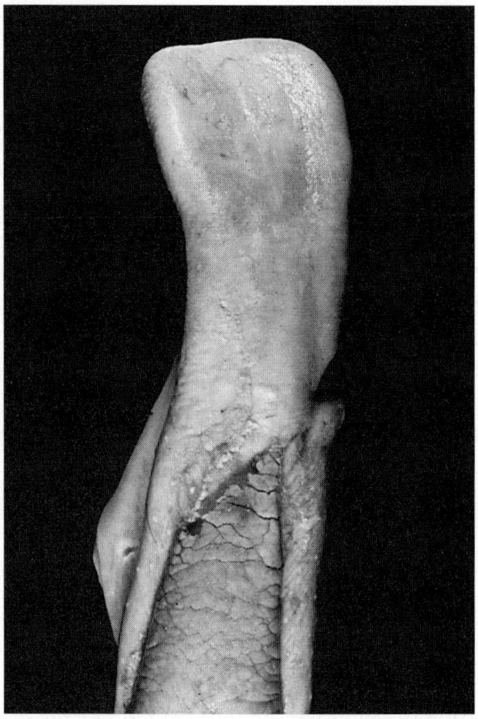

Figure 1-20 Tongue; foal. Thrush. A pseudomembrane of fungal hyphae is present on the lingual surface. It has been scraped off the rostral end of the tongue revealing normal mucosa beneath the fungal mat.

defect, or bird tongue of dogs, results in a pointed tongue that cannot wrap around a nipple and create the negative pressure required for nursing. Without intervention, starvation results.

Systemic Disease: Primary Involvement of the Tongue

Disease agents that principally target the tongue are relatively rare. The exception to this rule is *Actinobacillus lignieresii,* a normal inhabitant of the oral cavity. *A. lignieresii* is an opportunistic invader of damaged lingual tissue in cattle and occasionally small ruminants and horses. The granulomas resulting from infection have colonies of gram-negative bacilli at their centers that are surrounded by a zone of palisading, eosinophilic, club-shaped structures composed of immunoglobulin products of host inflammatory cells. Granulocytes, macrophages, epithelioid cells, and multinucleated Langhans' type giant cells often surround these rosettes (Splendore-Hoeppli phenomenon). Within and surrounding this granulomatous collar are lymphocytes and plasma cells. Depending on the duration of the disease, fibrous tissue can surround and be incorporated into the granulomas. Regional lymph nodes sometimes have similar granulomas or have abscesses that drain to the surface. The resulting lingual disease is called **wooden tongue;** the name is derived from the swelling, inflammation, and fibrosis that enlarge and firm the tongue.

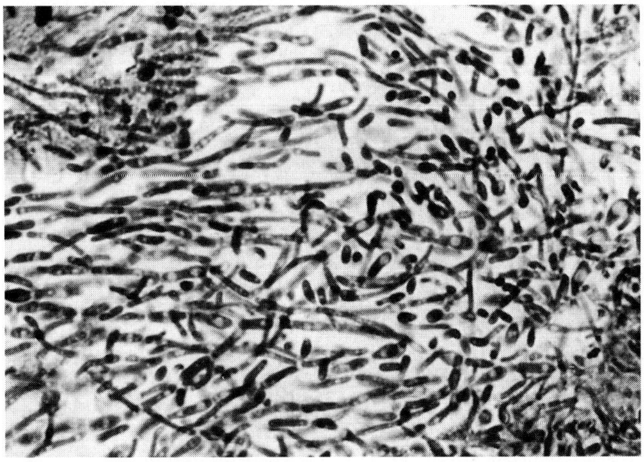

Figure 1-21 Esophagus; calf. Candidiasis. Yeast and pseudohyphal forms of *Candida albicans* in a tangled mat on the surface of the epithelium. Grocott's methenamine-silver (GMS) stain.

Systemic Disease: Secondary Involvement of the Tongue

Thrush is a *Candida albicans* (yeast) infection of the intact mucous membranes of the tongue and esophagus. It occurs principally in ungulates but has been seen in carnivores as well. Thrush is not a primary disease but often indicates an underlying debility, particularly in young animals. Thrush presents as a gray-green pseudomembrane that is easily scraped off the intact underlying mucosal surface (Figs. 1-20 and 1-21). Thrush occurs as a result of antibiotic treatment that kills normal flora, increased serum glucose concentrations as a result of diabetes mellitus, a high-sugar diet, or intravenous glucose therapy. The availability of iron is a limiting factor for the indigenous bacteria that compete with yeast for mucosal colonization. Immunodeficiency states also contribute to the development of thrush. All of these states provide tissue conditions suitable for the proliferation of yeast forms.

Oftentimes, lingual lesions are manifestations of systemic diseases such as bovine viral diarrhea (BVD), foot-and-mouth disease, and uremia. These diseases are discussed elsewhere.

Hyperplastic or Neoplastic Conditions

Epithelial hyperplasia of the lateral edges of the tongue is common in piglets before nursing when the fringelike epithelium is rubbed off (Fig. 1-22).

Lingual (glossal) neoplasms are rare but, when they occur, are generally of epithelial origin. **Squamous cell carcinomas** are most common, but rhabdomyomas, rhabdomyosarcomas, fibrosarcomas, melanomas, and granular cell tumors have been reported in domestic animals.

Parasites

Parasites of the tongue are uncommon with the exception of those that reside in muscles such as ***Sarcocystis*** spp. and ***Trichinella spiralis*** in pigs and occasionally in carnivorous wildlife such as polar bears. *Gongylonema* spp. can be present in the mucosa of pigs and ruminants and are of no clinical significance.

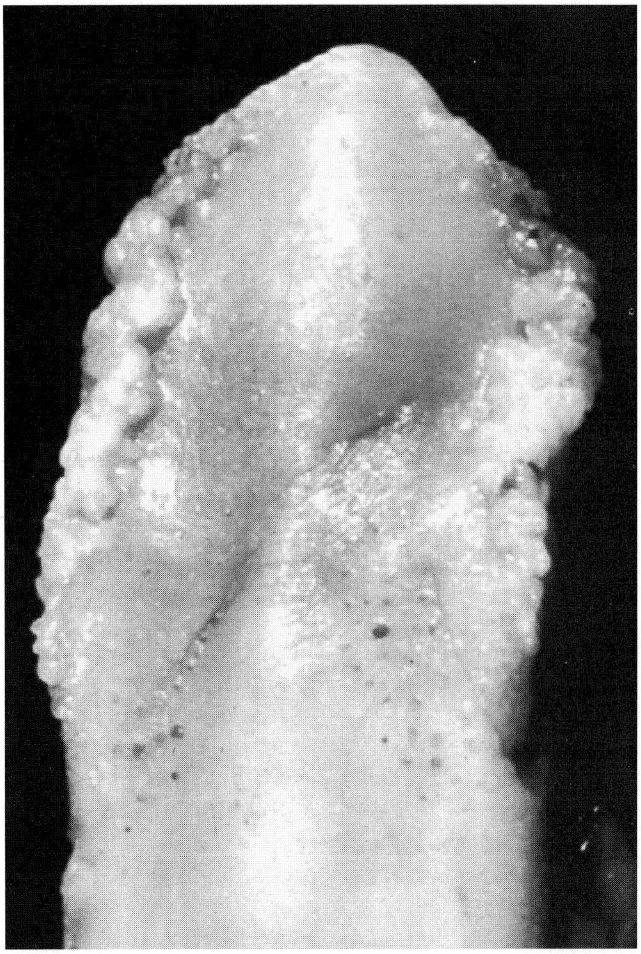

Figure 1-22 Tongue; neonatal pig. Lingual epithelial hyperplasia. The lateral surfaces of the tongue are covered by an epithelial fringe. This fringe will be mechanically removed by nursing.

ESOPHAGUS

Under normal circumstances the esophageal lumen is a potential space. The wall collapses when the esophagus is not transporting ingesta. The esophagus is lined by nonkeratinizing stratified squamous epithelium in carnivores and is keratinized in pigs, horses, and ruminants. Keratinization is greatest in ruminants, less in horses and least in pigs. Longitudinal and oblique epithelial folds are present to varying degrees. The tunica muscularis is completely striated in ruminants and dogs. In the horse, the distal third of the esophagus contains smooth muscle. The pig is similar to the horse, except the middle third of the esophagus contains a mixture of smooth and striated muscle. In the cat, opossum, and primates the distal two thirds of the esophagus is composed of smooth muscle. The smooth muscle is arranged as an inner circular layer and an outer longitudinal layer. It is important to remember that unlike the rest of the tubular digestive tract, the esophagus is unique in that it lacks a serosa. This means that sutures are not likely to seal an incision. Combine this with the strong muscular contractions that characterize this organ and it is easy to understand why esophageal surgery is not often performed and is even less often successful. For the same anatomic reason, perforating foreign bodies do not seal themselves off.

Developmental Anomalies

Cricopharyngeal achalasia, a congenital disorder of the upper esophageal sphincter, is recognized infrequently in dogs, but occurs most often in terriers, cocker spaniels, and miniature poodles. After weaning and before the animal is 6 months of age, dysphagia and regurgitation of ingesta characterize the disorder. After deglutition and failure of the sphincter to relax, short, sharp movements of the tongue, mandible, and neck are made by the dog in an attempt to dislodge the food bolus.

Acquired cricopharyngeal achalasia occurs rarely in the dog. The cause is unknown in both the congenital and acquired forms. The lesion, a grossly discernible deformity of the cricopharyngeus muscle, has been variously described as hypertrophy, fibrosis, myositis, or atrophy. Few specimens have been available for microscopic study, as surgeons perform simple myotomy as a treatment for the disease rather than a resection or biopsy.

Megaesophagus

Megaesophagus or esophageal ectasia is dilation of the esophagus due to insufficient or uncoordinated peristalsis in the mid and cervical esophagus. It has been described in dogs, cats, and horses. Causes range from motility problems related to innervation or denervation disorders to partial physical obstructions to stenosis secondary to inflammatory diseases of esophageal musculature. Many cases are idiopathic.

Congenital megaesophagus is due to partial blockage of the lumen of the esophagus by a persistent right fourth aortic arch. Because of the persistence of the arch, a vascular ring forms around the esophagus and trachea, preventing full dilation of the esophagus. The ring is formed by the aorta, pulmonary artery, and ductus arteriosus. This form of megaesophagus is unique in that the esophageal obstruction, and thus dilation, occurs cranial to the heart because of the location of the obstructing vascular ring. All other forms of megaesophagus result in dilation cranial to the stomach.

Congenital megaesophagus also occurs as an idiopathic denervation of the esophagus in great Danes, Irish setters, miniature schnauzers, Labrador retrievers, wire hair fox terriers, shar peis, Newfoundlands, and Siamese cats.

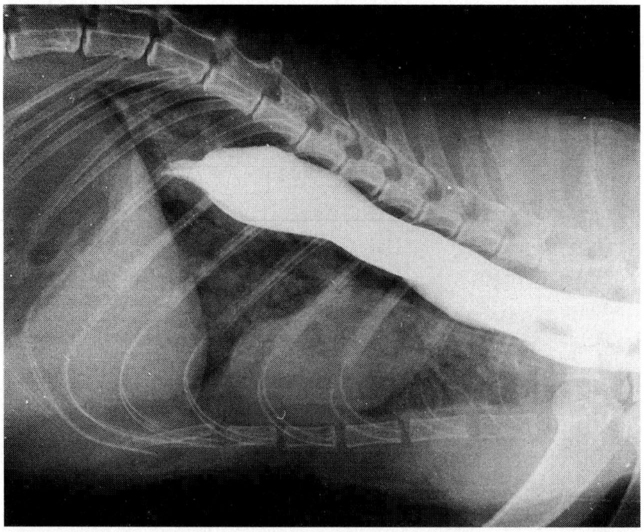

Figure 1-23 Esophagus; cat. Radiograph, lateral view of thorax. Megaesophagus. The contrast material within the esophagus demonstrates a dilation which is twice the diameter of normal esophagus. *Clifford DH, Soifer FK, Wilson CF, Waddel ED, Guilloud GL. J Am Vet Med Assoc 1971; 158:1554-1560.*

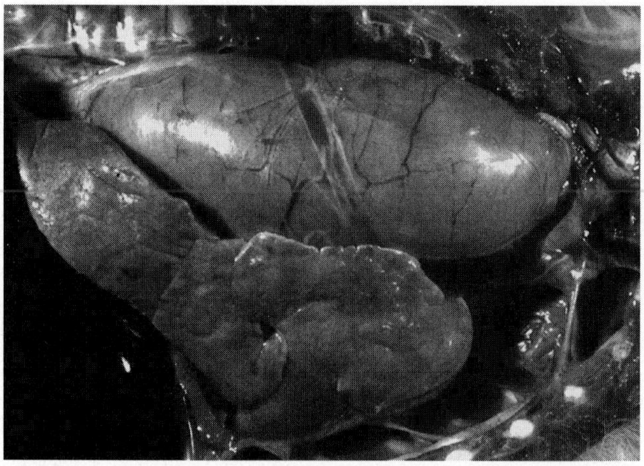

Figure 1-24 Thorax; dog. Megaesophagus. A markedly dilated esophagus has displaced the left lung caudally and ventrally.

Acquired megaesophagus or esophageal achalasia is the result of failure of relaxation of the cardiac sphincter of the stomach in human beings. The obstruction, and thus dilation, occurs cranial to the stomach. Although the gross appearance of acquired megaesophagus in animals is similar to that of human beings, the etiology of the condition in animals does not involve the cardiac sphincter. Causes are idiopathic or secondary to polymyositis (inflammation of the esophageal muscle), myasthenia gravis (an autoimmune disease directed against acetylcholine receptors of the neuromuscular junction), hypothyroidism (which can result in muscle atrophy), and to lead and thallium poisoning (via effect on innervation).

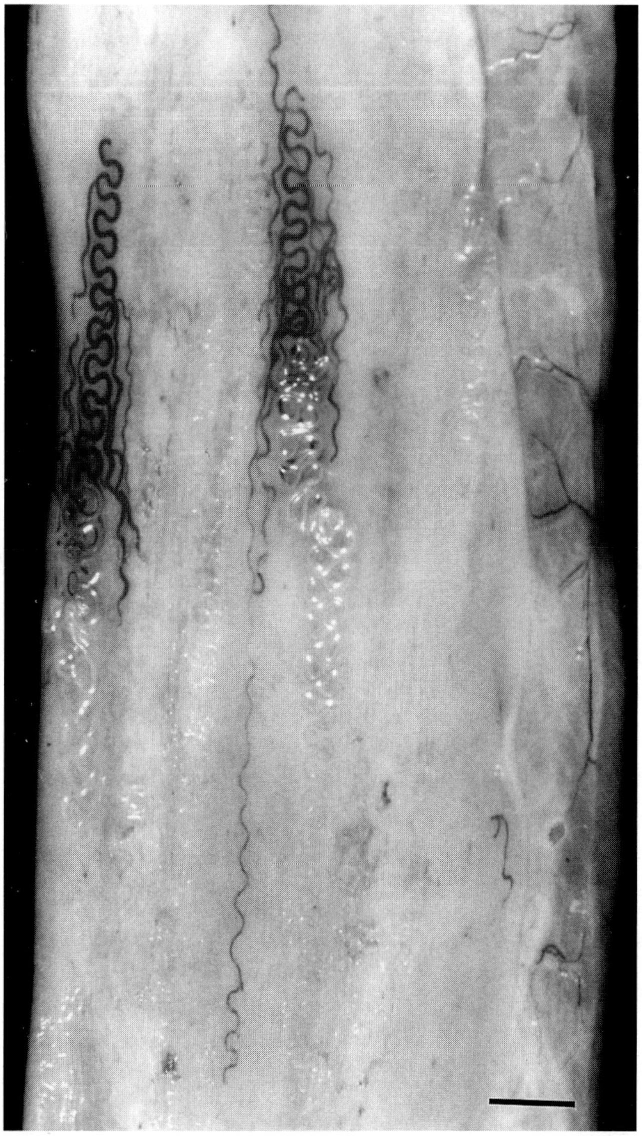

Figure 1-25 Esophagus; deer. Gonglyonemiasis. The gonglyonema are embedded within esophageal mucosa. Bar = 5 mm. *Courtesy Dr. M.D. McGavin.*

Megaesophagus is recognized clinically by regurgitation after ingestion of solid food. Thus congenital megaesophagus might not be recognized until weaning. Oftentimes animals are thin and can have aspiration pneumonia. Grossly, in megaesophagus the esophagus is flaccid, prominently dilated, and two to three times normal diameter (Figs. 1-23 and 1-24). There is uniform dilation along the length of the esophagus in some animals, but dilation can be quite eccentric in others. The dilated portions often contain a fetid fluid residue of ingesta. The lower esophageal sphincter, a zone 1 to 2 cm in length, proximal to the cardia, is unaffected. Microscopic examination and efforts to count myenteric ganglion cells are usually nondiagnostic. Vagus nerves sometimes contain degenerated nerve fibers.

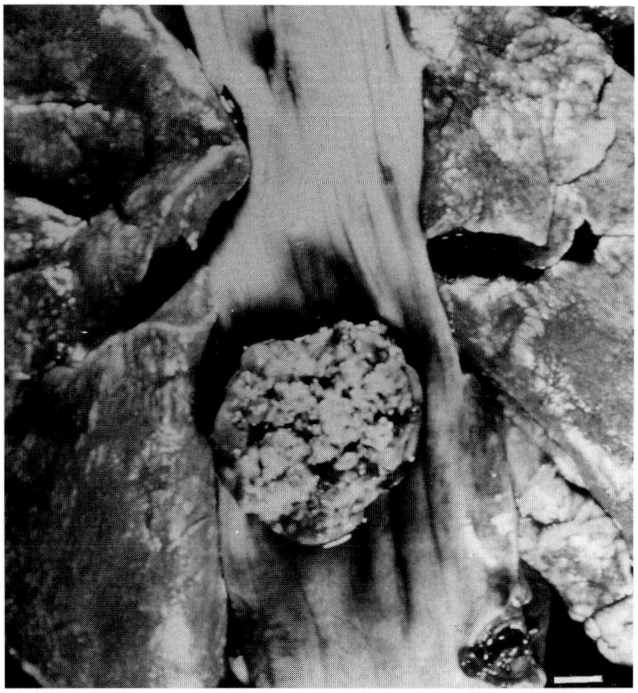

Figure 1-26 Esophagus; dog. Spirocercosis. A 4-cm diameter granulomatous nodule protrudes into the lumen of the distal esophagus. Bar = 1 cm. *Courtesy Department of Pathology and Parasitology, Auburn University.*

Esophageal Parasites

With notable exceptions, parasitic diseases of the esophagus are generally of no clinical importance. The more common parasites of the esophagus include *Gongylonema* spp., which affect ruminants, pigs, horses, primates, and occasionally rodents. These nematodes reside directly under the mucosa and are characteristically thin, red, and serpentine (Fig. 1-25). They can be 10 to 15 cm in length. The intermediate hosts are cockroaches and dung beetles.

Gastrophilus spp. occur in equids. These fly larvae have interesting life cycles, as their eggs are laid on the skin in varying locations. The warmth and moisture from licking activate them. The larvae burrow into the oral mucosa, molt, and then migrate down the esophagus. They occur both in the distal esophagus and stomach where they attach to the mucosa via oral hooks. They eventually detach, leaving craters at the site of attachment, and pass in the feces.

Hypoderma lineatum is the larvae of the warble fly of ruminants. These parasites eventually migrate to the esophageal adventitia and then to the subcutaneous tissues of the back.

Probably the most pathogenic of the esophageal parasites is ***Spirocerca lupi*** of canids. These nematodes reach the esophageal submucosa after migrating through the aortic wall. A passage forms between the esophageal lumen and the granuloma containing the parasite, allowing discharge of ova into the alimentary system and eventually into the feces (Fig. 1-26). Clinical sequelae of infestation include dysphagia, aortic aneurysms, and rarely esophageal fibrosarcomas or osteosarcomas. Spondylosis deformans sometimes occurs in the vertebral bodies adjacent to the aortic granulomas. *S. lupi* infestations occur in warmer climates. The intermediate hosts are dung beetles, and the paratenic hosts are rodents, chickens, and reptiles.

Miscellaneous Esophageal Lesions or Conditions

Idiopathic muscular hypertrophy of the distal esophagus is a peculiar lesion in horses that can be quite spectacular at necropsy (Fig. 1-27), but usually it is of no clinical significance. The esophageal musculature can be several centimeters thick, and the lesion can extend along the distal quarter of the esophagus. Rarely it plays a role in esophageal impaction.

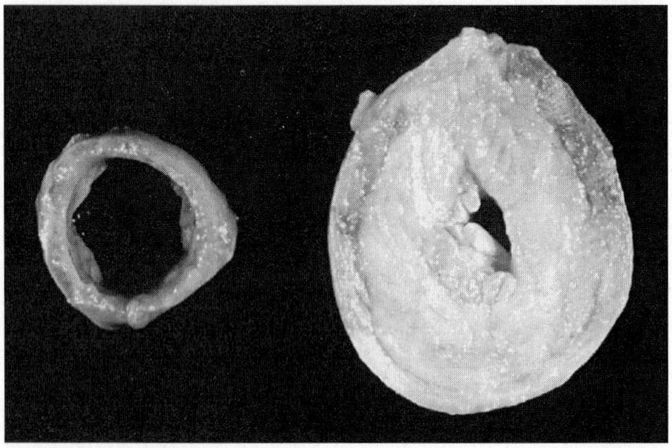

Figure 1-27 Esophagus; transverse sections; horse. Muscular hypertrophy of the distal esophagus. Cross sections of the proximal *(left)* and distal *(right)* esophagus demonstrate the marked increase in the thickness of the tunica muscularis of the distal esophagus.

Similarly, **dilation of the esophageal glands of aged dogs** can be a spectacular gross lesion of no clinical consequence. It is, therefore, important to carefully examine these lesions either at necropsy or during fiberoptic viewing in the live animal to determine whether what appear to be erosions and ulcers are rather mucosal elevations filled with mucus. Because the lesions are subepithelial, the overlying mucosa is smooth and shiny. Dilated esophageal glands vary in number and location but are generally only a few millimeters in diameter.

Esophageal erosions and ulcers are relatively common and have a variety of causes. One of the more common causes of esophageal erosions and ulcers is reflux of stomach acid. This reflux causes chemical burning of the lower esophagus and is commonly called **reflux esophagitis** (Fig. 1-28) or heartburn in human beings. Other causes of esophageal ulcers include improper use of stomach tubes, which cause linear scraping on the crests of the longitudinal folds of the esophageal mucosa (Fig. 1-29), and infectious diseases such as bovine viral diarrhea (Fig. 1-30), which cause mucosal injury in other locations as well.

Leukoplakia of the esophagus and stomach is characterized by discrete, flat, white mucosal elevations (epithelial plaques) of no clinical significance. They are sometimes mistaken for thrush lesions or neoplasia. Unlike thrush lesions, they do not scrape off easily, and their regularity, number, and location distinguish them from neoplasms.

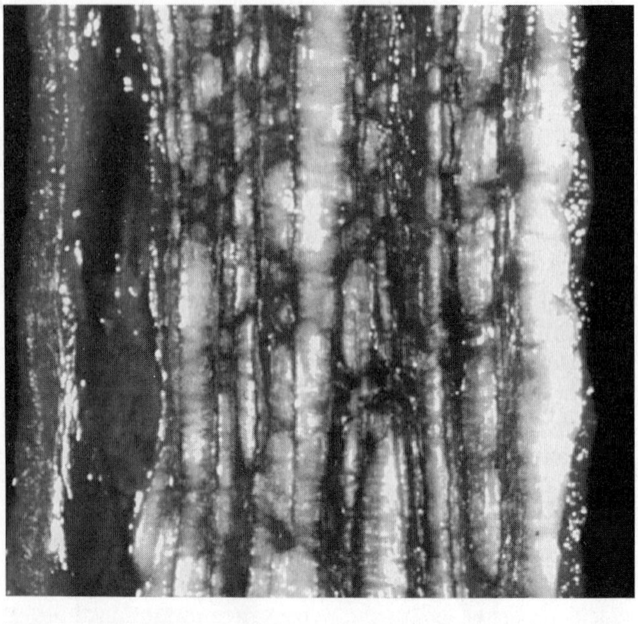

Figure 1-28 Esophagus; horse. Reflux esophagitis. The dark streaks on the surface of the esophagus are areas of epithelial loss secondary to gastric acid reflux.

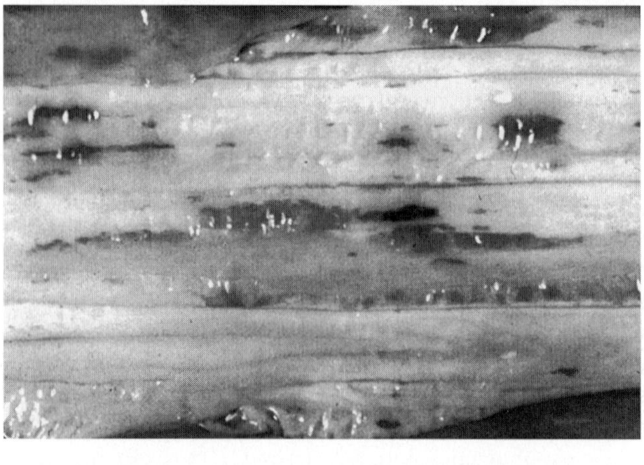

Figure 1-29 Esophagus; horse. Esophageal ulceration. Linear ulcers are the result of stomach tubing.

Choke

Choke is a clinical term referring to esophageal obstruction subsequent to stenoses that have a variety of causes. Choke most often occurs in those anatomic locations where the esophagus cannot fully expand. These locations are dorsal to the larynx, at the thoracic inlet, base of the heart, and at the diaphragmatic hiatus. Choke occurs most frequently as a result of ingestion of large bodies such as potatoes, apples, bones, or medicaments such as large gelatin-filled capsules or tablets (dry boluses). If these bodies are lodged against the epithelium for longer than 2 days, the interaction often results in circumferential pressure necrosis of the esophageal mucosa (Fig. 1-31), which forms strictures during healing. These strictures then can cause reflex regurgitation after ingestion of food.

In older horses, poor dentition causes feed to be incompletely masticated, resulting in impaction in the esophagus. Neoplastic or inflammatory lesions of the esophagus or periesophageal tissues also cause obstruction. Persistence of the right aortic arch has already been discussed as a cause of esophageal stenosis and megaesophagus.

Neoplasia

Neoplasms of the esophagus are rare in animals, but **squamous cell carcinomas** have been described in cats and horses and in cattle in Brazil and Great Britain, where consumption of bracken fern *(Pteridium aquilinum)* has been incriminated as a cause. Clinically, dysphagia, regurgitation, and dilation of the esophagus proximal to the mass, weight loss, and a palpable cervical mass accompany esophageal carcinoma. Esophageal squamous cell carcinomas often are not detected early because the neoplastic mass grows into the esophageal lumen. The surface is cauliflower-like and often ulcerated. With time, the mass obstructs the esophagus and produces a stenosis of the lumen. Spread to contiguous tissue occurs readily, and the neoplasms metastasize to regional lymph nodes, liver, and lungs.

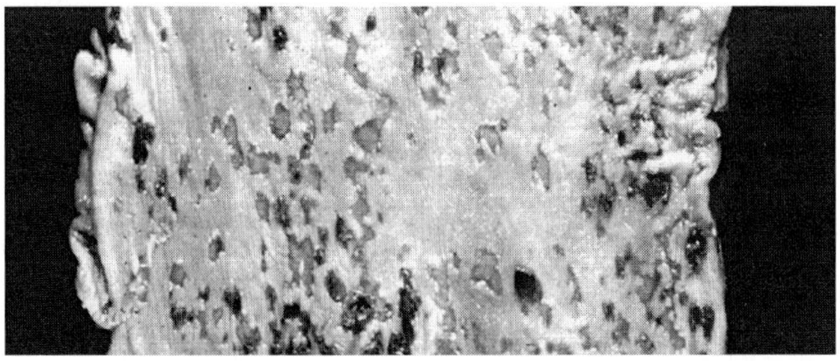

Figure 1-30 Esophagus; cow. Bovine viral diarrhea. Multiple variably sized and variably shaped esophageal ulcers are caused by the virus of bovine viral diarrhea.

RUMEN, RETICULUM, AND OMASUM

Ruminants have a three-part forestomach (reticulum, rumen, omasum). The forestomach is elaborately endowed with folds and subdivisions, a complex innervation and motility, and, most important, an extensive digestive, fermentative flora. The disorders of ruminant forestomachs are largely disorders of their flora and motility. Because of their fermentative functions, abrupt alterations in diet result in either cessation of bacterial actions or an exuberant and unstable proliferation by one species or another. Often, alterations in one member of the flora lead to a chain of events that can produce rumen acidosis at one extreme and rumen bloat at the other. The competition between flora and a steady availability of substrate keep the rumen healthy. It is not clear to what extent IgA or other antibodies have any role in this complex milieu of carbohydrate and cellulose-rich ingesta, bacteria, fungi, and protozoa. The stratified squamous mucosa of the reticulum, rumen, and omasum can be acutely inflamed when the contents have an acid pH and the abnormal milieu permits bacterial and mycotic overgrowth. Because the reticulo-omasal orifice is more dorsal than the floor of the compartments, the reticulum can trap foreign bodies as they exit the esophagus, and these can irritate or penetrate the mucosa. The motility disorders of the forestomachs are poorly understood.

Bloat (Ruminal Tympany)

Ruminal tympany or bloat is, by definition, an overdistension of the rumen and reticulum by gases produced during fermentation. Mortality of affected animals is approximately 50%. A hereditary predisposition to bloat might

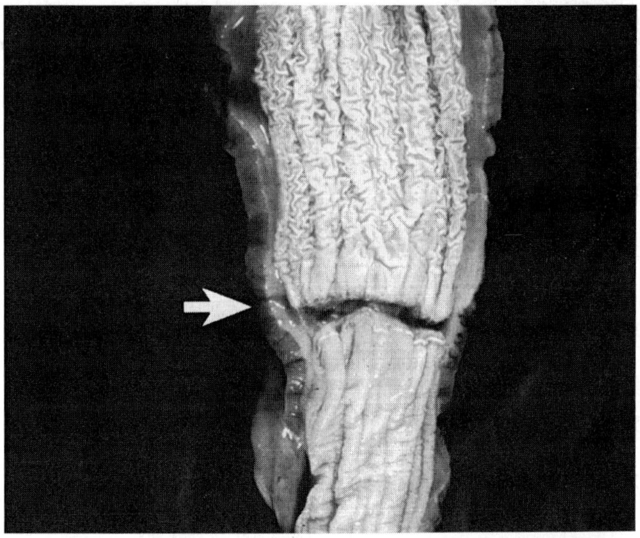

Figure 1-31 Esophagus; foal. Esophageal necrosis. The circumferential area of mucosal loss *(arrow)* with scarring occurred secondary to a lodged foreign body cranial to the thoracic inlet.

exist in cattle because cases are on record of bloat in monozygotic twins. Bloat can be divided into primary tympany and secondary tympany.

Primary tympany is also known as legume bloat, dietary bloat, or frothy bloat. It generally occurs 1 to 3 days after animals begin a new diet. Certain legumes such as alfalfa and ladino clover, as well as grain concentrates, promote the formation of a stable foam. The nonvolatile acids of legume and rumen origin lower the rumen pH to 5 to 6, which is optimal for formation of bloat. Foam, mixed with rumen contents, physically blocks the cardia causing the rumen to distend with the gases of fermentation. Clinical signs, therefore, include a distended left paralumbar fossa, a distended abdomen, increased respiratory and heart rates, and, late in the disease, decreased ruminal movements. Death, when it occurs, is attributable to distension of the abdomen and compression of the diaphragm with resultant decreased pleural cavity size, respiratory embarrassment, and increased intra-abdominal and intrathoracic pressure resulting in decreased venous return to the heart, which results in generalized congestion cranial to the thoracic inlet.

The lesions of primary tympany are often difficult to detect if there is an interval between death and postmortem examination because the foam can collapse. Conversely, fermentation can occur after death in a nonbloated animal resulting in the production of abundant gas. The most reliable postmortem indicator of antemortem bloat is the sharp line of demarcation between the pale, bloodless distal esophagus and the congested proximal esophagus at the thoracic inlet. This division is known as a **bloat line** (Fig. 1-32).

Secondary tympany is caused by a physical or functional obstruction or stenosis of the esophagus resulting in failure to eructate. Vagus indigestion or other innervation disorders, esophageal papilloma, lymphosarcoma, and esophageal foreign bodies are examples of potential causes of secondary tympany.

Foreign Bodies

Foreign bodies can collect or lodge in the rumen. These include **trichobezoars** and **phytobezoars:** hairballs and plant balls, respectively. Trichobezoars are a sometime sequela to a habit of bucket-fed calves of sucking on each other to satisfy their nursing instincts. Phytobezoars result from an excess of indigestible roughage.

Ingestion of nails and wire, common where straw and hay bales are packaged in wire, can result in perforation of the wall of the reticulum with resultant reticulitis, peritonitis, or pericarditis **(hardware disease).** Often in areas in the United States where ruminants are at high risk of hardware disease because of farming practices, magnets are placed in rumens to prevent the ingested ferrous wires and nails from penetrating the reticular mucosa. Occasionally, ruminants ingest parts from storage batteries and suffer lead poisoning.

Primary tympany (frothy bloat):
· Ingestion of legumes (alfalfa/clover) → formation of stable rumen foam → physical blockage of cardia → rumen gas distention → abdominal distention → compression of diaphragm → ↓ pleural cavity size → ↑ abdominal & thoracic pressure → ↓ venous return to heart → generalized congestion cranial to thoracic inlet

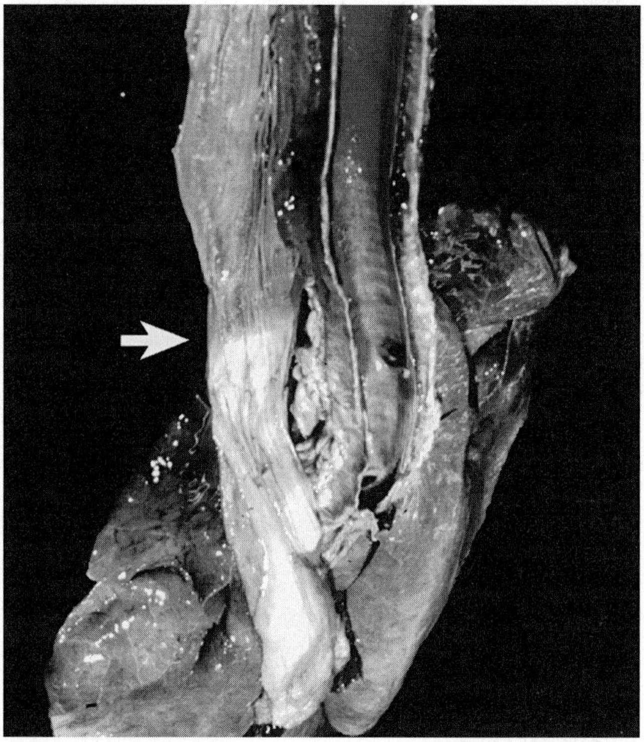

Figure 1-32 Esophagus; cow. Bloat line. There is a sharp line *(arrow)* of demarcation between the caudal (blanched) and the cranial (congested) esophagus. Agonal breathing resulted in tracheal hemorrhage. *Courtesy Department of Veterinary Pathology, Cornell University.*

Inflammatory Diseases

Inflammation of the rumen, **rumenitis,** is generally considered synonymous with **lactic acidosis.** Lactic acidosis is synonymous with grain overload, rumen overload, carbohydrate engorgement, and chemical rumenitis. All ruminants are susceptible. The pathophysiology of lactic acidosis usually involves a sudden dietary change to an easily fermentable feed or a change in the feed volume consumed. The latter scenario is most likely to occur during weather changes, especially among feedlot cattle when a sudden cooling rainstorm will stimulate food intake of cattle that had previously been inappetent due to high environmental temperatures and humidity.

Ruminal microflora are generally rich in cellulolytic gram-negative bacteria necessary for the digestion of hay. A sudden change to a highly fermentable, carbohydrate-rich feed promotes the growth of gram-positive bacteria, *Streptococcus bovis* and *Lactobacillus* spp. The lactic acid produced by the fermentation of these carbohydrates decreases the ruminal pH below 5 (normal = 5.5 to 7.5). This acidic pH eliminates normal ruminal flora and fauna and damages ruminal mucosa. Increased concentrations of dissociated fatty acids leads to ruminal atony. Death, when it occurs, is due to dehydration secondary to the increased osmotic effect of ruminal solutes' (organic acids) causing

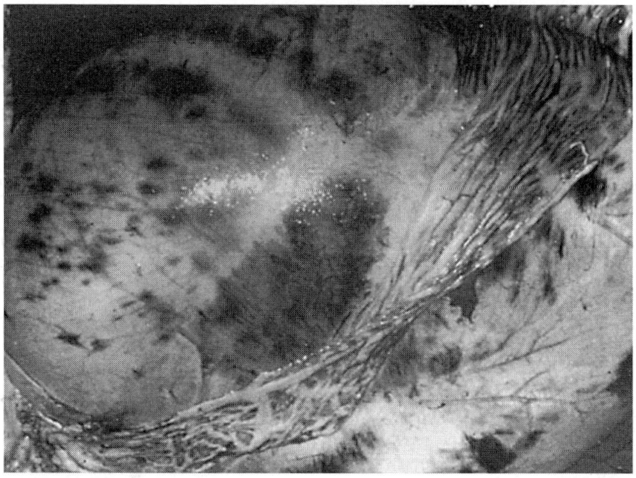

Figure 1-33 Rumen, serosal surface; cow. Mycotic rumenitis. Circular black foci and larger areas of infarction are present in the rumen wall as a result of mycotic vasculitis. *Courtesy Dr. M.D. McGavin.*

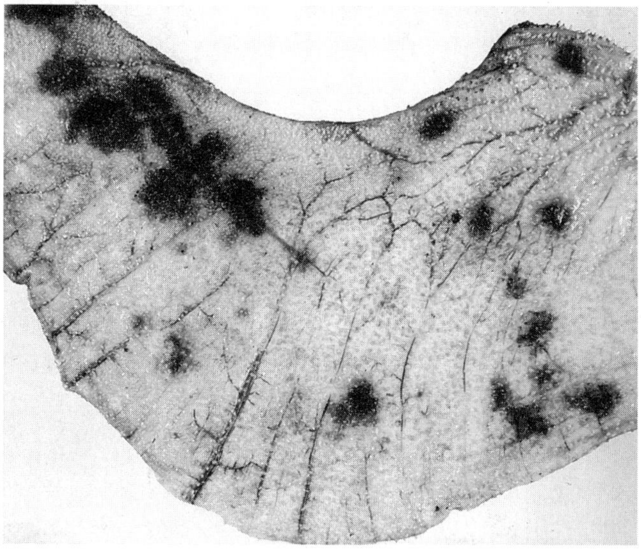

Figure 1-34 Omasum; cow. Mycotic omasitis. Well-delineated black focal infarcts are scattered over the laminae of the omasum. *Courtesy Dr. R.G. Thompson.*

movement of fluids across the damaged ruminal mucosa into the rumen, acidosis (from absorption of lactate from the rumen), and circulatory collapse. Mortality among animals with lactic acidosis ranges from 25% to 90% and usually occurs within 24 hours.

At necropsy the ruminal and intestinal contents are watery and acidic. Often abundant grain in found in the rumen. The mucosa of the ruminal papillae is brown and friable and detaches easily, especially from the ventral ruminal sac. Caution must be exercised in interpreting this latter finding as a lesion because the ruminal mucosa often detaches easily in animals that have been dead for even a few hours at high environmental temperatures. Hydropic change and coagulative necrosis of the ruminal epithelium followed by an influx of neutrophils are common microscopic lesions. Animals surviving lactic acidosis develop stellate scars, visible because of their color difference from the unaffected surrounding mucosa. The scars are pale; unaffected mucosa is dark brown to black.

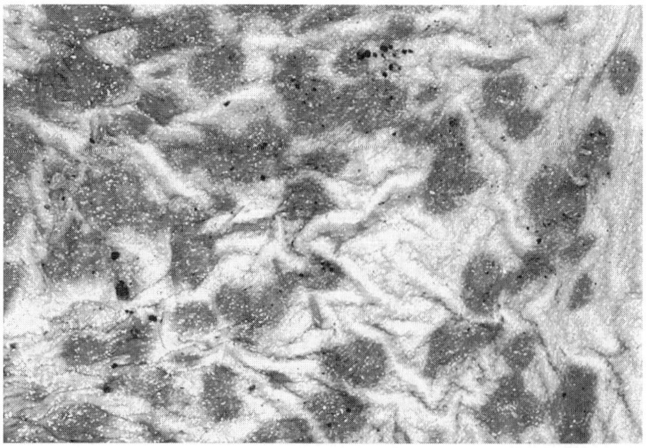

Figure 1-35 Rumen; calf. Mycotic rumenitis. Note the numerous well-demarcated foci of necrosis and hemorrhage in the rumenal mucosa.

Bacterial rumenitis generally occurs because of lactic acidosis or mechanical rumen injury. Bacteria that colonize the damaged rumen can be transported into the portal circulation and to the liver resulting in multiple abscesses. *Actinomyces pyogenes* is a common cause of bacterial abscesses in the liver. *Fusobacterium necrophorum,* also transported from the rumen to the liver, results in distinctive liver lesions that are termed necrobacillosis.

Mycotic infections of the rumen also occur because of damage to the ruminal mucosa caused by lactic acidosis and mechanical rumen injury. **Mycotic rumenitis** also results from the administration of antibiotics, usually in calves but in adult cattle as well. The antibiotics reduce the numbers of normal flora and allow fungi to proliferate. In cases of mycotic rumenitis, lesions are generally circular and well delineated and are due principally to infarction from thrombosis secondary to fungal vasculitis (Figs. 1-33 to 1-37). Offending fungi include *Aspergillus, Mucor, Rhizopus, Absidia,* and *Mortierella* spp. Certain fungi can spread to the placenta hematogenously and cause mycotic placentitis, which leads to abortions.

Ruminal candidiasis is seldom diagnosed during life. Severe candidiasis is seen at necropsy in calves that have failed to respond to treatment for a concomitant disease.

Miscellaneous Diseases or Conditions

Ruminal papilla vary in length, becoming longer with high-roughage diets. Such diets also can cause the papilla

Sudden Δ to highly fermentable, carbohydrate rich feed
→ ↑ G(+)(b) Strept. bovis & lactobacillus → ↑ lactic acid →
↓ rumen pH → ↓ normal flora, damage to ruminal mucosa, atony → mycotic rumenitis

dehydration, acidosis, circulatory collapse, death

survival: stellate mucosal scars

(b) rumenitis → liver abscesses/necrosis: Actinomyces pyogenes; Fusobacterium necrophorum

(F) invasion → vasculitis → thrombosis → rumenal infarcts
· Aspergillus, Mucor, Rhizopus, Absidia, Mortierella

to become tongue- or leaf-shaped. Animals consuming diets with less than 10% roughage can develop **ruminal parakeratosis.** These rumens have hard brown, often clumped, papillae. This lesion has little to no clinical consequence.

Ruminal papillomas are viral induced in some cases, but in certain countries, bracken fern has been implicated as a cause of rumen neoplasms (Fig. 1-38).

Vagus indigestion results in a functional outflow problem from the forestomachs. Damage to the vagus nerve can occur anywhere along its length and can result in functional pyloric stenosis. Causes of vagus indigestion vary from inflammation of the vagus nerve due to traumatic reticuloperitonitis, liver abscesses, volvulus of the abomasum, or bronchopneumonia. Mechanical obstruction of the forestomachs or abomasal outflow can be due to lymphosarcoma or papillomas or to blockage following ingestion of indigestible or foreign materials. Diet and dwarfism are sometimes associated with vagus indigestion. Many cases are idiopathic. Clinical signs include rumenoreticular distension; the presence of abomasal distension is dependent on the precise location of the damage to the vagus nerve.

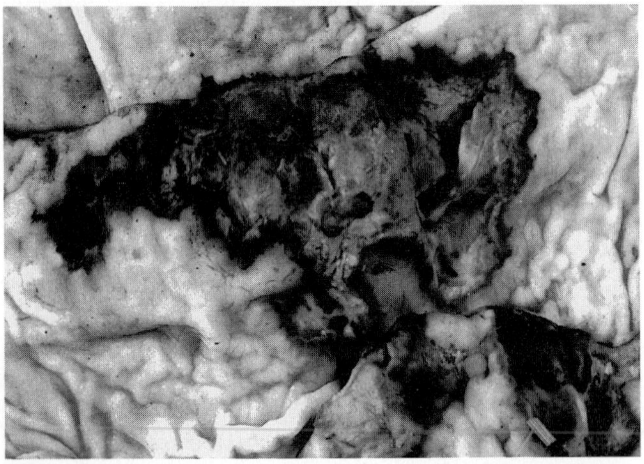

Figure 1-36 Omasum; cow. Mycotic omasitis. Note the large focus of necrosis and hemorrhage in the omasal mucosa.

STOMACH AND ABOMASUM

The acid-pepsin stomachs of the simple-stomached animals and the abomasum of ruminants are similar in function and in their response to injury. In each, the proximal portion is composed of the fundus and body, the acid and pepsin secretory organ; and the distal portion or antrum is lined by epithelium rich in gastrin-producing G cells and mucous glands. Simple stomachs have an indigenous flora. Protective features include the following:

1. Motility under normal circumstances clears the mucosa of substrate.
2. Foveolar mucus forms a protective blanket over the mucosa.
3. IgA inhibits bacterial attachment.
4. The stomach is acid-washed several times daily.

The stomach is protected from self-digestion during times of basal or maximal acid output by the gastric mucosal barrier, which includes a negative electric potential that prevents back-diffusion of hydrogen ions, cytoprotective prostaglandins, and foveolar and neck mucus secretions. Duodenal contents containing bile only infrequently reflux into the stomach in normal animals; normal antral peristalsis (4.5 contractions per minute in the dog) and a normal pylorus prevent more frequent refluxes, which would damage the gastric mucosal barrier.

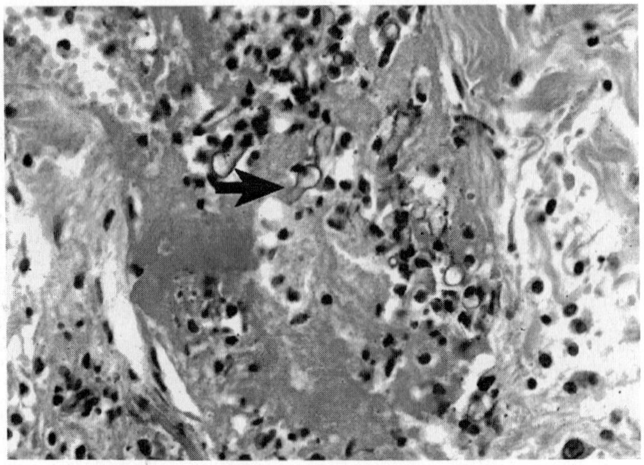

Figure 1-37 Rumen; cow. Mycotic rumenitis. Fungal hyphae (*arrow*) are present in a thrombosed vessel. H & E stain.

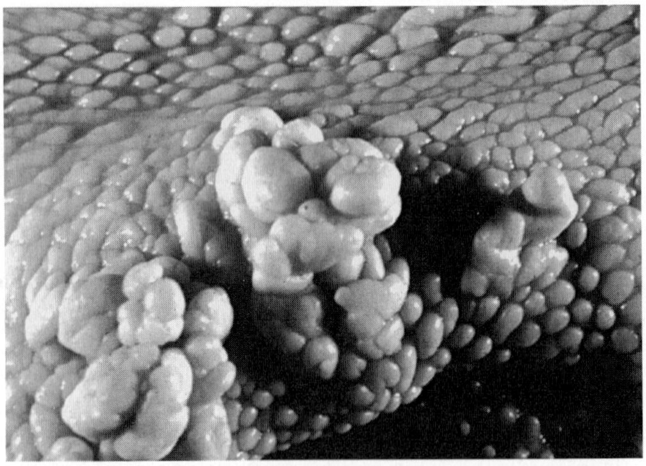

Figure 1-38 Rumen; cow. Ruminal papillomas. Smooth-surfaced epithelial-covered papillomas on ruminal papillae.

The mucosal surface of monogastric animals is thrown into convoluted folds called rugae, which are penetrated by the foveolae (numerous stellate-shaped crevices in the surface), through which gastric glands deliver their secretions to the surface. The rugal pattern is sparse and longitudinally arrayed along the lesser curve of the stomach and sparse and spirally arranged in the antrum. The mucosa of the body and fundus is composed of parallel tubular glands containing mucous neck cells, parietal cells (which secrete acid), chief cells (which secrete pepsin), and enterochromaffin cells, whereas the mucosa of the antrum has simple mucus-secreting glands. The submucosa of the antrum is rich in equidistantly spaced lymphoid follicles. Ruminants have a single lymphoid patch at the fold separating the omasum and abomasum.

In the horse and rat the stomach has a proximal stratified squamous epithelial portion and a caudal glandular portion. The pig has a small square area of stratified squamous epithelium surrounding the esophageal entrance to the stomach.

Gastric Dilatation and Volvulus Syndrome

Simple gastric dilation occurs in a variety of animals and in human beings. In dogs, particularly in the large, deep-chested breeds, the **acute gastric dilatation and volvulus syndrome** occurs. This lesion is life threatening and should not be confused with simple gastric dilation, which is common in young puppies after overeating. Predisposing factors to acute gastric dilation include a source of distending gas, fluid, or feed and obstruction of the cardia that prevents eructation and emesis and obstruction of the pylorus that prevents passage of gastric contents into the small intestine. The source of gas is not well understood. Theories include gas production by *Clostridium perfringens,* spores of which are present in the feed, CO_2 from physiologic mechanisms of digestion, or simple aerophagia (Figs. 1-39 and 1-40).

The result of repeated episodes of gastric dilation is stretching and relaxation of the gastrohepatic ligament. Recurrent dilation combined with overfeeding, postprandial exercise, and perhaps a hereditary predisposition to it results in gastric rotation. Gastric rotation is recognized by splenic displacement and a twisted esophagus and results in vascular compression and decreased venous drainage and hypoxemia (Figs. 1-41 and 1-42). The stomach generally is rotated clockwise on the ventrodorsal axis when the abdomen is viewed from the ventral surface. Rotation is 180, 270, or 360 degrees. The combination of gastric hypoxemia, acid-base imbalance, obstruction of the pylorus and cardia, and increased intragastric pressure leads to antiperistaltic waves followed by atony, cardiovascular ischemia, arrhythmias, and shock. Decreased portal venous return leads to pancreatic ischemia and release of myocardial depressant factor, cardiac collapse, and death.

Abomasal Displacement

Abomasal displacement is usually to the left side, although right-sided displacements also occur. Normally the abomasum lies on the xiphoid process at the abdominal ventral midline. Left-sided displacement of the abomasum is a generally nonfatal entity of high-producing dairy cattle during the 6 weeks following parturition. Strenuous activity can predispose nonpregnant cows to displacement. In the postcalving period, abomasal atony can occur as a result of heavy grain feeding (volatile fatty acids decrease motility) and hypocalcemia. Meanwhile, the gravid uterus

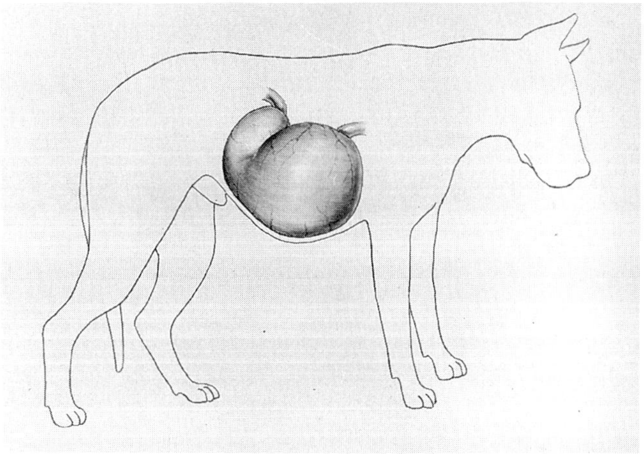

Figure 1-39 Stomach; dog. Acute gastric dilatation. This diagram drawn from postmortem photographs illustrates the position of the distended stomach in the live animal. *Van Kruiningen HJ, Gregoire K, Meuten DJ. J Am Anim Hosp Assoc 1974; 10:294-324.*

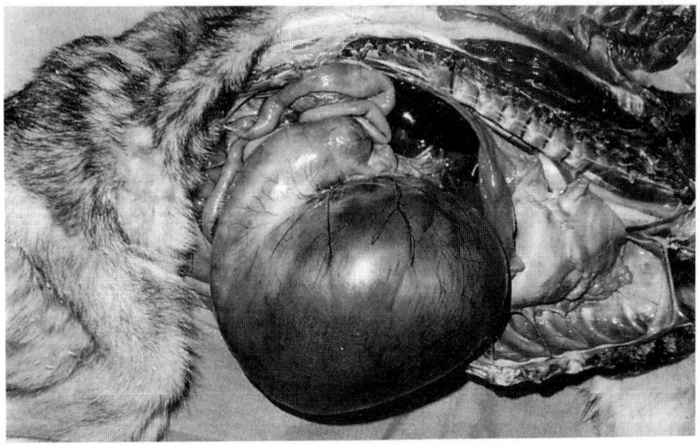

Figure 1-40 Stomach; dog. Acute gastric dilatation. The stomach is distended by ingesta and gas and its mucosal surface is red-violet from congestion and cyanosis. It has significantly displaced other abdominal viscera. Note the collapsed lung.

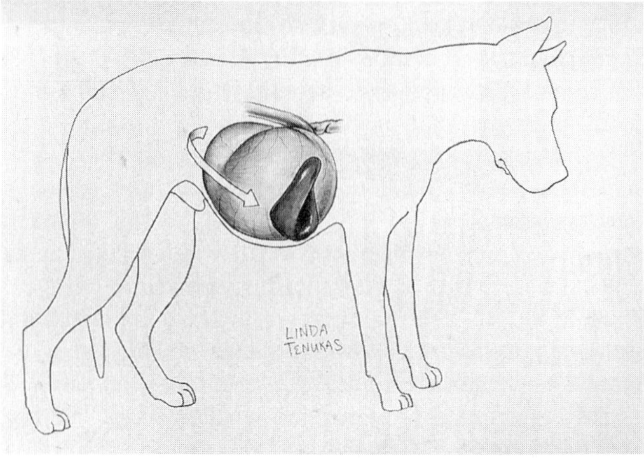

Figure 1-41 Stomach; dog. Acute gastric dilatation. This diagram made from postmortem photographs illustrates the 360-degree rotation and direction that occurs with volvulus. The spleen is folded and located in the right cranial abdomen against the diaphragm. *Van Kruiningen HJ, Gregoire K, Meuten DJ. J Am Anim Hosp Assoc 1974; 10:306.*

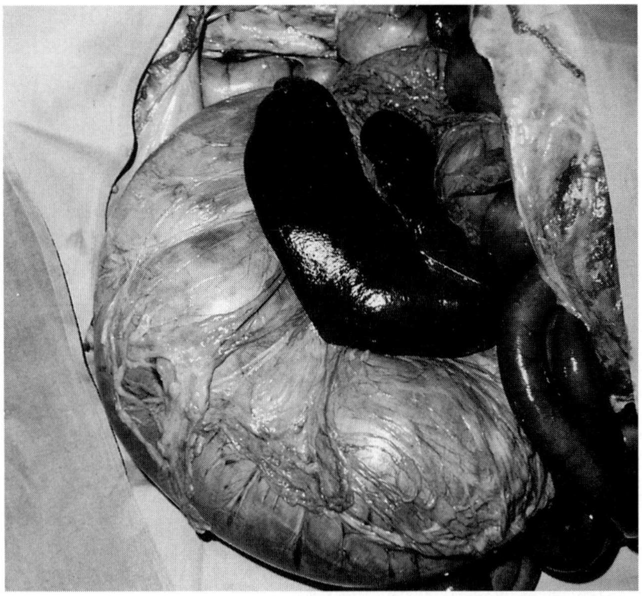

Figure 1-42 Stomach; dog. Acute gastric dilatation with a 360-degree volvulus. The stomach is greatly enlarged and distended, and the spleen is folded in a V, and located against the diaphragm adjacent to the last ribs on the right side of the abdomen. The intestines are dilated and congested secondary to vascular compromise.

might have displaced the rumen and abomasum forward and to the left, rupturing the attachment of the greater omentum to the abomasum (Figs. 1-43 and 1-44). The abomasum occupies the cranial left quadrant of the abdomen and displaces the rumen medially. This change leads to partial obstruction of abomasal outflow. Metabolic acidosis is due to rumen atony and impaired movement of ingesta. The associated hypochloremia is a result of HCl secretion and is common along with hypokalemia. Abomasal ulcers and peritoneal adhesions can result in chronic displacement.

Fifteen percent of abomasal displacements are right-sided. The abomasum can overdistend, curl dorsally, and twist on its mesenteric axis. Twenty percent of such cases lead to abomasal volvulus. Right-sided displacements occur in postparturient dairy cows and in calves.

Clinical features of displaced abomasum include partial anorexia, weight loss, dehydration, scant feces, and ketonuria. On auscultation a characteristic high-pitched ping can be heard over the distended, displaced abomasum, whether it is on the left or right side. Acute displacement of the abomasum to the right with volvulus is characterized by abomasal tympany and signs of abdominal pain such as grinding of the teeth (bruxism), abnormal posture, repeated getting up and lying down, and kicking at the belly. Other clinical signs include anorexia, restlessness, rapid heart rate, modest grunting or groaning, lack of abdominal peristalsis, and scanty feces.

Gastric Dilation and Rupture

Acute gastric dilation and rupture in the horse occurs most frequently as a terminal event in intestinal obstruction and displacement. **Gastric dilation** occurs in horses as a result of the ingestion of fermentable feeds or grain, a situation analogous to grain overload with lactic acidosis in cattle. Because gastric dilation and rupture can occur after death, the diagnostic challenge is to determine if the rupture occurred before or after death. The only reliable indicator of the time of rupture, in relation to the death of the animal, is the presence of hemorrhage and evidence of inflammation, such as fibrin strands, along the margins of the rupture, since such inflammatory responses occur only in live animals.

In Scotland, England, and Sweden, acute gastric dilation occurs in horses on pasture as part of a disease called **grass sickness.** Serologic evidence suggests an association of grass sickness with *Clostridium perfringens* type A enterotoxin.

Acute gastric dilation also occurs spontaneously in nonhuman primates. In captive monkeys an increased frequency of acute gastric dilation often occurs over weekends, when presumably there is a difference in the feeding pattern because of weekend caretakers. Evidence of the roles of *C. perfringens* and fermentable substrates comes from studies with monkeys and marmosets. *C. perfringens* was found in the gastric contents of 21 of 24 monkeys with acute gastric dilation but in few samples

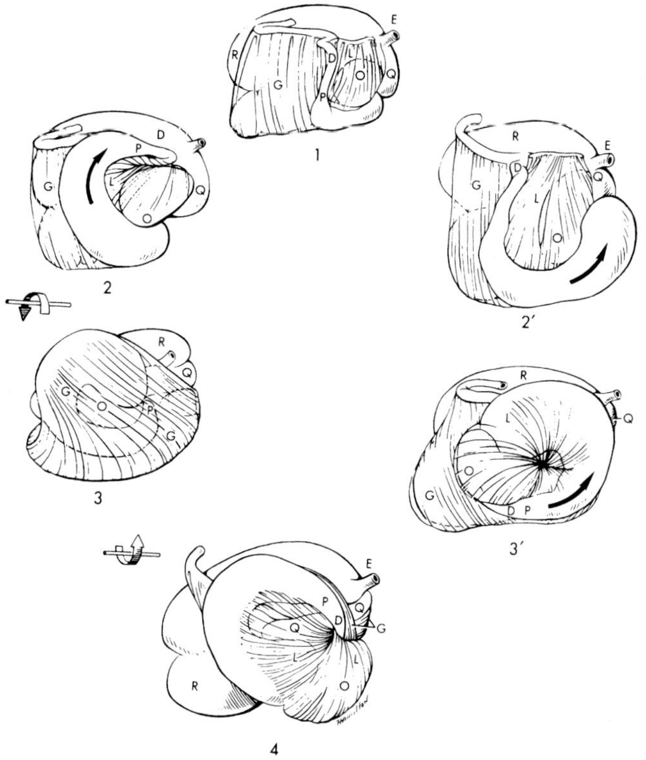

Figure 1-43 Abomasum; cow. Displaced abomasum with volvulus. Diagrams to illustrate two possible modes of rotation of the omasum, abomasum, and cranial part of the duodenum in volvulus. *1,* normal relations; *2,* simple dilatation and displacement on the right; *3,* 180-degree volvulus around the longitudinal axis of the lesser omentum, counterclockwise as seen from the rear; 2′, 90-degree rotation of the abomasum in a sagittal plane, counterclockwise as seen from the right; 3′, 180-degree rotation of the abomasum and omasum around the transverse axis of the lesser omentum, drawing the duodenum cranially, medial to the omasum; *4,* 360-degree counterclockwise volvulus, final stage resulting from either mode of rotation. *D,* duodenum; *E,* esophagus; *G,* greater omentum; *L,* lesser omentum; *O,* omasum; *P,* pylorus; *Q,* reticulum; *R,* rumen. *Habel RE, Smith DF. J Am Vet Med Assoc 1981; 179:447-455.*

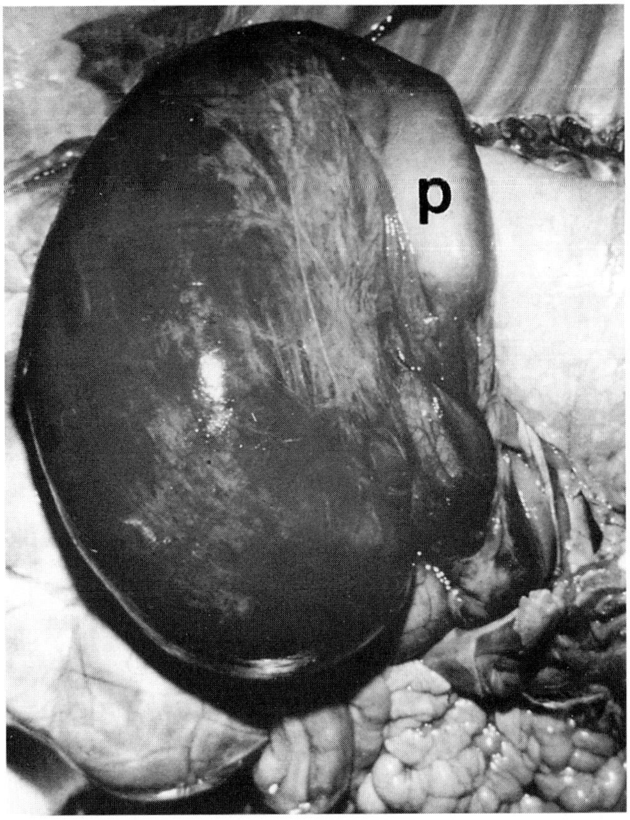

Figure 1-44 Abomasum; cow. Right displaced abomasum with volvulus. The abomasum is enlarged, and the wall is engorged with blood and edema fluid. *P,* pylorus.

(2 of 18) from normal monkeys. Twenty-nine cases of acute gastric dilation occurred in marmosets over a 5-week period after therapy with gentamicin and furoxone. *C. perfringens* type A was found in the gastric contents of all 25 animals that were necropsied, suggesting a link between the gas-forming bacteria and gastric dilation.

Chronic gastric dilation is almost always a secondary event. In the dog, it is due to gastric ulcer, lymphoma of the gastric wall, uremia, pyloric stenosis, acute gastric dilation, intervertebral disc disease, or vagotomy. In the horse, chronic gastric dilation occurs as a consequence of the consumption of nonnutritious feed, but it occurs more frequently in horses with the vice of cribbing and air swallowing. Chronic abomasal dilation occurs in cows with abomasal ulcers, abomasal malignant lymphoma, and vagal indigestion. Ruminants fed poorly nutritious feed such as straw, poor-quality hay, and frozen silage develop chronic gastric dilation. In ruminants, chronic dilation of the rumen occurs after engorgement, difficult parturition, transport fatigue, metabolic disorders, and vagus indigestion.

Clinically, animals with chronic gastric dilation have partial or complete anorexia, a lack of normal contraction sounds or peristaltic waves, a greater than normal gaseous bubble, and thus a noticeably distended abdomen. Chronic gastric dilation contributes to a slowing of the entire gastrointestinal system so that sounds and motility patterns of the small bowel are reduced and feces are scant. Lesions in chronic gastric dilation are few and consist of an enlarged stomach with an abnormal volume or character of feed residue. The dilated abomasum in vagus indigestion is enlarged and impacted with dry contents because of functional pyloric stenosis. Gastric trichobezoars and phytobezoars of monogastric animals are similar to those that occur in the rumen.

Impaction

Impaction of the monogastric stomach and abomasum has a variety of causes. Lesions of the thorax such as pneumonia, pleuritis, lymphadenopathy, and lymphosarcoma can infiltrate and damage the vagal nerves. Roughage, hairballs, and other foreign materials also cause impaction. **Abomasal emptying defect** is an idiopathic condition in Suffolk sheep.

Inflammatory Diseases

Inflammation of the simple stomach or abomasum, **gastritis** and **abomasitis,** respectively, must be distinguished from simple hyperemia and petechiae, which are often nonspecific agonal lesions. Gastritis is often associated clinically with vomiting, dehydration, and metabolic acidosis. Necrosis, hemorrhage, edema (Fig. 1-45), erosions, ulcerations, increased amounts of mucus, abscesses, granulomas, foreign body penetration, parasites, and inflammatory cells of various types characterize the changes in the mucosal surface and subsequent inflammatory reaction.

Acute phlegmonous gastritis occurs in the dog and is the result of infection of the gastric wall by bacteria. Infecting organisms include streptococci, staphylococci, *Escherichia coli, Proteus vulgaris,* or *Clostridium perfringens.* Clinically, phlegmonous gastritis is characterized by abrupt onset of mid epigastric pain, nausea, and vomiting accompanied by fever, chills, and prostration. Death usually ensues from circulatory collapse. Purulent emesis, a rare occurrence, is specific for this entity, and emesis of a necrotic cast of the gastric wall is pathognomonic.

Grossly, the stomach is dilated and has thickened walls, 1.5 cm in thickness, and a deep red to purple mucosa. The submucosa is usually edematous and might ooze pus. Less often, emphysema of the submucosa results in gas bubbles of varying sizes in the thickened gastric wall and imparts a cobblestone texture to the mucosa. **Emphysematous gastritis** is due to gas-forming organisms such as *C. perfringens* and sometimes occurs with acute gastric dilation with volvulus. Microscopically, the mucosa and submucosa are thickened and distended by edema and a diffuse, granulocytic inflammatory infiltrate. The mucosa has hemorrhage, congestion, and foci of coagulation necrosis. The causative bacteria usually can be seen enmeshed in a fibrinopurulent exudate in the gastric wall.

Clostridium septicum is a cause of hemorrhagic abomasitis with submucosal emphysema of sheep and cattle, a disease known as **braxy.** Although this disease is most common in the United Kingdom and Europe, it occurs in North America as well. Generally, the disease follows ingestion of frozen feeds contaminated with the causative *Clostridium* spp. The lesions are produced by the exotoxin of the bacteria, and death therefore is due to an exotoxemia.

In many septicemias of pigs, bacterial emboli lodge in the vessels of the submucosa and cause thrombosis resulting in infarction and ulceration. This occurs in salmonellosis, swine dysentery, Glasser's disease, and colibacillosis. Certain intoxicants such as vomitoxin produced by *Fusarium* spp. can cause similar lesions (Fig. 1-46).

Microorganisms that invade the deeper tissues of the gastric wall rather than just the mucosa and cause a **granulomatous gastritis** include *Histoplasma capsulatum* (see intestinal diseases of dogs and cats) and rarely *Mycobacterium tuberculosis.* Organisms gain access to the

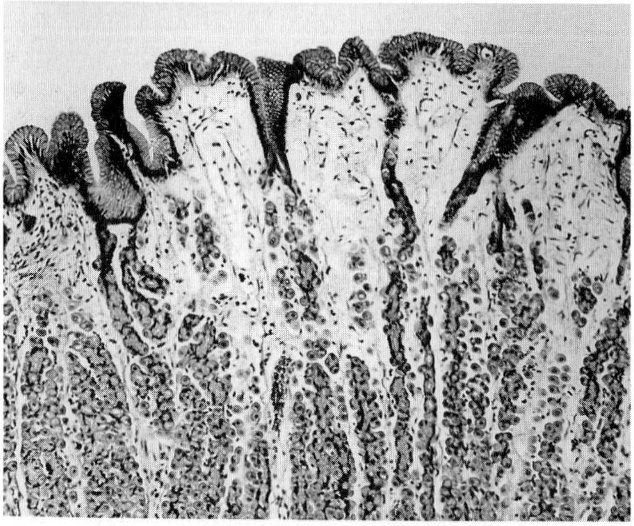

Figure 1-45 Stomach; dog. Gastric mucosal edema. The surface is raised, and foveolae are separated by edema fluid *(pale areas).* Gastric glands are similarly separated in the neck regions but appear normal at the base of the mucosa. H & E stain.

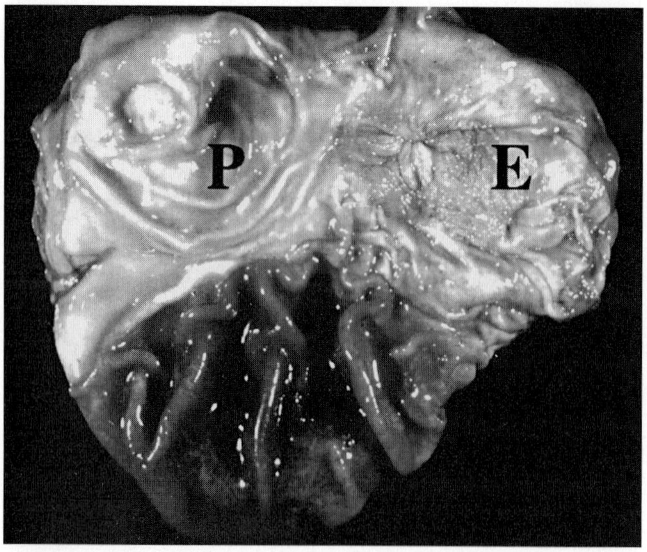

Figure 1-46 Stomach; pig. Acute necrohemorrhagic gastritis. The fundus of the stomach is hemorrhagic with multiple foci of mucosal necrosis. *E,* esophageal os; *P,* pylorus.

deeper tissues (i.e., the submucosa, the muscle layers, lymph vessels, subserosa, and adjacent lymph nodes) and cause a granulomatous inflammation. The wall of the stomach becomes increasingly thickened, and the stomach becomes less functional. Clinical features include postprandial epigastric pain, vomiting, weight loss, weakness, hematemesis, and gastric outlet obstruction. Microscopically, macrophages are the predominant cell type. Plasma cells, lymphocytes, fibroblasts, and variable numbers of neutrophils, eosinophils, and multinucleate giant cells are also present. Often, the causative organisms can be demonstrated with the granulomatous inflammation, but special stains such as acid fast or periodic acid Schiff are required.

Eosinophilic gastritis probably occurs, but rarely, in most species of animals but has been studied in dogs, cats, and human beings. In all three species, two forms of eosinophilic gastritis are recognized: a focal form caused by infiltrating eosinophils in response to trapped nematode larvae and a diffuse form, believed to be allergic in nature, affecting a large portion of the stomach. In the dog, focal eosinophilic gastritis occurs in response to the migration of larval *Toxocara canis*. Puppies are infected with *T. canis* larvae through the milk of the bitch or from eating feed contaminated by the eggs or larvae, presumably from the feces of the bitch. These larvae can remain in the tissues for years, attracting eosinophils because of their waste products, saliva, and sheath. The lesion is a polypoid or nodular mass on the surface of the gastric mucosa consisting of an embedded parasite surrounded by a collection of eosinophils and is often confined to the gastric antrum, where it can produce gastric outlet obstruction. A scirrhous eosinophilic gastritis occurs in dogs, and a similar disorder of the stomach and intestines is found in cats. The causes are not known. Scirrhous eosinophilic gastritis is characterized by weight loss, lethargy, recurrent vomiting, sometimes a pendulous abdomen, and a thickened stomach wall. Affected animals have peripheral eosinophilia, as great as 30% in the dog.

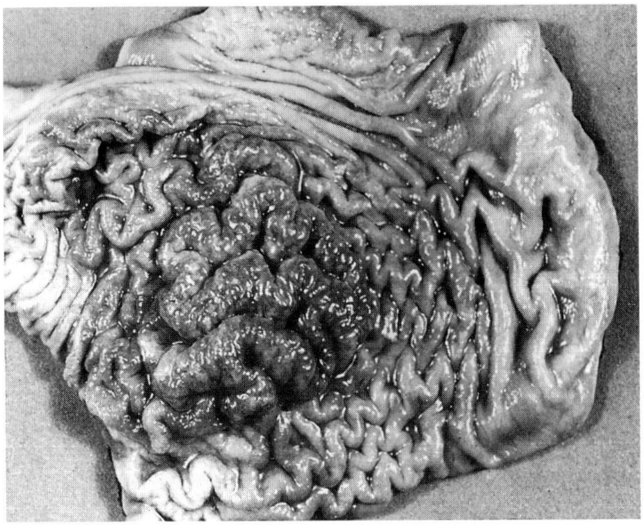

Figure 1-47 Stomach; dog. Hypertrophic gastritis. A circumscribed area of hyperplastic mucosa, composed of convoluted, reddened, and exaggerated rugae, occurs as a solitary mass several centimeters in diameter. *Van Kruiningen HJ. Vet Pathol 1977; 14:19-28.*

The microscopic lesions are characterized by infiltrates of eosinophils in the mucosa, the submucosa, and extensively through the muscle layers of the stomach and, sometimes, in segments of the small intestine and colon. In the dog, some of the small- and medium-sized arterioles of the submucosa of the affected antrum have medial necrosis, adventitial proliferation, and eosinophilic perivasculitis. The eosinophilic infiltrate is followed by fibroplasia of the lamina propria, submucosa, and muscle layers. Regional lymph nodes are enlarged with infiltrates of eosinophils and lymphoid hyperplasia.

Hypertrophic or Hyperplastic Diseases

The long-term outcome of chronic gastritis is **hypertrophic gastritis** characterized by thickened rugae, the result of hyperplasia of the gastric glands (Fig. 1-47). This effect is believed to be a response to retention of gastric fluid and reflux of intestinal bile. Similar mucosal glandular changes are seen in immune-mediated lymphoplasmacytic gastritis of dogs. Hypertrophic gastritis has also been described in primates, horses, and rodents. The gastric nematode *Nochtia nocti* causes this lesion in monkeys. In the horse, hypertrophic gastritis occurs in response to infection with *Habronema* spp. and *Trichostrongylus axei*.

Chronic giant hypertrophic gastropathy of dogs affects the basenji, beagle, boxer, and bull terrier breeds, among others. The disease is similar to Menétrier's disease of human beings. Clinically, observations include weight loss, diarrhea, vomiting, and hypoproteinemia. The chronic gastritis results in increased mucosal permeability to serum proteins with subsequent protein-losing gastropathy. Unlike normal gastric mucosal folds, in giant hypertrophic gastropathy the mucosa does not flatten with distension of the organ (Fig. 1-48). Microscopically, the mucosa is hypertrophic and hyperplastic. The incorporation of folds of submucosa and muscularis mucosa is variable, as is the presence of inflammatory cells. The etiology is unknown.

Fundic stomach

Ulcers and Erosions

An **ulcer** is a mucosal defect in which the entire epithelial thickness, down to or through the basement membrane, has been lost. Penetration through the remaining tissue layers to the abdominal cavity is termed a **perforating ulcer.** When focal coagulation necrosis produces excavation only partway through the depth of the epithelium, the lesion is termed an **erosion.** Ulcers are round, stellate, or linear. Acute stress ulcers are shallow, have soft hyperemic margins, and often occur in a diffusely congested mucosa. Ulcers that have been present for some time lack a

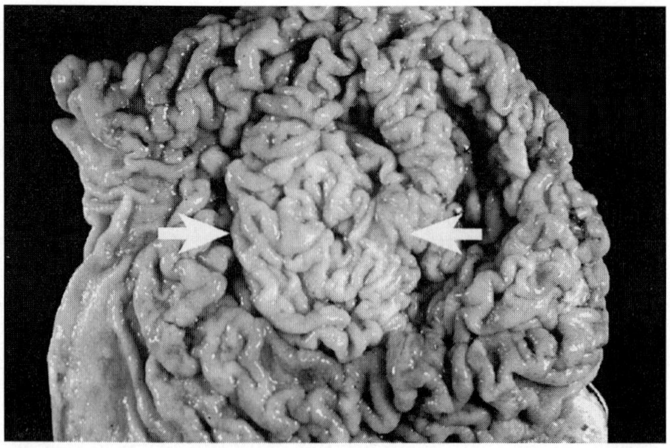

Figure 1-48 Stomach; basenji dog. Chronic giant hypertrophic gastropathy. A cerebreform mass of redundant mucosa is present in the center of the gastric mucosa *(arrows). Courtesy Department of Veterinary Pathology, Cornell University.*

hyperemic rim but have indurated fibrotic margins and are deeper. The crater is often coated with a gray or tan, fibrinopurulent pseudomembrane. Microscopically, ulcers appear as an abruptly marginated focal excavation in the mucosa, with or without fibrinopurulent exudate above and granulation tissue beneath. Thrombosis of blood vessels beneath the crater occurs in some ulcers, but this is usually not regarded as a cause of the ulcer except for those in ruminants with mycotic vasculitis, often secondary to lactic acidosis. Ulcers that penetrate through the submucosa into the tunica muscularis or to the subserosa are bordered by an acute inflammatory response.

The pathogenesis of most gastric and duodenal ulcers in human beings has been demonstrated to be due to a **helical bacterium.** Although similar gastric *Helicobacter*-like organisms (GHLO) are readily demonstrated in dogs and cats, their association with ulcer formation is not established. It appears that as many animals without gastritis or ulcers are as heavily colonized by these bacteria as are those animals with ulcers (Fig. 1-49). More than 90% of cats are infected with *Helicobacter* spp. *Helicobacter felis* can be cultured *in vitro,* but the noncultivatable *Helicobacter heilmannii* is present most often.

Theories abound as to the causes of most gastric ulcers in animals. None have been proved. The conditions necessary for **ulcer development** boil down to an imbalance between acid secretion and mucosal protection. This imbalance occurs as a result of:

- Local disturbances or trauma to the mucosal epithelial barrier. This injury can be due to back-flush of bile salts from the duodenum or ingestion of lipid solvents such as alcohol.
- Normal or high gastric acidity.
- Local disturbances in blood flow (i.e., stress-induced and sympathetic nervous system–mediated arteriovenous shunts) resulting in ischemia.

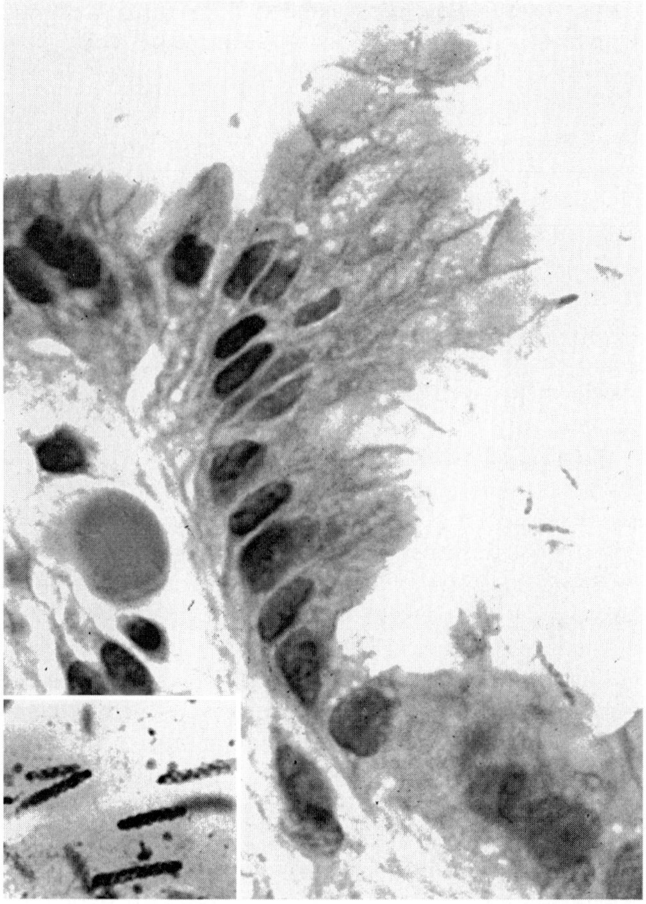

Figure 1-49 Stomach; cat. *Helicobacter pylori* infection. Numerous spiral bacteria are present in the superficial mucus layer. There is no inflammation in the adjacent mucosa. H & E stain. *Inset:* higher magnification of *Helicobacter* spp. Steiner's stain.

- Steroids and nonsteroidal anti-inflammatory drugs (NSAIDs) depress prostaglandin formation or concentration decreasing phospholipid secretions that are protective.

All of the above mechanisms allow pepsin and hydrochloric acid into the submucosa. There might be a heritable component to the susceptibility to ulcers.

In the dog, gastric ulceration is manifested clinically by vomiting, variable appetite, abdominal pain, anemia, and, occasionally, loss of weight. Foals with gastric ulcers have abdominal pain, bruxism (grinding of the teeth), salivation, and gastric reflux and lie in dorsal recumbency. Cattle with abomasal ulcers have partial or complete anorexia, decreased milk production, palpable discomfort to pressure applied to the right xiphoid area, and melena. In any species the vomiting of coffee grounds–like material (hematemesis) or melena is highly suggestive of gastric ulcer disease.

Abomasal ulcers of ruminants vary from subclinical to fatal (Fig. 1-50). In calves, ulcers are associated with dietary changes or mechanical irritation of the abomasum by roughage. Dietary changes involve substitution of

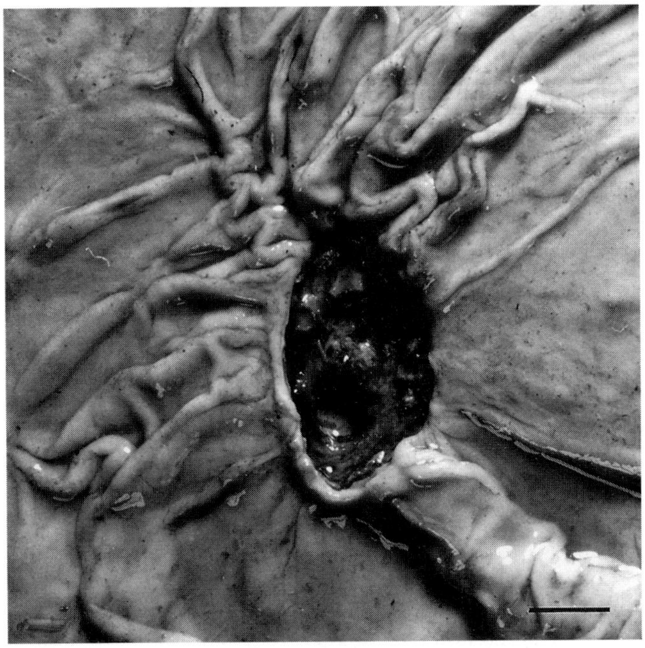

Figure 1-50 Abomasum; cow. Abomasal ulcer. This solitary, 4-cm diameter ulcer penetrated the abomasal wall causing diffuse peritonitis which resulted in death. Bar = 1 cm. *Courtesy Dr. M.D. McGavin.*

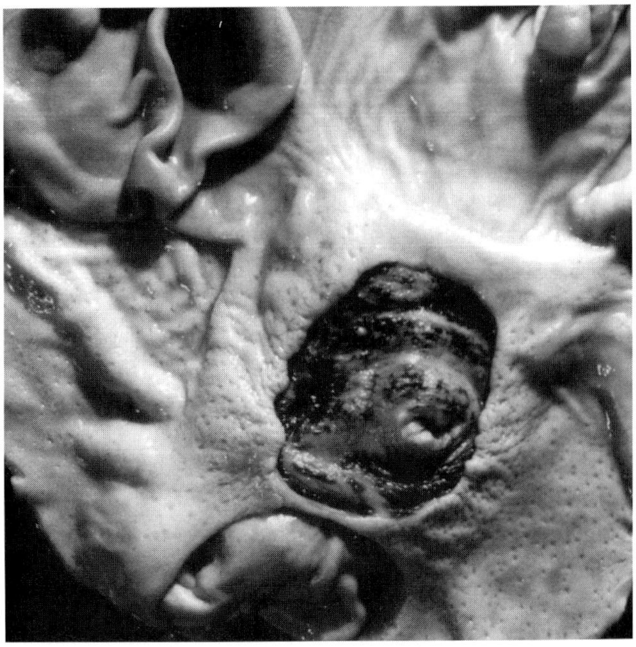

Figure 1-51 Stomach; pig. Ulcer of the nonglandular mucosa. This solitary chronic ulcer of the stratified squamous portion of the stomach surrounds the esophagus. *Courtesy Dr. M.D. McGavin.*

roughage for milk or milk replacer, together with the associated stress. In dairy cattle, ulcers are associated with heavy grain feeding (lactic acidosis) at the time of parturition, displacement of the abomasum, bovine viral diarrhea, impaction, torsion, and lymphosarcoma.

In pigs, gastric ulcers are common and occur in penned pigs fed finely ground grain. These ulcers always are limited to the stratified squamous epithelial esophageal portion of the gastric mucosa that surrounds the cardia (Fig. 1-51). Death can result from exsanguination into the gastric lumen. Evidence suggests that a high-carbohydrate diet is not sufficient to produce erosions and ulcers but rather that the appropriate diet in combination with fermentative commensal bacteria such as *Lactobacillus* and *Bacillus* spp. produce lesions.

Gastric ulcers in dogs and cats are generally idiopathic (Fig. 1-52) but can occur in animals with mast cell tumors. These neoplasms release histamine into the blood stream and it binds to receptors on parietal cells of the stomach increasing HCl secretion. Also, ulcers occur in the Zollinger-Ellison syndrome caused by pancreatic gastrinoma.

Ulcers are idiopathic in foals. Gastric ulcers associated with administration of NSAIDs are common in horses but are also described in other species given these drugs.

Miscellaneous Diseases and Conditions

Uremic gastritis occurs most frequently in carnivores as a result of chronic renal disease. In ungulates, it is a rare

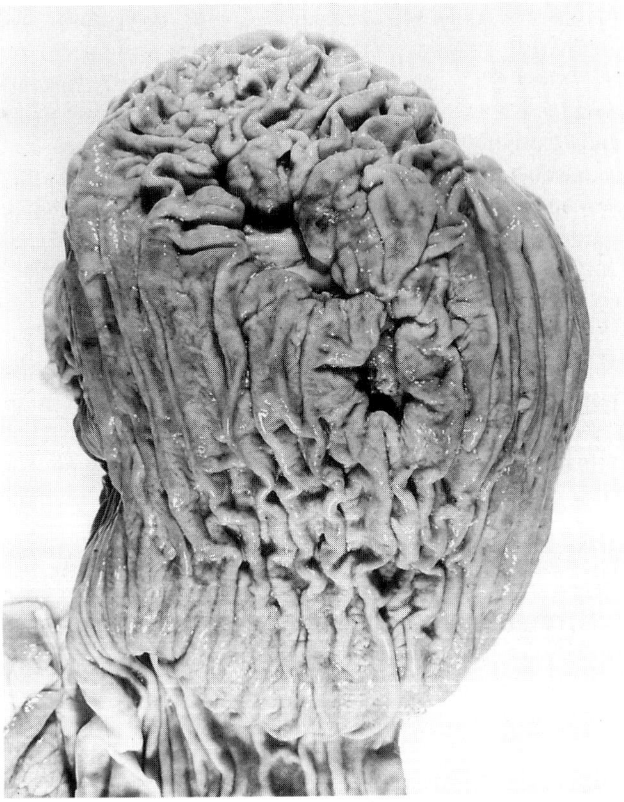

Figure 1-52 Stomach; dog. Chronic gastric ulcers. Three stellate ulcers are in the fundus, the upper two of which have perforated. Antrum is at the bottom. *Courtesy Dr. R.G. Thomson.*

event and is usually associated with obstructive kidney disease (postrenal uremia). Uremic gastritis is characterized by mineralization of the glands, vessels, and interstitium of the gastric mucosa and sometimes results in ulcer formation.

Pyloric stenosis can be due to an anatomic problem or an inability of the pyloric sphincter to function properly. This lesion occurs most often in brachycephalic dogs, especially the boxer, but is described in Siamese cats and occasionally in horses. The stenotic pylorus interferes with gastric emptying, and this results in projectile vomiting shortly after a meal, enlargement of the stomach, retention of a gastric residue, and accentuated peristaltic waves that can be heard, seen, or felt coursing from left to right across the abdomen. The hypertrophied pylorus can be palpated in animals that have a thin abdominal wall. The lesions of pyloric stenosis are grossly discernible enlargement and muscular hypertrophy of the pylorus, reduced lumen diameter, and accentuated mucosal folds. Microscopically, muscle hypertrophy is accompanied by variable submucosal edema, submucosal vascular ectasia, minimal leukocyte infiltrate, and variable degeneration of myenteric ganglion cells. Functional pyloric stenosis can be a feature of vagus indigestion.

Giant hypertrophic pyloric gastropathy, not to be confused with giant hypertrophic gastropathy of basenji and other dogs, is a lesion seen most often in older small-breed dogs. To the uninitiated, the gross and microscopic features of this pyloric lesion strongly imitate carcinoma (Fig. 1-53). Microscopically, there is marked foveolar and glandular hyperplasia with variable hypertrophy of smooth muscle, small mucosal erosions, and ulcerations. There is usually a lymphoplasmacytic infiltrate of variable degree. The cause of this condition is unknown.

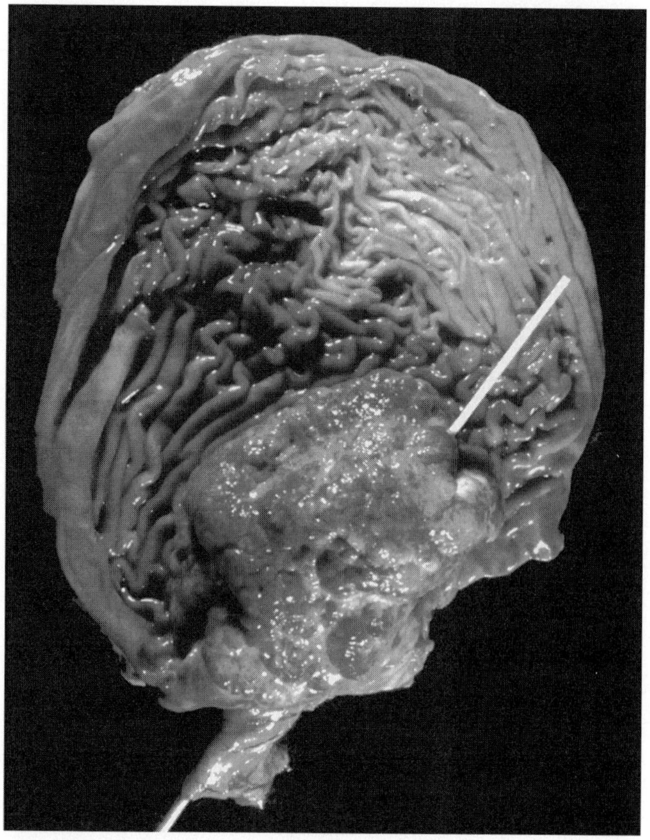

Figure 1-53 Stomach; dog. Giant hypertrophic pyloric gastropathy. The probe passes through the lumen of the pylorus into the unopened duodenum. The mass of hyperplastic glandular tissue should not be mistaken for a neoplasm.

Parasites

Horses

Many parasites cause disease of the stomach, especially of ungulates. Modern antihelmenthics have made these diseases relatively easy to control both in individual animals and in herds. **Equine bots,** *Gastrophilus intestinalis* and *Gastrophilus nasalis,* are commonly seen in animals on inadequate deworming regimens (Fig. 1-54). *G. intestinalis* colonizes the stratified portion of the stomach. The adult fly lays eggs on the hairs of the distal limbs of the horse. *G. nasalis* lays eggs around the nose of the horse and the larvae hatch after being licked. The larvae live in the glandular portion of the stomach. Both species attach to the mucosa via their anterior pincers. The larvae pass in the feces, pupate, and develop into flies.

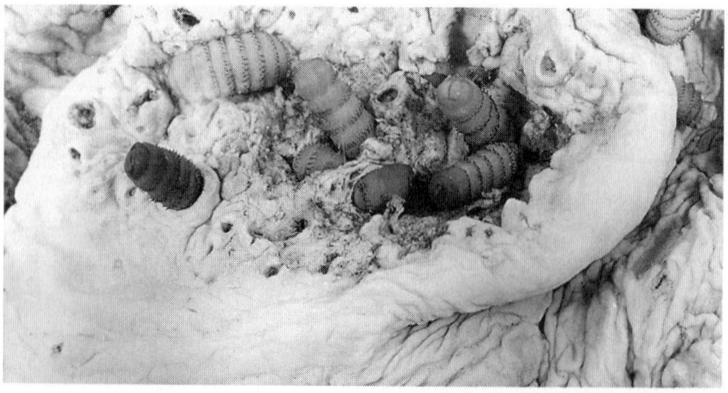

Figure 1-54 Stomach; horse. Gastric bots. *Gastrophilus* larvae and the craters produced by them are present in the squamous mucosa of the stomach. *Thomson RG. General Veterinary Pathology. Philadelphia: Saunders, 1978:398.*

Draschia megastoma is found in brood pouches in the glandular mucosa adjacent to the margo plicatus (Fig. 1-55). Infection is sometimes referred to as habronemiasis based on antiquated taxonomic nomenclature in which the nematodes were classified as *Habromena* spp. The adults in the cysts of the submucosal nodules release eggs through a pore. The eggs pass out with the feces from the animal and are consumed by larvae of a fly that serves as the appropriate intermediate host. Both *Draschia* spp. and

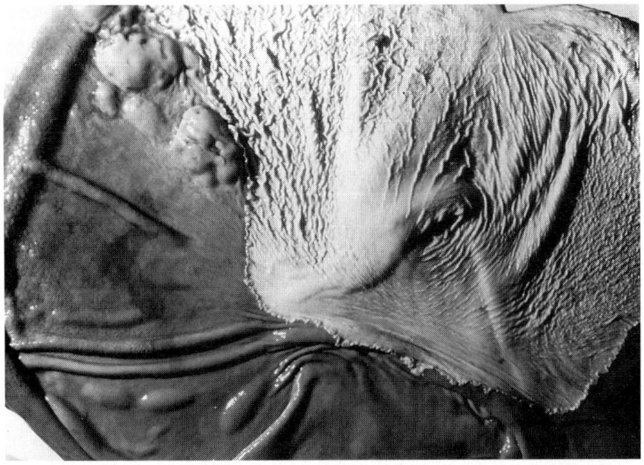

Figure 1-55 Stomach; horse. Draschiasis. Several raised parasitic nodules (brood pouches) are present in the glandular mucosa adjacent to the margo plicatus. *Courtesy Dr. M.D. McGavin.*

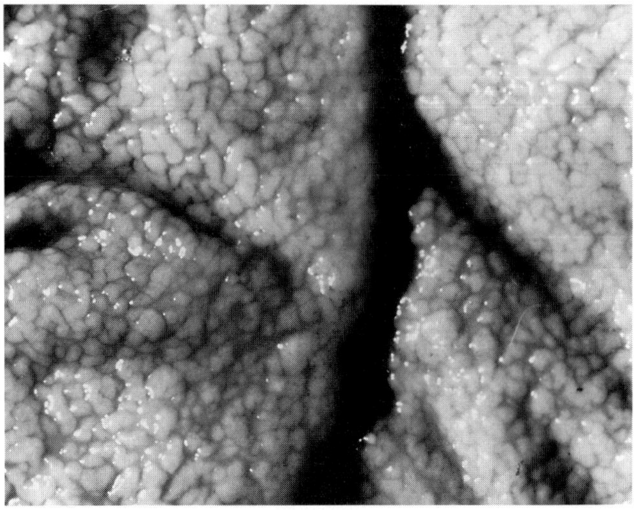

Figure 1-56 Abomasum; cow. Ostertagiasis. The granularity of the mucosa of the abomasal folds is due to mucus cell hyperplasia and the presence of lymphoid nodules. *Courtesy Dr. M.D. McGavin.*

Gastrophilus spp. can cause gastric ulcers. Considering their location and means of survival in the stomach, it is remarkable that they do not cause serious damage more often.

Ruminants

A common gastric parasite of sheep and other ruminants is *Haemonchus contortus,* the **barberpole worm.** The name is derived from the macroscopically visible entwining of the blood-filled intestine and white uterus in the female worm. These parasites are acquired on pasture when the third-stage larvae are consumed with pasture grasses. The ingested larvae enter the abomasum, where they reside within the gastric glands in a hypobiotic state, or they undergo development within the gastric glands to adults and move to the surface. Eggs of the nematode pass out in the feces, thereby completing the cycle. Haemonchosis is a serious problem when lambs on pasture ingest large numbers of larvae. These parasites feed on blood and can cause severe anemia as well as edema and hypoproteinemia, seen clinically as "bottle jaw" (marked submandibular edema). At necropsy, lesions are subcutaneous edema of the intermandibular space, pale conjunctiva and oral membranes, stunted growth, and liquid feces. Because of severe anemia, the organs are pale, the blood is watery, and the abomasal contents are fluid and brown. The abomasal folds have no lesions or have diffuse or patchy congestion and submucosal edema. Parasites are seen in the abomasal contents.

In cattle and small ruminants in temperate climates, **ostertagiosis** is considered the most important parasitic disease. Affected animals are unthrifty. In sheep and goats, the most common species is *Ostertagia circumcincta,* and in cattle it is *Ostertagia ostertagia.* These nematode parasites are approximately 1.5 cm long, have a direct life cycle similar to that of *Haemonchus* spp., and reside as third-, fourth-, and fifth-stage larvae in the gastric glands of the abomasum. *Ostertagia* spp. are often found in the company of other *trichostrongylus* spp. that reside in other gastrointestinal locations such as the small intestine. This combined parasitism results in failure to achieve adequate weight gains, inappetence, lassitude, diarrhea, and, in later stages, hypoproteinemia and attendant ventral edema. The abomasum of heavily infested animals takes on the appearance of Morocco leather (Fig. 1-56). This cobblestone appearance is due to mucous cell hyperplasia and lymphoid nodules in the abomasal submucosa elevating the overlying epithelium.

Abomasitis produced by *Ostertagia* spp. is characterized by an infiltration of chronic inflammatory cells (lymphocytes and plasma cells), some eosinophils, an increase in globule leukocytes in the mucosa, a decrease in the number of parietal and chief cells, and hyperplasia of mucous cells in the abomasum. The abomasal contents are fluid, brown-green, and fetid, as ingesta are partially putrefied because of large populations of bacteria. *Ostertagia* spp. can be demonstrated at necropsy. The worms are brown, smaller than *Haemonchus contortus,* and more difficult to see without magnification. The parasites occur within the gastric glands and in areas of chronic inflammation.

Hyostrongylus rubidus of pigs is a gastric parasite that causes a thickening of the mucosa with mucus accumulation similar to ostertagiosis of ruminants. The parasite is threadlike and red. Clinically, hyostrongylosis is associated with the "thin sow syndrome." Grossly, the gastric mucosa is thickened, catarrhal, and somewhat cobblestone. Microscopically, there is mucus metaplasia of parasitized and adjacent gastric glands. Submucosal lymphoid follicles develop in chronic infections.

Carnivores (Dogs and Cats)

Ollulaniasis and gnathostomiasis of the cat rarely produce gastritis. *Ollulanus tricuspis,* a minute nematode approximately 0.8 mm long, is transmitted in the vomitus of an infected cat and, rarely, causes mild gastritis or, sometimes, chronic fibrosing gastritis, indicated by mucosal nodularity or gastric rugal hypertrophy. The other parasite, *Gnathostoma* spp., is a Spiruroidea nematode with toothlike spines on the cephalic end that induces submucosal granulomatous masses that can exceed 5 cm in diameter.

Physaloptera spp. are often thought of as gastric parasites of carnivores because not infrequently they are found in the stomach on endoscopic examination or at necropsy. They are sometimes responsible for vomiting. They appear similar to ascarids but generally attach by anterior hooks to the proximal duodenal mucosa at the gastric valve. Intermediate hosts are coprophagous beetles.

Neoplasia

Gastric neoplasia, while uncommon, manifests in different ways in domestic animals. Leiomyoma and more rarely leiomyosarcoma arise from the tunica muscularis (Fig. 1-57). Lymphosarcoma can be primary, metastatic, or multicentric in origin. In cattle, it is often caused by the bovine leukemia virus and has a predilection for the abomasum as well as the right atrium and uterus. Squamous cell carcinoma of the stratified squamous (esophageal) portion of the stomach is relatively common in the horse. Glandular neoplasms, adenomas, and adenocarcinomas occur in all species but are seen most often in dogs and cats.

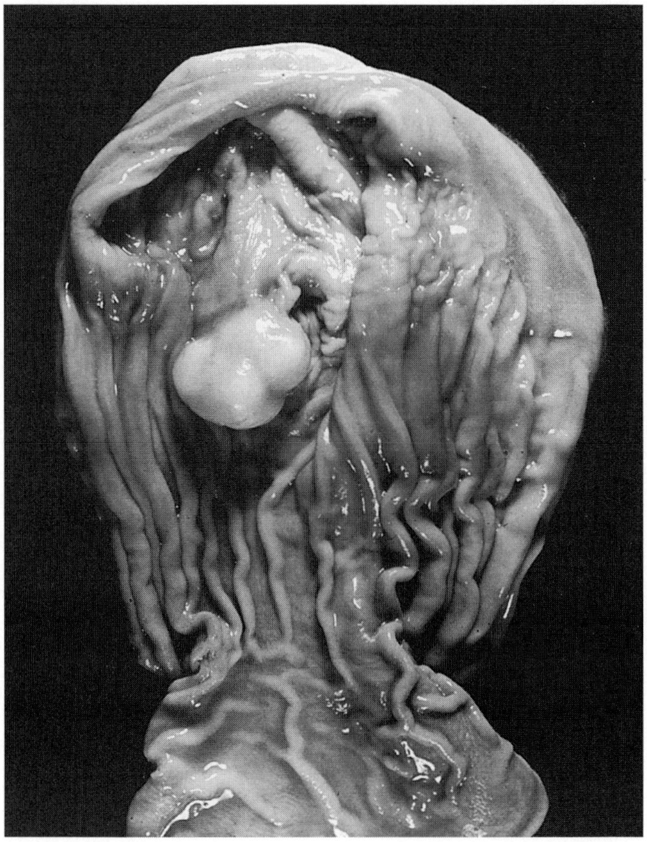

Figure 1-57 Stomach; dog. Leiomyoma. Note that this tumor is covered by intact mucosa. The tumor arose from the tunica muscularis.

INTESTINE

The intestines might be thought of as a tube within the body cavity that carries material (ingesta) through the body. By the action of enzymes and resident flora and added secretions, ingesta is broken down and useful substances are absorbed into the body and waste products are excreted. To perform these functions, the intestine needs a very large surface area. Creation of this surface area is accomplished by coiling the intestine in the abdomen. Herbivores have longer intestines than carnivores or omnivores and need a fermentation vat, either the rumen or cecum, to digest cellulose. In addition to its length, the intestinal mucosa is thrown into numerous folds that contain villi, which markedly increase the number of cells contacting the ingesta. Finally, each enterocyte has a microvillus border further increasing the surface area available for digestive and absorptive processes. Damage to any of these structures can result in malfunction and resultant diarrhea.

Cell Types of the Intestine

The intestinal mucosa is composed of epithelial cells lining the intestinal lumen and mesenchymal cells of the lamina propria and muscularis mucosa. An understanding of these cell types and their functional roles in digestion and absorption is important in understanding the mechanisms of intestinal disease. Similarly, an understanding of the biology of these cell types is important in predicting clinical outcomes and therapeutic strategies for intestinal disease.

Epithelial Cells

There are six types of epithelial cells lining the intestine. These are absorptive epithelial cells called enterocytes, undifferentiated or crypt epithelial cells, goblet cells, Paneth's cells, enterochromaffin cells, and M cells.

Enterocytes are tall and columnar with lumenal **microvilli.** They contain a surface glycocalyx that houses the digestive and absorptive enzymes. They do not proliferate but provide feedback inhibition of mitosis of the crypt cells by chalones. Many nutrients are absorbed through the lateral intercellular spaces between cells. Enterocytes move up the crypt and intestinal villus to the extrusion zone at the villus tip where effete enterocytes are discarded into the fecal mass. The turnover rate for enterocytes is the most rapid of any fixed cell population in the body. In neonatal pigs for instance, the turnover rate is 7 to 10 days. In 3-week-old pigs that have achieved climax flora, that rate accelerates to 2 to 3 days.

Undifferentiated **crypt epithelial cells** have little or no digestive capability. They are the progenitor cells that replace all of the other epithelial cell types. They have short sparse microvilli. Crypt cells are considered the source of secretory component that acts as a receptor for IgA and IgM produced by plasmacytes in the intestinal lamina propria. The migration rate of crypt cells up the villus is dependent on several factors, one of which is an adaptation to gut microflora. In germfree or gnotobiotic animals the enterocyte replacement rate is similar to that of the neonate. Crypt cells are considered a source of chloride ion secretion.

Goblet cells function in **mucous secretion.** They occur in both villus and crypt regions. Their numbers tend to increase caudad through the intestine.

Paneth's cells are located near the crypt base in some species, notably primates, horses, and rodents. They produce cryptdins and lyosins. These substances are toxic to bacteria and probably protect the proliferating crypt cells from infection. Paneth's cells are considered to have both secretory and phagocytic functions. Collectively, Paneth's cells comprise a cellular mass similar to that of the pancreas. It has been suggested that Paneth's cells play a role in elimination of heavy metals because they are selectively damaged by methylmercury.

Enterochromaffin cells, also known as argentaffin cells because of their affinity for silver, are enteroendocrine cells. They occur primarily in the crypts and produce serotonin, catecholamines, gastrin, secretin, and enteroglucagon. They secrete these products into the tissue rather than the gut lumen and, thus, are truly endocrine. Occasionally they form neoplasms called **carcinoids.**

M cells are so named because they have a microfolded or membranous surface. They form the dome epithelium, which covers the gut associated lymphoid tissue. They serve important functions in the uptake of antigens from the intestinal lumen and in the transport of these antigens to the gut-associated lymphoid tissue (GALT). M cells also serve as a portal of entry for some pathogens including bacteria such as *Salmonella, Yersinia,* and *Rhodococcus* spp. and some viruses such as bovine viral diarrhea virus.

Mesenchymal Cells

Mesenchymal cells reside in the lamina propria. **Theliolymphocytes** are of T cell origin. Their numbers increase with exposure to antigen, although there is a resident population of these cells in normal animals. The intestinal lymphoid tissue is 25% of the body's lymphoid mass (Fig. 1-58). This volume is larger than that of the spleen. In spite of the fact that the average person ingests 700 tons of antigens in a lifetime, the gut is adept at not responding to these food antigens. Data are beginning to accumulate identifying the different T lymphocyte types in the lamina propria.

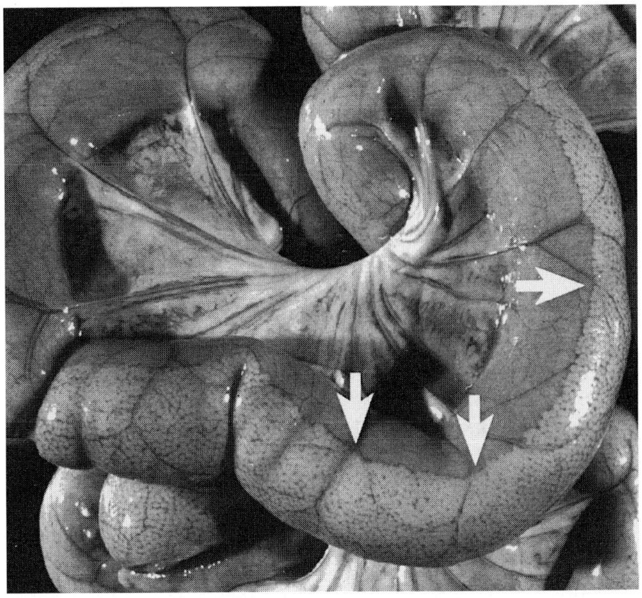

Figure 1-58 Intestine; pig. Ileum-associated lymphoid tissue. The outline of the intestinal lymphoid tissue is delineated by *arrows.*

Neutrophils are transient within the lamina propria of the intestine. Neutrophils are shortlived in the blood and tissues; their normal route of removal from the body is to migrate through the intestine to the lumen and be digested and excreted from the body via the feces.

Eosinophils, when present in the intestinal lamina propria and submucosa, indicate a hypersensitivity reaction, often to food antigens or parasites.

Globule leukocytes are large granular lymphocytes that are intraepithelial or within the lamina propria. They are found in all species and occasionally form neoplasms, most notably in the cat.

Defense Mechanisms of the Intestinal Tract

Defense mechanisms of the intestinal tract are diverse. They include indigenous (nonpathogenic) bacterial flora, intestinal and extraintestinal secretions, gastric acidity, intestinal motility, epithelial cell turnover, bile salts, immunologic mechanisms, and, although a secondary mechanism, the Kupffer cells of the liver.

- Secretions of the oral cavity, saliva, and intestine, called **mucins,** inhibit the adherence of organisms to the mucosa of the alimentary system.
- Normal **gastric acidity** kills many organisms before they have the chance to interact with enterocytes. Very young animals are achlorohydric and, thus, can be more susceptible to some organisms, such as pathogenic *E. coli.* It has recently been discovered that helical bacteria in the stomach are, in fact, the single greatest cause of gastric ulcers in human beings.

Although similar organisms occur in the stomachs of domestic animals, particularly carnivores, their role in gastritis of animals is less certain. Normal gastric acidity apparently does not kill all potentially pathogenic bacteria (helical bacteria) in the stomach and proximal small intestine of domestic animals.

- **Indigenous (nonpathogenic) bacterial flora** competitively bind to putative attachment sites on the enterocytes thus preempting pathogen attachment. They also compete for substrate with pathogens and alter the microenvironmental pH making competitive growth difficult. In addition, they produce inhibitory growth substances toxic to other bacteria called **bacteriocins.** Colicins are bacteriocins produced by *E. coli.*
- **Intestinal peristalsis** is protective in that loss of motility could lead to bacterial overgrowth in the intestine and increased susceptibility to toxins that are not moved out of the gut. Diarrhea can be, in part, a defense mechanism in that it rids the body of bacteria and toxins.
- As previously mentioned, epithelial cells of the intestine have the greatest turnover rate of any cell population in the body. In effect, this means that pathogens with a life cycle that exceeds that of the enterocytes will likely not be successful because their host cell will slough before the pathogen can reproduce.
- **Bile salts** inhibit the growth of many organisms, and the Kupffer cells of the liver act as a secondary line of defense. Since all the blood from the intestine percolates through the hepatic sinusoids, the Kupffer cells are perfectly positioned to phagocytose bacteria and endotoxins with which they come in contact.
- **Secretory IgA and IgM** constitute very important mechanisms of humoral immunity and function largely to prevent attachment of pathogens to intestinal epithelium. Crypt epithelial cells produce the secretory component of IgA.
- Bacterial growth is inhibited by lactoferin and peroxidase from the pancreas and lysozyme from Paneth's cells.

Diarrhea

Pathogenesis

Diarrhea is defined as secretion of abnormally fluid feces accompanied by an increased volume of feces and an increased frequency of defecation. Based on the various mechanisms of diarrhea just outlined, there are four major mechanisms by which diarrhea occurs:

- **Malabsorption** with or without bacterial fermentation leading to osmotic diarrhea. Generally, this is a problem of the small intestine, but secondary colonic malfunctions can occur due to malabsorption of bile salts and fatty acids, which stimulate fluid secretion in the large intestine.
- **Hypersecretion** by a structurally intact mucosa. This activity results in a net efflux of fluid and electrolytes independent of permeability changes, absorptive capacity, or exogenously generated osmotic gradients.
- **Exudation** due to increased capillary or epithelial permeability (protein-losing enteropathy).
- **Hypermotility** generally is involved in diarrhea but usually not as a primary mechanism in domestic animals. Hypermotility is defined as an increased rate, intensity, or frequency of peristalsis. Theoretically, with decreased mucosal contact time, digestion and absorption of nutrients should be less efficient. It is suspected that decreased motility in some diseases allows for increased bacterial proliferation. Conversely, some enterotoxins can stimulate intestinal motility.

As might be expected, the pathogenesis of diarrhea is much more complicated than as just explained. Involved are a complex interplay of cells and factors that are currently being elucidated by a variety of molecular techniques. For example, when a pathogen invades an enterocyte the pathogen can release an enterotoxin. This toxin causes the enterocyte to release cytokines, particularly interleukin 8. These cytokines activate resident macrophages and recruit new macrophages into the lamina propria from the blood. The activated leukocytes release soluble factors (histamine, serotonin, adenosine) that increase intestinal secretion of chloride ions and water and inhibit absorption.

Other factors (prostaglandins, leukotrienes, platelet-activating factor) act on enteric nerves to induce neurotransmitter-mediated intestinal secretion. Cell damage is possibly a consequence of inflammation mediated by T lymphocytes or proteases and oxidants secreted by mast cells. T lymphocytes also affect epithelial cell growth, causing villus atrophy and crypt hyperplasia. Cell death can result from pathogen invasion, multiplication, and extrusion. These changes lead to marked distortion of villus architecture accompanied by nutrient malabsorption and osmotic diarrhea.

Consequences

The consequence of excess fluid loss in the feces through diarrhea is dehydration. Dehydration results in hypovolemia. Hypovolemia results in hemoconcentration that results in inadequate tissue perfusion. Energy therefore is generated in the tissues by anaerobic glycolysis. The resultant hypoglycemia leads to ketoacidosis. Acidosis is, by definition, a reduction in blood and tissue pH. Acidosis leads to a reduction in pH-dependent enzyme system functions. Acidosis is compounded by fecal bicarbonate loss and the results of inadequate renal excretion of hydrogen ion and inadequate absorption of bicarbonate, which is a late effect of inadequate renal perfusion. The resultant electrolyte imbalance results in an increase in intracellular hydrogen ion concentration and a decrease in intracellular potassium ion concentration. The imbalances decrease neuromuscular control of myocardial contraction leading to a further decrease in tissue perfusion. A vicious cycle results, culminating in shock.

Developmental Anomalies

Occlusion of the intestinal lumen due to anomalous development of the intestinal wall is called **atresia.** Atresia is generally named for the part of the bowel that is occluded such as atresia ani or atresia coli. The causes of atresia in domestic animals are not completely understood but can be due to mechanical lesions in the blood vessels in a portion of the gut, such as malpositioning that compromises circulation and results in vascular accidents and ischemia. Release of meconium into the abdominal cavity of the fetus could result in sterile peritonitis and may be responsible for some cases of atresia such as in cystic fibrosis of human beings. In still other cases, a failure of the embryonic cells that occlude the lumen to break down could result in atresia. The end result is segmental atresia in which a segment of the bowel is either entirely missing or completely occluded due to lack of epithelial development and confluence between two contiguous portions (Fig. 1-59).

Meckel's diverticulum is a remnant of the omphalomesenteric duct. It is near the termination of the ileum and represents the stalk of the yolk sac. Generally, it disappears after the first trimester of gestation. It can persist in all mammalian species and, although blind ended, should not be confused with the cecum.

Megacolon, as its name implies, is a large, usually fecal-filled colon. It occurs in pigs, dogs, overo foals, and human beings. It may be caused by a congenital lack of myenteric plexuses (Hirschsprung's disease), the result of interference with the migration of neuroblasts from the embryonic craniocervical neural crest to the normal position of the myenteric plexus in the colon and rectum.

The equine overo pattern of spotting is characterized by white patches of skin on the ventral or lateral midsection and extend dorsally up to, but not including, the midline of the back. White skin also occurs on the lateral neck and flank. At least one, and usually all four legs are colored (i.e., not white). Affected foals appear normal at birth but fail to pass meconium, develop colic, and die. Such affected animals lack normal peristalsis because of absence of the myenteric (Auerbach's) plexus or submucosal (Meissner's) plexus. Thus these anomalies can be termed aganglionosis.

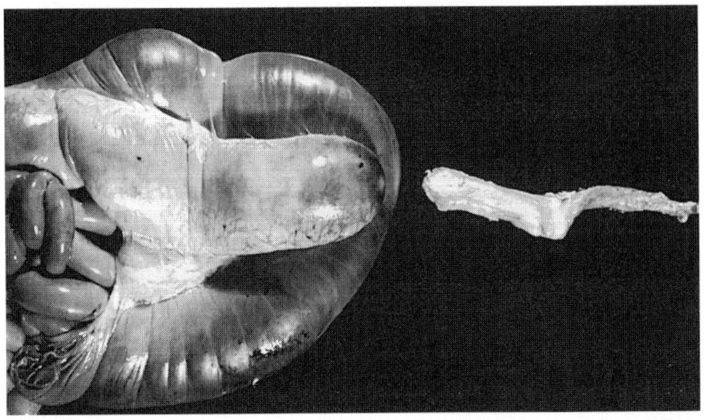

Figure 1-59 Colon; calf. Atresia coli. There is a blind-ended atresia of a segment of the spiral colon. The smaller segment at the right of the photomicrograph is the distal colon.

The gross lesion in congenital aganglionic megacolon is a contracted, nonperistaltic segment of rectum or rectum and contiguous colon, the so-called contracted distal segment. In foals, the abnormality is present in the rectum and small colon or rectum and the entire colon.

Megacolon when acquired is secondary to damage to the colonic innervation. Such events are usually traumatic. Atresia ani can also result in megacolon.

Intestinal Obstruction

Mechanical obstruction of the intestinal tract occurs in all species of domestic and wild animals. Although foreign bodies of all types have been removed from animals at surgery, the long-term systemic effects of some foreign bodies are also important. These include copper and zinc toxicosis from ingestion of coins in dogs, seals, ruminants, and horses, and lead poisoning in cattle from ingestion of old storage batteries. Primates caged in outdated facilities with leaded paint or lead bars can also succumb to lead poisoning.

Enteroliths

Enteroliths are rare in species other than the horse with an increased incidence in the Arabian breed. Generally, affected animals are older than 4 years. The stones are usually formed of ammonium magnesium phosphate (struvite) and form around a small central nidus or foreign body (Fig. 1-60). Enteroliths vary greatly in size from several centimeters in diameter to greater than 20 cm and can weigh several kilograms. They generally lodge at the pelvic flexure or transverse colon. Diets with large concentrations of magnesium and phosphorus enhance enterolith formation. In the past, miller's horses were frequently fed large amounts of bran and had an increased incidence of enteroliths. The frequency of enteroliths has been reduced by using magnets to remove metals from grain and by reducing the concentration of bran fed. The feeding of alfalfa hay, which is high in protein, and the greater-than-average magnesium content of California hay could contribute to the increased incidence of enteroliths in pleasure horses in that state.

Impaction of the intestine occurs in all species. It is especially common in horses following anthelminthic administration and is the result of rapid die-off of large numbers of nematodes, particularly ascarids (Fig. 1-61). Cecal impaction occurs in old horses because of a high-roughage diet, debility, or poor dentition. Fibrous ingesta can also result in ileal impaction. Large amounts of ingested sand can accumulate anywhere in the equine colon resulting in impaction.

Strictures with Obstruction

Strictures due to penetrating or nonpenetrating wounds of all kinds or to vascular injury can obstruct the intestine. For example, rectal stricture is a sequela to salmonellosis in pigs and is due in part to thrombosis of the cranial hemorrhoidal artery and lack of collateral circulation.

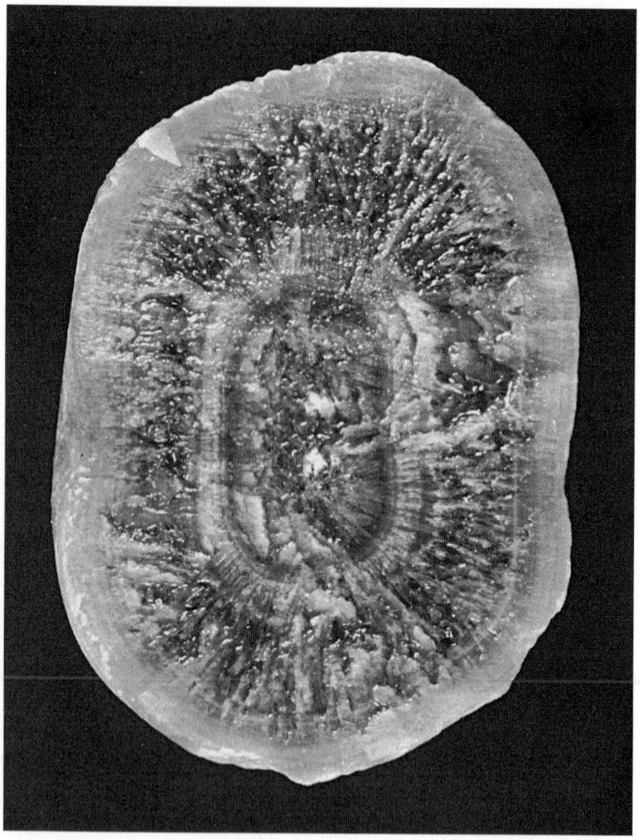

Figure 1-60 Enterolith, cross section; horse. The concentric laminations are visible on this incised specimen. A metal nidus was present at the center.

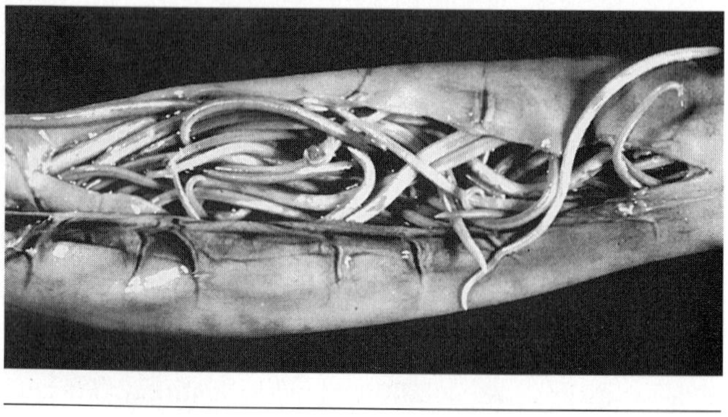

Figure 1-61 Intestine; horse. Ascarid impaction. Impaction occurred secondary to a rapid die-off of the ascarids; the result of administration of an anthelminthic.

Intussusception

When one segment of intestine becomes telescoped into the immediately distal segment of intestine, the lesion is called an **intussusception** (Fig. 1-62). The intussusceptum is the trapped segment and the intussuscipiens is the enveloping portion of the intestine. The etiology is generally unknown but is thought to be associated with intestinal irritability and hypermotility. Foreign bodies, neoplasms, and some parasites such as the nodular worm of sheep, *Oesophagostomum* spp., can provide a cause for the intestine to telescope into itself. In the dog, intussusception of the intestine has been related to, or caused by, the granulomas of visceral larva migrans and histoplasmosis, surgical exposure and manipulation of the small intestine, hypertrophied lymphoid nodules in salmon disease poisoning, *Yersinia pseudotuberculosis* infections, linear foreign bodies (e.g., string), and ascarids.

Causes of intussusception in the cat include foreign bodies and adenocarcinomas of the intestine. In cattle, papillomas, abscesses, fibromas, and lipomas are causes; and in the horse, ascarids, parasitic granulomas, verminous arteritis, and leiomyoma are identified as causes. Ileoileal, ileocecal, cecocecal, and cecocolic intussusceptions have been attributed to infestations with the horse tapeworm, *Anoplocephala perfoliata,* as the tapeworms can be found at the edge of the intussusceptum. Endoparasitism, malnutrition, protozoal infections, and the diarrheas that are often concomitant cause intussusception. Rarely, duodenogastric intussusception occurs.

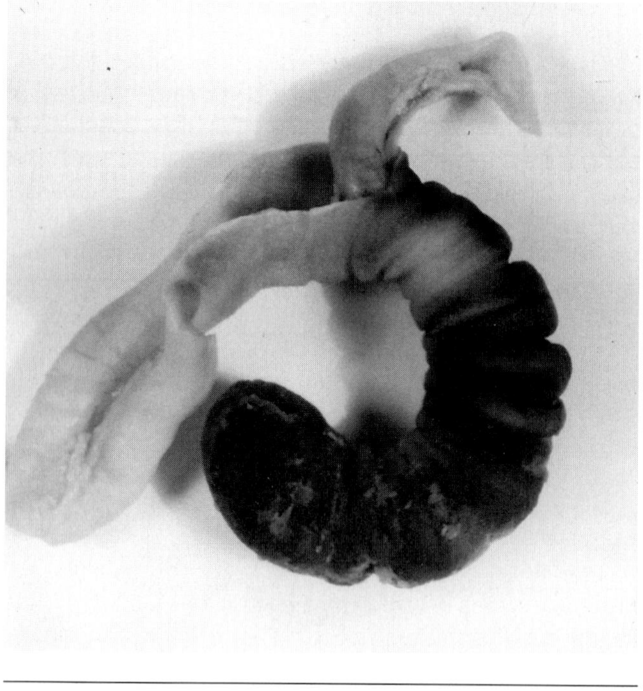

Figure 1-62 Small intestine; young dog. Compound intussusception. This intussusception within an intussusception is black from infarction and coated with tags of fibrin.

Because peristalsis continues after death, intussusceptions can occur after death. Before one attributes death to intestinal obstruction due to intussusception, one needs to determine if the intussusception took place before or after death. Since inflammation only occurs in the living organism, postmortem intussusceptions are easily reduced because there are no adhesions and they are not accompanied by hyperemia or fibrin on the peritoneal surfaces, which remain smooth and glistening. On rare occasions, antemortem intussusceptions spontaneously reduce by sloughing of the infarcted intussusceptum, which then passes in the feces. Often the site of sloughing is replaced with scar tissue, and a circumferential scar or stricture forms.

Clinical features of intussusception are those of intestinal obstruction and include abdominal distension, dilated bowel loops, palpable abdominal mass, signs of abdominal pain, complete anorexia, and vomiting. After 24 hours, melena is followed by a lack of feces. The intussusception is an enlarged, thickened segment of intestine that varies in length from several centimeters to a meter or more. The segment is grossly swollen, discolored, dark red or black because of congestion and hemorrhage, and heavy because of the mass within. At one end of the intussusception the invagination of the smaller segment is visible, and the mesentery of the intussuscepted portion is folded at the site of entry of the intussusceptum into the intussuscipiens and engorged with blood and edema. Microscopically, ischemic necrosis involves the mucosa of both segments, with congestion and edema of the submucosa, muscularis, and subserosa.

Paralytic Ileus

Paralytic ileus is a nonmechanical hypomotility resulting in a functional obstruction of the bowel. It can be due to paralysis of the bowel wall, generally the result of peritonitis, shock, severe painful stimuli elsewhere in the body, states of abnormal metabolism, toxemia, and electrolyte imbalance, such as hypocalcemia, hypomagnesemia, and hypokalemia, vitamin B deficiency, uremia, tetanus, diabetes mellitus, and lead poisoning. In the surgical manipulation of abdominal viscera, afferent and efferent limbs of the neurologic reflex are conducted through splanchnic nerves. Because chloride, potassium, and calcium are essential for neuromuscular conductivity, electrolyte deficits have been regarded as at least contributory in many cases of ileus.

Paralytic ileus also can occur with manipulation and handling of the bowel at surgery. In the latter case there are no morphologic lesions. The gut is not paralyzed but rather is adynamic because of sympathetic nerve inhibition. The stomach and intestines fail to respond to the presence of ingesta, cathartics, and enemas but can react to pharmacologic and electrical stimuli. Adynamic ileus represents a disease with a biochemical rather than a morphologic lesion. Clinical signs of adynamic ileus are anorexia, abdominal distension, absence of bowel sounds, fluid- and gas-filled loops (detected by palpation or radiography), failure to pass flatus and feces, vomiting, and large volumes of fluid aspirated by nasogastric tube. Laboratory findings often associated with the disorder include hypochloremia, hyponatremia, hypokalemia, and eosinopenia (apparently related to adrenal cortical output). Adynamic ileus is recognized in human beings, dogs, cats, cattle, and horses.

Intestinal Displacements

Intestinal displacements include herniations that lead to incarcerations and finally strangulations. Herniations are characterized as internal or external.

Internal herniations are displacements of intestine through a normal or pathologic foramen in the abdominal cavity. The most common of these displacements occur in horses. They include herniation through the epiploic foramen and through mesenteric tears. The dorsal border of the epiploic foramen is formed by the caudate lobe of the liver and the caudal vena cava. The ventral boundary is the right lobe of the pancreas, the gastropancreatic ligament, and the portal vein. The cranial boundary is the hepatoduodenal ligament, and the caudal boundary is the junction of the pancreas and mesoduodenum. The epiploic cavity is only a potential space. It is proposed that the caudate lobe of the liver atrophies in older animals enlarging the foramen and allowing loops of intestine to slip through, become incarcerated and then strangulated.

External hernias are formed when a hernial sac, formed by a pouch of parietal peritoneum, penetrates outside the abdominal cavity. Sites of external hernias include umbilical, ventral, diaphragmatic, hiatal, inguinal, scrotal (Fig. 1-63), and perineal. The latter hernia is seen in old male dogs with prostate gland enlargement and obstipation. Some of these herniations (e.g., diaphrag-

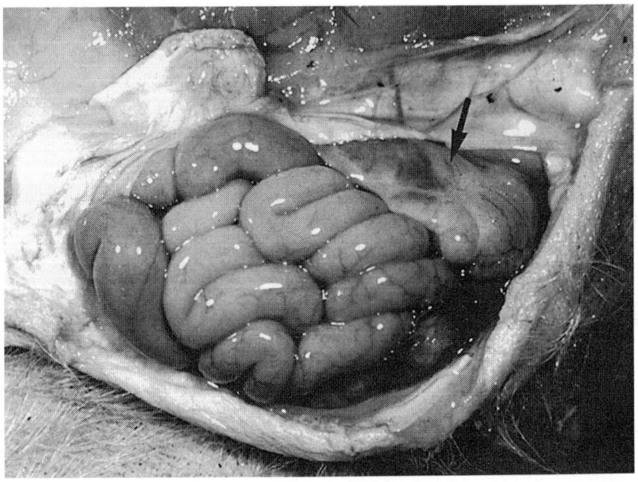

Figure 1-63 Scrotum; pig. Scrotal hernia. Loops of intestine present within the scrotum have displaced the testis *(arrow)* caudad.

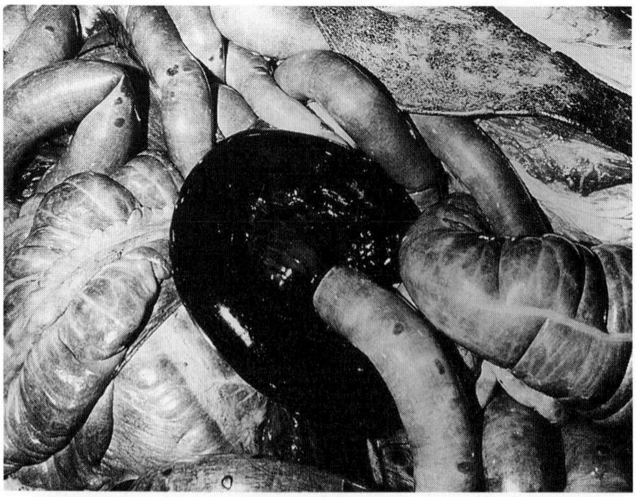

Figure 1-64 Intestines; horse. Intestinal incarceration and volvulus. The affected segment is black and gas-filled, and the mesenteric vessels are distended. The dark nodules in the serosa of the nonincarcerated small intestine are strongyle-induced hemomelasma ilei. *Thomson RG. General Veterinary Pathology. Philadelphia: Saunders, 1978:103.*

matic, perineal) are more correctly eventrations because they are not accompanied by a peritoneal pouch. Postoperative wound dehiscence also causes eventration.

It should be noted that umbilical hernias are generally caused by a defect in the abdominal wall and not by chewing of the umbilical cord by the dam. Umbilical hernias could have a genetic basis, so it may be a matter of some ethical concern whether to repair these hernias surgically in show and breeding animals.

Volvulus and Torsion

A **volvulus** is a twisting of the intestine on its mesenteric axis. A **torsion** is a rotation of a tubular organ along its long axis. The latter is most common in the cecum of cattle and horses and occasionally of the abomasum of calves. Both volvulus and torsion result in bowel obstruction and ischemic injury. The thin-walled veins of the mesentery are occluded first, while the nonoccluded arteries permit blood flow into the compromised segment. The mesentery is usually thickened, severely congested, and dark red. Lymph nodes adjacent to the intestine are congested and swollen. At necropsy the volvulus is usually a small or large twisted segment of small intestine, sometimes including the cecum or proximal colon, which is considerably distended with gas and fluid, and discolored dark red or black (Fig. 1-64). There is usually a sharp line of demarcation between the affected and normal intestine. A volvulus is often difficult to untangle; the twist can be 360 to 720 degrees, either clockwise or counterclockwise on its mesenteric axis. In some animals, a neoplasm, foreign body, incarceration, or intussusception is coexistent. Edema and severe congestion thicken the entire wall of the affected segment. Microscopically, the affected intestine has lesions of necrosis, congestion, and hemorrhage. The flora entrapped in blood-filled anoxic loops produce toxins and gas, which cause distension of the part and necrosis of the mucosa. This process leads to gangrene, intestinal rupture, peritonitis, and death.

The most common site of large bowel volvulus of the horse is the left colon. In this species, the colon extends from the cecum cranially on the right, then transversely across the ventral abdomen caudal to the diaphragm to form the (sacculated) left ventral colon, which at its caudal end turns dorsally at the pelvic flexure, to form the left dorsal (nonsacculated) colon. This left side loop of the left ventral and dorsal colon undergoes volvulus of 180 degrees or more. Although often referred to as torsion, the twist is actually around its mesenteric axis as the mesentery of the left ventral and left dorsal colons is horizontal. Thus it is analogous to volvulus that occurs in vertically suspended loops of intestine and has the same ischemic consequences. The twist is thought to be caused by overfilling, especially disproportionate filling, of the left dorsal colon with feces or sand. Most often in this disorder, the left dorsal colon is displaced medially, while the left ventral colon is moved laterally causing a clockwise twist of the axis. A counterclockwise twist occurs less frequently. At necropsy, that portion of the colon beyond the twist is black and its wall blood filled, the result of the occlusion of veins prior to the occlusion of arteries.

A peculiar type of intestinal strangulation occurs in horses in which lipomas, which are pedunculated, wrap around the intestinal mesentery or the bowel itself causing ischemia, colic, and death (Fig. 1-65). However, most mesenteric lipomas are of no clinical consequence. Although rare, intestinal strangulation by pedunculated lipomas has been reported in the dog.

Renosplenic Entrapment

Renosplenic entrapment of the large colon in horses is due to left dorsal displacement of the left dorsal or left ventral segments of the large colon between the spleen and left body wall. Entrapment occurs over the renosplenic ligament that runs between the left kidney and spleen. The cause of the displacement is unknown but could occur secondary to rolling behavior in horses or gaseous distension of the large colon.

Miscellaneous Diseases and Conditions

Cecal or large **intestinal rupture** occur most commonly in postparturient mares but can also result from impaction and as a complication of anesthesia. The sites of rupture vary, and the mechanism(s) are unknown.

Diverticula (singular, diverticulum) are epithelium-lined cavities that are derived from mucosal epithelium

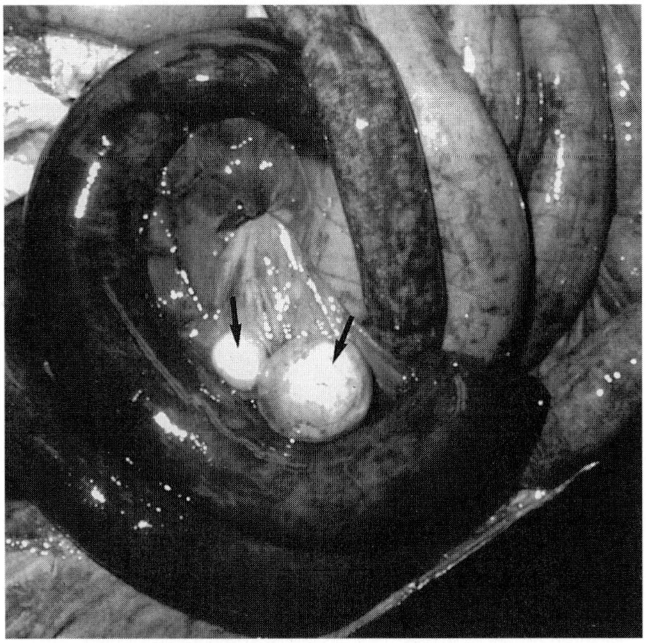

Figure 1-65 Intestines; horse. Intestinal strangulation by pedunculated lipomas. Two lipomas *(arrows)* have wrapped around the mesentery and strangled the bowel. *Courtesy Department of Veterinary Pathology, Cornell University.*

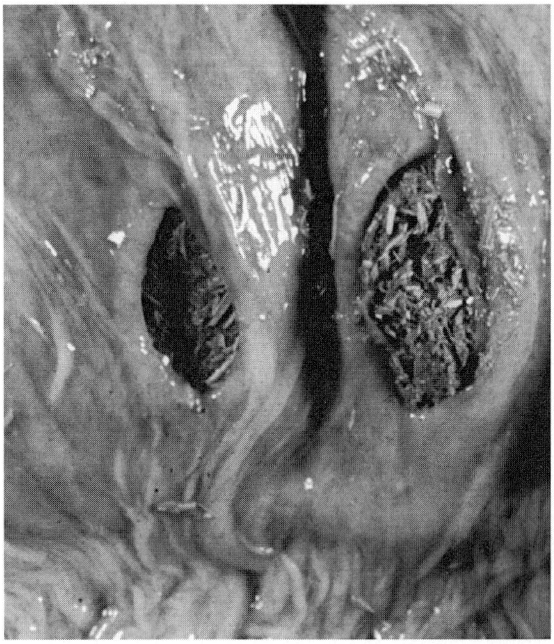

Figure 1-66 Cecum; lumenal surface; horse. Diverticula. Note the several mucosal outpouchings filled with ingesta and the rounded edges of the diverticula.

and that extend through the muscularis mucosa, submucosa, and muscularis and often reach the serosa, where they sometimes rupture, causing peritonitis (Fig. 1-66). Muscular hypertrophy of the tunica muscularis associated with diverticulosis has been recorded in young Yorkshire pigs and in Romney Marsh and Hampshire sheep.

Muscular hypertrophy of the distal ileum is an idiopathic condition of horses and pigs. Although generally an incidental finding, hypertrophy of the tunica muscularis can lead to impaction and rupture of the ileum. In some horses, it is an idiopathic segmental lesion affecting the ileum and progressing proximad to affect the jejunum and, subsequently, more cranial segments of the jejunum. In these cases, the lesion represents a work hypertrophy proximal to a damaged or stenotic ileocecal valve. In other horses, muscular hypertrophy affects the duodenum and jejunum and is associated with diverticula. Horses with muscular hypertrophy of the intestines have intermittent or subacute colic, a variable appetite, exaggerated bowel sounds, and, finally, cachexia. In some species, diarrhea is a feature. Associated signs include a "harsh" coat, "tucked-up" abdomen, depression, nasal discharge, and abnormal stance, with the hind limbs placed forward under the abdomen. An intestinal mass can be palpable caused by the thickened ileum, and, in small animals, vomiting has been a feature. Muscular hypertrophy of the ileum in pigs occurs either as a component of regional enteritis or as an independent disorder.

Cats can have a severe hypertrophy of the inner, circular layer of the tunica muscularis. This lesion appears to originate in the ileum and progress cranially. Segmental hypertrophy of the muscularis of the gastric antrum and variable segments of the small intestine occurs in cats with **hypereosinophilic syndrome,** a disease characterized by intramural eosinophil infiltrates. Muscular hypertrophy of the intestine and medial hyperplasia of the pulmonary arteries occur in cats given large oral doses of *Toxocara cati* larvae. The infected cases often have diarrhea and eosinophilic enteritis, and, later, variable fibrosis of the lamina propria of the mucosa and hypertrophy of the inner layer of the tunica muscularis.

Another unique lesion in the horse is **hemomelasma ilei.** These lesions are pink to black plaques that vary in length from several millimeters to many centimeters and can occur anywhere in the intestine, but are generally limited to the ileum. They are a result of the larval migrations of strongyles and are located on the antimesenteric surface of the serosa. These fibrovascular serosal plaques are formed in response to tissue damage caused by the migrating parasites. They are generally of no clinical consequence but can, on occasion, lead to intestinal strictures and intermittent colic. Proper deworming programs prevent their formation.

Intestinal lipofuscinosis or **leiomyometaplasia** is also called "brown dog gut." The brown, discolored small intestine occurs in bile duct occlusion, pancreatic insufficiency, chronic enteritis, vitamin E deficiency, or excess dietary lipids. Brown pigmentation of smooth muscle is a well-known lesion of vitamin E deficiency in several species of laboratory animals. The canine and human intestinal pigmentation is also the result of vitamin E deficiency. The dietary requirement for vitamin E is proportional to the concentration of polyunsaturated fatty acids in the diet. Intestinal lipofuscinosis probably does not cause clinical signs; however, the lesion is significant as an indicator of what has occurred previously in the patient. The small intestine, viewed from the serosal side, is brown. The color varies from tan to khaki in the mildly affected, to deep brown in the severely affected intestine. In severely affected dogs, portions of the stomach, cecum, or colon are also pigmented. Microscopically, the brown color results from the perinuclear lysosomal accumulation of lipofuscin granules in the cytoplasm of the smooth muscle cells of the intestine (Fig. 1-67). These granules vary from basophilic to brown with hematoxylin-eosin (H & E) stain and stain variably periodic acid–Schiff (PAS) positive and Sudan black positive depending on the age of the lesion. Older granules are acid-fast when stained by the special acid-fast technique for lipofuscin. Younger lesions have proportionally more carbohydrate and are thus PAS positive. Acid-fast granules are referred to as ceroid pigment.

Small Intestinal Intoxicants

Because most toxins enter the body through ingestion, those that are irritants can cause contact lesions in the esophagus, stomach, and intestine. The lesions that result are generally those of hemorrhage and inflammation. In many cases of intoxication, induction of vomiting is contraindicated since what burns going down will also burn coming up. The numbers and types of chemicals and intoxicants animals are exposed to makes a listing of them a monumental undertaking. A few examples are phosphorous, arsenic, bracken fern (cattle), mercury, oak, copper, nitrate, thallium, and blister beetles. The blister beetles are sometimes incorporated into crimped hay. They contain a topical irritant called cantharidin. Lesions include sloughing of the epithelium of the stomach and enterocytes of the proximal small intestine (Fig. 1-68). In addition, cantharidin can cause hemorrhagic ulcers of the urinary bladder and myocardial necrosis.

Although not generally considered an intoxicant, corticosteroids cause colonic perforation in some treated dogs. NSAIDs can cause **right dorsal colitis** in equids. This colitis is characterized by necrosis resulting in erosions and ulcers.

Vascular Diseases of the Intestine

Parasites

In horses, ***Strongylus vulgaris*** fourth-stage larvae are present in the wall of the cranial mesenteric artery, resulting in arteritis. So-called aneurysms and mural thrombosis develop. In many cases, even complete occlusion of the cranial mesenteric artery does not result in bowel infarction because collateral circulation will develop if the vascular occlusion develops slowly. Therefore, it is important to ascertain if the colonic arteries are thrombosed before assigning the cause of bowel death to *S. vulgaris*.

Eggs produced by *S. vulgaris* adults in the colon are discharged with the feces, embryonate on pasture, and, in

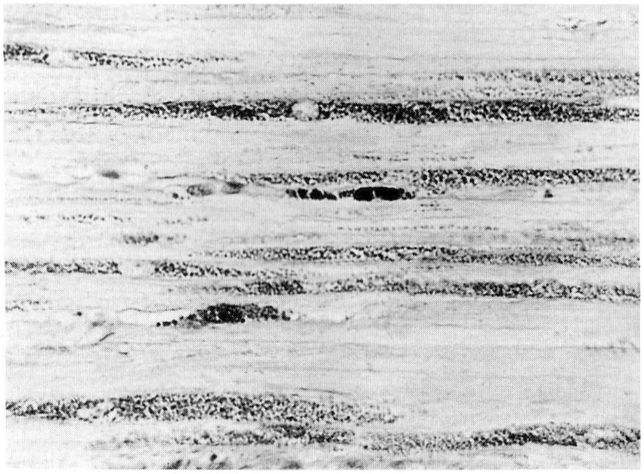

Figure 1-67 Intestine; dog. Intestinal lipofuscinosis. Myocytes of the inner muscle layer contain numerous PAS-stained cytoplasmic granules (lipofuscin). PAS-stain.

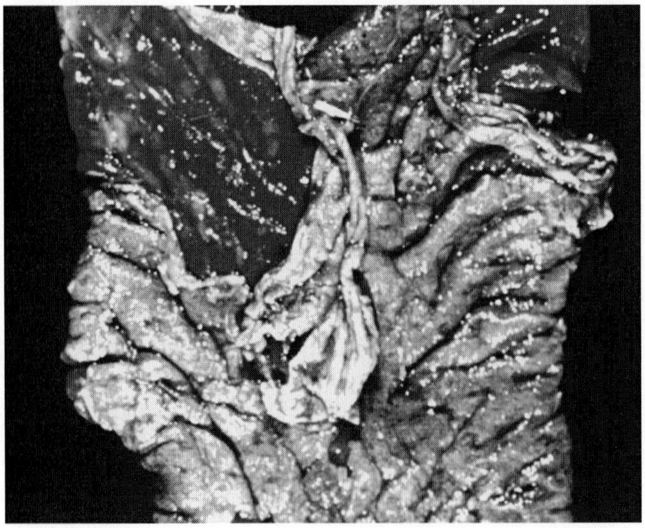

Figure 1-68 Intestine; horse. Acute necrohemorrhagic enteritis. The severe necrosis with sloughing of intestinal mucosa is the result of cantharidin, a toxin contained in ingested blister beetles. *Courtesy Department of Veterinary Pathology, Cornell University.*

less than 2 weeks, develop into third-stage infective larvae. These larvae, ingested with forage, penetrate the small and large intestinal mucosa to the submucosa, where they moult and gain access to submucosal arteries. In these arteries, they migrate along or under the intima to the cranial mesenteric artery. After a developmental period of 3 to 4 months, larvae exsheath and migrate as young adults down the lumen of arteries to the subserosa of the cecum and colon. Subsequently, young adults are trapped in intramural nodules that ultimately rupture into the intestinal lumen. Larvae that journey beyond the cranial mesenteric artery take up residence in the aorta or its major abdominal branches. Their prepatent period is 6 months or longer.

Wherever the larvae reside, they induce an arteritis that damages the intima causing mural thrombosis, mural thickening, and thick-walled outpouchings, the so-called aneurysms. This sequence of events is especially prominent in the cranial mesenteric artery. Larvae, 1 cm in length, adhere to or penetrate the intima and number from a few to several hundred. The intimal surface is rough and covered by layered thrombi in which the parasites are partially embedded. Chronically affected sites have degeneration of elastic laminae and muscle fibers. Until recently, the incidence of strongyle-induced vascular lesions in horses was 95%, and 90% to 95% of these horses had aneurysms. Earlier investigators estimated that 80% of colic cases were caused by *Strongylus* spp. larvae. Since the introduction and widespread use of ivermectin, an orally administered vermifuge with broad systemic larvacidal activity, these data no longer apply.

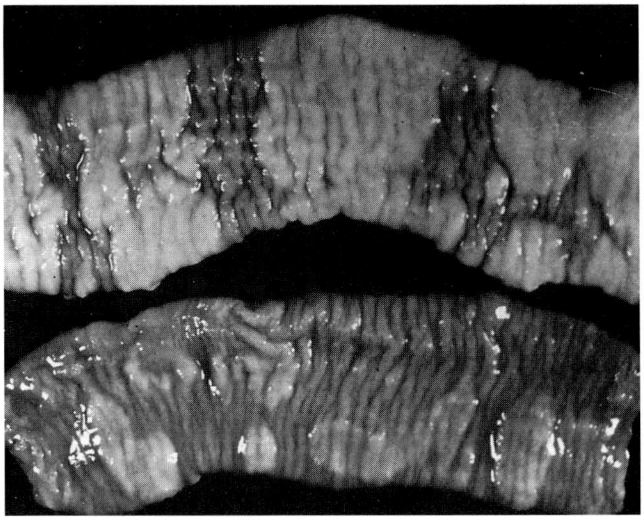

Figure 1-69 Small intestine; dog. Intestinal lymphangiectasia. Raised white zones and plaques are produced by mucosal edema and dilated lacteals. *Courtesy Dr. D.J. Meuten.*

Clinical signs include recurrent bouts of colic, failure to thrive, weight loss, variable appetite, and poor hair coat. Attacks of severe colic accompanied by fever are observed along with anorexia, dullness, sternal recumbency, looking at the flank, discomfort on lying down, kicking at the abdomen, sweating and rolling, increased intestinal sounds, and the passage of soft feces. On rectal examination, the detection of a large (6-cm diameter or greater), firm mass at the origin of the cranial mesenteric artery can be taken as evidence of parasitic arteritis. Laboratory findings include leukocytosis, neutrophilia, eosinophilia, normocytic anemia, hypoalbuminemia, and elevated β-globulins. Death occurs when strongyle-induced thrombi or emboli occlude branches of major arteries to the cecum, colon, or, less frequently, the small bowel, with resultant infarction. At necropsy, the affected bowel is black, blood-engorged, and friable. Often perforation has occurred and caused a terminal peritonitis.

Lymphangiectasia

Lymphangiectasia, or lacteal dilation, is the most commonly reported cause of protein-losing enteropathy in the dog (Fig. 1-69). Clinical signs include diarrhea, steatorrhea, hypoproteinemia, and ascites. Lymphangiectasia can be due to a congenital developmental disorder of the lymphatic vessels or it can be acquired secondary to lymph vessel obstruction caused by granulomatous or neoplastic diseases. A special case is lipogranulomatous lymphangiectasia of the dog, the name of which is descriptive of the lesions present (Fig. 1-70). Most cases of acquired lymphangiectasia are idiopathic. Microscopically, intestinal lymph vessels and lacteals are markedly dilated (Fig. 1-71). In some cases the lymphocyte and plasma cell

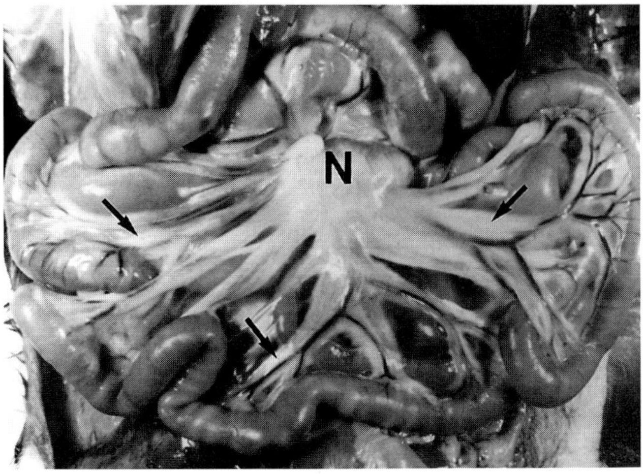

Figure 1-70 Small intestine; dog. Lipogranulomatous lymphangitis. Lymph vessels in the mesentery are distended and milky white *(arrows)* as they course toward the mesenteric lymph node *(N)*. The intestine is contracted and has caused the alternating light and dark bands.

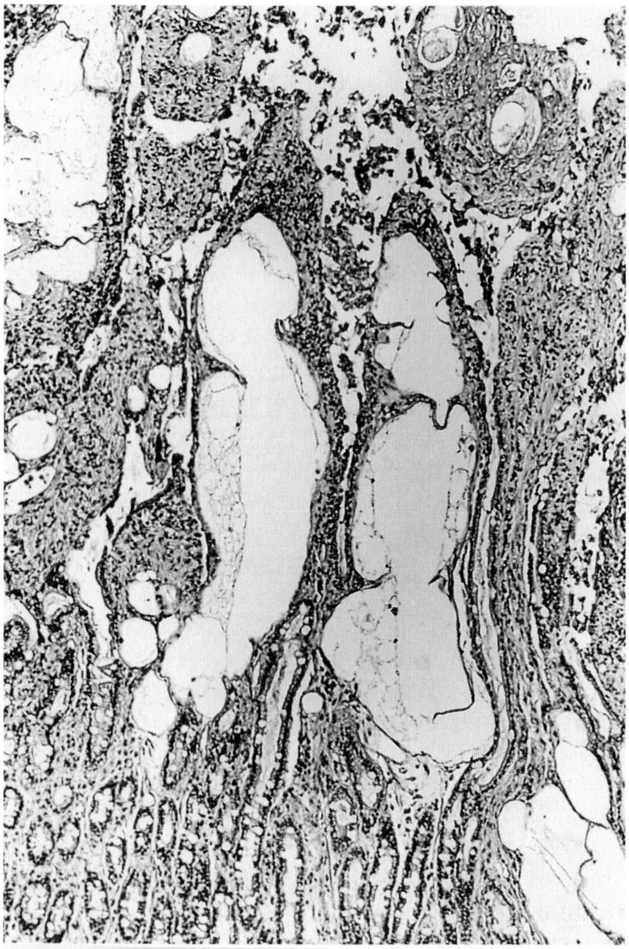

Figure 1-71 Small intestine; dog. Intestinal lymphangiectasia. Lacteals are dilated and distorted as a consequence of lipogranulomatous lymphangitis. H & E stain.

populations of the mucosa are increased. The lipogranulomas, when they occur, are located in submucosal, muscular, or subserosal lymph vessels, and are composed of a broad collar of lipophages surrounding centrally located amorphous lipid material.

DISEASES OF INTESTINAL EPITHELIUM

A number of diseases are characterized by colonization or destruction of the epithelial components of the intestinal mucosa. Although the disease-producing effects of pathogens are complex and multifactorial, a simplified understanding of the principal cell under attack is helpful in predicting disease outcome and managing treatment.

Diseases of the Absorptive Enterocytes

A number of agents have a tropism for the absorptive cells lining the intestinal villi. These agents include viruses such as rotavirus, enteric coronavirus, and the coronavirus of transmissible gastroenteritis virus of pigs. Intracellular bacteria and parasites can likewise invade and multiply in absorptive epithelial cells. Examples include the agent of swine dysentery *(Brachyspira hyodysenteriae)*, coccidia, and cryptosporidia.

Some pathogens with a tropism for absorptive lining cells of the intestine cause destruction of these cells. This mechanism results in loss of enterocytes and, at least temporary, villus atrophy. The loss of the absorptive-digestive villus enterocytes causes maldigestion, and malabsorption results. Furthermore, because ingesta and normal alimentary secretions are unabsorbed, they are degraded further and fermented in the intestine by bacteria increasing the osmolality of intestinal contents with subsequent increase in the fluid content of the bowel.

Because the regenerative crypt cells are not attacked by pathogens with tropism for villus enterocytes, diseases with villus enterocyte damage are not necessary fatal. The lost cells are replaced by the maturing cells migrating along the basement membrane from the crypt to the villus. The naked basement membrane contracts causing villus atrophy, and the functionally immature migrating crypt cells cover the villi. Often these immature cells become squamoid in an effort to cover the maximum area of basement membrane. If naked basement membranes contact each other, they will adhere resulting not only in villus blunting but also villus fusion preventing the formation of normal villi.

Diseases of Undifferentiated Crypt Cells

Loss of the undifferentiated epithelial cells in the base of the crypts means loss of the cells capable of rapid mitosis and thus regeneration of the epithelium. Therefore, the clinical effect of crypt cell loss can be delayed for several days because the villi are still covered by enterocytes. This type of loss is more severe, and often fatal, compared with villus enterocyte loss. Agents that target the crypt cells are called radiomimetic since they mimic the effects of radiation on the rapidly dividing enterocytes. Examples of these agents include the parvoviruses of carnivores, bovine viral diarrhea virus, rinderpest virus, and some mycotoxins.

Abnormalities of the Microvilli and Glycocalyx

Since the microvilli and glycocalyx on the villus enterocytes are largely responsible for the immense surface area and enzymes responsible for nutrient digestion and absorption, it follows that damage to either of these structures can result in intestinal malfunction and resultant diarrhea. A prime example of this is human lactose intolerance. Such persons lack lactase in the glycocalyx. Because of this lack, they are unable to digest lactose from dairy products. The lack of lactase results in failure of uptake and the lactose is fermented by bacteria in the colon. This results in an osmotic drain of fluid into the gut with resultant diarrhea. Thus, the malabsorption in this case is limited to a single substrate. Histologically, the intestine is normal.

Some bacteria such as attaching and effacing *Escherichia coli* damage the microvilli by their attachment. This attachment disrupts enzyme systems housed in the microvilli and glycocalyx and causes diarrhea. The antibiotic neomycin can similarly cause fragmentation of microvilli and destruction of the glycocalyx with resultant diarrhea. Cessation of neomycin therapy results in a return to normal.

Diseases in Which the Epithelial Targets are Unknown or Nonspecific

In a number of enteric diseases, the targeted epithelial cell is unknown or nonspecific. Many of the pathogens causing these diseases are of importance in the young of food-producing animals. Enterotoxic *E. coli* infection of neonatal pigs, calves, and lambs, as well as human beings, causes what is known as a secretory diarrhea. These bacteria are able to colonize the small intestinal enterocytes by way of their surface or pilis antigens that anchor them to the enterocytes. Different pilis antigens adhere to glycoconjugate receptors on enterocytes in different regions of the small intestine. Thus, these bacteria are not washed out by peristalsis. Because the enterocytes are not damaged, no lesions are observed, although microscopically the bacteria can be seen attached to the epithelial surface. The bacteria produce a toxin that causes enterocytes to secrete water and electrolytes. Although cyclic AMP (adenosine monophosphate) and GMP (guanosine monophosphate) mediate this process, the exact mechanism by which this secretion occurs is unknown. Some secretion, especially that of chloride ions, occurs via the cryptal cells. Intestinal secretion exceeds the ability of the colon to absorb the surplus fluid. The net result is diarrhea.

Clostridium perfringens type C is a pathogen of neonatal pigs, lambs, calves, and foals. Unlike the enterotoxic *E. coli,* which produces a toxin affecting enterocytes, *C. perfringens* produces a nonspecific cytotoxin. This toxin causes necrosis of villus absorptive cells that then extends to the lamina propria and blood vessels. The result is massive and acute necrohemorrhagic enteritis.

Separation of Apical Junctional Complexes

Apical junctional complexes, also called tight junctions or zona occludens, join enterocytes to each other. Normally, these junctions are a barrier to macromolecular transepithelial transport. In certain parasitic diseases, such as ostertagiosis, these tight junctions are pathologically opened allowing transport of macromolecules transport into the intestinal lumen. This opening of tight junctions is important in allowing macromolecules such as immunoglobulin into the lumen where the parasites can be attacked.

DISEASES OF THE LAMINA PROPRIA

Lesions within the lamina propria can be infiltrative, necrotizing, or vascular, all of which can cause diarrhea even though the epithelium is not the primary cell type injured.

Inflammation

Chronic inflammation of the lamina propria that results in dense cellular infiltration can cause diarrhea in a variety of ways, none of which are completely understood. These mechanisms include simple physical impairment of mucosal diffusion by space-occupying cells and disruption of the overlying epithelium causing increased permeability. Examples of these diseases in domestic animals are canine histiocytic ulcerative colitis (boxer colitis), Johne's disease (paratuberculosis) of cattle, amyloidosis, and lymphoma.

Necrotizing Processes

Primary necrotizing processes of the lamina propria generally involve necrosis of the gut-associated lymphoid tissue with extension to the overlying epithelium. Examples of such diseases with these lesions include bovine viral diarrhea and *Rhodococcus equi* infection.

Vascular Changes and Lymphangiectasia

Vascular changes and dilation of lacteals are idiopathic or secondary to obstruction of flow. These lesions are seen most commonly as part of the syndrome resulting from space-occupying lesions of the lamina propria such as occurs in Johne's disease and lymphoma. Endotoxemia resulting in vascular damage and disseminated intravascular coagulopathy can result in thrombi in small vessels, hemorrhage, necrosis, and ulceration of the intestine.

DISEASES DUE TO SPECIFIC PATHOGENS

A number of pathogens affect different animal species in similar ways. The mechanism of damage is similar among these animal species and pathogens. Therefore, it is useful to discuss the diseases caused by these organisms, across species. Specific diseases of the individual species that do not have analogs in other species are described later in this chapter.

Bacterial Diseases

Escherichia coli Diseases (Colibacillosis)

E. coli bacteria are among the first of the intestinal flora acquired after birth and comprise a part of that flora in virtually all animals. Various serotypes induce disease by a variety of means, especially in the young of each species. Genetic resistance, maternal antibodies, a high plane of hygiene, and high-quality nutrition can reduce the propensity for disease. In contrast, a heavily contaminated environment, failure to consume colostrum, formula feeding rather than maternal nursing, cold stress, and

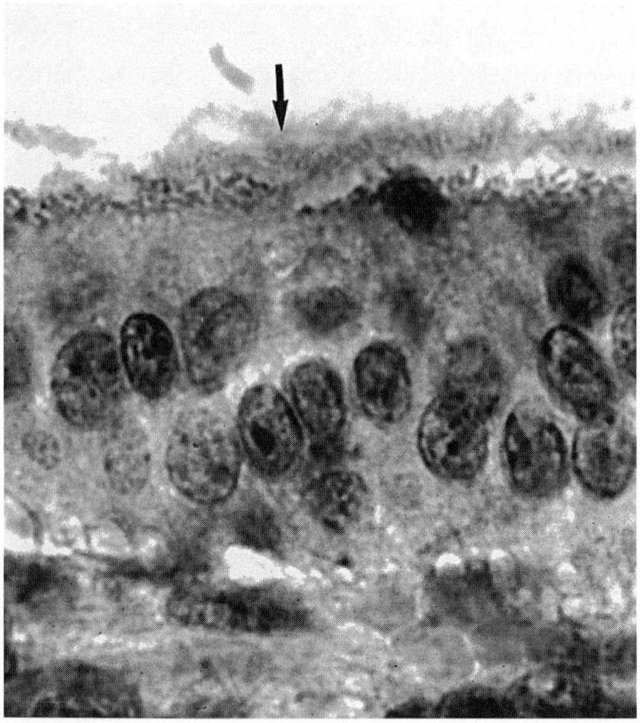

Figure 1-72 Jejunum; piglet. Enterotoxic colibacillosis. Mats of *E. coli (arrow)* are attached to the surface of the enterocytes. H & E stain.

crowding increase the susceptibility of animals for colibacillosis. *E. coli* infections often occur intercurrently with those due to rotavirus, coronavirus, or cryptosporidia. In farms and kennels, particular serotypes of *E. coli* sometimes become endemic seeming to increase in number of cases or pathogenicity, so that virtually no new offspring escape the disease. Under such circumstances, morbidity and mortality can approach 100%. Animals healthy through 3 weeks of age have, for the most part, survived the threat of neonatal colibacillosis.

Enterotoxic Colibacillosis. Enterotoxic colibacillosis is common in animals 2 days to 3 weeks of age. Why enterotoxic colibacillosis is a disease of neonates is not well understood. Some speculation is that enteric bacterial colonization is a function of gastric acidity and that the low pH of the stomach of postneonatal animals kills the bacteria.

The feces of affected animals are profuse, yellow to white, and watery to pasty. Affected animals are dehydrated, with their abdomen "tucked up" and eyeballs sunken. Animals that die of enterotoxic *E. coli* infection are severely dehydrated, often emaciated, and have diarrheic feces pasted over and around their perineum. The diarrhea is largely a function of secretion by enterocytes due to bacterial enterotoxin. Gross lesions include a small intestine that is dilated, flaccid, and filled with translucent fluid. Chyle is present in the mesenteric lymphatic vessels similar to animals without enteric disease. Unlike the malabsorptive diseases of the small intestine, absorption proceeds normally in cases of enterotoxic colibacillosis. Microscopically, the intestine is also normal. Diagnosis can be made by light microscopic examination in freshly dead animals by noting the presence of bacteria lining the lumenal surface of the enterocytes (Fig. 1-72).

Septicemic Colibacillosis. Septicemic colibacillosis is a disease of newborn calves, lambs, and occasionally foals that have not received sufficient colostral immunity. Although the lesions produced are generally those of septicemia similar to those caused by other organisms, infection can localize in the intestine causing enteritis. The bacteria gain entry to the body through the respiratory system, oral cavity, or umbilicus and become septicemic. Fibrinous arthritis, ophthalmitis, serositis, meningitis, and white-spotted kidneys (cortical abscesses) characterize the septicemia. Mixed bacterial infections often occur with enterotoxic *E. coli*.

Edema Disease. Edema disease, also known as enterotoxemic colibacillosis, is an *E. coli* infection that is specific for pigs. Edema disease is caused by a bacterial enterotoxin produced in the small intestine that spreads hematogeneously. It is generally a disease of pigs 6 to 14 weeks of age and is generally associated with dietary changes at weaning. It is often noted that the best pigs in a group are the ones affected. Edema disease is characterized by incoordination of the hind legs, sagging and swaying, difficulty in rising, irritability, muscle tremors, aimless wandering, and clonic convulsions.

Hemolytic *E. coli* proliferates in the small intestine subsequent to dietary changes and produces a heat-labile exotoxin, called the edema disease principle. This systemic toxin (angiotoxin) causes generalized vascular endothelial injury of arterioles and arteries resulting in fluid loss and edema. The edema can be found anywhere, but is most characteristic in the gastric submucosa, eyelids, gallbladder, and mesentery of the spiral colon (Figs. 1-73 to 1-75). In the brain, arterial damage causes malacia in the medulla, thalamus, and basal ganglia. These nervous tissue lesions are collectively known as focal symmetrical encephalomalacia or swine cerebral angiopathy. Death is due to an endotoxic shock–like syndrome. Some animals suffer from a Shwartzman-like bilateral renal cortical necrosis. Morbidity within a herd is approximately 35% and all affected animals die.

Postweaning Colibacillosis. Postweaning colibacillosis is another specific disease of pigs caused by a hemolytic *E. coli*. The disease appears identical to enterotoxic colibacillosis of the neonate in that it produces a secretory diarrhea and therefore no lesions. It is a distinct strain of

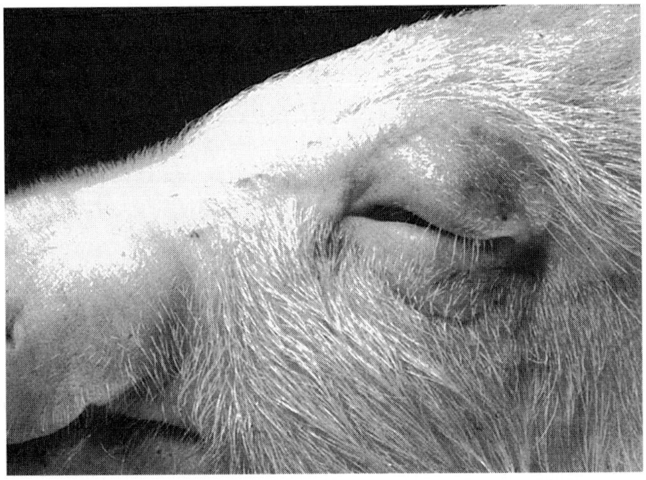

Figure 1-73 Head; pig. Edema disease. The skin of the eyelids and snout are edematous.

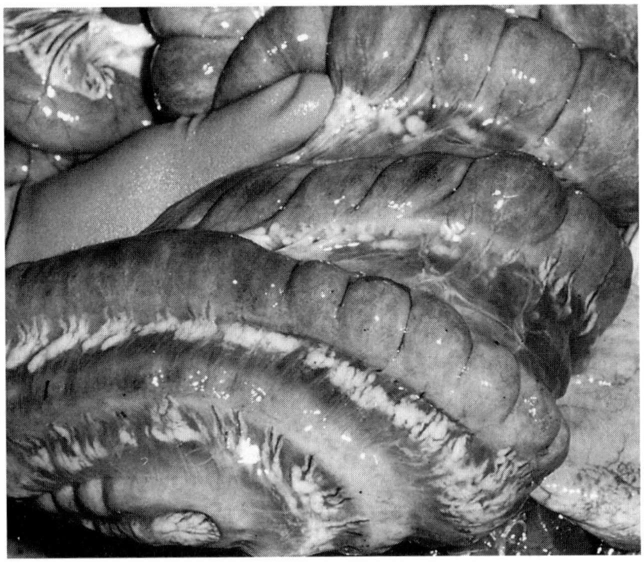

Figure 1-74 Spiral colon; pig. Edema disease. Gelatinous edema fluid is present in the mesocolon between loops of colon. *Courtesy Dr. M.D. McGavin.*

E. coli, however, and is associated with feed and management changes at weaning.

Enteroinvasive Colibacillosis. This disease is a relatively newly described condition of human beings, laboratory animals, and, occasionally, cattle and pigs. It has not been reported as a field problem in livestock. The pathogenesis of the disease is similar to that of other invasive bacteria

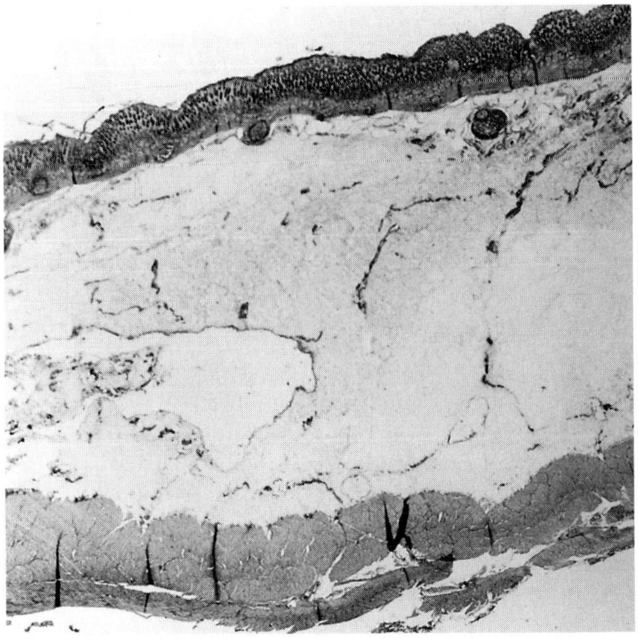

Figure 1-75 Stomach; pig. Edema disease. The submucosa is markedly distended by edema fluid. H & E stain. *Courtesy Dr. R.G. Thomson.*

such as *Salmonella* spp. In human beings, the colon is affected. A verotoxin is produced by the *E. coli* that results in hemorrhagic colitis and sometimes the hemolytic-uremic syndrome. Outbreaks of enteroinvasive colibacillosis in human beings are often a food-borne illness.

Attaching and Effacing E. coli. This disease has been infrequently reported in rabbits, calves, pigs, lambs, dogs, and human beings. The actual incidence of this disease in domestic animals is unknown. Lesions are characterized by *E. coli* attachment to the microvillus border of enterocytes via cups and pedestals (Fig. 1-76). Gross lesions are not present except that the intestine is dilated and fluid filled. Colonization of the epithelium by attaching and effacing *E. coli* is relatively common; disease occurs most often in association with other enteropathogens of calves of this age, namely rotavirus, *Cryptosporidium parvum,* enterotoxigenic *E. coli,* coronavirus, bovine viral diarrhea, and coccidia. In contrast to enterotoxic *E. coli* infection, in attaching and effacing *E. coli* infection the brush border of the enterocytes is disrupted and can be seen in H & E–stained tissue sections.

Salmonellosis

Salmonellae are enteroinvasive bacteria. All known species of *Salmonella* are pathogenic, and it is an important zoonosis and nosocomial infection. Salmonellosis is a significant cause of acute and chronic diarrhea and death in numerous animal species and in human beings. In veterinary medicine, salmonellosis can occur epizooti-

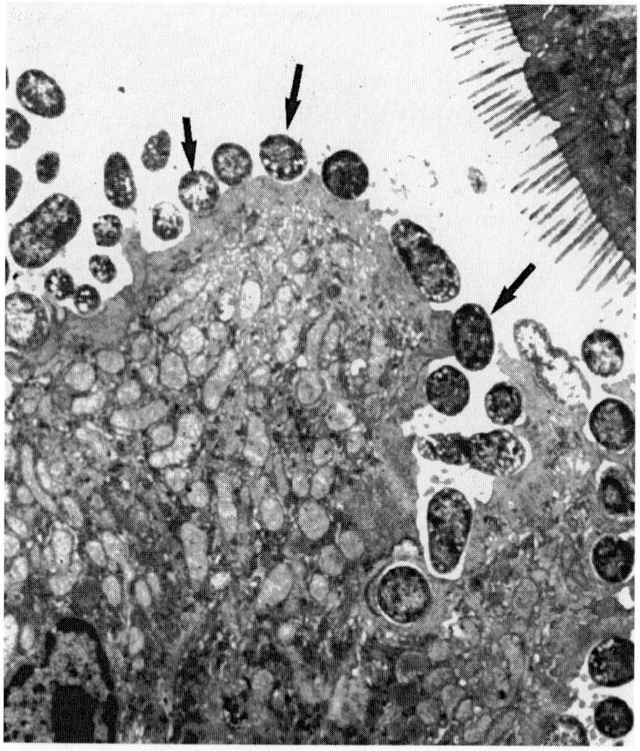

Figure 1-76 Jejunum; rabbit. Attaching and effacing *E. coli.* Electron micrograph. Bacterial rods *(arrows)* have attached to, and effaced, the microvillus border of enterocytes. *Thulin JD, Kuhlenschmidt MS, Gelberg HB. Lab Invest 1991;65:719-731.*

cally, enzootically, or sporadically. The species that are of major disease significance include *Salmonella typhimurium, Salmonella enteritidis, Salmonella dublin, Salmonella cholerasuis,* and *Salmonella typhosa.*

The salmonellae are gram-negative, motile bacilli, 0.5 to 0.8 μm in diameter and 1 to 3.5 μm in length. The bacteria are aerobes or facultative anaerobes. In carrier animals, salmonellae reside in the gallbladder, intestinal tract, and mesenteric lymph nodes. Fatal salmonellosis of horses and cats has occurred in veterinary hospitals following the stress of surgery and antibiotic treatment. The form of salmonellosis that occurs—septicemic, acute enteric, or chronic enteric—depends on the challenge dosage of the bacterium, previous exposure to the bacterium, and stress factors such as overcrowding, transport, cold temperatures, feed changes, pregnancy, parturition, surgery, anesthesia, and antibiotic administration. Some recovered animals become carriers and shed the organism in their feces, particularly after stress. Although dogs and cats rarely get clinical salmonellosis, 10% are carriers and can infect their human companions.

Salmonella infections are acquired by ingestion and contaminated feed and water are important sources of infection in all species. Contaminated fingers, flies, and fomites can transmit the disease. The tonsils and Peyer's patches are portals of entry for some species of *Salmonella,* whereas other species colonize the intestine, are invasive, and enter epithelial cells and, subsequently, macrophages of the mucosa. Salmonellae produce disease via enterotoxins, cytotoxins (Verotoxins), and endotoxins. Once in contact with macrophages of the lamina propria or Peyer's patches, the organisms are phagocytosed and transported to regional lymph nodes or, by way of the portal circulation, to the liver. The organisms colonize the small intestine, colon, mesenteric lymph nodes, and the gallbladder. Salmonellosis infects the young more frequently; the young are more severely affected than are adults; and the young are more likely to succumb to septicemia.

The clinical signs of salmonellosis vary from species to species and with age. The horse develops an acute fatal colitis. The cow has lingering febrile diarrhea with the passage of pseudomembranes, and calves have an acute diarrhea. Dogs develop sudden bouts of acute, but not life-threatening, diarrhea. Cats succumb to febrile enterocolitis. Pigs die of septicemia or enterocolitis. A sequel to salmonellosis in the pig is the "rectal stricture syndrome," a segmental scarring secondary to ulcerative proctitis and thrombosis of cranial hemorrhoidal artery. Such pigs are stunted and obstipated, and have a pendulous abdomen due to fecal retention.

Salmonellosis is often an enterocolitis. Lesions occur in the villi of the small intestine, lymphoid tissues, and colonic mucosa. The invasive salmonellae have a cytotoxic effect on epithelial cells, cause their dissociation and sloughing, and induce a granulocytic cellular infiltration of the lamina propria. Later, diphtheritic pseudomembranes form on the mucosal surface. Macrophages of the mucosa have the organisms in their cytoplasm and are accompanied by plasma cells and lymphocytes. In the basal mucosa and submucosa, lesions include perivasculitis and vasculitis that can cause thrombosis. The gross and microscopic hallmarks of salmonellosis are the enlargement of Peyer's patches and the lymphoid nodules of the cecum and colon with necrosis of surface epithelium. In the ileum of the pig, the oval, elongated Peyer's patches are ulcerated and coated with a necrotic pseudomembrane. In the colon, the solitary lymphoid nodules are raised and ulcerated, creating so-called button ulcers.

Mesenteric lymph nodes are enlarged, swollen, edematous and have foci of necrosis. The hepatic lesions, the result of bacteria being carried to the liver via the portal vein, are focal necrosis that progresses to microgranulomas; the latter are small clusters of macrophages (the "paratyphoid nodules or granulomas") that are a response to the seeding of *Salmonella* emboli. In the septicemic form, salmonellae disseminate to other tissues to produce, in some animals, focal meningoencephalitis, suppurative bacterial arthritis, or renal infarction. In pigs, septicemic salmonellosis is often accompanied by violet discoloration of the skin and extensive capsular petechiae of the kidneys ("turkey egg kidney").

↳ Salmonella septicemia
↳ CSF
↳ ASF

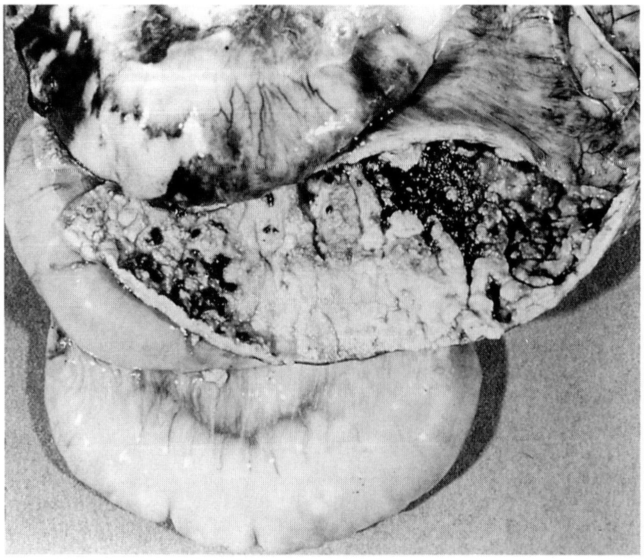

Figure 1-77 Colon; pig. Pseudomembranous colitis. A diffuse pseudomembrane coats the necrotic hemorrhagic mucosa. This animal had been inoculated with *Salmonella typhimurium* 6 days earlier. *Courtesy Dr. R.G. Thomson.*

Peracute Salmonella Septicemia. Peracute *Salmonella* septicemia is a disease of calves, foals, and pigs. Young animals are generally at greater risk than older animals, although the reasons for this difference are not understood. In foals, the feces of affected animals are typically green. The species of *Salmonella* most often involved in septicemic salmonellosis is *S. cholerasuis*. Gross lesions of animals dying of peracute salmonella septicemia are minimal and are due to fibrinoid necrosis of blood vessels. Necrosis of blood vessels causes a widespread petechiation and a blue discoloration (cyanosis) of the extremities and ventrum of white pigs. Peracute *Salmonella* septicemia is usually fatal in animals 1 to 6 months of age. Death is usually attributable to disseminated intravascular coagulopathy secondary to the generalized Shwartzman reaction.

Acute Enteric Salmonellosis. This disease is caused most frequently by *Salmonella typhimurium* and occurs in cattle, pigs, and horses. Carnivores are rarely affected. Characteristic of the disease is diffuse catarrhal enteritis with diffuse fibrinonecrotic ileotyphlocolitis (Fig. 1-77). Intestinal contents are malodorous and have mucus, fibrin, and occasionally, blood as components. The feces have a septic tank odor. Multiple foci of hepatocellular necrosis and hyperplasia of Kupffer cells **(paratyphoid nodules),** when present, are characteristic of acute enteric salmonellosis. Lymphadenopathy is usually present. Fibrinous **cholecystitis** at necropsy is pathognomonic for acute enteric salmonellosis in calves.

Chronic Enteric Salmonellosis. This disease occurs in pigs, cattle, and horses. Lesions are seen principally in pigs that have discrete foci of necrosis and ulceration, principally in the cecum and colon. These are termed **button ulcers** (Figs. 1-78 and 1-79). Additionally, since salmonellosis causes vascular thrombosis and pigs have poor or no collateral blood supply to the rectum (cranial hemorrhoidal artery), affected animals develop rectal strictures with

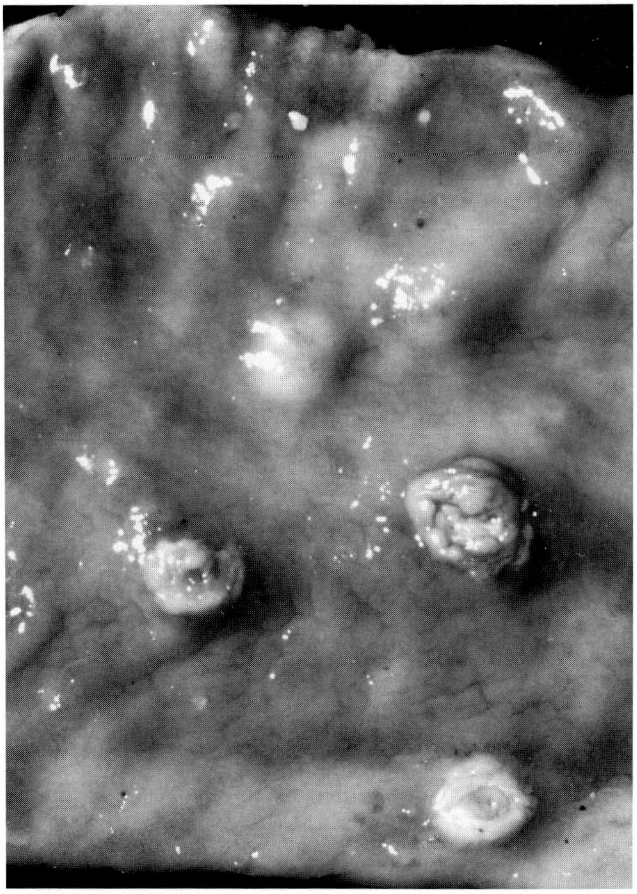

Figure 1-78 Colon; pig. Salmonellosis. Necrotic "button ulcers" are raised above the mucosal surface. *Courtesy Dr. M.D. McGavin.*

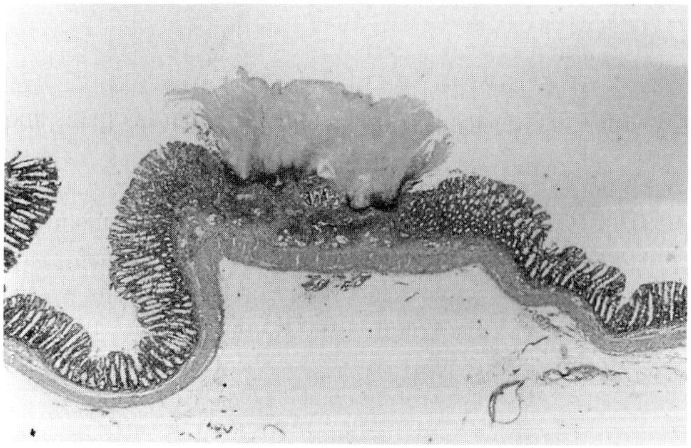

Figure 1-79 Colon; pig. Salmonellosis. Necrotic material protrudes from the "button ulcer." H & E stain. *Courtesy Dr. M.D. McGavin.*

resultant abdominal distension, secondary to fecal retention. Scar formation, secondary to ulcerative proctitis, also contributes to rectal stricture.

Clostridial Enteritis

Many diseases that affect animals and human beings are caused by clostridial organisms. This discussion is limited to those clostridia that produce diarrheal disease. All clostridial enteritides are enterotoxemias.

Clostridium perfringens is a gram-positive, anaerobic rod that is a normal inhabitant of the gastrointestinal tract. These bacilli are spore-formers under adverse circumstances and produce toxins in the presence of large quantities of nutrients that favor bacterial proliferation. The *C. perfringens* is a heterogeneous group of organisms divided into five types, from A to E, based on the production of one or more of the four major lethal toxins. *C. perfringens* type A produces the alpha toxin; type B produces alpha, beta, and epsilon toxins; type C produces alpha and beta toxins; type D produces epsilon toxin; and type E produces alpha and iota toxins. The toxins are protein exotoxins, some of which are proenzymes, and some have enzymatic activity. In addition, some strains of types A, C, and D produce an enterotoxin that is released upon lysis during sporulation.

Enterotoxigenic strains of *C. perfringens* are responsible for clostridial food poisoning. Most cases of clostridial food poisoning occur because of the consumption of cold or warmed-up poultry or other meat cooked the previous day or even a few hours before consumption and allowed to cool slowly. Cooking kills the vegetative cells of *C. perfringens,* but activates surviving spores that can eventually germinate and multiply in the low redox environment of the cooked food. Enterotoxin produced by sporulating *C. perfringens* is responsible for the poisoning.

Enterotoxemia. Enterotoxemia is produced by one of the five *C. perfringens* types elaborating the classic exotoxins, but *C. perfringens* type D is often incriminated. Clostridial enterotoxemia most often affects young fat animals. Outbreaks often follow a change in feed or an increase in its carbohydrate content, as when an animal is fed for sale or slaughter. In foals, it has been associated with increased feeding of readily available carbohydrates and soybeans found in high-protein feeds for pet horses. A change in feed or overfeeding precipitates an alteration in the balance in the bacterial flora of the intestine. When *C. perfringens* has an opportunity to overgrow, it produces abundant toxin. Clinical signs of enterotoxemia include diarrhea with brown, black, or bloody feces, anorexia, lethargy, increased heart rate, dilated atonic abdomen, dehydration, prostration, and death. Some animals die unexpectedly, without diarrhea. Affected lambs have glucosuria, a feature not seen in other species.

The small intestine is the target organ of clostridial enterotoxemia. Lesions include petechiae, ecchymoses, paintbrush hemorrhage, or diffuse hemorrhage of the serosa and mucosa and on gross examination can be mistaken for intestinal strangulation. The intestines are flaccid, thin-walled, dilated, and often gas-filled. Gas bubbles can also be present in the intestinal wall. The intestine can rupture as a result of the thinning of the wall and gas entrapment. There is often gastric hyperemia, excessive pleural and peritoneal fluid, and sometimes a cooked appearance of the skeletal musculature. The spleen is enlarged and pulpy because of congestion. The toxins produced by *C. perfringens* damage intestinal villi in a manner similar to an acid burn. Within a few minutes of exposure, epithelial cells at the villus tip undergo degeneration and separate from the basement membrane. These changes are followed by sloughing of cells and hemorrhage. This process extends down the villus toward the crypts. There is edema and transient leukocyte infiltration of the lamina propria, followed by necrosis. After 6 to 8 hours, more than a third of the villus is damaged. This damage results in exudation of serum, inflammatory cells, and blood. Villi that have been damaged by *C. perfringens* exotoxins stain poorly with H & E and are acellular. These lesions can resemble autolytic changes. The crypts usually remain intact but can be dilated. The intestinal submucosa can be edematous, hemorrhagic, or filled with leukocytes. Death occurs within 24 hours after the onset of clinical signs.

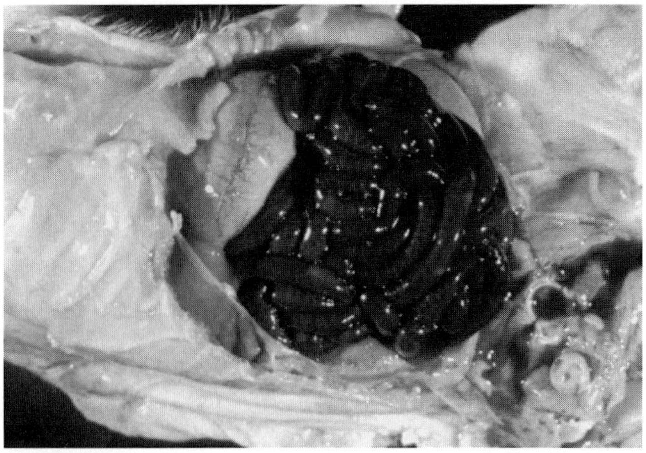

Figure 1-80 Small intestine; pig. Enterotoxemia. The entire small intestinal mucosa is hemorrhagic. Necrosis can extend through the muscularis mucosa. The entire litter was affected.

Clostridium Perfringens Type C. Enterotoxic hemorrhagic enteritis affects calves, lambs, and foals during the first few days of life and piglets during the first 8 hours of life. Clinical signs vary from none to bloody diarrhea. When piglets are affected, the whole litter dies. Lesions at necropsy include hemorrhagic or necrotizing enteritis of the small intestines, sometimes with gas in the lumen and within the walls of the intestine (Fig. 1-80). **Struck** is a disease affecting adult sheep and goats and feedlot cattle in winter and early spring. Also caused by *C. perfringens* type C, it is characterized by hemorrhagic enteritis with ulceration, ascites, and peritonitis.

Clostridium Perfringens Type D. This bacterium affects fattening sheep, goats, and calves. It is diet-related and associated with grain overload or "overeating disease." The sudden change in diet promotes growth of organisms in the small intestine. The disease is often characterized by unexpected death sometimes preceded by central nervous system signs or "blind staggers." Endothelial cell damage is produced by a bacterial toxin (angiotoxin). This lesion can result in bilateral symmetric encephalomalacia, which is similar in its regional distribution to edema disease of pigs (swine cerebral angiopathy). Lesions of *C. perfringens* type D infection are multisystem hemorrhages, particularly of serosal surfaces. Pericardial effusion is present as well as a mild gastroenteritis. The angiotoxin produces "pulpy kidney disease" of sheep.

Peracute Hemorrhagic Gastroenteritis of Dogs. Known as canine hemorrhagic gastroenteritis, the cause of this disease is undiscovered but is considered due to infection with *C. perfringens* type E. The disease most often occurs in dogs of toy breeds younger than 2 years. Blood is observed about the anal opening prior to death. As the name of the disease denotes, there is hemorrhagic necrosis of the mucosa anywhere from the stomach to the anus. Numerous clostridial organisms are present in the intestinal debris but are not attached to intact mucosa.

Lincomycin or Antibiotic Enteritis. This enteritis is associated with antibiotic administration and is seen most commonly in rabbits and horses. It has been suggested, but not proven, that antibiotic administration causes death of normal enteric flora that allows overgrowth of *C. perfringens* type A. Clinical signs and gross and microscopic lesions are similar to those observed in animals with *Clostridium* spp. enteritis but bacterial organisms are often lacking.

Clostridium Piliformis. Commonly called Tyzzer's disease, *C. piliformis* infects multiple mammalian species. The principal target is the liver (see Chapter 2), but lesions also occur in intestine and heart. Intestinal involvement is variable but is most common in rodents and rabbits (Fig. 1-81). Colitis occurs in some cats. The enteric manifestations of Tyzzer's disease are generally in the distal small intestine, particularly the ileum. Mucosal necrosis extends into the muscularis and is accompanied by edema. Definitive diagnosis is made microscopically by finding the causative bacillus (best done with silver stains) in the characteristic hepatic or intestinal lesions (Fig. 1-82). All of the characteristic lesions of Tyzzer's disease (i.e., segmental ileocolitis or ileotyphlitis and colitis, focal hepatic necrosis, and focal myocardial necrosis) are not present in every affected animal. The initial damage and entrance of the organism occur in the ileum, cecum, or colon; the liver is affected secondarily by bacteria carried via the portal circulation.

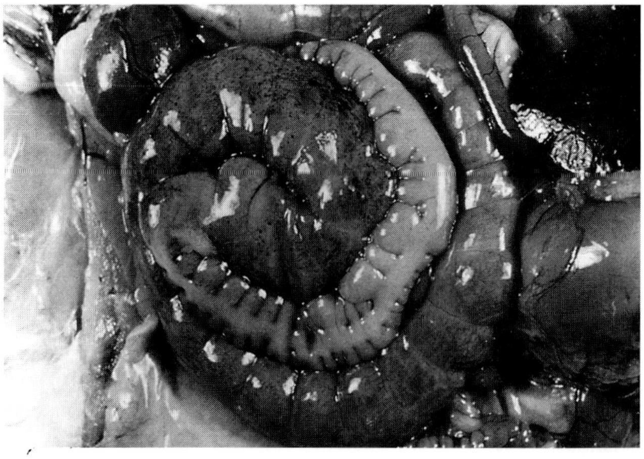

Figure 1-81 Intestines; rabbit. Tyzzer's disease. The cecum is congested, edematous, and speckled with foci of petechiae. The proximal 2 cm of sacculated colon is reddened because of hemorrhage, and there is an abrupt transition to normal colon. *Van Kruiningen HJ, Blodgett SB. J Am Vet Med Assoc 1971; 158:1205-1212.*

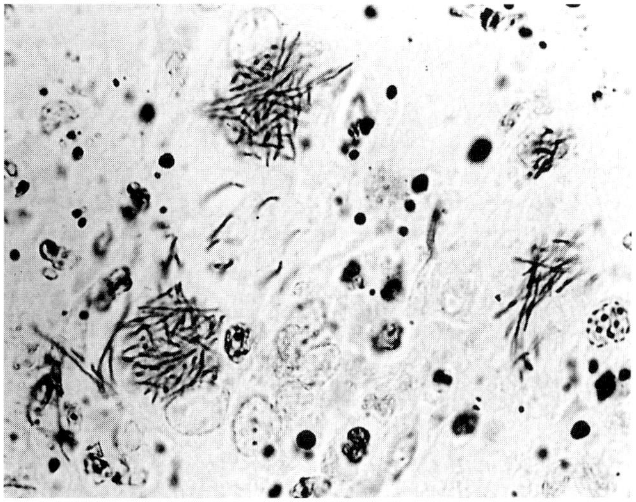

Figure 1-82 Liver; rabbit. Tyzzer's disease. Hepatocytes adjacent to foci of necrosis contain crisscrossed *Clostridium piliformis*. Warthin-Starry stain.

Clostridium Difficile. *C. difficile* spores are common in the environment and in the intestinal tract of many mammals. They cause disease in primates including human beings, enterocolitis in foals, typhlocolitis in horses, and enteritis in a variety of laboratory animals. *C. difficile* also affects suckling pigs in outbreaks characterized by mesocolonic edema and typhlocolitis. The induction of disease by *C. difficile* is likely dose related, but the reasons for bacterial overgrowth, apart from that caused by oral antibiotic administration, are not understood. The lesions are similar to those produced by *C. perfringens* infection.

Mycobacterial Enteritis

Intestinal Tuberculosis. *Mycobacterium tuberculosis* and *Mycobacterium bovis* enter most often by the respiratory or gastrointestinal route. Intestinal tuberculosis occurs rarely in cattle, in calves sucking infected mammary glands, nonhuman primates, and human beings ingesting unpasteurized milk. The portal of entry into the body is by ingestion and then via lymphoid tissue of the intestinal tract, where the bacilli are phagocytosed by M cells covering Peyer's patches. The most common site of disease is the distal ileum, and "skip" lesions occur, apparently corresponding to the location of Peyer's patches. Clinically, animals with intestinal tuberculosis suffer with chronic diarrhea, lower abdominal pain, and chronic weight loss. If a portion of the small intestine has become stenotic, vomiting is a clinical sign.

In some species, such as the dog, a thickened, firm, hoselike segment of intestine can be palpated through the abdominal wall. In large animals, thickened, firm loops of intestine are recognized at rectal examination. The affected segment of intestine is thickened, and the mucosa is corrugated and ulcerated. Regional lymph nodes have granulomas and calcification. The tuberculous lesion consists of numerous epithelioid granulomas with necrotic centers. Swirls of epithelioid and giant cells infiltrate the lamina propria and the submucosa. The affected mucosa and submucosa are distended by the caseating tuberculoid granulomatous lesion and have prominent infiltrates of lymphocytes and plasma cells. In some animals, *Mycobacterium avium* infections result in lesions similar to those of *M. tuberculosis,* complete with caseation, necrosis, and calcification. However, in most spontaneous *Mycobacterium avium-intracellulare*–induced diseases, a lepromatous (noncaseating) granulomatous inflammation occurs, similar to that of Johne's disease (see intestinal diseases of ruminants, paratuberculosis). Such lesions are described in dogs, pigs, horses, rhesus monkeys, AIDS patients, and exotic birds.

Pigs ingest the organisms along with the avian litter sometimes fed as an inexpensive source of dietary protein. In these cases, lesions also develop in the retropharyngeal lymph nodes. The early lesion consists of sheets of macrophages, 10 to 40 cells deep in the mucosa and up to 200 cells deep in the submucosa, and occurs over a large segment of the small intestine, colon, or both. Ziehl-Neelsen staining of these tissues demonstrates large numbers of intracellular acid-fast bacilli.

Viral Diseases

Rotavirus Enteritis

Rotaviruses are ubiquitous pathogens present everywhere in the environment including air and water. Each species of animal has its specific rotavirus, and although broad similarities exist in pathogenesis among viral infection of individual species, in general the viruses are not cross-infective among species. These viruses are important pathogens. Human group A rotavirus, for example, kills a million children a year in the developing countries of the world. However, in all species these viruses cause disease in association with other enteropathogens of neonates. In calves the disease is most important during the first week of life and in piglets in the first 7 weeks of life. These ages correspond to the reduction of colostral and milk-associated antirotavirus antibody titers that occur after weaning. Specific diagnosis of these diseases is difficult for a variety of reasons. The virus is ubiquitous and, therefore, can be isolated or detected in many animals, most of which do not have clinical disease. Additionally, since the viruses are cytolytic, some animals with viral diarrhea can be negative for viruses because the cells harboring virus have been shed previously in the feces.

Rotaviruses are around 70 nm in diameter and are trilayered. Only the complete triple-layered virion is infectious. Rotaviruses have double-stranded RNA at their core and protein spikes project from the surface. The complete particle looks like a wheel, thus the appellation rotavirus. Affected piglets and calves have a yellow, fluid diarrhea, are reluctant to stand and nurse, appear depressed, and sometimes have a few strings of thick saliva hanging from their lips. Calves that have died of rotavirus enteritis are often less than 72 hours old, are dehydrated, and have a "tucked-up" abdomen and sunken eyeballs. The intestines are moderately distended with yellow fluid, some loops appearing thin and transparent. Microscopically, the epithelial cells over the upper two thirds of the affected villi of the proximal small intestine are infected first (Fig. 1-83). Within hours, sloughing of villus cells is followed by blunting and fusion of villi and accelerated migration of remaining cells from the crypts toward the villus tips. The infection extends to the villus epithelial cells of the middle and distal small intestine. Within hours of the onset of diarrhea, all virus-containing cells (demonstrated by immunofluorescence) have been shed and replaced by cuboidal to squamoid cells (Fig. 1-84), which have migrated from the crypts in an attempt to cover the denuded basement membrane.

Coronavirus Enteritis

Coronaviruses responsible for calfhood enteritis are 100 to 120 nm in diameter and are composed of single-stranded RNA and have projecting peplomeres. Calves up to 21 days of age (usually 4 to 6 days old) are susceptible. Serotype of the virus, ingestion of colostral antibody, and the presence of concomitant disease influence the severity of infection. The incubation period is 36 to 60 hours. Clinically, the disease is characterized by yellow, fluid, sometimes bloody diarrhea, depression, reluctance to nurse, dehydration, and weakness. Lesions consist of

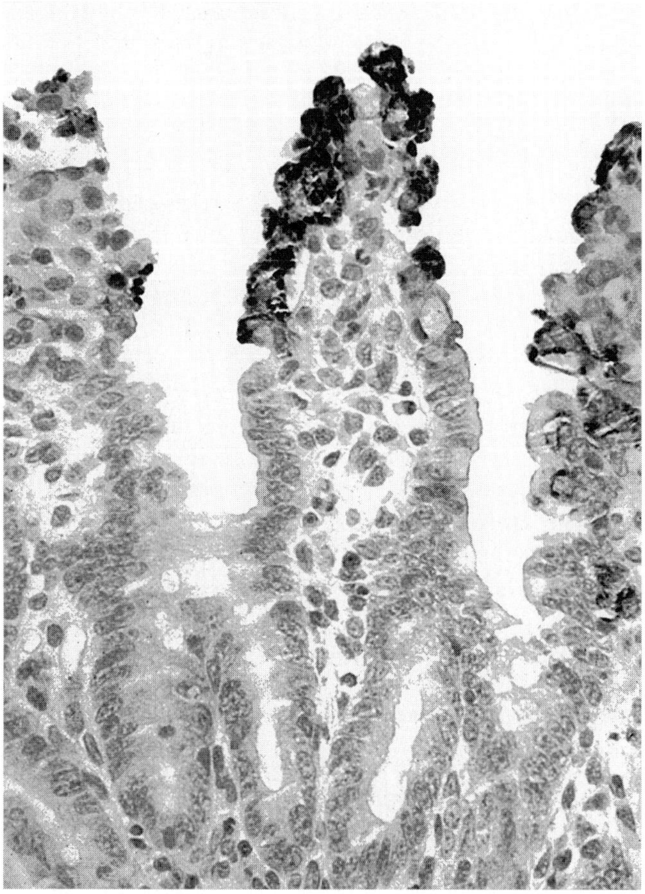

Figure 1-83 Jejunum; piglet. Rotavirus enteritis. Intestinal villi are shortened and villus enterocytes are sloughing. Infected enterocytes contain large amounts of viral antigen *(black)*. Immunoperoxidase stain. *Gelberg HB. Vet Pathol 1992; 29:161-168.*

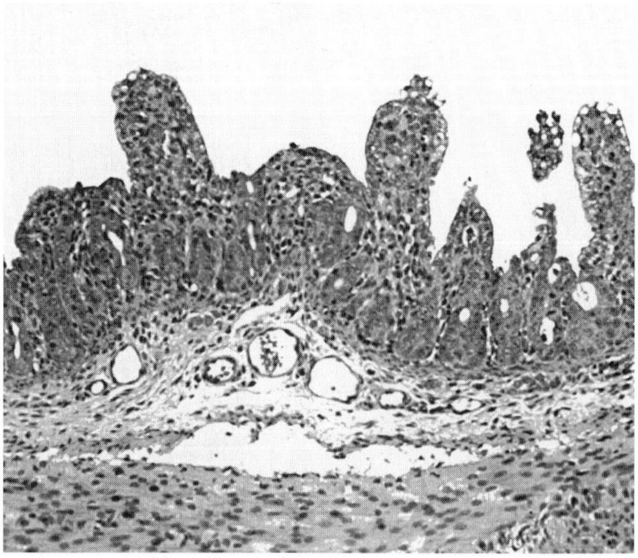

Figure 1-84 Jejunum; piglet. Rotavirus enteritis. There is marked blunting and fusion of intestinal villi secondary to virus-induced cytolysis of villus enterocytes. H & E stain.

enterocyte loss, blunting, and fusion of villi similar to rotavirus enteritis.

The course of infection, clinical signs, and tissue damage are more prolonged in coronavirus enteritis than in rotavirus-induced disease, and death occurs after 2 to 4 days of diarrhea. The gross lesions are indistinguishable from those of rotavirus enteritis or enterotoxigenic colibacillosis. The small and large intestines are moderately distended with yellow fluid. Microscopically, the coronavirus infection is first apparent in villus epithelial cells of the proximal small intestine and, subsequently, in the caudal small intestine and epithelial cells lining the colon. As determined by immunofluorescence, viral antigen is present in all the cells lining the villi at the onset of diarrhea. In the colon, virus is present in surface cells and cells in the crypts. Antigen persists in crypt cells for 3 to 4 days after the onset of diarrhea. During the first 48 to 96 hours after the onset of the illness, epithelial cells are necrotic and are replaced by immature cuboidal or squamous cells, covering markedly shortened or fused villi in the small intestine.

In the colon, surface cells are lost and replaced by less mature cuboidal and squamoid cells. Crypt lumens contain degenerate and necrotic cells. Focally, crypt epithelium is hyperplastic and the lamina propria near the surface contains increased numbers of lymphocytes and plasma cells. Cells of the lamina propria, including fibroblasts, histiocytes, and endothelial cells, are infected; these cells undergo necrosis, producing a focal loss of cells. The trabecular sinuses of regional lymph nodes are filled with lymphocytes, plasma cells, and macrophages. A hemorrhagic form of coronavirus enterocolitis is recognized in which virtually all colonic crypts are damaged throughout their length (Figs. 1-85 and 1-86). A bloody, fibrinonecrotic pseudomembrane covers the denuded colonic lamina propria. It is not known if this form of the disease represents infection with a more virulent strain of virus or an interaction of the virus with other pathogens. Although generally a mild and self-limiting disease of neonates, feline enteric coronavirus has been associated with fatal enteritis is a series of cats. Lesions consist of degeneration and loss of enterocytes from jejunal villus tips. Cats 2 months to 7 years old are affected.

Adenovirus Enteritis

Adenoviral infection occurs in cattle, sheep, pigs, and horses. Each species-specific virus cause inapparent respiratory disease and under some circumstances clinical disease. In horses of the Arabian and Arabian crossbreeds, adenovirus enteritis occurs in immunologically suppressed horses with combined immunodeficiency (CID) (see Chapter 7 for details). When enteritis is produced, characteristic basophilic to amphophilic intranuclear inclusion bodies are present in villus enterocytes, usually in

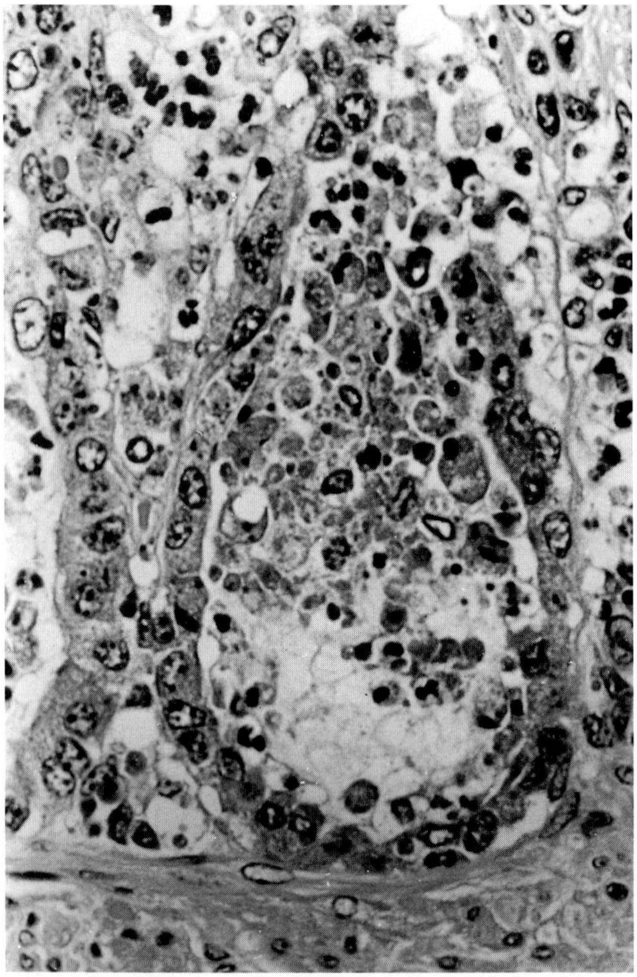

Figure 1-85 Colon; calf. Coronavirus enterocolitis. Crypt epithelium has undergone extensive degeneration and necrosis. H & E stain.

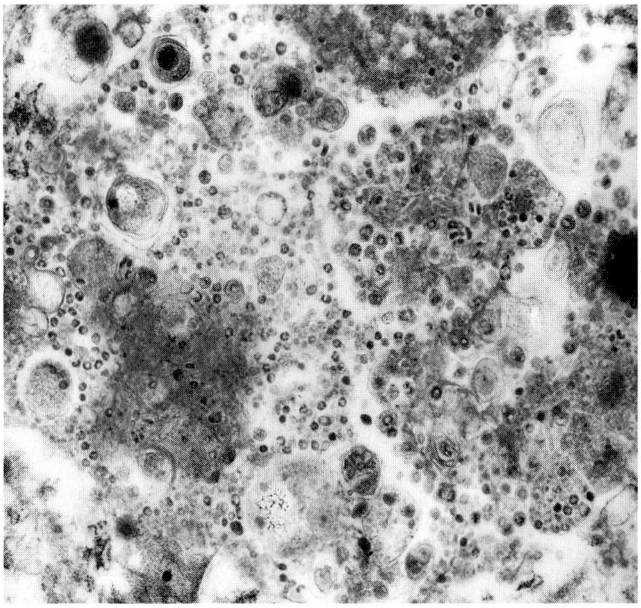

Figure 1-86 Colon; calf. Coronavirus enterocolitis. Electron micrograph. The cytoplasm of damaged epithelial cells is filled with 80- to 120-nm, doughnut-shaped coronavirus particles.

young animals that are immunosupressed (Fig. 1-87). Endothelial cells also are affected and have similar inclusions. Loss of enterocytes results in villus blunting and fusion. In general, adenovirus infection is subclinical.

INTESTINAL DISEASES OF PIGS

This listing of specific infectious causes of enteritis in pigs is exclusive of those agents already discussed. When formulating a differential diagnosis, all causes of enteritis must be considered including intestinal displacements, colibacillosis, rotavirus, *Salmonella*, parasites, toxins, and so on. Enteric diseases of pigs are an important cause of economic loss; rapid and accurate on-farm diagnosis is critical in controlling disease outbreaks. If one takes into account the epidemiology of the outbreak as well as the age of the affected animals and the location and nature of lesions, one can generally be fairly accurate in rendering an on-farm diagnosis pending laboratory confirmation.

Transmissible Gastroenteritis

Transmissible gastroenteritis (TGE) is an important disease in pigs younger than 10 days. The coronavirus that causes this disease cross-reacts with, but is distinct from, the coronavirus that causes feline infectious peritonitis. The virus is inactivated by sunlight; therefore this disease occurs mostly in winter. Piglets suffer from acute diarrhea, weight loss, vomiting, and dehydration. Morbidity and mortality, especially in neonates, approach 100% in susceptible herds. Target cells for the virus are villus enterocytes, and therefore lesions consist of marked atrophy of villi of the small intestine (Fig. 1-88). Sows are susceptible to the virus, and morbidity among the sows is 100%, but they suffer little clinically (vomiting, inappetence, agalactia), and none die. Immunity is complete. Diagnosis is by positive immunofluorescence of intestinal sections in piglets acutely ill with the disease.

Similar to rotavirus or non-TGE coronavirus infections, the virus is lytic and sloughed enterocytes carry virus into the feces. The difference in pathogenicity between rotavirus and non-TGE coronavirus infections and TGE is the number of villus enterocytes destroyed by virus. In TGE, most of the villus enterocytes are destroyed, and therefore the clinical disease is more severe. TGE is characterized by a sudden onset of vomiting and diarrhea. The diarrhea is profuse, contains white, undigested milk, and has an offensive odor. Dehydration is pronounced. Some young pigs have only a transitory fever, whereas affected sows are febrile for several days. Weakness and

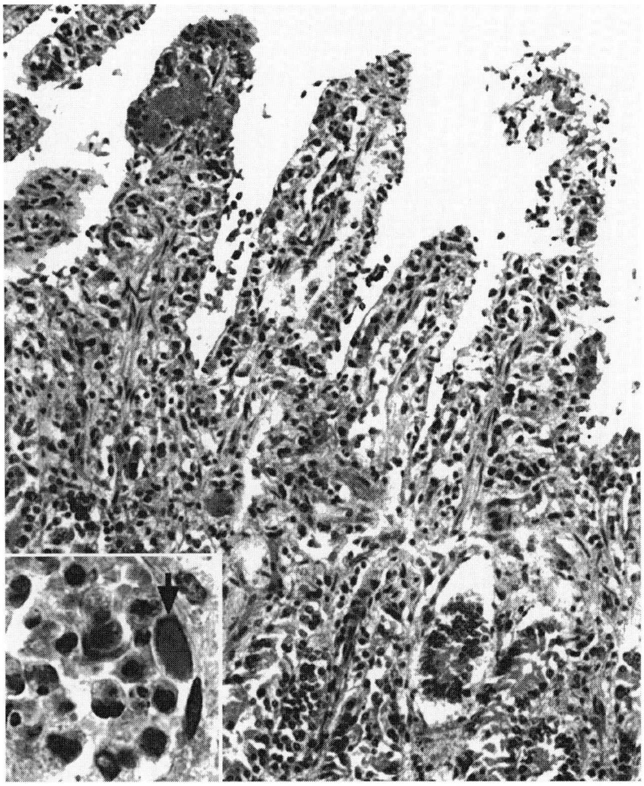

Figure 1-87 Small intestine; foal. Adenovirus enteritis. There is marked necrosis and loss of villus enterocytes. *Inset:* Intranuclear adenovirus inclusion body *(arrow)* in an endothelial cell. H & E stain.

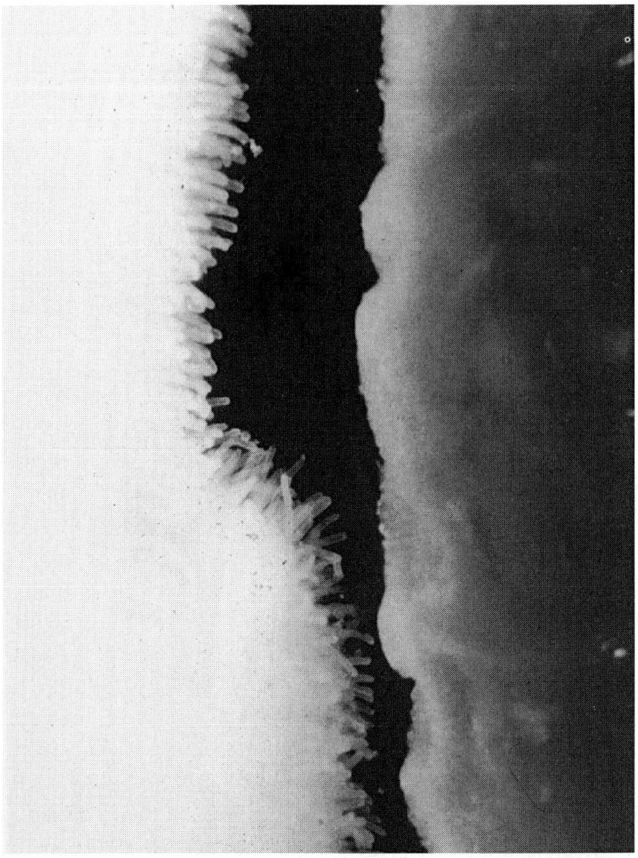

Figure 1-88 Intestine; piglet. Transmissible gastroenteritis. There is marked villus atrophy *(right)* compared with normal intestine *(left)*.

emaciation progress to death from the second to the fifth day of illness. Pigs that survive grow poorly because of continued intestinal malabsorption due to failure of the villi to regenerate completely, and some never recover completely. In growing and fattening pigs, TGE usually occurs as a transient, watery diarrhea, mild anorexia, some weight loss, and dehydration for 2 to 4 days. Laboratory findings include transient, mild leukopenia early in the disease and leukocytosis later.

Young pigs that have died of TGE are dehydrated, and their perineum is stained with fluid feces. The small intestine is ballooned, gas-filled, and contains a copious yellow fluid. The walls of the small intestine are thin and translucent. Piglets can have empty stomachs caused by vomiting. Mesenteric blood vessels are congested, giving variable light redness to some portions of the intestine. Mesenteric lymph vessels are notably empty of chyle. The stomach has patchy vascular engorgement. Microscopically, the diagnosis is partially based on the presence of villus atrophy (Fig. 1-89). The villus height:crypt depth ratio is reduced from 7:1 in normal pigs to 1:1 in infected

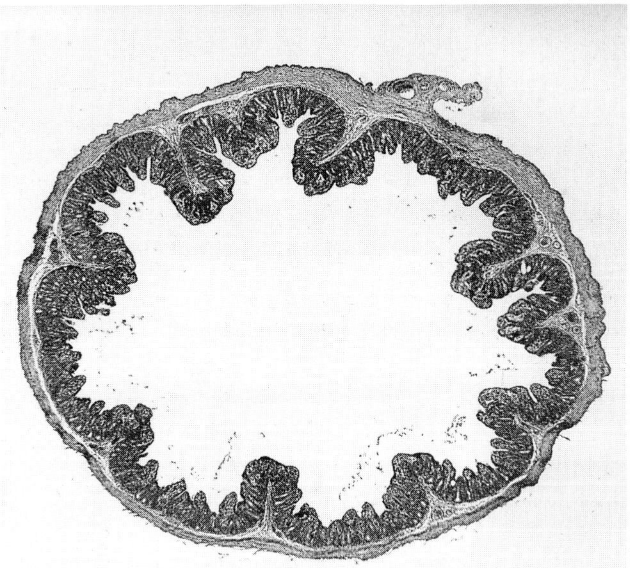

Figure 1-89 Proximal jejunum, transverse section; newborn pig. Transmissible gastroenteritis. Extensive villus atrophy is present throughout the mucosal circumference. *Moon HW. J Am Vet Med Assoc 1969; 155:1853-1859.*

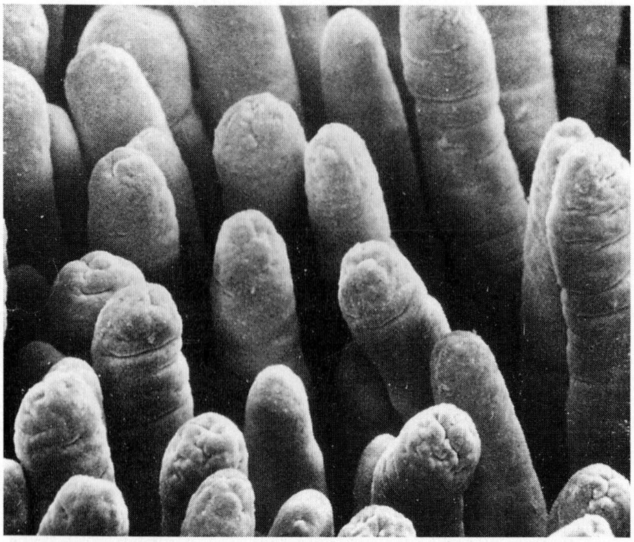

Figure 1-90 Small intestine; normal pig. Normal villi. Scanning electron micrograph. Note the tall, fingerlike villi with indented tips. *Moon HW. Intestine. In: Cheville NF, ed. Cell Pathology. 2nd ed. Ames, IA: Iowa State University Press, 1983:503.*

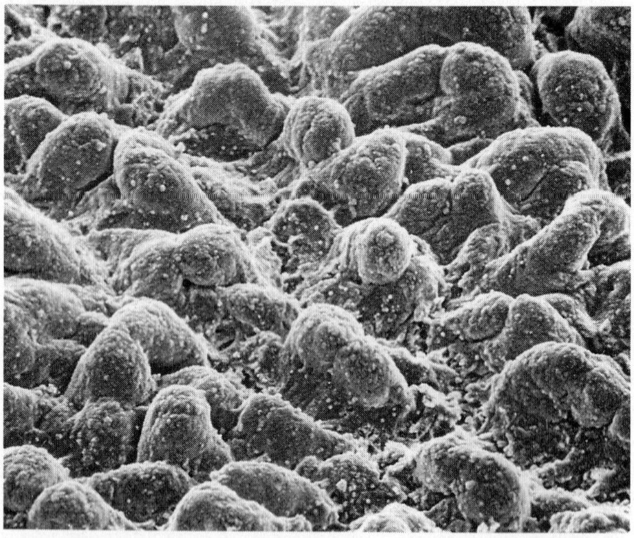

Figure 1-91 Small intestine; pig. Transmissible gastroenteritis. Scanning electron micrograph. Villi have atrophied as a sequella to viral epithelial damage. *Moon HW. Intestine. In: Cheville NF, ed. Cell Pathology. 2nd ed. Ames, IA: Iowa State University Press, 1983:503.*

pigs (Figs. 1-90 and 1-91). The atrophy is not accompanied by dense infiltration of inflammatory cells. The presence of inflammatory cells varies from one outbreak to the next and is influenced by secondary bacterial infections. Accumulations of neutrophils and lymphocytes occur in the lamina propria of the mucosa where it is denuded of enterocytes. Epithelial cell necrosis and villus atrophy are the principal lesions of TGE but are not pathognomonic. Colibacillosis, coccidiosis, cryptosporidiosis, rotavirus, and non-TGE coronavirus are among the differential diagnoses.

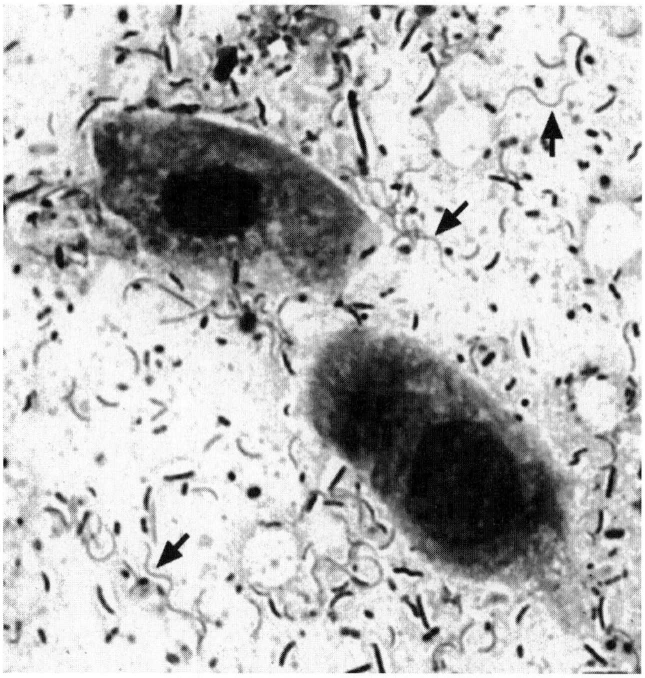

Figure 1-92 Colon; pig. Swine dysentery. This impression smear contains a few enterocytes and numerous bacteria. Note spiral bacteria consistent with *Brachyspira* spp. *(arrow).*

Swine Dysentery

Unlike most of the other diseases of the porcine gut, swine dysentery is generally confined to the large intestine. The gross lesions of the disease closely approximate those of acute enteric salmonellosis except that bloody feces are more usual in dysentery. Weanling pigs 8 to 14 weeks old are usually affected, and the disease spreads rapidly through a herd. Morbidity approaches 90%, and mortality is around 30%. Gross lesions include mucohemorrhagic colitis. Lesions are present in the spiral colon, colon, cecum, and rectum. The intestine often has a fibrinonecrotic pseudomembrane, which correlates with the severe diarrheic feces containing blood, mucus, and fibrin-noted clinically. The diarrhea and electrolyte loss that occur are due to colonic absorptive failure.

The causative bacterium, *Brachyspira hyodysenteriae,* previously known as *Treponema* and *Serpulina,* acts synergistically with anaerobic colonic flora such as *Fusobacterium necrophorum* or *Bacteroides vulgatus* to produce disease. This synergism is believed to be partially responsible for the age restriction (8 to 14 weeks old) of the disease since neonatal animals have not yet developed the appropriate anaerobic gut flora. *B. hyodysenteriae*

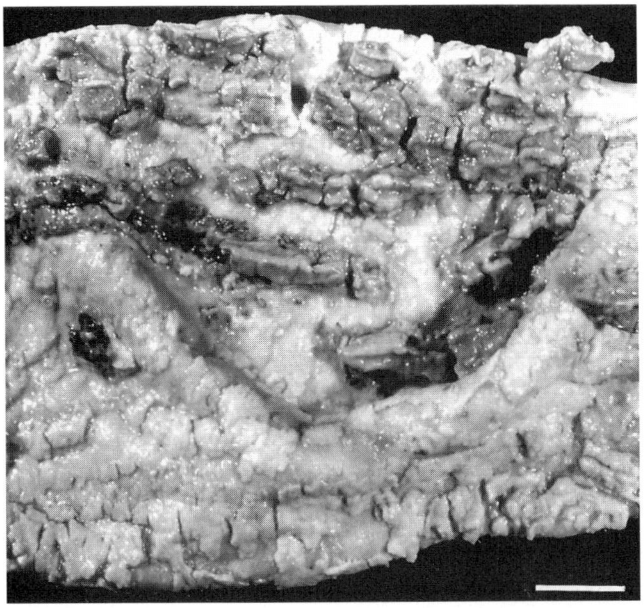

Figure 1-93 Ileum; pig. Necrotic proliferative ileitis. The mucosa is markedly hyperplastic. The dark areas are necrotic. Bar = 1 cm. *Courtesy Dr. M.D. McGavin.*

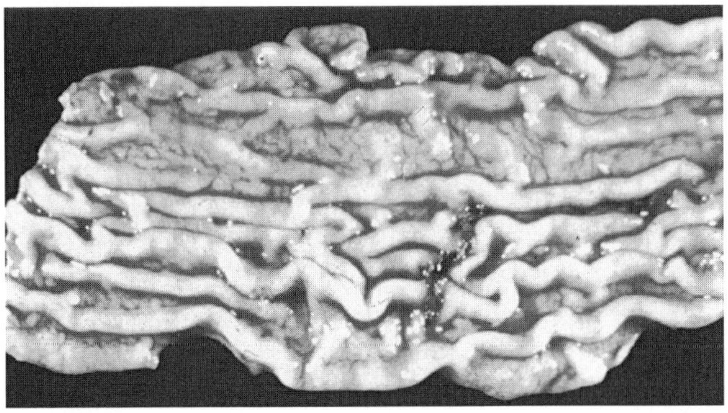

Figure 1-94 Ileum; pig. Proliferative enteritis. Note the marked epithelial ridges, the result of epithelial hyperplasia.

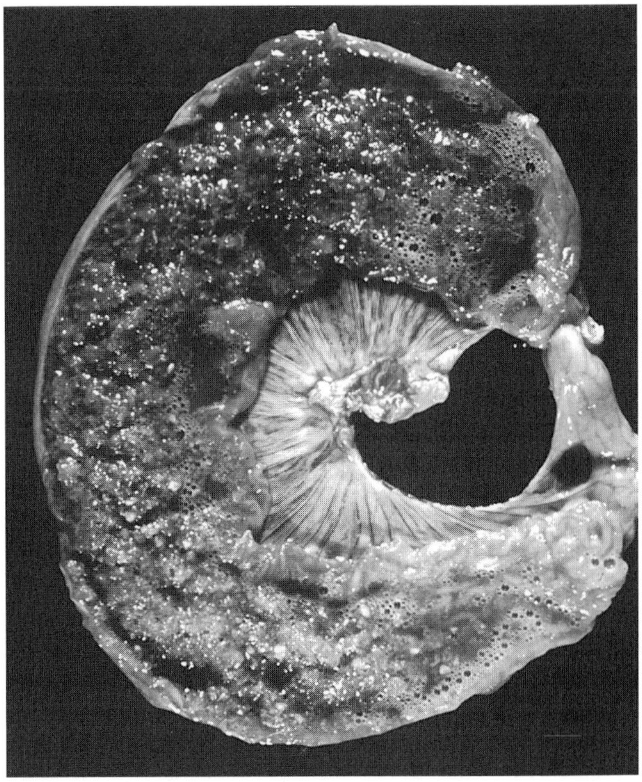

Figure 1-95 Ileum; pig. Necrotizing enteritis. There is marked necrosis and hemorrhage of the intestinal mucosa *(dark areas).*

produces a cytotoxic hemolysin, which is a virulence determinant. *B. hyodysenteriae* is identified by impression smear (Fig. 1-92), dark-field microscopy, and fluorescent antibody techniques, as well as by newer methods such as the polymerase chain reaction.

Lawsonia Enteritis

This disease manifests in a variety of ways as indicated by the number of names applied to it: **Proliferative enteropathy, proliferative ileitis, intestinal adenomatosis, distal ileal hypertrophy, terminal ileitis,** and **proliferative hemorrhagic enteropathy.** The genus of the causative agent has undergone several recent changes in nomenclature also. For many years, this disease was believed to be caused by *Campylobacter* spp. (*C. sputorum mucosalis, C. jejuni, C. hyointestinalis*). Newer methods of bacterial classification caused the name to be changed first to *Ileobacter* and now *Lawsonia.* Pigs older than 4 weeks of age are susceptible; thus this condition is a postweaning disease. The nature of the lesions is a function of the extent of intestinal mucosal necrosis. The disease begins as a bacteria-induced stimulation of intestinal crypt epithelial cell proliferation of the small intestine, particularly in the ileum (Fig. 1-93). Lesions are generally most severe in the ileum. With time, the lesions progress to necrosis with hemorrhage (Figs. 1-94 and 1-95). Thus the morphologic appearance of the lesions varies from case to case.

Morbidity within a herd is 10% to 15%; mortality is around 50%. In fatal cases, affected pigs usually die within a day of the appearance of clinical signs. Pigs that recover are generally "poor-doers." At clinical and necropsy examination, variable amounts of blood and intestinal casts are present in the feces. Microscopically, the comma-shaped bacteria are made visible with special stains within the mitotically active cells of the small intestinal the villus crypts (Fig. 1-96). Mitosis can be so intense that the histologic features suggest a neoplasm and a disease diagnosis of "intestinal adenomatosis." A similar organism and associated intestinal proliferation are found in horses, hamsters, ostriches, and macaques.

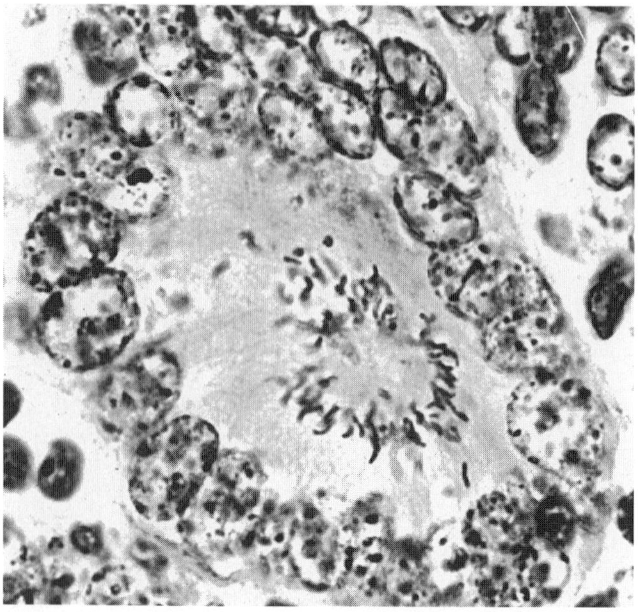

Figure 1-96 Ileum; pig. Proliferative ileitis. Curved *Lawsonia* spp. bacteria are present in the apical cytoplasm of enterocytes. There is proliferation of enterocytes. Warthin-Starry stain.

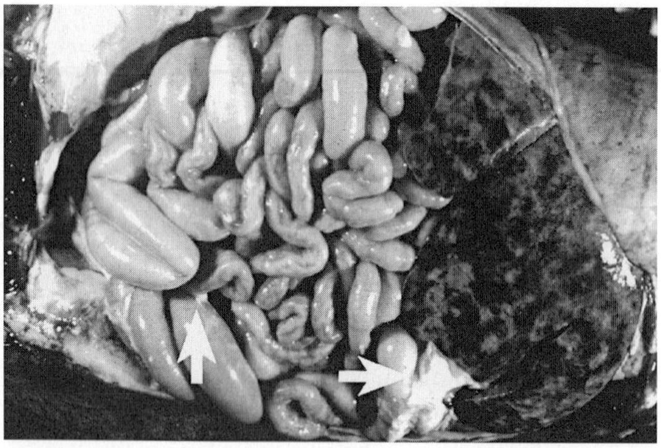

Figure 1-97 Abdomen; pig. Fibrinous polyserositis. Strands and clumps of fibrin are scattered throughout serosal surfaces (*arrows*). A milk-spotted liver is also present.

Glasser's Disease

Glasser's disease is characterized by fibrinous polyserositis. Although not generally a diarrheal disease, it does cause inflammation of the intestinal serosa (serositis). Lesions range from arthritis to peritonitis to leptomeningitis depending on the serous surface infected. Glasser's disease generally occurs in 5- to 12-week-old pigs. Mortality of affected animals within a herd is high, but morbidity is low. Although classic

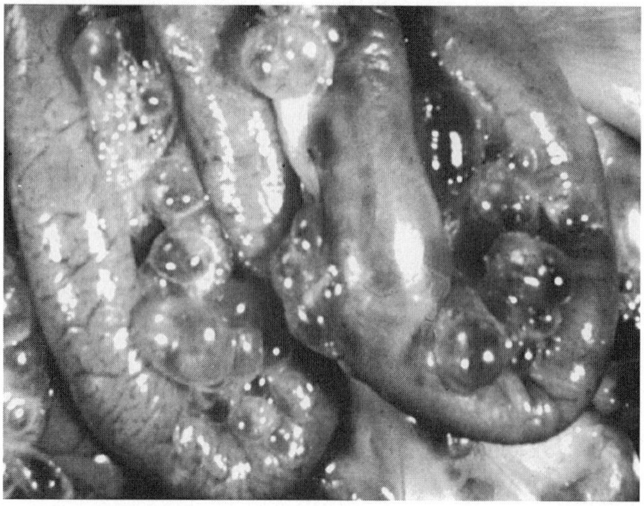

Figure 1-98 Intestines; pig. Intestinal emphysema. Gas bubbles dilate serosal and mesenteric lymphatics.

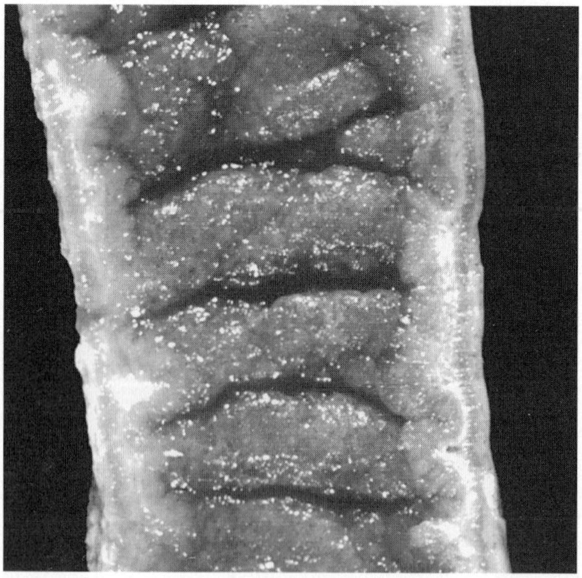

Figure 1-99 Ileum mucosa; sheep. Johne's disease. There is marked thickening of the lamina propria from macrophage infiltration.

Glasser's disease is caused either by *Haemophilus suis* or *Haemophilus parasuis,* porcine polyserositis can be caused by *Mycoplasma hyorhinis, Streptococcus suis* type II (zoonotic), and septicemic salmonellosis (Fig. 1-97).

Intestinal Emphysema

Intestinal emphysema of pigs translates to gas-dilated lymphatics of the intestinal serosa and mesentery. The

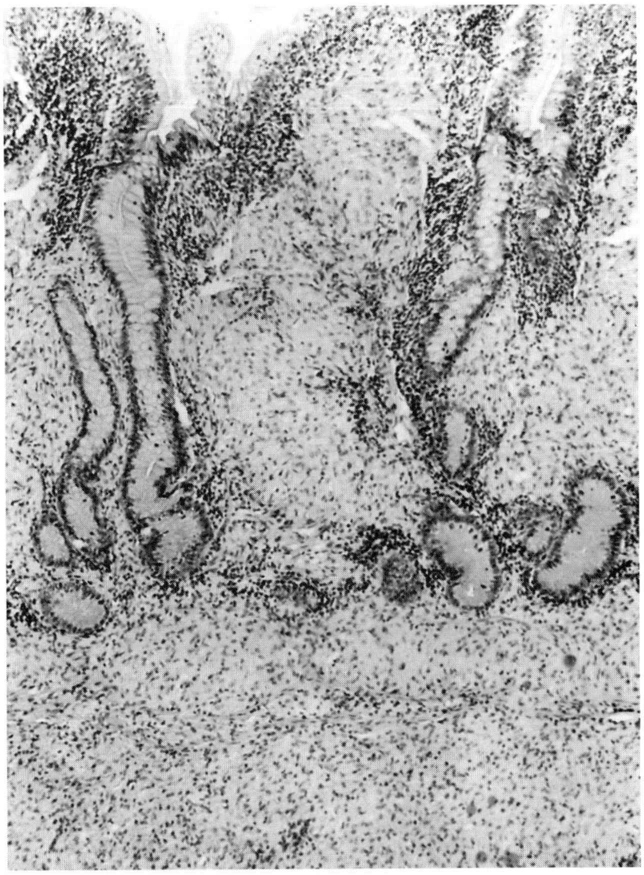

Figure 1-100 Small intestine; cow. Johne's disease. Macrophages distend the lamina propria of the villi and submucosa. A lepromatous (noncaseating) granulomatous response is present.

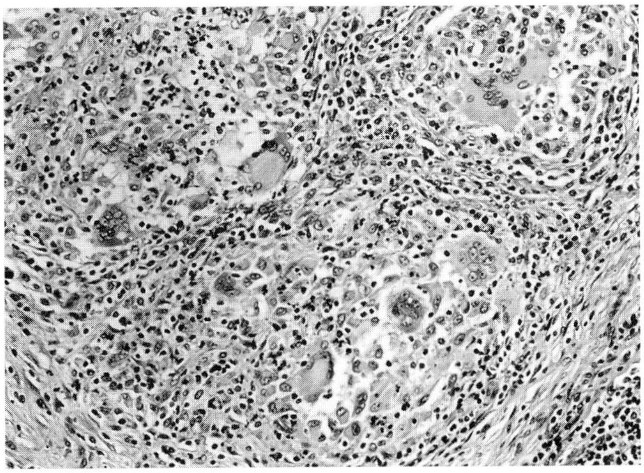

Figure 1-101 Small intestine; goat. Johne's disease. Tuberculoid, epithelioid, and giant cell granulomas, with collars of lymphocytes, in a Peyer's patch of a goat that had been inoculated with *Mycobacterium paratuberculosis* 5 months previously. These granulomas contained no acid-fast bacilli. H & E stain.

etiology of this condition is unknown, and it is not associated with clinical disease (Fig. 1-98).

INTESTINAL DISEASES OF RUMINANTS

Paratuberculosis

Paratuberculosis or Johne's disease has been described in numerous ruminant species. In cattle, the disease is characterized by intractable diarrhea, emaciation, and hypoproteinemia in animals older than 19 months. In the average infected herd, 32% to 42% of animals are infected. In small ruminants (sheep and goats) the clinical disease is similar to that observed in cattle except that diarrhea does not occur. The pygmy goat is an exception to the course of disease in other small ruminants in that some pygmy goats develop explosive diarrhea and die unexpectedly. In other ruminants, the disease has a protracted course and is considered a wasting disease due to the loss of body mass. Ruminants are infected with *Mycobacterium paratuberculosis (johnii)* from feces-contaminated soil. Newer methods of bacterial classification suggest that *M. johnii* is closely related to *Mycobacterium avium*.

The causative organisms are very resistant to environmental stressors, particularly in regions with acid soils. After ingestion, the bacilli penetrate the gastrointestinal mucosa and are taken up by macrophages. Lesions in the lamina propria of the intestines, particularly in the ileum, include the accumulation of macrophages. There is little correlation between the severity of the gross lesions and the severity of clinical disease. An age-related immune resistance to infection and disease develops in animals older than 2 months. Fetuses can be affected, but disease is delayed until the animals are much older. Isolation of newborns from fecal contamination is a useful measure to reduce the incidence of infection in a particular herd. Diagnosis is made by observing clinical signs together with the signalment. The gross lesion in Johne's disease is a chronic, segmental thickening of the caudal small intestine, cecum, and proximal colon (Fig. 1-99). Affected segments have a corrugated mucosa that is focally ulcerated. Mesenteric lymph nodes are greatly enlarged.

At microscopic examination, noncaseating granulomas consist of macrophages with foamy cytoplasm and large numbers of acid-fast organisms (Fig. 1-100). In contrast, sheep, goats, and deer can have a tuberculoid (caseating) granulomas in the intestines, lymphatics, and lymph nodes, sometimes with central mineralization. These lesions are composed of well-differentiated epithelioid cells in a whorled pattern and a variable number of Langhans-type giant cells (Fig. 1-101). Organisms are few. Granulomas of either type occur in the regional lymph nodes (Fig. 102).

Mycobacterium paratuberculosis can be isolated from feces of affected animals, from diseased intestines and regional lymph nodes, and, sometimes, from a variety of other tissues and fluids, including the liver, uterus, fetus, milk, urine, and semen. Acid-fast bacteria in rectal mucosal scrapings are found in 60% of the cases. Hepatic

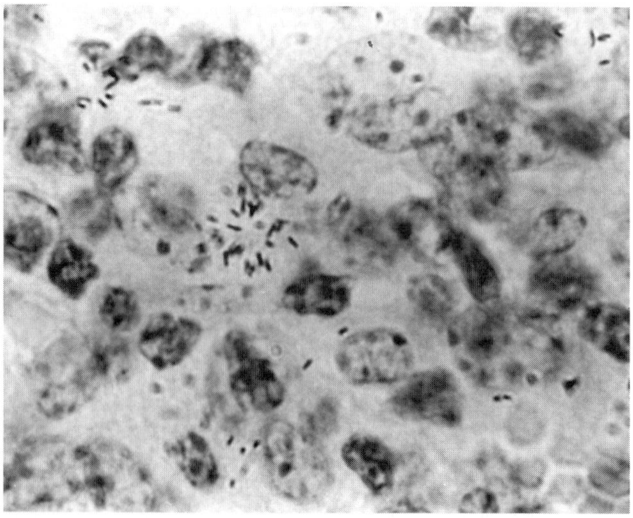

Figure 1-102 Mesenteric lymph node; cow. Johne's disease. Note the acid-fast mycobacteria within macrophages. Ziehl-Neelsen stain.

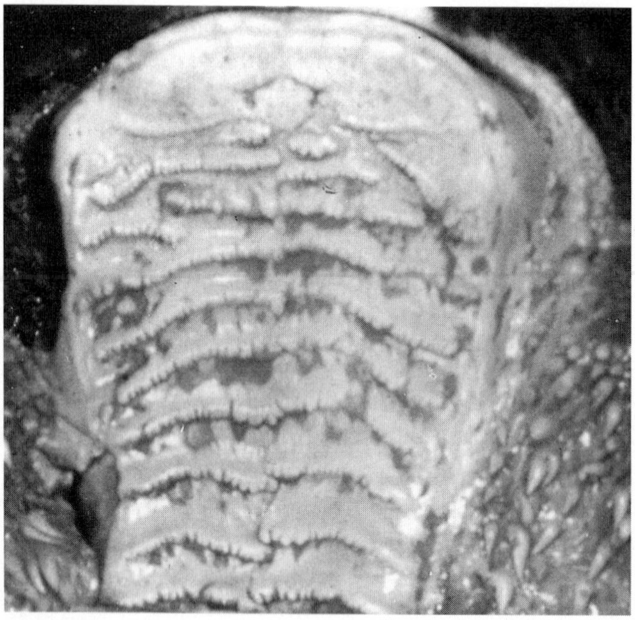

Figure 1-103 Hard palate; cow. Bovine viral diarrhea. Multiple, shallow, erosions are present among the mucosal ridges of the palate.

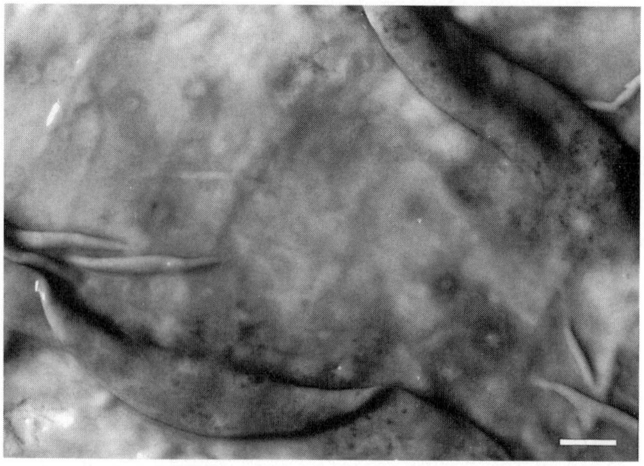

Figure 1-104 Abomasum; cow. Bovine viral diarrhea. The mucosa contains multiple, 2 to 3 mm, shallow ulcers with hyperemic rims. Bar = 1 cm. *Courtesy Dr. M.D. McGavin.*

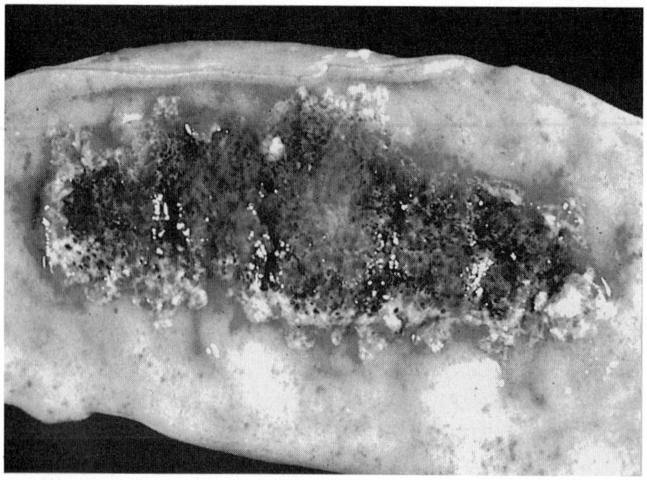

Figure 1-105 Ileum; cow. Bovine viral diarrhea. Peyer's patch and the overlying epithelium are necrotic and covered with suppurative exudate.

microgranulomas occur in about 25% of affected animals. Aortic mineralization (arteriosclerosis), when it occurs, is specific for Johne's disease in cattle. The pathogenesis of this vascular lesion is not well understood, but is associated with the severe cachexia associated with the disease. The epizootiology of Johne's disease leads many to believe it is one of the most important diseases facing the dairy industry.

Bovine Viral Diarrhea

Also known as mucosal disease, bovine viral diarrhea (BVD) affects cattle of all ages but is most common in animals 8 months to 2 years of age. In this respect, clinical cases are typically younger than animals susceptible to Johne's disease. Animals infected early in life with noncytopathic BVD virus develop a persistent infection. Later in life, if exposed to cytopathic virus, they develop

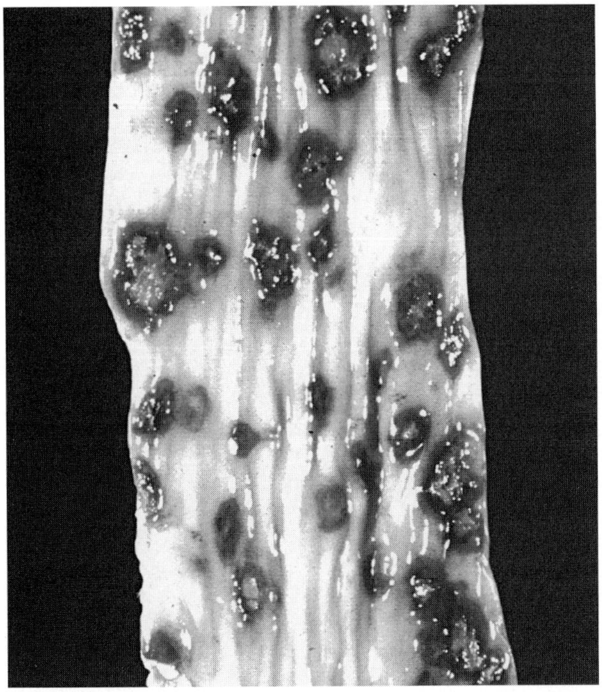

Figure 1-106 Colon; bison. Multifocal ulcerative colitis. Multiple mucosal ulcers were caused by bovine viral diarrhea virus.

disease. Clinical signs of BVD include anorexia, depression, profuse diarrhea, cessation of milk production, fever, rumen atony, salivation, lacrimation, and a mucopurulent nasal discharge. Multifocal, sharply demarcated, erosions and ulcers in the tongue, gingiva, palate, esophagus, rumen, abomasum, and coronary bands of the hooves characterize BVD (Fig. 1-103). In the intestine, the characteristic lesion is sharply demarcated areas of necrosis in the epithelium over the gut-associated lymphoid tissue (Figs. 1-104 to 1-106). Calves infected in utero develop cerebellar hypoplasia, cataracts, microophthalmia, renal dysplasia, and other congenital defects. Abortions, stillbirths, and mummified fetuses can also result from an in utero infection. BVD is caused by a pestivirus related to the virus of hog cholera. Morbidity in a herd varies from 2% to 50%. All affected animals die.

Microscopically, the lesions in the stratified squamous epithelium begin with focal hydropic degeneration and necrosis of the stratum spinosum. This change is followed by erosion and ulceration, with hyperemia and influx of granulocytes at the margins and base of the lesions. In the abomasum, small intestine, cecum, and colon, the villus, and crypt epithelium is necrotic. Loss of epithelium is extensive; cells that survive are spread thin, and there is dilation of some intact crypts. The lamina propria is collapsed and infiltrated by a variety of acute and chronic inflammatory cells. Necrosis of lymphocytes is extensive within the germinal centers of Peyer's patches. These lymphoid follicles often have acellular centers that have cystic crypt epithelium or necrotic debris and mucus. A fibrinonecrotic or fibrinohemorrhagic pseudomembrane can cover Peyer's patches, the ileum, and large intestine. A more common outcome from BVD infection occurs in immunocompetent animals that are seronegative at the time of exposure to either the cytopathic or noncytopathic virus. Variable signs develop, but they are mostly mild or subclinical. Most cattle in the United States have serologic evidence of exposure to nonvaccine BVD.

Rinderpest

Lesions similar to those of BVD occur in cattle with **rinderpest.** This morbillivirus disease of cattle, however, has characteristic multinucleate enterocytes in the intestinal lesions that do not occur in BVD. Rinderpest does not occur in the United States or Europe but is a significant disease in Africa and Asia.

Winter Dysentery

Winter dysentery is a somewhat enigmatic, acute, nonfatal disease of cattle. As the name implies, it is a seasonal disease and additionally occurs only in northern latitudes. Catarrhal ileitis and jejunitis characterize the disease.

Although its cause is unknown, a coronavirus has been implicated in the disease. Acute onset of profuse diarrhea, severe decrease in milk production, variable depression and anorexia, and, sometimes, a mild cough characterize the illness. Fever, leukocytosis, and leukopenia are notably absent at the onset of time of onset of diarrhea. The feces can be dark brown, dark green, or black (melena) and often are flecked or streaked with blood or mucus and have a characteristic fetid odor. At the onset of winter dysentery, 5% to 10% of a herd are ill. By the second day, 30% to 50% are affected; morbidity reaches 100% by the third day. The course of the illness is 1 to 4 days. Postparturient animals are affected most severely; heifers experience mild disease, and calves younger than 4 to 6 months apparently are unaffected. Mortality is less than 1%, but the reduction in milk production is severe. Cattle that have had the disease cannot be reinfected for several years.

At necropsy, the abomasal mucosa is reddened and the small intestine is segmentally hyperemic, dilated, and flaccid. The contents have the consistency of thin paint and are gray, tan, or olive-green. Peyer's patches have a variegated appearance. The cecum is unaffected. The spiral and distal colon are empty or contain a thin fluid. The mucosal surface is moist and shiny, without necrosis or pseudomembranes, and streaked segmentally with aggregates of petechiae. The latter lie irregularly over colonic lymphoid patches or in parallel rows along colonic ridges ("zebra striping") (Figs. 1-107 and 1-108). The lesions of the colon consist of focal crypt epithelial damage and necrosis of cells of the lamina propria.

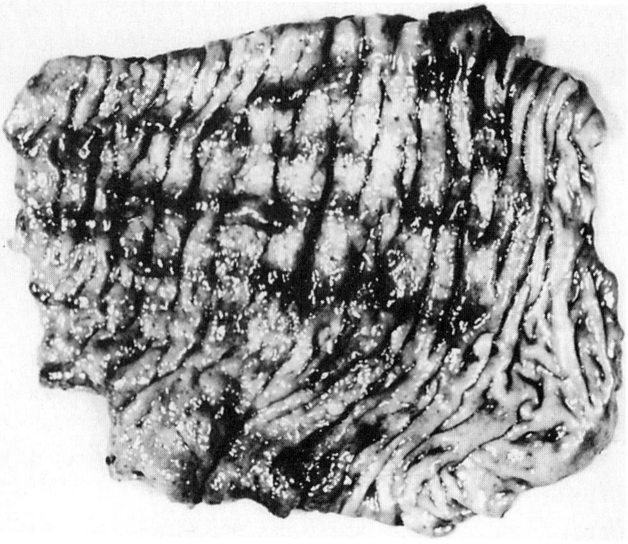

Figure 1-107 Colon; cow. Winter dysentery. Linear mucosal hemorrhages overlie a lymphoid patch of the proximal colon. *Van Kruiningen HJ, Hiestand L, Hill DL, Tilton RC, Ryan RW. Compend Cont Educ Pract Vet 1985; 7:5591-5598.*

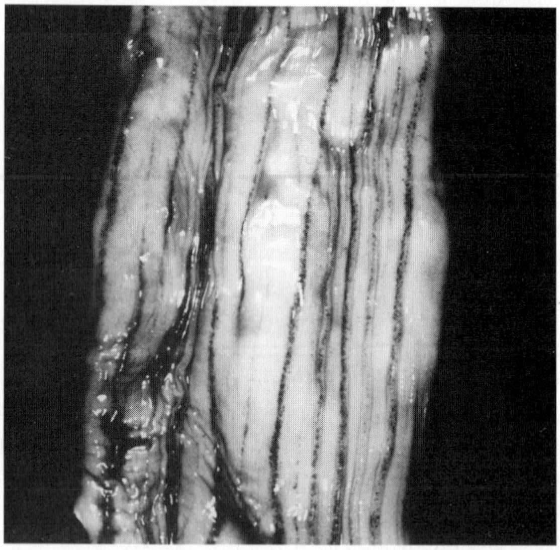

Figure 1-108 Distal colon; cow. Winter dysentery. Linear petechiae on the crests of colonic mucosal folds. *Van Kruiningen HJ, Hiestand L, Hill DL, Tilton RC, Ryan RW. Compend Cont Educ Pract Vet 1985; 7:5591-5598.*

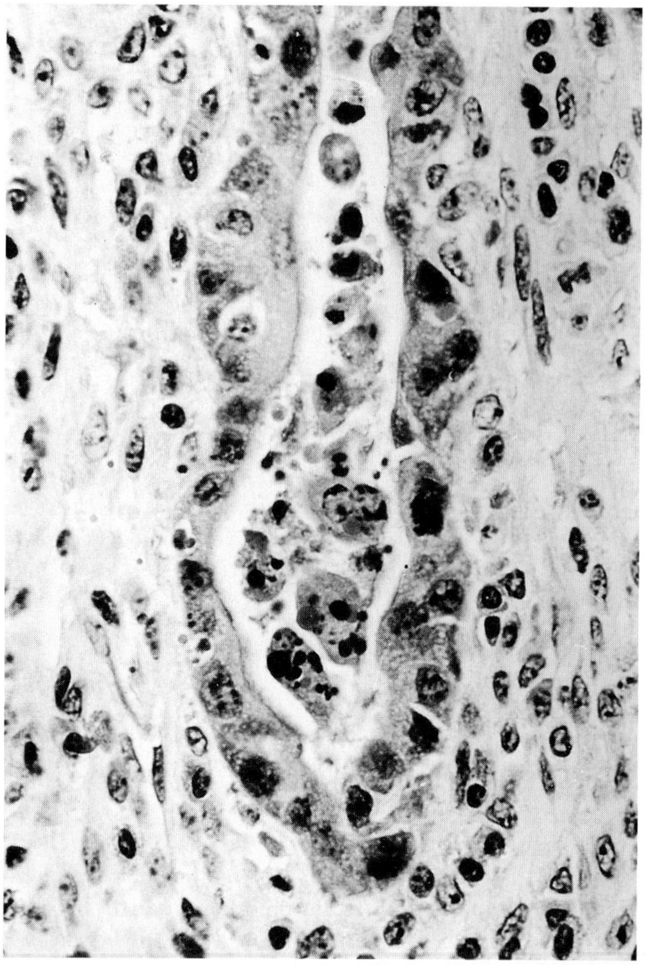

Figure 1-109 Colon; cow. Winter dysentery. Extensive virus-induced colonic crypt damage. Degenerate and necrotic cells in the lumen. H & E stain. *Van Kruiningen HJ, Hiestand L, Hill DL, Tilton RC, Ryan RW. Compend Cont Educ Pract Vet 1985; 7:5591-5598.*

Damaged crypts contain clusters of necrotic cells (Fig. 1-109). Similar fragmented and pyknotic nuclei occur in the lamina propria, where the lysis of cells creates a "moth-eaten" appearance. Capillary beds near the surface of colonic ridges are the source of petechiae and luminal bleeding. The putative coronavirus of winter dysentery can be demonstrated in damaged crypt epithelium by immunoperoxidase and electron microscopic methods (Fig. 1-110).

Chlamydiosis

Bovine chlamydias (strains of *Chlamydia psittaci*) have been recovered from spontaneous enteritis of young calves. Affected calves have diarrhea, fever, anorexia, and depression. Following experimental inoculation, newborn calves develop fever and diarrhea within 24 hours and become moribund within 4 to 5 days. Grossly, the ileum is most severely affected, but the jejunum and large intestine have lesions as well. In diseased segments the mucosa is congested and marked with petechiae. The intestinal wall and mesentery are edematous. The lumen contains watery, yellow fluid mixed with yellow, tenacious, fibrin-rich material attached to the surface. Colonic ridges are hyperemic and have small erosions. Bleeding from

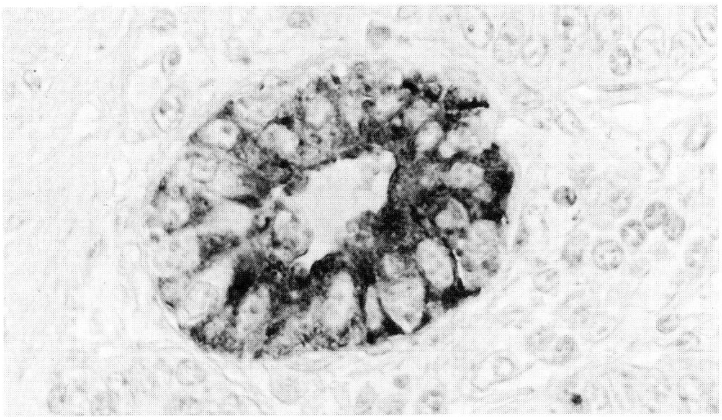

Figure 1-110 Spiral colon; cow. Winter dysentery. Immunoperoxidase reaction for coronavirus antigen in crypt epithelial cells.

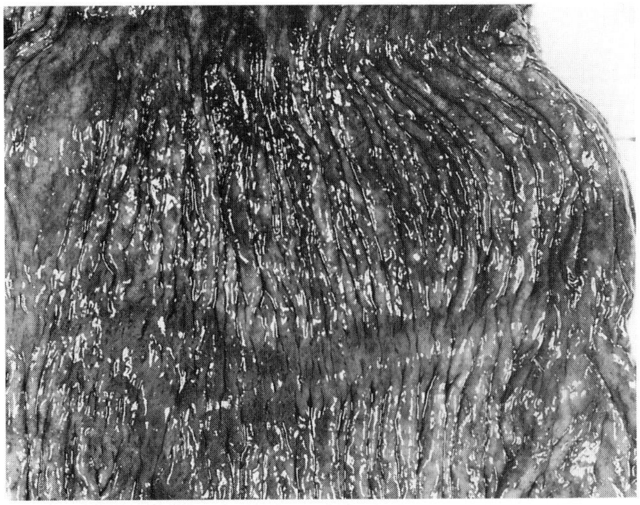

Figure 1-111 Colon; horse. Potomac horse fever. The mucosa has patchy areas of congestion and hyperemia. *John GA, Van Kruiningen HJ, Reim D, Wachtel AW. J Equine Vet Science 1989; 9:250-252.*

petechiae and ecchymoses of the colonic or rectal ridges occurs infrequently. Regional lymph nodes are enlarged.

Microscopically, villus epithelial cells, enterochromaffin cells, goblet cells, macrophages, and fibroblasts of the lamina propria and endothelial cells of lacteals are parasitized by the *Chlamydia*. In the epithelial cells the *Chlamydia* are located in the apical cytoplasm. The *Chlamydia* are adsorbed to the brush border, are taken up by endocytosis, and then multiply in epithelial cell apices. They subsequently are liberated into the lamina propria. Villi are enlarged by dilated lacteals and infiltrates of mononuclear cells and neutrophils. Crypts of both small and large intestine are dilated and have sloughed epithelial cells and inflammatory exudate (colitis cystica superficialis). The centers of lymphoid follicles of Peyer's patches are necrotic. The mucosa and submucosa of the intestine are thickened by a diffuse granulomatous reaction. The abomasum also has lesions, and, in some calves, foci of inflammation extend transmurally, thereby initiating focal peritonitis.

INTESTINAL DISEASES OF HORSES

Potomac Horse Fever

Although Potomac horse fever, also known as equine monocytic ehrlichiosis, was first reported in 1983, it appears that the disease was present for at least the previous 5 years. First described in the Potomac River valley of Maryland, Virginia, and Pennsylvania, it is now found throughout the United States. Fever, depression, severe diarrhea, dehydration, and laminitis characterize the disease.

Horses with Potomac horse fever have a mild necrotizing enterocolitis similar in distribution to colitis X and enteric salmonellosis. The nature of the gross lesions is somewhat controversial, since experimental infections produce variable results. Like hog cholera before it, Potomac horse fever is often associated with concurrent *Salmonella* infection, perhaps accounting for the *Salmonella*-like lesions.

The causative agent, *Ehrlichia risticii*, an intracytoplasmic rickettsial pathogen of epithelial cells, macrophages, and monocytes is found in association with trematodes in freshwater snails. Although rickettsia are often transmitted by arthropods and although this disease is seasonal in northern latitudes (May through September), an arthropod host has not been identified. Without treatment, one third of cases with diarrhea die as a result of dehydration.

The gross lesions of Potomac horse fever are subtle and occur primarily in the cecum and colon; however, the small intestine sometimes has lesions as well. The mucosa of diseased segments is bright pink and has petechiae. Small segments (4 to 8 cm) of the small intestine and large areas of the cecum or colon (5 to 20 cm) have patchy mucosal hyperemia with petechiae; less frequently seen are ecchymoses and scattered 1- to 2-mm ulcers (Fig. 1-111). Intestinal contents are fluid, pale brown, and fetid.

Microscopically, in the cecum and colon, the mucosa is reduced in thickness by loss of surface epithelium, marked decrease in the number of intestinal crypts, and collapse of the lamina propria (Fig. 1-112). Capillaries and veins of the mucosa are engorged with blood. The remaining intestinal crypts have intact epithelium, and a few have necrotic debris. Pseudomembranes are focal and consist of fibrin, necrotic cells, and bacteria covering the denuded surface. The lamina propria is hypercellular, most severely at the base of the intestinal crypts. Macrophages are prominent both in the lamina propria and in the edematous submucosa. The germinal centers of the lymphoid follicles are depleted of lymphocytes and contain karyorrhectic nuclei. Clusters of the ehrlichia are readily demonstrated in macrophages of the deep lamina propria and submucosa (Fig. 1-113) in sections stained with a modified Steiner's or Dieterle's silver stain.

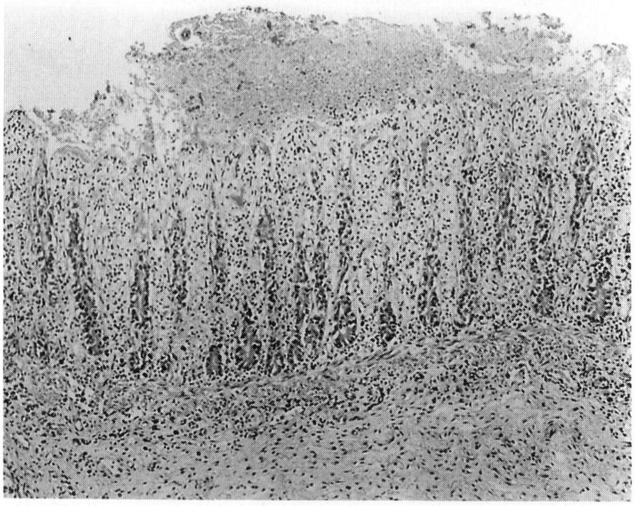

Figure 1-112 Cecum; horse. Potomac horse fever. The villi are covered by a pseudomembrane formed from necrotic enterocytes. H & E stain. *John GA, Van Kruiningen HJ, Reim D, Wachtel AW. J Equine Vet Science 1989; 9:250-252.*

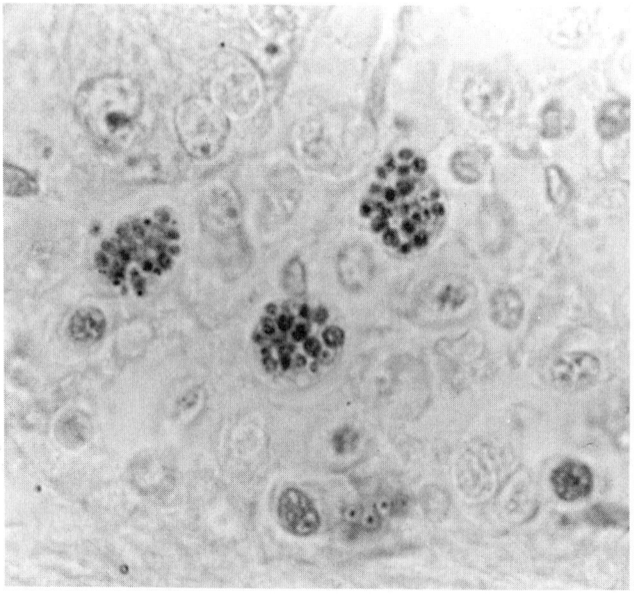

Figure 1-113 Cecum; horse. Potomac horse fever. Clusters of *Ehrlichia risticii* are present in macrophages of the lamina propria adjacent to intestinal crypts. Steiner's silver stain. *John GA, Van Kruiningen HJ, Reim D, Wachtel AW. J Equine Vet Science 1989; 9:250-252.*

Rhodococcus Equi Enteritis

Rhodococcus equi is a soil saprophyte and a normal inhabitant of the equine intestine. The disease caused by this large gram-positive rod is often characterized by pulmonary pyogranulomas. The frequent occurrence of helminths and *R. equi* infection together suggests that migrating larvae participate in distributing the bacterium through the body of the foal. Helminth control appears to bring about great reduction or elimination of *R. equi* infection. When coughed up and swallowed in large numbers, the bacteria enter the M cells of the intestine and cause pyogranulomas in the gut-associated lymphoid tissue and intestinal lymph nodes. The result is a pyogranulomatous, ulcerative enteritis of the cecum and colon and, sometimes, segments of the small intestine. About half of the cases of *R. equi* infection involve the intestine. *R. equi* is zoonotic, especially in immunocompromised human beings.

Affected intestinal segments have greatly thickened, corrugated mucosa, 2 to 5 cm thick, which is mottled red, white, and tan. Multiple, irregularly shaped, soft, well-defined, necrotic foci, 1 to 3 cm in diameter, occur in the mucosal surface of the colon along with multiple, small ulcers (Fig. 1-114). Mesenteric, cecal, and colonic lymph nodes are enlarged and firm (Fig. 1-115). On incision, the lymph nodes have areas of homogeneous gray tissue and abscesses. The mucosa of the small intestine, colon, and cecum is infiltrated by large macrophages filled with gram-positive bacilli 1 to 2 μm in length and 0.25 μm in diameter. The accumulations of large, bacteria-filled

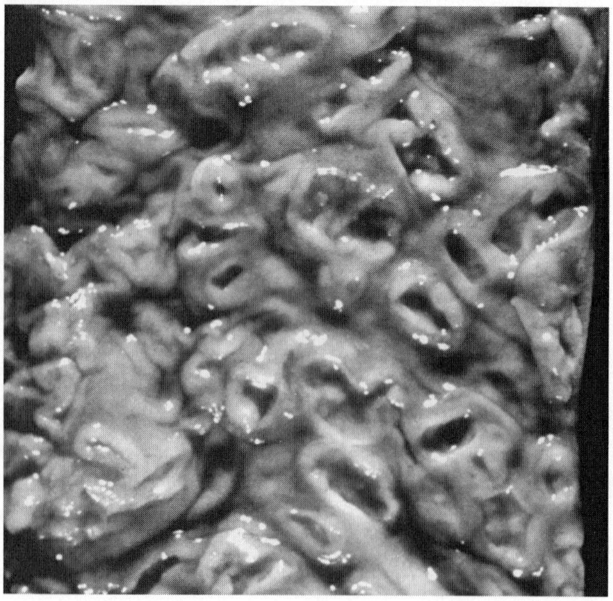

Figure 1-114 Colon; horse. Multifocal ulcerative colitis. *Rhodococcus equi* infection. There are multiple mucosal ulcers centered over lymphoid nodules.

macrophages and multinucleated giant cells in the lamina propria distort the shapes of villi in the small intestine and displace crypts in the small intestine, colon, and cecum. Sharply demarcated foci of coagulation necrosis occur, and the mucosal surface is ulcerated. Affected lymph nodes have masses of the bacteria-filled macrophages, as well as multinucleated giant cells.

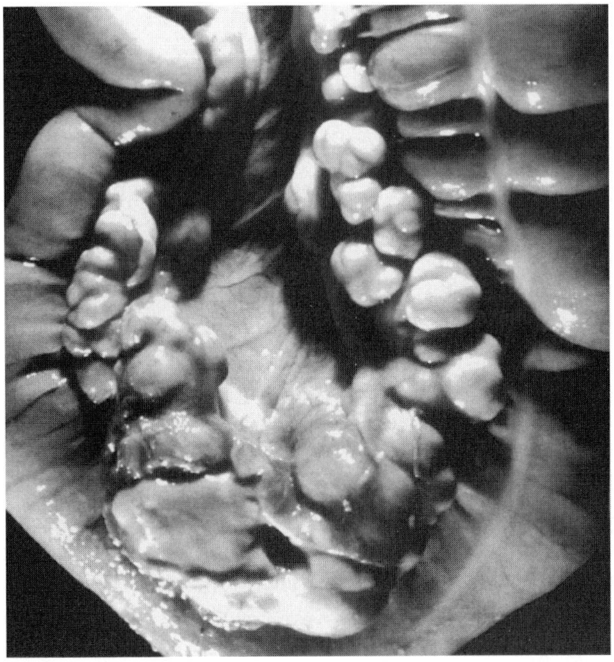

Figure 1-115 Colon; horse. Mesenteric lymphadenitis. *Rhodococcus equi* infection. Colonic lymph nodes are enlarged by pyogranulomatous inflammation.

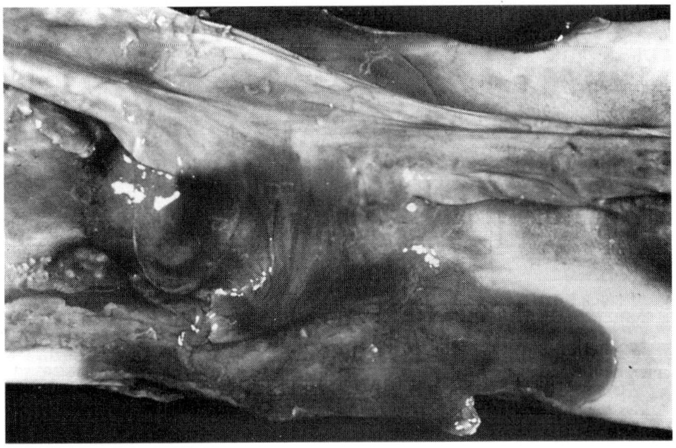

Figure 1-116 Small intestine, serosal surface; horse. Equine granulomatous enteritis. The serosal surface has irregular, thickened, dark red plaques of inflammatory tissue. *Courtesy Dr. D.J. Meuten.*

Equine Granulomatous Enteritis

This sporadic disease, characterized by wasting and hypoalbuminemia, has been reported most often in Thoroughbred and Standardbred horses younger than 5 years. The pathogenesis of the disease is unknown. In a few cases *Mycobacterium avium* was isolated from lesions. The disease is characterized by diffuse or segmental transmural noncaseating granulomatous inflammation of the small and occasionally large intestine. Giant cells are present in about half the cases. The result is a markedly thickened bowel (Figs. 1-116 to 1-119).

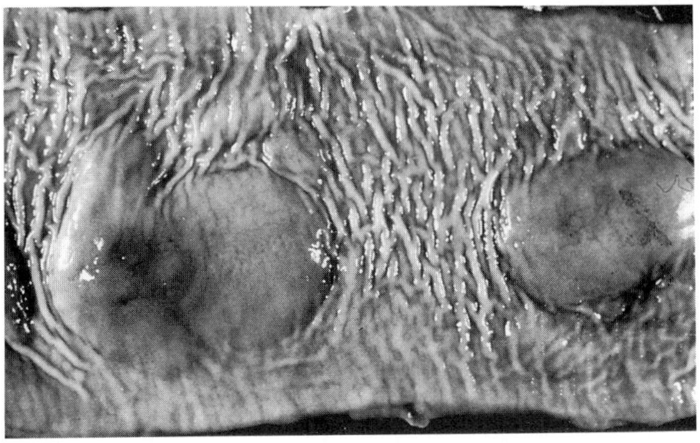

Figure 1-117 Small intestine; horse. Equine granulomatous enteritis. The lesions are firm gray or white. The left plaque has a central ulcer. *Courtesy Dr. D.J. Meuten.*

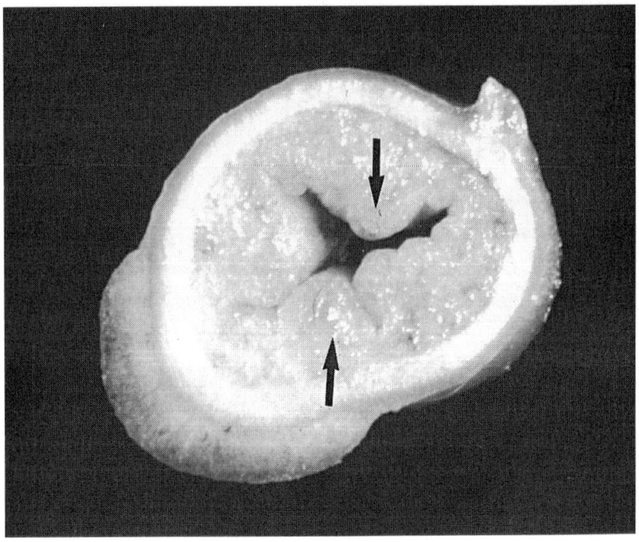

Figure 1-118 Small intestine; transverse section; horse. Equine granulomatous enteritis. The lamina propria *(arrows)* is greatly thickened by mononuclear inflammatory cells.

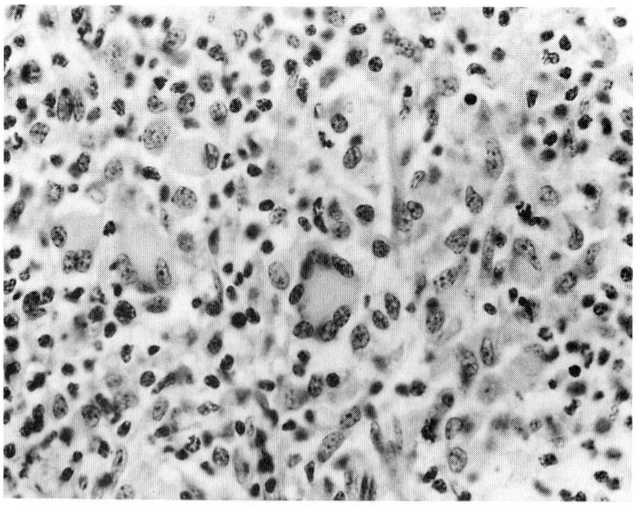

Figure 1-119 Intestine; horse. Equine granulomatous enteritis. A mixed cellular infiltrate of lymphocytes, plasma cells, macrophages, and giant cells are present in all layers of the intestine. *Meuten DJ, Butler DG, Thompson GW, Lumsden JH. J Am Vet Med Assoc 1978; 172:326-333.*

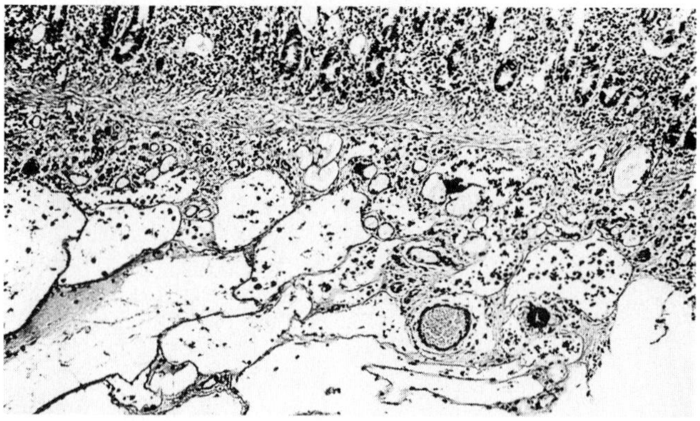

Figure 1-120 Colon; horse. Colitis X. There is loss of mucosal glands and an influx of neutrophils in the lamina propria. The submucosa is edematous. H & E stain.

Colitis X

The severe diarrhea seen in cases of colitis X contains no blood and is rapidly fatal. The etiology is unknown. However, the disease is associated with certain environmental and clinical variables. These include exhaustion shock or other stressors, enterotoxemia perhaps associated with overgrowth of *Clostridium perfringens* type A (antibiotic enteritis), or anaphylaxis. Lesions are limited to the mucosa of the cecum and colon and consist of edema, congestion, and hemorrhage (Fig. 1-120). The location and nature of these lesions overlap with those of acute enteric salmonellosis and Potomac horse fever. Therefore, elimination of *Salmonella* spp. and *Ehrlichia risticii* as causes is necessary before a diagnosis of colitis X can be made. Thus, colitis X is a diagnosis made by exclusion. At necropsy, in addition to the intestinal lesions, evidence of endotoxic shock such as disseminated intravascular coagulopathy, thrombosis, and hemorrhage of the adrenal cortices (Waterhouse-Friderichsen syndrome) can be present, as in salmonellosis.

Hemorrhagic Fibrinonecrotic Duodenitis–Proximal Jejunitis

Also known as anterior enteritis and gastroduodenojejunitis, the morphologic description of the lesions is the same as the name of this idiopathic disease. The disease is characterized microscopically by submucosal edema and a neutrophilic infiltrate of the submucosa and lamina propria. *Salmonella* and clostridial infections are suspected as the cause. This disease occurs in horses older than 9 years of age, and the definitive diagnosis is made at necropsy. The duodenum is always involved; jejunal involvement is variable.

Chronic Eosinophilic Gastroenteritis

Soft stools accompanied by weight loss characterize this uncommon condition in the horse. The inflammatory reaction consists of eosinophils among other inflammatory cells in both nodular and diffuse accumulations within all portions and layers of the gastrointestinal system and the mesenteric lymph nodes. The histology of the condition suggests a hypersensitivity reaction that in at least one instance was associated with *Pythium* spp. infection.

Anaphylactoid Purpura

Leukocytoclastic vasculitis associated with numerous discrete foci of necrosis and hemorrhage throughout the intestine, as well as in the mucosa of the larynx and skeletal muscles, is termed anaphylactoid purpura in the horse, and Henoch-Schönlein disease in human beings. Anecdotal evidence suggests an Arthus-like hypersensitivity reaction to a streptococcal respiratory infection.

INTESTINAL DISEASES OF CARNIVORES

Parvovirus Enteritis

Parvovirus enteritis of dogs and cats is a severe, usually fatal disease. Because the target cells are those that are rapidly dividing in the intestine, the crypt cells are principally affected. Initial virus replication occurs in lymphoid tissue. Although there is much overlap in the disease syndrome in dogs and cats, the dissimilarities warrant independent discussion of each species.

In the cat, mink, and raccoon, **panleukopenia,** cat distemper, feline enteritis, and mink enteritis are synonyms for this important disease. The clinical disease is characterized by dehydration, depression, and vomiting. Since the bone marrow is a rapidly dividing tissue, panleukopenia dominates the clinical pathologic findings.

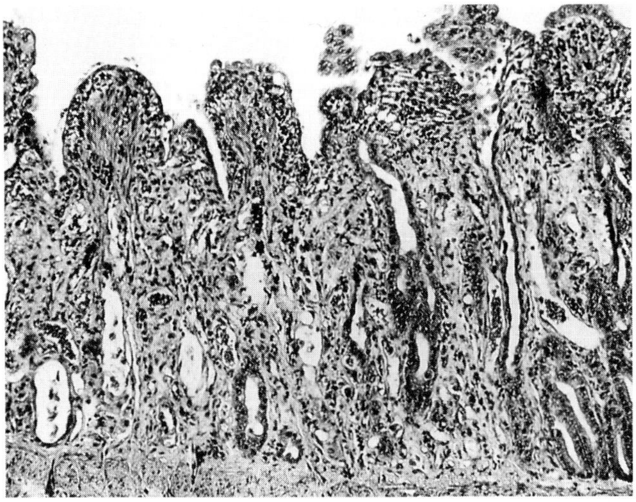

Figure 1-121 Small intestine; cat. Feline panleukopenia. Villi are denuded of epithelium. Some crypts are dilated. Note the squamoid epithelial cells in some crypts *(arrows)* and hyperplasia in others. H & E stain.

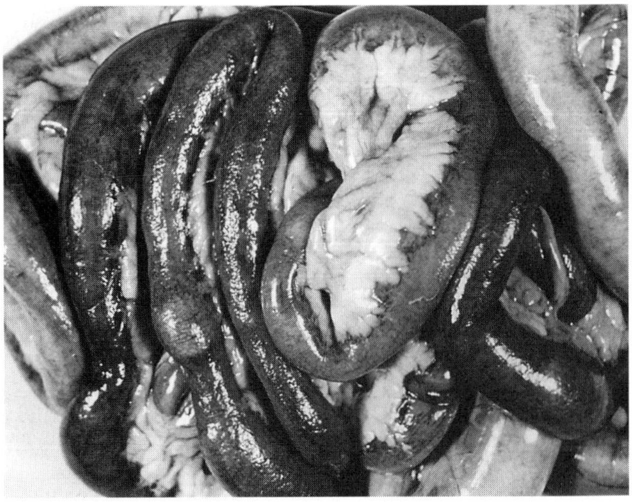

Figure 1-122 Small intestine; dog. Parvovirus enteritis. Affected segments of small intestine are diffusely reddened, and the serosa is faintly granular.

Early lesions in the course of the disease are lymphoid depletion and thymic involution. Later, lesions include flaccid, segmentally reddened intestine with serositis. Lesions are generally limited to the small intestine, but colitis occurs in some cats. Microscopically, villus atrophy occurs secondary to crypt cell destruction (Fig. 1-121). Basophilic intranuclear inclusion bodies are present in enterocytes and lymphocytes early in infection. In germ-free cats with a low enterocyte turnover, the disease caused by feline parvovirus is much less severe. Intrauterine infection causes congenital cerebellar hypoplasia of kittens. The virus, as described above, is cytolytic and infects dividing cells and thus alters the differentiation of layers in the cerebellum during organogenesis.

Canine parvovirus enteritis first appeared in Europe and the United States in 1978. The disease was initially recognized because of the gross and microscopic lesions that were identical to feline parvovirus enteritis. Panleukopenia vaccines were effective in preventing this disease in dogs and were used extensively until canine-specific parvovirus vaccines were developed. Rottweillers and Doberman pinschers, which are genetically related, are at increased risk for parvovirus disease, even if properly vaccinated.

Canine parvovirus disease initially was described as occurring in three distinct syndromes. Puppies younger than 2 weeks of age had generalized disease with focal areas of virus-induced necrosis in those tissues with rapidly dividing cells. Puppies 3 to 8 weeks of age would sometimes develop myocarditis for the same reason. Often initial infection would go undetected, and these animals would die unexpectedly up to 5 months later because of myocardial scarring and conduction failure. In puppies 8 weeks or older, the disease is identical to that in the cat. Cerebellar hypoplasia has not been induced in puppies.

At necropsy, the dilated, fluid-filled, flaccid small intestine is quite characteristic. The contents of the small intestine are brown to red-brown fluid and a fibrinous exudate, with or without hemorrhage. Mesenteric lymph nodes are enlarged and have a variegated red and white appearance. The bone marrow is semiliquid and yellow-gray.

Microscopically, the intestinal lesion is characterized by necrosis of crypt epithelial cells, with necrotic cell fragments in the crypts. Surviving epithelial cells become cuboidal or squamoid to cover the surface of the denuded crypt. After several days the epithelium over the villi is lost by normal extrusion as the crypts fail to supply replacement cells. Severe lesions consist of partially denuded small villi over a series of damaged crypts, some of which lack epithelial cells completely. Some crypts are lined by squamoid epithelial cells; others have a hyperplastic lining. Inclusion bodies are not present in lymphoid tissues. In bone marrow smears or sections, erythropoiesis appears normal but granulopoiesis is reduced. The colon has lesions as well, but these lesions are usually focal and less severe, and seldom receive much attention because of the more severe damage of the small intestine.

Dogs with the hemorrhagic form of parvovirus enteritis have bloody diarrhea and die a shocklike death within 24 hours. Canine parvovirus enteritis has many similarities to feline panleukopenia, and the sequence of tissue events is virtually the same. The gross lesion in the canine disease is a segmental or diffuse hemorrhagic enteritis. The affected segment is hyperemic, congested, and blood-filled (Fig. 1-122). It has not been possible to reproduce this form of the disease experimentally by giving canine parvovirus to young dogs. This lack of success in reproducing the disease suggests participation by another pathogen in those natural cases characterized by hemorrhagic diarrhea. The segmental vascular engorgement and mucosal hemorrhages are reminiscent of findings in *Clostridium perfringens* enterotoxemias. Coagulation necrosis of the lymphoid tissue of Peyer's patches and regional lymph nodes is present in canine parvovirus enteritis, but these lesions are not seen in panleukopenia. This latter change can be diagnostic, even when the intestinal mucosa has been effaced by autolysis.

Minute Virus of Canids

In addition to enteritis, canine parvovirus type 1 produces myocarditis and respiratory disease in young pups. The virus is widely distributed in the canine population but disease is only diagnosed sporadically. The virus is spread via the oronasal route. Fetal death and embryo absorption occur between 25 and 35 days of gestation. Microscopically, intestinal lesions consist of enterocyte hyperplasia with eosinophilic or amphophilic intranuclear inclusion bodies in cells of the intestinal villus tips. Crypt necrosis, characteristic of canine parvovirus type 2 infection is not present.

Inflammatory Bowel Disease

In dogs and cats this disease is microscopically determined to be a lymphoplasmacytic enteritis (Fig. 1-123). Diagnosis can be made by biopsy. Breeds with a predilection to this disease include the basenji and German shepherd. The cause is unknown, but the presence of numerous lymphocytes and plasma cells suggests an immune response problem. Malabsorption and chronic protein-losing enteropathy can be a result of the marked infiltrate of lymphocytes and plasmacytes in the lamina propria. In cats, but not dogs, dietary antigens cause some cases of inflammatory bowel disease; therefore, control of the disease can be achieved by regulation of the diet. Anecdotal evidence suggests that lymphocytic plasmacytic enteritis in the cat can be a prelude to intestinal lymphoma in some cases.

Histiocytic Ulcerative Colitis

Because of its occurrence in boxer dogs and the genetically related French bulldog, this disease has been called boxer colitis. It generally occurs in dogs younger than 2 years of age. Dogs can have soft feces, but often no diarrhea or weight loss are observed. In some cases, mucus and blood appear in the stool. The lesions, which are visible by proctoscopy, are raised ulcerative nodules (Fig. 1-124). Microscopically, the colon is ulcerated and has

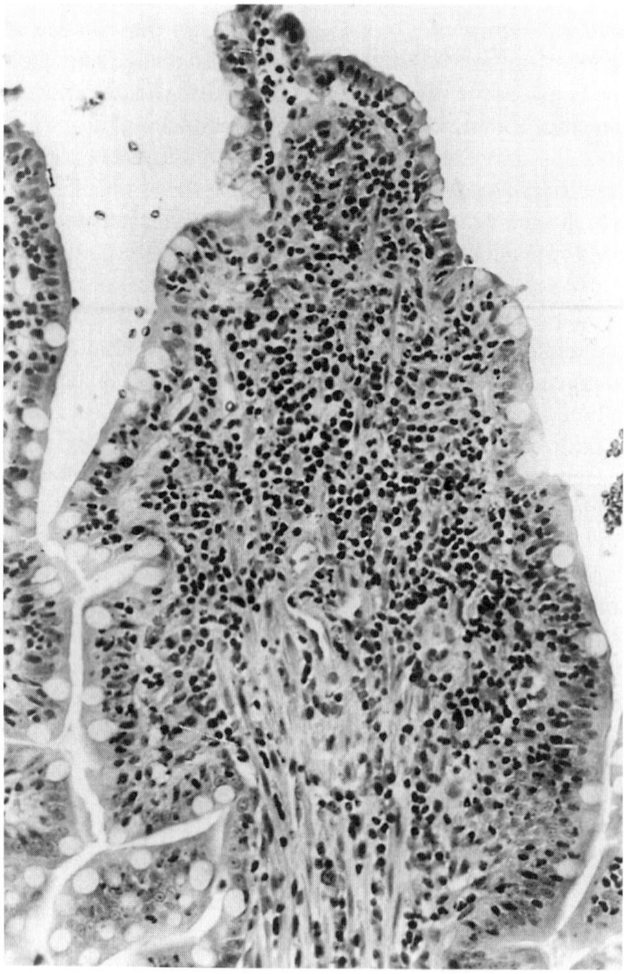

Figure 1-123 Intestine; dog. Lymphocytic plasmacytic enteritis. The lamina propria is infiltrated with lymphocytes and plasma cells. H & E stain.

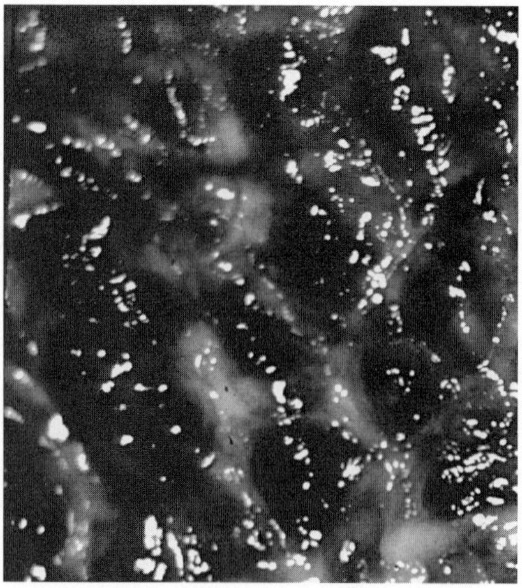

Figure 1-124 Colon; boxer dog. Histiocytic ulcerative colitis. There are numerous round and coalescing ulcers in the colon characteristic of this disease.

marked infiltration by macrophages containing PAS-positive material.

The earliest recognized lesion of histiocytic ulcerative colitis is the presence of large, foamy macrophages with abundant eosinophilic cytoplasm scattered in the basal lamina propria and superficial submucosa. In some dogs, lymphocytes and plasma cells of the mucosa are increased in number, but in most dogs the infiltrate is composed exclusively of macrophages. These cells apparently phagocytose bacteria to capacity and accumulate in numbers sufficient to distort the mucosa and submucosa. The colonic glands are obliterated by lateral compression or appear lifted from their basal attachments by a mantle of engorged macrophages in the basal lamina propria. In severe lesions the macrophages are 10 to 12 cells deep in the mucosa and 50 to 200 cells deep in the submucosa. The macrophages are 11 to 17 μm in diameter, are round to oval, and have abundant eosinophilic cytoplasm and prominent eccentric nuclei. The results of immunocytochemistry and electron microscopy studies have demonstrated that the macrophages in granulomatous colitis of boxer dogs are filled with *E. coli* antigen (Fig. 1-125).

Lymph nodes that drain the colon, cecum, or rectum and those that receive afferent lymphatics from colic lymph nodes are enlarged and have lymphoid hyperplasia. Macrophages aggregate in the cortex or medullary cords. In severely affected dogs, lymphadenopathy is generalized, and macrophages are found in many peripheral lymph nodes.

Feline Ulcerative Colitis

Feline ulcerative colitis is grossly and histologically analogous to its canine counterpart, histiocytic ulcerative colitis (Fig. 1-126). The causative agent is unknown.

Canine Histoplasmosis

Canine histoplasmosis occurs most often in the Ohio and Mississippi River valleys. This zoonotic systemic fungus can infect the intestine in some cases. The reservoir is believed to be soil and bird droppings. The organisms can be acquired by inhalation or by ingestion. The yeast invades tissue, causes necrosis, and replicates in macrophages, resulting in granulomatous lesions in the lungs, intestines, lymph nodes, liver, and other organs. Clinically, dogs with intestinal histoplasmosis suffer with intractable chronic diarrhea, progressive weight loss, anorexia, lassitude, poor hair coat, and anemia. Respiratory signs and peripheral lymphadenitis are present in some dogs. Pulmonary histoplasmosis is more common than the intestinal form. Grossly, the small intestine has a corrugated mucosa and ulcers. Mesenteric lymph nodes are enlarged and firm. The liver is enlarged and mottled. The lungs have areas of gray or red consolidation. The colonic wall is thickened, and colonic mucosal folds are prominent.

The lamina propria of the ileum and colon is thickened by macrophages containing the causative fungus, *Histoplasma capsulatum* (Fig. 1-127). The macrophages are unable to digest the phagocytosed fungi, and large numbers accumulate to cause corrugation of the mucosal surface. Extension of the inflammation occurs through the muscle layers and into lymph vessels and the subserosa. Regional lymph nodes have large masses of macrophages in the cortical and medullary sinuses. The liver has numerous clusters of yeast-filled macrophages.

Feline Infectious Peritonitis

Feline infectious peritonitis (FIP) is a uniformly fatal disease of cats. Although it affects cats of all ages, the disease is principally found in young and old cats. Twelve

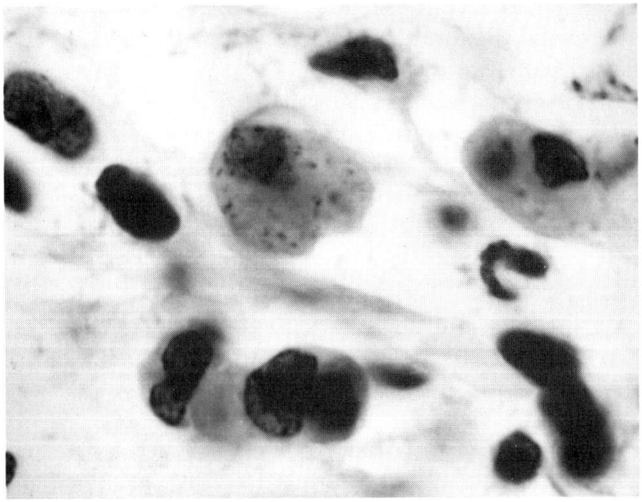

Figure 1-125 Colon; lamina propria; dog. Histiocytic ulcerative colitis. Some of the macrophages contain *E. coli*. Brown and Brenn (Gram) stain.

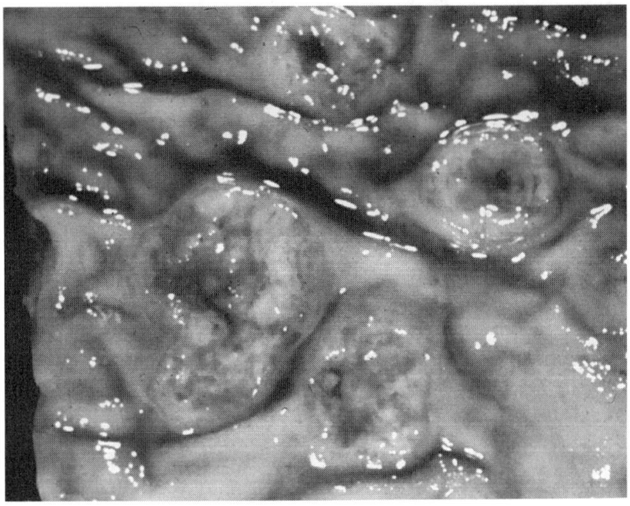

Figure 1-126 Colon; cat. Feline ulcerative colitis. There are numerous round ulcers in the mucosa.

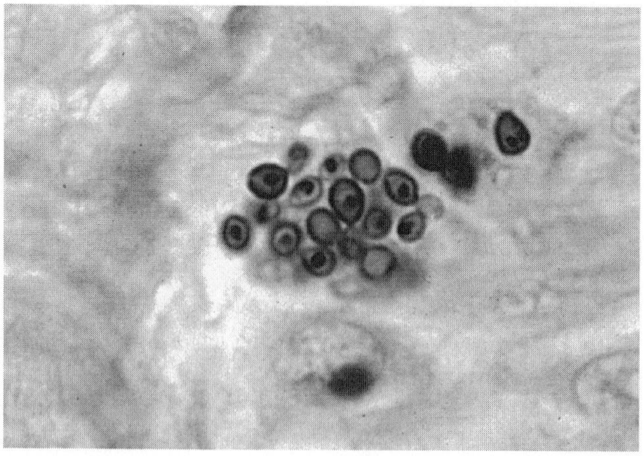

Figure 1-127 Intestine; lamina propria; dog. Histoplasmosis. Clusters of 3 to 5 μm *H. capsulatum* organisms with a central nucleoid are located within macrophages. Grocott Methanamine Silver stain.

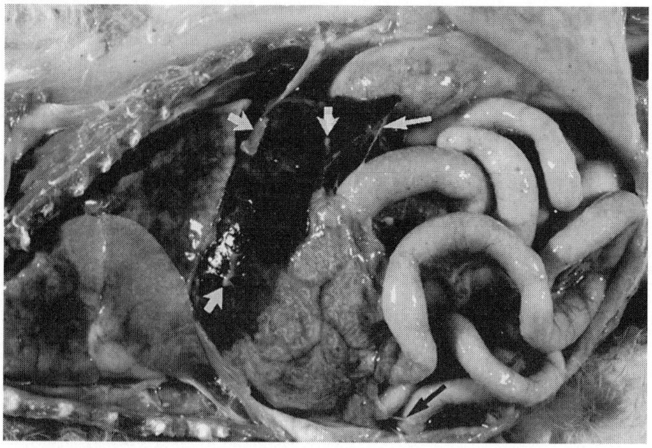

Figure 1-128 Abdomen; cat. Fibrinous polyserositis. Fibrin strands *(long arrows)* between viscera and mats of fibrin *(short arrows)* on organ surfaces are characteristic of the "wet form" of feline infectious peritonitis. Note the small nodules (pyogranulomas) (right) on the intestinal serosa.

percent of feline deaths are associated with FIP. The cause of the disease is a coronavirus that forms immune complexes that localize in the vasculature. Lesions are thus multifocal and most organs have lesions. The "wet form" of the disease is characterized by fibrinous polyserositis; the "dry form" is without the effusive process. Why one form develops rather than the other is not completely understood but may relate to the major type of immune effector cell. The disease often clusters in households, and virus spreads among cats by saliva on shared utensils or by mutation of an endogenous coronavirus.

An immune component to FIP is suggested by the observations that the disease occurs more rapidly and lesions are more severe in seropositive cats than in seronegative ones. In the presence of a strong immune response, phlebitis, thrombophlebitis, and thrombosis occur in several organ systems, including the intestine. Thus the disease is essentially an immune-mediated vasculitis with necrosis and pyogranulomas that occur secondary to vascular deposition of immune complexes. Pyogranulomatous lesions can occur anywhere, including the lungs, central nervous system, eyeballs, kidneys, liver, or visceral lymph nodes.

The "wet form" of FIP is characterized by large volumes of thick, yellow peritoneal transudate that contains flecks or strands of fibrin and by multiple granular, glistening vasocentric granulomas on the serosa of abdominal viscera (Fig. 1-128). The granulomas are translucent and less than 2 mm in diameter. The "dry form" of the disease, on the other hand, consists of vasocentric, firm, gray to white masses. These sometimes occur as 1 to 2 cm nodules in the kidneys. The localized "dry form" of FIP causes segmental granulomatous disease of the ileum, cecum, or colon. The affected bowel wall is thickened, firm, and fibrotic, and the lumen is stenotic. The granulomatous ileal or colonic lesions have insidious and progressive clinical effects on the cat. Signs include unthriftiness, weight loss, constipation, obstipation, vomiting, and palpable abdominal masses. Lesions caused by the dry form of FIP in the kidney and intestine must be differentiated from lymphosarcoma. Impression smears, aspirates, or biopsies can be diagnostic.

The microscopic lesions of colonic granulomatous FIP occur segmentally, originate in the submucosa or subserosa, and extend transmurally to the mucosa or along vascular channels through the tunica muscularis. The deeper layers of the colon are thickened by multifocal granulomas, accompanied by an intense mononuclear infiltration. Fibroplasia, lymphangiectasia, edema, and muscular hypertrophy are sequelae that contribute to the mural thickening. Mucosal glandular architecture is mostly preserved, although focally or segmentally the lamina propria contains excessive mononuclear cells. Focally, granulomatous nodules of the submucosa are confluent with areas of intense mononuclear reaction in the mucosa, with concomitant disruption of glandular architecture and occasional crypt abscesses.

The submucosal and subserosal granulomas are of three types. Some of the granulomas are composed of whorled, small, stellate or pleomorphic histiocytes with a few necrotic cell fragments at the center; others consist of whorled histiocytes surrounding lymphoid aggregates; and a third type has whorled histiocytes around a central microabscess (Fig. 1-129).

Canine Multifocal Eosinophilic Gastroenteritis

Canine multifocal eosinophilic gastroenteritis is a disease of young dogs, usually younger than 4 years of age, caused

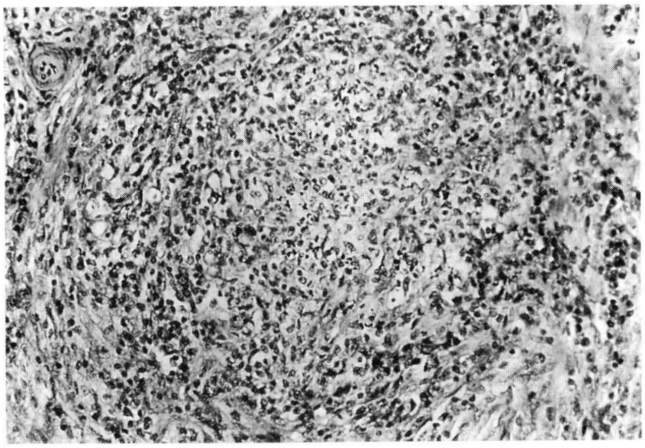

Figure 1-129 Colon; subserosa; cat. Feline infectious peritonitis. The central zone is formed by macrophages with a few granulocytes. H & E stain.

by migrating larvae of the ascarid, *Toxocara canis*. The incidence of this disease is low. The disease often originates in kennels that have less than satisfactory hygiene and parasite control. Clinically, chronic diarrhea, moderate weight loss, intermittent or persistent eosinophilia, and elevated serum β-globulin concentrations characterize this disorder. Serum albumin concentration, absorption tests, and small bowel contrast radiographs usually are normal.

T. canis larvae enter by the oral route, invade the mucosa of the stomach and small intestine, and then become trapped and localized by the inflammation they induce. Adult bitches often harbor significant larval parasite burdens in their tissues. Larvae migrate into the uterus and fetuses during late pregnancy. Shortly after birth, presumably in response to hormonal stimuli, larvae are directed to the mammary gland, where they are secreted in the milk of the bitch. Ascarid larvae also can be acquired from fecal contamination of the teats or the kennel environment. Larvae that are ingested by these puppies usually transit the mucosa of the stomach and small intestine and travel via intestinal lymph vessels or the portal vein to the liver and then to the lungs. Here they develop into third-stage larvae, which are then coughed up and swallowed. In the gastrointestinal tract, these larvae mature to adult roundworms. In the great majority of exposed dogs, ascarid larvae pass through tissues and complete the life cycle in several weeks, or the larvae are trapped and killed by granuloma formation, which results in necrosis of the parasite and calcification. Dogs that have developed multifocal eosinophilic gastroenteritis have *T. canis* larvae trapped in the gastrointestinal wall by an immune reaction and are surrounded by eosinophils, but still appear viable. These ascarid larvae can remain trapped and viable in the wall of the stomach and small intestine for as long as 4 years. Waste products of the parasites are chemotactic for eosinophils. The multifocal aggregates of eosinophils occur along pathways traveled by ascarid larvae and are found in the mucosa and submucosa of the stomach and small intestine, in the mesenteric lymph nodes, in the connective tissue of the pancreas, in the portal areas of the liver, and in the kidneys and lungs.

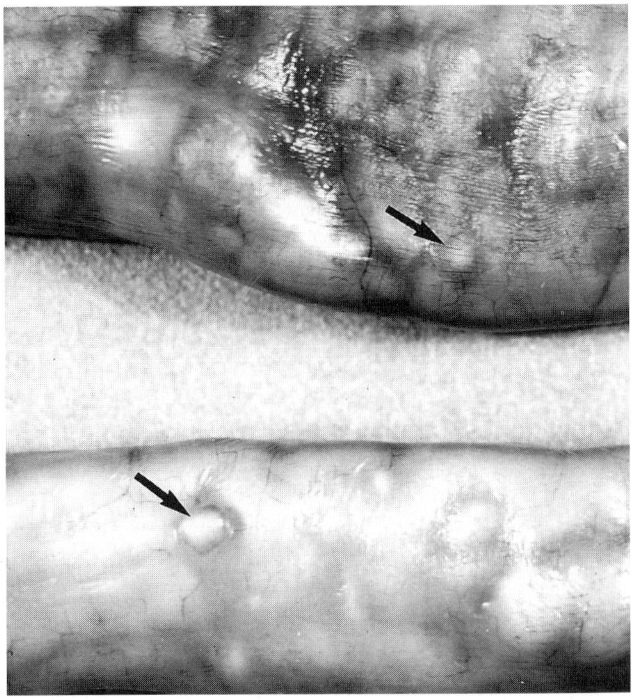

Figure 1-130 Jejunum; serosal surface; dog. Multifocal eosinophilic gastroenteritis (visceral larva migrans). Multiple intramural nodules *(arrows)*. *Courtesy Dr. D.W. Hayden.*

Focal eosinophilic lesions that occur in this disease are 1 to 4 mm in diameter and some are grossly visible (Fig. 1-130). In some dogs, as many as 40 to 80 white, firm nodules, the size of a pinhead, can be observed in the intestine from the serosa. Few nodules occur in the wall of the stomach and in the colon. Regional lymph nodes can be slightly enlarged and variegated, or they might contain grossly visible, 4- to 5-mm diameter, white nodules. Gross lesions occur in the renal cortex and are scattered throughout the pancreas, liver, and subpleurally. Microscopically, most of the lesions are composed of eosinophils; some lesions have plasma cells and macrophages, and some of the lesions are granulomas. Ascarid larvae can often be demonstrated in these aggregates. The larvae are surrounded by an eosinophilic, amorphous, fringed material, which stains PAS positive (the Splendore-Hoeppli phenomenon). The multifocal nature and size of these lesions produce little deformity to the mucosal surface.

Diffuse Eosinophilic Gastroenteritis

Although this type of eosinophilic gastroenteritis has a predilection for the German shepherd breed, it occurs in other breeds of dogs and in cats. It is characterized by recurrent episodes of diarrhea associated with tissue and circulating eosinophilia. The increased concentration of eosinophils in the circulation as well as within lesions suggests a hypersensitivity reaction to some ingested substance or to parasites. The cause has not been identified. There are no gross lesions. Histologically, eosinophils heavily infiltrate all layers of the stomach and intestine.

Proliferative Enteritis

This zoonotic condition occurs in all species of mammals. It is characterized by segmental proliferation of the intestinal epithelium of the ileum and large intestine. Causation is related to *Campylobacter* spp. infection. Diagnosis depends on characteristic histopathologic findings and demonstrating comma-shaped bacteria in the intestinal crypt epithelial cytoplasm. In the dog at least, the majority of cases occur in puppies younger than 3 months old. Clinically, diarrhea is of 5 to 15 days' duration. The diarrhea is mucus laden or watery, with or without blood, and accompanied by partial anorexia, vomiting, and slight fever.

Wheat-Sensitive Enteropathy of Irish Setters

This hereditary condition, similar to gluten-sensitive enteropathy of human beings, is the first described dietary-induced enteropathy of dogs. It is characterized initially by increased numbers of intraepithelial lymphocytes and goblet cells and later by partial villus atrophy, particularly of the jejunum.

Salmon Poisoning

Salmon poisoning is an acute granulomatous enterocolitis of the dog and fox. Animals that eat salmon carrying the fluke *Nanophyetus salmincola* are affected. This small trematode is the bearer of *Neorickettsia helminthoeca*, a 0.3 μm, coccoid rickettsia. Six to eight days after eating parasitized fish, dogs become acutely ill, febrile, and depressed. Affected animals have ocular and nasal discharge, severe diarrhea, vomiting, complete anorexia, and enlarged tonsils, spleen, and lymph nodes. Untreated animals die within 6 to 10 days of the onset of signs. Hemorrhagic inflammation of the wall of the intestine that can extend from the pylorus to the anus is the most characteristic gross lesion of salmon poisoning. The primary lesions are in the lamina propria and submucosa of the intestine and consist of hemorrhage, necrosis, and infiltrates of lymphocytes, plasma cells, macrophages, and neutrophils. The macrophages contain large numbers of rickettsial elementary bodies that can be demonstrated by using the Giemsa stain. Peyer's patches and solitary lymphoid follicles of the intestine are hyperplastic, as are the mesenteric, colic, portal, and iliac lymph nodes (Fig. 1-131). Lymphoid hyperplasia is characterized by enlarged cortical nodules and sinuses filled with neutrophils and macrophages. Peripheral lymph nodes are affected, but less severely than the regional nodes of the intestine. The characteristic macrophages containing Giemsa-stained elementary bodies occur in peripheral lymph nodes, spleen, liver, lungs, and blood cells, and in intracerebral lesions.

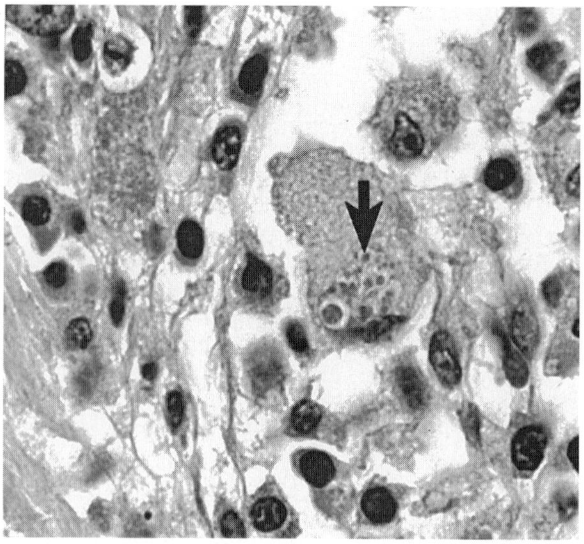

Figure 1-131 Lymph node; dog. Salmon poisoning. Macrophages contain elementary bodies *(arrow)*. H & E stain.

Canine Mucosal Colitis

Canine mucosal colitis occurs infrequently. It is recognized sporadically in such breeds as the Belgian Tervuren, dachshund, German shepherd dog, old English sheepdog, and collie. Adult dogs, 3 to 6 years of age, are affected, and males appear to be disproportionately affected. The cause of mucosal colitis is unknown. The character of the lesions indicates that an inciting agent damages colonic epithelium, and, subsequently, the lesion is perpetuated by continued presence of an antigen, the microbiologic flora, or immunologic events.

Dogs with mucosal colitis are usually afebrile, have chronic diarrhea, and pass fresh blood. There may not be weight loss. If the colitis is severe, however, secondary effects contribute to ill health and anorexia, and weight loss occurs. Tenesmus is a prominent clinical feature if the rectum is affected. Granulocytes can be demonstrated in the feces in some cases of mucosal colitis.

The gross lesions of the colon include hyperemia, granularity, friability, and multifocal mucosal ulceration. In some cases of canine mucosal colitis, the lesions have a diffuse distribution affecting the entire colon and rectum; whereas in other cases the lesions are segmental. Microscopic lesions of the colonic epithelial cells include degeneration and necrosis. Necrosis and resultant inflammatory debris occur in one, several, or many colonic

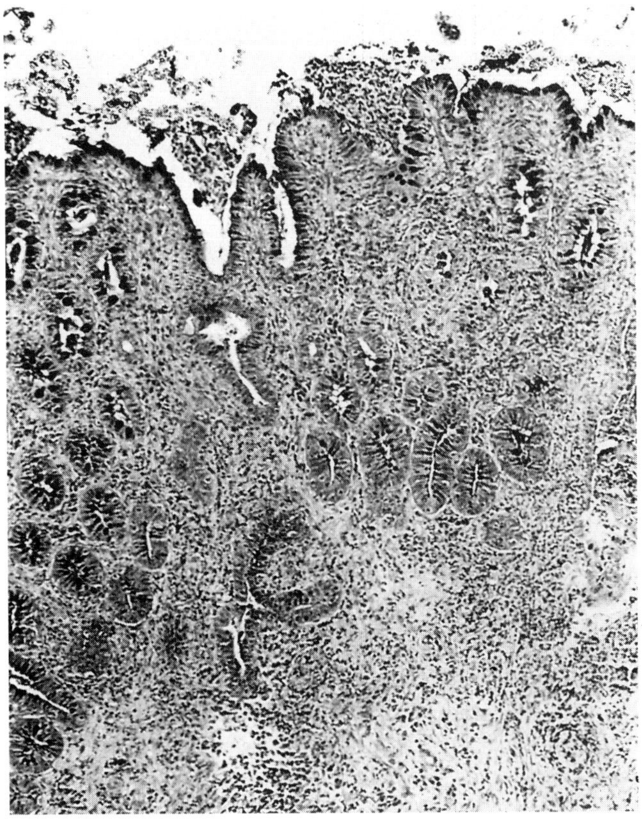

Figure 1-132 Colon; dog. Mucosal colitis. The colonic surface is irregular. Granulocytes occupy the crypts. Mucus glands are hyperplastic and surrounded by an acute inflammatory cell infiltrate. PAS stain.

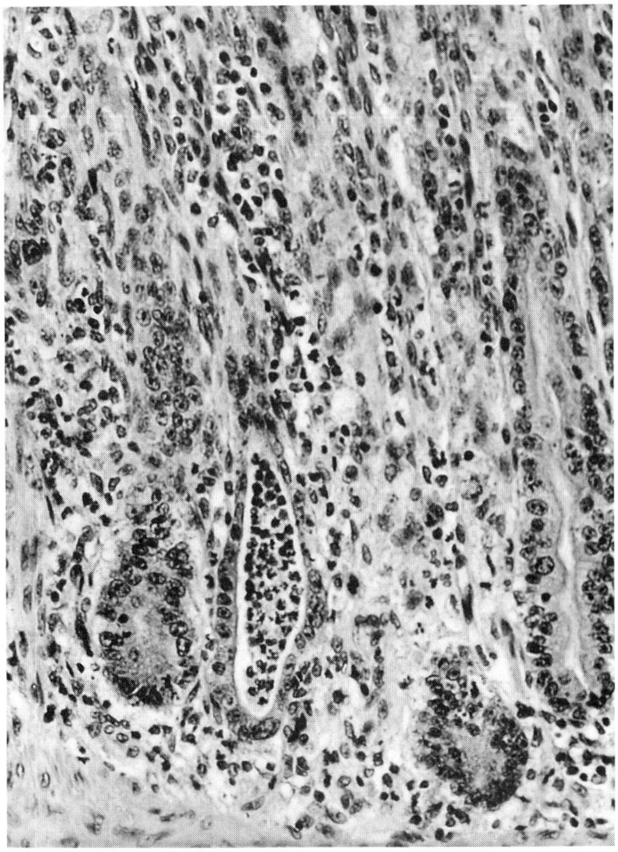

Figure 1-133 Colon; marmoset. Colitis. The area between colonic crypts is infiltrated by mononuclear leukocytes; one crypt contains an abscess. H & E stain.

crypts. Granulocytes are attracted into the colonic crypts and migrate onto the luminal surface (Fig. 1-132). A variety of inflammatory cells infiltrate the lamina propria between the crypts. The epithelium often undergoes regenerative hyperplasia (Fig. 1-133).

Other mucosal changes include congestion and hemorrhages in the lamina propria, increased numbers of lymphocytes and plasma cells in the lamina propria, and hyperplastic regenerative down growths of epithelium into the lymphoid follicles of the submucosa. Ulcers occur and are round, stellate, or serpiginous and coated with fibrinopurulent tags. The ulcers can coalesce, crisscross one another, and isolate islands of healthy mucosa. Eosinophils often comprise a moderate part of the inflammatory cell infiltrate in canine mucosal colitis, and increased numbers of mast cells occur in these areas as well. These forms of colitis are limited to the mucosa and superficial portions of the submucosa.

PARASITIC ENTERITIDES

Parasites of the intestinal tract are legion in the various domestic animal species. Refer to a parasitology textbook for specific information regarding the life cycles and identification of the various species. Diagnosis of enteric parasitism is generally performed via fecal flotation or intestinal scrapings.

Amebiasis

Amebiasis is an acute or chronic disease caused by the single-cell protozoan *Entamoeba histolytica*. Dogs, nonhuman primates, and human beings develop colitis and amebic abscesses. *E. histolytica* is found in intestinal contents; the trophozoites are transparent; contain an eccentric nucleus and, sometimes, erythrocytes; are three to five times the diameter of erythrocytes; and have an ameboid movement. Trophozoa parasitize intestinal mucosa; under unfavorable circumstances, the trophozoites encyst. The cysts, infectious forms of the agent, survive outside the body for as long as 10 days. A cyst ingested with feed or water undergoes cell division, which results in eight trophozoites that are liberated into the lumen of the intestine.

Amebae invade intact mucosa by means of lysozymes liberated at their surface. With continued cellular destruction, a punctiform ulcer with characteristic undermined edges is formed. Eventually, a flask-shaped ulcer extends into the submucosa and, sometimes, into the muscle layers. In the mucosa, the amebae create a colony, but do not stimulate an inflammatory response. Ulcers are covered by a small amount of yellow, fibrinopurulent exudate or have an exposed and bleeding surface. Amebae that enter the portal circulation become disseminated systemically. The organ most often secondarily infected is the liver, and it has amebic abscesses or granulomas.

Clinically, abdominal pain, intermittent diarrhea, anorexia, and malaise characterize amebiasis. These signs may wax and wane for weeks or months. Diarrhea is the most common feature, and the feces often contain blood and mucus. If the parasites have extended into the rectum, tenesmus is observed.

Grossly, the affected colon has numerous, randomly scattered punctate ulcers, varying from pinhead to 2 cm in diameter. In severe cases with greater denudation of the surface, pseudomembranes form.

Microscopically, punctiform ulcers with colonies of unicellular protozoa are diagnostic. Amebae are numerous in these areas and are accompanied by eosinophils or granuloma formation. In some individuals a mild lymphocytic-plasmacytic cell infiltrate is present. The protozoa are recognizable in H & E–stained sections, but they are more readily evaluated in Giemsa-stained sections.

Coccidiosis

Coccidia are exquisitely host- and tissue-specific protozoa. They are obligate intracellular pathogens. Lesions vary from proliferative in sheep and goats, to hemorrhagic in dogs, cats, and cattle. In pigs, a fibrinonecrotic pseudomembrane without blood in 5- to 7-day-old animals is characteristic of enteric coccidiosis. Most species of *Eimeria* and *Isospora* infect villus or crypt epithelial cells; some species reside in the endothelium of lacteals; other species occur in the lamina propria; and, on occasion, some organisms reach the regional lymph nodes. The coccidia undergo one or more asexual reproductive cycles, with the resulting sporozoites producing schizonts that contain from few to thousands of merozoites. The latter emerge and penetrate other cells.

Within the sexual cycle, merozoites yield gamonts that differentiate into microgametes and macrogametes; the microgametes fertilize the macrogametes to yield zygotes, which develop into oocysts. When a small number of coccidia parasitize the intestine of otherwise healthy young growing animals, little disease results. However, when animals are in crowded conditions and poor sanitation, fecal-oral transmission of large numbers of organisms can occur. Where such transmission is accompanied by feeding a marginally deficient diet or if concomitant parasitism is present, significant clinical disease can occur. With each cycle, sexual and asexual, epithelial cell lysis occurs; total damage is proportional to the environmentally acquired dose of oocysts and the numbers of various stages generated endogenously. Young animals are most susceptible.

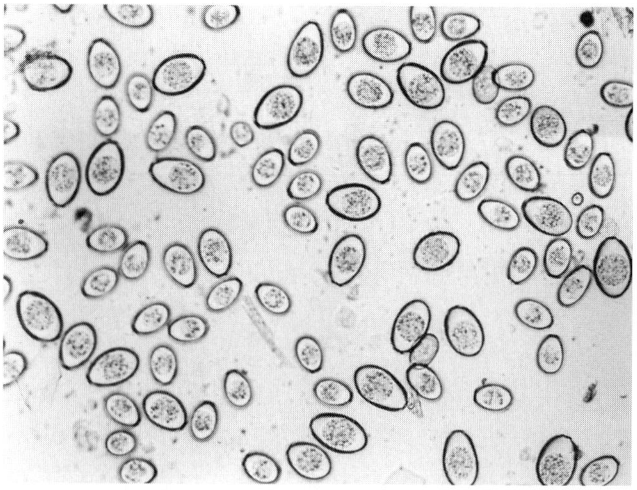

Figure 1-134 Feces; goat. Coccidiosis. Oocysts of *Eimeria* spp. are abundant in this fecal preparation.

Clinically, unthriftiness and diarrhea characterize coccidiosis. When the large intestine is infected, streaks of red blood color the feces, and the animal can have tenesmus. Diagnosis is made by demonstrating oocysts in the feces; the size and internal features enable species to be identified (Fig. 1-134).

The gross lesions of coccidiosis are variable hyperemia and fluid distension of affected intestinal segments, often caudal small intestine and/or cecum and colon. If the infecting *Eimeria* generate large schizonts, 300 μm in size, pinpoint white foci are visible from both serosal and mucosal surfaces. The mucosa could appear normal, be raised in convoluted hyperplastic patches, or be variably eroded, with or without a fibrinonecrotic pseudomembrane. Erosion and fissuring of the mucosa of the large intestine can be accompanied by bleeding. The severity of the hyperemia, segmental demarcation, and surface bleeding vary considerably among coccidial species.

Microscopically, coccidiosis is characterized by necrosis of villus or crypt epithelium, hyperemia, and a moderate inflammatory response in the lamina propria. The infiltrate usually consists of lymphocytes and plasma cells but, sometimes, eosinophils are numerous. Globule leukocytes increase in number. The loss of epithelial cells results in villus atrophy, collapse of the mucosa, or pseudomembrane formation. In some chronic infections, particularly of sheep and goats, the epithelium is hyperplastic, and this proliferation produces an adenomatous mucosal surface. The coccidia are readily recognized

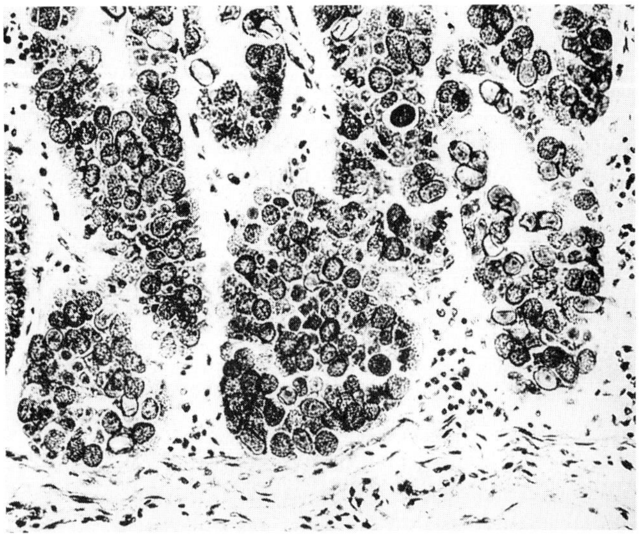

Figure 1-135 Intestine; goat. Coccidiosis. Virtually every epithelial cell contains a stage of the life cycle of *Eimeria* spp. H & E stain.

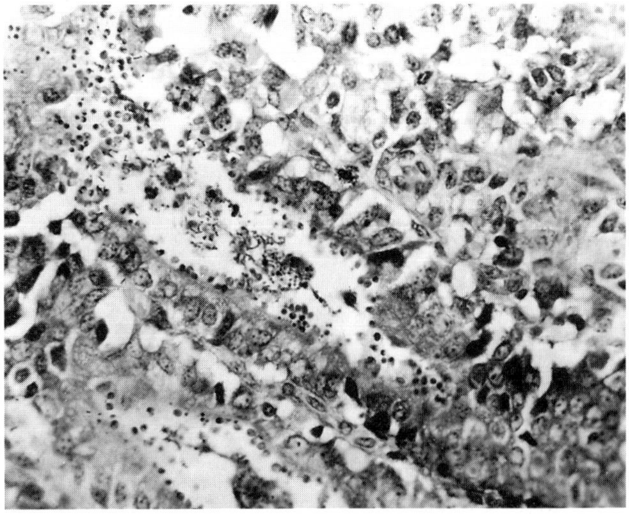

Figure 1-136 Small intestine; calf. Cryptosporidiosis. Numerous dot and ring forms are attached to the villus surface epithelium. Wolbach-Giemsa stain. *Courtesy Dr. D.J. Meuten.*

(Fig. 1-135). The schizonts are oval and filled with basophilic, banana-shaped merozoites; oocysts are oval and have refractile walls; macrogametes are large cells with refractile, eosinophilic, red "plastic granules"; and gamonts are round to oval with uniformly eosinophilic staining and a dotlike nucleus.

Cryptosporidiosis

Cryptosporidium parvum is a ubiquitous zoonotic protozoan pathogen of mammals. Often waterborne, it is a significant cause of municipal water contamination. Although it causes a self-limiting infection in immunocompetent animals, the very young or other immunocompromised individuals, such as AIDS patients, suffer from intractable diarrhea. Veterinarians and veterinary students are at particular risk for infection when treating bovine patients. The parasite lives in a unique environment described as intracellular but extracytoplasmic. Cryptosporidia attach to surface epithelial cells of the stomach, small intestine, or colon (Fig. 1-136). The protozoa attach to the epithelial cells, displace the microvilli (Fig. 1-137), and are enclosed by surface cell membranes. Microgametes, macrogametes, schizonts, trophozoites, meronts, merozoites and oocysts can be demonstrated in the intestine adjacent to or attached to epithelial cells. Oocysts are 4 to 5 μm in diameter and are shed in the feces (Fig. 1-138).

In fecal smears stained by the Giemsa method, the oocysts contain two to five dense red granules in a blue to blue-green cytoplasm. Oocysts can also be identified by Sheather's sucrose flotation and a modified acid-fast stain. Cryptosporidiosis causes subacute or chronic watery diarrhea, sometimes tinged with blood, with an associated dehydration, loss of electrolytes, and, subsequently, weakness. Although the disease can be fatal, particularly in

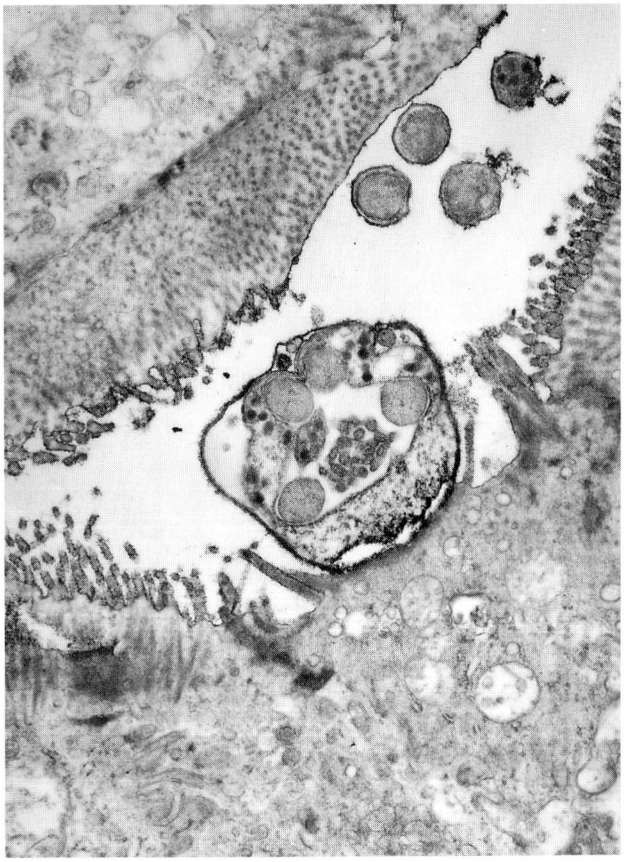

Figure 1-137 Small intestine; electron micrograph; calf. Cryptosporidiosis. Microvilli have disappeared at the site of attachment of the cryptosporidium. *Courtesy Dr. D.J. Meuten.*

the presence of other pathogens, it is often self-limiting in immunocompetent individuals, with the illness abating spontaneously in 6 to 8 days. Grossly, affected portions of the gastrointestinal tract are diffusely reddened and have fluid contents. Microscopically, in H & E–stained sections, the small organisms appear as tiny blue (hematoxylinophilic) dots attached to the epithelial cells of affected segments. In addition to the dot forms, ring- and banana-shaped organisms are readily seen in Giemsa-stained sections. The lesions of enteritis or colitis consist of decreased mucosal height, irregular mucosal thickness, crypt necrosis, hyperemia, and an increase in lymphocytes and plasma cells in the lamina propria. Villus atrophy and fusion of the small intestine is the end result.

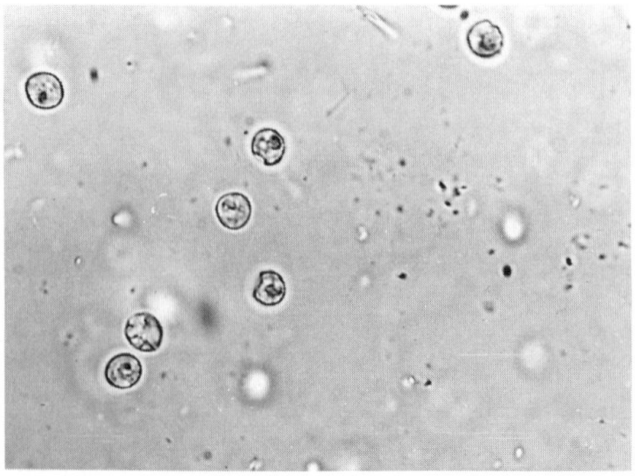

Figure 1-138 Feces; human being. Cryptosporidiosis. *Cryptosporidium parvum* oocysts, 4 to 5 μm in diameter, demonstrated in a sugar flotation medium (specific gravity 1.27). ×1280. *Anderson BC, Donndelinger T, Wilkins RM, Smith J. J Am Vet Med Assoc 1982; 180:408-409.*

Giardiasis

Giardiasis occurs in many species, including human beings, dogs, cats, horses, cattle, rabbits, guinea pigs, hamsters, rats, mice, chinchillas, and parakeets. In clinical veterinary medicine, giardiasis is frequently recognized in puppies and kittens. Giardiasis is caused by a unicellular flagellated protozoan. The pear-shaped organism has posterior flagella, a ventral sucker, and four nuclei, two of which resemble eyes (Fig. 1-139). *Giardia lamblia* inhabits the small intestine, particularly the duodenum, where the organisms attach to the microvillus border of epithelial cells producing membrane damage. When *Giardia* organisms are present in small numbers, they produce no clinical illness. However, when present in great numbers or in an immunologically deficient individual, diarrhea occurs.

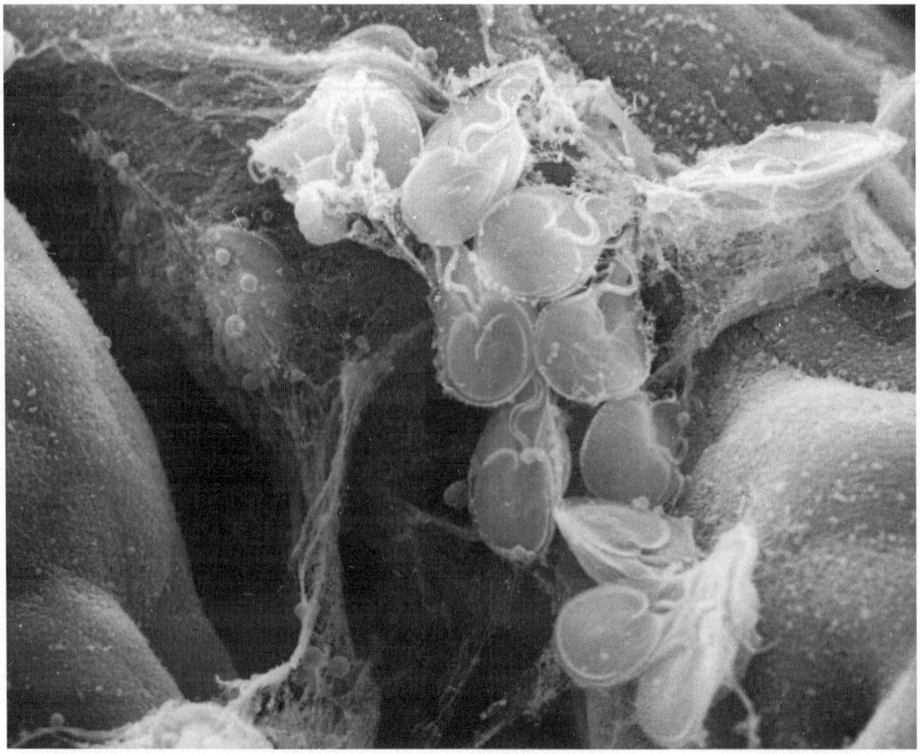

Figure 1-139 Small intestine; human being. Scanning electron micrograph. Giardiasis. *Giardia* trophozoites (round bodies) are attached to the surface of villus epithelium. *Poley JR, Rosenfield, S. J Pediatr Gastroenterol Nutr 1982; 1:63-80.*

In large numbers the parasites decrease the absorption of simple sugars and disaccharides, which are then fermented by bacterial flora, creating intestinal gas. The sugars also have an osmotic effect and draw water into the lumen. The result is distension of the small intestine with fluid and gas. Clinically, animals with giardiasis have brown, fluid diarrhea, signs of abdominal discomfort without fever, weight loss, melena, or steatorrhea. The diagnosis is made by demonstrating *Giardia* in preparations of fresh feces. Diagnosis in histologic sections is made by searching the periphery of duodenal and jejunal villi, as the organisms are seen attached to villus epithelial cells and sometimes are free between villi. In H & E–stained tissue sections the parasites are pear shaped with flagella. They are more readily seen in Giemsa-stained sections.

Ascariasis

Ascarids are long, smooth, white nematodes that vary in length from 3 to 4 cm in small animals up to 40 to 50 cm in pigs and horses. They reside in the upper small intestine. Common species include *Ascaris suum* of pigs, *Parascaris equorum* of horses, *Toxocara canis* of dogs, *Toxocara cati* of cats, and *Toxocara lumbricoides* of human beings. Young animals acquire ascarids by one of several routes. Intrauterine transmission of larvae occurs during the last 7 to 10 days of gestation. Larvae can be transmitted via the milk of the dam, and, later in life, embryonated eggs are ingested as a consequence of fecal contamination of the mammary gland, through feed, or via coprophagy. Transmission can also occur via paretenic hosts. Infective larvae penetrate the intestine and migrate to the liver via the portal circulation. From the liver, the larvae travel via the caudal vena cava to the lungs, where they break out of alveolar capillaries into the alveoli, undergo development, and migrate up the trachea or are coughed up, swallowed, and pass to the intestine for development to adults. Ova are passed in the feces.

Toxascaris leonina, another ascarid of dogs, is transmitted via ingestion and through an intermediate host; hepatopulmonary migration does not occur. The larvae of ascarids produce eosinophilic gastroenteritis when trapped in the submucosa of the stomach or intestine; they are responsible for eosinophilic granulomas of mesenteric lymph nodes, kidneys, and, rarely, the retina or other tissues. Larvae produce tracts, granulomas, and portal inflammatory infiltrates that contain abundant eosinophils, as well as focal fibrosis in the liver. The larvae also cause focal hemorrhages, infiltrates of eosinophils, and granulomas of the lungs. In aberrant hosts, the larvae appear to wander with less direction, often producing larval migration tracts (necrosis) in the brain, ocular granulomas, visceral larva migrans, and acute interstitial pneumonia. Adult ascarids apparently produce clinical disease by their physical presence and by inducing moderate malabsorption. Affected animals have less-than-normal weight gains, lassitude, pendulous abdomen, partial anorexia, and intermittent vomiting or diarrhea. Coughing and labored respiration called "thumping" are signs of pulmonary larva migrans. Eosinophilia occurs during the larval migration.

Adult ascarids are readily observed in the upper small intestine at necropsy (Fig. 1-140). They produce no gross lesions other than an occasional perforation or intussusception, but large masses can occlude the lumen. Sometimes, the ascarids find their way into the bile duct or pancreas, where they can cause obstruction and inflammation. Microscopically, parasites in the lumen of the intestine produce no lesions and do not increase the numbers of mucosal eosinophils or globule leukocytes. Some pigs with ascariasis develop hypertrophy of the intestinal tunica muscularis.

Hookworm Disease

Hookworms are short, stocky worms, 1 to 1.5 cm long, that inhabit the proximal small intestine of a number of animal species. Some of the common species include *Ancylostoma caninum* and *Uncinaria stenocephala* of dogs, *Bunostomum* spp. of ruminants, and *Ancylostoma duodenale* and *Necator americanus* of human beings. The canine hookworm, *A. caninum,* is transmissible to human beings, causing eosinophilic enteritis and obscure abdominal pain. Hookworm eggs, discharged from females living in the small intestine, are passed in the feces. Under satisfactory environmental conditions, development outside the host progresses to third-stage infective larvae that enter the host by cutaneous penetration or by ingestion. Depending on species and portal of entry, the larvae move directly to the small intestine, or they follow a transpulmonary route. Development continues through fourth- and fifth-stage larvae to adults that attach to the intestinal mucosa. Larvae of the canine hookworm, *A. caninum,* are transmitted in utero and via mammary secretion. These routes of transmission are responsible for the unusual occurrence of hookworm larvae in premature or stillborn puppies and the presence of hookworm eggs in the feces of puppies.

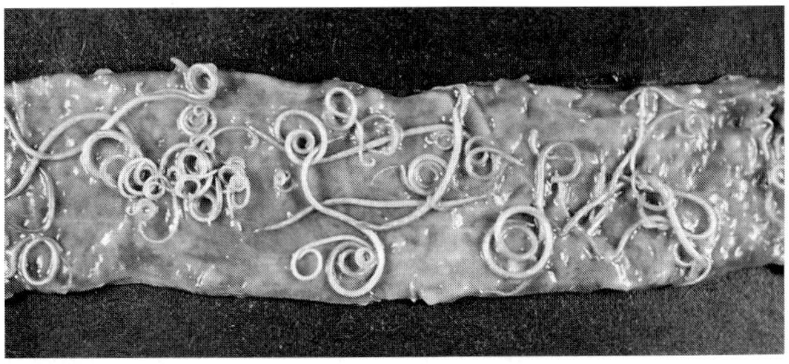

Figure 1-140 Proximal jejunum; dog. Ascariasis. Abundant ascarids in the lumen.

Hookworms are prevalent in animals occupying a warm, wet climate, particularly climates that are above freezing for most of the year. Larval development is inhibited by temperatures below 10° C or above 40° C, by sunlight, by abrupt changes in temperature, and by desiccation. Some species of hookworms have seasonal variation in egg output, an adaptation favoring survival.

Hookworm disease affects primarily the young of all host species. The young also are at risk from intrauterine or mammary transmission and are most likely to encounter oral or cutaneous contact with feces. Infections occur more commonly and are more severe under circumstances of poor sanitation, malnutrition, and multiple parasitisms. The housefly, *Musca domestica,* can disseminate the canine hookworm, *A. caninum.* Once larval migration has been completed, adult hookworms reside in the small intestine, the organ generally considered the site of hookworm disease. However, in at least a few species, adults are found in the caudal intestine to the level of the colon and rectum and make their way cranially. In the colon, cecum, and rectum, ulcerations with hemorrhages, usually 2 to 3 mm, where the parasites have attached occur focally or in rows on mucosal folds. The ulcerations are frequently present in the mucosa around solitary lymphoid follicles and along the edge of the ileocolic valve. This latter lesion, an ileocolic valvulitis, has been observed in young dogs at necropsy, sometimes in several puppies of a litter. The edge of the ileocolic valve contains several raised, glistening, black-red mucosal nodules, 2 to 4 mm in diameter; a hookworm is rarely found attached.

Microscopically, the colonic mucosa lining the edge of the valve is moderately hyperplastic, and the lamina propria contains a few aggregates of lymphocytes and plasma cells, and sometimes a few eosinophils, a few siderocytes, and hemorrhage. Hookworms coil in preparation for attachment and then thrust their heads into the villus (Fig. 1-141). The worm penetrates the epithelium and sucks up a wedge-shaped portion of the villus core. Vessels of the lamina propria immediately engorge, and a red disc appears at the point of attachment. The worm makes vigorous sucking movements, ingesting tissue fluid, mucus, and boluses of mucosa, as well as blood. The wound left by the bite, after the worm shifts from one point of attachment to another, continues to ooze blood for as long as 30 minutes. The blood loss that occurs in hookworm disease is the result of blood ingestion by the parasites and multifocal intestinal ulceration. The magnitude of the blood loss varies among species, from 0.07 ml per worm per day for *A. caninum* up to 0.2 ml per worm per day for *A. duodenale.* Boring, twisting movements help the worm to thrust its head deeper along the villus margin toward the intestinal crypts. The hookworm usually produces damage over an area of two to three villi but can injure many more. Grossly, the points of attachment can be seen as punctiform hemorrhages or ulcerations. Microscopically, mucosal lymphocytes are increased in the vicinity of hookworms, and granulocytes occur at the sites of attachment. There are increased numbers of intestinal goblet cells and surface mucus.

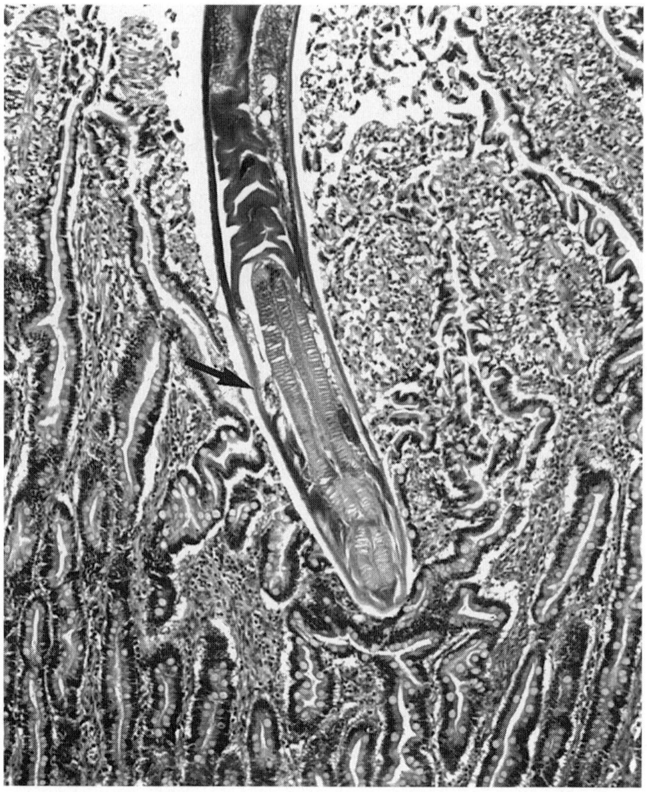

Figure 1-141 Intestine; dog. Hookworm enteritis. A hookworm *(arrow)* has burrowed deep into the mucosa. H & E stain. *Courtesy Department of Veterinary Pathology, Cornell University.*

Clinically, canine hookworm disease is characterized by unthriftiness, lethargy, weight loss, poor hair coat, anemia, diarrhea, variable appetite, and dehydration. Death commonly follows heavy infections in puppies. The feces are dark brown, olive-green, or black and variable in consistency. Infrequently, dogs with hookworms pass red blood. Laboratory findings include hypochromic, microcytic anemia, eosinophilia, hypoalbuminemia, occult fecal blood, and characteristic ova. Rectal involvement can provoke rectal pruritus or tenesmus. Ileocolic valvulitis is manifested by streaks of red blood mixed with, or on the surface of, formed feces. Cats, cattle, sheep, and pigs have lethargy, weight loss, poor hair coat, diarrhea, and weakness.

Trichuriasis

Trichuriasis occurs worldwide among several animal species and in human beings. The parasites most commonly involved in disease are *Trichuris vulpis* of the dog, *Trichuris suis* of the pig, and *Trichuris trichiura* of human beings. The trichurids, 3 to 5 cm in length, are whip-shaped parasites, with a long and slender anterior two thirds, like the lash of a whip, joined to the stouter hind end, the whip handle. The life cycle is direct. Eggs, discharged in the feces of a parasitized host, embryonate in damp, shady environments, and infection is acquired by ingestion. In the digestive tract, larvae emerge from the eggs and penetrate the small intestinal mucosa, where they reside for a short time. They emerge, undergo several stages of development, and then attach to the mucosa of the cecum and colon. The prepatent period is 4 to 5 weeks.

The trichurids damage the mucosa of cecum, colon, and rectum by the tunneling produced as the parasites burrow into the superficial lamina propria. The tunnels are lined by greatly attenuated surface epithelial cells that form a thin covering. The tunnels have an undulating pattern consistent with the way the worm burrows through the superficial mucosa. When few parasites are present, the animal has no clinical signs. When great numbers of parasites are present, diarrhea results.

Trichuris infection in the dog causes chronic diarrhea, which most often is bloodless. Less frequently, the feces contain blood and mucus. Weight loss is minimal, but some dehydration occurs. Laboratory findings include hypoalbuminemia, hyperglobulinemia, anemia, and electrolyte disturbances. The eggs of *Trichuris* spp. are characteristic: lemon shaped with an operculum on both ends. Dogs with trichuriasis sometimes have clinical signs indicative of typhlitis. They suck their flank or turn in circles trying to gnaw at their flank. In the pig, trichuriasis is characterized by anorexia, diarrhea, mucus, and blood in the feces, anemia, fever, labored respiration, incoordination, emaciation, retardation of growth, and death.

The entire surface of the cecum can be covered by these parasites; they can extend to cover the surface of the proximal colon; and in some species such as the dog, the parasites, when numerous, can extend to the rectum (Fig. 1-142). Microscopically, thin-walled tunnels encase the esophageal end of the trichurids, but little tissue damage is evident. The parasites induce little leukocytic infiltration and no necrosis. In heavy infections, a few parasites migrate into the deeper layers of the intestine and incite a granulomatous inflammation.

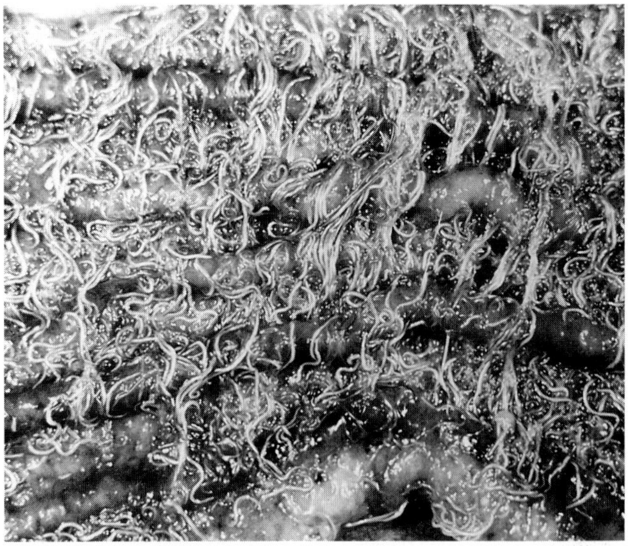

Figure 1-142 Colon; dog. Trichuriasis. *Trichuris vulpis* coat the entire mucosal surface.

Strongyloidosis

Strongyloides enteritis can be severe; larvae or larvated eggs are in the feces of infected animals. The canine and primate parasite, *Strongyloides stercoralis,* is transmissible to human beings. Other species of *Strongyloides* infect horses, pigs, and cats. Parasitism occurs in the upper small intestine, where 2- to 9-mm long females that can reproduce by parthenogenesis, reside in shallow epithelial tunnels at the base of villi. In the case of *S. stercoralis,* "autoinfection" is possible—eggs discharged from females develop into larvae without exiting the host and, in turn, reinfect the intestine of their host. Larvae (rhabditiform) that leave the host with the feces develop into free-living males and females, the offspring of which can become parasitic (filariform), or they can develop into infective (filariform) larvae directly. Infective larvae penetrate the skin or are ingested and penetrate the gastrointestinal mucosa. The larvae travel in the circulation to the lungs, enter the alveoli, are coughed up and then swallowed, and come to reside in the small intestine.

Some species of *Strongyloides* are transmitted in utero and through mammary secretions for several weeks post partum. Clinically, affected animals have diarrhea, weight loss, dehydration, hypoproteinemia, eosinophilia, anorexia, and debility. Larvae or eggs are demonstrable in the feces. Grossly, the affected anterior intestine may be hyperemic and fluid filled. Microscopically, the nematodes occur in the epithelium near the base of the villi or in the upper crypts, which is ulcerated or hyperplastic (Fig. 1-143). Villi are atrophied, cells of the crypts are proliferating, and the lamina propria has increased numbers of lymphocytes and plasma cells, as well as eosinophils. Serum components and granulocytes are lost into the lumen.

Trichostrongylosis

Trichostrongyles are small nematodes that parasitize the duodenum and jejunum of sheep, goats, cattle, and other ruminants. Three genera of the family Trichostrongylidae are significant: *Nematodirus,* which are 2 to 3 cm long; *Cooperia,* 1 cm long; and *Trichostrongylus,* 5 to 8 mm long. These nematodes all have a direct life cycle; eggs are passed in the feces and larvae are acquired by ingestion. Prepatent periods are 3 to 4 weeks, 2 to 3 weeks, and 2 to 3 weeks, respectively. Young animals are most susceptible;

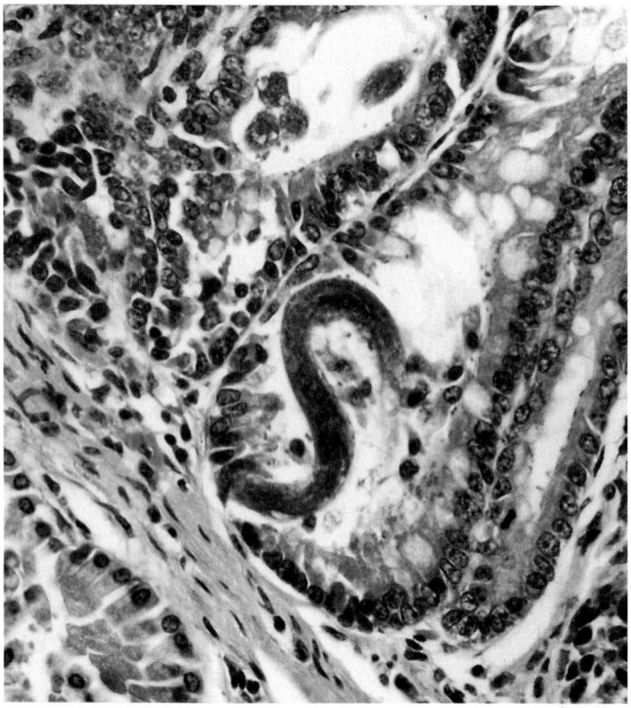

Figure 1-143 Small intestine; patas monkey. Strongyloidosis. *Strongyloides stercoralis* in an intestinal crypt. *Courtesy Dr. J.S. Harper III.*

crowding, poor sanitation, and inadequate nutrition increase susceptibility. Clinically, trichostrongylosis is characterized by weight loss, diarrhea, poor hair coat, dehydration, sunken eyeballs, anorexia, anemia, intermandibular edema, and recumbency. Malabsorption and enteric protein loss are variable. The feces can be formed but more commonly are fluid and dark. Laboratory findings include decreased hemoglobin concentrations and hypoalbuminemia. Parasite eggs can be identified in the feces. An animal that is heavily parasitized has stunted growth, a pendulous abdomen, and fecal staining of the hair or wool of the perineum.

Intermandibular edema, pale tissues, and serous atrophy of fat can be present at necropsy. The intestines have variable hyperemia, dark brown or green fluid contents, and a delicate, gray-white film of exfoliated cells, albumin, and fibrin on the mucosal surface. The parasites can be seen on the mucosal surface, but screening of intestinal contents enhances detection. Microscopically, adults of the *Trichostrongylus* species are found in shallow epithelium-lined tunnels, whereas the adults of *Nematodirus* and *Cooperia* are entwined among the villi. How the parasites induce damage is not totally clear. They cause tunnels and creases in the margins of villi; damage microvilli and reduce activity of brush border enzymes in enterocytes. Erosions can develop. Crypt epithelium has increased numbers of globule leukocytes and mitotic figures

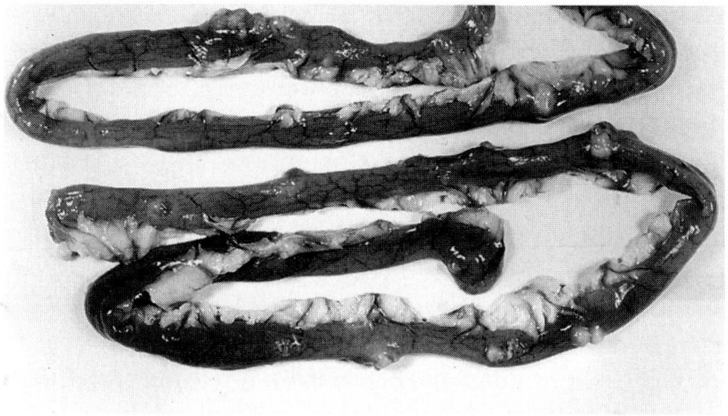

Figure 1-144 Small intestine; sheep. Oesophagostomiasis. Multiple, firm nodules protrude from the serosal surface.

indicating regeneration, and the lumens of the crypts are deeper than normal. Lymphocytes, plasma cells, and eosinophils infiltrate the lamina propria. Villus atrophy varies in severity.

Oesophagostomum

Oesophagostomum columbianum, Oesophagostomum radiatum, and *Oesophagostomum dentatum* the nodular worms of ruminants and pigs, cause subserosal mineralized nodules that are quite characteristic of the disease. These nodules generally are of no clinical significance but they do make the intestines unsuitable for use as sausage casings. Occasionally, they are associated with, and can be the cause of, intussusceptions.

Third-stage larvae are ingested, penetrate the mucosa of the distal small intestine or cecum and colon, reside there for a time, and then exit to develop into adults, 1 to 2 cm in length, that live on the mucosal surface of the cecum and colon. Here, they stimulate a response of eosinophils and globule leukocytes. Clinically, *Oesophagostomum* spp. are responsible for moderate electrolyte and protein loss, diarrhea, anemia, and unthriftiness.

The lesion seen most frequently at necropsy is a granulomatous nodule, 0.5 to 1.5 cm in diameter, produced by fourth-stage larvae penetrating the cecal and colonic walls. Very few sheep are free of these lesions; the nodules protrude from the serosal surface of the intestines (Fig. 1-144) and, on incision, contain a gritty, yellow to green, necrotic center. Nodules number 50 to 100; some occur in the mesentery, mesenteric lymph nodes, liver, and lungs as well. Microscopically, the oesophagostomum nodules contain parasite fragments and central, caseous, necrotic debris, and eosinophils that are surrounded by granulomatous inflammation, including Langhans' giant cells.

Pinworms

Oxyuris equi is the most common pinworm of domestic animals. The parasites occupy the lumen of the distal intestine of horses and occasionally cause rectal pruritus by laying their eggs on the perineal region. *Enterobius vermicularis* is the pinworm of primates and great apes. It is not zoonotic and is generally of little clinical consequence.

Cestodes

Tapeworms, although frequently found in the alimentary system, are generally of little clinical significance. They require two and sometimes three hosts to complete their life cycles. Tapeworms attach to the gut wall by means of their anterior scolex, which can have hooks in addition to four suckers. Although they can cause some damage at the site of attachment, generally they compete with the host for nutrients. Lacking an alimentary system, they absorb nutrients through their surface. Tapeworms are flat, segmented, and hermaphroditic, reproducing by addition of segments or proglottids. Examples of tapeworms are *Anoplocephala* spp. in the horse, *Moniezia* spp. in ruminants, and *Diphyllobothrium* and *Dipylidium* spp. in dogs and cats. *Mesocestoides* spp. can infect dogs. In some cases, this latter parasite can perforate through the intestine and proliferate in the peritoneal cavity.

Taenia and *Echinococcus* spp. are the most destructive of the cestodes. Although carnivores are the definitive hosts, the larval forms reside in the viscera and body cavities of the intermediate hosts, usually ruminants, pigs, horses, or rodents. Human beings can also become infected, sometimes taking 20 or 30 years for clinical disease to appear. The damage in the intermediate hosts can be quite severe.

Trematodes

Trematodes are uncommon parasites of the alimentary tract. *Nanophyetus salminicola* uses a snail and a fish as intermediate hosts. It carries the rickettsia responsible for salmon poisoning in the northwestern United States (see page 68 in this chapter). Lesions of the intestine are hemorrhagic enteritis.

Paramphistomiasis is a fluke infestation of ruminant forestomachs in warmer latitudes around the world. Although adult organisms residing in the forestomachs are usually of no clinical significance, heavy infestations of larvae in the proximal small intestine, before migration to the rumen and reticulum, can cause hypoproteinemia, anemia, and death. Larvae burrow deeply into, and sometimes through, the wall of the small intestine and can be found in the peritoneal cavity. The intermediate host is a snail. Cercariae encyst on aquatic vegetation eaten by the ruminant.

Alaria spp. can attach to the small intestine of dogs and cats but are generally innocuous. The mesocercariae can cause tissue damage during their organal migrations. Paratenic hosts are frogs, snakes, and mice.

Schistosomiasis of ruminants, pigs, horses, and dogs can cause granulomatous intestinal lesions with protein loss secondary to the parasite's presence in mesenteric veins after migration through the liver. Parasites are acquired by direct penetration of the skin by cercariae.

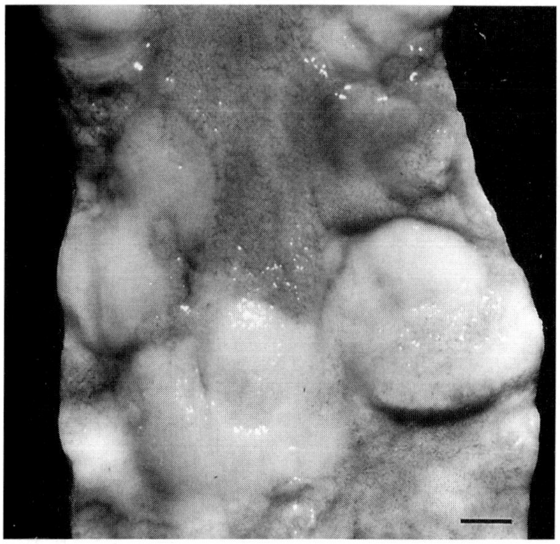

Figure 1-145 Ileum; dog. Intestinal lymphosarcoma. Multiple white nodules of lymphosarcoma protrude from the mucosal surface. Bar = 5 mm. *Courtesy Dr. M.D. McGavin.*

Acanthocephalans

The thorny-headed worm of pigs, *Macracanthorhynchus hirudinaceus,* is a small intestinal parasite with an arthropod intermediate host. They are occasionally misidentified as tapeworms, which they superficially resemble. However, they are not truly segmented parasites. They occasionally penetrate the bowel wall at the site of parasite attachment, causing peritonitis.

Prosthenorchis spp. are acanthocephalids of primates. Cockroaches are the intermediate hosts.

INTESTINAL NEOPLASIA

Neoplasms of various types occurs in the gastrointestinal system of domestic animals. Those of the oral cavity and stomach have already been discussed. Intestinal neoplasms are diagnosed most frequently in dogs and cats in large part due to their longer lifespan. Additionally, pets live in close harmony with their human companions and thus it is possible that some of the same environmental factors that cause human cancer could also cause similar problems in animals.

In dogs, benign neoplasms of the intestinal tract are most commonly adenomas or polyps, and their malignant counterparts adenocarcinomas. Smooth muscle neoplasms termed leiomyomas and leiomyosarcomas arise from existing muscular layers. In cats, the most common neoplasms include alimentary lymphosarcoma (Fig. 1-145), mastocytomas which are associated with ulceration, adenomas, adenocarcinomas, and carcinoids. In sheep, adenocarcinomas of the intestine are fairly common and are virus induced. In cows, alimentary lymphosarcoma is most common. Horses rarely develop intestinal neoplasms.

Suggested Readings

Baird AN, Cohen ND, Taylor TS, Watkins JP, Schumacher J. Renosplenic entrapment of the large colon in horses: 57 cases (1983-1988). J Am Vet Med Assoc 1991; 198:1423-1426.

Baker GJ. Oral anatomy of the horse. In: Harvey CE, ed. Veterinary Dentistry. Philadelphia: Saunders, 1985:203-216.

Batt RM, McLean L, Carter MW. Sequential morphologic and biochemical studies of naturally occurring wheat-sensitive enteropathy in Irish Setter dogs. Dig Dis Sci 1987; 32:184-194.

Batte EG, McLamb RD, Muse KE, Tally SD, Vestal TJ. Pathophysiology of swine trichuriasis. Am J Vet Res 1977; 38:1075-1079.

Bentinck-Smith J. Feline panleukopenia (feline infectious enteritis): A review of 574 cases. North Am Vet 1949; 30:379-384.

Bland AP, Frost AJ, Lysons RJ. Susceptibility of porcine ileal enterocytes to the cytotoxin of *Serpulina hyodysenteriae* and the resolution of epithelial lesions: An electron microscopic study. Vet Pathol 1995; 32:24-35.

Bowman DD. Georgi's Parasitology for Veterinarians, 7th ed. Philadelphia: Saunders, 1999.

Brown PJ, Clayton HM. Hepatic pathology of experimental *Parascaris equorum* infection in worm-free foals. J Comp Pathol 1979; 89:115-123.

Burrows CF. Canine hemorrhagic gastroenteritis. J Am Anim Hosp Assoc 1977; 13:451-458.

Carpenter JL, Roberts RM, Harpster NK, King NW. Intestinal and cardiopulmonary forms of parvovirus infection in a litter of pups. J Am Vet Med Assoc 1980; 176:1269-1273.

Cheville NF, Olson C. Cytology of the canine oral papilloma. Am J Pathol 1964; 45:849-872.

Chiodini RJ, Van Kruiningen HJ, Merkal RS. Ruminant paratuberculosis (Johne's disease): The current status and future prospects. Cornell Vet 1984; 74:218-262.

Cimprich RE. Equine granulomatous enteritis. Vet Pathol 1974; 11:535-547.

Cimprich RE, Rooney JR. *Corynebacterium equi* enteritis in foals. Vet Pathol 1977; 14:95-102.

Cordes DO, Perry BD, Rikihisa Y, Chickering WR. Enterocolitis caused by *Ehrlichia* sp. in the horse (Potomac horse fever). Vet Pathol 1986; 23:471-477.

Cordy DR, Gorham JR. The pathology and etiology of salmon disease in the dog and fox. Am J Pathol 1950; 26:617-637.

Croese J, Loukas A, Opdebeeck J, Prociv P. Occult enteric infection by *Ancylostoma caninum:* A previously unrecognized zoonosis. Gastroenterology 1994; 106:3-12.

Doughri AM, Young S, Storz J. Pathologic changes in intestinal chlamydial infection of newborn calves. Am J Vet Res 1974; 35:939-944.

Dubielzig RR, Adams WM, Brodey RS. Inductive fibroameloblastoma: An unusual dental tumor of young cats. J Am Vet Med Assoc 1979; 174:720-722.

Dubielzig RR, Goldschmidt MH, Brodey RS. The nomenclature of periodontal epulides in dogs. Vet Pathol 1979; 16:209-214.

Dubielzig RR, Higgins RJ, Krakowka S. Lesions of the enamel organ of developing dog teeth following experimental inoculation of gnotobiotic puppies with canine distemper virus. Vet Pathol 1981; 18:684-689.

Dubielzig RR, Thrall DE. Ameloblastoma and keratinizing ameloblastoma in dogs. Vet Pathol 1982; 19:596-607.

Dubielzig RR, Wilson JW, Beck KA, Robbins T. Dental dysplasis and epitheliogenesis imperfecta in a foal. Vet Pathol 1986; 23:325-327.

Eisner ER. Chronic subgingival tooth erosion in cats. Vet Med 1989; 84:378-387.

Fox JG, Krakowka S, Taylor NS. Acute-onset *Campylobacter*-associated gastroenteritis in adult Beagles. J Am Vet Med Assoc 1985; 187:1268-1270.

Gebhart CJ, Barns SM, McOrist S, Lin GF, Lawson GHK. Ileal symbiont intracellularis, an obligate intracellular bacterium of porcine intestines showing a relationship to *Desulfovibrio* species. Int J Syst Bacteriol 1993; 43:533-538.

Gelberg H, Lewis RM. The pathogenesis of vesicular exanthema of swine virus and San Miguel sea lion virus in swine. Vet Pathol 1982; 19:424-443.

Gelberg HB, Lewis RM, Felsburg PJ, Smith CA. Antiepithelial autoantibodies associated with the feline eosinophilic granuloma complex. Am J Vet Res 1985; 46:263-265.

Griesemer RA, Cole CR. Bovine papular stomatitis. II. The experimentally produced disease. Am J Vet Res 1961; 22:473-481.

Griesemer RA, Cole CR, Bovine papular stomatitis. III. Histopathology. Am J Vet Res 1961; 22:482-488.

Gunson DE, Rooney JR. Anaphylactoid purpura in a horse. Vet Pathol 1977; 14:325-331.

Hall EJ, Batt RM. Development of wheat-sensitive enteropathy in Irish setters: Morphologic changes. Am J Vet Res 1990; 51:978-982.

Harris DL, Alexander TJL, Whipp SC, Robinson IM, Glock RD, Matthews PJ. Swine dysentery: Studies of gnotobiotic pigs inoculated with *Treponema hyodysenteriae, Bacteriodes vulgatus,* and *Fusobacterium necrophorum.* J Am Vet Med Assoc 1978; 172:468-471.

Harvey CE, Dubielzig RR. Anatomy of the oral cavity in the dog and cat. In: Harvey CE, ed. Veterinary Dentistry. Philadelphia: Saunders, 1985:11-22.

Hayden DW, Fleischman RW. Schirrous eosinophilic gastritis in dogs with gastric arteritis. Vet Pathol 1977; 14:441-448.

Hayden DW, Van Kruiningen HJ. Eosinophilic gastroenteritis in German shepherd dogs and its relationship to visceral larva migrans. J Am Vet Med Assoc 1973; 162:379-384.

Holland CJ, Ristic M, Cole AI, Johnson P, Baker G, Goetz T. Isolation, experimental transmission, and characterization of causative agent of Potomac horse fever. Science 1985; 227:522-524.

Hooper BE, Haelterman EO. Lesions of the gastrointestinal tract of pigs infected with transmissible gastroenteritis. Can J Comp Med 1969; 33:29-36.

Janke BH, Francis DH, Collins JE, Libal MC, Zeman DH, Johnson DD, Neiger RD. Attaching and effacing *Escherichia coli* infection as a cause of diarrhea in young calves. J Am Vet Med Assoc 1990; 196:897-901.

Jarplid B, Johansson H, Carmichael LE. A fatal case of pup infection with minute virus of canines (MVC). J Vet Diag Invest 1996; 8:484-487.

Jergens AE, Moore FM, Haynes JS, Miles KG. Idiopathic inflammatory bowel disease in dogs and cats: 84 cases (1987-1990). J Am Vet Med Assoc 1992; 201:1603-1608.

Jonsson L, Martinsson K. Regional ileitis in pigs: Morphological and pathogenetical aspects. Acta Vet Scand 1976; 17:223-232.

Kipar A, Kremednahl J, Addie DD, Leukert W, Grant CK, Reinacher M. Fatal enteritis associated with coronavirus infection in cats. J Comp Pathol 1998; 119:1-14.

Krakowka S, Eaton KA, Rings DM, Argenzio. Production of gastroesophageal erosions and ulcers (GEU) in gnotobiotic swine monoinfected with fermentative commensal bacteria and fed high-carbohydrate diet. Vet Pathol 1998; 35:274-282.

Krook L, Maylin GA, Lillie JH, Wallace RS. Dental fluorosis in cattle. Cornell Vet 1983; 73:340-362.

Lindberg R. Pathology of equine granulomatous enteritis. J Comp Pathol 1984; 94:233-247.

Lloyd K, Hintz HF, Wheat JD, Schryver JF. Enteroliths in horses. Cornell Vet 1987; 77:172-186.

McOrist S, Jasni S, Mackie RA, MacIntyre N, Neef N, Lawson GHK. Reproduction of porcine proliferative enteropathy with pure cultures of *Ileal Symbiont intracellularis*. Infect Immun 1993; 61:4286-4292.

Mebus CA, Stair EL, Rhodes MB, Twiehaus MH. Pathology of neonatal calf diarrhea induced by a coronavirus-like agent. Vet Pathol 1973; 10:45-64.

Mebus CA, Stair EL, Underdahl NR, Twiehaus MJ. Pathology of neonatal calf diarrhea induced by a reo-like virus. Vet Pathol 1971; 8:490-505.

Meunier PC, Cooper BJ, Appel MJG, Lanieu ME, Slauson DO. Pathogenesis of canine parvovirus enteritis: Sequential virus distribution and passive immunization studies. Vet Pathol 1985; 22:617-624.

Montali RJ, Strandberg JD. Extraperitoneal lesions in feline infectious peritonitis. Vet Pathol 1972; 9:109-121.

Moon HW. Intestine. In: Cheville NF, ed. Cell Pathology. 2nd edn. Ames, IA: Iowa State University Press, 1983;503-529.

Morin M, Morehouse LG, Solorzano RF, Olson LD. Transmissible gastroenteritis in feeder swine: Clinical, immunofluorescence, and histopathological observations. Can J Comp Med 1973; 37:239-248.

Morton L, Morton D, Gelberg HB, Baker GI. Chronic eosinophilic enteritis attributable to *Pythium* sp. in a horse. Vet Pathol 1991; 28:542-544.

Murray M, Robinson PB, McKeating FJ, Baker GJ, Lauder IM. Peptic ulceration in the dog: A clinico-pathological study. Vet Rec 1972; 91:441-447.

Navin TR, Juranek DD. Cryptosporidiosis: Clinical, epidemiologic, and parasitologic review. Rev Infect Dis 1984; 6:313-327.

Pass DA, Bolton JR. Chronic eosinophilic enteritis in the horse. Vet Pathol 1982; 19:486-496.

Patnaik AK, Hurvitz AI, Johnson GF. Canine gastric adenocarcinoma. Vet Pathol 1978; 15:600-607.

Pospischil A, Mainil JG, Baljer G, Moon HW. Attaching and effacing bacteria in the intestines of calves and cats with diarrhea. Vet Pathol 1987; 24:330-334.

Rings DM, Welker FH, Hull BL, Kersting KW, Hoffsis GF. Abomasal emptying defect in Suffolk sheep. J Am Vet Med Assoc 1984; 185:1520-1522.

Rikihisa Y, Perry BD, Cordes DO. Ultrastructural study of ehrlichial organisms in the large colons of ponies infected with Potomac horse fever. Infect Immun 1985; 49:505-512.

Robertson JM. Left displacement of the bovine abomasum: Epizootiologic factors. Am J Vet Res 1968; 29:421-434.

Sander CH, Langham RF. Canine histiocytic ulcerative colitis. Arch Pathol 1968; 85:94-100.

Seiler RJ. Colorectal polyps of the dog: A clinical pathologic study of 17 cases. J Am Vet Med Assoc 1979; 174:72-75.

Sheaser TR, Kostad DL, Suttie JW. Bovine dental fluorosis: Histologic and physical characteristics. Am J Vet Res 1978; 39:597-602.

Songer JG. Clostridial enteric diseases of domestic animals. Clin Microbiol Rev 1996; 9:216-234.

Strand EA, Sommers SC, Petrak M. Regional enterocolitis in Cocker Spaniel dogs. Arch Pathol 1954; 57:357-362.

Toombs JP, Collins LG, Graves GM, Crowe DT, Caywood DD. Colonic perforation in corticosteroid-treated dogs. J Am Vet Med Assoc 1986; 188:145-150.

Torres-Medina A, Schlafer DH, Mebus CA. Rotaviral and coronaviral diarrhea. Vet Clin North Am Food Anim Pract 1985; 1:471-493.

Turk MAM, Gallina AM, Perryman LE. *Bacillus piliformis* infection (Tyzzer's disease) in foals in Northwestern United States: A retrospective study of 21 cases. J Am Vet Med Assoc 1981; 178:279-281.

Van Der Gaag I, Tribboel D. Intestinal atresia and stenosis in animals: A report of 34 cases. Vet Pathol 1980; 17:565-574.

Van Kruiningen HJ. Canine colitis comparable to regional enteritis and mucosal colitis in man. Gastroenterology 1972; 62:1128-1142.

Van Kruiningen HJ, Gregoire K, Meuten DJ. Acute gastric dilatation: A review of comparative aspects, by species, and a study in dogs and monkeys. J Am Anim Hosp Assoc 1974; 10:294-324.

Van Kruiningen HJ, Hiestand L, Hill DL, Tilton RC, Ryan RW. Winter dysentery in dairy cattle: Recent findings. Comp Cont Educ Pract Vet 1985; 7:S591-S598.

Van Kruiningen HJ, Lees GE, Hayden DW, Meuten DJ, Rogers WA. Lipogranulomatous lymphangitis in canine intestinal lymphangectasia. Vet Pathol 1984; 21:377-383.

Van Kruiningen HJ, Montali RJ, Strandberg JD, Kirk RW. A granulomatous colitis of dogs with histologic resemblance to Whipple's disease. Path Vet 1965; 2:521-544.

Van Kruiningen HJ, Wojan LD, Stake PE, Lord PF. The influence of diet and feeding frequency on gastric function in the dog. J Am Anim Hosp Assoc 1987; 23:145-153.

Van Kruiningen HJ, Khairallah LH, Sasserville VG, Wyand MS, Post JE. Calfhood coronavirus enterocolitis: A clue to the etiology of winter dysentery. Vet Pathol 1987; 24:564-567.

Verstraete, FJM, Ligthelm AG, Weber A. The histological nature of epulides in dogs. J Comp Path 1992; 106:169-182.

Vonderfecht SL, Trommershausen Bowling A, Cohen M. Congenital intestinal aganglionosis in white foals. Vet Pathol 1983; 20:65-70.

Walker RI, Caldwell MB, Lee EC, Guerry P, Trust TJ, Ruiz-Palacios GM. Pathophysiology of *Campylobacter enteritis*. Microbiol Rev 1986; 50:81-94.

Wilcock BP, Olander HJ. The pathogenesis of porcine rectal stricture. I. The naturally occurring disease and its association with salmonellosis. Vet Pathol 1977; 14:36-42.

Waters EH, Orr JP, Clark EG, Schaufele CM. Typhlocolitis caused by *Clostridium difficile* in sucking piglets. J Vet Diagn Invest 1998; 10:104-108.

CHAPTER 2

Liver, Biliary System, and Exocrine Pancreas

JOHN M. CULLEN
N. JAMES MACLACHLAN

LIVER AND BILIARY SYSTEM

Anatomy

The liver is the largest gland in the body, but its relative size varies in different species. In adult carnivores, the liver comprises 3% to 4% of the body weight. It is about 2% in omnivores and about 1% to 1.5% of the body weight of herbivores. In the neonate of all species, the liver is a larger percentage of body weight than in adults and it may atrophy in aged animals. The liver is reddish to mahogany brown and has a soft and friable consistency.

In monogastric animals, the liver occupies the central area of the cranial abdomen, slightly shifted to the right, and abuts the diaphragm. In ruminants, the liver is displaced to the right side of the cranial abdominal cavity. A series of ligaments maintain the liver in its position. The coronary ligament and the right and left triangular ligaments attach the liver to the diaphragm near the esophagus. The falciform ligament attaches the midline of the liver to the ventral midline of the abdomen. The round ligament, a remnant of the umbilical vein, is embedded within the falciform ligament. The liver is supplied with blood from two sources. The portal vein drains the digestive tract, pancreas, and spleen and provides 60% to 70% of the total hepatic blood flow. The hepatic artery provides the remainder of hepatic blood flow. Blood leaves the liver via the hepatic vein, which is very short, and enters the caudal vena cava. The liver has a smooth capsular surface, and the parenchyma consists of friable red-brown tissue that is divided into lobes. Gross subdivision of the liver into lobes differs among the domestic species. At the periphery, the lobes taper to a sharp edge.

The traditional functional subunit of the liver is the hepatic lobule, a hexagonal structure, 1 to 2 mm wide. The lobule has a central vein (also termed the terminal hepatic venule), which is a tributary of the hepatic vein, at the center, and portal areas at the angles of the hexagon (Fig. 2-1). The portal areas contain bile ducts, branches of the portal vein, the hepatic artery, nerves, and lymph vessels, all supported by a collagenous stroma. The limiting plate, a discontinuous border of hepatocytes, forms the outer boundary of the portal area.

Alternatively, when the liver is viewed as a bile-secreting gland, the acinus is the anatomic subunit of the hepatic parenchyma. Terminal afferent branches (penetrating vessels) of the portal vein and hepatic artery project into the parenchyma, like branches from the trunk of a tree, forming the long axis of the diamond-shaped acinus (Fig. 2-1). Thus, terminal afferent branches of the portal vein and hepatic artery are at the center of the acinus and the terminal hepatic venule (central vein) is located at the periphery. Each terminal hepatic venule (central vein) receives blood from several acini. There are three zones in each acinus. Zone 1 is closest to the afferent blood coming from the distributing branches of the hepatic artery and portal vein. It corresponds roughly to the periportal area of the hepatic lobule. Zone 2 is peripheral to zone 1, and zone 3 borders the terminal hepatic venule (central vein). Zone 3, farthest from the source of oxygen and nutrients, corresponds roughly to the centrilobular region of the hepatic lobule. In this anatomic unit, bile flows from the hepatocytes through the bile canaliculi in zone 3 into the bile ducts at the termination of zone 1 at the portal area.

The ultrastructural appearance of the hepatocyte reflects the cell's active metabolism, bile secretion, and close contact with the plasma (Fig. 2-2). The cytoplasm contains glycogen, numerous mitochondria, lysosomes, and abundant smooth and rough endoplasmic reticulum. There are several specialized features of the hepatocyte membranes. These include the bile canaliculi, modified portions of the cell membrane in two adjacent hepatocytes that form a lumen for bile secretion, and the microvilli on the luminal face of the hepatocytes.

Within the liver, hepatocytes are arranged in branching plates that radiate from the terminal hepatic venule (central vein). Hepatic plates are separated by vascular sinusoids. Blood from the terminal afferent branches of the hepatic artery and portal vein mixes in the hepatic sinusoids and

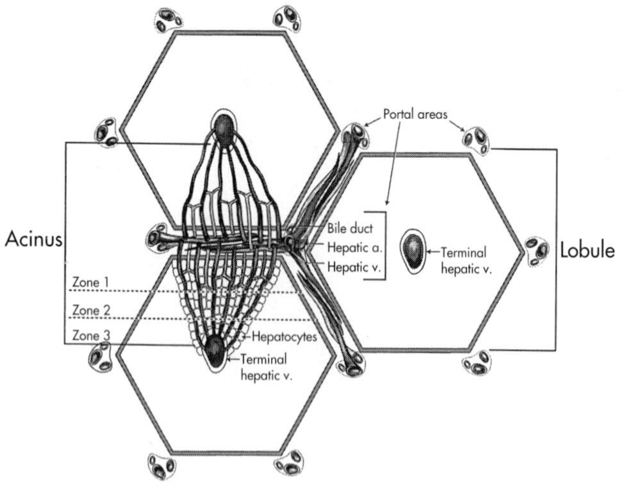

Figure 2-1 Schematic view of the microscopic organization of the liver. Both the lobule and the acinus are represented. The lobule is a hexagonal unit with portal areas at the margin and a terminal hepatic vein (central vein) at the center. The lobule is divided into the periportal, midzonal, and centrilobular areas. The acinus is a diamond-shaped structure with the distributing branches of the vessels from the portal areas as the center of the structure. Zone 1 of the acinus is closest to the afferent blood supply, and zone 3 is at the tip of the diamond-shaped structure, close to the terminal hepatic vein. Zone 2 is between the zones 1 and 3.

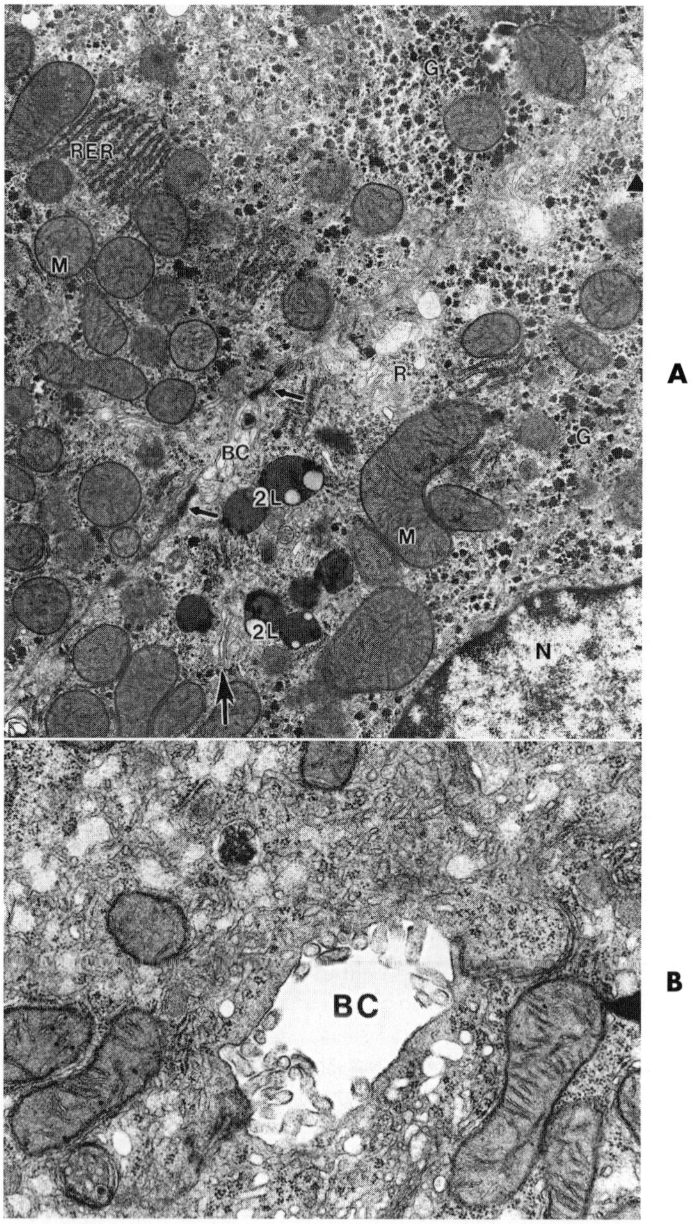

Figure 2-2 **A,** A transmission electron micrograph. Liver; normal dog. Hepatocyte ultrastructural features. Note nucleus *(N)*, mitochondria *(M)*, secondary lysosomes *(2L)*, glycogen *(G)*, rough endoplasmic reticulum *(RER)*, golgi *(large arrow)*, bile canaliculus *(BC)*, and free ribosomes. Note desmosomes on both sides of the bile canaliculus *(small arrows)*. **B,** Higher magnification of bile canaliculus. Note the microvilli projecting into the lumen of the canaliculus. *Courtesy Dr. V. Meador.*

flows to the terminal hepatic venule (central vein). Hepatic sinusoids differ from capillaries in that they are lined by greatly fenestrated endothelial cells that have a markedly reduced and modified basement membrane, whereas capillaries have a continuous endothelial lining and are ensheathed in basement membrane (Fig. 2-3). The sinusoidal endothelial cells are supported by a fine scaffold of electron-lucent basement membrane that contains collagen types IV and XVIII and many other extracellular matrix components, including laminin, proteoglycans, and fibronectin. These elements collectively compose the fine fibers that are evident when the liver is stained with silver stains that demonstrate the "reticulin" of the liver.

The fenestrated endothelial cells of the sinusoid do not lie in direct contact with hepatocytes. The gap between these cells is termed the space of Disse (Figs. 2-3 and 2-4). The fenestrations are small enough to keep red blood cells within the lumen of the sinusoid but permit passage of plasma into the space of Disse. Within this space, plasma constituents, such as albumin-bound unconjugated bilirubin, are in close contact with hepatocyte microvilli. These microvilli dramatically expand the surface area of the hepatocytes and increase the efficiency of the uptake of plasma constituents and the secretion of products of hepatocellular synthesis. Any damage, such as fibrosis, within the space of Disse has serious consequences for hepatic function, since loss of the close association between the hepatocytes and the plasma impairs the ability of hepatocytes to function normally.

Within the lumen of the sinusoids a population of macrophages termed Kupffer cells is attached to endothelial cells. These Kupffer cells are members of the monocyte-macrophage system; they clear particulate material, endo-

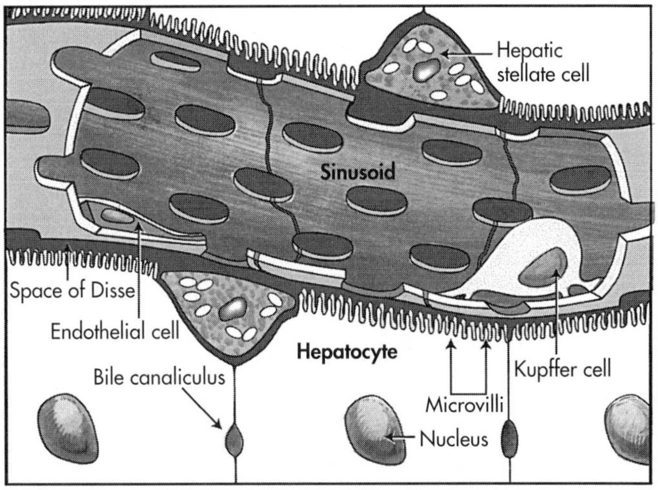

Figure 2-3 Diagram of the hepatic sinusoid. One side of the wall of the sinusoid has been removed to reveal the lumen lined by fenestrated endothelial cells. Kupffer cells rest on the endothelial cells and project into the sinusoid. Between the endothelial cells and the hepatocytes is a gap called the space of Disse. Microvilli extending from the luminal aspect of the hepatocytes are found in this space. Hepatic stellate cells are situated within the space of Disse and extend between hepatocytes.

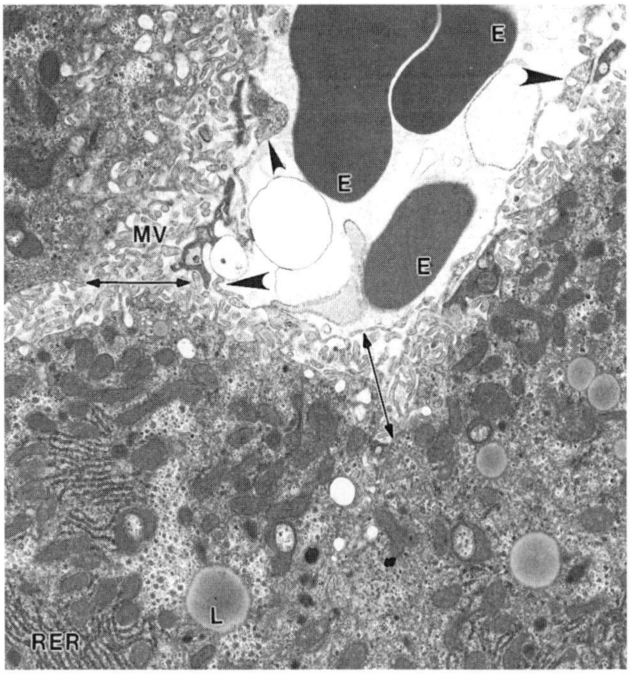

Figure 2-4 Transmission electron micrograph. Liver; normal dog. A sinusoid containing erythrocytes *(E)* is in the upper right hand portion of the figure. The margins of the sinusoid are lined by fenestrated endothelial cells *(arrowheads).* The space of Disse *(double-headed arrows)* lies between the endothelial cells and the hepatocytes. Microvilli *(MV)* project from the hepatocytes into the space of Disse. Rough endoplasmic reticulum *(RER)* and lipid droplets *(L)* can be seen in the hepatocyte cytoplasm. *Courtesy Dr. V. Meador.*

toxin, and other substances from the sinusoidal blood. They are a source of a variety of inflammatory mediators that influence adjacent cells. For example, Kupffer cells release transforming growth factor-β, which is a mitoinhibitor of hepatocytes.

Hepatic stellate cells (also termed lipocytes or Ito cells) are found within the space of Disse and between hepatocytes at the edge of the space of Disse (Figs. 2-3 and 2-5). Normally, hepatic stellate cells have a low rate of replication and are primarily responsible for storing vitamin A in cytoplasmic vacuoles. These vacuoles are a characteristic of the resting stellate cell. During hepatic injury, stellate cells are the principal source of hepatic fibrosis. Activated hepatic stellate cells release their vitamin A content, alter their morphology to a myofibroblast conformation, and develop a proliferative capability. In addition, they begin to synthesize collagen (collagen type I primarily) and other extracellular matrix components (laminin, fibronectin, proteoglycans) that lead to hepatic fibrosis in the perisinusoidal space or in larger areas of injury. The influence of inflammatory cytokines and changes in the underlying extracellular matrix—for example, a change from collagen type IV to collagen type I—are known stimuli for this change.

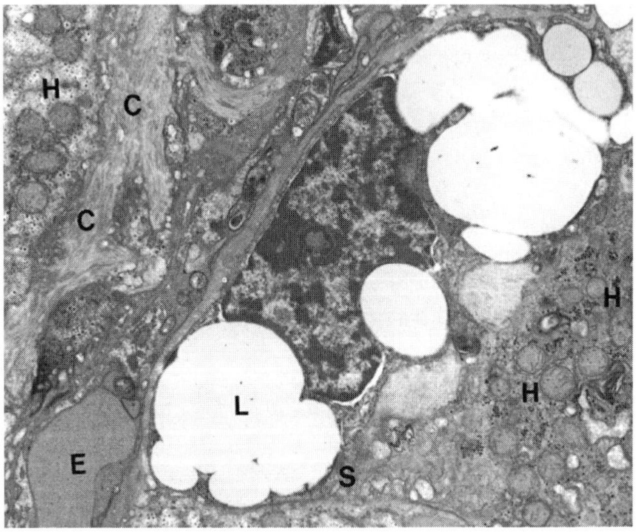

Figure 2-5 Transmission electron micrograph. Liver; normal dog. A hepatic stellate cell *(S)* with its characteristic cytoplasmic lipid vacuoles *(L)* is adjacent to hepatocytes *(H)* and within the space of Disse. Bundles of collagen *(C)* are at the margins of the stellate cells. An eryrthrocyte *(E)* is within the sinusoidal lumen. *Courtesy Dr. V. Meador.*

Bile flows within the lobule in the opposite direction to blood flow, which facilitates the concentration of bile. The biliary system commences as canaliculi within the centrilobular (periacinar) areas of the hepatic lobule. The walls of canaliculi are formed entirely by the cell membranes of adjacent hepatocytes (Fig. 2-2). Just outside the limiting plate, canaliculi drain into cholangioles (also known as the canals of Hering) that are lined by low cuboidal epithelium. The cholangioles converge into interlobular bile ducts lined by cuboidal epithelium, located in the portal areas. Bile then flows into the main hepatic ducts that unite to form the common bile duct by which bile is carried to the duodenum. The gallbladder, upstream of the common bile duct, is responsible for storage and concentration of bile in those species that have a gallbladder. It is absent in the horse and rat.

Function

The liver performs many critical functions that maintain homeostasis. These functions occur in the following microanatomic regions of the liver:

1. The smooth endoplasmic reticulum. This is the site of the synthesis of cholesterol and bile acids and the generation and utilization of glycogen. It is also the site for metabolism of various substances in preparation for their excretion from the body via the bile or urine. These substances include bile pigments, xenobiotics or ingested substances, and steroid hormones.
2. The rough endoplasmic reticulum. This is the site of production of plasma proteins such as albumin and fibrinogen, lipoproteins, and a variety of α- and β-globulins. It is also the site of production for all of the clotting factors with the possible exception of factor VIII, which is primarily produced in endothelial cells.
3. The bile canaliculus, a modified region of hepatocyte cell membranes forming a lumen between hepatocytes. This is the site where bile, which is formed in the liver, is actively transported to begin the process of bile secretion.
4. The hepatic sinusoids. Within the sinusoids, Kupffer cells attached to endothelial cells filter blood through their ability to phagocytose infectious agents and foreign material absorbed from the intestines before they gain access to the systemic circulation. Most blood-borne foreign material is cleared by Kupffer cells in all domestic species except swine, goats, and cattle (members of the family Artiodactyla), where this function is performed primarily by intravascular macrophages in the pulmonary alveolar capillaries.
5. Hepatic mitochondria. Energy is produced by oxidative phosphorylation and β-oxidation of fatty acids in hepatic mitochondria. This energy is used to sustain the activities of the liver and to provide a reservoir of glycogen for the body.

Hepatic Dysfunction and Failure

Only after severe injury or repeated significant insults does prolonged hepatic dysfunction or failure occur because the liver has considerable functional reserve and regenerative capacity. In healthy animals, more than two thirds of the hepatic parenchyma can be removed without significant impairment of hepatic function, and normal hepatic mass is regenerated by proliferation of hepatocytes, bile duct epithelium, and endothelial cells in the remaining liver lobes within 5 to 7 days. This process of tissue removal and regeneration can be repeated more than five times, particularly in younger animals, and normal function is retained. In all species, clinical signs from hepatic derangement, including icterus, hepatoencephalopathy, and clotting disorders, are similar, regardless of their cause. These signs are manifest, however, only when the liver's considerable reserve and regenerative capacity are depleted or when biliary outflow is obstructed. Only lesions that affect the majority of the hepatic parenchyma are likely to produce the signs of hepatic failure because focal lesions rarely destroy sufficient parenchyma to deplete the liver's reserve. The term **hepatic failure** implies loss of adequate hepatic function as a consequence of either acute or chronic hepatic damage; however, all hepatic functions are not usually lost at the same time. The potential consequences of hepatic dysfunction and failure include (1) disturbances of bile flow with a resultant hyperbilirubinemia; (2) hepatic encephalopathy; (3) a variety of metabolic disturbances including hyperammonemia and possibly hypoglycemia and acidosis; (4) vascular and hemodynamic alterations, such as shunting of portal blood into the systemic circulation, thus bypassing the hepatocytes; and (5) cutaneous manifestations such as epidermal necrosis syndrome in dogs and photosensitization in herbivores.

Disturbances of Bile Flow and Icterus

Bile is composed of water, bile acids, bilirubin, cholesterol, inorganic ions, and other constituents. There are two major purposes for bile synthesis. The first purpose is excretory; bile is the major route of excretion of many of the body's waste products such as surplus cholesterol, bilirubin, and metabolized xenobiotics. The second purpose is the facilitation of digestion; bile acids are the major metabolite of cholesterol metabolism and the predominant organic solute in the bile. Bile acids are effective detergents that assist in the digestion of lipids within the intestine, as well as increasing the solubility of lipids secreted into the bile. The rate of synthesis of bile acids is relatively low, and to meet the body's need for bile acids, they are avidly conserved by the body through a process of recycling. Secreted bile acids are reabsorbed from the intestine in a process known as enterohepatic circulation that takes place primarily in the ileum. Enterohepatic circulation is quite efficient and recycles as much as 95% of the bile acids that are secreted into the intestines.

Bilirubin is produced from the metabolic degradation of hemoglobin, and to a lesser extent, other heme proteins including myoglobin and the hepatic hemoproteins such as cytochromes. The majority of bilirubin is derived from the hemoglobin in senescent erythrocytes after they have been phagocytosed by the mononuclear phagocytic system of the spleen, bone marrow, and liver. Within the phagocyte, the globin portion is degraded and the constituent amino acids are returned to the amino acid pool. The heme iron is transferred to iron-binding proteins such as transferrin for recycling. The remaining portion of the heme molecule is oxidized by heme oxygenase to biliverdin. In the next metabolic step, biliverdin reductase converts biliverdin to bilirubin. Subsequently, bilirubin is released from the phagocytes into the blood. Before bilirubin is conjugated in the liver, it is poorly soluble in the aqueous environment of the plasma and is bound to albumin to make it more soluble. The process of bilirubin elimination can be divided into three phases: uptake, conjugation, and secretion. **Uptake** refers to the process by which hepatocytes remove the bilirubin bound to albumin from the circulation. Once in the hepatocyte, the lipid soluble bilirubin undergoes **conjugation;** it is combined with a polar molecule such as glucuronic acid to make bilirubin diglucuronide, which is water soluble and more easily secreted into the bile. In the final phase, termed **secretion,** conjugated bilirubin is transported into the bile canaliculus for delivery into the bile ductular system.

Within the gastrointestinal tract, conjugated bilirubin is converted to urobilinogen by bacteria, and a fraction of urobilinogen is reabsorbed from the ileum into the portal blood and returned to the liver by the enterohepatic circulation. The majority of urobilinogen that is absorbed from the gastrointestinal tract is resecreted into bile. Urobilinogen has a low molecular weight and is freely filtered through the glomerulus; low concentrations are normally found in the urine. Urobilinogen that is not absorbed from the intestine becomes oxidized to stercobilin, which is responsible for the color of the feces.

Increased concentrations of conjugated or unconjugated bilirubin in blood is called hyperbilirubinemia. High concentrations of bilirubin can produce icterus (jaundice), a yellow discoloration of tissues especially evident in those tissues rich in elastin such as the aorta and sclera.

The causes of hyperbilirubinemia include the following:

1. Intravascular hemolysis (prehepatic icterus): Overproduction of bilirubin as a consequence of hemolysis, particularly severe intravascular hemolysis, which overwhelms the liver's capacity to remove bilirubin from the plasma and to secrete conjugated bilirubin into bile.
2. Extravascular hemolysis (prehepatic icterus): The destruction of damaged red blood cells by extravascular hemolysis can also increase the burden of bilirubin presented to the liver. Secretion of conjugated bilirubin into bile canaliculi is an energy-dependent process and is the rate-limiting step in bilirubin excretion in most species.
3. Severe hepatic disease (hepatic icterus): Decreased uptake, conjugation, or secretion of bilirubin by hepatocytes arising as a consequence of severe, diffuse hepatic disease, whether acute or chronic.
4. Biliary obstruction (posthepatic icterus): Reduced outflow of bile **(cholestasis).** Cholestasis refers to reduced canalicular flow of bile, which occurs as a consequence of either obstruction of the biliary ducts (extrahepatic cholestasis) or impairment of bile flow within canaliculi (intrahepatic cholestasis).

Intrahepatic cholestasis is commonly associated with a variety of disorders of hepatocytes, because hepatocyte cytoplasm forms the wall of the canaliculus. Intrahepatic cholestasis commences where bile flow originates, that is, in centrilobular areas, and as bile accumulates, the canaliculi become distended and bile pigments discolor the cytoplasm of adjacent hepatocytes (Fig. 2-6). In domestic animals, intrahepatic cholestasis can occur as the consequence of a variety of insults (hepatotoxins, such as endotoxin or toxic chemicals, viral or bacterial infections, and ischemia), all of which can inhibit membrane-bound and cytoplasmic enzymes that facilitate metabolism of either bile acids or bilirubin and secretion of bile across the hepatocyte's membrane into the bile canaliculus.

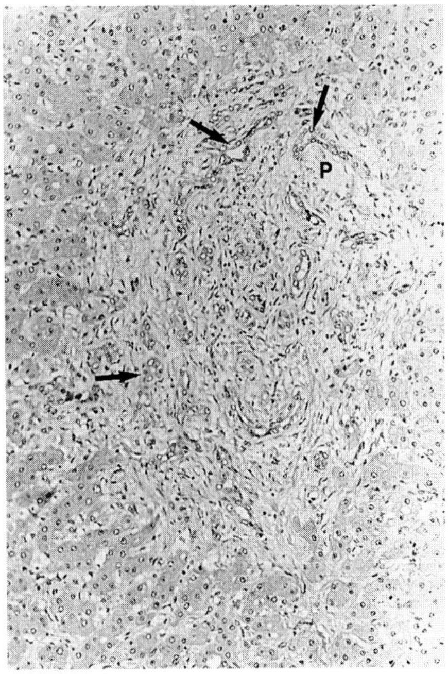

Figure 2-6 Liver; horse. Chronic extrahepatic cholestasis caused by cholelithiasis. There is reduplication of bile ducts *(arrows)* and extensive fibrosis (biliary fibrosis) throughout the portal tract *(P)* as a consequence of prolonged stasis and subsequent leakage of bile. Hematoxylin-eosin (H & E) stain.

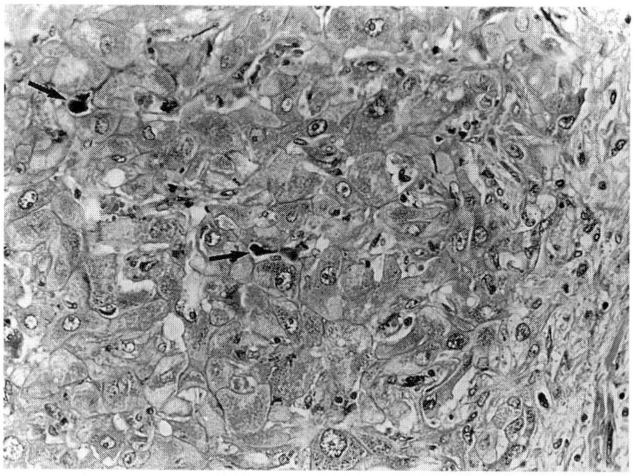

Figure 2-7 Liver; horse. Intrahepatic cholestasis associated with pyrrolizidine alkaloid intoxication. Note that the canaliculi are grossly distended with bile *(arrows)*. H & E stain.

Extrahepatic cholestasis (posthepatic) is a consequence of mechanical obstruction of bile flow, as can occur with choleliths or foreign body obstructions (such as a parasite within the bile duct), neoplasms that compress or constrict the common bile duct, or inflammatory or reparative processes that result in fibrosis that subsequently constricts the lumen of the duct and reduces or prevents outflow of bile. Extrahepatic obstruction initially leads to distension of the bile ducts proximal to the obstruction, and progressive retrograde distension of the intrahepatic bile ductal system. Within the lobule, changes are first obvious within the portal areas, and only later does plugging of canaliculi and stasis of bile occur within the cytoplasm of hepatocytes. Chronic extrahepatic cholestasis may result in extensive hepatic fibrosis (biliary fibrosis) that is centered on the portal areas (Fig. 2-7). On occasion, distension of canaliculi may lead to rupture and extravasation of bile, thereby resulting in focal hepatocellular necrosis.

Obviously, hepatic dysfunction is not the only cause of hyperbilirubinemia and icterus. In fact, icterus in ruminants is usually a consequence of severe intravascular hemolysis and, less often, a sequel to hepatic damage. Horses often manifest icterus with acute hepatic dysfunction, but icterus may or may not occur in horses with chronic hepatic disease. Interestingly, "physiologic icterus" is also common in the horse, and horses deprived of feed for several days can become icteric because uptake of bilirubin from the plasma by hepatocytes is decreased. Icterus in carnivores occurs as a consequence of either hemolysis or hepatic dysfunction. Complete obstruction of bile outflow in any species can lead to extrahepatic cholestasis and icterus. However, in the dog, obstruction of the common duct does not always lead to icterus because supernumerary ducts allow the bile to flow into the duodenum.

Hepatic Encephalopathy

Hepatic failure can result in a metabolic disorder of the central nervous system termed hepatic encephalopathy (synonym: hepatic coma or **portosystemic encephalopathy**). Neurologic manifestations vary from depression and other behavioral changes to mania and convulsions. The central feature of this disorder is abnormal neurotransmission in the central nervous system, as well as the neuromuscular system. Undetermined as yet are the specific metabolites that cause the neurologic dysfunction, but increased concentrations of plasma ammonia derived from amines absorbed from the gastrointestinal tract may be responsible. Normally, amines are absorbed from the intestines into the portal blood and metabolized by the liver. If they bypass the liver and gain access to the systemic circulation, they can exert toxic effects on the brain. These toxic products can enter the systemic circulation by two mechanisms. Blood can be shunted to the systemic circulation before it reaches the liver because of congenital portosystemic shunts or because of portal vein hypertension. Shunting of more than 10% to 15% of portal flow away from the liver is considered abnormal. Alternatively, the toxic products may not be fully eliminated by the liver if there is sufficient liver disease. Hepatic encephalopathy is common in ruminants and horses with hepatic failure, dogs and cats with congenital portosystemic shunts, and animals with end-stage liver disease (hepatic fibrosis and nodular regeneration) that leads to shunting of blood within regenerative nodules.

Metabolic Disturbances of Hepatic Failure

Hepatic failure can be manifested by a variety of metabolic disturbances. The type and duration of the hepatic disorder may influence the nature of the metabolic perturbation.

Bleeding Tendencies. Bleeding tendencies (hemorrhagic diathesis) sometimes accompany hepatic failure. Impaired synthesis of clotting factors, reduced clearance of the products of the clotting process, and metabolic abnormalities affecting platelet function can affect normal clotting, individually or in combination. All clotting factors, with the possible exception of factor VIII, are synthesized in the liver. In acute hepatic failure, diminished synthesis of clotting factors with a short half-life, such as factors V, VII, IX, and X, impairs the coagulation of blood. In chronic liver disease, factor II (prothrombin) deficiency also contributes to diminished coagulation of blood. Diminished clearance of fibrin degradation products (FDP), activated coagulation factors, and plasminogen factors by the damaged liver also perturbs clotting. Metabolic disturbances resulting from hepatic failure can affect platelet function and lead to synthesis of abnormal fibrinogen, termed dysfibrinogenemia. Obstruction of the biliary system prevents the release of bile into the intestinal tract. The resulting impaired fat absorption limits vitamin K uptake from the intestine, which leads to an inactivity of factors II, VII, IX, and X. Acute hepatic failure may also precipitate disseminated intravascular coagulation that can itself cause hemorrhagic diathesis. Acute hepatic failure in the horse, and, perhaps other species, is sometimes accompanied by severe intravascular hemolysis, the cause of which is undetermined.

Hypoalbuminemia. Hypoalbuminemia, as a consequence of hepatic dysfunction, usually reflects severe chronic hepatic disease, because of the relatively long half-life of plasma albumin (which ranges from 8 days in the dog to 21 days in cattle) and the time necessary for portal hypertension to develop. Hypoalbuminemia can occur as a consequence of severe, diffuse chronic hepatic disease that results in both decreased hepatic production of albumin and, because of portal hypertension, increased loss of albumin in ascitic fluid or into the intestinal tract.

Vascular and Hemodynamic Alterations of Hepatic Failure. Chronic hepatic injury typically is accompanied by extensive diffuse fibrosis of the liver, which increases resistance to blood flow through the liver. This, in turn, elevates pressure within the portal vein (portal hypertension). With time, collateral vascular channels open to allow blood in the portal vein to bypass the abnormal liver (acquired portosystemic vascular anastomoses, which connect the portal vein and its tributaries to the systemic venous circulation). In addition, the increased pressure within the hepatic vasculature causes transudation of fluid (modified transudate) into the peritoneal cavity to produce ascites in several species, except, in most cases, horses. Transudation of fluid into the peritoneal cavity can be enhanced by hypoalbuminemia because colloid osmotic pressure of plasma is decreased. Hypoalbuminemia and reduced plasma colloid osmotic pressure arise as a consequence of accelerated albumin loss into the lumen of the intestines and reduced hepatic synthesis of albumin and other plasma proteins. Ascites associated with hepatic fibrosis in chronic liver disease (end-stage liver) or other causes of portal hypertension, such as right-sided heart failure, occurs most commonly in dogs and cats, occasionally in sheep, and is unusual in horses and cattle.

Cutaneous Manifestations

Superficial necrolytic dermatitis (Toxic epidermal necrolysis) is a disease process recognized in some dogs with severe hepatic disease that is characterized by crusting, ulceration, and full-thickness necrosis of the epidermis of the skin. The mechanism of cutaneous injury is not understood. It seems likely that this distinctive cutaneous disorder results from abnormal hepatic metabolism.

Photosensitization is an injury to the cutaneous tissues resulting from activation of photodynamic pigments by ultraviolet light present in the sun's rays. Photodynamic pigments cause injury via the production of oxygen radicals. Cutaneous lesions typically are limited to hairless skin, particularly to lightly or nonpigmented areas of skin. The sources of photodynamic pigments that can induce photosensitization are from plants and certain drugs, and only in hepatogenous (secondary) photosensitization is hepatic dysfunction responsible for photosensitization.

1. **Primary photosensitization** is the disease that occurs after some primary (preformed) photodynamic agent is deposited in tissues following its absorption into the blood after ingestion. Certain plants, such as *Hypericum perforatum* (St. John's wort), *Fagopyrum sagittatum* (buckwhcat), and *Cymopterus watsonii* (spring parsley) contain compounds that are photodynamic. Some pharmaceutical agents, such as phenothiazine, tetracyclines, thiazides, and sulfonomides can cause photosensitization through their photodynamic activity. Lesions are described in Chapter 11.
2. **Hepatogenous** or **secondary photosensitization** occurs in herbivores when hepatic dysfunction or biliary obstruction impairs normal excretion of phylloerythrin in bile. Phylloerythrin, a photodynamic agent, is produced from the chlorophyll contained in ingested plants by microflora of the gastrointestinal tract of herbivores. Phylloerythrin is normally absorbed from the intestines and excreted in bile, using the same pathway as bilirubin; thus, hepatocellular dysfunction or biliary obstruction prevents normal excretion and allows high concentrations of phylloerythrin to accumulate in blood and cutaneous tissues. Hepatic photosensitivity is a consequence of the increased serum concentration of phylloerythrin, and this may occur in either acute or chronic hepatic disease.
3. **Inherited photosensitization** occurs in a variety of species including cattle, sheep, and cats as the result of metabolic disorders that lead to an accumulation of photodynamic substances. Cattle and cats have inherited abnormalities of porphyrin metabolism, and accumulated porphyrins lead to cutaneous injury. In mutant Corriedale and Southdown sheep, a syndrome of photosensitization becomes evident in lambs once they begin to ingest plant material. An abnormality in the uptake of bilirubin and phylloerythrin inhibits normal excretion of these substances and results in photosensitization.

Developmental Anomalies and Incidental Findings

Developmental anomalies of the liver occur in domestic animals, although most are of little consequence.

Congenital Cysts

These cysts can be found within the livers of all domestic species, and are usually an incidental finding. The potential origins of congenital cysts include the intrahepatic bile ducts and the hepatic capsule. Although these cysts are considered to be congenital anomalies, they can

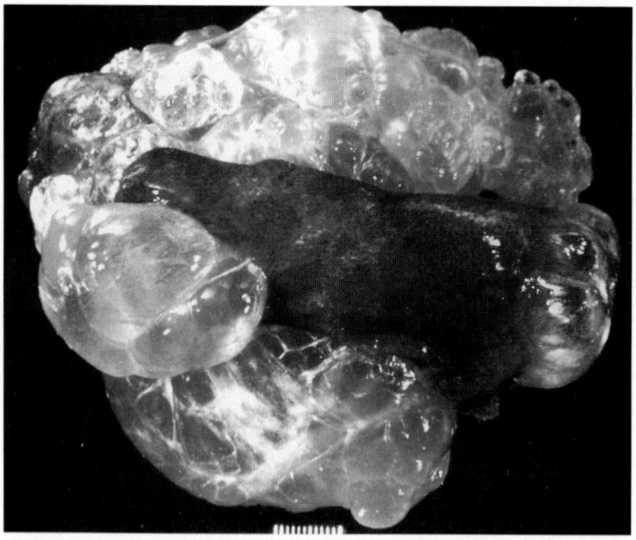

Figure 2-8 Liver; cat. Multilobular biliary cysts have replaced much of the parenchyma in the affected portion of liver. Bar = 1 cm.

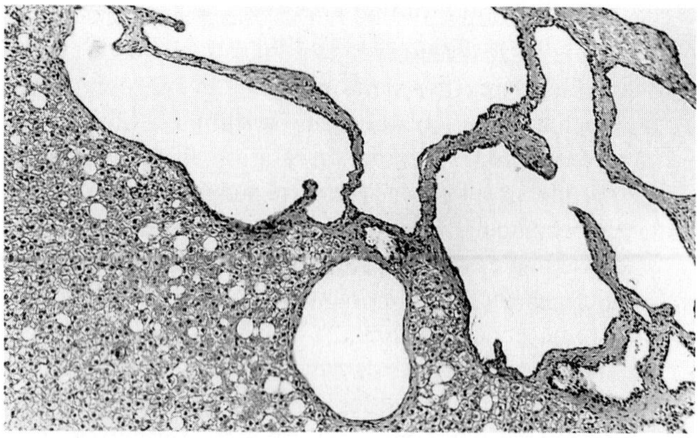

Figure 2-9 Liver, biliary cysts; cat. Note that the biliary cysts are lined by a single layer of biliary epithelium. H & E stain.

be found in animals of any age. There is some uncertainty as to whether cysts that occur within the liver of adult cats, which typically are multiple and affect extensive areas of the liver, are developmental anomalies or benign cystic neoplasms (Figs. 2-8 and 2-9). Congenital polycystic hepatic disease, characterized by numerous epithelial-lined cysts in the liver and kidneys, occurs in the dog, and the Cairn terrier is predisposed. Congenital cysts must be distinguished from parasitic cysts, particularly cysticerci.

Hepatic Displacement

Displacement of the liver into the thoracic cavity, called a diaphragmatic hernia, can occur when there is a defect in the diaphragm. A congenital malformation that leaves an opening in the diaphragm or trauma that ruptures the

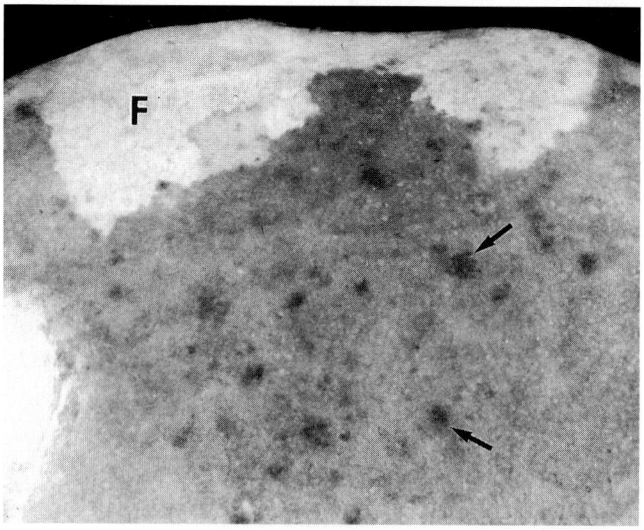

Figure 2-10 Liver, capsular surface; cow. Tension lipidosis. Note the pale area of fatty infiltration *(F)* and scattered areas of telangiectasis *(arrows)*.

diaphragm can result in herniation of the liver into the thoracic cavity.

Tension Lipidosis

Discrete, pale areas of parenchyma at the liver margins are common in cattle and horses (Figs. 2-10 and 2-11). These foci typically occur adjacent to the insertion of a ligament (serosal) attachment, and it is proposed that these attachments impede blood supply to the subjacent hepatic parenchyma by exerting tension on the capsule. Affected hepatocytes most probably accumulate fat within their cytoplasm (lipidosis) as a consequence of hypoxia. These lesions are of no functional significance to the liver.

Capsular Fibrosis

Discrete fibrous tags or plaques are frequently present on the diaphragmatic surface of the liver and on the adjacent diaphragm of the horse (Fig. 2-12). Resolution of nonseptic peritonitis, rather than of parasitic nematode migration tracts, has been proposed as the cause of this capsular fibrosis.

Postmortem Change

Autolysis of the liver occurs rapidly and can be advanced before it is obvious in most other tissues. Bacteria released from the gastrointestinal tract agonally into the portal circulation reach the liver, where they proliferate rapidly after death. This process is especially rapid in large animals during hot weather, particularly cattle, in which fermentation in the adjacent rumen produces heat, and pigs, which are often well insulated by fat. Pale areas appear on the capsular surface as bacterial degradation begins. In time,

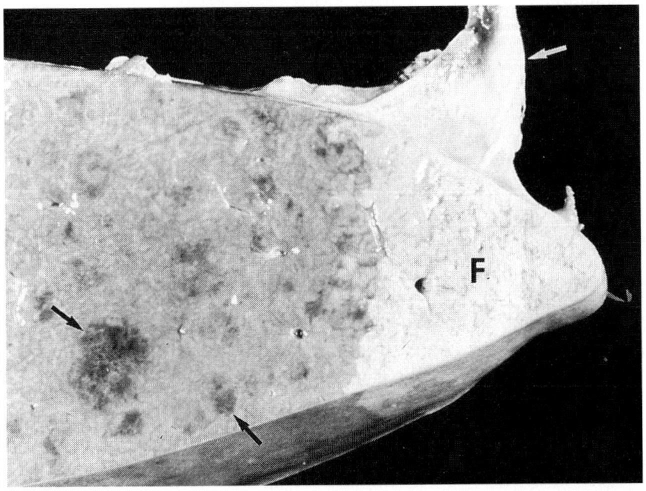

Figure 2-11 Liver, cut surface; cow. Tension lipidosis. Area of fatty infiltration *(F)* adjacent to mesenteric attachment adjacent to the affected portion *(white arrow)*. Areas of telangiectasis are indicated by the black arrows.

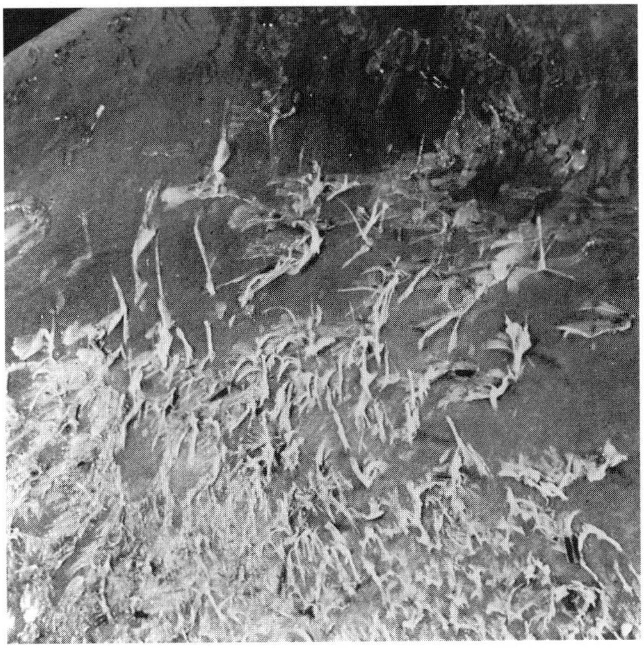

Figure 2-12 Liver, diaphragmatic surface; horse. Capsular fibrosis. Note the fibrous tags scattered across the capsule.

the organ becomes green-blue as bacteria degrade blood pigments to hydrogen sulfide. The liver in contact with the gallbladder is quickly discolored by bile pigment that has passed through the wall of the gallbladder. The consistency of the organ becomes puttylike, and gas bubbles may form beneath the capsule and in the parenchyma from bacterial fermentation.

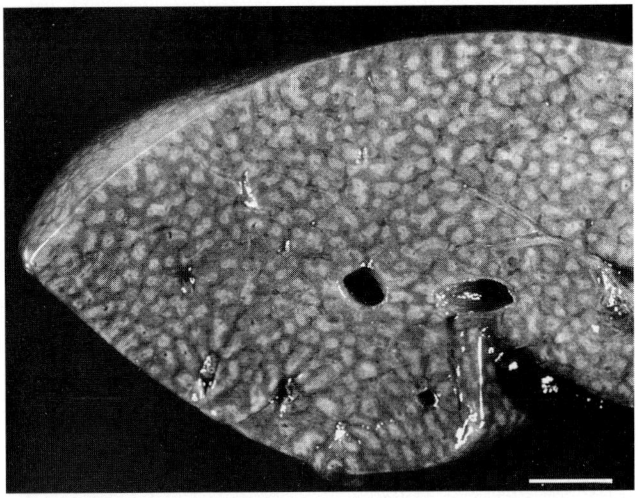

Figure 2-13 Liver, cut surface; cat. Enhanced lobular pattern. Note accentuation of the normal lobular pattern. Bar = 5 mm. *Courtesy Dr. R. Fairley.*

Hemodynamic and Vascular Disorders

The Liver and Anemia

The centrilobular (periacinar) region of the lobule receives blood last; thus, it is the least oxygenated and the effects of hypoxia are usually manifested first in this area. Acute severe anemia, regardless of cause, can cause centrilobular degeneration and even necrosis of hepatocytes. This typically occurs in severe anemias of precipitous onset. Chronic anemia can cause atrophy of centrilobular hepatocytes, which results in dilation and congestion of sinusoids. Livers from animals with severe anemia, whether acute or chronic, typically have an enhanced lobular pattern (Figs. 2-13 and 2-14) that is evident on both the capsular and cut surfaces of the organ (see description of enhanced lobular pattern in the next section).

Congenital Portosystemic Shunts

Congenital portosystemic shunts are abnormal vascular channels that allow blood within the portal venous system to bypass the liver and to drain into the systemic circulation. Congenital shunts can be either intra- or extrahepatic in location, but are usually limited to a single vessel. A variety of shunts have been described. One type involves failure of closure of the ductus venosus, a normal vessel during fetal development that carries blood from the portal vein to the caudal vena cava, that occurs most often in large breed dogs. Other types of congenital shunts, such as portal vein to caudal vena cava and portal vein to azygous vein, occur more often in small breeds of dogs. Shunts have been described in several species, but occur most commonly in the dog and cat. Affected animals are typically stunted and frequently have signs of hepatic encephalopathy. The liver is small and may have a characteristic histologic appearance. Affected livers have lobular atrophy, and portal areas are characterized by reduplication of arterioles and portal veins may be small or absent (Fig. 2-15). Typically, the portal vein pressure is normal in congenital shunts and ascites is not associated with these lesions. The vascular anastomoses are often difficult to identify without benefit of antemortem imaging studies.

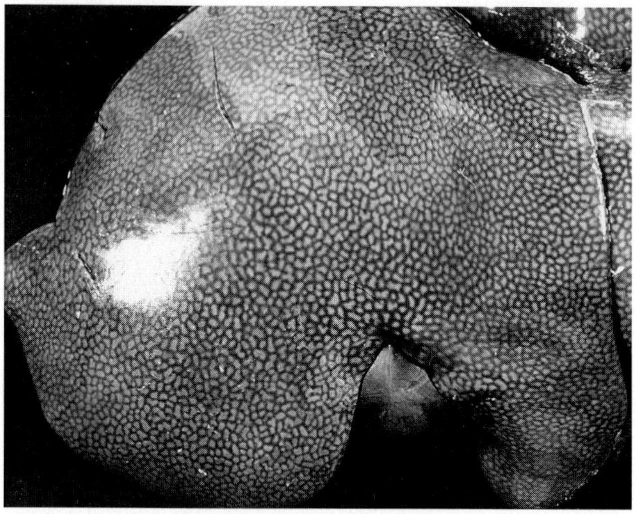

Figure 2-14 Liver, diaphragmatic surface; cat. Enhanced lobular pattern. This is not a specific change, as it may be associated with zonal hepatocellular degeneration or necrosis (regardless of lobular location), passive congestion, and diffuse cellular infiltration within the liver (often reflecting disseminated cholangitis, diffuse portal hepatitis, or hepatic involvement with hematopoietic neoplasms, such as lymphosarcoma and myeloproliferative disorders).

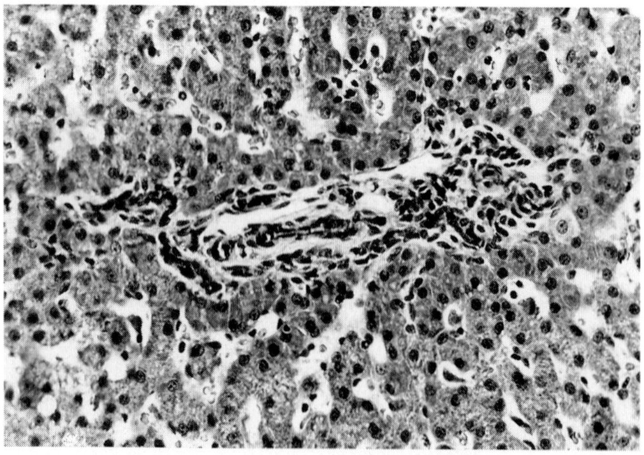

Figure 2-15 Liver; dog. Congenital portosystemic vascular anastomosis. Portal areas are abnormal because they lack a portal vein and contain numerous small-caliber arterioles. H & E stain.

Portal Hypertension and Its Causes

Increased pressure within the portal vein can arise from disturbances of venous blood flow in any of three sites. Increased resistance to venous outflow in the hepatic vein (as discussed previously in passive hepatic congestion) is termed **posthepatic.** Chronic passive congestion is the most common posthepatic cause of portal hypertension. Far less common is portal hypertension occurring as a result of partial or complete occlusion of the hepatic veins (Budd-Chiari syndrome), or the adjacent caudal vena cava. **Intrahepatic** portal hypertension arises from increased resistance to blood flow within the sinusoids. Chronic hepatic disease that typically results in increased collagen and loss of normal lobular architecture is the most common intrahepatic cause of portal hypertension. Arterioportal shunts (discussed later) in the hepatic parenchyma can also cause portal hypertension. **Posthepatic** portal hypertension occurs when blood flow through the portal vein is impaired. This may occur from thrombosis, invasion by neoplasms, or other causes.

Regardless of cause, persistent portal hypertension can lead to acquired portosystemic shunts. These shunts are usually numerous and composed of distended thin-walled veins that may connect the mesenteric veins and the caudal vena cava (Fig. 2-16). Ascites is common with these types of shunts because of the associated portal hypertension.

Passive Congestion. Right-sided heart failure increases the pressure within the caudal vena cava, which later extends to the hepatic vein and its tributaries. Passive congestion may be either acute or chronic, and the appearance of the liver differs with the duration and severity of the congestion. Passive congestion is initially seen as distension of

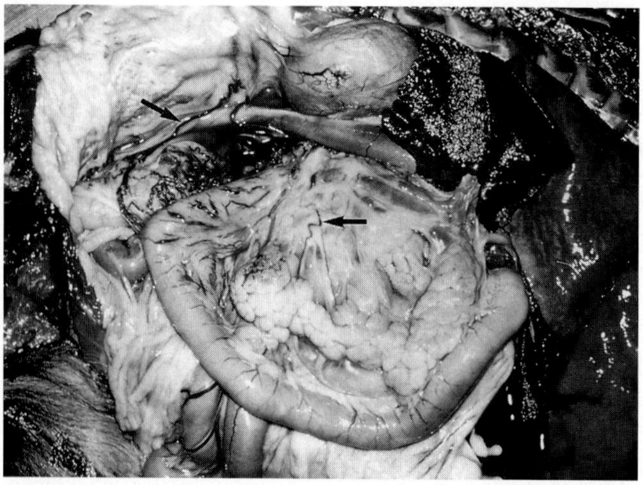

Figure 2-16 Abdomen; dog. Acquired portosystemic anastomoses secondary to portal hypertension and subsequent to chronic passive congestion. Numerous prominent veins *(arrows)* within the mesentery allow blood in the portal venous system to bypass the liver and directly enter the systemic circulation. *Courtesy Dr. R. Fairley.*

central veins and centrilobular sinusoids. Persistent centrilobular hypoxia leads to atrophy or loss of hepatocytes and, eventually, to fibrosis about central veins. Fibrosis of the central vein (phlebosclerosis) may also occur.

Acute congestion of the liver produces slight enlargement of the organ, and blood flows freely when the liver is incised. The intrinsic lobular pattern of the liver may be slightly more pronounced, particularly on the cut surface, because centrilobular areas are congested (dark red) in contrast to the more normal color of the remainder of the lobule.

Chronic passive congestion leads to persistent hypoxia in centrilobular areas and, because of oxygen and nutrient deprivation, the centrilobular hepatocytes atrophy, degenerate, or eventually undergo necrosis. As a result, sinusoids in these areas are dilated and congested and grossly appear red, whereas periportal hepatocytes frequently undergo lipidosis (fatty degeneration) because of hypoxia, thereby causing this area of the lobule to appear yellow. The result is accentuation of the lobular pattern of the liver, referred to as an enhanced lobular or reticular pattern. It is especially evident on the cut surface of the liver; the enhanced lobular pattern that occurs with severe chronic passive congestion has been likened to the appearance of the cut surface of a nutmeg, and so is termed the **nutmeg liver.** This pattern is not unique to passive congestion, however, and is encountered with other processes, such as zonal hepatic necrosis. In addition to an enhanced lobular pattern, chronic passive congestion is characterized by focal fibrous thickening of Glisson's capsule, and, in severe cases, widespread hepatic fibrosis, particularly around central veins. Central veins are also fibrosed, which reduces their luminal diameters (Figs. 2-17 to 2-19).

Passive congestion of the liver can occur in any species and is almost always the consequence of cardiac dysfunction. Chronic passive congestion is particularly common in aged dogs and often occurs as a consequence of valvular insufficiency from endocardiosis (mucoid degeneration) of the right atrioventricular valve. Acute

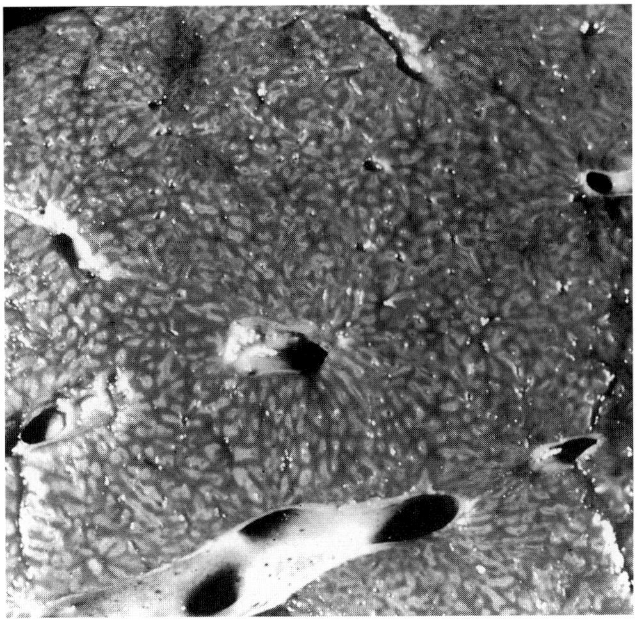

Figure 2-18 Liver, cut surface; cow. Chronic passive hepatic congestion secondary to severe fibrinous pericarditis. Note enhanced lobular (nutmeg) pattern. The irregular light gray foci are portal tracts. The hepatic parenchyma between the portal tracts is congested. *Courtesy Dr. C. Miller.*

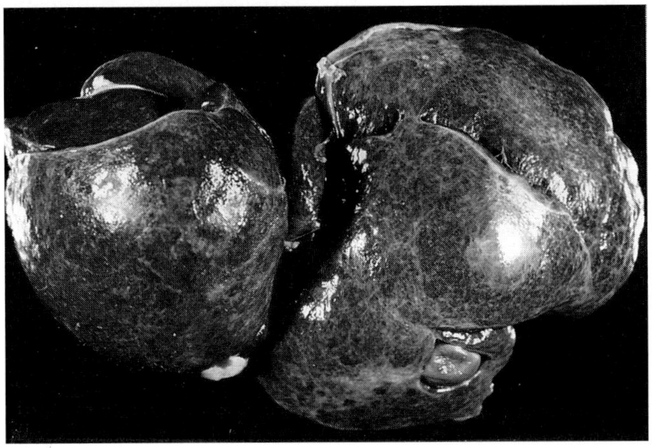

Figure 2-17 Liver, diaphragmatic surfaces, dog. Chronic passive hepatic congestion. The liver is enlarged and has rounded margins. *Courtesy Dr. K. Sokoe.*

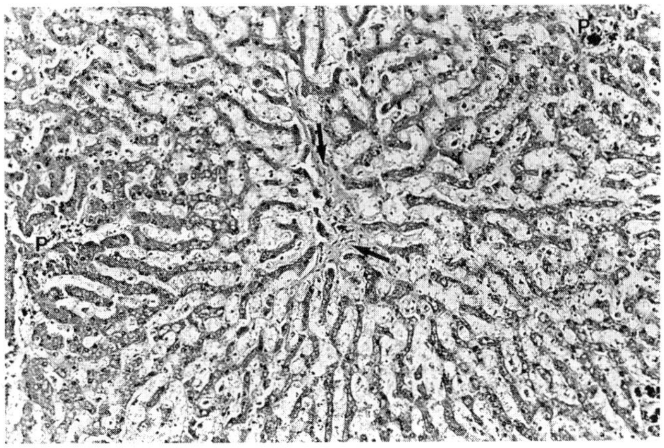

Figure 2-19 Liver; dog. Chronic passive hepatic congestion. Hepatic fibrosis is most severe in centrilobular areas *(arrows)*. The central vein is encircled with connective tissue. Adjacent hepatic plates are atrophic, and sinusoids are excessively dilated. Hepatic plates are of relatively normal thickness around the portal tracts *(P)*. H & E stain.

passive congestion, on the other hand, can occur as a consequence of acute right heart failure, which has a wide variety of causes.

Arterioportal Shunts (Anastomoses)

Arterioportal shunts, either acquired or congenital, occur in the dog and cat, are direct communications between the hepatic artery and branches of the portal vein, and may occur anywhere within the liver. Shunting of blood may lead to portal hypertension and subsequent development of acquired portocaval shunts and ascites; clinical signs are probably the result of the portosystemic shunting of blood.

Hepatic Venoocclusive Disease

The distinctive lesion of this syndrome is characterized by intimal thickening and occlusion of the central vein by fibrous connective tissue. The consequence is passive hepatic congestion and resultant hepatic injury, which may progress to hepatic failure and its associated constellation of signs. The lesion is not etiologically specific, but can follow pyrrolizidine alkaloid– or aflatoxin-induced hepatic injury. An extremely high incidence is recognized in captive exotic cats such as cheetahs, possibly because of the ingestion of large amounts of vitamin A.

Telangiectasis

Telangiectasis means the marked dilatation of sinusoids in areas where hepatocytes have been lost. Grossly, these areas appear as variably sized (from 1 to 5 mm) dark blue (from unoxygenated blood) foci within the liver (Figs. 2-10 and 2-11). Telangiectasis is particularly common in cattle and, apparently, is of no clinical significance. It also occurs in old cats where it can be mistaken for vascular tumors such as hemangioma or hemangiosarcoma.

Infarction

Infarction of the liver occurs infrequently because of the organ's dual blood supply from the hepatic artery and portal vein. Infarcts are usually sharply delineated and may be either dark red or pale. They tend to occur at the margins of the liver. Torsion of individual lobes of the liver, which occurs infrequently, can cause vascular occlusion and infarction of the affected lobe.

Metabolic Disturbances and Hepatic Accumulations

Hepatic Lipidosis or Fatty Liver

Lipids are normally transported to the liver from adipose tissue and the gastrointestinal tract in the form of free fatty acids and chylomicrons, respectively. Within hepatocytes, free fatty acids are esterified to triglycerides that are complexed with apoproteins to form low-density lipoproteins, and these are released into the plasma as a readily available energy source for a variety of tissues. Some oxidation of fatty acids for energy production occurs within hepatocytes and some fatty acids are converted to phospholipid and cholesterol esters. With the exception of ruminants, the liver also actively produces lipids from amino acids and glucose.

The presence of excessive lipid within the liver is termed hepatic lipidosis or fatty liver and occurs when the rate of triglyceride accumulation within hepatocytes exceeds either their rate of metabolic degradation or their release as lipoproteins. Hepatic lipidosis is obviously not a specific disease entity, but can occur as a sequel to a variety of perturbations of normal lipid metabolism. The potential mechanisms responsible for excessive accumulation of lipids within the liver include the following:

1. Excessive entry of fatty acids into the liver, which occurs as a consequence of excessive dietary intake of fat or increased mobilization of triglycerides from adipose tissue as a result of increased demand (e.g., lactation, starvation, and endocrine abnormalities).
2. Abnormal hepatocyte function leads to accumulation of triglycerides within hepatocytes as a result of decreased energy for oxidation of fatty acids within hepatocytes.
3. Excessive dietary intake of carbohydrates results in the synthesis of increased amounts of fatty acids with formation of excessive triglycerides within hepatocytes.
4. Increased esterification of fatty acids to triglycerides in response to increased amounts of glucose and insulin, which stimulate the rate of triglyceride synthesis from glucose or from prolonged increases in dietary chylomicrons.
5. Decreased apoprotein synthesis and subsequent decreased production and export of lipoprotein from hepatocytes.
6. Impaired secretion of lipoprotein from the liver caused by secretory defects produced by hepatotoxins or drugs.

It must be stressed that these are potential mechanisms (some being more significant than others depending on the condition of the animal) and that more than one defect might occur in any given hepatic disorder. Regardless of cause, the gross appearance of hepatic lipidosis is highly characteristic. With progressive accumulation of lipid, the liver enlarges and becomes yellow (Fig. 2-20). In mild cases, lipids may only accumulate in specific portions of each lobule, such as centrilobular regions, thereby imparting an enhanced lobular pattern to the liver. In extreme cases, the entire liver is affected, and the organ becomes considerably enlarged and has a markedly greasy texture. The parenchyma of severely affected livers bulges from the cut surface when incised and liver sections float in formaldehyde solutions. Lipid vacuoles are readily detected within the cytoplasm of hepatocytes (Fig. 2-21).

Specific causes and syndromes of hepatic lipidosis in domestic animals include the following.

1. Dietary causes of hepatic lipidosis include simple dietary excess in monogastric animals such as a high-fat or high-cholesterol diet. Hepatic lipidosis is

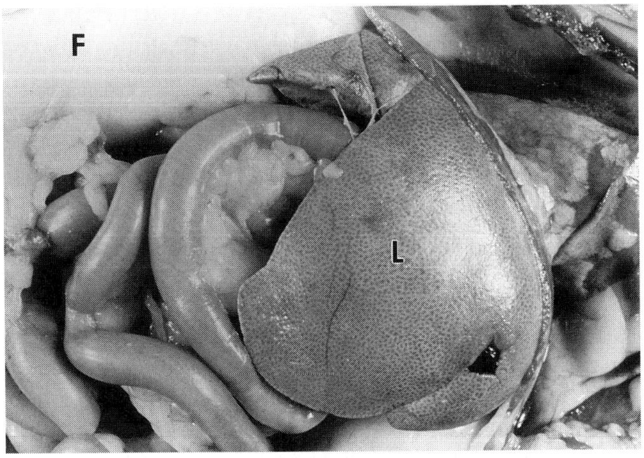

Figure 2-20 Abdomen; cat. Idiopathic fatty liver syndrome. The liver *(L)* is swollen and yellow, and the animal has extensive fat deposits *(F)*.

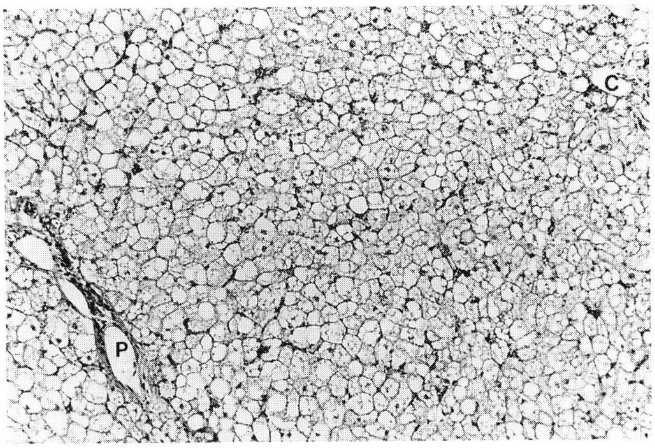

Figure 2-21 Liver; cow. Ketosis. Diffuse cytoplasmic accumulation of lipid is evident within the hepatocytes throughout the liver. Terminal hepatic venule *(C)*; portal tract *(P)*. H & E stain.

especially common in ruminants with high-energy demands, such as those in peak lactation or late gestation, and reflects increased entry of lipids into the liver as a result of increased mobilization of lipids from adipose tissue. Obese animals are particularly predisposed to develop hepatic lipidosis when dietary intake is restricted.

2. Toxic and anoxic causes of hepatic lipidosis are common. Sublethal (reversible) injury to hepatocytes frequently results in accumulation of lipid within the affected cell. Injury to hepatocytes can lead to accumulation of lipids because of decreased formation or export of lipoproteins by hepatocytes and decreased oxidation of fatty acids within hepatocytes.
3. Ketosis is a metabolic disease that results from impaired metabolism of carbohydrate and volatile fatty acids. Ketone bodies are derived from acetyl-acetyl coenzyme A (CoA), which is a normal intermediate in the oxidation of fatty acids. In pregnant and lactating animals, there is a continuous demand for glucose and amino acids, and ketosis results when fat metabolism, which occurs in response to the increased energy demands, becomes excessive. Ketosis is characterized by increased concentrations of ketone bodies in blood (hyperketonemia), hypoglycemia, and low concentrations of hepatic glycogen. Ketosis is common in ruminants and usually occurs during peak lactation, whereas ketosis of sheep usually occurs in late gestation, particularly in ewes carrying twins; this latter disease is known as pregnancy toxemia.
4. **Bovine fatty liver syndrome,** also known as **fatty liver disease,** is mechanistically similar to ketosis. In dairy cattle, the disease is usually encountered in obese animals within a few days after parturition and is often precipitated by an event that causes anorexia such as retained placenta, metritis, mastitis, abomasal displacement, or parturient paresis. Affected beef cattle are typically obese, and the disease occurs within a few days before parturition. Accumulation of lipid within the liver is the result of both increased mobilization of lipids from adipose tissue that results in increased influx of fatty acids to the liver and defective hepatocytic function, which results in decreased export of lipoprotein from the liver.
5. **Feline fatty liver syndrome** is a distinct syndrome of idiopathic hepatic lipidosis recognized in cats. Typically affected cats are obese and anorectic and have no other diseases that could cause hepatic lipidosis. Cats with this type of hepatic lipidosis (Fig. 2-20) frequently develop hepatic failure, icterus, and subsequently hepatic encephalopathy.
6. Hepatic lipidosis occurs in ponies and miniature horses, and Shetland ponies are predisposed. The condition usually occurs in pregnant or lactating mares, characteristically after an event that causes anorexia. In addition to marked hepatic lipidosis, affected ponies may also manifest signs of hepatic encephalopathy or terminal disseminated intravascular coagulation and hemorrhagic diathesis.
7. **White liver disease** is a syndrome in sheep and goats that is caused by dietary deficiencies in vitamin B_{12} and cobalt. Affected animals sustain damage to their livers, but the characteristic hepatic lipid accumulation is believed to be secondary to anorexia and anemia.
8. Endocrine disorders, such as diabetes mellitus and hypothyroidism, can produce hepatic lipidosis in a variety of species. In these cases, hepatic lipidosis is obviously but one manifestation of abnormal metabolism. The accumulation of lipids in the liver in the diabetic animal is the result of increased fat

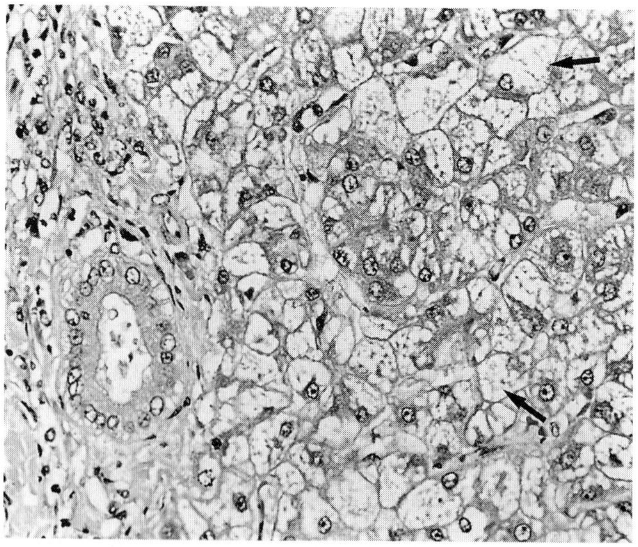

Figure 2-22 Liver; dog. Glucocorticoid-induced hepatopathy. The swollen hepatocytes *(arrows)* have extensive cytoplasmic vacuoles. H & E stain.

mobilization and decreased utilization of lipids by injured hepatocytes.

Glycogen Accumulation

Glucose is normally stored within hepatocytes as glycogen and is often present in large amounts after feeding. Excessive hepatic accumulation of glycogen occurs with the metabolic perturbations associated with diseases such as diabetes mellitus and the glycogen storage diseases. In these instances, hepatic involvement is just one manifestation of a systemic disease process.

Glucocorticoid-induced hepatocellular degeneration is a specific disorder characterized by excessive hepatic accumulation of glycogen. Excessive amounts of endogenous or exogenous glucocorticoids cause extensive swelling of hepatocytes from the accumulation of glycogen. Glucocorticoids induce glycogen synthetase and so enhance hepatic storage of glycogen. Glycogen accumulation leads to pronounced swelling of hepatocytes (up to 10 times normal volume), particularly those in the midzonal areas (Fig. 2-22). In severe cases of glucocorticoid-induced hepatocellular degeneration (often referred to as steroid-induced hepatopathy) the liver is enlarged and pale, but otherwise unremarkable. The disorder occurs in dogs, and frequently is iatrogenic, but can also be a consequence of hyperadrenocorticism. The diagnosis can be confirmed on the basis of the characteristic microscopic appearance of the liver and identification of the source of the excess glucocorticoids.

Amyloidosis

Hepatic amyloidosis occurs in most species of domestic animals. Amyloidosis is not a single disease entity, but a term used for various diseases that lead to the deposition of proteins that are composed of β-pleated sheets of nonbranching fibrils. The physical properties of amyloid are responsible for its birefringence and characteristic apple green appearance in Congo red–stained sections viewed under polarized light. As many as 15 distinct amyloid proteins have been identified, but hepatic amyloid is usually derived from one of three types. In primary amyloidosis, the amyloid protein AL (amyloid light chain) is derived from immunoglobulin light chains synthesized by plasma cell neoplasms. In secondary amyloidosis, by far the most common type seen in veterinary medicine, a serum protein synthesized by the liver, called serum amyloid–associated (SAA) protein is the precursor to AA (amyloid-associated) fibrils. Secondary amyloidosis occurs as a consequence of prolonged inflammation such as chronic infection or tissue destruction. The third type, inherited or familiar amyloidosis, is uncommon in animals but occurs in shar-pei dogs and Abyssinian and Siamese breeds of cats.

Regardless of the cause, amyloid usually accumulates in the space of Disse and impairs the normal access of plasma to hepatocytes. Amyloid deposits can produce varying degrees of hepatomegaly, and extensive accumulations cause the liver to appear pale. In severe cases, affected animals may have clinical signs of either hepatic dysfunction or failure, and because the liver is more fragile, liver rupture and exsanguination may occur, especially in the horse. Frequently, amyloid is also deposited within the kidneys, particularly the glomeruli. Renal failure often occurs before signs of hepatic dysfunction are manifested.

Copper Accumulation

Copper poisoning is included as a metabolic disorder because hepatic injury in copper poisoning of domestic animals frequently is the result of progressive accumulation of copper within the liver. This occurs in domestic animals, especially sheep, in which storage of copper is poorly regulated. Also, hereditary disorders of copper metabolism have been described in dogs.

Copper is an essential trace element of all cells, but even a modest excess of copper can be life threatening because copper must be properly sequestered to avoid toxicosis. Normally, serum copper is bound to ceruloplasmin and hepatic copper is bound to metallothionein. In cases of excess, the copper distribution is initially diffuse throughout the hepatic cytoplasm, but in later stages it is concentrated within lysosomes. Excess copper, like excess iron, can lead to the production of reactive oxygen species that initiate destructive lipid peroxidation reactions that affect the mitochondrial as well as other cellular membranes. In domestic animals, copper toxicosis usually occurs as a consequence of one of the following:

1. Simple dietary excess in ruminants, occurring, for example, from excessive dietary supplementation as

an overcorrection for copper deficiency or from contamination of pasture with copper from sprays or fertilizer. It also occurs in sheep that have access to copper-containing mineral blocks formulated for cattle.

2. Animals grazing on pastures with normal concentrations of copper but inadequate concentrations of molybdenum in the soil, which antagonizes copper uptake by the plant.
3. Pasturing herbivores on fields with plants that contain hepatotoxic phytotoxins, usually pyrrolizidine alkaloids. *Heliotropium, Crotalaria,* and *Senecio* species are common examples of such plants. Copper is excreted in the bile, and hepatic diseases that result in cholestasis are particularly likely to produce excessive accumulation of copper within the liver, even when dietary intake of copper is not excessive. Pyrrolizidines prevent hepatocellular proliferation by their toxic action on the spindle during mitosis. This failure to replace necrotic hepatocytes leads to ever-increasing copper load in surviving hepatocytes, as these hepatocytes take up the copper released by the dying cells.
4. Hereditary disorders of copper metabolism, as occur in Bedlington and West Highland white terriers. The disorder is best characterized in Bedlington terriers that have an autosomal recessive inheritance of abnormal copper binding by metallothionein that leads to impaired biliary excretion of copper, which results in progressive accumulation within the liver.

The consequences of excessive accumulation of copper within the liver of domestic animals are species-dependent. In ruminants, particularly sheep, copper accumulates within the liver over a period of time (for one of the first three reasons listed above), but some event triggers sudden release of copper, which is followed by acute, severe intravascular hemolysis and hepatocellular necrosis. Necrosis of the liver is extensive and affects centrilobular and midzonal regions most consistently, but massive necrosis can occur. Despite the acute and fulminant nature of the terminal event, this process is referred to as **chronic copper poisoning** to distinguish it from disease associated with simple copper intoxication, which causes gastroenteritis. In contrast, in the livers of Bedlington terriers and to a lesser extent, in West Highland white terriers, both of which have hereditary metabolic disorders of copper metabolism, copper continues to accumulate, leading to ongoing necrosis of hepatocytes, chronic inflammation, replacement fibrosis, and eventually to an end-stage liver and signs of hepatic failure. Excessive concentrations of hepatic copper may be present in other breeds of dog including the Doberman pinscher, Skye terrier, American and English cocker spaniel, Dalmatian, and Labrador retriever, although the significance of copper in the hepatic disease of these breeds of dog is uncertain. These diseases are discussed in the section on canine chronic hepatitis.

Pigment Accumulation

Pigments are colored substances, some of which are normal cellular constituents, while others accumulate only in abnormal circumstances.

1. **Bile pigments** may accumulate in excessive amounts as a consequence of either extrahepatic or intrahepatic cholestasis and typically produce icterus and yellow to green discoloration of the liver.
2. **Hemosiderin** is an iron-containing, golden-brown, granular pigment. In macrophages, hemosiderin is derived from the breakdown of erythrocytes that have been phagocytosed. Iron bound to a plasma glycoprotein called transferrin is the primary source of hemosiderin in hepatocytes. Other sources of iron include hemoglobin bound to haptoglobin or free hemoglobin as in cases of intravascular hemolysis. Within the hepatocyte, iron complexes with apoferritin to form ferritin, the initial iron storage protein. As iron accumulates within the hepatocyte, aggregates of ferritin molecules form hemosiderin. Most hemosiderin in Kupffer cells and other macrophages located in tissues throughout the body is derived from breakdown of erythrocytes, whereas most hepatocellular hemosiderin is derived from iron present in transferrin and to a lesser extent hemoglobin. Hemosiderin forms in the liver when there is local or systemic excess of iron, such as when erythrocytic breakdown is excessive (e.g., hemolytic anemia), and within areas of hepatic necrosis. An excessive systemic load of iron that is characterized by abundant hemosiderin in a variety of tissues without impairment of organ function is called hemosiderosis. In contrast, hemochromatosis is an abnormal increased storage of iron within the body associated with hepatic dysfunction. Marked accumulation of iron can produce a dark brown or even a black liver.
3. **Lipofuscin** is an insoluble pigment that is yellow-brown to dark brown and is derived from incomplete oxidation of lipids such as those in cell membranes. Lipofuscin is progressively oxidized with time; thus, it actually is a group of lipid pigments, all of which consist of polymers of lipid, phospholipid, and protein (and minimal carbohydrate in early forms). **Ceroid** is the earliest form of lipofuscin and the least oxidized. Amounts of lipofuscin present in the liver tend to increase with age, hence the appellation "wear and tear" pigment.
4. **Melanin** is an endogenous pigment that is dark brown or black. Benign disorders of melanin pigmentation are usually designated as **melanosis.** Congenital melanosis of the liver occurs in swine

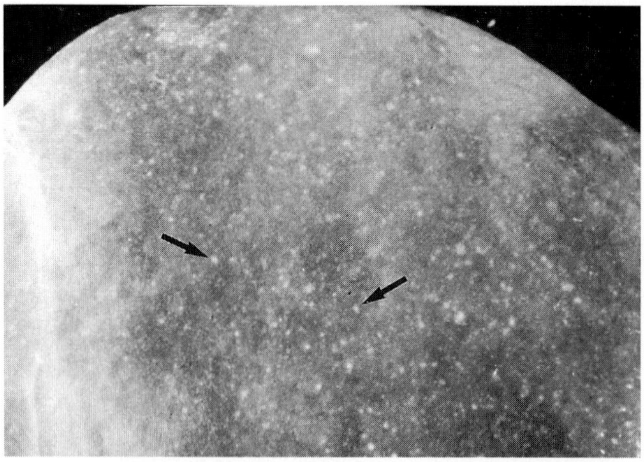

Figure 2-23 Liver; foal. Random hepatic necrosis in a foal with septicemia caused by *E. coli*. Multiple pale foci of necrosis are evident on the capsular surface *(arrows)*. *Courtesy Dr. K. Thompson.*

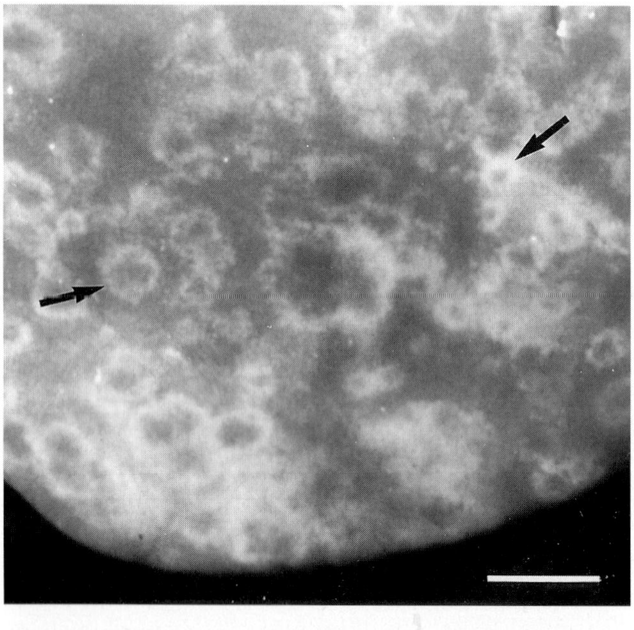

Figure 2-24 Liver; lamb. Random hepatic necrosis in an aborted lamb caused by *Campylobacter fetus* infection. Arrows indicate areas of necrosis. Bar = 1 cm. *Courtesy Dr. B. Johnson.*

and ruminants and produces variably sized areas of discoloration of the liver. Acquired "melanosis" of sheep has been described in Australia and is associated with the ingestion of certain plants.

5. **Liver flukes** specifically produce a very dark excreta that contains a mixture of iron and porphyrin. These excreta produce the characteristic discoloration of bile that occurs in fascioliasis *(Fasciola hepatica)*, and is especially pronounced in the migratory tracts produced by *Fascioloides magna* in bovine livers.

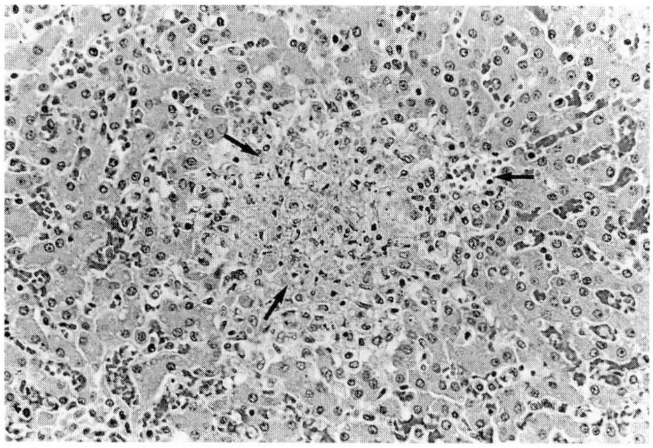

Figure 2-25 Liver; horse. Random hepatic necrosis in an aborted fetus caused by equine herpesvirus. A focal area of necrosis is outlined by the arrows. H & E stain.

Hepatic Injury and Inflammation

The high metabolic rate of hepatocytes renders them highly susceptible to metabolic disturbances that lead to cellular degeneration and necrosis. This section considers the patterns of hepatic degeneration, responses of the liver to injury, and inflammation of the liver and concludes with descriptions of various infectious and toxic disorders of the liver in domestic animals.

Patterns of Hepatocellular Degeneration and Necrosis

Although the liver is subjected to a wide variety of different insults, the cellular degeneration or necrosis that results invariably occurs in one of three morphologic patterns.

Random hepatocellular degeneration or necrosis is characterized by the presence of either single-cell necrosis throughout the liver or multifocal aggregates of necrotic hepatocytes. These areas are scattered randomly throughout the liver; there is no predictable location within lobules. This pattern is typical of many infectious agents, including viruses, bacteria, and certain protozoa, that arrive at the liver hematogenously. Gross lesions are discrete pale or, less often, dark red foci that are sharply delineated from the adjacent parenchyma (Figs. 2-23 to 2-25). The size of such foci is variable, ranging from tiny (<1 mm) to several centimeters. Hepatocytes in affected areas either degenerate or become necrotic as a result of the injurious effects of the infectious agents.

Zonal hepatocellular degeneration or necrosis or, as it is more simply termed, zonal change, affects hepatocytes within defined areas of the hepatic lobule. The zones are centrilobular (periacinar), midzonal (between centrilobular and periportal areas), or periportal (centroacinar) areas. Extensive zonal change within the liver, regardless of

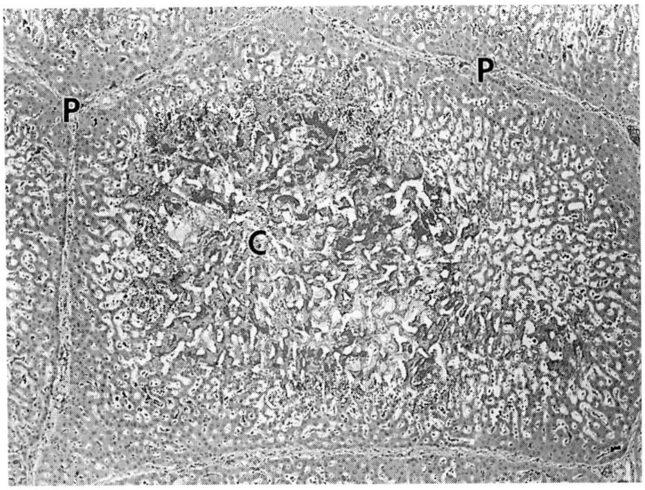

Figure 2-26 Liver; pig. Centrilobular necrosis. Hepatocytes in centrilobular and midzonal areas have undergone coagulation necrosis *(C)*, whereas those adjacent to portal tracts *(P)* appear normal. H & E stain.

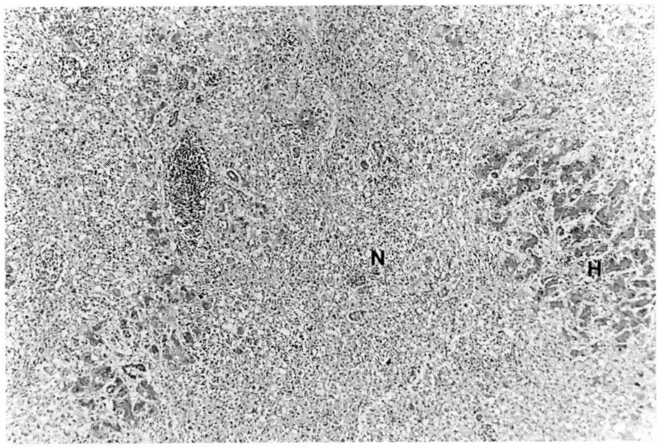

Figure 2-27 Liver; dog. Massive hepatic necrosis in a dog with caval syndrome. Areas of complete hepatocellular necrosis *(N)* affecting entire lobules are adjacent to areas of viable hepatocytes *(H)*. H & E stain.

location within the lobule, typically produces a liver that is pale and modestly enlarged with rounded margins, has increased friability, and, characteristically, an enhanced lobular pattern on the capsular and cut surface of the organ (Figs. 2-13 and 2-14). Degenerated hepatocytes swell, and when the majority of hepatocytes in a zone are affected, that portion of the lobule appears pale. In contrast, necrosis of hepatocytes in a particular zone of the lobule results in loss of hepatocytes and the consequent dilation and congestion of sinusoids so that the affected zone appears red. Although zonal change typically produces an enhanced lobular pattern, microscopic examination is usually required to determine the type of zonal change. Specific forms of zonal change are described below.

1. **Centrilobular** degeneration and necrosis of hepatocytes is particularly common (Fig. 2-26), as this portion of the lobule receives the least oxygenated blood and is, therefore, susceptible to hypoxia, and it has the greatest enzymatic activity (mixed-function oxidases) capable of activating compounds into toxic forms. Centrilobular necrosis can result from a precipitous and severe anemia or right-sided heart failure. Similarly, passive congestion of the liver results in hypoxia due to stasis of blood and produces atrophy of centrilobular hepatocytes.
2. **Paracentral (periacinar)** cellular degeneration involves only a wedge around the central vein because only the periphery of one acinus is affected. As several acini border on a single central vein (terminal hepatic venule), changes induced by hypoxia (usually anemia-induced) may not be present equally in all acini and, thus, hepatocytes at the periphery of one acinus can have more severe change than those in adjacent acini. Unequal metabolism of toxins by different acini can also cause necrosis to be evident in a paracentral distribution.
3. **Midzonal** degeneration and necrosis are unusual lesions in domestic animals but have been reported in pigs and horses with aflatoxicosis and cats exposed to hexachlorophene.
4. **Periportal** degeneration and necrosis are also uncommon, but may occur following exposure to toxins, such as phosphorus, that do not require metabolism by mixed-function oxidases to cause injury.
5. **Bridging** necrosis is the result of confluence of areas of necrosis. Bridging may link centrilobular areas (central bridging) or centrilobular areas to periportal areas.

Massive necrosis is not necessarily, as the name might imply, necrosis of the entire liver; rather the term describes necrosis of an entire hepatic lobule or contiguous lobules. All hepatocytes within affected lobules are necrotic. The gross appearance of the liver varies with the maturity of the lesion. If, in acute cases, the majority of the parenchyma is affected, the liver might be modestly enlarged and have a smooth external surface and dark parenchyma because of extensive congestion. Microscopically, affected areas consist of blood-filled spaces within a connective tissue stroma devoid of hepatocytes (Fig. 2-27). Later in the course of the process, necrotic hepatocytes lyse without regeneration and the residual stroma becomes condensed. Stellate cells may survive and contribute new collagen (collagen I, in particular) to the sites of injury. The final result is collapse of the lobule and replacement of the lost hepatic parenchyma with a scar composed of condensed stoma, including variable amounts and types of collagen. Grossly, the liver typically is small with a wrinkled capsule. Partial involvement of the liver is characterized by depressed areas of parenchymal necrosis and vascular congestion scattered throughout the organ.

Response of the Liver to Injury

Following destruction of hepatic parenchyma, regeneration of parenchyma, replacement by fibrosis, and biliary hyperplasia may occur. The outcome of a given hepatic insult depends on the nature and duration of the insult, and survival of the host.

Regeneration. A characteristic feature of the liver is the ability to rapidly and efficiently regenerate lost hepatic mass. Experimentally, as much as two thirds of the liver can be excised from a healthy animal without signs of hepatic dysfunction, and the liver is rapidly regenerated. In addition to replication of hepatocytes, there is a wave of replication in bile duct epithelium, endothelium, and sinusoidal lining cells that is coordinated with hepatocyte replication.

Regeneration does not involve the production of new lobules. Following removal of liver lobes, the remaining liver responds by increasing the size of the lobules to replace the lost mass. Individual cell necrosis leads to local proliferation of adjacent hepatocytes. Zonal necrosis in the lobule leads to a wave of hepatocyte proliferation in the hepatocytes left in the remaining areas of the lobule. In some circumstances, such as exposure to chemical toxins, in which the mature hepatocytes are unable to divide, replacement of hepatocytes lost by tissue removal or necrosis occurs through proliferation of hepatocyte stem cells or **oval cells.** These cells reside in the connective tissue of the portal areas and have the ability to differentiate into hepatocyte or bile duct epithelium. Histologically, they are identified as small basophilic cells with an oval shape. They are not apparent in most circumstances of hepatic regeneration, but can be abundant in experimental studies.

The body carefully orchestrates hepatic regeneration to replace lost hepatocyte mass along with bile ducts and vessels without producing excess liver. A variety of growth factors, including transforming growth factor-α and hepatocyte growth factor, stimulate hepatocyte replication. Once normal hepatic mass has been established, macrophages release transforming growth factor-β, which stops hepatic parenchymal cell proliferation.

Extensive hepatic necrosis is usually followed by parenchymal regeneration without scarring as long as the normal extracellular matrix (reticulin) scaffolding of the affected portion remains intact and has not collapsed as in massive hepatic necrosis. However, repetitive injury or massive necrosis can disrupt the normal lobular architecture through parenchymal collapse on removal of the dead hepatocytes and stromal collapse with repair by collagen synthesis (postnecrotic scarring). Even when necrosis of hepatocytes is continuous, the liver will attempt to regenerate its functional mass. However, prolonged regenerative effort with damage to the normal extracellular matrix scaffolding (reticulin framework) of the liver often results in nodular proliferations of parenchyma that architecturally distort the liver. Although regenerative nodules may reconstitute a proportionately large amount of hepatic mass, adequate function is rarely attained. Blood flow into the regenerative nodules and bile flow out of the nodules are abnormal; as a result, hepatic function cannot be reestablished. As the nodules grow, the portal areas and the central vein can be moved closer to each other, creating vascular shunts that allow blood to bypass hepatocytes.

Fibrosis. Fibrosis is one of the more common manifestations of chronic hepatic injury. The pattern of fibrosis can be a useful indicator of the type of insult that produced the lesion in the early stages of fibrosis, but this is not the case in the late stages of hepatic fibrosis, when no distinctive pattern is apparent. The significance of fibrosis depends on its effect on hepatic function and its reversibility. Early fibrosis may respond to treatment or removal of the source of injury, but more advanced fibrosis is generally irreversible with the therapies currently available. Despite the considerable regenerative capacity of the liver, hepatic fibrosis, when sufficiently severe, can be lethal.

In the normal liver, fibrillar collagens, collagen I and III, are confined primarily to the connective tissue of the portal areas and immediately around the terminal hepatic venule (central vein). Collagen IV is the most abundant collagen in the sinusoids, but it is present in small amounts. Small amounts of collagen and other extracellular matrix components, produced by hepatic stellate cells, endothelial cells, and hepatocytes, comprise the normal reticular framework of the sinusoid. This stroma supports the endothelial cells and separates them from the underlying hepatocytes and thereby maintains the shape of the space of Disse.

Hepatic fibrosis is an overall increase in the amount of extracellular matrix, as well as a change in the types of hepatic collagen and their site of deposition. Severely fibrotic liver can contain up to six times as much collagen and other extracellular matrix components as normal liver. In fibrotic livers there is an increase of fibrillar collagens, type I and type III, and nonfibrillar collagen XVIII within the parenchyma, in the space of Disse, or in areas of hepatic injury. Along with the collagen deposition, there is also a commensurate increase in proteoglycans, fibronectin, and hyaluronic acid.

The hepatic stellate cells (Ito cells, lipocytes) have a

central role in hepatic fibrosis. In the normal liver, hepatic stellate cells occupy a subendothelial position in the sinusoid, nestled between hepatocytes, and are characterized by the presence of large lipid-containing vacuoles in their cytoplasm (Figs. 2-3 and 2-5). The vacuoles are a primary storage site for retinyl esters, including vitamin A. Hepatic stellate cells are positioned around the circumference of the sinusoids and have been likened to pericytes in other organs, such as the mesangial cells of the renal glomerulus. Hepatic stellate cells have been shown to have a role in the control of the diameter of the sinusoids and consequently the flow of blood through the sinusoids. When activated, they express smooth muscle actin. In the dog and rat, but not human beings, they express desmin, a marker usually found in muscle cells.

When the liver is injured, these cells proceed through a progressive phenotypic change from the typical lipid-storing cell to a cell with a myofibroblastic appearance (Fig. 2-28). These cells develop the ability to synthesize collagen, which leads to hepatic fibrosis.

Once these cells have switched phenotype to the myofibroblast phenotype, they begin synthesis of collagen types I, III, and IV. They also produce other extracellular matrix components, including laminin and chondroitin sulfate, and other proteoglycans. Hepatocytes synthesize few or no matrix proteins, and the large sum of matrix is derived from the hepatic stellate cells.

Hepatic fibrosis can be produced by a variety of types of hepatic injury. Chemical injury, biliary obstruction, and

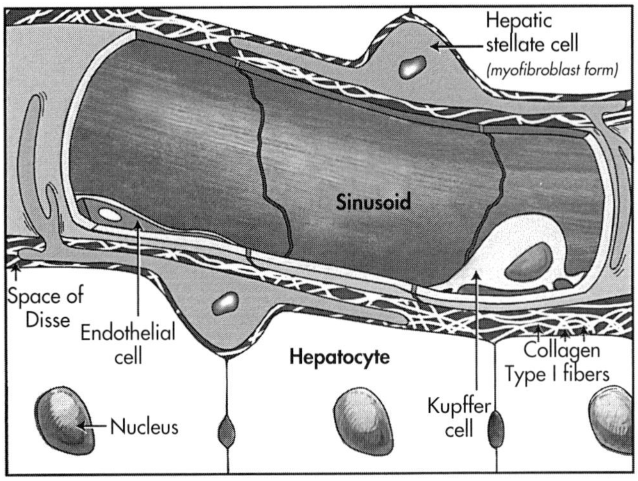

Figure 2-28 Diagram of a fibrotic hepatic sinusoid. Contact between the plasma and the hepatocytes is dramatically reduced. The sinusoidal endothelial cells have lost their fenestrations. The space of Disse contains abundant collagen type I fibers that have been synthesized by activated hepatic stellate cells. The hepatic stellate cells have eliminated the lipid vacuoles and assumed a myofibroblastic morphology with cell extensions surrounding the endothelial cells. Hepatocyte microvilli have been lost.

iron overload produce similar patterns of activation of hepatic stellate cells. Hepatic stellate cells can be activated by various cytokines produced either by inflammatory cells that infiltrate damaged hepatic parenchyma or by constituent cells of the liver (Kupffer cells, endothelial cells, hepatocytes, and biliary epithelium). Damage to the extracellular matrix also stimulates hepatic stellate cell activation, as do various toxins.

The site in which collagen is deposited in the liver has a significant impact on hepatic function. **Perisinusoidal fibrosis** can have a severe effect on hepatic function. In addition to collagen and extracellular matrix deposits, a loss of fenestrations in the endothelial cells accompanies these changes. These changes have been termed capillarization of the sinusoids because the alterations in the sinusoids result in a vascular structure that more closely resembles that of a capillary than a sinusoid. Also, there is a loss of microvilli on the luminal surface of the hepatocytes. The functional effect of these microanatomic changes is profound. The loss of fenestrations and the presence of collagen in the space of Disse prevent plasma's coming in contact with hepatocytes, and thus the ability of the liver to carry out its synthetic, catabolic, and excretory roles is severely compromised.

The site of fibrosis within the hepatic lobule can be indicative of the type of insult, but often, chronic injury, depending on severity of injury and the timing of the episodes of injury, produces fibrosis affecting all parts of the liver. The genesis of the morphologic pattern of hepatic fibrosis is complex and not completely understood. Long-standing right-sided heart failure can cause **centrilobular (periacinar)** fibrosis. Chronic toxic injury can also produce **centrilobular (periacinar)** fibrosis because this region is the site of metabolism for most drugs. However, repeated injury with chemicals that produce centrilobular injury, such as diethylnitrosamine and carbon tetrachloride, often result in fibrosis that involves portal tracts, and from here fibrous septae extend into the parenchyma and to the centrilobular areas of the liver (Fig. 2-29). The loss of hepatocytes in the affected areas leads to collapse and condensation of the residual extracellular matrix of the liver. Activated stellate cells proliferate in these damaged areas and synthesize collagen and other extracellular matrix proteins, producing a zonal pattern of fibrosis. **Periportal (centroacinar) fibrosis** can result from chronic inflammatory lesions or a small group of toxins that affect the periportal hepatocytes. Fibrosis may be limited to individual lobules, but when injury is more severe, the areas of fibrosis can be more extensive. **Bridging fibrosis,** which is similar in location to bridging necrosis, implies fibrosis that extends from one portal area to another, or from portal areas to central veins (Fig. 2-29). Bridging fibrosis is more likely to be associated with impaired hepatic function than focal forms of hepatic fibrosis; however, all forms of hepatic fibrosis, if

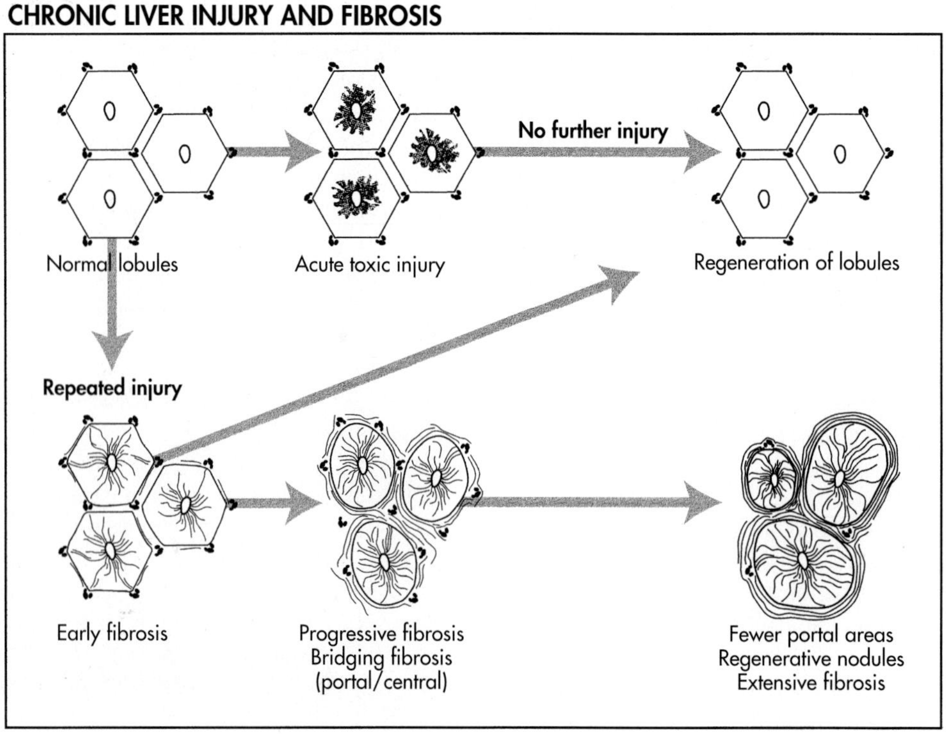

Figure 2-29 Diagram of the effects of hepatic injury on the development of fibrosis. Acute hepatic centrilobular injury that occurs only once usually resolves and normal liver architecture returns. Repeated bouts of injury or severe injury can initiate hepatic fibrosis. In the earliest stages, fibrosis may be reversible, but as fibrosis progresses it reaches a point that repair is not likely. Fibrosis starts as fine branches of collagen deposition between portal areas or central areas or dissecting into the hepatic parenchyma. Over time greater amounts of collagen and extracellular matrix are deposited and the lobular architecture becomes progressively distorted. In the end-stage liver, nodular regeneration and extensive, circumferential fibrosis are typical.

sufficiently severe, are associated with impaired hepatic function.

A single event of widespread (usually centrilobular to massive) hepatocellular necrosis, sometimes is followed, not by the usual regenerative response, but by fibrosis and condensation of the preexisting connective tissue stroma that results in formation of bands of dense connective tissue. This process is referred to as **postnecrotic scarring** (Fig. 2-29).

Other patterns of hepatic fibrosis can occur, including **biliary fibrosis** (centered on bile ducts in the portal areas), focal or **multifocal hepatic fibrosis** (randomly scattered throughout the hepatic parenchyma), and **diffuse hepatic fibrosis** (affects all regions of the lobule and is present throughout the liver). Marked diffuse fibrosis with hyperplastic nodule formation is, by definition, cirrhosis. Different hepatic insults may produce different patterns of fibrosis, but when fibrosis is severe (end-stage liver disease), it frequently is impossible to determine either the cause or the initial pattern of fibrosis.

Biliary Hyperplasia. Biliary hyperplasia, proliferation of new biliary ducts within the portal areas and periportal regions, can be a relatively nonspecific response to a variety of insults to the liver. The mechanism responsible for this proliferation is unknown. Biliary hyperplasia can occur swiftly, particularly in young animals, but is usually regarded as a lesion seen in long-standing hepatic injury. Biliary hyperplasia occurs in particular after diseases that obstruct normal bile drainage.

End-Stage Liver or Cirrhosis

The end-stage or cirrhotic liver is characterized by loss of normal hepatic architecture due to nodular regeneration of parenchyma, fibrosis, and often, biliary duct hyperplasia (Figs. 2-30 and 2-31). Profound vascular abnormalities with serious consequences for the health of affected patients occur in cirrhosis, including multiple abnormal vascular anastomoses between the portal vein and the systemic vasculature as a consequence of the increased portal pressure. Also, venous shunts between the

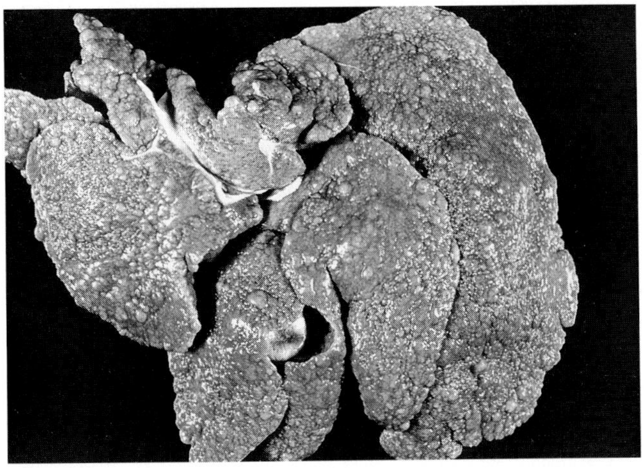

Figure 2-30 Liver; dog, Doberman pinscher. End-stage liver with chronic hepatitis. The liver is small, firm, and irregular with nodules of regenerative parenchyma separated by tracts of connective tissue. *Courtesy Dr. S. Smith.*

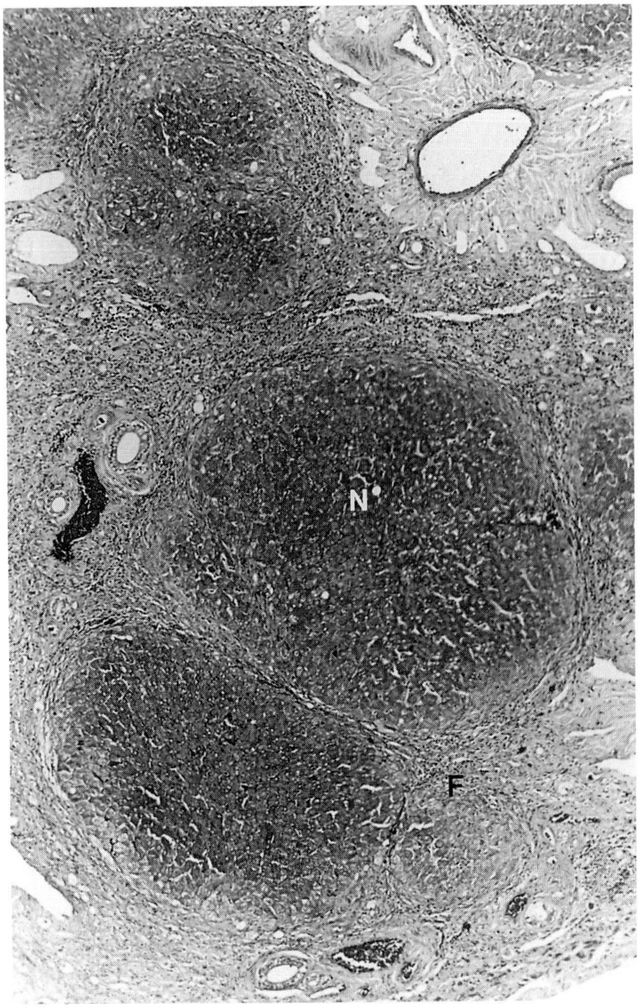

Figure 2-31 Liver; dog. End-stage liver induced by chronic anticonvulsant therapy. Nodules of regenerative parenchyma *(N)* are separated by tracts of collapsed reticulin and fibrous connective tissue *(F),* which also contain numerous blood vessels and bile ducts. H & E stain.

central veins and the portal veins and arteriovenous shunts between the hepatic arteries and the central veins can occur within the regenerative nodules. As it is the final, irreversible result of any one of several different hepatic diseases, the term end-stage liver is appropriate, particularly since the term cirrhosis is neither descriptive nor precise in meaning and originally meant "tawny yellow." However, "cirrhosis" is still widely used, and one definition is that it is "a diffuse process characterized by fibrosis and conversion of normal liver architecture into structurally abnormal lobules." Another authority states that the hallmark is the total absence of any normal lobular architecture. The architecture of the liver is altered by loss of hepatic parenchyma, condensation of reticulin framework, and formation of tracts of fibrous connective tissue. Regeneration of hepatic tissue between fibrous bands leads to the formation of variably sized regenerative nodules. The entire liver is, thus, distorted and consists of nodules of regenerating parenchyma separated by fibrous bands that appear as depressions on the surface. The potential causes of an end-stage (cirrhotic) liver are numerous.

Chronic toxic insult results from the continued ingestion of any hepatotoxin (e.g., herbivores ingesting toxic plants such as those that contain pyrrolizidine alkaloids) and the long-term administration of anticonvulsant drugs such as primidone to dogs. Following chronic toxic insult and depending on the degree of injury, fibrosis can be evident in portal areas, centrilobular areas, and in anastomotic tracts that connect these structures. Chronic extrahepatic **biliary obstruction** and cholestasis leads to extensive portal fibrosis that primarily affects the portal triads, but the fibrosis can eventually extend into the adjacent hepatic parenchyma. Chronic inflammation of the liver (hepatitis) or biliary tract (cholangitis) may lead to an end-stage liver. Although infection of the liver typically is focal or multifocal, diffuse hepatitis and subsequent fibrosis occur in disease entities such as so-called **canine chronic (chronic-active) hepatitis. Chronic passive hepatic congestion** eventually leads to fibrosis around central veins, which can progress to **cardiac cirrhosis,** although the actual amount of fibrosis is usually small. Abnormal storage or metabolism of metals such as copper, as occurs in Bedlington and West Highland white terriers with hereditary copper accumulations, may produce an end-stage liver. A variety of more poorly defined disease entities can lead to progressive hepatocellular injury and hepatic fibrosis resulting in end-stage hepatic disease.

The end-stage liver obviously cannot perform its normal functions, so the clinical manifestations of hepatic failure invariably occur in affected animals. However, the cause of the hepatic damage that leads to the end-stage liver frequently cannot be determined at the time signs of hepatic failure are observed.

Inflammation of the Liver (Hepatitis)

Inflammation of the liver parenchyma is termed **hepatitis,** whereas inflammation of the biliary ducts (either intrahepatic or extrahepatic) is **cholangitis.** Inflammation that affects the biliary ducts and adjacent hepatic parenchyma is termed **cholangiohepatitis.** Other terms are occasionally used. Pericholangitis implies inflammation that surrounds, but does not encroach on, the biliary ducts, whereas **portal hepatitis** refers to accumulation of inflammatory cells within the portal areas.

Routes of infection into the liver are hematogenous, direct penetration, and ascending via the biliary system. The most common route is hematogenous because the liver receives both arterial blood via the hepatic artery and venous blood from the gastrointestinal tract via the portal vein. Ascending biliary infections and direct penetration are less common. The nature and distribution of inflammatory lesions in the liver are usually dictated by the nature of the infectious agent (e.g., virus, bacterium, fungus), the route of entry, and any predilection for a cell type in the liver. The pattern of inflammation often reveals the route of infection. Hematogenous infection, viral, bacterial, fungal, or protozoal, tends to cause a random multifocal distribution of lesions. Infections, usually bacterial (i.e., *Salmonella* spp.), that ascend the biliary tract produce cholangitits initially, but eventually become most evident as cholangiohepatitis as severe infections extend into the adjacent parenchyma. Penetrating wounds from external sources or from foreign bodies in the digestive tract (reticulum) can cause discrete areas of inflammation with or without necrosis. These foci develop into abscesses that are visible on the capsule and extend into the hepatic parenchyma.

Acute hepatitis is characterized by inflammatory cells, initially neutrophils, and, subsequently, lymphocytes, plasma cells, particularly if an infectious agent is present. Infectious agents, particularly bacteria and protozoa, supply chemotactic stimuli for inflammatory cells, causing them to accumulate. In time, if the animal survives, areas of acute hepatitis in which hepatocytes were killed are replaced by regenerating hepatocytes or fibrous tissue. If antigen persists, as occurs with some infectious agents (see below), chronic inflammatory lesions, such as an abscess or granuloma, may form. In most circumstances, toxin-induced necrosis does not produce much inflammatory response other than an influx of phagocytes to remove cell debris and a mononuclear cell infiltration limited to the portal areas. Similarly, acute viral infections in animals often produce multifocal necrosis, but scant inflammation.

Grossly, small foci of acute inflammation are usually detected only if accompanied by hepatocellular necrosis. Characterization of the type of inflammation usually requires microscopic evaluation. A variety of patterns occur. Viral infection tends to produce a random pattern of necrosis with scant inflammation, if there is any. Random foci of neutrophilic hepatitis as a consequence of embolic localization of bacteria are relatively common in all species. In neonates, especially calves, lambs, and foals, bacteria usually seed the liver via the umbilical veins or the portal venous or hepatic arterial systems. Neutrophilic cholangitis and cholangiohepatitis typically result from ascending bacterial infection of the biliary system, often as a consequence of biliary obstruction by parasites or compression of the duct either by fibrous tissue or a neoplasm.

Chronic hepatitis results when there is continued inflammation due to persistence of an antigenic stimulus. In the absence of such a stimulus, inflammation rapidly resolves. Certain species of bacteria (e.g., *Mycobacterium, Salmonella*) and fungi (e.g., *Histoplasma capsulatum*) are particularly resistant to killing by phagocytic cells and induce chronic inflammation and granuloma formation. Other causes of chronic inflammation of the liver include chronic cholangiohepatitis from persistent infection of the biliary system, and so-called chronic (chronic-active) hepatitis of the dog (see Canine Chronic Hepatitis). Chronic inflammation is obvious grossly if it produces a discrete granuloma or abscess. Also, when chronic inflammation occurs throughout the liver, loss of hepatic parenchyma produces architectural distortion of the liver as a consequence of fibrosis and nodular parenchymal regeneration. Whereas acute hepatitis usually is characterized by accumulation of neutrophils, chronic hepatitis is characterized by fibrosis and accumulation of mononuclear inflammatory cells including lymphocytes, macrophages, and plasma cells. Neutrophils often are present in chronic unresolved hepatic inflammation such as that which characterizes some forms of canine chronic hepatitis. Focal lesions such as abscesses or granulomas often are sufficiently localized that they do not alter hepatic function. In contrast, diffuse and severe chronic hepatitis usually leads to end-stage hepatic disease with hepatic failure and its associated constellation of clinical signs. The form of chronic hepatitis that has been referred to as chronic active hepatitis is discussed in a separate section.

Viral Diseases

Infectious Canine Hepatitis

This disease is caused by canine adenovirus 1 and now is uncommon in much of the world, probably because of widespread vaccination. The majority of infections are asymptomatic, and infections that result in disease may not be fatal. The virus has a predilection for vascular endothelium and hepatocytes; fulminant disease is characterized by hepatic necrosis and widespread hemorrhage that can affect a variety of organs. Virus-induced endothelial damage may lead to disseminated intravascular coagulation and hemorrhagic diathesis.

Gross lesions of infectious canine hepatitis include widespread petechiae and ecchymoses, accumulation of clear fluid in the peritoneal and other serous cavities, the presence of fibrin strands on the surface of the liver, and enlargement and reddening of the tonsils and lymph nodes. The liver is moderately enlarged, friable, and may contain small foci of hepatocellular necrosis centered on centrilobular areas. The predilection for centrilobular necrosis is more likely to be related to the virus's penchant for infection and necrosis of endothelial cells that may lead to vascular stasis and local hypoxia, than any increased propensity for the virus to damage centrilobular hepatocytes. An enhanced lobular pattern is sometimes evident as a result of the centrilobular hepatic necrosis. Characteristically, the wall of the gallbladder is thickened by edema.

The severity of microscopic lesions present in individual dogs may reflect the duration of the disease. Susceptible puppies rapidly succumb to infection and have only scattered foci of hepatocellular necrosis, whereas fulminant disease in older dogs often produces both randomly scattered foci of hepatocellular necrosis and widespread centrilobular necrosis. Large amphophilic intranuclear inclusions are found in vascular endothelium and hepatocytes. Zonal necrosis may reflect ischemic injury and not direct virus-mediated destruction of hepatocytes. Some dogs recovering from infectious canine hepatitis develop an immune complex uveitis (type III hypersensitivity), which produces degeneration of the corneal endothelium and corneal edema clinically known as "blue eye."

Rift Valley Fever

This is an acute, arthropod-transmitted zoonotic viral disease that principally affects ruminants, causing extensive mortality among calves and lambs, and abortion of pregnant ewes and cows. The causative virus is a member of the family Bunyaviridae, genus *Phlebovirus*. The disease occurs throughout much of Africa and is especially prevalent after periods of unusually abundant rainfall. Hepatic involvement is consistent in fulminant cases and is characterized by hepatic enlargement and orange-brown discoloration. Pale foci of hepatocellular necrosis that are randomly scattered throughout the parenchyma impart a mottled appearance, and, sometimes, the lobular pattern is enhanced because of the centrilobular hepatic necrosis. Diffuse petechiae and ecchymoses are also characteristic of the disease, as are edema and hemorrhages of the wall of the gallbladder. Disseminated intravascular coagulation probably contributes to the hemorrhagic diathesis and perhaps to the zonal hepatic necrosis.

Microscopic lesions are characterized by the presence of both randomly distributed foci of hepatocellular necrosis and more widespread zonal necrosis that ranges from centrilobular to massive. These lesions, particularly random hepatic necrosis, are more severe and widespread in young animals and aborted fetuses. Eosinophilic intranuclear inclusion bodies may be present in degenerated hepatocytes in areas of necrosis.

Wesselsbron Disease

This disease, like Rift Valley fever, is a zoonotic arthropod-transmitted viral disease that occurs in Africa; the virus occasionally causes disease in newborn lambs and abortion in ewes. The causative agent is a member of the Flaviviridae. Affected lambs have multifocal areas of hepatocellular necrosis, and icterus develops occasionally. Infected adult sheep usually survive infection, although they may develop focal areas of hepatocellular necrosis.

Herpesvirus Infections

A variety of abortogenic herpesviruses are described; each animal species is affected by a specific virus. The abortogenic herpesviruses characteristically induce multifocal, randomly distributed, small (<1 mm) areas of necrosis in several fetal organs, including the liver (Fig. 2-25). Similar lesions occasionally are present in neonates infected with abortogenic herpesviruses. Examples of these viruses include the abortogenic equine herpes virus (equine herpesvirus 1), infectious bovine rhinotracheitis virus (bovine herpesvirus 1), caprine herpesvirus, feline viral rhinotracheitis virus, and pseudorabies virus. Canine herpesvirus can produce multifocal hepatic necrosis in neonatal pups, but foci of necrosis are more consistently present in the kidneys, lungs, and spleen.

Other Viral Infections

Certain viral diseases may involve the liver, but the hepatic involvement either does not occur invariably or is but one manifestation of a systemic process. Such diseases include feline infectious peritonitis, which is characterized by foci of pyogranulomatous vasculitis or perivascular accumulations of lymphocytes and plasma cells within multiple organs sometimes including the liver. Subacute and chronic forms of equine infectious anemia are characterized by cellular infiltration, particularly lymphocytes, in portal areas of the liver. Systemic adenoviral infection of lambs, calves, and goat kids may produce multifocal areas of hepatocellular necrosis, cholangitis, and necrosis of biliary epithelium.

Bacterial Diseases

Liver Abscess

Bacteria can reach the liver via a number of different routes and induce the formation of abscesses. Routes include the portal vein, the umbilical veins from umbilical infections in newborn animals, as part of a generalized bacteremia reaching the liver via the hepatic artery, as an ascending infection of the biliary system, by parasitic migration, and as a direct extension of an inflammatory process from tissues such as the reticulum, immediately adjacent to the liver.

Bacterial infections of the liver and subsequent formation of hepatic abscesses are especially common in feedlot cattle. Hepatic abscesses are usually a sequela to toxic rumenitis because damage to the ruminal mucosa allows ruminal microflora, particularly *Fusobacterium necrophorum,* to enter the portal circulation. After initially localizing within the liver, bacteria proliferate and produce focal areas of hepatocellular necrosis and hepatitis that can, in time, develop into hepatic abscesses. Hepatic abscesses of cattle frequently are incidental lesions, but affected cattle can have weight loss and decreased milk production. Less commonly, a hepatic abscess encroaches on the lumen of either a hepatic vein or the caudal vena cava. This can cause a phlebitis that results in mural thrombosis and, because of the obstruction of the outflow to the venous drainage of the liver, passive congestion of the liver and portal hypertension. Detachment of portions of these mural thrombi can produce septic thromboemboli that lodge in the lungs. Rupture of hepatic abscesses directly into the hepatic vein or into the caudal vena cava occurs sporadically in cattle and may result in death of the affected animal because of fatal septic embolization of the lungs. Sometimes death can be sudden from the blockage of large areas of pulmonary capillaries by the exudate. Hepatic abscesses derived from bacteria arriving via the portal vein are not evenly distributed throughout the liver possibly because of portal streaming. Occasionally, fungi such as *Mucor* that proliferate in areas of ruminal ulceration invade the portal circulation and are carried to the liver and there cause extensive areas of necrosis.

Bacillary Hemoglobinuria

This acute and highly fatal disease of cattle and sheep occurs in various areas of the world, typically in those regions in which liver fluke *(Fasciola hepatica)* infection also occurs. Spores of *Clostridium haemolyticum,* the causative agent of bacillary hemoglobinuria, are ingested and come to reside within Kupffer cells, but they proliferate only in areas of low oxygen tension. Migration of immature liver flukes, or, less commonly, other parasites, or an event, such as liver biopsy, produces a nidus of necrotic hepatic parenchyma in which bacterial spores can germinate. Bacteria proliferate and release toxins, the most important of which is phospholipase C, that induce the hepatocellular necrosis and intravascular hemolysis that characterize the disease. Affected animals have icterus, hemoglobinemia, and hemoglobinuria. The liver contains one or more discrete foci of hepatic necrosis in which causative organisms are visible in histologic sections. Grossly, these foci are sharply delineated from the adjacent parenchyma and usually are pale and surrounded by an intensely hyperemic zone. Migration tracts of the immature flukes that typically precipitate the disease are present. Serous cavities (pleura, peritoneum, and pericardium) often contain excessive accumulation of red or straw-colored fluid that is sometimes flecked with fibrin.

Infectious Necrotic Hepatitis

Also known as black disease, infectious necrotic hepatitis is most common in sheep and cattle, but occurs in swine and horses. This disease is somewhat analogous to bacillary hemoglobinuria in that dormant spores of *Clostridium novyi* (usually type B) germinate in areas of lowered oxygen tension and release toxins that produce discrete foci of coagulation necrosis within the liver and eventually death of the host. Germination of spores is usually initiated by hepatic necrosis caused by the migration of immature liver flukes; however, a variety of other initiating factors have been described. Affected animals typically have one or more areas of hepatocellular necrosis, which grossly manifest as discrete, pale areas of variable size. A zone of intense hyperemia often surrounds these foci. Parasitic migration tracts are also usually present within the affected liver. Other lesions include diffuse venous congestion and accumulation of fluid within the pericardial sac and pleural and peritoneal cavities. The carcass of affected animals typically putrefies rapidly because of high fever before death.

Tyzzer's Disease

This disease, caused by *Clostridium piliformis,* is well recognized in laboratory animals but occurs only sporadically in domestic animals. It is most common in foals, but has been described in calves, cats, and dogs and many other species. Typically, only very young or immunocompromised animals are affected. The disease is characterized by enlarged, edematous, and hemorrhagic abdominal lymph nodes, hepatic enlargement, and the presence of randomly distributed, pale foci of hepatocellular necrosis. Diagnosis requires the demonstration of the characteristic, elongated large bacilli within viable hepatocytes at the margins of necrotic foci.

Leptospirosis

The liver is often involved in acute, severe leptospirosis of all domestic species because of ischemic injury to centrilobular areas as a consequence of the intravascular hemolytic anemia that accompanies infection with some serovars. Furthermore, organisms are present in large numbers in the liver, although the direct effects of leptospira on hepatocytes are less well established. Infection of dogs with *Leptospira grippotyphosa* has been associated with chronic (chronic-active) hepatitis, but it is unlikely that leptospira are involved in the pathogenesis of the majority of spontaneous cases of chronic hepatitis.

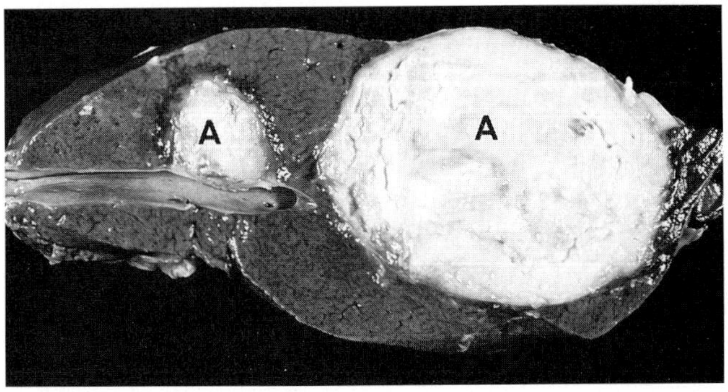

Figure 2-32 Liver, cut surface; sheep. Two abscesses *(A)* caused by *Corynebacterium pseudotuberculosis. Courtesy of Dr. M. Leach.*

Other Bacterial Infections

These include infections that accompany bacteremia associated with systemic infection. A comprehensive list of systemic infections that produce hepatocellular necrosis and hepatitis is beyond the scope of this chapter, but examples include *Yersinia tularensis (Francisella tularensis), Yersinia pseudotuberculosis, Haemophilus agni,* and *Pasteurella haemolytica* infection of sheep; *Salmonella* infection in many species (lesions present within the liver are discrete accumulations of mixed mononuclear inflammatory cells which often are referred to as "paratyphoid nodules"); *Actinomyces pyogenes (Arcanobacterium pyogenes)* infection of the bovine fetus and neonate; *Campylobacter fetus* subsp. *fetus* in fetal and neonatal lambs; *Actinobacillus equuli* infection of neonatal foals; and *Nocardia asteroides* infection of dogs. Bacterial infections such as these may produce lesions within the liver that range from small foci of hepatic necrosis to multiple, large abscesses (Figs. 2-23, 2-24, 2-32, and 2-33). Determination of the specific causative agent is often dependent on bacterial isolation and characterization.

Parasitic Diseases

Nematodes

Migration of nematode larvae through the liver is a common occurrence in domestic animals. As larvae travel through the liver, they produce local tracts of hepatocellular necrosis that are accompanied by inflammation. These tracts are eventually replaced with connective tissue to produce fibrous scars, which are especially prominent on the capsular surface (Fig. 2-34). These capsular scars appear as pale areas, and the term "milk spotted liver" has been used to describe livers in pigs scarred by migrating larvae of *Ascaris suum.* Larvae occasionally become entrapped within the liver or its capsule and are walled off within abscesses or granulomas. Examples of chronic hepatitis or hepatic scarring as a consequence of larval migration include that from migration of ascarids in several species of domestic animals, such as *Stephanurus dentatus* in swine, and *Strongylus* sp. in the horse. Infestation of the liver with adult nematodes is considerably less common than larval migration. *Capillaria hepatica* occasionally may be found in the liver of dogs and cats.

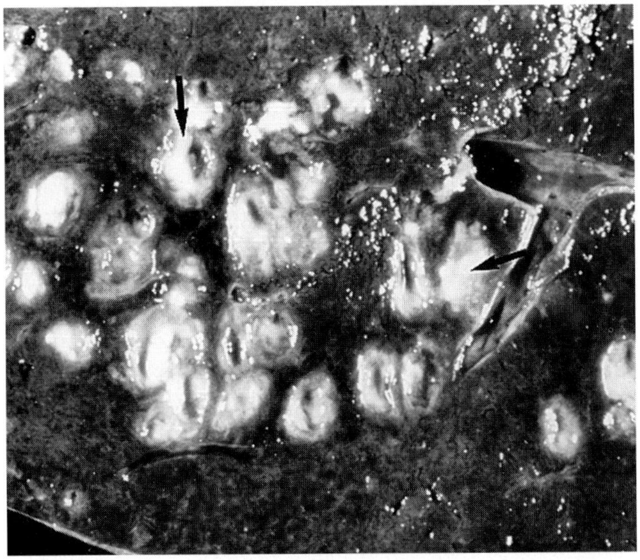

Figure 2-33 Liver, cut surface; horse. Disseminated hepatic abscesses *(arrows)* caused by *Corynebacterium pseudotuberculosis. Courtesy of Dr. M. Leach.*

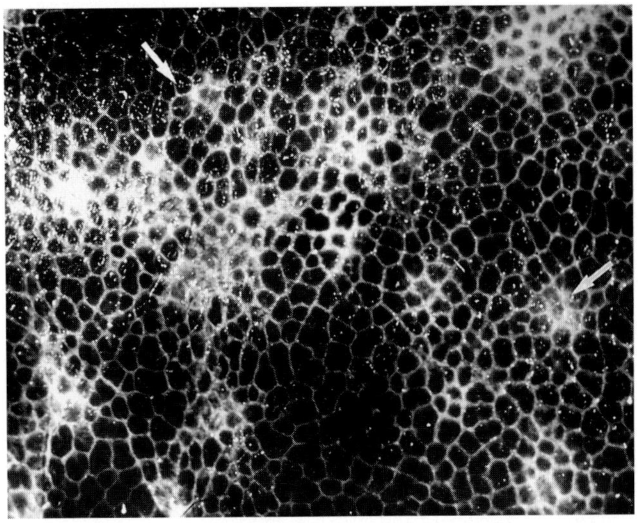

Figure 2-34 Liver, diaphragmatic surface; pig. Capsular and portal fibrosis from parasitic migration (milk-spotted liver). Migration tracks and the fibrosis of adjacent portal areas are identified with arrows. *Courtesy Dr. M.D. McGavin.*

Dogs with heartworm infection *(Dirofilaria immitis)* occasionally develop **vena caval syndrome,** also known as postcaval syndrome, which is characterized by disseminated intravascular coagulation, intravascular hemolysis, and acute hepatic failure. The syndrome typically occurs in dogs with large numbers of adult worms in the vena cava, as well as the more usual location within the right heart and pulmonary artery. The liver is engorged with blood as a consequence of severe passive congestion from the partial blockage of the caudal vena cava. It is proposed that mechanical factors associated with the presence of large numbers of worms in the right atrium or caudal vena cava are the cause of intravascular hemolysis that characterizes vena caval syndrome.

Cestodes

A number of cestodes occur within the hepatobiliary system of domestic animals. Those of greatest significance are the encysted forms of cestode parasites within the tissues of the intermediate hosts. The most important are larval cestodes of the genus *Taenia,* adults of which inhabit the gastrointestinal tract of carnivores and which usually are innocuous to their definitive host. The ova ingested by an intermediate host develop into embryos, which penetrate the wall of the gut and then are distributed through the blood to virtually any site in the body. Parasitic cysts develop within the tissues of the intermediate host, and the life cycle of the parasite is completed when the cysts are ingested by the definitive host. Although the liver is but one organ in the intermediate host that may be affected, hepatic involvement is common since portal blood, in which embryos migrate, drains into the liver before flowing to the systemic circulation.

The cestode *Taenia hydatigena* occurs in dogs, whereas its intermediate stage, *Cysticercus tenuicollis,* occurs in the peritoneal cavity of a variety of species including horses, ruminants, and swine. Immature cysticerci migrate in the liver and can induce extensive damage if infection is heavy; lesions present are comparable to those induced by migration of immature *Fasciola hepatica.*

Hydatid liver disease is common in some countries. *Echinococcus granulosus* is a cestode that parasitizes canids, and hydatid cysts can develop in many different animal species, including human beings. The dog-sheep cycle is most important in many geographic areas. Pastured cattle are also commonly affected in other geographic locations. Embryos may develop into hydatid cysts in virtually any organ in the intermediate host, but the liver and lungs are commonly affected. These cysts are usually less than 10 cm in diameter, but can attain quite spectacular size, particularly in human beings. Hydatid cysts, even when present in large numbers, rarely cause overt clinical signs of disease in domestic animals.

Cestode worms that can occur within the hepatobiliary system include *Stilesia hepatica, Stilesia globipunctata,* and *Thysanosoma actinoides,* all of which can inhabit the bile duct of ruminants. Infections with these parasites may result in chronic inflammation of the biliary tract, but they usually are not associated with clinical signs of hepatic dysfunction.

Trematodes

Liver fluke disease of sheep and cattle, and occasionally other species, most commonly is due to *Fasciola hepatica.* Hepatic fascioliasis occurs throughout the world in areas where climatic conditions (low swampy areas) are suitable for the aquatic snails that serve as intermediate hosts for the parasites. Adult *F. hepatica* are leaf-shaped parasites that inhabit the biliary system; their eggs pass via the bile to the intestinal tract and eventually are passed in the feces. Larvae then must develop in the snail intermediate host (genus *Lymnaea*). Cercariae that leave the snail encyst on herbage, where they develop into infectious metacercariae. Metacercariae are ingested by the ruminant host and penetrate the wall of the duodenum to enter the peritoneal cavity and, subsequently, enter the liver. They migrate within the liver before taking up residence within the biliary ducts. Migration of immature flukes through the liver produces hemorrhagic tracts of necrotic liver parenchyma. These tracts are grossly visible and, in acute infestation, are dark red, but with time become paler than the surrounding parenchyma. Resolution is often by fibrosis. A variety of untoward sequelae can follow these migrations including acute peritonitis, hepatic abscesses, death of the host as a consequence of acute, widespread hepatic necrosis associated with massive infiltration of immature flukes, and the proliferation of spores of *Clostridium haemolyticum* or *Clostridium novyi* in necrotic tissue and the subsequent development of bacillary hemoglobinuria or infectious necrotic hepatitis.

Mature flukes reside in the larger bile ducts and cause cholangitis or cholangiohepatitis. Chronic cholangitis and bile duct obstruction lead to ectasia and stenosis of the ducts and to periductular fibrosis that thickens the walls so the ducts become increasingly prominent. Bile within the distended ducts is brown. Obstruction of the ducts leads to extrahepatic cholestasis. Animals with chronic liver fluke disease are often in poor bodily condition.

Fasciola gigantica and *Fascioloides magna* are important causes of liver fluke disease of ruminants in some parts of the world. The adults of *F. gigantica* and *F. hepatica* reside in the bile ducts. In contrast, adult *F. magna,* whose normal host is elk, continue to migrate in the liver, causing widespread damage in aberrant hosts such as cattle and sheep. In cattle, the immature *F. magna* flukes cause extensive tissue damage as they migrate through the liver (Fig. 2-35), but the adults are enclosed by fibrous connective tissue in cysts containing a black fluid. In sheep, the flukes continuously migrate through the liver, causing extensive damage to the organ.

Other trematodes that inhabit the bile ducts include *Dicrocoelium dendriticum* in horses, ruminants, swine, dogs, and cats; *Eurytrema pancreaticum* and *Eurytrema coelomaticum* in ruminants; *Opisthorchis tenuicollis* in pigs, dogs, and cats, and *Opisthorchis viverrini* in dogs and cats; *Pseudamphistomum truncatum, Metorchis conjunc-*

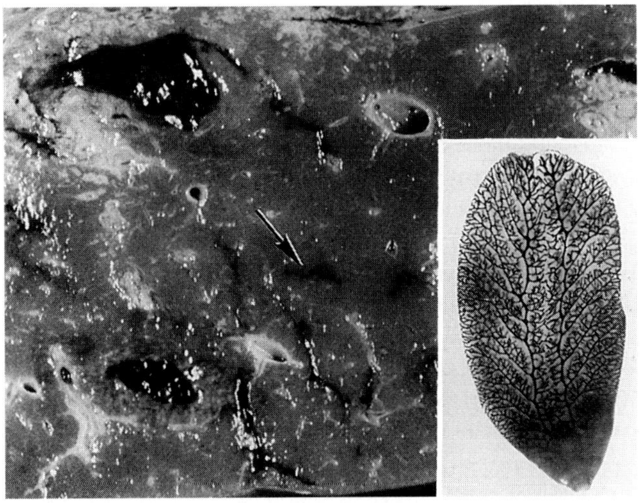

Figure 2-35 Liver, cut surface; cow. Fascioliasis. Migration of *Fascioloides magna* through this bovine liver produced characteristic dark tracks *(arrow)* of hepatocellular necrosis. *Inset:* Adult *F. magna. Courtesy Dr. M. McEntee.*

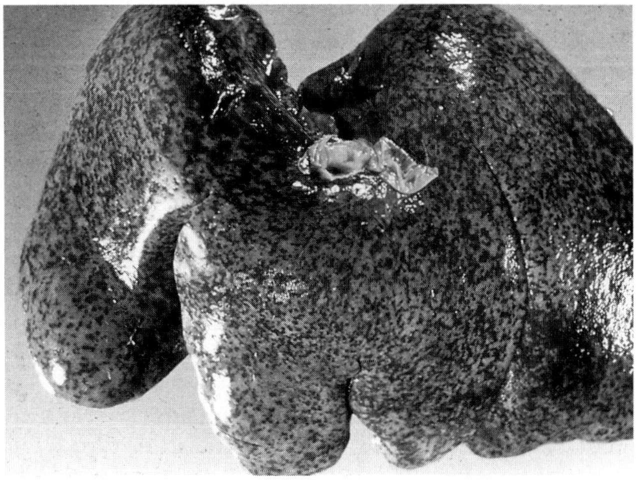

Figure 2-36 Liver; pig. Hepatosis dietitica. Foci of massive necrosis appears as dark regions of different size that are scattered throughout the liver. *Courtesy Dr. R.L. Michel.*

tus, Metorchis albidus, Parametorchis complexus, Concinnum procyonis, and *Platynosum fastosum* in dogs and cats. All are capable of inducing changes similar, but usually considerably milder than those associated with *Fasciola hepatica.* In addition, they occasionally cause obstruction of the biliary ducts.

Nutritional Diseases: Hepatosis Dietetica

Hepatosis dietetica (nutritional hepatic necrosis) is a syndrome of acute hepatic necrosis that occurs in young, rapidly growing swine. This is but one manifestation of a variety of disorders that are, at least in part, caused by a deficiency of either vitamin E or selenium (Chapter 9). The pathogenesis of hepatosis dietetica is incompletely defined, although it is established that vitamin E– and selenium-containing enzymes are antagonists of free radical formation and are, therefore, important for the maintenance of stability and integrity of cellular membranes.

Hepatosis dietetica is characterized by hemorrhagic centrilobular to massive hepatic necrosis (Figs. 2-26 and 2-36). The appearance of the liver of individually affected swine reflects the extent of hepatic necrosis, the severity of the hemorrhages, and the duration of the deficiency. Regions of massive necrosis in the affected liver initially are distended, deep red, and friable and later collapse to form dense tracts of connective tissue (postnecrotic scarring) in some animals that survive the acute disease.

Toxic Liver Disease

The liver is the most common site of toxic injury for two reasons. First, the liver receives approximately 70% of its blood supply from the portal vein, which drains blood from the gastrointestinal tract. Thus, ingested toxic substances, including plant, fungal, and bacterial products, as well as metals, minerals, and other chemicals that are absorbed into the portal blood, are transported to the liver. Second, the liver possesses enzymes capable of metabolizing a variety of endogenous and exogenous substances for elimination from the body; this process may also activate some substances to a more toxic form, thereby causing hepatic injury.

The conversion of lipid-soluble substances into water-soluble substances for elimination from the body is known as **biotransformation.** Many exogenous chemicals (xenobiotics) are absorbed by the skin, lungs, or digestive tract more readily because they are lipophilic and cross cell membranes easily. In order for these compounds to be eliminated, they must be made water-soluble to facilitate their excretion into bile or urine. There are two stages or phases to the process of biotransformation. During phase 1 metabolism, functional groups are introduced or existing polar groups are exposed on the substrate xenobiotic by oxidation, hydrolysis, or reduction. In phase 2, the product of phase 1 metabolism is conjugated with glucuronic acid, sulfate, or other groups, and this water-soluble form is then excreted in bile or urine. Phase 1 metabolism is primarily performed by the mixed-function oxidase (MFO) system or, as it is also known, the cytochrome P-450 system. This is the major enzyme system of the liver involved with drug metabolism and is located in the smooth endoplasmic reticulum. Activity of this enzyme system is greatest in hepatocytes in centrilobular regions. The MFOs are a collection of isoenzymes with different substrate specificities and can, therefore, oxidize a variety of chemicals. This enzyme system is inducible, that is, activities of these enzymes increase in response to frequent exposure to substrates metabolized by this system, such as insecticides or phenobarbital. Amounts of smooth endoplasmic reticulum, and thus MFO activity, also vary between the sexes (males of some species have more MFO activity than females) and with age (neonates have less activity than adults). Enzymes involved in phase 2 metabolism are found primarily in the cytoplasm.

Although hepatic biotransformation is a means of detoxifying and eliminating chemicals, it can also generate toxic metabolites. This process in which relatively inert compounds are metabolized to toxic metabolites, often free radicals, occurs during phase 1 metabolism and is termed **bioactivation.** Free radicals can react with hepatocellular DNA, RNA, and proteins as well as producing oxidative stress within cells. Antioxidants, particularly reduced glutathione and vitamin E, afford some protection against oxidative injury to cell membranes or organelles. Animals deficient in antioxidants are especially predisposed to hepatocellular injury. Hepatocyte injury was once considered to result primarily from lipid peroxidation, but other factors such as oxidative stress, disruption of calcium homeostasis, and direct effects of certain chemicals on cellular and organelle membranes have come to be recognized as additional important pathways of cellular injury.

An individual compound may be simultaneously metabolized by several different pathways; some of these pathways produce toxic intermediates, whereas others produce nontoxic compounds. The proportion of a compound metabolized by a particular pathway influences the degree of injury caused by the compound. For example, chemicals such as phenobarbital that induce formation of smooth endoplasmic reticulum and associated oxidases influence the toxicity of other compounds by altering the proportion of those compounds metabolized by MFOs versus other metabolic pathways. A variety of factors influence the severity of injury induced by a toxin; these factors include age, sex, diet, endocrine function, genetic constitution, and diurnal factors. It is, therefore, not surprising that responses of individual animals exposed to the same toxin can vary considerably.

Toxic hepatic injury is best understood in terms of the acinus concept of hepatic microanatomy, although the site of injury is usually denoted based on the zones of the hepatic lobule. The site of toxic cellular injury within the hepatic acinus reflects the site of bioactivation of the chemical. For instance, carbon tetrachloride is metabolized by MFOs to $CCl_3^{\cdot}$, a free radical. Lesions induced by carbon tetrachloride are most severe in the periacinar (centrilobular) areas, because this is the area where the smooth endoplasmic reticulum is most abundant, and, therefore, where the active form of the chemical is present in greatest concentration. Conversely, allyl alcohol is activated by alcohol dehydrogenase, a cytosolic enzyme that is most abundant in centroacinar (periportal) areas; hepatocellular injury induced by allyl alcohol consequently is most severe periportally.

Toxic chemicals can be divided into two groups: those that cause predictable hepatic injury (**predictable hepatotoxins**) and those that do not, the latter being referred to as **idiosyncratic toxins.** Predictable hepatotoxins are those that, if given in a sufficient dose, produce hepatic injury in virtually all susceptible animals. The majority of recognized hepatotoxins in veterinary medicine fall into this category; carbon tetrachloride and pyrrolizidine alkaloids are examples of predictable hepatotoxins. Idiosyncratic toxins are those chemicals that cause hepatic injury in a minority of exposed individuals, usually only after prolonged or repeated exposure. The pathogenesis of idiosyncratic toxic injury to the liver is not well understood, and proof of the toxic effect of these chemicals is obviously more difficult to establish. An example of an idiosyncratic hepatotoxin is the inhalation anesthetic halothane.

The morphology of toxin-induced hepatic injury varies considerably with the type, dose, and duration of exposure to toxin, as well as other factors described above. Hepatocytic responses to acute toxic injury usually involve cellular swelling and accumulation of lipid (lipidosis or fatty degeneration) with or without cholestasis. This may progress to necrosis if the toxicosis is sufficiently severe. Continuous or repetitive toxic injury to the liver is characterized by the three stereotypical responses of fibrosis, biliary hyperplasia, and parenchymal regeneration. Toxic hepatic injury can lead to an end-stage liver and, with toxins such as aflatoxins, to hepatic neoplasia. Both acute and chronic toxic injury to the liver can cause hepatic failure. Liver failure can occur in acute intoxications if sufficient functional hepatic mass is lost from degeneration or necrosis of hepatocytes. Chronic liver injury is more likely to lead to liver failure as a result of fibrosis and disruption of hepatic architecture and vascular perfusion.

Toxic Plants. Toxic plants of great variety cause hepatic injury in domestic animals. A comprehensive discussion of each is beyond the scope of this chapter. The phytotoxins (Table 2-1) to be discussed represent three distinct types. The first of these are the preformed hepatic phytotoxins such as occur in blue-green algae. The second type, represented by pyrrolizidine alkaloids, must be metabolized to an active form in the liver. The third types are toxins that are deconjugated by bacteria within the digestive tract to release a factor that is subsequently bioactivated in the liver.

Blue-green algae are now considered protists and no longer members of the plant family, but are grouped with the plants for convenience. Several genera of blue-green algae, including *Anabaena, Aphanizomenon,* and *Microcystis,* have been associated with lethal poisoning of livestock and, less commonly, small animals such as dogs

Table 2-1 Common Hepatotoxic Plants of Veterinary Importance

PLANT FAMILY	SPECIES AFFECTED	TOXIC PRINCIPLE	CHARACTERISTIC INJURY	MISCELLANEOUS
Compositae *Xanthium* spp	Cattle, pigs	Carboxyatractyloside	Periacinar necrosis	Hypoglycemia and ascites in acute intoxication in pigs.
Myoporaceae *Myoporum* spp	Sheep, cattle, horses, pigs	Furanosesquiterperiod oils (ngaione)	Usually periacinar to variable zonal necrosis	Pulmonary injury also occurs in sheep.
Verbenaceae *Lantana camara* *Lippia* spp	Cattle, sheep, goats occasionally	Triterpens (lentadene A & B)	Megalocytosis, canalicular cholestasis, focal hepatocellular necrosis	Icterus and photosensitization common. Renal and myocardial injury also occur.
Compositae *Senecio* spp Leguminosae *Crotalaria* spp Boraginaceae *Heliotropium* spp *Echium* spp *Amsinki* spp	Pigs, horses, cattle, sheep, goats	Pyrrolizidine alkaloids	Megalocytosis, fibrosis, biliary hyperplasia	Pulmonary and renal injury also.
Leguminosae *Cassia* spp	Cattle	Unknown	Periacinar necrosis	Myocardial and skeletal muscle injury predominate in *Cassia occidentalis* intoxication.
Zygophyllaceae *Tribulus terrestris*	Sheep	Unknown	Crystalline material in bile ducts	Interaction with mycotoxin sporidesmin necessary to produce characteristic photosensitization (geeldikkop).
Ulmaceae *Trema aspera*	Cattle, sheep, goats	Trematoxin	Periacinar necrosis	Neuromuscular toxins also. Usually acute disease.
Solanaceae *Cestrum parqui*	Cattle, sheep	Unknown	Periacinar necrosis	Gallbladder edema and hemorrhage. Usually acute disease.
Asteroceae *Tetradymia glabrata*	Sheep	Tetradymol	Periacinar necrosis	Photosensitization is common.
Cyanophyceae (Blue-green algae) *Microcystis* *Aphanizomenon*	Cattle, sheep, horses, goats, dogs	Toxic polypeptide(s)	Periacinar to massive necrosis	Multiple toxins present. Can also cause death by neuromuscular injury.
Cycadales Zamiacea Cycadaceae Stangeriaceae	Cattle, sheep, goats	Methylazoxymethanol	Periacinar necrosis, megalocytosis, cholestasis	Toxin split from nontoxic glycoside. Neurotoxins also present. Chronic ingestion can cause paralysis in cattle.

and cats. Algal blooms usually occur in late summer or early fall, because of the warm temperatures, long hours of sunlight, and abundance of essential nutrients. Dead and dying algae that contain preformed toxins such as microcystin LR, a cyclic heptapeptide, accumulate on the surface of bodies of water and are ingested by livestock. Secondary bacterial growth in dying algae may contribute to toxin formation. Signs develop rapidly and include diarrhea, prostration, and death. Gross lesions include hemorrhagic gastroenteritis and zonal, or even massive, hepatic necrosis. Animals that survive the acute manifestations develop signs of chronic liver disease. Other preformed toxins that affect different organ systems, including the nervous system, have also been identified in blue-green algae.

Pyrrolizidine alkaloids are found in many plant families, including Compositae, Leguminosae, and Borgaginaceae, that occur throughout much of the world. The most important genera are *Senecio, Cynglossum, Amsinckia, Crotolaria, Echium, Trichodesma,* and *Heliotropium.* Approximately 100 different alkaloids are recognized; toxic effects depend on which alkaloids are present within ingested plants. Ingested alkaloids are converted to pyrrolic esters by the hepatic MFO system. These esters are alkylating agents, which react with cytosolic and nuclear constituents. Swine are particularly susceptible to pyr-

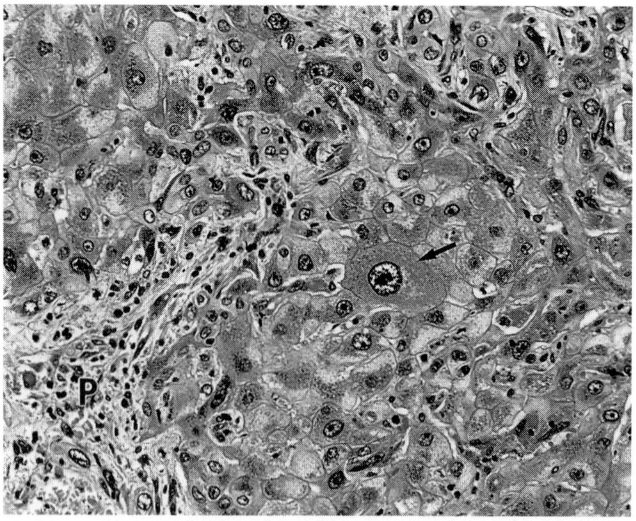

Figure 2-37 Liver; horse. Pyrrolizidine alkaloid intoxication. Note the fibrosis and associated proliferation of bile ducts in portal tracts *(P)* and presence of a greatly enlarged hepatocyte (megalocyte) in the remaining lobular parenchyma *(arrow)*. H & E stain.

rolizidine alkaloid intoxication, sheep considerably less so, and cattle and horses are intermediate in susceptibility. The characteristic lesion of pyrrolizidine alkaloid intoxication is the presence of megalocytes, which are hepatocytes with enlarged nuclei and increased cytoplasmic volume. Megalocytes may be many times the size of normal hepatocytes (Fig. 2-37). Megalocytes are the result of the antimitotic effects of pyrrolizidine alkaloids, which prevent cell division but not DNA synthesis as the hepatocytes attempt to divide to replace those that have undergone necrosis. This change, although indicative of pyrrolizidine alkaloid intoxication, is not pathognomonic, since it occurs with other toxins such as aflatoxins and nitrosamines. Typically, chronic intoxication is accompanied by hepatic fibrosis, biliary duct proliferation, and, in some circumstances, nodular regeneration of parenchyma. Nodular regeneration does not always occur, because hepatocyte proliferation can be inhibited by pyrrolizidines; however, exposure is not likely to be constant and there may be periods during which hepatocyte replication can occur. Species differences also have an impact on the hepatic response to pyrrolizidine alkaloids as cattle have regenerative nodules more often than horses. Chronic hepatic damage can lead to hepatic failure and its associated constellation of signs (described in detail earlier).

Cycads are primitive, palmlike plants that inhabit tropical and subtropical regions. They contain cycasin, a nontoxic glycoside that, following ingestion, is deconjugated by intestinal microflora to release a toxic metabolite, methylazoxymethanol. Hepatic metabolism of this compound produces alkylating agents leading to chronic hepatic lesions in cattle characterized by hepatocellular megalocytosis and nuclear hyperchromasia, and varying degrees of hepatic fibrosis. Acute intoxication is more common in sheep than other species and produces acute gastrointestinal dysfunction and periacinar hepatic necrosis. Chronic cycad poisoning in cattle causes a nervous disease with progressive proprioceptive deficits in the hind legs due to "dying back" of axons in the dorsal funiculus and the spinocerebellar and corticospinal tracts. Dogs can also be intoxicated by cycads. Table 2-1 summarizes some hepatotoxic plants of veterinary importance.

Mycotoxins. Mycotoxins are secondary metabolites of fungi; that is, their production is not necessary for the survival of the fungus. The amount of toxin synthesized by a given strain of fungus reflects the genetic constitution of the particular strain, presence of appropriate substrate, temperature, humidity, and available nutrients. Several hepatotoxic mycotoxins are of significance in veterinary medicine.

Aflatoxins are produced by the fungi *Aspergillus flavus* and *A. parasiticus.* There are four major naturally occurring aflatoxins, B_1, B_2, G_1, and G_2. Aflatoxin B_1 is the most commonly occurring of the group and is also the most potent toxin and carcinogen. Aflatoxins are usually elaborated during storage of fungal-contaminated feed and may be present in many crops, including corn, peanuts, and cottonseed. Aflatoxins are converted to toxic intermediates by the smooth endoplasmic reticulum of hepatocytes. Carcinogenic, toxic, and teratogenic effects of aflatoxins reflect binding of the toxic intermediates to cellular DNA, RNA, or proteins. Pigs, dogs, horses, cattle and ducks, especially younger animals, are sensitive to the toxic effects of aflatoxins, whereas sheep are more resistant. Acute intoxication is rare in domestic animals except dogs, because of the inordinately large amounts of contaminated feed that an animal would have to ingest at one time. Acute aflatoxicosis in dogs is characterized by hemorrhage and centrilobular to massive hepatocellular necrosis. Lipidosis and biliary proliferation also occur. Chronic intoxication is more common and results in ill-thrift, increased susceptibility to infection, and, occasionally, signs of hepatic failure. Affected livers are firm and pale, and, microscopically, are characterized by lipidosis and necrosis of hepatocytes, biliary hyperplasia, fibrosis, and cellular atypia of hepatocytes.

Facial eczema is caused by the mycotoxin sporidesmin, which is produced by *Pithomyces chartarum,* a fungus that grows particularly well in dead rye grass *(Lolium perenne),* a common pasture plant in New Zealand and Australia. Ingestion of sufficient amounts of the toxin produces necrosis of the epithelium of large intrahepatic and extrahepatic biliary ducts and subsequent cholangiohepatitis. Cholestasis with a concurrent failure to excrete phylloerythrin frequently leads to photosensitization with lesions of the head, thus the common name facial eczema. The disease is common in sheep and less so in cattle. Acute cases are characterized by a bile-stained liver with prominent biliary ducts due to dilation, the presence of bile in the lumen and periductual edema. In chronic cases of facial eczema the biliary ducts become thickened secondary to biliary epithelial necrosis and subsequent inflammation (chronic cholangitis and cholangiohepatitis). Perhaps because of streaming of blood in the portal vein, the left lobe (although this lobe occupies the ventral area of the ruminant liver) of the liver is usually most severely affected and, in severe cases, undergoes atrophy and fibrosis. A similar disease, **Geeldikkop,** which is characterized by hepatogenous photosensitization, occurs in sheep in South Africa. It is associated with ingestion of the plant *Tribulus terrestris* and, perhaps, concurrent exposure to sporidesmin.

Phomopsins are products of the fungus **Phomopsis leptostromiformis,** which grows on lupins and produces hepatic injury in cattle, sheep, and occasionally horses that graze contaminated lupin stubble. Hepatic dysfunction is usually chronic and is characterized by hepatic atrophy and fibrosis. Signs of hepatic failure, including photosensitization, occur in affected animals. This mycotoxicosis should not be confused with the poisoning known as lupinosis, which is caused by naturally occurring alkaloids in lupins that are capable of inducing skeletal deformities, but not obvious hepatic injury.

Poisonous mushrooms such as *Amanita* species and others can cause acute fatal liver necrosis. Toxic octapeptides, α-amanitin, in particular, are responsible for hepatocellular necrosis caused by the inhibition of messenger RNA synthesis.

Hepatotoxic Therapeutic Drugs

Various drugs have proven therapeutic application but can cause significant hepatic injury in some animals. Clearly, these drugs would not be used if the proportion of injured animals was high, but it is important to keep in mind that many drugs have the potential to cause hepatic injury in some patients. The mechanisms by which these drugs can cause injury varies by species and by individual, but hepatic metabolism of these compounds is likely to be involved since the site of hepatic injury is typically centrilobular. Cats are more susceptible than dogs to intoxication by many chemicals because they are relatively deficient in hepatic glucuronyl-transferase activity. This phase II enzyme forms conjugates between bioactivated (phase I) xenobiotics and glutathione. When phase II metabolism is overwhelmed, injurious bioactivated products cause hepatic injury. Cats are more sensitive to acetaminophen intoxication than dogs because of this relative enzyme deficiency. The tranquilizer diazepam can cause acute fatal hepatic injury in some cats, but the majority of treated cats are unaffected. The mechanism of injury is not known, but may be a consequence of inherited differences in hepatic enzyme content and activity. Acute hepatic injury can occur in dogs following treatment with trimethoprim-sulfonamide antibiotic preparations. The anti-inflammatory drug carprofen can cause acute hepatic necrosis in dogs. Its toxicity may be more pronounced in certain breeds of dogs, since Labrador retrievers have been affected more often than other breeds.

Chronic hepatic toxicity has been described in dogs receiving any of the anticonvulsants, primidone, phenytoin, and phenobarbital, for prolonged periods. The mechanism of hepatotoxicity is unknown. Only a small proportion of dogs receiving these drugs are affected, and these dogs frequently have signs of hepatic failure. The liver is small and has widespread hepatic fibrosis and nodular regeneration (end-stage liver).

Hepatotoxic Chemicals

Phosphorus occurs in two forms, red phosphorus and white phosphorus. Red phosphorus is unimportant as a toxin, but white phosphorus is occasionally used as a rodenticide. The mechanism of phosphorus toxicity is unclear, although it apparently is directly toxic. Poisoning is first indicated by signs of gastroenteritis and, subsequently, by microscopic lesions of lipidosis of hepatocytes and centroacinar (periportal) necrosis. **Carbon tetrachloride** is the classic example of a compound that must be bioactivated by MFO system in order to become toxic. Although once used widely, it is only occasionally used as an anthelmintic. Carbon tetrachloride produces centrilobular hepatic necrosis and lipidosis of surviving hepatocytes.

Cresols once were incorporated in clay pigeons and asphalt shingles. If swine ingest cresols, centrilobular to massive hepatic hemorrhage and necrosis results.

Metals also can cause toxic hepatic injury. Copper toxicity may present as an acute intravascular hemolytic anemia in ruminants or as chronic hepatic injury and end-stage hepatic disease in dogs. Two specific syndromes of iron poisoning are iron-dextran intoxication of piglets and ferrous fumarate intoxication of newborn foals. Severe cases of these two toxicities are characterized by massive hepatic necrosis. Intoxication of foals with ferrous fumarate occurred following its use as a component of a specific dietary supplement, and was characterized by biliary hyperplasia, despite the short clinical course of the disease. Iron-dextran is frequently administered intramuscularly to suckling pigs to prevent anemia, but administration of iron-dextran has occasionally resulted in significant mortality and affected pigs die soon after infection. Excessive iron supplementation of dogs and cats may result in excessive storage of iron and subsequently hepatic disease associated with iron overload, termed hemochromatosis.

Diseases of Uncertain Etiology

Equine Serum Hepatitis

This disease was first described by Theiler in South Africa at the beginning of the 20th century, but now is recognized in many countries. It occurs in horses frequently, but not invariably in those that have received an injection of a biologic that contains equine serum, for instance, equine antisera such as tetanus antitoxin or pregnant mare serum gonadotropin. It appears that an infectious agent is responsible, although none has been identified. The incubation period is prolonged, but the clinical course of the disease is very rapid and is invariably fatal. Affected horses typically present with hepatic failure that manifests as hepatic encephalopathy and icterus. Intravascular hemolysis occurs in the terminal stages of the disease. The liver of affected animals is small and friable with an enhanced lobular pattern, because of diffuse centrilobular degeneration and necrosis of hepatocytes and subsequent congestion of these necrotic areas. Frequently, only a narrow rim of hepatocytes around portal areas (periportal hepatocytes) survive, and these sometimes are accompanied by proliferating cholangioles.

Canine Chronic Hepatitis (Chronic-Active Hepatitis)

Chronic-active hepatitis is a descriptive term that has been used to identify a particular pattern of inflammation in human liver. There has been considerable debate over the histologic features of chronic-active hepatitis. Emphasis has been placed on the presence of "piecemeal necrosis," which is the destruction of hepatocytes in the limiting plate, those hepatocytes at the border of the hepatic parenchyma and the connective tissue of the portal area. Close contact between hepatocytes, lymphocytes, and macrophages is a characteristic histologic feature. Originally, the purpose of this classification was to identify hepatic lesions, regardless of cause, that were predictive of a progressive course of inflammation and fibrosis. This term was adopted by veterinary pathologists and used to indicate hepatic disorders of the dog that have microscopic changes similar to those seen in human livers. There have been no studies in animals to assess the risk of subsequent hepatic fibrosis in chronically inflamed livers. Based on usage, the term has incorrectly evolved from a morphologic description into a disease entity. The appropriateness and utility of this designation is conjectural in human beings and in dogs. Recent publications in the medical literature have argued that this terminology be abandoned because it was no longer regarded as useful in predicting the course of hepatic disease and it ignored the etiology of the hepatic inflammation.

The term chronic hepatitis, with modifiers indicating the type and degree of inflammation and fibrosis, is used to fully characterize the lesion. If the cause of the inflammation is known, it should be included in the diagnosis. The cause of most spontaneous cases of canine chronic (chronic-active) hepatitis is undetermined, although some cases have been associated with leptospire infection and experimental infectious canine hepatitis virus infection. Progressive chronic hepatitis has been described in cases of hereditary copper toxicosis of Bedlington and West Highland white terriers and has been described previously (see Metabolic Disturbances and Hepatic Accumulations). Familial chronic hepatitis also is associated with excessive hepatic accumulation of copper in the Doberman pinscher (females are predisposed), Skye terrier, cocker spaniel, and Labrador retriever. Abnormal concentrations of hepatic copper in affected dogs of at least some of these breeds has been attributed to cholestasis and decreased hepatic excretion of copper. Many dogs with chronic (chronic-active) hepatitis do not have increased concentrations of hepatic copper, and a wide range of hepatic copper concentrations are present in clinically normal dogs. Thus, the precise role of copper in mediating chronic hepatic disease in breeds of dogs other than the Bedlington and West Highland white terrier remains uncertain. Given the uncertainties regarding etiology and the fact that many cases of chronic (chronic-active) hepatitis in dogs and cats are diagnosed purely on microscopic criteria (i.e., they are not proven to be either chronic or progressive), the use of the term may not be appropriate.

Chronic hepatitis, depending on the duration of inflammation and injury, is characterized by portal and periportal mononuclear cell inflammation, fibrosis of portal areas that may extend into adjacent periportal areas of the lobule, and intrahepatic cholestasis (Fig. 2-38). The liver in cases of chronic hepatitis is usually small, often with an accentuated lobular pattern; severely affected livers are characterized by architectural distortion that ranges from a coarsely nodular texture to an end-stage liver (Fig. 2-30).

Chronic Lymphocytic Cholangitis of Cats

Affected cats are usually older than 4 years and often present with icterus as a consequence of intrahepatic cholestasis. The inflammatory cells can involve bile ducts

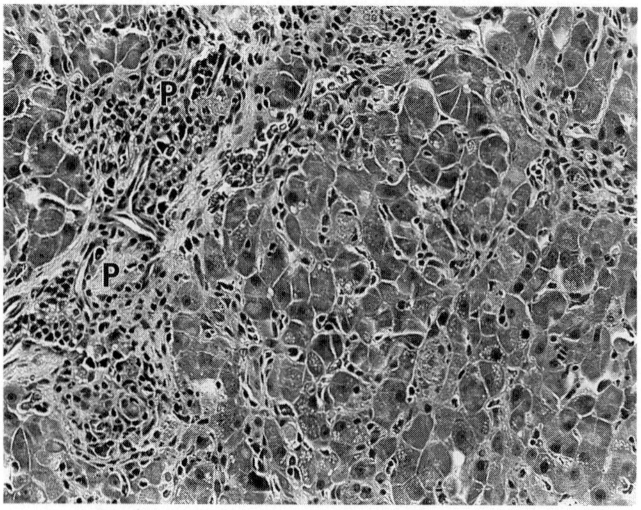

Figure 2-38 Liver; dog, Doberman pinscher. Chronic hepatitis. Note the fibrosis and accumulation of mononuclear and polymorphonuclear inflammatory cells within portal tracts *(P)*. Inflammation and fibrosis also extend into the adjacent hepatic lobule. H & E stain.

directly, making it difficult to identify the original bile duct within an affected portal area. Often by the time a biopsy is obtained, the liver is characterized by extensive aggregations of inflammatory cells, typically lymphocytes and plasma cells, that are present in portal areas, particularly around numerous small biliary ducts (Fig. 2-39). Inflammation usually is accompanied by biliary duct proliferation, hepatic or biliary fibrosis, and intrahepatic cholestasis. The cause or causes of this syndrome are unknown. It can usually be distinguished from cholangitis and cholangiohepatitis from ascending infection of the biliary system secondary to obstruction of the biliary system by cholelithiasis, pancreatitis, and parasitism by the absence of neutrophils. The disease might have an immunologic basis and has been compared with primary biliary cirrhosis of human beings.

Hepatic Injury as a Consequence of Systemic Disease

A variety of extrahepatic disorders can result in hepatocellular injury and hepatic dysfunction. Acute hemorrhagic pancreatitis of dogs, for example, sometimes is accompanied by icterus and increased activities of hepatic enzymes in serum. Release of various toxins and inflammatory mediators from the injured pancreas into the portal vein showers the liver with a variety of injurious substances. Similarly, hepatotoxic substances, such as endotoxin, enter the portal vein as a consequence of diseases that disrupt the mucosal barrier of the intestine. Accumulation of inflammatory cells within the portal areas may be in response to blood-borne infection or abdominal sepsis.

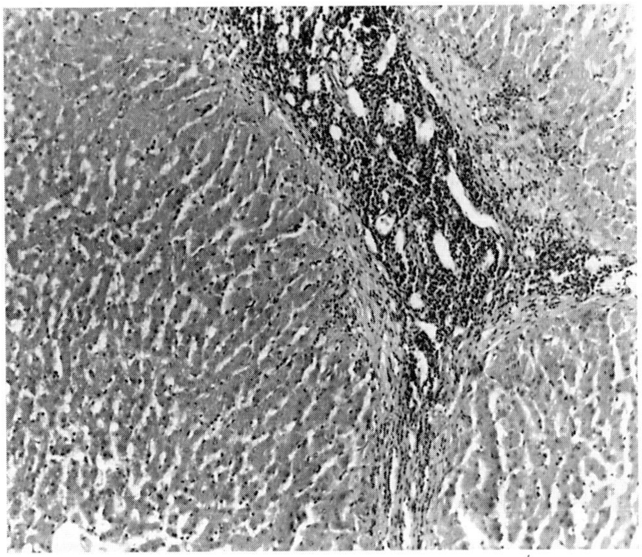

Figure 2-39 Liver; cat. Feline lymphocytic cholangitis. Accumulation of large numbers of lymphocytes and plasma cells within the portal tracts. H & E stain.

The liver is particularly susceptible to the effects of hypoxia; thus, any disease that causes anemia can produce centrilobular (paracentral) degeneration and necrosis. Also, the hepatocytes, in hemolytic anemias, must remove and conjugate the increased amounts of circulating bilirubin and hemoglobin, and Kupffer cells remove either erythrocytes during extravascular hemolysis or erythrocytic fragments during intravascular hemolysis.

Proliferative Lesions of the Liver

Hepatocellular Nodular Hyperplasia

Hepatic nodular hyperplasia is common only in the dog. Incidence increases with age, without predilection for either sex or breed. Nodular hyperplasia is not associated with significant hepatic dysfunction, but hyperplastic nodules must be distinguished from regenerative nodules and hepatic neoplasms, with which they are often confused. Multiple nodules are frequently present. Nodules that can be seen on the capsular surface are typically raised and hemispherical, yellow to tan, 0.5 to 3.0 cm in diameter, and are more friable than normal liver. On incision, the hyperplastic nodules are well demarcated from normal parenchyma and usually compress adjacent parenchyma (Figs. 2-40 and 2-41). Hyperplastic nodules contain all the elements of normal liver, but the lobular pattern is distorted. The lobules in areas of nodular hyperplasia contain an increased proportion of hepatocytes and decreased numbers of portal areas and central veins compared with normal liver. Hepatocytes are variably sized and frequently contain cytoplasmic lipid or glycogen-containing vacuoles.

Regenerative Nodules

Regenerative nodules are another type of nodular hepatic lesion. Regenerative nodules are unlikely to be related to

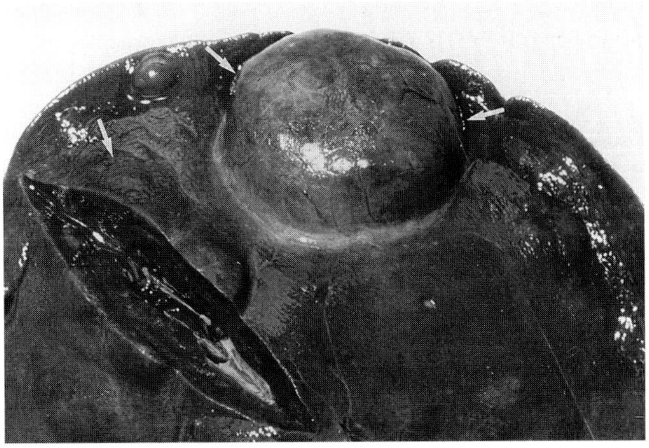

Figure 2-40 Liver, visceral surface; dog. Nodular hyperplasia. Two nodules *(arrows)* protrude above the surface of the adjacent, normal parenchyma. *Courtesy Dr. M.D. McGavin.*

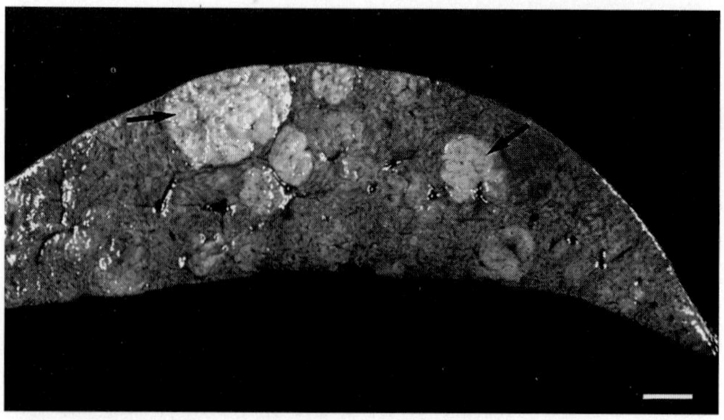

Figure 2-41 Liver, cut surface; dog. Nodular hyperplasia. Several hyperplastic nodules are indicated by arrows. Bar = 5 mm. *Courtesy Dr. R. Fairley.*

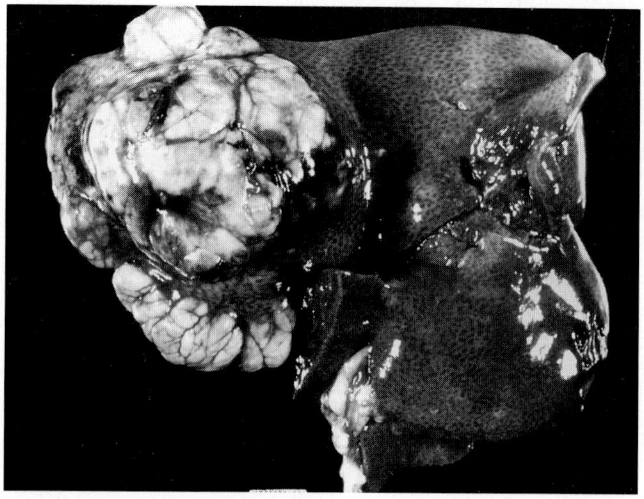

Figure 2-42 Liver; cat. Hepatocellular carcinoma. Multilobular mass that has replaced much of the normal liver.

nodular hyperplasia, since regenerative nodules arise from the proliferation of hepatocytes in response to loss of hepatocytes and the incidence is not related to age. Often the insult is unknown, but the response of some dogs to anticonvulsant drugs such as phenobarbital or phenytoin is a well-recognized cause. Regenerative nodules are readily distinguished from nodular hyperplasia since the process occurs in the presence of significant fibrosis and disruption of normal hepatic parenchymal architecture. Because these lesions result from the outgrowth of surviving hepatocytes, there is usually only a single portal area apparent in sections of the regenerative nodules.

Cholangiocellular (Bile Duct) Hyperplasia

Hyperplasia of biliary ductules commonly occurs as a nonspecific response to a variety of hepatic injuries and has been described previously (see Response of the liver to injury). Reactive proliferation of the ductular elements of the liver must be distinguished from neoplastic proliferations.

Hepatic Neoplasia

Primary neoplasms of the hepatobiliary system can arise from epithelial elements such as hepatocytes and biliary epithelium of bile ducts or the gallbladder and from mesenchymal elements such as connective tissue and blood vessels. The liver is a common site of metastasis for many malignant tumors; in fact, the majority of neoplasms within the liver are metastases from other organs.

Hepatocellular Adenoma

Hepatocellular adenomas are benign neoplasms of hepatocytes. Hepatocellular adenomas have been described most commonly in young ruminants. The neoplasms usually are single, unencapsulated, variably sized, red or brown masses that compress adjacent parenchyma. They are typically spherical but may be pedunculated. They are composed of well-differentiated hepatocytes that form uniform plates that may be two to three cells thick. Hepatic plates in adenomas tend to abut normal adjacent hepatocytes at right angles. Portal areas and central veins are scarce within the neoplasm, if they can be found at all. Diagnostic criteria to distinguish hepatocellular adenomas and hepatocytic nodular hyperplasia are not well established and confusion persists in classification schemes. In other cases, it may also be difficult to distinguish adenomas from well-differentiated hepatocellular carcinomas.

Hepatocellular Carcinoma

Hepatocellular carcinomas are malignant neoplasms of hepatocytes. They are uncommon in all domestic species but occur more frequently in ruminants, particularly sheep. Neoplasms are usually solitary, often involving an entire lobe, and are well demarcated. They typically consist of friable, gray-white or yellow-brown tissue that is subdivided into lobules by multiple fibrous bands (Fig. 2-42). Malignant hepatocytes characteristically form irregular plates (trabeculae) three or more cells thick, and vascular spaces are present between the trabeculae (Fig.

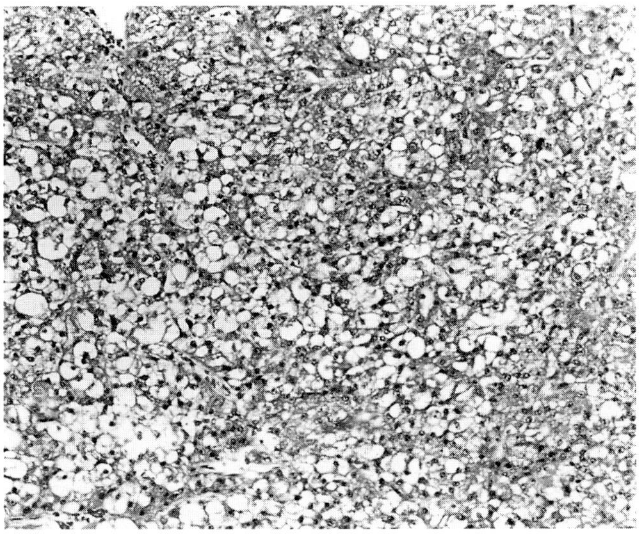

Figure 2-43 Liver; dog. Hepatocellular carcinoma. Note the irregular lobules of hepatocytes that lack the normal microanatomic appearance of liver tissue. H & E stain.

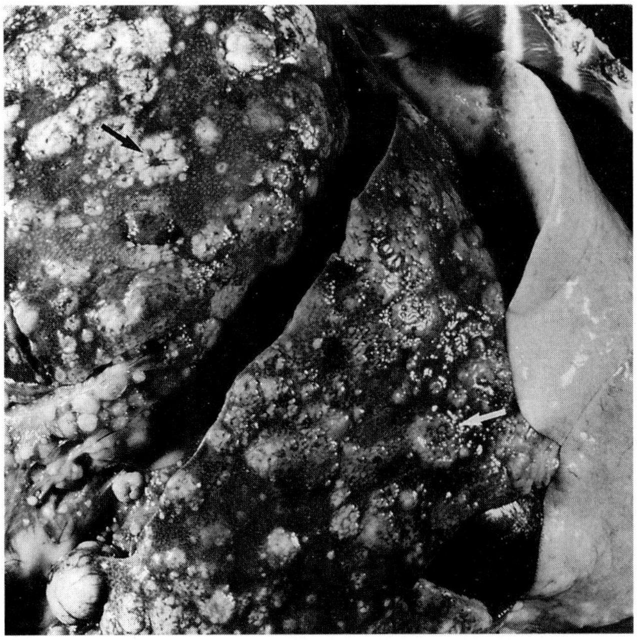

Figure 2-44 Liver; dog. Cholangiocellular carcinoma. Multiple nodules of tumor, some of which have an umbilicated appearance *(arrows)*. H & E stain. *Courtesy Dr. M.D. McGavin.*

2-43). Crude acini or aggregates of neoplastic cells are sometimes present. Cells present in the neoplasm range from well-differentiated hepatocytes to atypical or bizarre forms. In the absence of metastasis, which is obviously indicative of malignancy, distinction of well-differentiated carcinoma and adenoma can be difficult, although invasion of malignant hepatocytes at the margin of the compressed normal hepatocytes is a useful indicator of malignancy. Metastasis to a variety of sites occurs, particularly to lymph nodes within the cranial abdomen, lungs, and seeding into the tissues lining the peritoneal cavity. Some hepatocellular carcinomas spread extensively within the liver (intrahepatic metastasis).

Cholangiocellular (Bile Duct) Adenoma

Adenomas of the biliary ducts are uncommon in most species, but may be the most common primary hepatic neoplasm in cats. They are usually discrete, firm, gray or white masses composed of well-differentiated biliary epithelium. Cholangiomas are glandlike structures formed by tubules lined with cuboidal epithelium and moderate amounts of stroma. The tubules may have narrow lumens or be distended by fluid, forming cystic structures of variable sizes. Cystic variants, biliary cystadenomas, typically have a nonencapsulated, multilocular cystic structure. Hepatocytes are usually compressed at the margins, but may be entrapped by expanding cysts. The stroma of the cyst wall consists of fibrovascular tissue with moderate amounts of collagen. Cysts are lined with benign biliary epithelium, simple cuboidal to flattened. The lining epithelium tends to be more flattened in the biliary cystadenomas, presumably as a result of compression. Biliary epithelial cells may form papillary projections extending into the cystic spaces.

In cats, large cystic cavities that are lined by flattened biliary epithelium are regarded as adenomas by some investigators, whereas others consider them to be congenital malformations (Figs. 2-8 and 2-9). Some of these lesions are multiloculated and can involve extensive areas of the liver. A similar, but clearly congenital polycystic hepatic disease also occurs in dogs. It is likely that the proliferative ductular elements in affected dogs and cats represent abnormal cellular proliferations, rather than simple congenital anomalies of the ductular system.

Cholangiocellular (Bile Duct) Carcinoma

Cholangiocellular carcinomas are malignant neoplasms of biliary epithelium that usually arise from the intrahepatic ducts. These neoplasms occur in all species. A large single mass or multiple nodules may be present within the liver. These neoplasms typically are firm, raised, often with a central depression (umbilicated), pale gray to tan, and unencapsulated (Fig. 2-44). The tumors are composed of cells that retain a resemblance to biliary epithelium. Characteristically, well-differentiated carcinomas are organized into a tubular or acinar arrangement. In less-differentiated neoplasms, some acinar arrangements can be

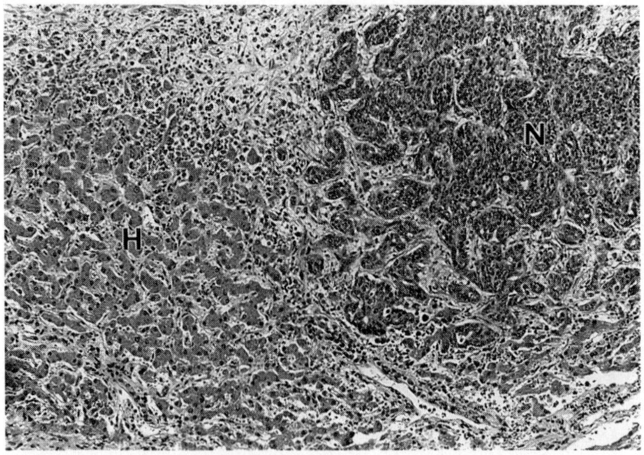

Figure 2-45 Liver; cat. Cholangiocellular carcinoma. Cords and acini of neoplastic cells *(N)* are adjacent to persisting hepatic parenchyma *(H)*. H & E stain.

detected among solid masses of neoplastic cells. Poorly differentiated carcinomas are composed of packets, islands, or cords, and areas of squamous differentiation can occur. The epithelial components of the neoplasms are usually separated by fibrous connective tissue (Fig. 2-45). The amount of the connective tissue varies among tumors, but an abundant deposition of collagen, termed a scirrhous response, is relatively common and is responsible for the firm texture of these neoplasms. The margins of cholangiocarcinomas are characterized by multiple sites of local invasion by tumor cells of surrounding hepatic parenchyma. Multiple sites of hepatic necrosis are also common in the adjacent parenchyma.

Metastasis to extrahepatic sites is common, particularly to the adjacent lymph nodes of the cranial abdomen, lungs, or by seeding into the abdominal cavity. Metastasis into the peritoneal cavity can produce variably sized nodules within the mesentery and on the serosal surface of the abdominal viscera.

Miscellaneous Primary Neoplasms of the Liver

Primary neoplasms can arise from any of the cellular constituents of the liver, including carcinoids, which are neoplasms of neuroendocrine cells; mesenchymal neoplasms derived from the liver's connective tissue (fibrosarcoma, osteosarcoma); muscle (leiomyosarcoma); and endothelium (hemangioma and hemangiosarcoma). Hemangiosarcoma primary to the liver is well recognized in dogs, although it is a relatively uncommon site of origin for this neoplasm compared with the skin and spleen. Primary mesenchymal neoplasms of the liver must be distinguished from metastases; the presence of disseminated masses throughout the liver is more typical of metastatic sarcomas than of primary hepatic sarcomas.

Metastatic Neoplasms

The liver and the lungs are the two most common sites for metastatic spread of malignant neoplasms. Metastatic neoplasms must be distinguished from primary hyperplasia or neoplasia of the hepatobiliary tissues. It is important, therefore, when examining a neoplasm within the liver to determine whether a neoplasm is present at some extrahepatic site that might be the primary neoplasm. Malignant lymphoma is the most common metastatic neoplasm found in the liver of most, if not all, species.

Some metastatic neoplasms have a typical appearance within the liver; for example, melanomas frequently are black because of the presence of melanin, and hemangiosarcomas are usually dark red to brown. Hematopoietic neoplasms such as lymphoma and the myeloproliferative disorders can diffusely expand the liver, thereby producing hepatomegaly and an enhanced lobular pattern on the cut surface. This characteristic appearance is attributable to centrilobular hepatocellular degeneration because of anemia in both malignant lymphoma and myeloproliferative disorders and because of different sites of accumulation of neoplastic cells within the hepatic lobule. In malignant lymphoma, neoplastic lymphocytes tend to infiltrate portal tracts and expand their margins with extension into the adjacent parenchyma in severe cases. Sarcomas of the myeloid cell series are more often characterized by a distribution of neoplastic cells within the sinusoids. Metastatic carcinomas often have an umbilicated appearance, similar to that seen with cholangiocellular carcinomas, but umbilication is rarely a feature of sarcomas.

GALLBLADDER

Structure and Function

The structure of the gallbladder and major ducts of the biliary system is similar in most species (the gallbladder is absent in the horse, the rat, and the elephant). It consists of a muscular wall (tunica muscularis) and a mucosa lined by simple columnar epithelium. The epithelium and muscularis are separated only by the lamina propria as the gallbladder lacks a muscularis mucosae. Hepatic bile ducts carry bile from different lobes of the liver; these ducts and the cystic duct from the gallbladder unite to form the common bile duct. Location of the opening of the common bile duct into the intestine differs somewhat among the domestic species; it is as little as 2 cm from the pylorus in the pig to as much as 70 cm from the pylorus in the cow.

The gallbladder stores and concentrates bile. Considerable concentration (20- to 30-fold) of bile by active transport of sodium and anions across the gallbladder epithelial cells occurs in dogs and cats, whereas little concentration occurs in swine and ruminants. The horse lacks a gallbladder and continuously releases bile into the duodenum.

Bile consists of water, bile acids, bilirubin, cholesterol, inorganic ions, and a variety of other constituents. Bile formation is continuous, but the rate of secretion can vary significantly. Active secretion of bile acids into the bile canaliculi is the most important physiologic stimulus for bile production. Secretion of bile provides (1) bile acids that are necessary for digestion of dietary fats, (2) an excretory route for various metabolites and drugs, and (3) buffers to neutralize the acid pH of the ingesta.

Bile acids are critical for normal digestion and absorption of fats and fat-soluble vitamins; however, the quantities of bile acids required far exceed the liver's capacity to produce them. For this reason, bile acids are reabsorbed from the intestine and resecreted into bile. This process is referred to as the **enterohepatic circulation of bile acids.** This is a very efficient system, and the proportion of reabsorbed bile acids in the liver greatly exceeds recently synthesized bile acids. Interruption of this process results in fat malabsorption and a deficiency of fat-soluble vitamins.

Biliary Obstruction, Cholelithiasis, and Inflammatory Disorders

Biliary Obstruction

Obstruction of the bile ducts in domestic animals is usually caused by choleliths, foreign bodies such as parasites within the bile ducts, and stenosis of the ducts as a consequence of external compression by a neoplasm or periductular fibrosis; the latter may follow pancreatic inflammation. Complete obstruction of the common bile duct leads to extrahepatic cholestasis and jaundice. Obstruction of the individual intrahepatic hepatic ducts is usually asymptomatic. Prolonged extrahepatic cholestasis causes dilation of bile ducts, biliary hyperplasia in the portal areas with extension into the parenchyma, and hepatocellular injury due to retention of bile constituents. Bile may be evident within distended canaliculi or within bile ducts. Rupture of canaliculi can lead to hepatocyte death and formation of areas of pooled bile (bile lakes). The leakage of bile into portal areas causes inflammation and fibrosis that can progress to extensive scarring of these areas, termed biliary fibrosis (Fig. 2-6).

Cholelithiasis

Choleliths, or gallstones as they are commonly called, occur infrequently in all the domestic species, but they are especially well described in ruminants. Choleliths are concretions of normally soluble components of bile. They form when these components become supersaturated and precipitate. Choleliths in the gallbladder usually do not become clinically significant unless they migrate and obstruct the biliary system.

Cholecystitis

Cholecystitis is inflammation of the gallbladder and can be acute or chronic. Acute inflammation of the gallbladder occurs in viral infections such as Rift Valley fever in ruminants and infectious canine hepatitis, which produces a characteristic edema and hemorrhages in the gallbladder. Fibrinous cholecystitis occurs in calves with acute salmonellosis, particularly that caused by *Salmonella enteritidis,* serotype *dublin*. Other bacteria, either derived from the blood or ascended from the intestine, can cause acute or chronic cholecystitis. Chronic cholecystitis typically accompanies prolonged bacterial infection of the biliary tree, or ongoing irritation from choleliths or parasites of the gallbladder. Rupture of the gallbladder is rare, but can occur as a result of acute or chronic infection. The resultant release of bile, with or without accompanying bacteria, can cause life-threatening peritonitis because of the irritating effect of bile on the serosal surfaces of the abdomen.

Hyperplastic and Neoplastic Lesions of the Gallbladder

Cystic Mucinous Hyperplasia of the Gallbladder

Cystic mucinous hyperplasia of the gallbladder mucosa has only been reported in dogs and sheep. There are no apparent abnormalities evident from the exterior of the gallbladder, and the features of cystic hyperplasia can only be appreciated by opening the gallbladder and draining residual bile that may obscure the mucosa. When the bile is rinsed away, the affected mucosa is gray-white and has a diffusely thickened, spongelike consistency. Sessile or polypoid masses are occasionally found, and occasionally large cysts occur and are evident as papillary projections into the lumen of the gallbladder. Numerous 1- to 3-mm cysts within the hyperplastic mucosa impart the characteristic appearance. The hallmark of cystic hyperplasia of the gallbladder is the abundance of variably sized cystic spaces that distort and thicken the entire mucosa of the gallbladder. Most of the cysts contain a copious amount of mucus. The majority of the lining epithelial cells are typical of the normal gallbladder epithelium, i.e., tall columnar with abundant apical cytoplasmic mucus. The entire mucosa may be affected (Fig. 2-46). These lesions are usually of no significance to the host. In all likelihood, cystic hyperplasia of the gallbladder frequently goes undetected clinically. The cause is not known.

Adenoma

Adenomas of the gallbladder are rare neoplasms but are most common in young cattle and have also been described in dogs, cats, and sheep. They are multinodular or papillary masses that protrude from the mucosal surface and consist of a loose connective tissue stalk that is lined by well-differentiated biliary epithelium.

Carcinoma

Malignant neoplasms of the gallbladder epithelium are rare in domestic animals, but have been described in dogs, cats, and cattle. They typically are composed of mucin-secreting epithelial cells and often have a papillary

A

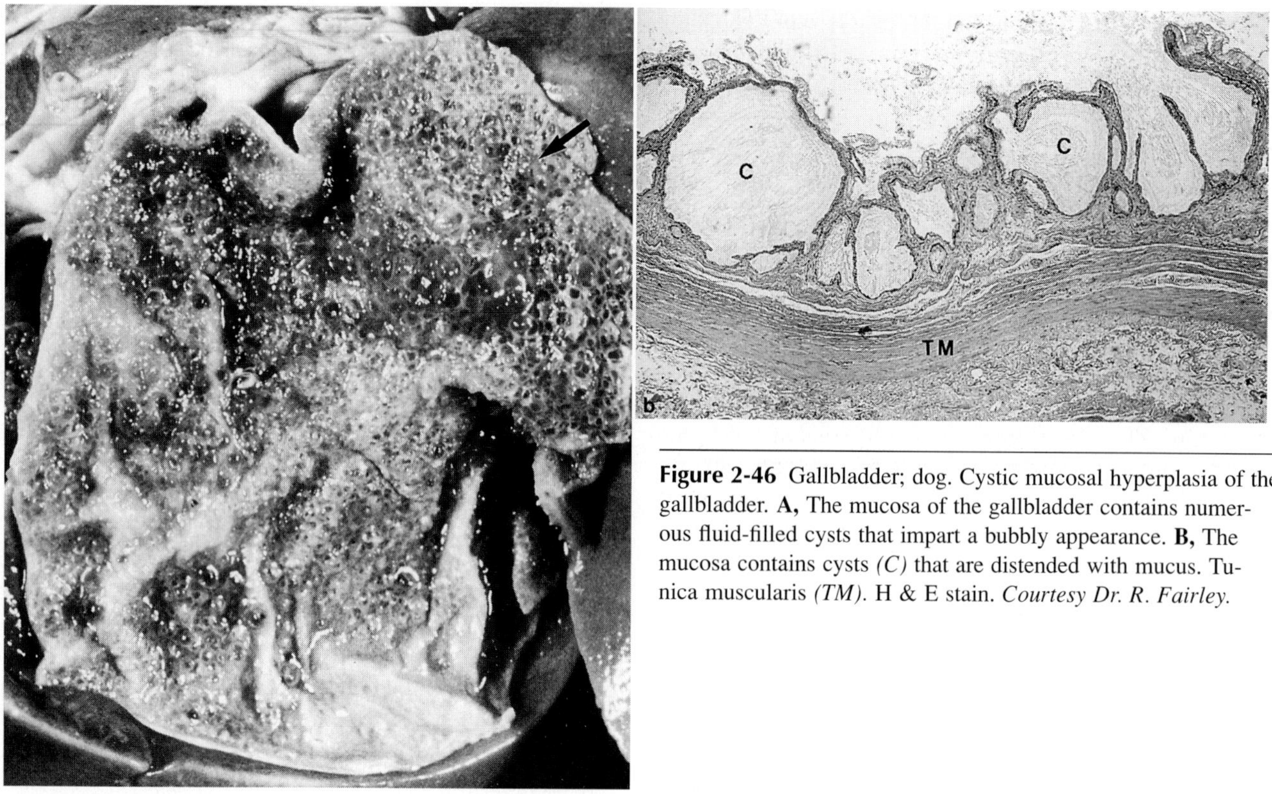

B

Figure 2-46 Gallbladder; dog. Cystic mucosal hyperplasia of the gallbladder. **A,** The mucosa of the gallbladder contains numerous fluid-filled cysts that impart a bubbly appearance. **B,** The mucosa contains cysts *(C)* that are distended with mucus. Tunica muscularis *(TM)*. H & E stain. *Courtesy Dr. R. Fairley.*

arrangement. Carcinoma of the gallbladder may invade the liver by direct extension and may metastasize to the hepatic lymph nodes and to more distant sites.

EXOCRINE PANCREAS

Structure and Function

The pancreas is a lobulated, pink to gray, tubuloalveolar gland, a large portion of which is located immediately adjacent to the duodenum. The blood vessels, nerves, and lymph vessels that serve the pancreas are located within the delicate connective tissue septa that separate the lobules of pancreatic tissue. The pancreas contains both endocrine and exocrine elements, the endocrine portion being the islets of Langerhans. The exocrine portion constitutes the majority of the pancreas and consists of acini composed of secretory cells. The ductal system, in which secretions of the exocrine pancreas are conveyed to the intestinal tract, commences as fine radicals within acini and progresses to intralobular and interlobular ducts. These small ducts eventually drain into the main pancreatic duct or ducts. The arrangement of the major pancreatic ducts and how they empty into the duodenum varies among the domestic species, and is particularly variable in the dog in which at least five different anatomic arrangements are recognized.

The exocrine pancreas produces secretions that contribute to digestion in that they contain a variety of enzymes that break down dietary lipids (lipase and phospholipase), proteins (trypsin and chymotrypsin), and carbohydrates (amylase). The secretions also contain electrolytes that maintain the pH of the intestinal contents within a range that is optimal for enzymatic activity. Pancreatic enzymes act on the products of gastric digestion after they enter the duodenum. These enzymes often are released into secretions as inactive precursors (proenzymes), which helps prevent degradation of the pancreas by its own digestive enzymes. These are activated within the intestine. In addition, inhibitors of pancreatic enzymes are present in the pancreatic tissue. Secretion is controlled by both neural and humoral factors.

Consequences of Dysfunction of the Exocrine Pancreas

The exocrine pancreas has considerable functional reserve; thus, only disorders that affect large portions of this organ can cause the maldigestion that characterizes failure of exocrine pancreatic function. Maldigestion as a consequence of exocrine pancreatic insufficiency is most common in the dog, in which it usually is associated with either pancreatic atrophy or chronic pancreatitis. However, the disorder does occur sporadically in other species including cattle, specifically calves with pancreatic hypoplasia, and in cats. Exocrine pancreatic insufficiency in small animals and calves is characterized by steatorrhea, diarrhea, and weight loss despite polyphagia. In contrast, horses with very little functional pancreatic tissue may develop hypoinsulism, but rarely develop the clinical signs that characterize exocrine pancreatic insufficiency in other species.

Developmental Anomalies

Pancreatic Hypoplasia

Hypoplasia of the exocrine pancreas occurs sporadically in calves and is characterized by signs of exocrine pancreatic insufficiency. Pancreatic hypoplasia has also been described in the dog, but this disease entity is usually considered as pancreatic atrophy rather than true hypoplasia (described under juvenile pancreatic atrophy). In cases of pancreatic hypoplasia, pancreatic tissue is difficult to identify; the amount is small and the persisting parenchyma is neither discrete nor lobulated like the normal gland. The distinction between atrophy and hypoplasia can be difficult to determine because both processes lead to abnormally small organ with diminished function. Parenchymal cells of the hypoplastic exocrine pancreas do not usually contain lipofuscin, which can be seen in atrophic cells.

Anomalies of the Duct System

The arrangement of the major pancreatic duct or ducts varies between and within species, so a variety of normal arrangements occurs. Sheep, for instance, have only one pancreatic duct that drains into the common bile duct, whereas cattle and horses typically have two ducts, and several distinct arrangements of the pancreatic ducts have been described in dogs. Specific anomalies include congenital stenosis of the pancreatic ducts and cystic dilation of the ducts. Congenital cysts within the pancreas occasionally occur in lambs.

Incidental Findings

Ectopic Pancreatic Tissue

Nodules of ectopic pancreatic tissue sometimes are present in the duodenum, stomach, spleen, gallbladder, and mesentery of the dog and cat. This typc of anomaly, normal tissue in an abnormal location, is termed a choristoma.

Pacinian Corpuscles

Pacinian corpuscles are normally present within the interlobular connective tissue of the pancreas and mesentery of the cat, and appear as discrete 1- to 3-mm nodules (Fig. 2-47). The corpuscles should not be mistaken for abnormal structures.

Autolysis

Autolysis of the pancreas is very rapid after death, particularly if the pancreas is traumatized. Postmortem release and activation of pancreatic proteolytic enzymes within the pancreas can hasten tissue breakdown. Thus, autolysis may be advanced in the pancreas before it is evident in other organs. As autolysis progresses, the color of the gland changes from its normal pink to dark red or green. The metabolic activity of intestinal bacteria, which can easily gain access to the pancreas, can contribute to the discoloration of the pancreas through hemolysis and tissue decomposition.

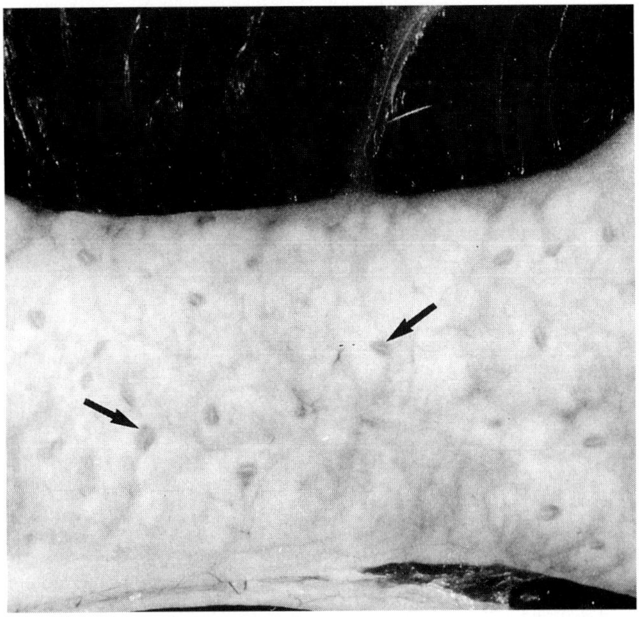

Figure 2-47 Pancreas; cat. Pacinian corpuscles *(arrows)*. The feline pancreas contains numerous pacinian corpuscles, which may be visible grossly.

Pancreatic Calculi

The formation of concretions or "stones" within the pancreatic duct system is termed **pancreolithiasis,** and occurs uncommonly in cattle. It is usually an incidental finding at slaughter, and apparently is slightly more common in cattle greater than 4 years of age.

Stromal Fat Cell Infiltration

Fat cell infiltration of the interstitial connective tissue of the pancreas occurs occasionally, especially in obese cats. The pancreas itself is usually unaffected, so exocrine pancreatic function is normal, but the dispersion of the parenchyma creates the impression that the pancreas has been replaced by adipose tissue.

Pancreatic Degeneration, Necrosis, Inflammation, and Response to Injury

Pancreatic Degeneration

Degeneration of the acinar cells of the exocrine pancreas is a nonspecific process that can occur as a consequence of a variety of local and systemic diseases. For instance, starvation results in loss of zymogen granules within the cytoplasm of acinar cells of the exocrine pancreas because the rate of synthesis of the granules is diminished and available protein is used to maintain serum protein concentrations when dietary protein is limited. Obstruction of the pancreatic ducts, whatever the cause, can also cause degeneration and atrophy of the exocrine pancreas. Obstruction of the pancreatic duct(s) can be caused by neoplasms or chronic inflammation and associated fibrosis, which compress the duct, or by foreign bodies such as parasites or pancreoliths, which occlude the ductal lumen. Exocrine pancreatic atrophy also may occur secondary to widespread interstitial fibrosis of the pancreas, as occurs for example in dogs with chronic pancreatitis.

Juvenile Pancreatic Atrophy

A distinct syndrome characterized by atrophy of the exocrine pancreas has been recognized in several breeds of dog. It is particularly common in the German shepherd dog, in which it appears to be inherited as an autosomal recessive trait. Young animals are affected, usually between 6 and 12 months of age. This lesion may be one of hypoplasia or atrophy, although recent studies suggest the latter process. Affected dogs have signs typical of maldigestion secondary to exocrine pancreatic insufficiency and rapidly lose weight despite a voracious appetite. The pancreas in affected dogs is small (Fig. 2-48), but islands of normal exocrine pancreatic tissue usually remain.

Pancreatic Necrosis, Pancreatitis, and Response to Injury

Pancreatic necrosis and pancreatitis has been described in a variety of species, although the cause usually is different in each species. Specific causes of necrosis of acinar cells of the exocrine pancreas include *Cassia occidentalis* intoxication and T-2 toxin (a trichothecene mycotoxin) toxicosis of swine, as well as zinc toxicosis of veal calves and sheep. Undoubtedly, however, spontaneous (idiopathic) necrosis and inflammation of the pancreas is most common in the dog and, to a lesser extent the cat. Pancreatic necrosis and pancreatitis may occur as either an acute or chronic disease process and, although the pathogenesis is similar, the clinical signs and lesions of acute and chronic pancreatitis are distinct.

Acute Pancreatitis. Acute pancreatitis is particularly common in the dog, and obese sedentary bitches are especially predisposed. A similar process occurs less often in cats. Pancreatitis in dogs occurs as a consequence of release of activated pancreatic enzymes into the pancreatic parenchyma and adjacent tissues. These activated enzymes, particularly phospholipase A and elastase, digest pancreatic tissue, which in turn results in release of inflammatory mediators, which further amplify the process and attract inflammatory cells. The mechanism responsible for the release of the potent pancreatic enzymes into these tissues is incompletely characterized and may involve more than one initiating event. Acute pancreatitis commonly occurs after dogs have consumed a meal high in fat.

Signs of acute pancreatitis include anorexia, vomiting, and abdominal pain. The lesions of acute pancreatitis are referable to proteolytic degradation of pancreatic parenchyma, vascular damage and hemorrhage, and necrosis of peripancreatic fat by lipolytic enzymes. Inflammation, characterized by the accumulation of leukocytes around the affected tissue, rapidly follows the initial tissue necrosis. Mild cases of pancreatitis are characterized by edema of the interstitial tissue of the pancreas. Acute

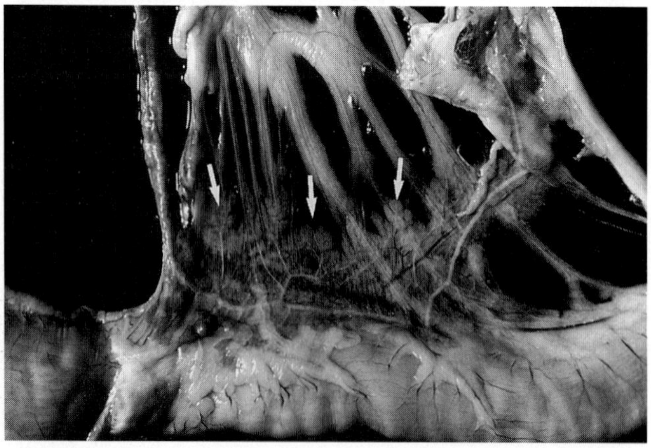

Figure 2-48 Pancreas; dog. Pancreatic atrophy/hypoplasia. Virtually no pancreatic tissue is present in this case. Pancreatic remnant is identified with arrows. *Courtesy Dr. M.D. McGavin.*

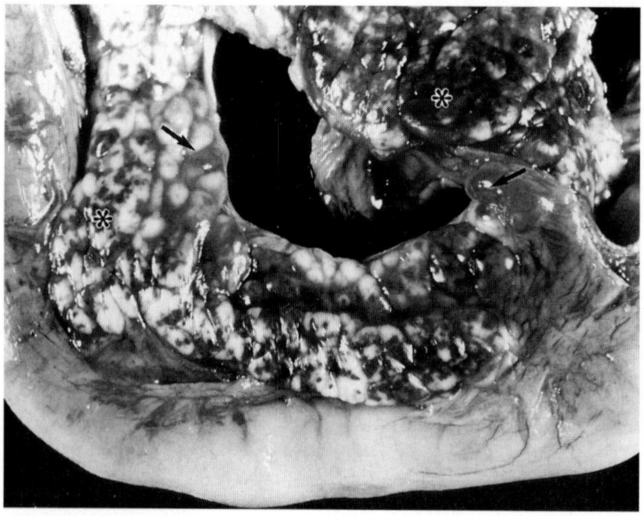

Figure 2-49 Pancreas; dog. Acute hemorrhagic pancreatitis. Note areas of hemorrhage *(asterisks)* and edema *(arrows)* present throughout the pancreas. *Courtesy Dr. R. Fairley.*

hemorrhagic pancreatitis is more severe. Characteristically the pancreas is edematous and contains areas that are gray-white, the result of coagulation necrosis, and other dark red or blue-black areas that are hemorrhagic (Fig. 2-49). Areas of fat necrosis are manifest as chalky-white foci as a result of saponification of necrotic adipose tissue in the mesentery adjacent to the pancreas. Portions of normal pancreatic parenchyma may be interspersed between affected portions. The peritoneal cavity frequently contains blood-stained fluid, which may contain droplets of fat. Peritonitis is manifest by fibrinous adhesions between the affected portions of the pancreas and adjacent tissues.

The microscopic appearance of acute hemorrhagic pancreatitis reflects the gross lesions just described. Characteristic lesions include focally extensive areas of hemorrhage, influx of leukocytes and coagulation necrosis of the pancreatic parenchyma, accumulation of fibrinous exudate in the interlobular septa, and necrosis and inflammation of fat in the mesentery adjacent to the affected portions of pancreas (Figs. 2-50 and 2-51).

Acute, severe pancreatitis produces systemic effects in affected dogs. The release of inflammatory mediators and activated enzymes from the damaged pancreas may produce widespread vascular injury and subsequent widespread hemorrhage, shock, and disseminated intravascular coagulation. The liver also is affected in many cases of pancreatitis, as indicated by increased concentrations of serum hepatic enzymes (such as alanine aminotransferase), and sometimes focal hepatic necrosis.

Pancreatitis is occasionally initiated by trauma, usually in dogs and cats as a consequence of some crushing or impact trauma to the abdomen. Leakage of enzymes from the pancreas initiates necrosis followed by trauma and inflammation of the pancreas and adjacent tissues in the same manner as previously described for pancreatitis in the dog.

Acute pancreatitis sufficient to cause clinical disease apparently is considerably less common in species other than the dog and cat. Acute pancreatic necrosis and pancreatitis have been described in the horse; but the pathogenesis of pancreatitis in this species differs from that in the dog and cat. Necrosis and inflammation are the result of migration of strongyle larvae through the pancreas, which results in the release of pancreatic enzymes and enzymatic digestion of the pancreas, and surrounding tissues.

Chronic Pancreatitis. Chronic pancreatitis is often accompanied by fibrosis and parenchymal atrophy. It can occur in all species as a consequence of obstruction of the pancreatic ducts. Chronic inflammation of the pancreas is most common and important in the dog, but does occur in the cat, horse, and cattle, in which it is rarely of clinical significance. In the dog, pancreatic fibrosis and chronic pancreatitis are the result of progressive destruction of the pancreas by repeated mild episodes of acute pancreatic necrosis and pancreatitis. The pancreas has poor regenerative capacity and responds to injury with replacement fibrosis and atrophy of persisting parenchyma. Thus, ongoing destruction of pancreatic tissue causes progressive loss of glandular tissue without replacement (Fig. 2-52). If a significant portion of the pancreas is affected, dogs develop signs of exocrine pancreatic insufficiency, with or without signs of endocrine pancreatic insufficiency (diabetes mellitus). Grossly, the pancreas in

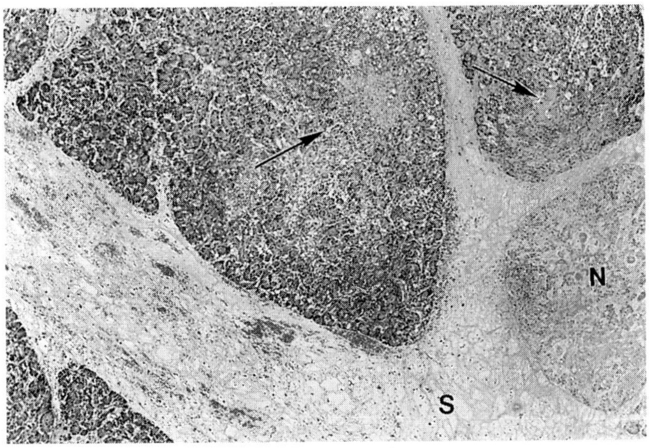

Figure 2-50 Pancreas; dog. Acute hemorrhagic pancreatitis (histologic appearance of the pancreas depicted in Fig. 2-49). Note the accumulation of fibrinous exudate within the interlobular septa *(S)* and coagulation necrosis of one lobule *(N)* and portions of others *(arrows)*. H & E stain.

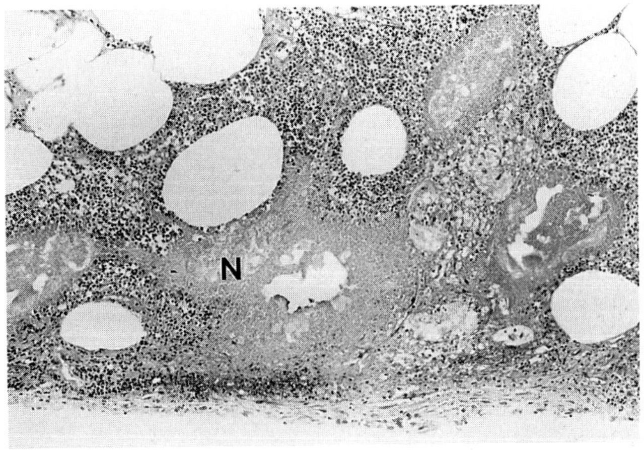

Figure 2-51 Pancreas; dog. Acute hemorrhagic pancreatitis. Necrotic fat *(N)* in the mesentery adjacent to the pancreas is surrounded by degenerated neutrophils. H & E stain.

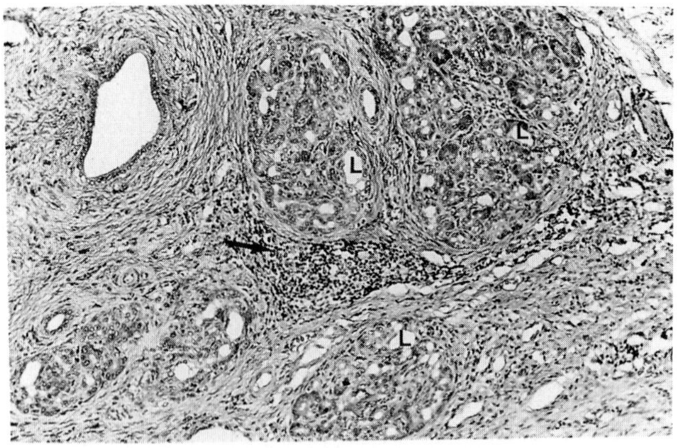

Figure 2-52 Pancreas; cat. Chronic pancreatitis. Note the atrophic lobules *(L)* separated by fibrous connective tissue that contains lymphocytes *(arrow)*. H & E stain.

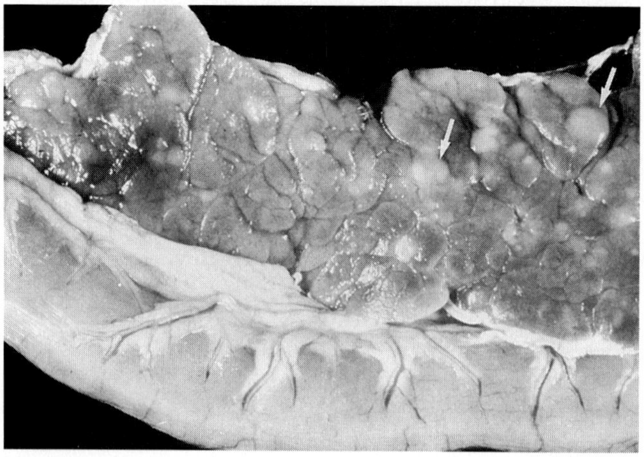

Figure 2-53 Pancreas; dog. Nodular hyperplasia of exocrine pancreas. Hyperplastic nodules *(arrows)* are pale and project above the surface.

affected animals is a distorted, shrunken, and nodular mass with fibrous adhesions to adjacent tissues. Destruction of pancreatic tissue frequently is not of sufficient magnitude to cause exocrine pancreatic insufficiency, and pancreatic fibrosis is sometimes found as an incidental lesion at necropsy of dogs with apparently normal digestive function. Fibrosis of the exocrine pancreas also occurs with some frequency in cats and following necrosis of exocrine pancreatic cells from zinc toxicosis in sheep.

Chronic pancreatitis and replacement fibrosis occur sporadically in the horse, usually as a consequence of either parasitic migration or from ascending bacterial infection of the pancreatic ducts. In addition, pancreatitis may occur in horses with chronic eosinophilic gastroenteritis. However, chronic pancreatitis usually is not clinically apparent in the horse, as signs of exocrine pancreatic insufficiency rarely, if ever, occur in this species.

Pancreatic cysts are fluid-filled fibrous sacs that occur as a sequela to pancreatitis in some dogs and cats. Ectasia of the pancreatic ducts with cyst formation also is relatively common in cats with interstitial pancreatic fibrosis.

Parasitic Infections

A variety of parasites inhabit the pancreatic ducts of domestic animals. Parasitic infections of the pancreatic ducts are important if they occlude the ducts, either by direct physical obstruction or by inducing inflammation within and around ducts. Examples include flukes of the families Opisthorchidae *(Opisthorchis tenuicollis, Opisthorchis viverrini, Clonorchis sinensis, Metorchis albidus, Metorchis conjunctus)* and Dicrocoelidae *(Eurytrema pancreaticum, Concinnum procyonis, Dicrocoelium dendriticum)* that may inhabit the pancreatic ducts of a variety of animal species. Nematodes, particularly ascarids, and cestodes are common gastrointestinal parasites of the domestic species; occasionally, they lodge within the pancreatic ducts.

Hyperplasia and Neoplasia

Pancreatic Nodular Hyperplasia

Nodular hyperplasia of the exocrine pancreas occurs in dogs, cats, and cattle. It is especially common in older dogs and cats. The lesion is of no clinical significance, but it must be distinguished from neoplasms of the endocrine and exocrine pancreas.

These hyperplastic nodules typically are multiple, raised, smooth, and a uniform gray or white on cut surface (Fig. 2-53). The nodules are firmer than adjacent normal pancreas. Microscopically, these nodules consist of unencapsulated aggregates of acinar cells. The distinction between hyperplasia and adenoma of the exocrine pancreas is poorly defined in domestic animals.

Pancreatic Adenoma

Adenomas of the exocrine pancreas are rare, but have been described in the cat (Fig. 2-54). Those of acinar cell origin share all the features of hyperplastic nodules, but are single and larger than normal pancreatic lobules, whereas hyperplastic nodules are not larger than normal lobules; this distinction clearly is somewhat arbitrary.

Pancreatic Carcinoma

Carcinoma of the ductular epithelium or acinar cells of the exocrine pancreas is uncommon in all species. It is most often reported in the dog and cat. The neoplasms are single or multiple nodules of variable size within the pancreas, each of which consists of gray or yellow tissue. Areas of hemorrhage or necrosis may be present within the neoplasm. The neoplasm is usually firmer than the

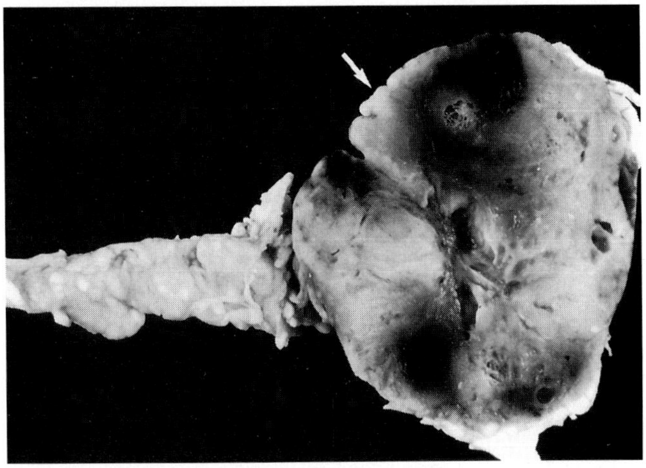

Figure 2-54 Pancreas; cat. Pancreatic adenoma. This is a single large mass within the pancreas *(arrow)*.

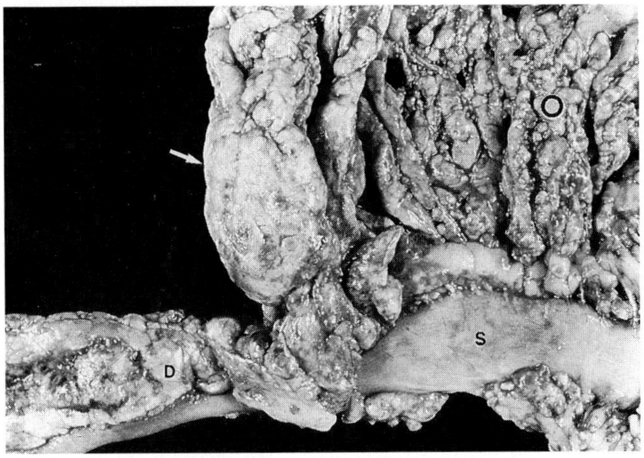

Figure 2-55 Pancreas; dog. Pancreatic carcinoma with metastasis into the peritoneal cavity. The primary tumor is present in the pancreas *(arrow)*, and tumor implants are present on the serosal surface of the stomach *(S)*, duodenum *(D)*, and omentum *(O)*.

adjacent pancreas because of proliferation of fibrous connective tissue. Adhesion of the affected pancreas to adjacent tissues occurs. This neoplasm often invades adjacent tissues and the peritoneal cavity. Peritoneal implants are nodules over the mesentery, omentum, and serosa of the abdominal viscera (Fig. 2-55). Metastasis to the abdominal lymph nodes adjacent to the pancreas is also common, and some carcinomas metastasize widely.

Microscopic features of carcinomas of the exocrine pancreas range from well-differentiated adenocarcinomas with tubular patterns to undifferentiated carcinomas with a solid pattern. The amount of fibrous stroma varies considerably and usually is greatest in poorly differentiated neoplasms. Zymogen granules similar to those present in normal acinar cells of the pancreas are often absent within the cytoplasm of the neoplastic cells.

Acknowledgments

The authors gratefully acknowledge the following individuals who have generously contributed photographs or material used in the figures contained in this text: Drs. R. Fairley, B. Johnson, J. King, M. Leach, M. McEntee, M.D. McGavin, R. Michel, S. Smith, and K. Sokol.

GLOSSARY

Acinus the functional unit of the liver. The acinus is a diamond-shaped structure formed by the terminal (distributing) branches of the portal vein and hepatic artery that extend from the portal areas at the center and the terminal hepatic venules (central veins) that are at the periphery.

Bioactivation process by which hepatic biotransformation of chemicals produces reactive metabolites that mediate hepatic injury.

Biotransformation process by which endogenous and exogenous substances are metabolized by the liver for excretion.

Bridging hepatic necrosis or fibrosis necrosis or fibrosis that connects portal areas to terminal hepatic venules, or other portal areas.

Centroacinar the portion of the acinus that centers on the portal triad.

Centrilobular the portion of the hepatic lobule that surrounds the terminal hepatic venule.

Cholangiohepatitis inflammation that often centers on the bile ducts of the portal areas, but extends into the hepatic parenchyma.

Cholecystitis inflammation of the gallbladder.

Cholelithiasis the presence of "stones" within the biliary system.

Cholestasis interruption in the flow of bile. Cholestasis can arise from intrahepatic or extrahepatic causes. In cases of cholestasis, bile may be evident in canaliculi, bile ducts, or infrequently, in the cytoplasm of hepatocytes and Kupffer cells.

Cirrhosis synonymous with end-stage liver; a liver characterized by diffuse fibrosis and nodular parenchymal regeneration leading to severe architectural distortion of the liver.

Enterohepatic circulation reabsorption of materials, particularly bile acids, from the intestine for resecretion into the intestine via the hepatobiliary system.

Hemochromatosis iron overload disorder. A condition characterized by abnormal accumulation of iron in hepatocytes, associated with liver dysfunction.

Hemosiderosis a condition characterized by excess hemosiderin in the liver.

Hepatic encephalopathy metabolic disorder of the central nervous system that occurs as a consequence of liver failure.

Hepatic lipidosis (synonym: fatty liver) excessive accumulation of lipid within hepatocytes.

Hepatitis inflammation of the liver.

Icterus (synonym: jaundice) yellow discoloration of tissues, especially those rich in elastin, as a consequence of hyperbilirubinemia.

Idiosyncratic toxic hepatic injury that does not occur in the majority of animals exposed to a particular agent.

Massive necrosis hepatic necrosis that affects all the hepatocytes in entire lobules.

Midzonal necrosis that affects only the portion of the lobule between the periportal and centrilobular regions.

Mixed-function oxidases hepatic enzymes responsible for much of the biotransformation of chemicals that occurs in the liver.

Mycotoxin toxin produced by a fungus.

Pancreatitis inflammation of the pancreas; term often is used interchangeably with acute hemorrhagic necrosis of the canine pancreas.

Paracentral synonymous with periacinar; however, not all acini bordering a central vein are necessarily affected.
Passive hepatic congestion hepatic congestion secondary to increased pressure within the hepatic vein.
Periportal area of the hepatic lobule adjacent to the portal triad.
Periacinar area of the acinus adjacent to the central vein.
Photosensitization cutaneous injury resulting from the action of ultraviolet light on accumulated photodynamic pigments in the plasma.
Phytotoxin plant toxin.
Reticular pattern enhancement of the liver's normal lobular pattern reflecting any one of a variety of different causes (ischemia, toxic injury, lipid accumulation, etc.). This may arise from processes that make the portal areas more prominent, as seen with neoplastic infiltrates, such as malignant lymphoma, or by processes such as passive hepatic congestion, centrilobular lipidosis, or necrosis, that accentuate the centrilobular zone or the central vein. Also known as "nutmeg liver" if associated with passive hepatic congestion.
Tension lipidosis focal accumulation of fat at the margins of the liver, typically at the sites of mesenteric attachments. The condition likely is the result of impaired blood flow to the affected portion of the liver.
Zonal change degeneration or necrosis affecting one or more zones of the hepatic lobule or acinus throughout the liver.

References

Acland HM, Mann PC, Robertson JL, Divers TJ, Lichensteiger CA, Whitlock RH. Toxic hepatopathy in neonatal foals. Vet Pathol 1984; 21:3-9.

Anthony PP, Ishak KG, Nayak NC, Poulsen HE, Scheuer PJ, Sobin LH. The morphology of cirrhosis: definition, nomenclature, and classification. Bull WHO 1977; 55:521-540.

Bergman JR. Nodular hyperplasia in the liver of the dog: An association with changes in the Ito cell population. Vet Pathol 1985; 22:427-438.

Bunch SE, Castleman WL, Hornbuckle WE, Tennant BC. Hepatic cirrhosis associated with long-term anticonvulsant therapy in dogs. J Am Vet Med Assoc 1982; 181:357-362.

Buoro IBJ, Atwell RB. Development of a model of caval syndrome in dogs infected with *Dirofilaria immitis*. Aust Vet J 1984; 61: 267-268.

Center SA. Feline liver disorders and their management. Comp Cont Educ Pract 1986; 8:889-901.

Cornwell HJC, Wright NG. The pathology of experimental infectious canine hepatitis in neonatal puppies. Res Vet Sci 1969; 10:156-160.

Cullison RF. Acetaminophen toxicosis in small animals: Clinical signs, mode of action and treatment. Comp Cont Educ Pract 1984; 6:315-321.

Dillon R. The liver in systemic disease. Vet Clin North Am 1985; 15:97-117.

Ewing GO, Suter PF, Bailey CS. Hepatic insufficiency associated with congenital anomalies of the portal vein in dogs. J Am Anim Hosp Assoc 1974; 10:463-476.

Fittschen C, Bellamy JEC. Prednisone-induced morphologic and chemical changes in the liver of dogs. Vet Pathol 1984; 21:399-406.

Haywood S, Rutgers HC, Christian MK. Hepatitis and copper accumulation in Skye terriers. Vet Pathol 1988; 25:408-414.

Higgins R. A minireview of the pathogenesis of acute leptospirosis. Can Vet J 1981; 22:277-278.

Hill RC, Van Winkle TJ. Acute necrotizing pancreatitis and acute suppurative pancreatitis in the cat: a retrospective study of 40 cases (1976-1989). J Vet Intern Med 1993; 7:25-33.

Kelly WR. The liver and biliary system. In: Jubb KVF, Kennedy PC, Palmer N, eds. Pathology of Domestic Animals. 4th ed. New York; Academic Press, 1985:239.

Kingsbury JM. Poisonous Plants of the United States and Canada. Englewood Cliffs, NJ: Prentice-Hall, 1964.

Kircher CH, Nielsen SW. Tumors of the pancreas. Bull WHO 1976; 53:195-202.

Moore PF, Whiting PG. Hepatic lesions associated with intrahepatic arterioportal fistulae in dogs. Vet Pathol 1986; 23:57-62.

Moore RP. Pathophysiology of canine exocrine pancreatic insufficiency. Comp Cont Educ Pract 1980; 2:657-660.

Newberne PM, Butler WH. Acute and chronic effects of aflatoxin on the liver of domestic and laboratory animals: A review. Cancer Res 1969; 29:236-250.

Ponomarkov V, Mackey LJ. Tumors of the liver and biliary system. Bull WHO 1975; 53:187-194.

Popp JA. Tumors of the liver, gall bladder, and pancreas. In: Moulton JE, ed. Tumors in Domestic Animals. 3rd. ed. Berkeley, Calif: University of California Press, 1990.

Prentice DE, James RW, Wadsworth PF. Pancreatic atrophy in young beagle dogs. Vet Pathol 1980; 17:575-580.

Rowe LD, Corrier DE, Reagor JC, Jones LP. Experimentally induced *Cassia roemeriana* poisoning in cattle and goats. Am J Vet Res 1986; 48:992-997.

Scarratt WK, Saunders GK. Cholelithiasis and biliary obstruction in a horse. Comp Cont Educ Pract 1985; 7:S428-S431.68.

Schiff L, Schiff ER. Diseases of the Liver. 6th ed. Philadelphia: JB Lippincott, 1987.

Seawright AA. Animal Health in Australia. Vol. 2. Chemical and plant poisons. Canberra: Australian Government Printing Service, 1982.

Seawright AA, Allen JE. Pathology of the liver and kidney in Lantana poisoning of cattle. Aust Vet J 1972; 48:323-331.

Sherding RG. Acute hepatic failure. Vet Clin North Am 1985; 15:119-133.

Sipes IG, Gandolfi AJ. Biotransformation of toxicants. In: Klassen CD, Amdur MO, Doull J, eds. Casarett and Doull's Toxicology. 3rd ed. New York: MacMillan, 1986:64.

Stogdale L, Booth AJ. Bacillary hemoglobinuria in cattle. Comp Cont Educ Pract 1974; 6:S284-290.

Tennant B, Evans CD, Schwartz LW, Gribble DH, Kanecko JJ. Equine hepatic insufficiency. Vet Clin North Am 1973; 3:279-289.

Thompson KG, Lake DE, Cordes DO. Hepatic encephalopathy associated with chronic facial eczema. N Z Vet J 1979; 27:221-223.

Thomson GW, Wilson RW, Hall EA, Physick-Sheard P. Tyzzer's disease in the foal: Case reports and review. Can Vet J 1977; 18:41-43.

Thornburg LP, Shaw D, Dolan M, Raisbeck M, Crawford S, Dennis GL, Olwin DB. Hereditary copper toxicosis in West Highland white terriers. Vet Pathol 1986; 23:148-154.

Trigo FJ, Thompson H, Breeze RG, Nash AS. The pathology of liver tumors in the dog. J Comp Pathol 1982; 92:21-39.

Twedt DC, Sternlieb I, Gilbertson SR. Clinical, morphologic and chemical studies on copper toxicosis of Bedlington terriers. J Am Vet Med Assoc 1979; 175:269-275.

VanEnkevort BA, O'Brien RT, Young KM. Pancreatic pseudocysts in 4 dogs and 2 cats: Ultrasonographic and clinicopathologic findings. J Vet Intern Med 1999; 13:309-313.

Wigton DH, Kociba GJ, Hoover EA. Infectious canine hepatitis: animal model for viral-induced disseminated intravascular coagulation. Blood 1976; 47:287-296.

CHAPTER 3

Respiratory System, Thoracic Cavity, and Pleura

Alfonso López

Diseases of the respiratory system are some of the leading causes of morbidity and mortality in animals and a major source of economic losses. Thus, veterinarians are routinely called to diagnose, treat, and implement health management practices to reduce the impact of these diseases. In companion animals, diseases of the respiratory tract are also common and, although of little economic significance, are important to clinicians and owners.

STRUCTURE AND FUNCTION

To facilitate the understanding of the structure and function, it is convenient to arbitrarily divide the respiratory system into **conductive, transitional,** and **gas exchange** systems. The **conductive system** includes nasal cavity, pharynx, larynx, trachea, and bronchi, all of which are largely lined by pseudostratified, ciliated columnar cells plus a variable proportion of secretory goblet (mucous) and serous cells (Figs. 3-1 and 3-2). The **transitional system** of the respiratory tract is composed of bronchioles, which serve as a transition zone between the conductive system (ciliated) and the gas exchange (alveolar) system (Fig. 3-3). The disappearance of cilia in the transitional system is not abrupt; the ciliated cells in the proximal bronchiolar region become scarce and progressively attenuated until the point where distal bronchioles no longer have ciliated cells. Normal bronchioles also lack goblet cells, but instead have other types of secretory cells, notably the Clara cell (Fig. 3-4). Actively metabolic, Clara cells play an important role in detoxification of xenobiotics (foreign substances), similar to the role of hepatocytes. In carnivores and monkeys, and to a much lesser extent in horses and human beings, the terminal portions of bronchioles are not only lined by cuboidal epithelium but also by segments of alveolar capillaries. These unique bronchioloalveolar structures are known as respiratory bronchioles. The **gas exchange system** of the respiratory tract in all mammals is formed by millions of alveoli (Fig. 3-3). Alveoli are superficially lined by two distinct types of epithelial cells known as pneumonocytes type I (membranous) and pneumonocytes type II (granular).

All three—the conductive, transitional and exchange systems of the respiratory system—are vulnerable to injury due to constant exposure to a myriad of microbes, particles and fibers, and toxic gases and vapors present in the air. Vulnerability of the respiratory system to aerogenous (airborne) injury is primarily due to (1) the extensive area of the interface between the respiratory system and inspired air, (2) the large volume of air passing continuously into the lungs, and (3) the high concentration of noxious elements that can be present in the air (Table 3-1). For human beings, it has been estimated that the surface of the respiratory tract is approximately 200 m^2, roughly the area of a tennis court. It has also been estimated that the volume of air reaching the human lung every day is around 10,000 L. The surface of the equine lung is estimated to be around 2,000 m^2.

Lungs are also susceptible to hematogenously borne microbes, toxins, and emboli. This fact is not surprising since the pulmonary capillary bed is the largest in the body, with a surface area of 70 m^2 in the adult human being; this area is equivalent to 2400 km of capillaries, with 1 ml of blood occupying up to 16 km of capillary bed.

NORMAL FLORA OF THE RESPIRATORY SYSTEM

The respiratory system has its own normal bacterial flora, as does any other body system in contact with the external environment. If a swab is passed deep into the nasal cavity of any healthy animal and cultured for microbes, many species of bacteria are recovered. The organisms that constitute the normal flora of the respiratory tract are restricted to the most proximal region of the conductive system (nasal cavity, pharynx, larynx). The thoracic portions of the trachea, bronchi, and lungs are considered to be sterile. The types of bacteria present in the nasal flora vary considerably among animal species and in different geographic regions. Some bacteria present in the nasal flora are pathogens and are associated with important respiratory infections. For instance, *Pasteurella haemolytica* is part of the bovine nasal flora, yet this bacterium causes a devastating disease in cattle, pneumonic pasteurellosis (shipping fever pneumonia). Experimental

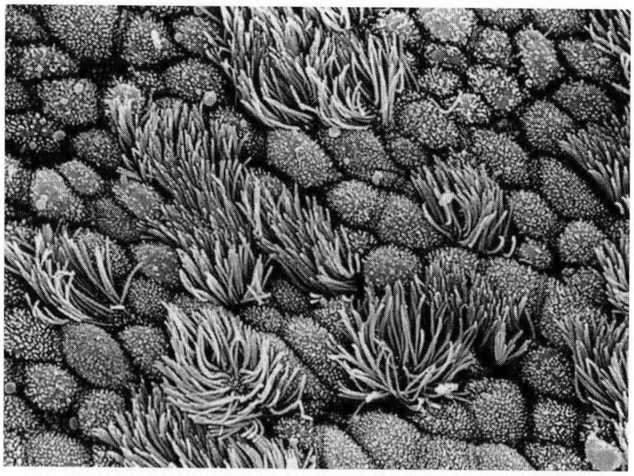

Figure 3-1 Scanning electron micrograph. Bronchus; rat. Normal bronchial mucosa. Mucous layer was removed before fixation to expose the external surface of the epithelium. Mucosa is composed of ciliated and nonciliated secretory cells. Ciliated cells have numerous slender cilia. Nonciliated secretory cells have a dome-shaped surface with abundant microvilli. The proportion of ciliated to nonciliated cells varies depending on the level of airways. Ciliated cells are more abundant in proximal airways, whereas secretory cells are more numerous in distal portions of the conductive and transitional systems.

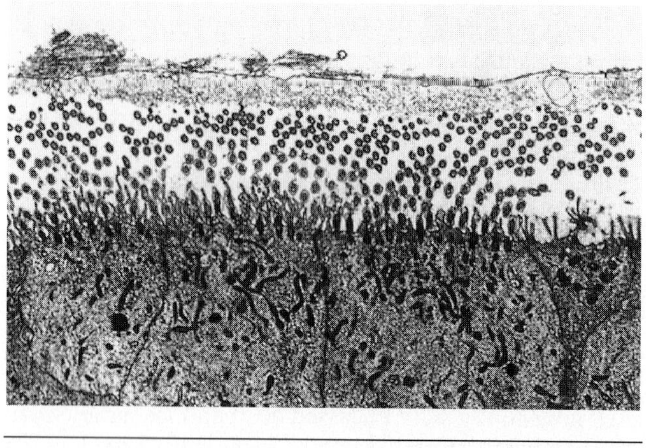

Figure 3-2 Transmission electron micrograph. Trachea; cow. Cross-sectioned view of cilia. Normal ciliated epithelium. This trachea was specially fixed in order to preserve the mucous lining. The mucuous layer is composed of an internal, clear, hypo-phase-fluid layer (not visible) surrounding microvilli and kinocilia and an external mucous epiphase at the level of the tips of the kinocilia (×5000). *Sims et al. Biotechnol Histochem 1991; 66:173-180.*

studies have established that microorganisms from the nasal flora are continuously carried into the lungs via tracheal air. In spite of this constant bacterial bombardment from the nasal flora and from contaminated air, normal lungs remain sterile due to their remarkably effective defense mechanisms.

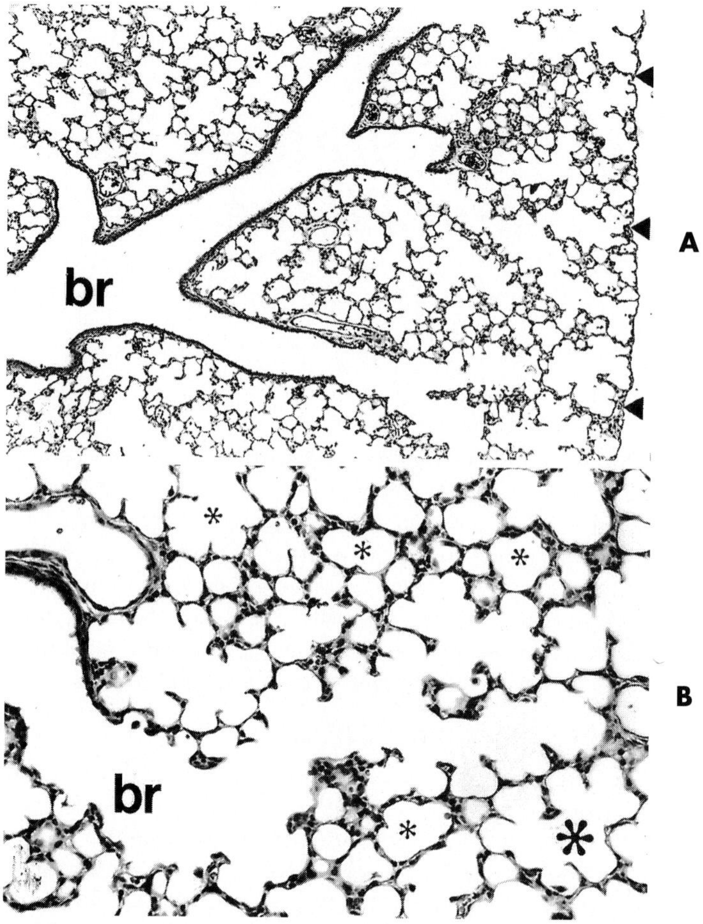

Figure 3-3 Lung; rat. Lungs were fixed by intratracheal perfusion of fixative to retain normal distension of airways. **A,** Branching bronchioles *(br),* alveoli (✻), and visceral pleura (▲). **B,** Higher magnification of terminal bronchiole *(br)* and alveoli (✻).

DEFENSE MECHANISMS OF THE RESPIRATORY SYSTEM

A particle, microbe, or toxic gas must first gain entry to a vulnerable region of the respiratory system before it can have a pathologic effect. The characteristics of size, shape, and distribution of particles present in inspired air are studied in **aerobiology.** It is important to recognize the difference between deposition and retention of inhaled particles. **Deposition** is the process by which particles of various sizes and shapes are trapped within specific regions of the respiratory tract. **Clearance** is the process by which deposited particles are destroyed, neutralized, or removed from the mucosal surfaces. The main mechanisms involved in clearance are sneezing, coughing, mucociliary transport, and phagocytosis. The difference between what is deposited and what is cleared from the respiratory tract is referred to as **retention.** Abnormal retention of particles resulting from increased deposition, decreased clearance, or a combination of both is the

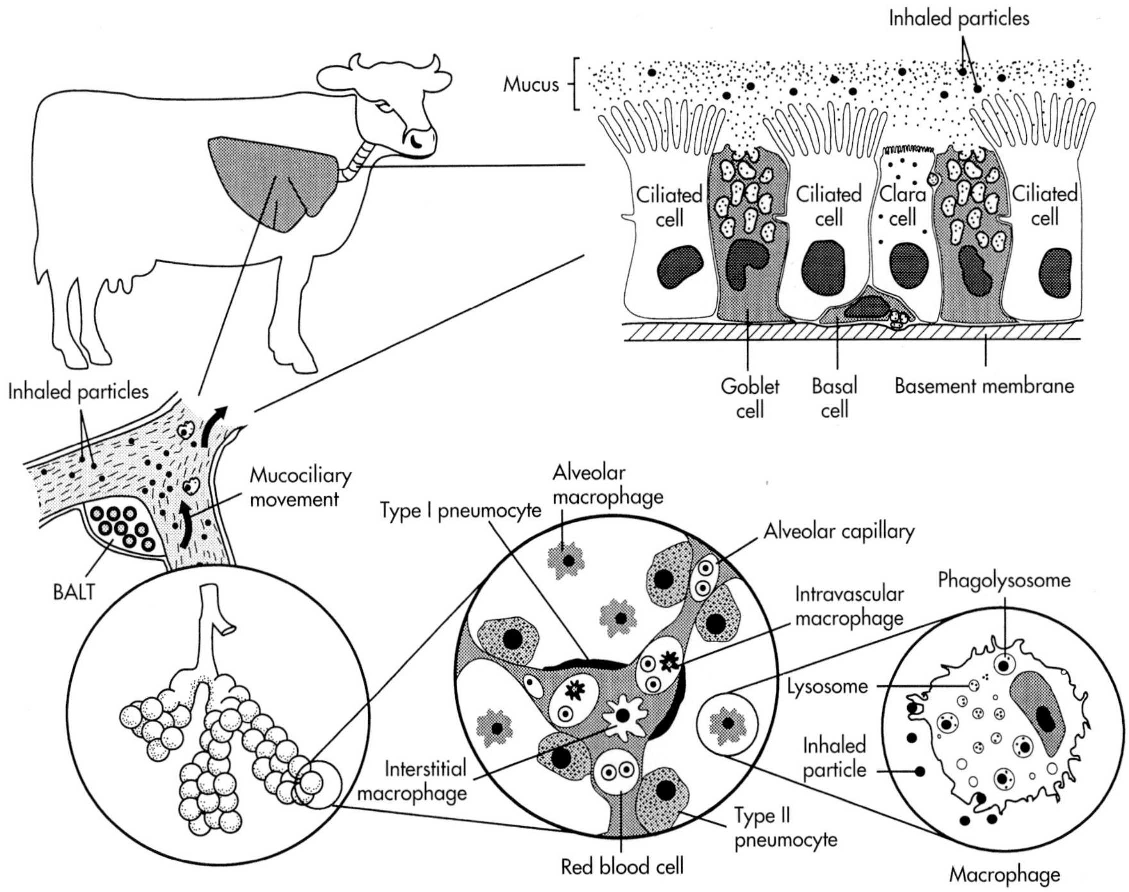

Figure 3-4 Respiratory tract, schematic representation. The conductive system extending from nasal cavity to bronchi is lined by the mucociliary escalator, which is comprised of ciliated and nonciliated secretory cells and mucus. The large dots (•) represent particles trapped by mucus. Bronchial associated lymphoid tissue (BALT) is strategically located at the bifurcation of airways. Particles reaching the transitional and exchange systems (bronchioles and alveoli) are ingested by the pulmonary alveolar macrophages, which exit the lung via the mucociliary escalator. The alveolar wall is comprised of capillaries, interstitium, and alveolar lining (type I and II pneumonocytes).

Table 3-1 Common Pathogens, Allergens, and Toxic Substances Present in Air

Microbes	Viruses, *Chlamydia,* bacteria, fungi, protozoa
Plant dust	Grain, flour, cotton, wood
Animal products	Dander, feathers, mites, insect chitin
Toxic gases	Ammonia (NH_3), hydrogen sulfide (H_2S), nitrogen dioxide (NO_2) , sulfur dioxide (SO_2), chlorine
Chemicals	Organic and inorganic solvents, herbicides, asbestos, nickel, lead

underlying pathogenetic mechanism involved in many pulmonary diseases.

The anatomic configuration of the conductive system (nasal cavity and bronchi) plays a unique role in preventing or reducing the penetration of noxious material into the lungs, especially into the alveolar region, which is the most vulnerable portion of the respiratory system. The coiled arrangement of the nasal conchae creates enormous turbulences of airflow and, as a result, centrifugal forces are created that forcefully impact particles larger than 10 μm onto the surface of the nasal mucosa. Although particles smaller than 10 μm could escape trapping in the nasal cavity, these medium-sized particles meet a second barrier at the bifurcation of the trachea and in the lumen of the bronchi. Here, abrupt changes in the direction of air (inertia), which occurs at the bifurcation of major airways, cause particles in the 2- to 10-μm size range to collide with the surface of bronchial mucosa (Fig. 3-4). Since the velocity of inspired air at the level of small bronchi and bronchioles has become rather slow, inertial and centrifugal forces no longer play a significant role in process by which inhaled particles contact the mucosal surface. Here, in the transitional (bronchiolar) and exchange (alveolar) regions, particles, 2 μm or smaller, may come into contact with the mucosa by means of sedimentation due to gravitation or by diffusion due to Brownian movement. Infective aerosols containing bacteria and viruses are within the size range to gain access to the bronchioloalveolar region.

In addition to size, other factors such as shape, length, electrical charge, and humidity play an important role in mucosal deposition, retention, and pathogenicity. For instance, particles longer that 200 μm may also reach the lower respiratory tract, provided the mean aerodynamic diameter of the airway is less than 1 μm. Asbestos is a good example of a large but slender fiber that can bypass the filtrating mechanisms by traveling parallel to the airstream. Once in the lungs, asbestos fibers cause **asbestosis,** a serious pulmonary disease in human beings. In summary, the anatomic features of the nasal cavity and airways provide an effective barrier, preventing the penetration of most large particles into the lungs.

Once larger particles are trapped in the mucosa of conductive airways and small particles are deposited on the surface of the bronchioalveolar mucosa, it is crucial that these exogenous materials be removed to prevent or minimize injury to the respiratory system. For these purposes, the respiratory system is equipped with several defense mechanisms, all of which are provided by specialized cells operating in a remarkably well-coordinated manner.

Defense Mechanisms of the Conductive System (Nose, Trachea and Bronchi)

Mucociliary clearance is the physical unidirectional movement and removal of deposited particles and gases dissolved in the mucus from the respiratory tract. Mucociliary clearance is provided by the **mucociliary blanket (mucociliary escalator)** and is the main defense mechanism of the conductive system (nasal cavity, trachea, and bronchi) (see Figs. 3-2 and 3-4). Mucus is a complex mixture of water, glycoproteins, immunoglobulins, lipids, and electrolytes produced by goblet (mucous) cells, serous cells, submucosal glands, and fluid from transepithelial ion and water transport. Once serous fluid and mucus are secreted onto the surface of the respiratory mucosa, a thin, double-layer film of mucus is formed on top of the cells. The outer layer of this film is in a viscous, gel phase, while the inner layer, which is in fluid or sol phase, is directly in contact with cilia (see Fig. 3-2). A healthy human being produces around 100 ml of mucus per day. Each ciliated cell in the conductive system has around 250 cilia (6 μm long) beating spontaneously and harmoniously at approximately 1000 strokes per minute and producing in a horse, for instance, an estimated longitudinal movement of up to 20 mm per minute. Rapid and powerful movement of cilia creates a series of waves that, in a continuous and harmonious manner, propel the mucus, on whose surface any particles and exfoliated cells are trapped, out of the respiratory tract. The mucus is finally swallowed, or when present in large amounts, it is coughed out of the conductive system. If mucus flow were to move at the same rate in all levels of conductive system, a "bottleneck" effect would be created in major airways to which the minor but more numerous airways converge. For this reason, the mucociliary transport in proximal airways is physiologically faster than that of the distal ones.

The mucociliary blanket of the nasal cavity, trachea, and bronchi also plays an important role in preventing injury from toxic gases. If a soluble gas contacts the mucociliary blanket, it mixes with the mucus, thus reducing the concentration of gas reaching deep into the alveolar region. In other words, mucus acts as a "scavenger system" whereby gases are solubilized and subsequently cleared from the respiratory tract via mucociliary transport. If ciliary transport is reduced (loss of cilia) or mucus production is excessive, coughing becomes an important mechanism for clearing the airways.

In addition to the physical transport provided by the mucociliary escalator, other cells closely associated with ciliated epithelium contribute to the defense mechanism of the conductive system. Among the most notable ones are the **M cells** ("microfold cells"), which are modified epithelial cells covering the **bronchial associated lymphoid tissue (BALT).** M cells are strategically located at the corner of the bifurcation of bronchi and bronchioles, where inhaled particles often collide onto the mucosa due to inertial forces (see Fig. 3-4). From here, inhaled particles and soluble antigens are phagocytosed and transported by macrophages, dendritic cells, and other professional **"antigen-processing cells" (APC)** into the BALT, thus providing a unique opportunity for B and T lymphocytes to enter into close contact with potentially pathogenic substances. Pulmonary lymphocytes are not quiescent in the BALT but are in continual traffic to other organs and contribute to both cellular (cytotoxic, helper, suppressor T cells) and humoral immune responses. IgA, and to a lesser extent, IgG and IgM play important roles in the local immunity of the conducting system, especially with regard to preventing attachment of pathogens to the mucociliary blanket. Chronic airway diseases, especially those of infectious etiology, are often accompanied by severe hyperplasia of the BALT.

The mucociliary clearance terminates at the pharynx, where mucus, propelled caudally from the nasal cavity and cranially from the tracheobronchial tree, is eventually swallowed and thus eliminated from the conductive system of the respiratory tract.

Defense Mechanisms of the Exchange System (Alveoli)

Alveoli lack ciliated and mucus-producing cells; thus, the defense mechanism against inhaled particles in the alveolar region cannot be provided by mucociliary clearance. Instead, the main defense mechanism of alveoli (exchange system) is phagocytosis provided by the **pulmonary alveolar macrophages** (Fig. 3-4).

These highly phagocytic cells are derived largely from blood monocytes and, to a much lesser extent, from a slowly dividing population of interstitial macrophages. After a temporary adaptive stage within pulmonary interstitium, blood monocytes reduce their glycolytic and increase their oxidative metabolisms to function in aerobic rather than in an anaerobic environment. Pulmonary alveolar macrophages rapidly attach and ingest bacteria and other particles reaching the alveolar region (see Fig. 3-4). The number of macrophages in the alveolar space is closely related to the number of particles reaching the lungs. This ability to increase the number of available phagocytic cells within hours is vital in protecting the distal lungs against foreign material, particularly when the latter is excessive. Unlike that of tissue macrophages, the lifespan of alveolar macrophages in the alveoli is short, only a few days. Alveolar phagocytosis plays a prominent role in the defense mechanism against inhaled bacteria without the need of an inflammatory reaction. Bacteria reaching the alveoli are rapidly ingested, and bactericidal enzymes present in lysosomes are discharged into the phagosome containing the bacteria (see Fig. 3-4). Except for some facultative organisms that are resistant to intracellular killing (e.g., *Mycobacterium tuberculosis, Listeria monocytogenes*), most bacteria are rapidly destroyed by activated alveolar macrophages. Similarly, inhaled particles such as dust, pollen, spores, carbon, or erythrocytes from intraalveolar hemorrhage are all phagocytosed and eventually removed from alveoli by pulmonary alveolar macrophages.

Generally, most alveolar macrophages leave the alveoli by migrating toward the bronchiolar (transitional) region until the mucociliary blanket is reached. Once there, pulmonary macrophages are removed in the same way as any other particle, that is, along the mucociliary flow to the pharynx and swallowed.

Pulmonary clearance by alveolar macrophages operates in a well-orchestrated manner with other cells and secretions of the distal lungs. These cell-to-cell interactions are complex and involve many cells, including pulmonary alveolar macrophages, pneumonocytes, lymphocytes, dendritic cells, and surfactant. A humoral immune response also plays an important role in protecting the lungs against inhaled pathogens. Although IgA is the most abundant antibody in the nasal and tracheal secretions, IgG is the most abundant antibody in the alveolar surface and acts as an opsonizing antibody to promote uptake and destruction of inhaled pathogens by alveolar macrophages and neutrophils. In addition to antibodies, there are several secretory products locally released into the alveoli that constitute the alveolar lining material and contribute to the pulmonary defense mechanisms. The most important of these antimicrobial products are transferrin, anionic peptides, and pulmonary surfactant (Table 3-2).

To facilitate phagocytosis and discriminate between "self" and "foreign" antigens, pulmonary alveolar macrophages are furnished with a wide variety of specific receptors on their cell surfaces. Among the most important ones are IgG, Fc and complement (C3b, C3a, C5a), tumor necrosis factor (TNF), and CD40 receptors, which facilitate the phagocytosis of opsonized particles. "Scavenger receptors," which prompt recognition and uptake of foreign particulates such as dust and fibers, are also present on pulmonary alveolar macrophages.

Defense Mechanisms Against Blood-Borne Pathogens (Intravascular Space)

Lungs are also susceptible to hematogenously borne microbes, toxins, or emboli. In dogs, laboratory rodents, and human beings, the hepatic (Kupffer cells) and splenic macrophages are the primary cells responsible for

Table 3-2 Defense Mechanisms Provided by Some Cells and Secretory Products Present in the Respiratory System

Cell/Secretory Product	Action
Alveolar macrophage	Phagocytosis, main line of defense against inhaled particles and microbial pathogens in the alveoli
Intravascular macrophage	Phagocytosis, removal of particles, endotoxin, and microbial pathogens in the circulation
Ciliated cells	Expel mucus and inhaled particles and microbial pathogens by ciliary action
Clara cells	Detoxification of xenobiotics (mixed function oxidases)
Mucus	Trap inhaled particles, microbial pathogens, and neutralizes soluble gases
Surfactant	Protects alveolar walls and enhances phagocytosis
Lysozyme	Antimicrobial enzyme
Transferrin and lactoferrin	Suppression of bacterial growth
α_1-Antitrypsin	Protects against the noxious effects of proteolytic enzymes release by phagocytic cells; also inhibits inflammation
Interferon	Antiviral and modulator of the immune and inflammatory responses
Antibodies	Prevent microbe attachment to cell membranes, opsonization
Complement	Chemotactasis and enhance phagocytosis
Antioxidants*	Prevent injury caused by superoxide anion, hydrogen peroxide, and free radicals generated during phagocytosis, inflammation, or by inhalation of oxidant gases (ozone NO_2, SO_2)

*Superoxide dismutase, catalase, glutathione peroxidase, oxidant free radical scavengers (tocopherol, ascorbic acid).

removing circulating bacteria and other particles from the blood. In contrast, removal of circulating pathogenic bacteria and particles from the blood of ruminants, cats, and pigs is mainly dependent on **pulmonary intravascular macrophages,** a distinct population of phagocytes normally residing within the pulmonary capillaries (Fig. 3-4). In pigs, 16% of the pulmonary capillary surface is lined by pulmonary intravascular macrophages. In ruminants, 95% of intravenously injected tracer particles or bacteria are rapidly phagocytosed by these intravascular macrophages.

Defense Mechanisms Against Oxidant-Induced Lung Injury

Existing in an oxygen-rich environment and being the site of numerous metabolic reactions, the lungs also require an efficient defense mechanism against oxidant-induced cellular damage. This form of damage can be caused by inhalation of oxidant gases (e.g., nitrogen dioxide, ozone, sulfur dioxide), by xenobiotic toxic metabolites produced locally or reaching the lungs via the bloodstream (e.g., 3-methylindole, paraquat), or by free radicals released by phagocytic cells during inflammation. Oxygen and free radical scavengers such as catalase, superoxide dismutase, and vitamin E are largely responsible for protecting pulmonary cells against peroxidation and are present in the intracellular and extracellular spaces of the lung.

In summary, the defense mechanisms are so effective in trapping, destroying, and removing bacteria that, under normal conditions, animals can be exposed to aerosols containing massive numbers of bacteria without any ill effects. If defense mechanisms are impaired, inhaled bacteria colonize, multiply, and produce infection, which, in some instances, results in fatal pneumonia. Similarly, when air-borne and blood-borne pathogens, inhaled toxicants, or free radicals overwhelm the protective defense mechanisms, cells of the respiratory system could be injured, often causing serious respiratory diseases.

IMPAIRMENT OF DEFENSE MECHANISMS IN THE RESPIRATORY SYSTEM

For many years, factors such as stress, viral infections, and pulmonary edema have been implicated in predisposing human beings and animals to secondary bacterial pneumonia. There are many pathways by which the defense mechanisms can be impaired; only those relevant to veterinary species are discussed.

Viral Infections

Viral agents are notorious in predisposing human beings and animals to secondary bacterial pneumonias by what is known as viral-bacterial synergism. A good example of this synergistic effect of combined virus-bacterial infections is documented from epidemics of human beings with influenza virus in which the mortality rate significantly increased due to secondary bacterial pneumonia. The most common viruses incriminated in predisposing animals to secondary bacterial pneumonia include influenza virus in pigs and horses; *bovine herpesvirus* 1 (BHV-1), *parainfluenza*-3 (PI-3), and *bovine respiratory syncytial virus* (BRSV) in cattle; and *canine distemper virus* in dogs. The mechanism of the synergistic effect of viral-bacterial infections was considered to be the destruction of mucociliary blanket and a concurrent reduction of mucociliary clearance. However, in experimental studies, viral infections do not significantly reduce the physical removal of particles or bacteria out of the lungs. Instead, it is now known that 5 to 7 days after a viral infection, the phagocytic function of pulmonary alveolar macrophages is notably impaired. The mechanisms by which viruses impair defense mechanisms are multiple and remain poorly understood (Table 3-3). Immunization against viral infections in many cases prevents or reduces the synergistic effect of combined viral-bacterial pneumonia.

Table 3-3 Postulated Mechanisms by Which Viruses May Impair the Defense Mechanisms of the Respiratory Tract

Changes in mucociliary clearance
Injured epithelium enhances attachment for bacteria
Enhanced bacterial attachment predispose to colonization
Decreased mucociliary clearance prolongs resident time of bacteria favoring colonization
Injured epithelium prevent mucociliary clearance and physical removal of bacteria
Lack secretory products facilitate further cell injury
Break down the antimicrobial barrier in mucus and cells (β-defensins and anionic peptides)
Ciliostasis caused by inflammation or by some pathogenic organism (mycoplasmas)
Dysfunction of pulmonary alveolar macrophages and lymphocytes
Consolidation of lung cause hypoxia resulting in decreased phagocytosis
Infected macrophages fail to release chemotactic factors for other cells
Infected macrophages fail to attach and ingest bacteria
Lysosomes become disoriented and fail to fuse with phagosome-containing bacteria
Intracellular killing or degradation is decreased because of biochemical dysfunction
Reduced cytokines and secretory products impair bacterial phagocytosis
Viral induced apoptosis of alveolar macrophages
Altered CD4 and CD8 lymphocytes

Toxic Gases

Certain gases also impair respiratory defense mechanisms, rendering animals more susceptible to secondary bacterial infections. For instance, hydrogen sulfide and ammonia, frequently encountered in the farming environment, especially in areas with poor ventilation, can impair pulmonary defense mechanisms and increase susceptibility to bacterial pneumonia. The effects of environmental pollutants on the defense mechanisms of human beings and animals living in crowded and polluted cities remain to be determined.

Other Conditions that Predispose to Secondary Bacterial Pneumonia

Uremia, endotoxemia, dehydration, starvation, hypoxia, acidosis, pulmonary edema, anesthesia, ciliary dyskinesia, and stress are only some of the many conditions that have been implicated in impairing the respiratory defense mechanism and consequently predisposing animals to develop secondary bacterial pneumonia. The mechanisms by which each of these factors suppresses pulmonary defenses are diverse and sometimes not well understood. For instance, hypoxia and pulmonary edema decrease phagocytic function of pulmonary alveolar macrophages and alter the production of surfactant by type II pneumonocytes; dehydration is thought to increase the viscosity of mucus, which reduces or stops mucociliary movement; anesthesia induces ciliostasis with concurrent loss of mucociliary function; ciliary dyskinesia, an inherited defect in cilia, causes abnormal mucociliary transport; starvation, hypothermia, and stress can reduce humoral and cellular immune responses.

Immunodeficiency

This disorder, whether acquired or congenital, is often associated with increased susceptibility to viral, bacterial, and protozoal pneumonias. For instance, human beings with acquired immunodeficiency syndrome (AIDS) are markedly susceptible to the development of pneumonia caused by proliferation of *Pneumocystis carinii.* This ubiquitous organism, which under normal circumstances is not considered pathogenic, is also found in the pneumonic lungs of immunosuppressed pigs, foals, dogs, and rodents. Pigs infected with the porcine reproductive and respiratory syndrome (PRRS) virus frequently develop *P. carinii* infection. Arabian foals born with combined immunodeficiency disease easily succumb to infectious diseases, particularly adenoviral pneumonia. Also, large doses of chemotherapeutic drugs cause immunosuppression in dogs, cats, and other animals, increasing susceptibility to secondary bacterial infections.

EXAMINATION OF THE RESPIRATORY TRACT

Postmortem

The respiratory tract should always be examined in a systematic fashion. To determine whether negative pressure is present in the thoracic cavity, the diaphragm is punctured through the abdominal cavity before the thorax has been opened. In an animal that has not been dead for more than a few hours, the act of puncturing it results in loss of negative pressure, which causes the cupula of the diaphragm to drop back toward the abdominal cavity and at the same time to make an audible sound due to the inrush of air. Lack of this movement may be an indication of advanced pneumothorax, pleural effusion, or presence of noncollapsible lungs due to pulmonary edema, pneumonia, fibrosis, or emphysema.

The rib cage must be removed in such a way that pleural adhesions and abnormal thoracic contents can be observed and grossly quantified (e.g., 200 ml of clear, yellow fluid). The tongue, pharynx, larynx, trachea, and thoracic viscera (lungs, heart, and thymus) should be removed as a unit and placed on the postmortem table.

The pharynx and esophagus are each opened by a single cut with scissors along the dorsal midline and inspected for ulcers, foreign bodies, and neoplasms. The larynx and trachea must be examined by opening both along the dorsal midline from cranial to caudal ends and then extending the incision into the large bronchi of the caudal lung lobes. Normal tracheobronchial mucosa has a smooth and glistening pearl-colored surface with empty lumina of airways. Presence of foamy fluid in airways indicates pulmonary edema. Feed particles may suggest aspiration; however, careful examination of the mucosa is required since aspiration of ingesta from stomach or rumen into the lungs commonly takes place at death or can be displaced into these areas when the carcass is moved.

The lungs should be examined before incision. External changes include presence of rib imprints on the pleural surface. In addition, the lungs should be inspected for changes in color and texture and distribution of lesions. **Color** changes can be various shades of red, indicating hypostatic congestion, hyperemia (acute pneumonia), and hemorrhage; dark collapsed lobules are indicative of atelectasis; pale pink to white lungs indicate fibrosis or emphysema. Lungs from exsanguinated and anemic animals are generally paler than normal due to reduced blood in the pulmonary tissue. A covering of yellowish material on the pleural surface indicates accumulation of fibrin. Since it is impossible to describe the texture of normal lungs, repeated palpation is required to understand the actual feeling of a normal lung. **Texture** is determined by gently palpating the surface and parenchyma of the lungs. Abnormal textures of the lungs include firm, hard, rubbery (elastic), or crepitant. Palpation of the lungs, which should be gentle, also permits detection of nonvisible nodules or abscesses in the parenchyma. Knowing the **distribution** of a lesion in the lungs also facilitates diagnosis as particular etiologic agents cause lesions with specific distribution. Distribution of lesions is generally described as focal, multifocal (embolic), locally extensive, or diffuse. According to their topography, pulmonary lesions can also be classified as cranioventral, dorsocaudal, and so on.

Postmortem reports must also contain an estimate of the extent of the pulmonary lesions, preferably expressed as a percentage (%) of the lungs affected. For instance, a report may read "cranioventral consolidation involving 40% of the lungs." If the lungs have focal lesions, a rough estimate of the number should also be included in the report. For instance, "numerous (approximately 25), small (1 to 2 cm in diameter), hard nodules were randomly distributed in all lung lobes."

Two methods are used to examine the nasal structures. The first is by making a midsagittal cut through the head and removing the nasal septum; the second is by making several transverse sections of the nose. This latter method is preferred when examining pigs suspected of having atrophic rhinitis or in animals with suspected nasal neoplasms.

Histopathology and Biopsies

Microscopic examination of pulmonary tissue is routinely done in diagnostic laboratories. Samples of normal and abnormal lungs, along with other appropriate tissues, should always be submitted in formalin for histopathologic examination. **Lung biopsy specimens** are taken only sporadically because complications often outweigh the diagnostic value. However, the use of new techniques such as endoscopic-directed biopsies has notably reduced some of these complications. Biopsies of the lungs are recommended in cases of chronic persistent pulmonary disease unresponsive to treatment or intrathoracic masses of undetermined origin. Endoscopic-directed biopsies of the nasal and bronchial mucosa are routinely used in clinical practice and generally have a much better diagnostic value.

Bronchoalveolar Lavage

A valuable diagnostic tool in human medicine, bronchoalveolar lavage (BAL) has in recent years become more widely used in veterinary clinical diagnosis of respiratory ailments in animals. The basis of BAL is sampling of the cellular and biochemical composition of the lung in a live animal by injecting and retrieving sterile fluid. BAL is done intratracheally by inserting a tube directly into the larynx and bronchi, or transtracheally by inserting a tube through a needle percutaneously inserted into the trachea. Microscopic examination of properly collected, stored, and processed BAL fluid may reveal many erythrocytes and siderophages in pulmonary hemorrhage or left heart failure, inclusion bodies or syncytial cells in viral pneumonias, increased number of leukocytes in pulmonary inflammation, abundant mucus in asthma or equine heaves (chronic obstructive pulmonary disease [COPD]), presence of pulmonary pathogens such as parasites, fungi and bacteria, or tumor cells in cases of pulmonary neoplasia.

NASAL CAVITY AND SINUSES

Pattern of Injury and Host Response in the Nasal Mucosa

The conductive portion of the respiratory system is lined by pseudostratified columnar ciliated epithelium (most of the nasal cavity and larynx, trachea, and bronchi), olfactory epithelium (nasal mucosa, particularly ethmoidal conchae), and squamous epithelium (nasal vestibulum and parts of the larynx). The pattern of injury, inflammation, and host response is characteristic for each of these three types of epithelium, independent of its anatomic location.

Pseudostratified ciliated epithelium, which lines most of the nasal cavity and nasopharynx, part of the larynx, and all of the trachea and bronchi, is exquisitely sensitive to injury. When cell injury becomes biochemically irreversible, whether caused by a viral infection, trauma, or inhalation of toxic gases, ciliated cells swell, typically lose their attachment to underlying basement membrane, and rapidly exfoliate (Fig. 3-5). A transient and mild exudate of plasma proteins and neutrophils covers the ulcer. In the absence of complications or secondary bacterial infec-

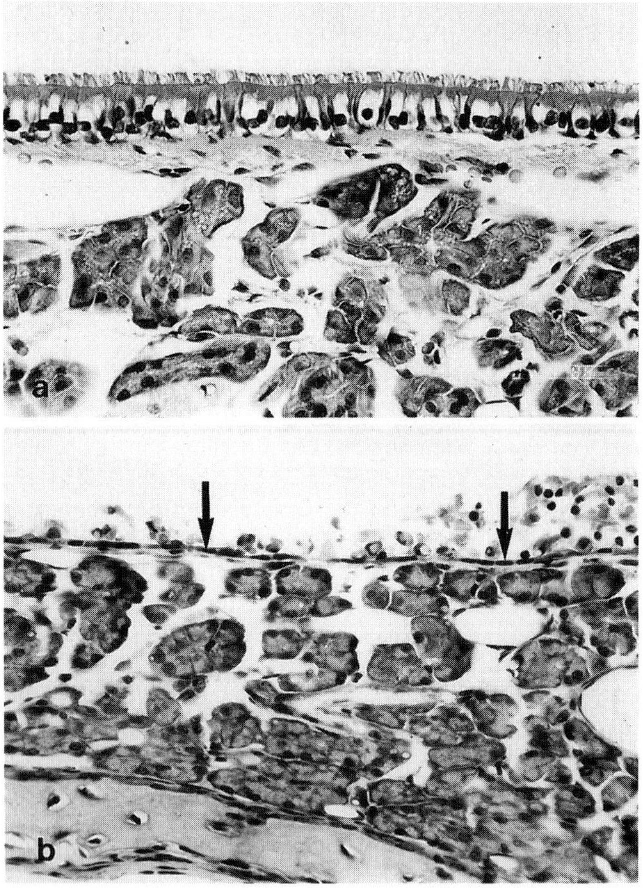

Figure 3-5 Nasal conchae; rats. **A,** Ciliated epithelium, nasal mucosa; rat. The normal mucosal lining is predominantly comprised of tall columnar cells with numerous cilia projecting to the lumen. **B,** Histologic section of nasal mucosa; rat. Rat was exposed to an atmosphere containing an irritant gas (hydrogen sulfide) and euthanatized 2 hours after exposure. Note how extensive detachment and exfoliation of ciliated cells have left a denuded basement membrane *(arrows)*. This same type of lesion is seen in viral or mechanical injury to the mucosa of the conductive system. *López et al. Am J Vet Res 1988; 49:1107-1111.*

tions, a specific type of progenitor cell known as "nonciliated secretory cells" undergoes mitosis and moves to cover the denuded basement membrane, eventually differentiating into new ciliated epithelial cells. Cellular proliferation, movement, and attachment is regulated by locally released growth factors and extracellular matrix proteins such as collagen, integrins, and fibronectin. The capacity of ciliated epithelium to repair itself is remarkably effective. For instance, repair of an uncomplicated ulcer of the tracheal mucosa can be completed in only 10 days. This sequence of cell degeneration, exfoliation, ulceration, mitosis, and repair is typically present in many viral infections in which viruses replicate in nasal, tracheal, and bronchial epithelium. Examples of transient infections of this type include human colds (rhinoviruses), infectious bovine rhinotracheitis (*bovine herpesvirus* 1), feline rhinotracheitis (*feline herpesvirus* 1), and canine infectious tracheobronchitis (*canine adenovirus* 2 and *canine parainfluenza*-2).

If damage to the mucociliary blanket becomes chronic, goblet cell hyperplasia results in excessive mucus production, and when there is loss of basement membrane, repair is hampered resulting in mucosal scars. In the most severe cases, prolonged injury causes squamous metaplasia and interference with the mucociliary clearance. Hyperplastic and metaplastic changes (squamous metaplasia) from persistent mucosal injury are considered a prelude to neoplasia in laboratory rodents.

The second type of epithelium lining the conductive system is the sensory **olfactory epithelium,** present in parts of the nasal mucosa, notably in the ethmoidal conchae. The patterns of degeneration, exfoliation, and inflammation in the olfactory epithelium are similar to those of the ciliated epithelium, except that olfactory epithelium has only limited capacity for regeneration. When olfactory epithelium has been irreversibly injured, olfactory cells swell, separate from adjacent sustentacular cells, and finally exfoliate into the nasal cavity. Once the underlying basement membrane of the olfactory epithelium is exposed, cytokines are released, and inflammatory cells move into the affected area. When damage is extensive, ulcerated areas of olfactory mucosa are replaced by ciliated and goblet cells or squamous epithelium, or by fibrous tissue, all of which eventually cause reduction or loss of olfactory function (anosmia).

Squamous epithelium, located in the vestibular region of the nose (mucocutaneous junctions), is the third type of epithelium present in the nasal passages. Compared with ciliated and olfactory epitheliums, nasal squamous epithelium is quite resistant to all forms of injury.

Anomalies of the Nasal Cavity

Localized congenital anomalies of the nasal cavity are rare in domestic animals and are often merely part of a more extensive craniofacial deformity (e.g., cyclops) or a component of generalized malformation (e.g., chondrodysplasia). Congenital anomalies involving the nasal cavity and sinuses such as choanal atresia, some types of chondrodysplasia, and osteopetrosis are incompatible with life. Examples of nonfatal congenital anomalies include cystic nasal conchae, nasal and sinus cysts, deviation of nasal septum, cleft upper lip (harelip, cheiloschisis), hypoplastic turbinates, and cleft palate (palatoschisis). Bronchoaspiration and aspiration pneumonia are common sequelae to cleft palate. As in other organs or systems, it is extremely difficult to determine the actual cause (genetic versus congenital) of anomalies based on pathologic examination.

Metabolic Disturbances of the Nasal Cavity

Metabolic disturbances affecting the nasal cavity and sinuses are also rare in domestic animals. **Amyloidosis,** the deposition of amyloid protein (fibrils with a β-pleated configuration) in various tissues, has been sporadically reported in the nasal cavity of horses. Affected horses have difficultly in breathing, epistaxis, and show reduced athletic performance; on clinical examination, large, firm nodules can be observed in the alar folds, rostral nasal septum, and floor of nasal cavity. Microscopic lesions are similar to those seen in other organs and consist of a deposition of hyaline material (Congo red–positive) in nasal mucosa. Unlike amyloidoses in other organs of domestic animals where amyloid is generally of the reactive type (amyloid AA), equine nasal amyloidosis appears to be of the immunocytic type (amyloid AL).

Circulatory Disturbances of the Nasal Cavity

Congestion and Hyperemia

The nasal mucosa is well vascularized and is capable of rather dramatic variation in blood flow, whether passively due to interference with venous return (congestion) or actively due to vasodilation (hyperemia). Congestion of the mucosal vessels is a nonspecific lesion commonly found at necropsy and presumably associated with the circulatory failure preceding death (e.g., heart failure, bloat in ruminants). Hyperemia of the nasal mucosa is also associated with early stages of inflammation, whether caused by irritations (e.g., ammonia, regurgitated feed), viral infections, secondary bacterial infections, allergy, or trauma.

Hemorrhage

Epistaxis is the clinical term used to denote blood flow from the nose (nosebleed) regardless of whether blood originates from the nasal mucosa or from deep in the lungs. Unlike blood in the digestive tract, where the approximate anatomic location of the bleeding can be estimated by the color the blood imparts to fecal material, blood in the respiratory tract always is red. This fact is due to the rapid transport of blood out of the respiratory tract by the mucociliary blanket. Hemorrhages into the nasal cavity can originate from local trauma, erosions of submucosal vessels by inflammation (e.g., guttural pouch mycosis), or neoplasms.

Ethmoidal (progressive) hematomas are important in older horses and are characterized clinically by chronic, progressive, often unilateral nasal bleeding. Grossly or endoscopically, an ethmoidal hematoma appears as a single, soft, tumorlike, pedunculated, dark red mass arising from the mucosa of the ethmoidal conchae. Microscopic examination reveals a capsule lined by epithelium and hemorrhagic stromal tissue infiltrated with abundant macrophages, some of which are siderophages.

Inflammation

Inflammation of the nasal mucosa is called **rhinitis** and that of the sinuses, **sinusitis.** These conditions usually occur together, although mild sinusitis can be undetected.

The occurrence of infectious rhinitis presupposes an upset in the balance of the normal microbial flora of the nasal cavity. Innocuous bacteria are present normally, protecting the host through a process called **competitive exclusion,** whereby the numbers of potential pathogens are kept at harmless numbers. Disruption of this protective mechanism can be caused by respiratory viruses, pathogenic bacteria, irritant gases, environmental changes, immunosuppression, local trauma, stress, or prolonged antibacterial therapy.

Based on the nature of exudate, rhinitis can be classified into **serous, catarrhal, purulent, fibrinous,** or **granulomatous.** Microscopic examination of impression smears and bacterial cultures are generally required in establishing the cause of the exudate. Other changes such as **hemorrhage, ulcers,** and **mucosal hyperplasia** can also be found in inflamed nasal mucosa. Rhinitis also can be classified according to the age of the lesions as acute, subacute, or chronic; to the severity of the insult as mild, moderate, or severe; and to the etiologic agent as viral, allergic, bacterial, mycotic, or toxic.

Serous Rhinitis

Serous rhinitis is the mildest form of inflammation and is characterized by hyperemia and increased production of a clear fluid locally manufactured by serous glands present in the submucosa. Serous rhinitis is of clinical interest only. It is caused by mild irritants or cold air, and it occurs during the early stages of viral infections, such as the common cold in human beings and upper respiratory tract infections in animals, or in mild allergic reactions.

Catarrhal Rhinitis

Catarrhal rhinitis is a slightly more severe process and has, in addition to serous secretions, a substantial increase in mucus production by increased activity of goblet cells and mucous glands. A mucus exudate is a thick, translucent or slightly turbid viscous fluid, sometimes containing a few leukocytes and cellular debris. In chronic cases, catarrhal rhinitis is characterized microscopically by marked hyperplasia of goblet cells. As the inflammation becomes more severe, the mucus is infiltrated with neutrophils that have a cloudy appearance. This exudate is referred to as mucopurulent.

Purulent (Suppurative) Rhinitis

This inflammation, characterized by a neutrophilic exudate, occurs when the nasal mucosa suffers a more severe injury that generally is accompanied by mucosal necrosis and secondary bacterial infection. Cytokines, leukotrienes, complement activation, and bacterial products cause exudation of leukocytes, especially neutrophils, which mix with nasal secretions including mucus. Grossly, the exudate in suppurative rhinitis is thick and opaque, but can vary from white to green to brown, depending on the types of bacteria and type of leukocytes present in the exudate. In severe cases, the nasal passages are completely blocked by the exudate. Microscopically, neutrophils can be seen in the submucosa and mucosa and form plaques of exudate on the mucosal surface. Neutrophils are commonly found attached to the vessels and between epithelial cells in their migration to the surface of the mucosa.

Fibrinous Rhinitis

This reaction occurs when nasal injury causes a severe increase in vascular permeability, resulting in abundant exudation of plasma fibrinogen, which coagulates into fibrin. Grossly, fibrin appears like a yellow, tan, or grey rubbery mat on nasal mucosa. Fibrin accumulates on the surface and forms a distinct film of exudate sometimes referred to as pseudomembrane (Fig. 3-6). If this fibrinous exudate can be removed, leaving an intact underling mucosa, it is termed a **croupous** or **pseudodiphtheritic**

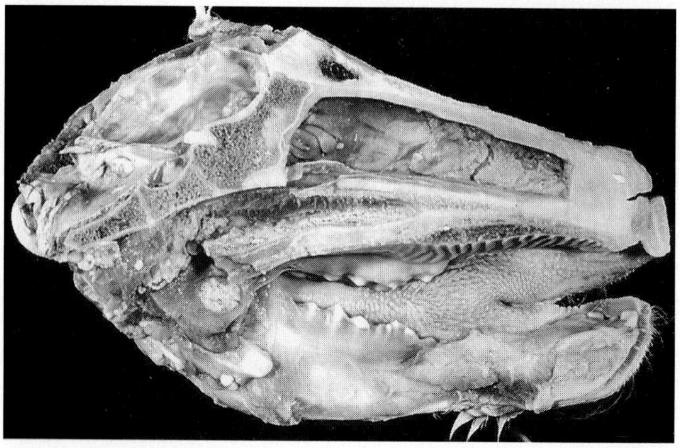

Figure 3-6 Midsagittal section of head; neonatal calf. Infectious bovine rhinotracheitis (bovine herpesvirus 1). The nasal septum was removed to expose nasal conchae. The nasal mucosa is covered by diphtheritic membranes (fibrinonecrotic exudate). There is a large, round ulcer in the nasopharynx. *Courtesy of Dr. Scott McBurney.*

rhinitis. Conversely, if removal of this pseudomembrane leaves an ulcerated mucosa, it is referred to as **diphtheritic** or **fibrinonecrotic rhinitis.** The term diphtheritic was derived from human diphtheria, which causes a severe and destructive inflammatory process of the respiratory mucosa. Microscopically, the lesions include a perivascular edema with fibrin, a few neutrophils infiltrating the mucosa, and plaques of exudate consisting of fibrin strands mixed with leukocytes and cellular debris covering a necrotic and ulcerated epithelium.

Granulomatous Rhinitis

This reaction is characterized by infiltration of macrophages, lymphocytes, and plasma cells in the mucosa and submucosa. In some cases, inflammation leads to the formation of polypoid nodules that, in severe cases, are large enough to cause obstruction of the nasal passages. Granulomatous rhinitis is generally associated with specific organisms such as those of systemic mycoses (see Lungs), tuberculosis, and with foreign bodies. In some cases, the etiology of granulomatous rhinitis is less specific such as in allergic rhinitis; in others, the etiology cannot be determined.

Inflammatory processes in the nasal cavity are not life-threatening and usually resolve completely. However, some adverse sequelae in cases of infectious rhinitis include bronchoaspiration of exudate leading to bronchopneumonia and pulmonary abscesses. Also, nasal inflammation may extend into the sinuses causing sinusitis, into facial bones causing osteomyelitis, through the cribriform plate causing meningitis, along the eustachian tubes causing otitis media and interna, and vestibular syndrome (abnormal head tilt and abnormal gait), which in severe cases, may lead to emaciation.

Sinusitis

Sinusitis occurs sporadically in domestic animals and is frequently combined with rhinitis or occurs as a sequela to septic wounds, improper dehorning in cattle (frontal sinus), or tooth infection in horses and dogs (maxillary sinus). Paranasal sinuses have poor drainage; therefore, exudate tends to accumulate, causing **mucocele** (accumulation of mucus) or **empyema** (accumulation of pus). Chronic sinusitis may extend into the adjacent bone (osteomyelitis) or through the bone into the meninges and brain (meningitis and encephalitis).

SPECIFIC DISEASES OF THE NASAL CAVITY AND SINUSES

Equine Nasal Diseases

Viruses such as equine *viral rhinopneumonitis virus, influenza virus, adenovirus,* and *rhinovirus* cause mild and generally transient respiratory infections in horses. All these infections are indistinguishable clinically; signs consist mainly of malaise, fever, coughing, and nasal discharge varying from serous to purulent. Viral respiratory infections are common medical problems in adult horses.

Equine Viral Rhinopneumonitis (EVR)

This disease, caused by equine herpesvirus (EVH), may be manifested as a mild respiratory disease in weanling foals and racehorses (EHV-4) or as abortion in mares (EHV-1). The respiratory form of EVR is generally transient; thus, the primary viral-induced lesions in the nasal mucosa and lungs are rarely seen at necropsy unless complicated by secondary bacterial rhinitis, pharyngitis, or bronchopneumonia. Studies with polymerase chain reaction (PCR) techniques have demonstrated that, like other herpesvirus, EHV-4 persists latently in the trigeminal ganglia after infection.

Equine Influenza

This disease is a common, highly contagious, self-limiting upper respiratory infection of horses caused by type A strains of influenza virus (A/equi-1 and -2). Equine influenza has high morbidity (outbreaks) but low mortality, and it is clinically characterized by fever, conjunctivitis, and nasal discharge. It occurs mainly in 2- to 3-year-old horses at the racetrack. As with human influenza, equine influenza is usually a mild disease, but occasionally it can cause severe bronchointerstitial pneumonia with pulmonary edema. In some horses, viral infection is complicated by a secondary bacterial bronchopneumonia caused by opportunistic organisms (*Streptococcus zooepidemicus; Staphylococcus aureus; Bacteroides* sp.) found in the normal flora of the upper respiratory tract. Uncomplicated cases of equine influenza are rarely seen in the postmortem room.

Other Equine Respiratory Viruses

Equine rhinovirus, adenovirus, and **parainfluenza virus** produce mild and transient upper respiratory infections in horses, unless complicated by secondary pathogens. In addition to reduced athletic performance, infected horses may have a temporary suppression of cell-mediated immunity. Fatal adenoviral infections with severe pneumonia or enteritis occur commonly in immunocompromised horses, particularly in Arabian foals with inherited combined immunodeficiency disease.

Strangles, Glanders, and Melioidosis

Strangles, glanders, and melioidosis of horses are all systemic bacterial diseases that cause purulent rhinitis and suppuration in various organs. These diseases are grouped as upper respiratory diseases because nasal discharge is often the most notable clinical sign.

Strangles. This infectious disease of equidae is caused by *Streptococcus equi* subsp *equi (S. equi).* It is characterized by suppurative rhinitis and lymphadenitis (mandibular and retropharyngeal) with occasional hematogenous dissemination to internal organs. Unlike *S. equi* subsp *zooepi-*

demicus (S. zooepidemicus) and *Streptococcus equisimilis, S. equi* is not part of the normal nasal flora; infection occurs when susceptible horses come into contact with feed, exudate, or air droplets containing the bacterium. After penetrating through the nasopharyngeal mucosa, *S. equi* drains to mandibular and retropharyngeal lymph nodes via lymphatic vessels. Clinically, the disease is characterized by nasal discharge, conjunctivitis, and marked swelling of lymph nodes.

The gross lesions correlate with clinical findings and consist of copious amounts of mucopurulent exudate in the nasal passages with notable hyperemia of nasal mucosa. Affected lymph nodes are enlarged, painful, warm, and contain thick purulent exudate (purulent lymphadenitis). The term "bastard strangles" is used in cases where hematogenous dissemination of *S. equi* results in metastatic abscesses in such organs as the lungs, liver, spleen, kidneys, brain, or in the joints.

Common sequelae to strangles include bronchopneumonia due to aspiration of exudate; laryngeal hemiplegia ("roaring"), resulting from compression of the recurrent laryngeal nerves by enlarged retropharyngeal lymph nodes; facial paralysis and Horner's syndrome due to compression of cranial nerves; and purpura hemorrhagica as a result of vasculitis presumably caused by deposition of *S. equi* antigen-antibody complexes in arterioles, venules, and capillaries. In severe cases, nasal infection extends directly into the paranasal sinuses or to the guttural pouches via the Eustachian tubes causing inflammation and accumulation of pus (empyema). Rupture of abscesses in the mandibular and retropharyngeal lymph nodes leads to suppurative inflammation of adjacent subcutaneous tissue (cellulitis).

Glanders. This infectious disease of equidae is caused by *Pseudomonas mallei (M. mallei [Malleomyces mallei])* and can be transmitted to carnivores by consumption of infected horse meat. Human beings are also susceptible, and the infection is often fatal. In the past, it was found throughout the world, but today glanders has been eradicated from most countries, except for some areas in North Africa, Asia, and Eastern Europe. The pathogenesis of glanders is not fully understood. Results from experimental infections suggest that infection with *P. mallei* occurs via the ingestion of contaminated feed and water and, very rarely, via inhalation of infectious droplets. At the portal of entry, presumably the oropharynx or intestine, bacteria penetrate the mucosa and spread via lymph vessels to lymph nodes, then to the bloodstream, thus hematogenously to the internal organs, particularly the lungs. Lesions in the nasal cavity start as pyogranulomatous nodules in the submucosa; these lesions subsequently ulcerate, releasing copious amounts of *P. mallei*–containing exudate into the nasal cavity. Finally, ulcerative lesions in conchal mucosa are replaced by typical stellate (star-shaped), fibrous scars. In some cases, the lungs also contain numerous gray, hard, small (2 to 10 mm), miliary nodules, randomly distributed because of the hematogenous route, in one or more pulmonary lobes. Microscopically, these nodules are typical granulomas composed of a necrotic center, with or without calcification, surrounded by a thick band of connective tissue infiltrated with numerous macrophages, some giant cells, lymphocytes, and plasma cells. Cutaneous lesions, often referred to as ***equine farcy,*** are characterized by nodular thickening of extended segments of lymph vessels in the subcutaneous tissue of the legs and ventral abdomen. This thickening of lymph vessels is the result of severe suppurative lymphangitis. Eventually affected lymph vessels rupture and release large amounts of purulent exudate through sinuses to the surface of the skin.

Melioidosis (Pseudoglanders). This important, life-threatening disease of human beings, horses, cattle, sheep, goats, pigs, dogs, cats, and rodents is caused by *Burkholderia pseudomallei (B. pseudomallei [Pseudomonas pseudomallei; Malleomyces pseudomallei]).* This disease in horses is clinically and pathologically similar to glanders, hence the name pseudoglanders. In human beings, this infection can be fatal. Melioidosis is currently present in Southeast Asia and, to a much lesser extent, in some European countries and Australia, where the causative organism is frequently found in rodents, feces, soil, and water. Ingestion of contaminated feed and water appears to be the main route of infection; direct transmission between infected animals and insect bites has also been postulated as a possible mechanism of infection. After gaining entrance to the animal, *B. pseudomallei* is disseminated by the bloodstream and causes suppuration and abscesses in most internal organs, nasal mucosa, joints, brain and spinal cord, liver, spleen, and lymph nodes. The exudate is creamy or caseous and yellow to green. The pulmonary lesions in melioidosis are those of an embolic bacterial pneumonia with formation of pulmonary abscesses. Focal adhesive pleuritis develops where abscesses rupture through the pleura and heal.

Other Equine Rhinitis

Rhinosporidium seeberi causes nasal infection in horses, cattle, and dogs. Gross lesions vary from barely visible granulomas to large polypoid nodules that are easily detected by rhinoscopy. The offending organism, *R. seeberi,* is readily visible in impression smears appearing as a large (400 μm), oval sporangium containing thousands of endospores.

Bovine Nasal Diseases

Infectious Bovine Rhinotracheitis (IBR or "Rednose")

This disease is of great importance in the cattle industry because of the synergism of the IBR virus with *Pasteurella haemolytica* in producing pneumonia and its association with bovine abortion, systemic infections of calves, and infectious pustular vulvovaginitis (IPV). The causative agent, bovine herpesvirus-1 (BHV-1), has probably existed as a mild venereal disease of cattle in Europe since at least the mid-1800s, but the respiratory form was not reported until intensive management feedlot systems were first introduced in North America around the 1950s. Typically, the disease is manifested as a transient, acute, febrile illness that only in very severe cases results in inspiratory dyspnea due to obstruction of airflow by exudate. Other forms of BHV-1 infection include nonsuppurative encephalitis, enteritis in calves, infertility, and, in experimental infections, mastitis, mammillitis, and necrosis of the ovaries. Except for the encephalitic form, the type of disease caused by BHV-1 depends more on the site of entry than the viral strain. Like other herpesviruses, BHV-1 also can remain latent in nerve ganglia, with recrudescence following stress or immunosuppression.

The respiratory form of IBR is characterized by severe hyperemia and focal necrosis of nasal, pharyngeal, laryngeal, tracheal (Figs. 3-6 and 3-7), and, sometimes, bronchial mucosa. As in other respiratory viral infections, IBR lesions generally consist of necrosis and exfoliation of ciliated cells followed by repair. Secondary bacterial infection in areas of necrosis result in the formation of a thick layer of fibrinonecrotic material (diphtheritic) in the airway. Intranuclear inclusion bodies, commonly seen in herpesvirus infections, are rarely seen in field cases since inclusion bodies only occur during the early stages of the disease.

The most important sequela to IBR is pneumonia, which is caused either by direct aspiration of exudate from airways or as a result of an impairment in pulmonary defense mechanisms, thus predisposing the animal to secondary

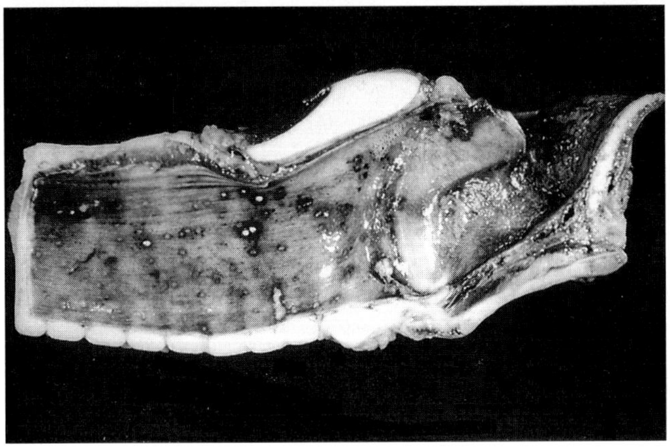

Figure 3-7 Larynx and proximal trachea, mucosal surface; cow. Infectious bovine rhinotracheitis (IBR), multifocal necrotizing laryngitis, and tracheitis. Ten days before, this calf was exposed experimentally to an aerosol of bovine herpesvirus 1. *Courtesy of Dr. G.A. Gifford.*

bacterial infection, most frequently *P. haemolytica* (see pneumonic pasteurellosis, p 45). Postmortem diagnosis of IBR is confirmed by isolation of the virus or its identification by immunohistochemistry or polymerase chain reaction (PCR).

Other Bovine Rhinitis

Nasal granulomas occur in cattle presumably as a result of repeated exposure to as-yet unidentified inhaled antigens. Nasal granulomas (atopic rhinitis) are reported mainly in cattle in Australia, South Africa, and the United Kingdom, where affected cattle develop multiple, small, pink or red, polypoid nodules, starting in the nasal vestibule and, in time, extending into the caudal aspect of the nasal septum. These nodules are composed of fibrovascular tissue mixed with lymphocytes (granulation tissue) superficially lined by hyperplastic epithelium with abundant mast cells and eosinophils in the lamina propria (nasal eosinophilia). The microscopic features suggest that hypersensitivity type I, type III (immune complex), and IV (delayed) may be involved in nasal granulomas of cattle. Bovine (idiopathic) nasal granuloma must be differentiated from nasal mycetomas, nasal rhinosporidiosis, and nasal schistosomiasis, which also cause the formation of nodules in the nasal mucosa of cattle.

Ovine and Caprine Nasal Disease

***Oestrus ovis* (nasal bot)** is the brownish fly, about the size of a honeybee, that deposits its first-stage larvae in the nostrils of sheep raised in most parts of the world. Microscopic larvae mature into large bots that spend most of their larval stages in nasal passages and sinuses, causing irritation, inflammation, and obstruction of airways. Matured larvae drop to the ground and pupate into flies. This type of parasitism in which living tissues are invaded by larvae of flies is known as myiasis. Although *O. ovis* is primarily a myiasis of sheep, it sporadically affects goats, dogs and, sometimes, human beings (shepherds). The presence of the larvae in nasal passages causes chronic irritation and erosive mucopurulent rhinitis; bots of *O. ovis* can be found easily if the head is cut to expose the nasal passages. Rarely, larvae of *O. ovis* penetrate the cranial vault through the ethmoidal plate, causing direct or secondary bacterial meningitis.

Rhinitis is only sporadically reported in goats; most cases are associated with infections with *Pasteurella multocida* or *P. haemolytica*. The lesions range from a mild serous to catarrhal or mucopurulent inflammation.

Porcine Nasal Diseases

Inclusion Body Rhinitis

This disease of young pigs, with high morbidity and low mortality, is caused by a porcine cytomegalovirus (herpesvirus) and is characterized by a mild rhinitis. This virus commonly infects the nasal epithelium of piglets younger than 5 weeks and produces a mild and transient rhinitis, causing sneezing, nasal discharge, and excessive lacrimation. Since this disease is seldom fatal, lesions are seen only incidentally or in euthanized animals. In uncomplicated cases, the gross lesion is hyperemia of the nasal mucosa, but, with secondary bacterial infections, mucopurulent exudate can be abundant. Microscopic lesions are typical and consist of a necrotizing, nonsuppurative rhinitis with giant, basophilic, intranuclear inclusion bodies in the epithelial cells of the mucosa and glands (Fig. 3-8). Immunosuppressed piglets can develop a systemic cytomegalovirus infection characterized by necrosis of the liver, lungs, adrenal glands, and brain with intralesional inclusion bodies.

Atrophic Rhinitis

A common worldwide disease of pigs, atrophic rhinitis is clinically characterized by sneezing, coughing, and nasal discharge as a result of inflammation and atrophy of nasal conchae (turbinates). In severe cases, atrophy of the conchae may cause a striking facial deformity due to deviation of the nasal bones. The etiopathogenesis of atrophic rhinitis is complex and has been a matter of controversy for many years. Pathogens historically associated with atrophic rhinitis include *Bordetella bronchiseptica, Pasteurella multocida, Haemophilus parasuis,* and viral infections such as porcine cytomegalovirus (inclusion body rhinitis). In addition, predisposing factors have included genetic makeup, environment, and nutritional deficiencies. Currently, the etiology of atrophic rhinitis is believed to be combined infection of specific strains of *B. bronchiseptica* and some toxigenic strains of *P. multocida* (types D and A). The only lesion associated with infection with *B. bronchiseptica* alone is a mild to moderate turbinate atrophy, but this bacterium actively promotes the colonization of the nasal cavity by *P. multocida*. The toxigenic strains of *P. multocida* produce potent cytotoxins that inhibit osteoblastic activity and promote osteoclastic reabsorption in nasal bones, particularly in the ventral nasal conchae, where abnormal bone remodeling results in atrophy of conchae.

The degree of conchal atrophy in pigs with atrophic rhinitis varies considerably, and, in most pigs, the severity of the lesions does not correspond to the severity of the clinical signs. The best diagnostic method of evaluating this disease is to make a transverse section of the snout between the first and second premolar teeth. In normal pigs, conchae are symmetric and fill most of the cavity, leaving only narrow air spaces (meatuses) between coiled conchae. The normal nasal septum is straight and divides the cavity into two mirror-imaged cavities. In contrast, the septum in pigs with atrophic rhinitis is generally deviated and the conchae appear smaller and asymmetric (Fig. 3-9). Conchal atrophy causes dorsal and ventral meatuses to appear rather enlarged, and, in the most advanced cases, the entire nasal conchae may be missing, leaving a large, empty space. It may seem logical to assume that, after loss of conchae in an obligate nasal breather like the pig, the

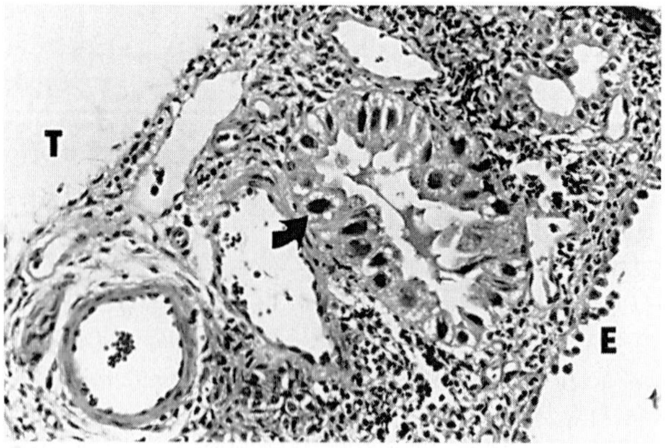

Figure 3-8 Nasal conchae; 4-week-old pig. Inclusion body rhinitis. Note the large intranuclear inclusion bodies *(arrow)* caused by cytomegalovirus infection in epithelial cells. The inclusions are in a submucosal gland between the epithelial surface *(E)* and the turbinate *(T)*, which was removed during tissue processing. Hematoxylin-eosin (H & E) stain. *Courtesy of Western College of Veterinary Medicine.*

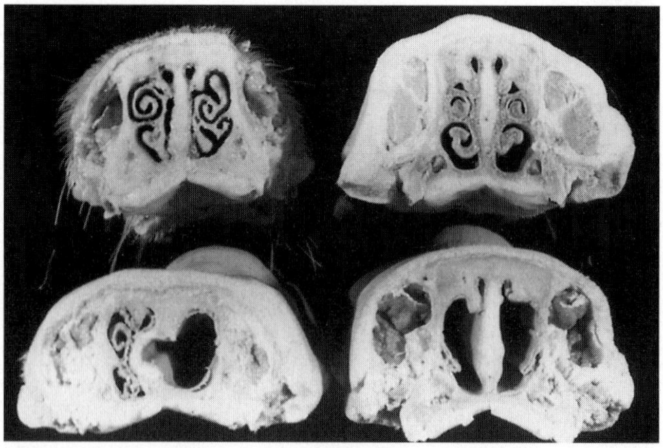

Figure 3-9 Cross-section of nasal passages and sinuses at the level of the first and second premolar teeth; atrophic rhinitis; pigs. Normal nasal cavity with complete conchae (turbinates) filling most of the nasal cavity and forming narrow air passages or meatuses *(top left)*. Three pigs with atrophic rhinitis. Mild, symmetric atrophy of nasal conchae *(top right)*. Severe, unilateral atrophy of right ventral nasal conchae with deviation of the nasal septum and widening of the ventral meatuses *(bottom left)*. Severe, bilateral atrophy with complete loss of nasal conchae and vast enlargement of the meatuses *(bottom right)*.

filtration defense mechanism of the nasal cavity would be impaired. However, the relationship between atrophic rhinitis, pneumonia, and growth rates in pigs is still controversial.

Obstruction of the nasolacrimal duct is common in pigs with atrophic rhinitis and results in accumulation of dust and dried lacrimal secretions on the skin below the medial canthus of the eye. Osteopenia is the key microscopic lesion in atrophic rhinitis. Depending on the stage of the disease, mucopurulent exudate may be found on the surface of the conchae, hyperplastic or metaplastic changes can occur in the nasal epithelium and glands, and infiltrates of lymphoplasmacytic cells can be present in the lamina propria. In summary, atrophic rhinitis is an important disease of swine worldwide; morphologic diagnosis is simple, but additional understanding of the pathogenesis will be necessary before effective preventive measures can be established.

Canine Nasal Diseases

Dogs have no specific viral infectious affecting exclusively the nasal cavity or sinuses. Acute rhinitis occurs as part of general respiratory disease caused by several distinct viruses such as *canine distemper virus, canine adenovirus 1* and *2, canine parainfluenza virus, reovirus,* and *canine herpesvirus*. The viral lesions in the respiratory tract are generally transient, but the effect of the virus on other tissues and cells can be fatal, as in distemper encephalitis in dogs. As in other species, secondary bacterial rhinitis, sinusitis, and pneumonia are possible sequelae of respiratory viral infections; *Bordetella bronchiseptica, Escherichia coli,* and *Pasteurella multocida* are the most common isolates in dogs with bacterial rhinitis. **Immotile cilia syndrome** (ciliary dyskinesia), a congenital disease, reduces mucociliary clearance and is an important factor in recurrent canine rhinosinusitis, bronchitis, bronchiectasis, and pneumonia.

Other Canine Rhinitis

Aspergillus sp. and *Penicillium* sp. cause mycotic rhinitis in dogs; the infection is clinically characterized by mucopurulent nasal discharge. Nasal biopsies reveal extensive necrosis of the nasal epithelium and thick plaques of fibrinopurulent exudate mixed with many fungal hyphae. *Cryptococcus neoformans* and *Rhinosporidium seeberi* infections of the nasal cavity occur sporadically in dogs. Lesions are characterized by formation of granulomas in the nasal mucosa.

LINGUATULA SERRATA. This highly specialized arthropod (pentastomid) parasite occurs primarily in carnivores, although herbivores and human beings have become aberrant hosts. The adult parasite is found throughout the nasal passages and, sometimes, can reach the sinuses and middle ear by moving through the eustachian tubes. In common with other nasal parasites, *L. serrata* acts as an irritant, causing catarrhal inflammation.

CAPILLARIA AEROPHILA. This nematode is a parasite of the nasal passages, sinuses, trachea, and bronchi of carnivores. Although generally asymptomatic, some dogs cough because of the local irritation caused by the parasites on the airway mucosa. When present, the lesions are catarrhal to mucopurulent inflammation of airway mucosa.

The nasal cavity and sinuses of dogs can occasionally be infested with other parasites, including mites *(Pneumonyssus caninum)*.

Allergic rhinitis (*hay fever;* nasolacrimal urticaria), which is so common in human beings sensitized to pollens or allergens, has been reported only sporadically in dogs and cats. "Hay fever" in human beings and animals is a type I hypersensitivity reaction in which degranulation of mast cells results in an acute rhinitis and conjunctivitis clinically characterized by profuse serous nasal discharge and lacrimation. Microscopically, the nasal mucosa is edematous and infiltrated with numerous eosinophils, neutrophils, and some macrophages.

Feline Nasal Diseases

Feline Viral Rhinotracheitis (FVR)

This common and worldwide respiratory disease of cats is caused by a feline herpesvirus (FHV-1) and is characterized by lethargy, oculonasal discharges, severe rhinitis, and conjunctivitis. The disease causes an impairment of pulmonary defense mechanisms, predisposing cats to secondary bacterial pneumonia. The virus also can remain latent in ganglia. The vast majority of cats that recover from FVR become carriers and shed FHV-1, either spontaneously or following stress. Susceptible animals, particularly kittens with low maternal immunity, become infected following exposure to a diseased or a carrier cat. Replication of FHV-1 in the nasal, conjunctival, pharyngeal, and, to a lesser extent, tracheal epithelium causes degeneration and exfoliation of cells. Lesions caused by FHV-1 are fully reversible, but secondary infections with bacteria such as *Pasteurella multocida, Bordetella bronchiseptica, Streptococcus* sp., and *Mycoplasma felis* can cause a chronic, severe suppurative rhinitis and conjunctivitis. Intranuclear inclusion bodies are rarely seen in cats with FVR, because inclusions are only present during the early stages of infection and have already disappeared by the time the cat is presented for diagnosis.

Respiratory sequelae to FVR can include chronic bacterial rhinitis and sinusitis with persistent purulent discharges; lysis of conchal bone, which can lead to complete loss of the conchae; permanent damage to the olfactory epithelium; and secondary bacterial pneumonia. In addition to respiratory lesions, FVR also causes ulcerative keratitis, hepatic necrosis, emaciation, abortion, and stillbirths.

Feline Calicivirus (FCV)

This disease is caused by different strains of feline calicivirus. It is an important infection of the respiratory tract of cats, and, depending on the virulence of the strain, lesions vary from a mild oculonasal discharge to severe rhinitis, mucopurulent conjunctivitis, and ulcerative stomatitis. Clinical and pathologic features of FCV disease are strikingly similar but not identical to those of FVR; these two viral infections account for 80% of all cases of feline respiratory diseases. The lesions, in addition to rhinitis and conjunctivitis, include acute, diffuse interstitial pneumonia with necrotizing bronchiolitis and prominent ulcers of the tongue and hard palate. Primary viral lesions are generally transient, but secondary bacterial infections (*Bordetella bronchiseptica; Pasteurella multocida; Escherichia coli*) are a common complication. Some kittens develop lameness following infection or vaccination with calicivirus due to an acute and self-limiting arthritis ("limping kitten syndrome"). Carrier state and virus shedding from oronasal secretions and feces are natural sequelae following recovery from the acute phase of the disease.

Feline Chlamydiosis

This disease is a persistent respiratory infection of cats caused by feline strains of *Chlamydia psittaci (felis)*. Infection results in a mild conjunctivitis (similar to that of human trachoma) and serous or mucopurulent rhinitis, but, in severe cases, can also produce a mild, transient bronchointerstitial pneumonia referred to as feline pneumonitis (see "Pneumonias of cats").

Mycoplasma felis can also cause conjunctivitis and a mild upper respiratory infection, with clinical signs and lesions overlapping those seen with chlamydiosis, FVR, and feline calicivirus infections. Respiratory tract infections in cats may also be associated with the immunosuppressive effects of feline retroviruses such as **feline leukemia virus** (FeLV) and **feline immunodeficiency virus** (FIV).

Other Feline Rhinitis and Sinusitis

Mycotic Rhinitis. The most common mycotic infection in the feline nasal cavity is caused by *Cryptococcus neoformans*. The lesions vary from discrete nasal granulomas to large masses of mucopurulent exudate filling the entire nasal cavity. Allergic rhinitis is also reported in cats (see Other Canine Rhinitis).

Neoplasia of the Nasal Cavity and Sinuses

Neoplasms of the nasal cavity and sinuses may arise from any of the tissues forming these structures, including bone (osteoma or osteosarcoma), cartilage (chondroma or chondrosarcoma), connective tissue (fibroma or fibrosarcoma, myxoma or myxosarcoma), blood vessels (hemangioma or hemangiosarcoma), and from all the different types of cells of glands and lining epithelium (adenoma or adenocarcinoma). In general, nasal neoplasms are rare in domestic animals, except for endemic ethmoidal neoplasms of sheep and cattle that can occur in several animals of a flock or herd.

In companion animals, nasal neoplasms are seen most commonly in dogs, particularly in breeds such as the collie and German shepherd. The cat and the horse are significantly less affected. The most common sites are the nasal passages for dogs, the nasal vestibule for cats, and the maxillary sinus for horses.

Nasal neoplasms become secondarily infected by bacteria, and clinical signs often overlap those of infectious rhinitis, including catarrhal or mucopurulent nasal discharge, periodic hemorrhage, increased lacrimation due to obstruction of nasolacrimal ducts, and sneezing. In some instances, it is not possible to clinically or grossly differentiate neoplasms from hyperplastic nodules or granulomatous rhinitis. Some neoplasms may infiltrate adjacent structures and produce notable facial deformities, loss of teeth, exophthalmus, and nervous signs. Large neoplasms also interfere with airflow, causing stertorous breathing (Fig. 3-10). Brush and imprint cytology have proven effective in the antemortem diagnosis of nasal neoplasms, particularly in those of epithelial lineage.

The majority of neoplasms in the nasal cavity are malignant. Benign nasal neoplasms (papilloma and adenoma)

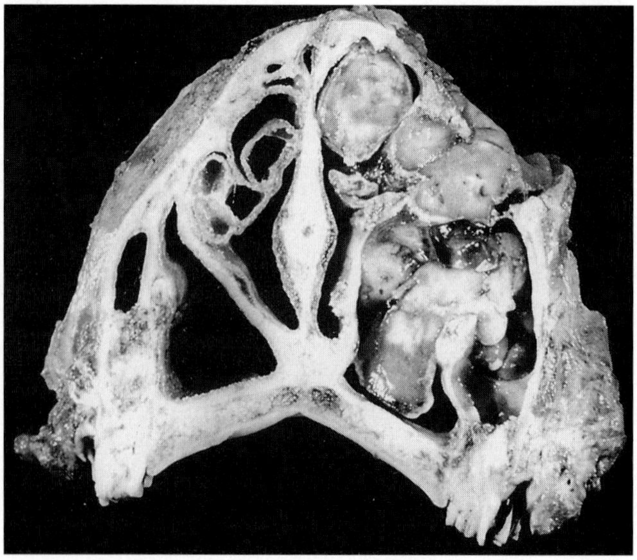

Figure 3-10 Cross-section of nasal passages and sinuses; cow. Nasal neurofibroma. A swelling on the lateral aspect of the head was visible before slaughter. The tumor has destroyed bone dorsolaterally and has not yet invaded beyond the cartilaginous nasal septum. *Courtesy of Western College of Veterinary Medicine.*

are rare and generally are either solitary or multiple, well-delineated nodules. In contrast, **nasal carcinomas** and **nasal sarcomas** are generally of larger but variable size, often pale and multilobulated masses composed of fleshy to friable tissue. Malignant neoplasms are locally invasive and tend to infiltrate sinuses, brain, nerves, and vessels, resulting in hemorrhage. Carcinomas vary from anaplastic (poorly differentiated) to more differentiated, in which cell and tissue morphology retains some glandular (adenocarcinoma) or squamous cell patterns. Because nasal tumors in dogs and cats are usually large and invasive at the time of diagnosis, survival times are usually short.

Enzootic Ethmoidal Neoplasms

A unique group of nasal carcinomas of sheep, goats, and cattle arise from the ethmoidal conchae and are associated with viral infections of the respiratory epithelial cells. A retrovirus has been postulated as the oncogenic agent, and tumors have been successfully transmitted with the virus or infected tissues. Enzootic nasal tumors are typically invasive but do not metastasize (Fig. 3-11).

Nasal Polyps and Nasal Cysts Resembling Neoplasia

Nonneoplastic masses that resemble neoplasms are common sequelae to chronic rhinitis in horses, cats, and, to a lesser extent, other species. In horses, polyps tend to form in the ethmoidal region, whereas in cats, polyps are most frequently found in the nasopharynx and Eustachian tubes. Grossly, polyps appear as firm, pedunculated nodules of various sizes protruding from the nasal mucosa into the air passages; the surface may be smooth, ulcerated, secondarily infected, and hemorrhagic. Microscopically, polyps are characterized by a core of well-vascularized stromal tissue that contains inflammatory cells and is covered by pseudostratified or squamous epithelium.

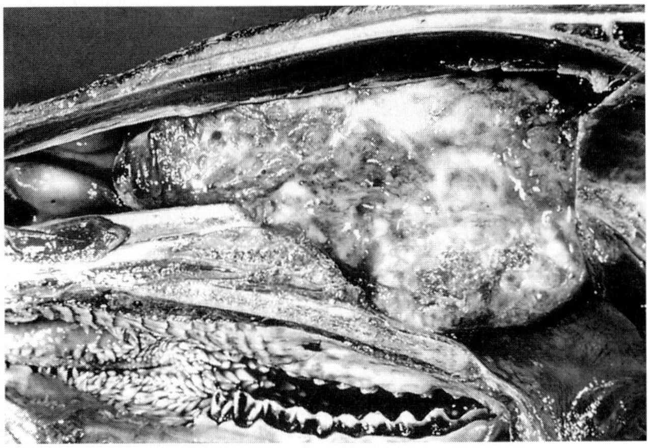

Figure 3-11 Midsagittal section of the head; 2-year-old ewe. Nasal adenocarcinoma. The tumor has occluded the right nasal passage and posterior nares. The location and type of tumor are typical of a retrovirus-induced "enzootic nasal carcinoma." *Courtesy of Western College of Veterinary Medicine.*

Nasal and paranasal sinus cysts are common in horses and are of great medical importance because they clinically mimic neoplasms or infections. Although not considered a neoplastic growth, cysts are expansive and cause deformation or destruction of the surrounding bone. These cysts are typically composed of an epithelial cell capsule filled with yellow or hemorrhagic fluid, and do not recur after surgical removal. Ethmoidal hematomas also resemble nasal tumors in horses (see Nasal Cavity and Sinuses, Hemorrhage).

PHARYNX, LARYNX, AND TRACHEA

Anomalies

Congenital anomalies of this region are rare in all species. Depending on their location and severity, they may be inconsistent with postnatal life, pose little or no problem, or manifest themselves in later life. If clinical signs of respiratory distress do occur, they are usually exacerbated by excitement, heat, stress, or exercise.

Brachycephalic Airway Syndrome

This clinical term refers to respiratory impairment caused by stenotic external nostrils and an excessive length of soft palate. These abnormalities are present in brachycephalic canine breeds such as bulldogs, boxers, Boston terriers, pugs, Pekingese, and others. The defects are due to a mismatch of the ratio of soft tissue to cranial bone and the obstruction of air flow by excessive palatine soft tissue. Secondary changes, such as nasal and laryngeal edema caused by forceful inspiration, eventually lead to severe upper airway obstruction and respiratory distress.

Hypoplastic Epiglottis

This anomaly of horses leads to respiratory noise associated with dorsal displacement of the soft palate. An undersized epiglottis is prone to entrapment below the arytenoepiglottic fold, causing an equine syndrome known as **epiglottic entrapment,** clinically characterized by airway obstruction, exercise intolerance, respiratory noise, and cough. Epiglottic entrapment also occurs in horses with lateral deviation and deformity of epiglottis, epiglottic cysts, or necrosis of the tip of the epiglottis. Hypoplastic epiglottis also occurs in pigs.

Subepiglottic and Pharyngeal Cysts

These types of anomalous lesions are occasionally seen in horses. These cysts vary in size (1 to 10 cm) and occur most commonly in the subepiglottic area and to a lesser extent in the upper pharynx, larynx, and soft palate. Cysts are lined by squamous or pseudostratified epithelium and contain thick mucus. Large cysts cause airway obstruction or dysphagia, predisposing to bronchoaspiration of food.

Tracheal Agenesis and Tracheal Hypoplasia

Tracheal hypoplasia occurs most often in English bulldogs; the tracheal lumen is decreased throughout its length.

Tracheal Collapse

This lesion occurs in toy and miniature breeds of dogs, in which it is also called **tracheobronchial collapse** or **central airway collapse.** The defect also occurs in horses, cattle, and goats. Grossly, there is dorsoventral flattening of the trachea with concomitant widening of the dorsal tracheal membrane, which may then prolapse ventrally into the lumen. Most commonly, the defect involves the entire length of the trachea and only rarely affects the cervical portion alone. Affected segments with a reduced lumen contain froth and even be covered by a diphtheritic membrane. Tracheal collapse is presumed to be associated with reduced glycoproteins and loss of elasticity in tracheal cartilages.

Other tracheal anomalies include **scabbard trachea** in horses, in which there is lateral flattening, so the tracheal lumen is a narrow vertical slit, and **tracheoesophageal fistula** in dogs and cattle.

Degenerative Diseases: Laryngeal Hemiplegia (Paralysis)

This disease, sometimes called *roaring,* is a common, but obscure, disease of horses characterized by atrophy of the dorsal and lateral cricoarytenoid muscles (abductor and adductor of the arytenoid cartilage), particularly on the left side. Atrophy is due to denervation as a result of either a primary axonal disease (idiopathic) or secondary nerve damage caused by compression or inflammation of the left recurrent laryngeal nerve. The cranial laryngeal nerve and medial retropharyngeal lymph nodes are located immediately ventral to the floor of the guttural pouches. As a result of this close anatomic relationship, swelling or inflammation of the guttural pouches and retropharyngeal lymph nodes often results in secondary damage to the laryngeal nerve. Common causes of secondary nerve damage (Wallerian degeneration) include guttural pouch mycosis, retropharyngeal abscesses, inflammation due to iatrogenic injection into the nerves, neck injury, and metastatic neoplasms involving the lymph nodes (e.g., lymphosarcoma). The abnormal inspiratory sounds (roaring) noted during exercise in horses with laryngeal hemiplegia are due to paralysis of the left dorsal and lateral cricoarytenoid muscles, which cause incomplete dilation of the larynx, obstruct airflow, and loose vocal cords vibrate. Grossly, affected laryngeal muscle is pale and smaller than normal (muscle atrophy). Microscopically, muscle fibers have lesions of denervation atrophy (see Chapter 9, Muscle). Atrophy of laryngeal muscles also occurs in dogs as an inherited condition (Siberian husky and Bouvier des Flandres), as a degenerative neuropathy in older dogs, or secondary to laryngeal trauma (e.g., choke chain damage).

Circulatory Disturbances

Laryngeal and Tracheal Hemorrhages

Hemorrhages in these sites usually occur as mucosal petechiae in coagulopathies or septicemias such as hog cholera and porcine salmonellosis. Similarly, hemorrhages can be seen in slaughtered cattle and pigs as incidental findings. Severe dyspnea, especially in cattle, prior to death can cause congestion, ecchymosis, and petechiae in the tracheal mucosa; this lesion must be differentiated from postmortem imbibition of hemoglobin in autolysed carcasses.

Laryngeal Edema

This lesion is a common feature of acute inflammation, but it is of particular importance because of its potential to obstruct the laryngeal orifice resulting in asphyxiation. Laryngeal edema occurs in pigs with edema disease, in horses with purpura hemorrhagica, in cattle with acute interstitial pneumonia, systemic anaphylaxis in cats, and in all species as a result of trauma, inhalation of irritant gases (e.g., smoke), local inflammation, and allergic reactions. Grossly, the laryngeal mucosa is thickened and swollen, often protrudes dorsally onto the epiglottis, and has a gelatinous appearance.

Tracheal Edema

Also known as the **"honker syndrome"** or **"tracheal edema syndrome of feeder cattle,"** this entity is a poorly documented, acute disease of unknown etiology, most often seen during the summer months. Clinical signs include inspiratory dyspnea that can progress to oral breathing, recumbency, and death by asphyxiation in less than 24 hours. Severe edema and a few hemorrhages are present in the mucosa and submucosa of the dorsal surface of the trachea, extending caudally from the midcervical area to as far as the tracheal bifurcation. On cut section, the tracheal mucosa is diffusely thickened and gelatinous.

Patterns of Injury and Host Response in Pharynx, Guttural Pouches, Larynx, and Trachea

The laryngeal mucosal is formed by columnar ciliated epithelium with goblet cells (mucociliary blanket) and squamous epithelium, whereas the trachea is exclusively lined by columnar ciliated epithelium. The pattern of injury and host response in the larynx and trachea is similar to the nasal mucosa (see Defense Mechanisms of the Conductive System). The pharyngeal mucosa, composed of squamous epithelium, has similar patterns of necrosis and inflammation as the oral mucosa (see Chapter 1, Alimentary System).

Inflammation

Pharyngitis, Laryngitis, and Tracheitis

Inflammation of the pharynx, larynx, and trachea are important because of their potential to obstruct airflow and to lead to aspiration pneumonia. The pharynx is vulnerable to the maladies of both the upper respiratory and upper digestive tracts, and the trachea can be involved by extension from both the lungs and upper respiratory regions.

Intraluminal foreign bodies in the pharynx such as medicinal boluses, apples, or potatoes can obstruct the laryngeal and tracheal airways. Also, pharyngeal obstruction can be caused by masses in surrounding tissues such as neoplasms of the thyroid gland, thymus, and parathyroid glands, tonsils, lymph nodes, and esophagus. Other esophageal lesions include those caused by *Spirocerca lupi,* retropharyngeal and cervical lymph nodes swollen by hyperplasia, neoplasia, or lymphadenitis, cysts, polyps, and abscesses. **Chronic polypoid tracheitis** occurs in dogs and cats, probably secondary to chronic infection. Laryngeal abscesses involving the mucosa and underlying cartilage occur as a herd or flock problem in calves and sheep, presumably caused by a secondary infection with *Arcanobacterium pyogenes (Actinomyces pyogenes; Corynebacterium pyogenes).*

Equine Pharyngeal Lymphoid Hyperplasia

This lesion is the most common cause of partial upper airway obstruction in horses, particularly in 2- and 3-year-old racehorses. Lymphoid hyperplasia tends to regress with age in older horses. The etiology is undetermined, but chronic bacterial infection combined with environmental factors may cause excessive antigenic stimulation and lymphoid hyperplasia with clinical signs of stertorous inspiration, expiration, or both. The gross lesions, visible endoscopically or at necropsy, consist of variably sized white foci located on the dorsolateral pharynx and extending into the openings of the guttural pouches and onto the soft palate. Microscopically, the lesion is hyperplasia of lymphoid cells within the pharyngeal nodules.

Pharyngeal Perforation

A number of nonspecific insults can cause lesions and clinical signs. Trauma may take the form of penetrating wounds in any species, perforation of the caudodorsal wall of the pharynx from the improper use of drenching or balling guns in sheep, cattle or pigs, choking injury due to use of collars in dogs and cats, and the shearing forces of bite wounds. The results of the trauma may be minimal (local edema) and inflammation or as serious as fatal cellulitis. Foreign bodies may occur anywhere in the region; the location and size determine the occurrence of dysphagia, regurgitation, dyspnea, or asphyxiation. Pigs have a unique structure known as the pharyngeal diverticulum (4 cm long in adult pigs), which is located in the pharyngeal wall rostral and dorsal to the esophageal entrance. It is important because barley awns may lodge in the diverticulum, causing an inflammatory swelling that affects swallowing. The diverticular wall may be perforated by awns or drenching syringes, which results in a cellulitis that can extend down the tissue planes of the neck. The pharynx of the dog may also be damaged by trauma from chicken bones, sticks, and needles, resulting in the formation of a pharyngeal abscess.

Inflammation of Guttural Pouches

The guttural pouches of horses are large diverticula (300 to 500 ml) of the ventral Eustachian tubes. They are, therefore, exposed to the same pathogens as is the pharynx and have drainage problems similar to those of sinuses. Although it is probable that various pathogens, including viruses, infect them, the lesions that are most often diagnosed are guttural pouch mycosis and guttural pouch empyema. Because of the close anatomic proximity of guttural pouches to the internal carotid arteries, cranial nerves (VI, IX, X, XI, and XII) and atlantooccipital joint, disease of these diverticula may involve these structures and cause a variety of clinical signs in horses.

Guttural pouch mycosis occurs primarily in stabled horses and is caused by *Aspergillus fumigatus* and other *Aspergillus* species. Infection is usually unilateral, and presumably starts with the inhalation of spores from moldy hay. Grossly, the dorsal and lateral aspects of the guttural pouch mucosa are covered by a diphtheritic, fibrinonecrotic exudate. Microscopically, the lesions are severe necrotic inflammation of the mucosa and submucosa with widespread vasculitis and intralesional fungal hyphae. The characteristic necrosis of this mycotic disease and its proximity to the internal carotid artery explain why guttural pouch mycosis can lead to vascular erosion and epistaxis. Erosion of the internal carotid artery can also lead to formation of an aneurysm and fatal bleeding into the guttural pouches. In other cases, the fungi may be angioinvasive, leading to the release of mycotic thromboemboli into the carotid, generally resulting in multiple cerebral infarcts. Dysphagia, another clinical sign seen in guttural pouch mycosis, is associated with damage to the pharyngeal branches of the vagus and glossopharyngeal nerves, which lie on the ventral aspect of the pouches. Horner's syndrome results from damage to the cranial cervical ganglion and sympathetic fibers located in the caudodorsal aspect of the pouches. Finally, equine laryngeal paralysis (hemiplegia) can result from involvement of the laryngeal nerves (previously described under Degenerative Disease: Laryngeal Hemiplegia [Paralysis]).

Empyema of guttural pouches is a sequela to suppurative inflammation of the nasal cavities, most commonly from *Streptococcus equi* infection (strangles). It is clinically characterized by nasal discharge, enlarged retropharyngeal lymph nodes, parotitis, dysphagia, and respiratory distress. In severe cases, the entire guttural pouch can be filled with purulent exudate. With the exception of erosion of the internal carotid artery, empyema of guttural pouches has sequelae similar to those of guttural pouch mycosis.

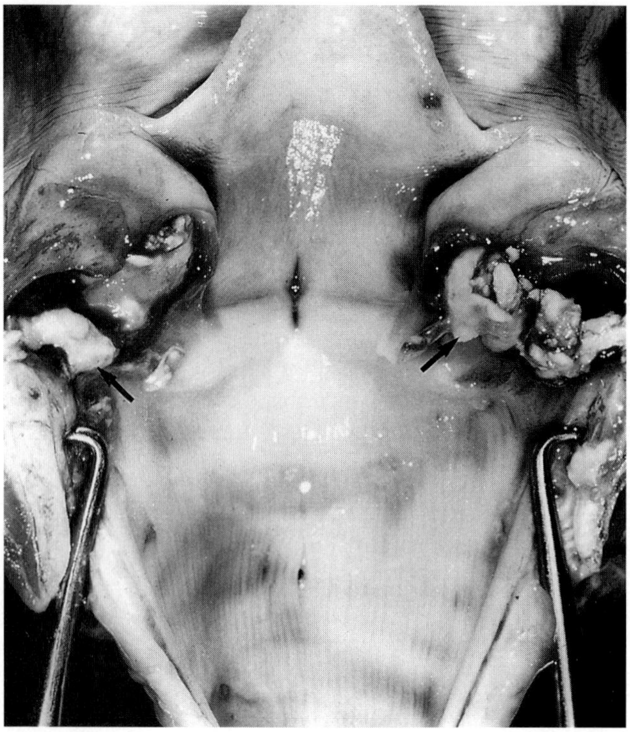

Figure 3-12 Larynx and trachea; calf. Necrotic laryngitis, calf diphtheria *(Fusobacterium necrophorum)*. Plaques of fibrinonecrotic exudate *(arrows)* are present on the mucosal surface of the arytenoid cartilages. *Courtesy of Dr. M.D. McGavin.*

Necrotic Laryngitis (Calf Diphtheria, Laryngeal Necrobacillosis)

Necrotic laryngitis is a common disease of feedlot cattle and cattle affected with other diseases, with nutritional deficiencies, or housed under unsanitary conditions. It also occurs in sheep. Necrotic laryngitis, caused by *Fusobacterium necrophorum,* is part of the syndrome termed orolaryngeal necrobacillosis, which can include lesions of the tongue, gingiva, cheeks, palate, and pharynx. An opportunistic pathogen, *F. necrophorum* produces several exotoxins and endotoxins after gaining entry either through lesions of viral infections such as IBR and papular stomatitis in cattle and contagious ecthyma in sheep, or after traumatic injury produced by feed or careless use of specula or balling guns.

The clinical signs of necrotic laryngitis are fever, anorexia, depression, halitosis, moist painful cough, dysphagia, and inspiratory dyspnea and ventilatory failure due to fatigue of the respiratory muscle.

The gross lesions, regardless of location in the mouth or larynx (most common in arytenoid cartilages), consist of well-demarcated, dry, yellow-gray, thick-crusted, necrotic areas (Fig. 3-12) that, in the early stages, are bounded by a zone of hyperemia. Deep ulceration develops, and, if the lesion is not fatal, healing is by granulation tissue formation. Microscopically, large necrotic foci initially have hyperemic borders. Later these areas are replaced by a band of leukocytes and, still later, by granulation tissue and collagen (fibrosis). The lesions can extend deep into the submucosal tissues, with bacteria evident at the advancing edge.

There are numerous important sequelae to calf diphtheria, the most serious being death due to toxemia or fusobacteremia. The exudate may be copious enough to cause asphyxiation or be aspirated and cause bronchopneumonia.

Laryngeal Contact Ulcers

These lesions, found in feedlot cattle, grossly, are unilateral or bilateral circular ulcers (up to 1 cm in diameter) deep enough to expose the underlying arytenoid cartilages. The cause has not been established; viral, bacterial, and traumatic etiologies have been proposed. These ulcers may be caused by increased frequency and rate of closure of the larynx (excessive swallowing and vocalization) when cattle are exposed to market and feedlot stresses, such as dust, pathogens, and interruption of feeding. Contact ulcers predispose calves to diphtheria and laryngeal papillomas. Ulceration of the mucosa and necrosis of the laryngeal cartilages have also been described in calves, sheep, and horses under the term **laryngeal chondritis.**

Canine Infectious Tracheobronchitis (Kennel Cough)

This highly contagious infection is clinically characterized by an acute onset of coughing notably exacerbated by exercise. The term is nonspecific, much like "common cold" in human beings or "shipping fever" in cattle. The infection occurs commonly as a result of mixing dogs from different origins, such as occurs at commercial kennels, animal shelters, and veterinary clinics.

The etiology of canine infectious tracheobronchitis is complex, and many pathogens and environmental factors have been incriminated. *Bordetella bronchiseptica,* canine adenovirus 2 (CAV-2), and canine parainfluenza virus (CPV) are most commonly implicated. The severity of the disease is increased when more than one agent is involved or extreme environmental conditions (e.g., poor ventilation) add additional stresses. For example, dogs asymptomatically infected with *B. bronchiseptica* are more severely affected by superinfection with CAV-2 than those not carrying the bacterium. Other agents, sometimes isolated but of lesser significance, include CAV-1 (infectious canine hepatitis virus), reovirus type 1, canine herpesvirus, and *Mycoplasma* species.

Between bouts of coughing, most animals appear normal, although some have rhinitis, pharyngitis, tonsillitis, or conjunctivitis; and some with secondary pneumonia become quite ill.

Depending on the agents involved, gross and microscopic lesions are completely absent, or they vary from catarrhal to mucopurulent tracheobronchitis with enlargement of the tonsils and retropharyngeal and tracheobronchial lymph nodes. In dogs with *B. bronchiseptica* infection, the lesions are exudative suppurative rhinitis, tracheobronchitis, and bronchiolitis. In contrast, when lesions are purely viral, microscopic changes are focal necrosis of the tracheobronchial epithelium. Sequelae can include spread either proximally or distally into the respiratory tract, the latter possibly inducing chronic bronchitis and bronchopneumonia.

Parasitic Diseases

Parasitic infections of the pharynx, larynx, and trachea can have dramatic obstructive consequences, but burdens sufficient to cause such effects are not commonly seen.

Besnoitia bennetti

This coccidian, whose life cycle is still unknown, can cause papilloma-like lesions in the larynx, skin, and sclera of horses. Besnoitiosis has been reported from Africa, Central and South America, and Britain. Grossly, nodules up to 2 cm in diameter occur on most surfaces of the larynx. These nodules microscopically consist of thick-walled parasitic cysts overlain by fingerlike projections covered by hyperplastic and sometimes, ulcerated epithelium.

Mammomanogamus laryngeus (Syngamus laryngeus)

This nematode is found in the larynx of cattle in tropical Asia and South America, and cats (gapeworm) in the Caribbean and Southern United States. Occasionally, human beings with a persistent cough or asthma-like symptoms carry the parasite in the larynx or bronchi.

Oslerus (Filaroides) osleri

This parasite of dogs and other canidae forms characteristic protruding nodules into the lumen at the tracheal bifurcation. They are readily seen on endoscopic examination or at necropsy. In severe cases, these nodules can extend 5 cm cranially or caudally from the tracheal bifurcation and even into primary and secondary bronchi. The disease occurs worldwide, and *O. osleri* is considered the most common respiratory nematode of dogs. Clinically, it can be asymptomatic, although it most often causes a chronic cough that can be exacerbated by exercise or excitement. Severe infestations can result in dyspnea, exercise intolerance, cyanosis, emaciation, and even death in young dogs.

The gross lesions are variably sized, up to 1 cm, submucosal nodules that extend up to 1 cm into the tracheal lumen (Fig. 3-13). Microscopically, a mild mononuclear cell reaction is present when parasites are alive, but with the death of the parasite, an intense foreign body reaction develops with neutrophils and giant cells.

Neoplasms of Guttural Pouches, Larynx, and Trachea

Neoplasms of the Guttural Pouches

These occur rarely in horses and are usually squamous cell carcinomas.

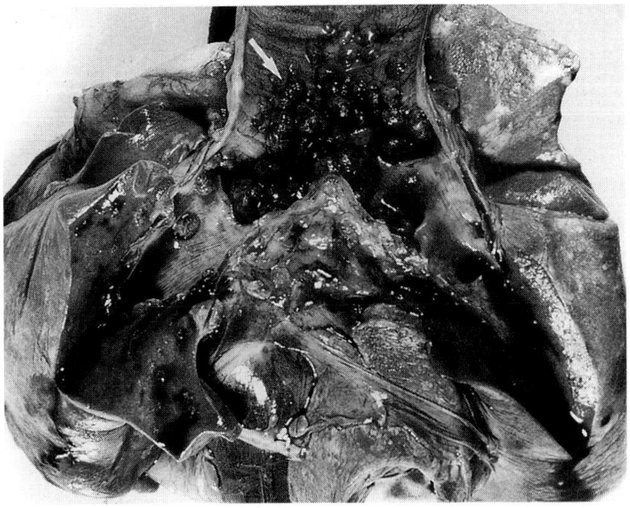

Figure 3-13 Trachea, bronchi, and lungs; dog. Parasitic tracheobronchitis *(Filaroides osleri).* Note the numerous dark parasitic nodules *(arrow)* on the mucosal surface of distal trachea and bronchi. *Courtesy Dr. M.D. McGavin.*

Neoplasms of the Larynx and Trachea

Laryngeal neoplasms are rare in dogs and extremely so in other species, although they have been reported in cats and horses.

When large enough to be obstructive, neoplasms may cause a change or loss of voice, cough, or respiratory distress with cyanosis, collapse, and syncope. Other signs include dysphagia, anorexia, and exercise intolerance. The neoplasm is sometimes visible from the oral cavity and causes swelling of the neck. The prognosis is poor, as most lesions recur after excision.

The most common laryngeal neoplasm in dogs is **squamous cell carcinoma.** Others include **laryngeal oncocytoma, "granular cell tumor," rhabdomyoma, rhabdomyosarcoma, mastocytoma, melanoma, leiomyoma, adenoma, adenocarcinoma, osteosarcoma,** and **chondrosarcoma.**

Tracheal neoplasms are even more uncommon than those of the larynx, but are similarly significant in clinical terms when they do arise. Giant cell tumor has been reported in the horse and adenocarcinoma in the dog. Tracheal cartilages can be the site of chondromas. **Lymphosarcomas** in cats can extend from the mediastinum to involve the trachea.

LUNGS

Species Differences

Each lung is subdivided into various numbers of **pulmonary lobes.** In the past, these were defined by anatomic fissures. However, in current anatomy, lobes are defined by the ramification of the bronchial tree. Following this criterion, the left lung of all domestic species is composed of cranial and caudal lobes, while the right lung, depending on species, is composed of cranial, middle (absent in horse), caudal, and accessory lobes. Each pulmonary lobe is further subdivided by connective tissue into **pulmonary lobules,** which in some species are rather prominent and in others are much less conspicuous. From a practical point of view, identification of the lungs among different species could be achieved by carefully observing the degree of lobation (external fissures) and the degree of lobulation (connective tissue between lobules). Cattle and pigs have well-lobated and well-lobulated lungs; sheep and goats have well-lobated but poorly lobulated lungs; horses have both poorly lobated and poorly lobulated lungs and resemble human lungs; finally, dogs and cats have well-lobated but not well-lobulated lungs. The degree of lobulation determines the degree of air movement between the lobules. In pigs and cattle, movement of air between lobules is practically absent because of the thick connective tissue wall separating individual lobules. This movement of air between lobules and between alveoli (pores of Kohn) constitutes what is referred to as collateral ventilation. This collateral ventilation is poor in cattle and pigs and good in dogs. The functional implications of collateral ventilation are discussed under Pulmonary Emphysema.

The lungs have an interconnecting network of stromal tissue supporting the blood and lymphatic vessels, nerves, bronchioles, and alveoli. For purposes of simplicity, the pulmonary interstitium can be anatomically divided into contiguous compartments: (1) **bronchovascular interstitium,** where main bronchi and pulmonary vessels are situated, (2) **interlobular interstitium** separating pulmonary lobules and supporting small blood and lymph vessels, and (3) **alveolar interstitium** supporting pulmonary capillaries and alveolar epithelial cells (no lymphatic vessels here). Pulmonary changes such as edema and emphysema may affect one or more of these interstitial compartments.

Congenital Anomalies

Congenital anomalies of the lungs are rare in all species but are most commonly reported in cattle. Compatibility with life largely depends on the type of structures involved and the proportion of functional tissue present at birth. **Accessory lungs** are one of the most common anomalies and consist of distinctively lobulated masses of incompletely differentiated pulmonary tissue present in the thorax, abdominal cavity, or subcutaneous tissue virtually anywhere in the trunk. Large accessory lungs can cause dystocia. **Ciliary dyskinesia (immotile cilia syndrome)** is characterized by deficient ciliary movement due to a defect in the microtubules of all ciliated cells and, most importantly, in the ciliated respiratory epithelium and spermatozoa. Ciliary dyskinesia has been reported in dogs with chronic recurrent pneumonia and infertility, often associated with *situs inversus.* **Pulmonary agenesia, pulmonary hypoplasia, abnormal lobulation, congenital emphysema, lung hamartoma,** and **congenital bronchiectasis** are occasionally seen in domestic animals. **Congenital melanosis** is a common incidental finding in pigs and ruminants and is usually seen at slaughter. It is characterized by black spots, often a few centimeters in diameter, in various organs, mainly the lungs, meninges, intima of aorta, and caruncles of the uterus. Melanosis has no clinical significance and the texture of pigmented lungs remains unchanged.

Metabolic Disturbances

Pulmonary Calcification ("Calcinosis")

Calcification of the lungs occurs in some hypercalcemic states, generally associated with hypervitaminosis D or from ingestion of toxic plants such as *Solanum malacoxylon* (Manchester wasting disease) that contain vitamin D analogs. It is also a common sequela to uremia in dogs and to pulmonary necrosis (dystrophic calcification) in most species. Calcified lungs may fail to collapse when the thoracic cavity is opened and have a characteristic "gritty" texture. Microscopic lesions vary from mild calcification of the alveolar basement membranes to heterotopic ossification of lungs. In most cases, pulmonary calcification in itself has little clinical significance, although its cause (e.g., uremia or vitamin D toxicosis) may be very important.

Abnormalities of Inflation

To achieve gaseous exchange, a balanced ratio of air to capillary blood must be present in the lungs (ventilation/perfusion ratio), and the air and capillary blood must be in close proximity across the alveolar membrane. A ventilation-perfusion mismatch occurs if pulmonary tissue is either collapsed (atelectasis) or overinflated (emphysema).

Atelectasis

The term atelectasis means incomplete distension of alveoli and is used to describe lungs that have failed to expand with air at the time of birth (congenital atelectasis) or lungs that have collapsed after inflation has taken place (acquired atelectasis).

During fetal life, lungs are not fully distended, contain no air, and are partially filled with a locally produced fluid known as **fetal lung fluid.** Not surprisingly, lungs of aborted and stillborn fetuses sink when placed in water, whereas those from animals that have breathed float. At the time of birth, fetal lung fluid is rapidly reabsorbed and replaced by inspired air, leading to the normal distension of alveoli. **Congenital atelectasis** occurs in newborns who fail to inflate their lungs after taking their first few breaths of air; it is caused by obstruction of airways, often as result of aspiration of amniotic fluid and meconium (described under Meconium Aspiration Syndrome) (Fig. 3-14).

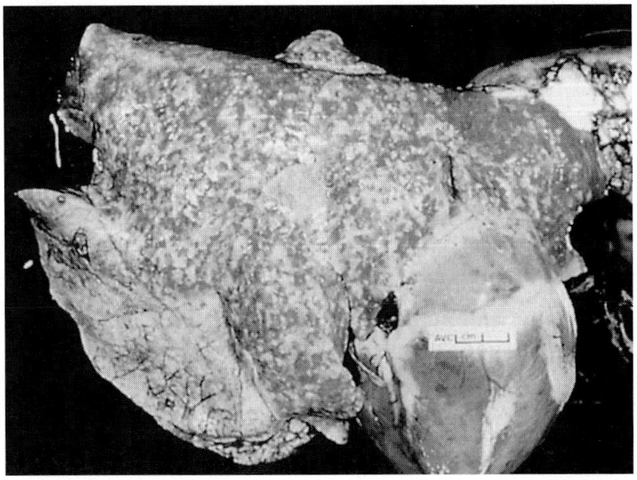

Figure 3-14 Lung; 1-day-old calf. Multifocal neonatal atelectasis. Prominent mosaic pattern of normally inflated *(light)* and atelectatic, uninflated *(dark)* lobules. Atelectasis is due to aspiration of amniotic fluid, meconium, and squamous epithelial cells. All pulmonary lobes are involved. *López et al. Vet Pathol 1992; 29:104-111.*

Congenital atelectasis also develops when alveoli cannot remain distended following initial aeration because of a defect in pulmonary surfactant produced by type II pneumonocytes. This form of congenital atelectasis is referred to in human neonatology as **"acute respiratory distress syndrome"** or as **"hyaline membrane disease"** because of the clinical and microscopic features of the disease. It commonly occurs in babies who are premature or born to diabetic or alcoholic mothers and is occasionally found in animals, particularly in foals and piglets. The pathetic, gasping attempts to breathe have prompted the use of the name "barkers" for affected foals and pigs; foals that survive may have brain damage from cerebral hypoxia and are referred to as "wanderers," owing to their aimless behavior and lack of a normal sense of fear.

Acquired atelectasis occurs in two main forms: compressive and obstructive. The simple physical presence of fluids, masses, or transferred pressures to the pleural space can cause **compressive atelectasis.** Examples include pneumothorax, hydrothorax, hemothorax, chylothorax, empyema, neoplasms (e.g., thymic lymphoma, pulmonary carcinoma), and bloat. Another form of compressive atelectasis occurs when the negative pressure in the thoracic cavity is lost because of pneumothorax. This form is generally massive atelectasis and thus is also referred to as lung collapse.

Obstructive (absorption) atelectasis occurs when an airway is blocked by mucosal edema, exudates, aspirated foreign material, parasites, or neoplasms and the trapped air in the lung is reabsorbed. Unlike the compression type, obstructive atelectasis often has a lobular pattern and is more common in species with poor collateral ventilation such as cattle and sheep. Atelectasis also occurs when large animals are kept recumbent for prolonged periods, such as during anesthesia (hypostatic atelectasis). The factors contributing to hypostatic atelectasis are a combination of blood-air imbalance, shallow breathing, airway obstruction due to drainage failure of mucus and fluid from alveoli and bronchioles, and inadequate surfactant production. Atelectasis can also be a sequela to the prolonged use of respirators in intensive care.

In general, the lungs with atelectasis of any type appear dark blue and collapsed and may be flabby or firm; they are firm if there is concurrent edema or other processes such as can occur in "shock" lungs (see Pulmonary Edema). Distribution and extent vary with the process, being patchy (multifocal) in congenital atelectasis, lobular in the obstructive type, and of various degrees in between in the compressive type. Microscopically, the alveoli are collapsed or slitlike, giving prominence to the interstitial tissue even without any superimposed inflammation.

Pulmonary Emphysema

Pulmonary emphysema, simply referred to as emphysema, is an extremely important primary disease in human beings, whereas in animals it is always a secondary lesion resulting from other types of pulmonary lesions. In human medicine, emphysema is strictly defined as an abnormal permanent enlargement of airspaces distal to the terminal bronchiole, accompanied by destruction of alveolar walls (alveolar emphysema). This definition separates it from simple airspace enlargement or hyperinflation, in which there is no destruction of alveolar walls and which can occur congenitally (Down syndrome) or be acquired with age (aging lung, sometimes misnamed "senile emphysema"). The pathogenesis of emphysema in human beings is still controversial, but current thinking overwhelmingly suggests that destruction of alveolar walls is largely the result of an imbalance between proteases released by phagocytes and antiproteases produced in the lung as a defense mechanism (the protease-antiprotease theory). The destructive process is markedly accelerated by any factor such as cigarette smoking, pollution, or defects in the synthesis of antiproteases in human beings that increases the recruitment of macrophages and leukocytes in the lungs. This theory originated when it was found that human beings with homozygous α_1-antitrypsin deficiency were remarkably susceptible to emphysema and that proteases (elastase) inoculated intratracheally into the lungs of laboratory animals produced lesions similar to those found in the disease. More than 90% of the problem relates to cigarette smoking. Airway obstruction is no longer considered to play a major role in the pathogenesis of emphysema in human beings.

Primary emphysema does not occur in animals, and, thus, no animal disease should be called simply emphysema. In animals, this lesion is always secondary to obstruction of outflow of air or agonal at slaughter. Secondary pulmonary emphysema occurs frequently in animals with bronchopneumonias in which exudate plugging bronchi and bronchioles causes an airflow imbalance where the volume of air entering exceeds the volume leaving the lung.

Depending on the area of the lung affected, emphysema can be classified into alveolar or interstitial. **Alveolar emphysema** occurs in all species, and it is characterized by distension and rupture of the alveolar walls forming variably sized air bubbles in pulmonary parenchyma (Fig. 3-15). **Interstitial emphysema** occurs mainly in cattle, presumably because thick interlobular septa and lack of collateral ventilation in these species does not permit air to move freely into adjacent pulmonary lobules. As a result, accumulated air disrupts and forces its way into connective tissue, causing notable distension of the interlobular septa. It is also suspected that forced respiratory movements predispose to interstitial emphysema when air at high pressure breaks into the loose connective tissue of the interlobular septa (Fig. 3-15). Sometimes these bubbles of trapped air become confluent, forming large (several centimeters in diameter) pockets of air that are referred to as **bullae** (singular: bulla); the lesion is called **bullous emphysema.** This lesion is not a specific type of emphysema and does not indicate a different disease process, but rather is a larger accumulation of air at one focus. It should be noted that mild alveolar emphysema is difficult to judge at necropsy and by light microscopy unless special techniques are used to prevent collapse of the lung when the thorax is opened. These techniques include plugging of the trachea before opening the thorax to prevent collapse of the lungs when the thorax is opened or intratracheal perfusion of fixative (10% neutral-buffered formalin).

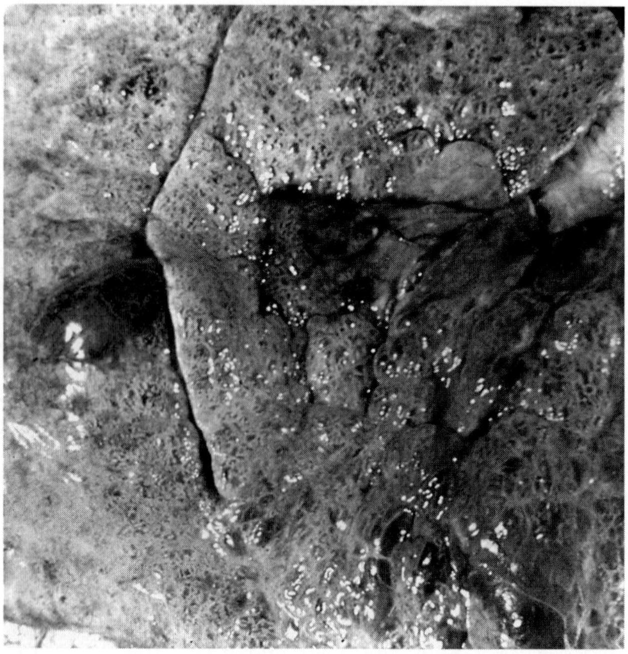

Figure 3-15 Lung; cow. Bovine pulmonary edema and emphysema (fog fever). Emphysema, edema, and interstitial pneumonia involving all pulmonary lobes. Note variably sized air bubbles in pulmonary parenchyma and interlobular septa.

Important diseases that cause secondary pulmonary emphysema in animals include **small airway obstruction** (such as **heaves**) in horses and **pulmonary edema and emphysema (fog fever)** in cattle.

Circulatory Disturbances of the Lungs

Lungs are extremely well vascularized organs with a dual circulation provided by pulmonary and bronchial arteries. Disturbances in pulmonary circulation have a notable effect on gaseous exchange, which may result in life-threatening hypoxemia and acidosis. In addition, circulatory disturbances in the lungs can have an impact on numerous organs due to passive congestion and generalized edema (anasarca).

Hyperemia and Congestion

Hyperemia is an active process that is part of acute inflammation, whereas congestion is the passive process resulting from decreased outflow of venous blood, as occurs in congestive heart failure. In the acute stages of pneumonia, the lungs appear notably red, and, microscopically, blood vessels and capillaries are engorged with blood from hyperemia. Pulmonary congestion is most frequently caused by heart failure, which results in stagnation of blood in pulmonary vessels, leading to edema and egression of erythrocytes into the alveolar spaces. As with any other foreign particle, erythrocytes in alveolar spaces are rapidly phagocytosed (erythrophagocytosis) by pulmonary alveolar macrophages. When extravasation of erythrocytes is severe, large numbers of macrophages with brown cytoplasm may accumulate in the bronchoalveolar spaces. The brown cytoplasm is the result of accumulation of considerable amounts of hemosiderin; these macrophages (siderophages) are generally referred to as "heart failure cells." The lungs of animals with chronic heart failure usually have a patchy red appearance with foci of brown discoloration due to accumulated hemosiderin. In severe and persistent cases of heart failure, the lungs fail to collapse due to edema and pulmonary fibrosis. Terminal pulmonary congestion (acute) is frequently seen in animals euthanized with barbiturates and should not be mistaken for an antemortem lesion.

Pulmonary Hemorrhage

Pulmonary hemorrhages can occur as a result of trauma, coagulopathies, pulmonary thromboembolism due to jugular thrombosis or hepatic abscess that has ruptured into the vena cava (cattle), disseminated intravascular coagulation, vasculitis, or septicemia. There is growing evidence that ultrasonography can produce pulmonary hemorrhage in small domestic mammals. A finding that resembles pulmonary hemorrhage and often leads to an erroneous diagnosis is the aspiration of blood after the carotid arteries and trachea have been cut at the time of slaughter. Grossly, affected lungs have numerous, focal (1 to 10 mm) areas of red discoloration scattered throughout the pulmonary lobes.

Rupture of a major pulmonary vessel with resulting massive hemorrhage occurs occasionally in cattle when a growing abscess in a lung invades and disrupts the wall of a major pulmonary vessel. In most cases, animals die rapidly, often with spectacular hemoptysis, and on postmortem examination, the airways are filled with blood.

"Exercise-induced pulmonary hemorrhage" (EIPH) is a specific form of pulmonary hemorrhage in racehorses following exercise and clinically is characterized by epistaxis. Since only a small percentage of horses with bronchoscopic evidence of hemorrhage have clinical epistaxis, it is likely that EIPH goes undetected in many cases. The pathogenesis is still controversial, but current literature suggests alveolar hypoxia, bronchiolitis, laryngeal paralysis, extremely high pulmonary vascular pressures during exercise, and preexisting pulmonary injury as possible causes. EIPH is seldom fatal; postmortem lesions in affected horses are large areas of dark brown discoloration, largely in the caudal lung lobes. Microscopically, lesions are alveolar hemorrhage, abundant macrophages containing hemosiderin (siderophages), and mild interstitial fibrosis.

Pulmonary Edema

In normal lungs, fluid from the vascular space slowly but continuously passes into the interstitial tissues where it is rapidly drained by the lymph vessels. Recent investigations demonstrated that alveolar fluid clearance across the alveolar epithelium is also a major mechanism of fluid removal from the lung. Edema develops when the rate of fluid transudation from pulmonary vessels into interstitium or alveoli exceeds that of lymph and alveolar removal. **Pulmonary edema** can be classified into hemodynamic or permeability types.

Hemodynamic pulmonary edema develops when there is an elevated rate of fluid transudation due to increased hydrostatic pressure in the vascular compartment or decreased osmotic pressure in the blood. Once the lymph drainage has been overwhelmed, fluid accumulates in the perivascular spaces, causing distension of the bronchovascular bundles and alveolar interstitium, and eventually leaking into the alveolar spaces. Causes of hemodynamic pulmonary edema include congestive heart failure (increased hydrostatic pressure), iatrogenic fluid overload, disorders in which blood osmotic pressure is reduced such as in the hypoalbuminemia seen in some hepatic diseases, nephrotic syndrome, and protein-losing enteropathy. Hemodynamic pulmonary edema also occurs when lymph drainage is impaired and is generally associated with neoplastic invasion of lymph vessels.

Permeability edema occurs when there is excessive opening of endothelial gaps or damage to the air-blood barrier (type I pneumonocytes or to endothelial cells). This type of edema is an integral and early part of the inflammatory response, primarily due to the effect of inflammatory mediators such as leukotrienes, platelet activator factor, cytokines, and vasoactive amines that increase the permeability of pulmonary vessels. In other cases, permeability edema results from direct damage to the endothelium and pneumocytes, allowing plasma fluids to move freely from the vascular space into the alveolar lumen. Since type I pneumonocytes are highly vulnerable to some pneumotropic viruses (influenza, BRSV), toxicants (NO_2, SO_2, H_2S, 3-methylindole), and particularly to free radicals, it is not surprising that alveolar edema commonly accompanies many viral or toxic pulmonary diseases. A permeability edema also occurs when endothelial cells in the lung are injured by bacterial toxins (endotoxemia, sepsis, disseminated intravascular coagulation), anaphylactic shock, milk allergy, paraquat toxicity, and adverse drug reactions.

The concentration of protein in edematous fluid is greater in permeability edema (exudate) than in hemodynamic edema (transudate); this difference has been used clinically in human medicine to differentiate one type of pulmonary edema from another. Microscopically, edematous fluid tends to stain more intensely eosinophilic in lungs with inflammation or damage to the air-blood barrier than the fluid present in hemodynamic edema related to heart failure.

Acute respiratory distress syndrome (ARDS; shock lung) is an important condition in human beings characterized by intravascular aggregation of neutrophils in the lungs, diffuse alveolar damage, permeability edema, and formation of hyaline membranes. The pathogenesis is complex and multifactorial but in general terms can be defined as diffuse alveolar damage that results from lesions occurring in distant organs, from generalized systemic diseases, or from direct injury to the lung. Sepsis, multiple trauma, aspiration of gastric contents, extensive burns, and pancreatitis are some of the disease entities known to trigger ARDS. All these conditions provoke "hyperreactive macrophages" to generate overwhelming amounts of cytokines (mainly TNF-α) and prime neutrophils stationed in the lung capillaries to release enzymes and free radicals, thus causing diffuse endothelial and alveolar damage and fulminating pulmonary edema. A syndrome analogous to ARDS occurs in domestic animals and explains why pulmonary edema is one of the most common lesions found in many animals dying of sepsis, toxemia, and pancreatitis as examples.

Neurogenic pulmonary edema is another distinctive but poorly understood form of lung edema in human beings that follows increased intracranial pressure (i.e.,

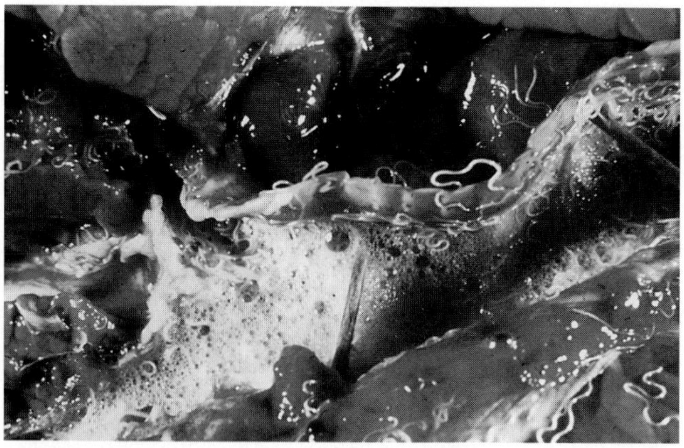

Figure 3-16 Bronchus; calf. Verminous pneumonia *(Dictyocaulus viviparus).* The bronchus contains large amounts of foamy edematous fluid and numerous slender lungworms.

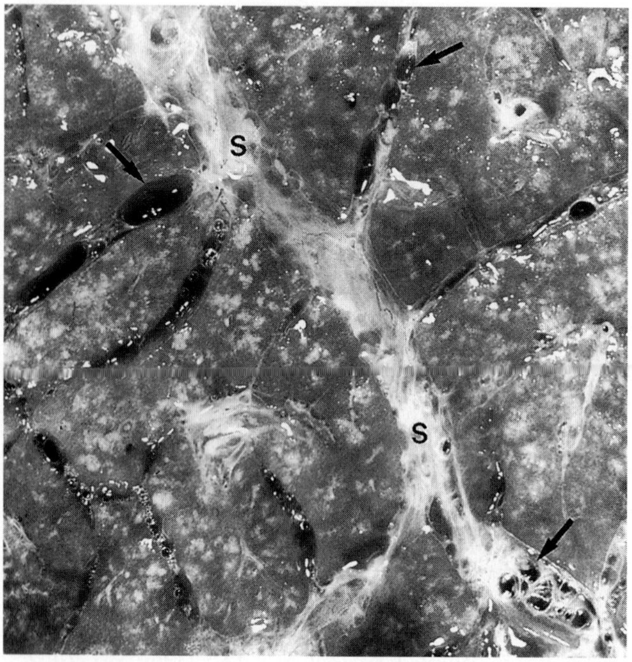

Figure 3-17 Lung, cut surface; calf. Pulmonary edema. The lungs have a "wet appearance," because of the white froth exuding from the bronchioles, and the interlobular septa *(S)* are distended by accumulation of edematous fluid and emphysema *(arrows).* *Courtesy Dr. M.D. McGavin.*

head injury). It involves both hemodynamic and permeability pathways and has sporadically been reported in animals with brain injury or severe seizures.

Grossly, the edematous lungs independent of etiology, are wet and heavy; the color varies depending on the degree of congestion or hemorrhage; and fluid may be present in the pleural cavity. If edema is severe, bronchi and trachea contain considerable amounts of foamy fluid,

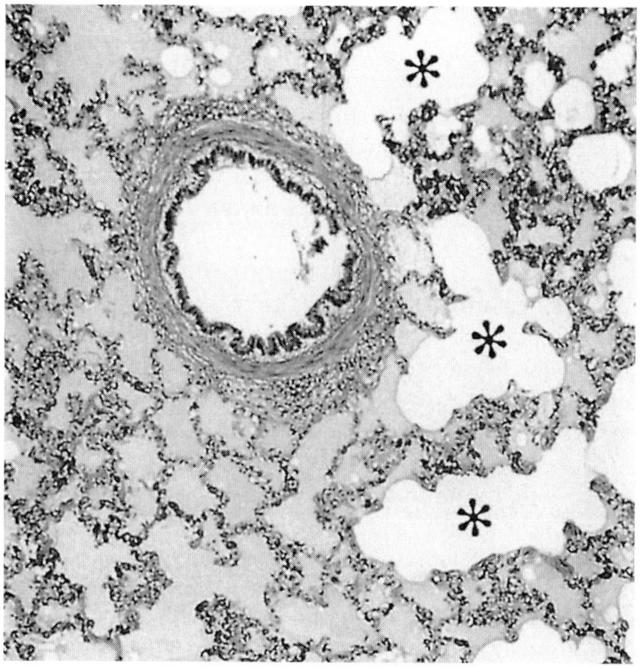

Figure 3-18 Lung; horse. Pulmonary edema in the lungs of a healthy horse euthanatized with intravenous barbiturate. Note darker appearance of alveoli containing edematous fluid as compared with that of the alveoli filled with air *(asterisks).* H & E stain.

which originates from the mixing of edema fluid and air (Fig. 3-16). On cut surfaces, the lung parenchyma oozes fluid like a wet sponge. In cattle and pigs, the lobular pattern becomes rather accentuated due to edematous distensions of interlobular septa (Fig. 3-17). Severe pulmonary edema may be impossible to differentiate from peracute pneumonia; this fact is not surprising since pulmonary edema occurs in the very early stages of inflammation. Careful observation of lungs at the time of necropsy is critical, since diagnosis of pulmonary edema cannot be reliably performed microscopically. This is due in part to the loss of the edema fluid from the lungs during fixation with 10% neutral, buffered formalin and in part to the fact that the fluid itself stains very poorly because of its low protein content (hemodynamic edema). A protein-rich (permeability) edema is easier to visualize microscopically because it is deeply eosinophilic in hematoxylin and eosin (H & E)–stained sections (Fig. 3-18), particularly if a fixative such as Zenker's solution, which precipitates protein, is used.

Pulmonary Embolisms

With its vast capillary bed and position in the circulation, the lungs act as a safety net to catch emboli before they reach the brain and other tissues. However, this positioning is often to its own detriment. The most common emboli found in domestic animals include thromboemboli, septic (bacterial) emboli, fat emboli, and tumor cell emboli.

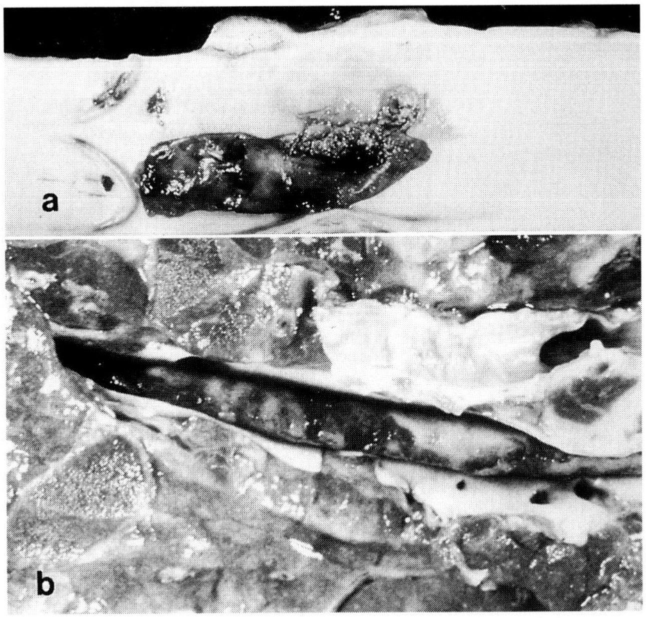

Figure 3-19 Jugular vein and lung, cut surface; cow. Jugular thrombophlebitis and pulmonary thromboembolism. **A,** The jugular vein shows a large thrombus attached to the wall. **B,** The pulmonary artery contains a large, well-organized thrombus. These lesions are the consequence of prolonged catheterization of the jugular vein.

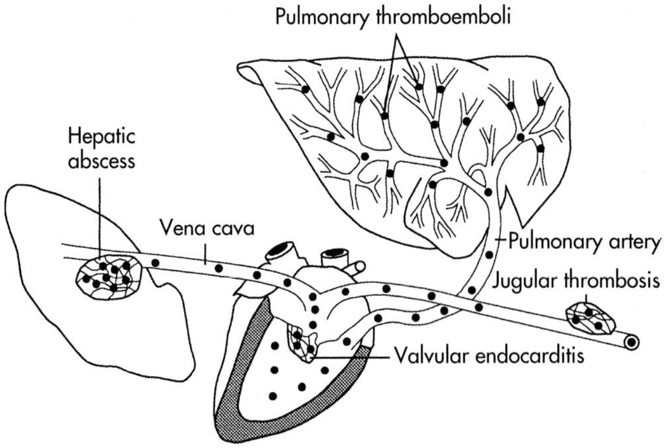

Figure 3-20 Diagram of pulmonary emboli arising from rupture of a hepatic abscess into the caudal vena cava; emboli arising from vegetative valvular endocarditis (tricuspid valve); emboli arising from jugular thrombosis.

Pulmonary **thromboembolism** generally originates from a thrombus present elsewhere in the venous circulation. Fragments released inevitably reach the lungs and become trapped in pulmonary vasculature. Sterile thromboemboli are generally of little clinical or pathologic significance since they can be rapidly degraded and disposed of by the fibrinolytic system. Parasites such as *Dirofilaria immitis* and *Angiostrongylus vasorum,* endocrinopathies such as hyperadrenocortisism and hypothyroidism, glomerulopathies, and hypercoagulable states can be responsible for pulmonary arterial thrombosis and pulmonary thromboembolism in dogs. Pieces of thrombi breaking free from a jugular vein thrombus can cause pulmonary thromboembolism. This outcome is particularly evident in animals undergoing long-term intravenous catheterization (Figs. 3-19 and 3-20).

Septic emboli, pieces of thrombi contaminated with bacteria and broken free from infected mural thrombi in heart and vessels, eventually become entrapped in the pulmonary circulation. These emboli originate most commonly from bacterial endocarditis (right side) and jugular thrombophlebitis in all species, hepatic abscesses that have eroded and discharge their contents into caudal vena cava in cattle, and septic arthritis and omphalitis in farm animals (Fig. 3-20). When present in large numbers, septic emboli may cause unexpected death due to massive pulmonary edema; survivors generally develop arteritis, thrombosis, embolic (suppurative) pneumonia, that may lead to pulmonary abscesses.

Fat emboli can occur after bone fractures but are not as significant a problem in domestic animals as they are in human beings. **Brain emboli** into the pulmonary vasculature reported in severe cases of head injury in human beings has recently been recognized in the bovine lung following pneumatic stunning at slaughter. Although obviously not important as an antemortem pulmonary lesion, brain emboli are intriguing as a potential risk for public health in bovine spongiform encephalopathy (BSE). **Hepatic emboli** occur after severe trauma and hepatic rupture. **Tumor emboli** (e.g., osteosarcoma and hemangiosarcoma in dogs, uterine carcinoma in cattle) can be numerous and striking and the ultimate cause of death in malignant neoplasia. In experimental studies, cytokines released during pulmonary inflammation are chemotactic for tumor cells and promote pulmonary metastasis.

Because of a dual arterial supply to the lung, **pulmonary infarction** is rare and generally asymptomatic. However, pulmonary infarcts can be readily caused when pulmonary thrombosis and embolism are superimposed on an already compromised pulmonary circulation, such as occurs in congestive heart failure. It also occurs in dogs with torsion of a lung lobe. The gross features of

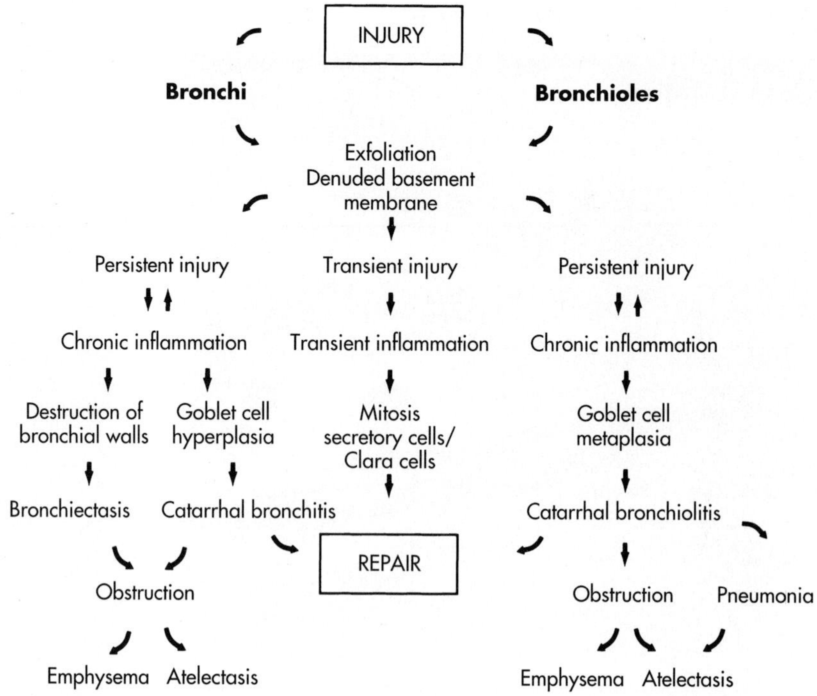

Figure 3-21 Patterns of host response and possible sequelae to bronchial and bronchiolar injury.

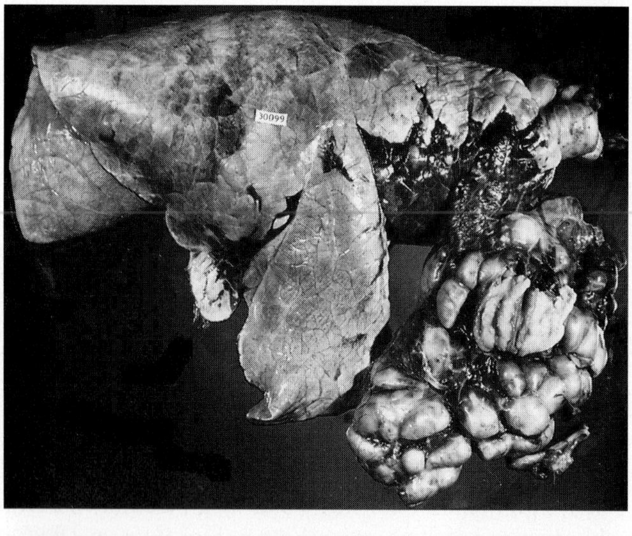

Figure 3-22 Right lung; calf. Chronic suppurative bronchopneumonia with severe bronchiectasis. Note markedly distended (bosselated) cranioventral bronchi. The cut surfaces of affected bronchi are filled with purulent exudate. The surrounding parenchyma is partially atelectatic.

infarcts vary considerably depending on the stage, and they can be red to black, swollen, firm, and cone or wedge shaped. In the acute stage, microscopic lesions are severely hemorrhagic with necrosis. In 1 to 2 days, a border of inflammatory cells develops, and a few days later, a large number of siderophages are present in the infarcted lung. If sterile, pulmonary infarcts heal as fibrotic scars; if septic, an abscess may form.

Patterns of Injury and Host Response in the Lungs

Bronchi

The patterns of necrosis, inflammation, and repair in intrapulmonary bronchi are similar to those previously described for the nasal and tracheal epithelium. In brief, injury to ciliated bronchial epithelium may result in degeneration, detachment, and exfoliation of these cells. Under normal circumstances, this loss is promptly followed by exudative inflammation and repair. Depending on the type of exudate, **bronchitis** can be **fibrinous, catarrhal, purulent, fibrinonecrotic** (diphtheritic), and, sometimes **granulomatous.** When epithelial injury becomes chronic, production of mucus is increased via **goblet cell hyperplasia** (chronic catarrhal inflammation). This form of chronic bronchitis is well illustrated by habitual smokers who continuously need to cough out excessive mucous secretions (sputum). Unfortunately, in some cases excessive mucus cannot be effectively cleared from airways, and this leads to **chronic obstructive bronchitis** (Fig. 3-21). Chronic bronchial irritation can also cause **squamous metaplasia,** in which highly functional but vulnerable ciliated epithelium is replaced by a poorly functional, but more resistant, squamous epithelium. Squamous metaplasia has a calamitous effect on pulmonary clearance as it causes a break in the mucociliary escalator.

Bronchiectasis is one of the most devastating sequela that follows chronic bronchitis. It consists of a pathologic and permanent dilation of a bronchus as a result of the accumulation of exudate in the lumen and partial rupture of bronchial walls. Destruction of walls occurs, in part, when proteolytic enzymes released from phagocytic cells during chronic inflammation degrade and weaken the smooth

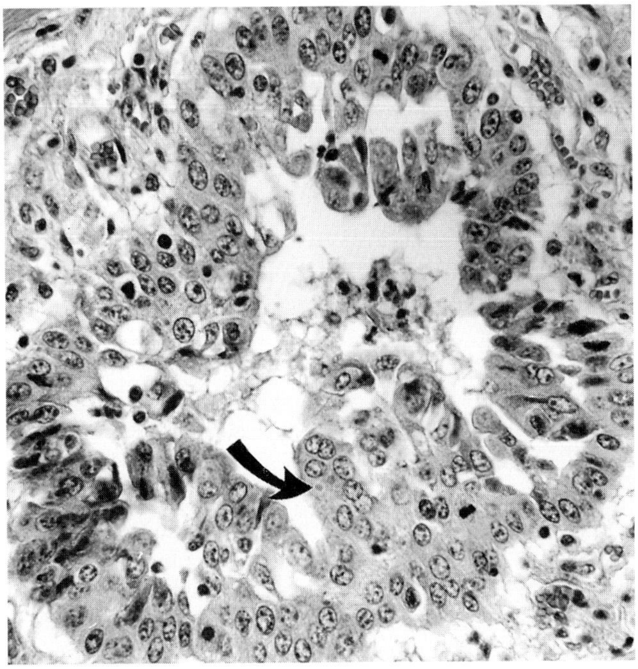

Figure 3-23 Lung; 5-week-old calf. Acute necrotizing bronchiolitis. Bovine respiratory syncytial virus (BSRV). Bronchiolar cells are swollen and sloughed into the lumen. Inclusion bodies surrounded by a clear halo are present in the cytoplasm of bronchilar epithelial cells *(arrow)*. H & E stain.

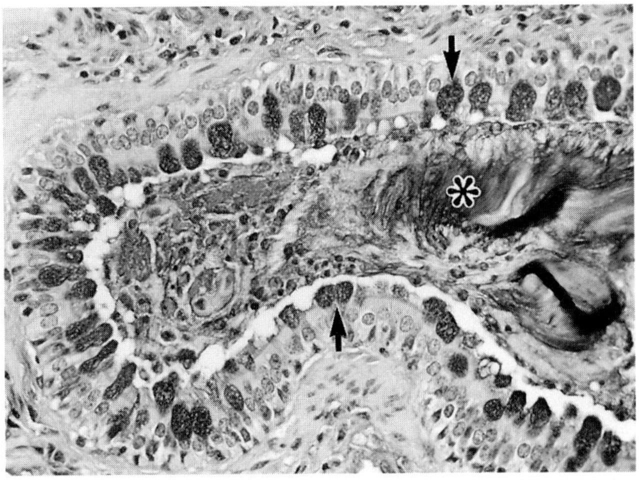

Figure 3-24 Lung; horse. A 3-year history of recurrent dyspnea and terminal pulmonary emphysema. Chronic obstructive pulmonary disease (COPD; heaves). Numerous goblet cells *(arrows)* in the bronchiolar epithelium (goblet cell metaplasia) are discharging mucus (*) into the lumen, causing complete obstruction of the bronchiole. PAS–Alcian blue stain.

muscle and cartilage that help to maintain normal bronchial diameter (Fig. 3-21). Bronchiectasis may be **saccular** when destruction affects only a small localized portion of the bronchial wall or **cylindrical** when destruction involves a large segment of a bronchus. Grossly, bronchiectasis is manifested by prominent lumps in the lungs (bosselated appearance) resulting from distension of bronchi and concurrent obstructive atelectasis of surrounding parenchyma. The cut surfaces of dilated bronchi are filled with purulent exudate; for this reason, bronchiectasis is often mistaken for pulmonary abscesses (Fig. 3-22). Careful inspection, usually requiring microscopic examination, will confirm that bronchiectatic exudate is contained and surrounded by remnants of a bronchial wall and not by a pyogenic membrane (connective tissue) as it is in the case of a pulmonary abscess.

Bronchioles

The epithelial lining of the bronchiolar region (transitional zone) is exquisitely susceptible to injury, particularly to that caused by some respiratory viruses (PI-3, adenovirus, BRSV) (Fig. 3-23), oxidant gases (NO_2, SO_2, O_3), and toxic substances (3-methylindole). The precise explanation as to why bronchiolar epithelium is so prone to injury is still not clear, but it is presumably due in part to (1) its high vulnerability to oxidants and free radicals; (2) the presence of Clara cells rich in mixed-function oxidases, which locally generate toxic metabolites; and (3) the tendency for pulmonary alveolar macrophages and leukocytes to accumulate in this region of the lungs.

Once injury becomes irreversible, bronchiolar ciliated cells degenerate and exfoliate into the bronchiolar lumen, leaving a denuded basement membrane. Repair in the bronchiolar region is similar to, but less effective than that in the tracheal or nasal mucosae. Under normal circumstances, recruited phagocytic cells remove exudate and cell debris from the lumina of affected bronchioles, thus preparing the basement membrane to be repopulated with new, undifferentiated cells originating from a rapidly dividing pool of Clara cells. After several days, these proliferating cells fully differentiate into normal bronchiolar ciliated cells (Fig. 3-21).

In severe injury, exudate cannot be removed from the basement membrane of bronchioles. The exudate becomes infiltrated by fibroblasts, which form small masses of fibrovascular tissue and develop into well-organized, microscopic polyps inside the bronchiolar lumen. Their external surface eventually becomes covered by ciliated cells. This lesion is referred to as **bronchiolitis obliterans.**

On the other hand, if bronchiolar injury is mild but persistent, goblet cells normally absent from bronchioles proliferate from basal cells, resulting in **goblet cell metaplasia** and causing an alteration in the physicochemical properties of bronchiolar secretions (Fig. 3-24). The normally serous bronchiolar fluid released by Clara cells becomes a tenacious material when mucus produced by goblet cells is added. As a result of increased viscoelasticity of the mucus, bronchiolar secretions cannot be removed effectively by ciliary action, leading to plugging and obstruction of distal airways. Under such conditions, often grouped as **chronic obstructive pulmonary disease,** cough is required to clear mucus from obstructed bronchioles. Further sequelae to bronchiolar obstruction depending on the extent of the obstruction are pulmonary emphysema and atelectasis. These two inflation abnormalities are characteristically present in chronic obstructive pulmonary disease, such as "heaves" in horses.

Chronic obstructive pulmonary disease (COPD) of horses (chronic bronchiolitis-emphysema complex, heaves, chronic small airway disease, alveolar emphysema, "broken wind") is a common asthmalike, clinical syndrome of horses and ponies, characterized by recurrent respiratory distress, chronic cough, and poor athletic performance. The pathogenesis is still obscure, but genetic predisposition and airways exceptionally sensitive to environmental allergens (hyperreactive airways disease) have been postulated as the basic underlying mechanisms. What makes small airways hyperreactive to allergens is still a matter of controversy. Epidemiologic and experimental studies suggest that it could be the result of preceding bronchiolar damage caused by viral infections, ingestion of pneumotoxicants (3-methylindole), or prolonged exposure to environmental allergens (molds). Most recently, it has been postulated that sustained inhalation of dust particles, whether antigenic or not, up-regulates the production of cytokines (interleukin 8 [IL-8] and monokine-inducible protein [MIP-2]) by alveolar macrophages attracting neutrophils into the bronchioloalveolar region and promoting leukocyte-induced bronchiolar injury.

Grossly, lungs are unremarkable, except for extreme cases in which alveolar emphysema may be present. Microscopically, the lesions include goblet cell metaplasia in bronchioles, plugging of bronchioles with mucus mixed with a few eosinophils (Fig. 3-24), peribronchiolar infiltration with lymphocytes, plasma cells and variable numbers of eosinophils, and hypertrophy of smooth muscle in bronchi and bronchioles. In severe cases, accumulation of mucus leads to the complete obstruction of bronchioles and alveoli, and resultant alveolar emphysema.

"Airway hyperresponsiveness" (hyperreactive airway disease) is another sequela to bronchiolar injury. It develops in human beings and animals (experimentally) following a transient and often innocuous viral infection of the lower respiratory tract or from exposure to certain allergens. Airway hyperresponsiveness is characterized by an exaggerated bronchoconstriction following exposure to mild stimuli such as cold air or after a challenge with aerosols of histamine or methacholine. Hyperreactive animals typically have an increased number of mast cells, eosinophils, and T lymphocytes in the airway mucosa. Whether airway hyperreactivity is specifically associated with postviral bronchiolitis or is a nonspecific sequela to some types of bronchiolar injury remains to be elucidated.

Feline Asthma (Feline Asthma Syndrome; Feline Allergic Bronchitis). Feline asthma, also known as feline allergic bronchitis, is a clinical syndrome in cats of any age characterized by recurrent episodes of bronchoconstriction, cough, or dyspnea. The pathogenesis is not well understood but is presumed to originate, as in human asthma, in a type I hypersensitivity (IgE–mast cell reaction) to inhaled allergens. Dust, cigarette smoke, plant and household materials, and parasitic proteins have been incriminated as possible allergens. This self-limited allergic disease responds well to steroid therapy; thus it is rarely implicated as a primary cause of death except when suppressed defense mechanisms result in secondary bacterial pneumonia. Bronchial biopsies from affected cats at the early stages reveal mild to moderate inflammation characterized by mucosal edema and infiltration of leukocytes, particularly eosinophils. Increased number of circulating eosinophil leukocytes (blood eosinophilia) is present in some, but not all cats with feline asthma. In the most advanced cases, chronic bronchoconstriction and excess mucus production may result in smooth muscle hyperplasia and obstruction of the bronchi and bronchioles. A syndrome known as **canine asthma** has been reported in dogs but is not as well characterized as the feline counterpart.

Alveoli

Due to their extremely delicate structure, alveoli are quite vulnerable to injury once defense mechanisms have been overwhelmed (Fig. 3-3). The alveolus has a thin, three-layered wall composed of **vascular endothelium, alveolar interstitium,** and **alveolar epithelium.** These three layers of cells constitute what is customarily referred to as the **air-blood barrier.** The epithelial side of the alveolus is primarily lined by rather thin **type I pneumonocytes,** which are arranged as a very delicate continuous membrane extending along the alveolar surface (see Fig. 3-4). Type I pneumonocytes are particularly susceptible to noxious agents that reach the alveolar region. Injury to type I pneumonocytes causes swelling and vacuolation of these cells. When cellular damage has become irreversible, type I cells detach, resulting in denudation of the basement membrane and increased alveolar permeability. Alveolar repair is possible as long as the basement membrane remains intact and lesions are not complicated by further injury or infection. Within 3 days, cuboidal **type II (granular) pneumonocytes,** which are the precursor cell and more resistant to injury, undergo mitosis and provide a large pool of new undifferentiated cells. These new cells repave the denuded alveolar basement membrane and finally differentiate in type I pneumonocytes. When alveolar injury is diffuse, proliferation of type II pneumonocytes becomes so spectacular that the microscopic appearance of the alveolus resembles that of a gland or fetal lung; the lesion has been termed **epithelialization** or **fetalization.** In uncomplicated cases, type II pneumonocytes eventually differentiate into type I pneumonocytes, thus completing the last stage of alveolar repair.

Type I pneumonocytes are one of the three structural components of the air-blood barrier (endothelium–basement membrane–pneumonocyte), so when these epithelial cells are damaged, there is an increase in alveolar permeability and transient leakage of plasma fluid, proteins, and fibrin into the alveolar lumen. Under normal circumstances, these fluids and necrotic pneumonocytes (type 1) are rapidly cleared from the alveolus by alveolar reabsorption and by pulmonary alveolar macrophages.

On a minute-to-minute basis, the pulmonary defense mechanisms deal effectively with noxious stimuli and mild tissue injury without the need for an inflammatory response. However, if normal defense mechanisms are ineffective or insufficient (overwhelmed), the inflammatory process is rapidly turned on as a second line of defense.

General Aspects of Lung Inflammation

In the past two decades, an information explosion has increased the overall understanding of pulmonary inflammation with so many pro- and anti-inflammatory mediators described to date that it would be impossible to review them all here.

Pulmonary inflammation is a highly regulated process that involves a complex interaction between cells imported from the blood (neutrophils, eosinophils, mast cells, lymphocytes) and pulmonary cells (pneumonocytes type I and II, endothelial, Clara, and stromal interstitial cells). Blood-borne leukocytes, platelets, and plasma proteins are brought into the areas of inflammation by an elaborate network of chemical signals emitted by pulmonary cells and resident leukocytes. Long-distance communication between pulmonary cells and blood cells is largely done by soluble cytokines; once in the lung, imported leukocytes communicate with pulmonary and vascular cells through adhesion and other inflammatory molecules. The best-known inflammatory mediators are the complement system (C3a; C3b; C5a), coagulation factors (factors V, VII), arachidonic acid metabolites (leukotriens and prostaglandins), cytokines (interleukins, monokines, chemokines), adhesion molecules, enzymes and enzyme inhibitors (elastase, antitrypsin), oxygen metabolites ($O_2^{\bullet}$, $OH^{\bullet}$, H_2O_2), antioxidants (glutathione), and nitric oxide (Table 3-4). Acting in concert these and many other molecules

Table 3-4 Main Chemical Mediators Involved in Pulmonary Inflammation

Name	Source	Function in the Lung
Prostaglandins and leukotrienes	Cell membranes	Increase permeability, platelet aggregation, vasoconstriction or vasodilation, lung edema
L-Selectin	Neutrophils, monocytes	Leukocyte attachment and migration, homing to areas of pulmonary inflammation
P-, E-Selectins; ICAM-1, ELAM-1	Venules and capillary endothelium	Leukocyte attachment and migration to areas of pulmonary inflammation
Interleukin 1 (IL-1)	Alveolar Macrophages	Endothelial-leukocyte adherence, leukocyte chemotaxis
Interleukin 6 (IL-6)	Macrophages	Lymphocyte and fibroblast activation in the lung; down-regulates TNF and reduces inflammation
Interleukin 8 (IL-8)	Macrophages, fibroblasts	Leukocyte and lymphocyte chemotaxis
Interleukin 10 (IL-10)	Macrophages, alveolar cells	Decreases cytokine production in pulmonary alveolar macrophages
Tumor necrosis factor (TNF-α)	Alveolar macrophages	Endothelial-leukocyte attachment, vascular permeability, lung edema; fever and acute-phase proteins
Eotaxin and IL-5	Lymphocytes	Eosinophil chemotaxis
Epithelial secretory proteins	Pneumonocytes type I and II, Clara Cells	Modulation of lung inflammation; regulation of fibroblasts-fibrosis and NO
Surfactant A, B (collectins)	Pneumonocyte type II	Chemotaxis, phagocytosis, immunomodulation, regulation of nitric oxide
Nitric oxide (NO)	Pneumonocytes, macrophages, endothelium	Decreases cytokine production in pulmonary alveolar macrophages

ICAM, Intercellular adhesion molecule; *ELAM*, endothelial adhesion molecule.

send positive or negative signals to initiate, maintain, and hopefully resolve the inflammatory process without causing injury to the lung.

The pulmonary macrophages (alveolar, intravascular, and interstitial), furnished with an immense biological armamentarium, are the single most important effector cell and source of cytokines for all stages of pulmonary inflammation. These all-purpose phagocytic cells modulate the recruitment and trafficking of blood-borne leukocytes in the lung through the secretion of chemokines (Table 3-4).

Before reviewing how inflammatory cells are recruited in the lungs, three significant features in pulmonary injury must be remembered. (1) Leukocytes can exit the vascular system through the alveolar capillaries, unlike other tissues, where postcapillary venules are the sites of leukocytic diapedesis (extravasation). (2) The intact lung contains within alveolar capillaries a large pool of resident leukocytes (marginal pool). (3) Additional neutrophils are sequestered within alveolar capillaries within minutes of local or systemic inflammatory response. These three pulmonary idiosyncrasies, along with the enormous length of the capillary network in the lung, explain why recruitment of leukocytes into alveolar spaces develops so rapidly. Experimental studies with aerosols of endotoxin or gram-negative bacteria have shown that within minutes of exposure, there is a significant increase in capillary leukocytes, and by 4 hours the entire alveolar lumen is filled with cellular exudates. Not surprisingly, the BAL fluid collected from patients with acute pneumonia contains large amounts of TNF-α, IL-1, and IL-8 as examples. Also, the capillary endothelium of patients with acute pneumonia has increased "expression" of adhesion molecules, which facilitate the migration of leukocytes from capillaries into the alveolar interstitium and lumen. In allergic pulmonary diseases, eotaxin and IL-5 are primarily responsible for recruitment and trafficking of eosinophils in the lung (Table 3-4).

Movement of plasma proteins into the pulmonary interstitium and alveolar lumen is a common but poorly understood phenomena in pulmonary inflammation. In addition to direct physical damage to the air-blood barrier (endothelium and type I pneumonocytes), leakage of fibrinogen and plasma proteins is promoted by cytokines that also enhance and reduce the procoagulant and fibrinolytic activities, respectively. Excessive exudation of fibrin in the lung is particularly common in ruminants and pigs. In some cases, plasma proteins leaked into the alveoli mix with pulmonary surfactant forming microscopic eosinophilic bands (membranes) along the lining of alveolar septa. These membranes, known as **"hyaline membranes"** are found in specific types of pulmonary diseases, particularly in cattle with acute interstitial pneumonias such as **bovine pulmonary edema and emphysema and extrinsic allergic alveolitis.**

In the last few years, nitric oxide has been identified as a major regulatory molecule of inflammation in a variety of tissues including the lung. Locally produced by macrophages, pulmonary endothelium and pneumonocytes, nitric oxide regulates the vascular and bronchial tone, modulates the production of cytokines, and the recruitment and trafficking of neutrophils in the lung. Recent investigations suggest that pulmonary surfactant up-regulates the production of nitric oxide in the lung, supporting the current view that pneumonocytes are also pivotal in amplifying and down-regulating the inflammatory and immune responses in the lung (Table 3-4).

As the inflammatory process becomes chronic, the cell types making up the cellular infiltrates in the lung change from mainly neutrophils to largely mononuclear cells. This shift in cellular composition is accompanied by an increase in specific cytokines such as IL-4, interferon gamma (IFN-γ), and interferon-inducible protein (IP-10), which are chemotactic for lymphocytes and macrophages. Under appropriate conditions, these cytokines activate T lymphocytes, regulate granulomatous inflammation, and induce the formation of multinucleated giant cells.

Inflammatory mediators locally released from inflamed lungs also have a biological effect in other tissues. For instance, pulmonary hypertension and heart right failure **(cor pulmonale)** often follows chronic alveolar inflammation, not only as a result of increased blood pressure, but from the effect of inflammatory mediators on the contractibility of smooth muscle of the pulmonary and systemic vasculature. Cytokines, particularly TNF-α, which are released during inflammation are associated, both as cause and effect, with the **systemic inflammatory response syndrome** (SIRS), **sepsis, severe sepsis** with **multiple organ dysfunction,** and **septic shock** (cardiopulmonary collapse).

As any other sentinel system where many biological promoters and inhibitors are involved (coagulation, the complement and immune systems), the inflammatory cascade could go into an "out-of-control" state, causing severe damage to the lungs. Adult respiratory distress syndrome, extrinsic allergic alveolitis, pulmonary fibrosis, and asthma are archetypical diseases that ensue from an uncontrolled production and release of cytokines.

As long as alveolar injury is transient and there is no interference with the normal host response, the entire process of injury, degeneration, necrosis, inflammation, and repair can occur in less than 1 week. On the other hand, when alveolar injury becomes persistent or when the capacity of the host for repair is impaired, lesions can progress to an irreversible stage where restoration of alveolar structure is no longer possible. In diseases such as extrinsic allergic alveolitis, the constant release of proteolytic enzymes and free radicals by phagocytic cells perpetuates alveolar damage in a vicious circle. In other cases, such as in paraquat toxicity, the magnitude of alveolar injury can be so severe that type II pneumonocytes, basement membranes, and alveolar interstitium are so disrupted that the capacity for lung repair is lost. Fibronectins released from macrophages and other mononuclear cells at the site of chronic inflammation regulate the recruitment, attachment, and proliferation of fibroblasts. In turn, these cells synthesize and release considerable amounts of extracellular matrix (collagen, elastic fibers, proteoglycans), eventually leading to fibrosis and total obliteration of normal alveolar architecture. In summary, in diseases in which there is chronic and irreversible alveolar damage, lesions invariably progress to a stage of terminal alveolar fibrosis.

Classification of Pneumonias

Few subjects in veterinary pathology have caused so much debate as the classification of pneumonias. Historically, pneumonias in animals have been classified or named based on (1) **presumed etiology,** with names such as viral pneumonia, pasteurella pneumonia, distemper pneumonia, verminous pneumonia, chemical pneumonia, and hypersensitivity pneumonitis; (2) **type of exudation,** with names such as suppurative pneumonia, fibrinous pneumonia, and pyogranulomatous pneumonia; (3) **morphologic features,** with names such as gangrenous pneumonia, proliferative pneumonia, and embolic pneumonia; (4) **distribution of lesions,** with names such as focal pneumonia, cranioventral pneumonia, diffuse pneumonia, and lobar pneumonia; (5) **epidemiologic attributes,** with names such as enzootic pneumonia, contagious bovine pleuropneumonia, and shipping fever pneumonia; (6) **geographic regions,** with names such as Montana progressive pneumonia; and finally, (7) **miscellaneous attributes,** with names such as atypical pneumonia, cuffing pneumonia, progressive pneumonia, aspiration pneumonia, pneumonitis, farmer's lung, and extrinsic allergic alveolitis. Until a universal and systematic nomenclature for animal pneumonias are established, veterinarians should be acquainted with this heterogenous list of names and should be well aware that one disease may be known by different names. In pigs, for instance, enzootic pneumonia, virus pneumonia, and mycoplasma pneumonia all refer to the same disease caused by *Mycoplasma hyopneumoniae.*

The word pneumonitis has been used by some as a synonym for pneumonia; however, others have restricted this term to chronic proliferative inflammation generally involving the alveolar interstitium and with little or no evidence of exudate. In this chapter, the word pneumonia is used for any inflammatory lesion in the lungs, regardless of whether it is exudative or proliferative, alveolar, or interstitial.

Pneumonias in domestic animals can be classified into four morphologically distinct types: **bronchopneumonia, interstitial pneumonia, embolic pneumonia,** and **granulomatous pneumonia.** By using this classification, it is possible to predict with some degree of certainty the likely etiology (virus, bacteria, fungi, parasites), routes of entry (aerogenous *versus* hematogenous), and possible sequelae to which each of these types of pneumonia may progress if the animal were to survive. However, overlapping of these four types of pneumonias is possible, and, sometimes, two morphologic types may be present in the same lung.

The criteria used to classify pneumonias into bronchopneumonia, interstitial pneumonia, embolic pneumonia, and granulomatous pneumonia are based on morphologic changes, including distribution, texture, color, and appearance of the affected lungs (Table 3-5). According to **distribution** of the inflammatory lesions in the lungs, pneumonias can be **cranioventral,** as in most bronchopneumonias; **focal,** as in embolic pneumonias; **diffuse,** as in interstitial pneumonias; or **locally extensive,** as in granulomatous pneumonias. **Texture** of pneumonic lungs can be **firmer** or **harder** (bronchopneumonias), more **elastic** (rubbery) than normal lungs (interstitial pneumonias), or have a nodular feeling (granulomatous pneumonias). Describing in words the palpable difference between the texture of a normal lung compared with the firm or hard texture of a consolidated lung can be a difficult undertaking. An analogy illustrating this difference based on touching the parts of the face with the tip of your finger has been advocated by some pathologists. The texture of a normal lung is comparable to the texture of the center of the cheek. Firm consolidation is comparable to the texture of the tip of the nose, and the hard consolidation is comparable to the texture of the forehead.

Changes in the **appearance** of pneumonic lungs include abnormal color, presence of nodules or exudate, fibrinous or fibrous adhesions, and presence of rib imprints on serosal surfaces. On cut surfaces, pneumonic lungs may have exudate, hemorrhage, edema, necrosis, abscesses, bronchiectasis, granulomas or pyogranulomas, and fibrosis.

Palpation and careful observation of the lungs are essential in the diagnosis of pneumonia. (For details, see the section on postmortem examination of the respiratory tract.)

Bronchopneumonia

Bronchopneumonia is undoubtedly the most common type of pneumonia seen in domestic animals and is, with few exceptions, characterized by cranioventral consolidation of the lungs. The reason why bronchopneumonias in animals are almost always restricted to the cranioventral portions of the lungs is not well understood. Possible factors contributing to this topographic selectivity within the lungs include (1) shortness and abrupt branching of airways; (2) greater deposition of infectious organisms; (3) inadequate defense mechanisms; (4) reduced vascular perfusion; (5) gravitational sedimentation of the exudate; and (6) regional differences in ventilation.

Table 3-5 Different Types of Pneumonias in Domestic Animals

Type of Pneumonia	Port of Entry (e.g., Pathogens)	Distribution of Lesions	Texture of Lung	Grossly Visible Exudate	Disease Example	Common Pulmonary Sequelae
Bronchopneumonia						
Suppurative (lobular)	Aerogenous (bacteria and mycoplasmas)	Cranioventral consolidation	Firm	Purulent exudate in bronchi	Enzootic pneumonia	Cranioventral abscesses, adhesions bronchiectasis,
Fibrinous (lobar)	Aerogenous (bacteria and mycoplasmas)	Cranioventral consolidation*	Hard	Fibrin in lung and pleura	Pneumonic pasteurellosis	BALT hyperplasia, "sequestra," pleural adhesions, abscesses
Interstitial pneumonia	Aerogenous or hematogenous (virus, toxin, allergen, sepsis)	Diffuse	Elastic with rib imprints	Not visible, trapped in alveolar septa	Influenza, extrinsic allergic alveolitis, PRRS, ARDS	Edema, emphysema, type II alveolar hyperplasia, alveolar fibrosis
Granulomatous pneumonia	Aerogenous or hematogenous (*Mycobacteria*, systemic mycoses)	Multifocal	Nodular	Pyogranulomatous, caseous necrosis, calcified nodules	Tuberculosis, blastomycosis, cryptococcosis	Dissemination of infection to lymph nodes and distant organs
Embolic pneumonia	Hematogenous (septic emboli)	Multifocal	Nodular	Purulent foci surrounded by hyperemia	Vegetative Endocarditis, ruptured liver abscess	Abscesses randomly distributed in all pulmonary lobes

*Porcine pleuropneumonia is an exception because it often involves the caudal lobes.
Porcine reproductive and respiratory syndrome (PRRS); adult respiratory distress syndrome (ARDS).

Bronchopneumonias are generally caused by bacteria and mycoplasmas or by bronchoaspiration of feed or gastric contents. As a rule, the bacterial pathogens causing bronchopneumonias arrive in the lungs via inspired air (aerogenous), either from infected aerosols or from the nasal flora. Before establishing infection, pathogens must overwhelm or evade the pulmonary defense mechanism. The initial injury in bronchopneumonias is centered on the mucosa of bronchioles and alveoli; from there, the inflammatory process can spread downward to distal portions of the alveoli and upward to the bronchi. Typically for bronchopneumonias, the inflammatory exudate collects in the bronchial, bronchiolar, and alveolar lumina leaving the alveolar interstitium reasonably unchanged. Through the pores of Kohn, the lesions and exudates can spread centripetally to adjacent alveoli until part or all of the alveoli in an individual lobule are involved. If the inflammatory process cannot control the inciting cause of injury, the lesions spread rapidly from lobule to lobule through alveolar pores and destroyed alveolar walls, until an entire lobe or large portion of a lung is involved.

At the early stages of bronchopneumonia, the pulmonary vessels are engorged with blood (active hyperemia) and the bronchi, bronchioles, and alveoli contain some fluid (permeability edema). In cases where pulmonary injury is mild to moderate, cytokines cause rapid recruitment of neutrophils and alveolar macrophages into bronchioles and alveoli. When pulmonary injury is much more severe, proinflammatory mediators induce more pronounced vascular changes by further opening endothelial gaps, thus, increasing vascular permeability resulting in fibrinous inflammation or sometimes hemorrhage. Alterations in permeability can be further exacerbated by structural damage to pulmonary capillaries and vessels directly caused by microbial toxins. The final result of these functional and structural changes is that blood vessels become markedly permeable and allow substantial leakage of plasma fluid and proteins (fibrinogen) into the alveoli. Filling of alveoli, bronchioles, and small bronchi with inflammatory exudate progressively obliterates airspaces, and as a consequence of this process, portions of severely affected (consolidated) lungs sink to the bottom of the container when placed in fixative. The replacement of air by exudate also changes the texture of the lungs, and depending on the severity of bronchopneumonia, the texture varies from firmer to harder than normal.

The term "consolidation" is used when the texture of pneumonic lung becomes firmer or harder than normal as a result of loss of airspaces due to exudation and atelectasis. (For details, see the discussion of lung texture in classification of pneumonias.) Inflammatory consolidation of lungs has been referred to in the past as "hepatization," because the affected lung had the appearance and texture of liver. The process was referred to as "red hepatization" in acute cases in which there was marked active hyperemia with little exudation of neutrophils; conversely, the process was referred to as "gray hepatization" in those chronic cases in which hyperemia was no longer present. This terminology, although used and applicable to human pneumonias, is rarely used in veterinary medicine primarily because the evolution of pneumonic processes in animals does not necessarily follow the red-to-gray hepatization pattern.

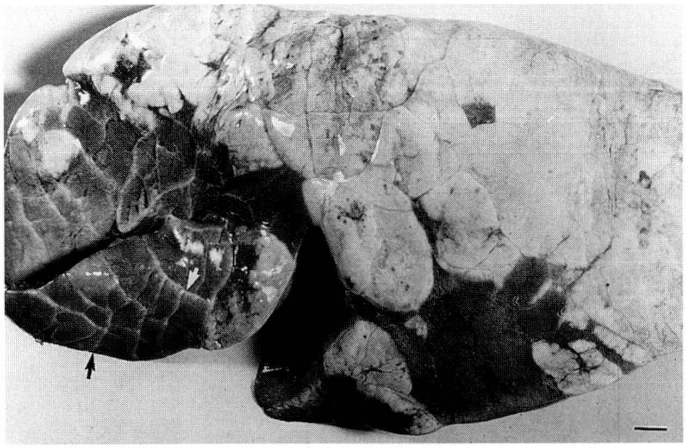

Figure 3-25 Left lung; pig. Suppurative bronchopneumonia. Porcine enzootic pneumonia. Cranioventral consolidation of the lung involves approximately 40% of pulmonary parenchyma. The lobular pattern is accentuated by widening of the interlobular septa *(arrows)*. Bar = 1 cm. *Courtesy Dr. M.D. McGavin.*

Bronchopneumonias can be arbitrarily subdivided into **suppurative bronchopneumonia** if the exudate is predominantly composed of neutrophils and **fibrinous bronchopneumonia** if fibrin is the predominant component of the exudate (see Table 3-5). It is important to note that some pathologists use the term "fibrinous pneumonia" or "lobar pneumonia" as a synonym for fibrinous bronchopneumonia, and "bronchopneumonia" or "lobular pneumonia" as a synonym for suppurative bronchopneumonia. Currently, the term "bronchopneumonia" is widely used for both suppurative and fibrinous consolidation of the lungs, since both forms of inflammation have essentially the same pathogenesis. It must be emphasized that it is the severity and not the type of pulmonary injury that largely determines whether bronchopneumonia becomes suppurative or fibrinous. In some instances, however, it is difficult to discriminate between suppurative and fibrinous bronchopneumonia since both types can coexist (fibrinosuppurative bronchopneumonia) and one type can progress to the other.

Suppurative bronchopneumonia is characterized by cranioventral consolidation of lungs (Fig. 3-25), with typical presence of purulent or mucopurulent exudate in the airways. This exudate can be best demonstrated by

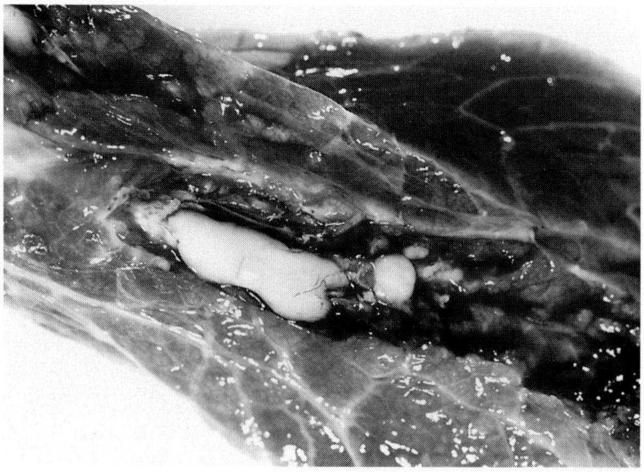

Figure 3-26 Intrapulmonary bronchus; calf. Suppurative bronchopneumonia. Abundant purulent exudate appears in the bronchus when the lung is compressed.

expressing intrapulmonary bronchi, thus forcing exudates out of the bronchi (Fig. 3-26). The inflammatory process in suppurative bronchopneumonia is generally confined to individual lobules, and, as a result of this distribution, the lobular pattern of the lung becomes markedly emphasized. This pattern is particularly obvious in cattle and pigs, since these species have prominent lobulation of the lungs. The gross appearance often resembles an irregular checkerboard due to an admixture of normal and abnormal (consolidated) lobules (Fig. 3-25). Because of this typical lobular distribution, suppurative bronchopneumonias are also referred to as lobular pneumonias.

The color of consolidated lungs in suppurative bronchopneumonia varies considerably depending on the age of the lesion. In acute cases (few days), pneumonic lobules are red due to the active hyperemic response that occurs during the early stages of inflammation. In longer duration cases, the purulent exudate and the collapsed alveoli cause the lungs to be gray-pink. Finally, in the most chronic cases, the lungs take on a rather pale gray appearance similar to that of fish flesh. "Enzootic pneumonias" of ruminants and pigs are typical examples of chronic suppurative bronchopneumonias.

Microscopically, suppurative bronchopneumonias are characterized by abundant neutrophils, macrophages, and cellular debris within the lumen of bronchi, bronchioles, and alveoli (Fig. 3-27). Recruitment of leukocytes is promoted by cytokines, complement, and other chemotactic factors that are released in response to alveolar injury or by the chemotactic effect of bacterial toxins, particularly endotoxin. In most severe cases, purulent or mucopurulent exudates completely obliterate the entire lumen of bronchi, bronchioles, and alveoli.

If suppurative bronchopneumonia is merely the response to a transient pulmonary injury or a mild infection,

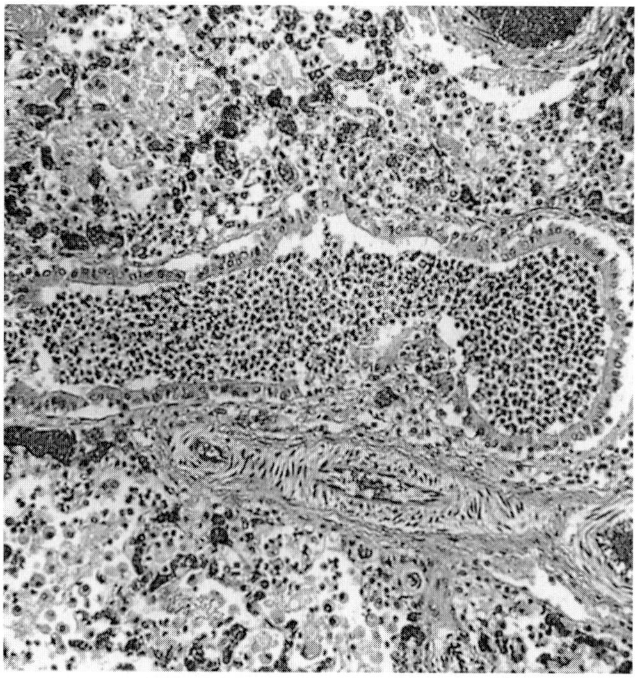

Figure 3-27 Lung; calf. Suppurative bronchopneumonia. Note the extensive loss of airspaces due to infiltration of neutrophils and macrophages into the bronchoalveolar spaces. H & E stain.

lesions resolve uneventfully. Within 7 to 10 days, cellular exudate can be removed from the lungs via the mucociliary escalator, and complete resolution may take place within 4 weeks. In other cases, if injury or infection is persistent, suppurative bronchopneumonia can become chronic with goblet cell hyperplasia, an important component of the inflammatory process. Depending on the proportion of pus and mucus, the exudate in chronic suppurative bronchopneumonia varies from mucopurulent to mucoid. A mucoid exudate is found in the more chronic stages when consolidated lung has a "fish flesh" appearance.

Hyperplasia of BALT is another change commonly seen in chronic suppurative bronchopneumonias; it appears grossly as conspicuous white nodules (cuffs) around bronchial walls (cuffing pneumonia). Further sequelae to chronic suppurative bronchopneumonia include bronchiectasis (Fig. 3-22), pulmonary abscesses, and pleural adhesions (from pleuritis), as well as atelectasis and emphysema from completely or partially obstructed bronchi or bronchioles (e.g., bronchiectasis).

Clinically, suppurative bronchopneumonias can be acute and fulminating, but are often chronic, depending on the etiologic agent, stressors affecting the host, and immune status. The most common pathogens causing suppurative bronchopneumonia in domestic animals include *Pasteurella multocida, Bordetella bronchiseptica, Arcanobacterium (Actinomyces) pyogenes, Streptococcus*

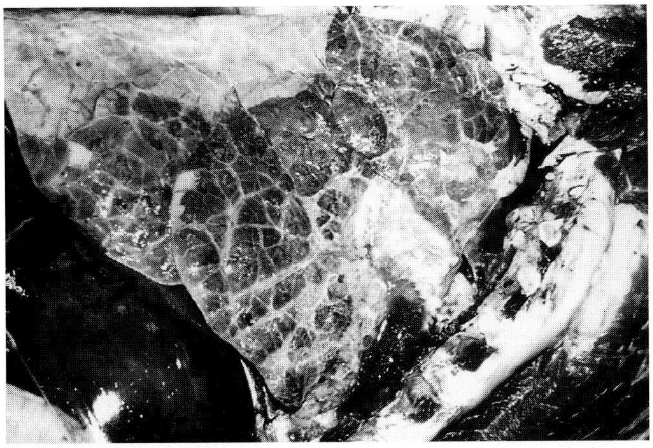

Figure 3-28 Right lung; steer. Fibrinous bronchopneumonia (pleuropneumonia). Pneumonic pasteurellosis *(P. haemolytica).* Note the cranioventral distribution that affects approximately 80% of the lung parenchyma. The lung is firm, swollen, and covered with fibrin, and interlobular septa are distended by edema and exudate. *Courtesy of Western College of Veterinary Medicine.*

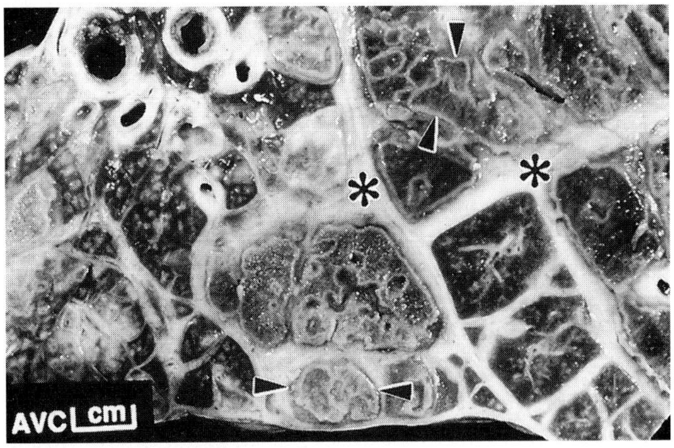

Figure 3-29 Lung, cut surface; steer. Pneumonic pasteurellosis *(P. haemolytica).* Interlobular septa *(asterisks)* are distended by edema and fibrin. Lung parenchyma has irregular areas of coagulative necrosis *(arrowheads)* surrounded by a rim of inflammatory cells.

spp., *E. coli* and several species of mycoplasmas. Most of these organisms are secondary pathogens requiring a preceding impairment of the pulmonary defense mechanisms to colonize the lungs and establish an infection. Suppurative bronchopneumonia can also result from aspiration of bland material (e.g., milk).

Fibrinous bronchopneumonia is similar to suppurative bronchopneumonia except that the predominant exudate is fibrinous rather than neutrophilic. With only a few exceptions, fibrinous bronchopneumonias also have a cranioventral distribution (Fig. 3-28). However, exudation is not restricted to the boundaries of individual pulmonary lobules, as is the case in suppurative bronchopneumonias. Instead, the inflammatory process in fibrinous pneumonias involves numerous contiguous lobules and the exudate moves quickly through pulmonary tissue until the entire pulmonary lobe is affected. Because of the involvement of the entire lobe, fibrinous bronchopneumonias are also referred to as lobar pneumonias. In general terms, fibrinous bronchopneumonias are the result of more severe pulmonary injury and, thus, are more life threatening than suppurative bronchopneumonias. Even in cases where fibrinous bronchopneumonia involves 30% or less of the total area, clinical signs and death can occur as a result of severe toxemia.

The gross appearance of fibrinous bronchopneumonia depends on the age and severity of the lesion and on whether the lung is observed externally or on cut surface. Externally, early stages of fibrinous bronchopneumonias are characterized by severe congestion and hemorrhage, giving the affected lungs a characteristically intense red discoloration. A few hours later, fibrin starts to accumulate on the surface, giving the pleura a ground glass appearance and eventually forming plaques of fibrinous exudate over a red dark lung. At this stage, a yellow fluid starts to accumulate in the thoracic cavity. The color of fibrin deposited over the pleural surface is also variable depending on the proportion of red blood cells, hemoglobin, and leukocytes. It can be yellow when the exudate is formed primarily by fibrin, tan when fibrin is mixed with blood, and gray when a large number of leukocytes are part of the fibrinous plaque. Because of the tendency of fibrin to deposit on the pleural surface, some pathologists use the term pleuropneumonia as a synonym for fibrinous bronchopneumonia.

On the cut surface, early stages of fibrinous bronchopneumonia appear as simple red consolidation. In more advanced cases (24 hours), fibrinous bronchopneumonias are generally accompanied by marked dilation and thrombosis of lymph vessels and edema of interlobular septa. This distension of the interlobular septa gives affected lungs a typical marbled appearance. Distinct focal areas of coagulative necrosis in the pulmonary parenchyma are also common in fibrinous bronchopneumonia (Fig. 3-29). In animals that survive the early stage of fibrinous bronchopneumonia, pulmonary necrosis often develops into pulmonary "sequestra," which are pieces of necrotic lung encapsulated by connective tissue.

Microscopically, in the initial stage of fibrinous bronchopneumonia there is massive exudation of plasma proteins into the bronchioles and alveoli, and, as a result, most of the airspaces become obliterated by fluid and fibrin. Movement of fibrin and fluid into alveolar lumena is due to extensive disruption of the integrity and increased permeability of the blood-air barrier. Since fibrin is chemotactic for neutrophils, these types of leukocytes are always present a few hours after the onset of fibrinous inflammation. As inflammation progresses (3 to 5 days), fluid exudates are gradually replaced by a fibrinocellular exudate composed of fibrin, neutrophils, macrophages, and necrotic debris (Fig. 3-30). In chronic cases (after 7 days) there is notable fibrosis of the interlobular septa and pleura.

In contrast to suppurative bronchopneumonia, fibrinous bronchopneumonia rarely resolves completely, thus leaving noticeable scars in the form of pulmonary fibrosis and pleural adhesions. The most common sequelae found in animals surviving an acute episode of fibrinous bronchopneumonia include bronchiolitis obliterans, gangrene, pulmonary sequestra, pulmonary fibrosis, abscesses, and chronic pleuritis with pleural adhesions. In some cases, pleuritis can be so extensive that fibrous adhesions extend onto the pericardial sac. Pathogens causing fibrinous bronchopneumonias in domestic animals include *Pasteurella haemolytica* (pneumonic pasteurellosis), *Haemophilus somnus, Actinobacillus pleuropneumoniae* (porcine pleuropneumonia), and *Mycoplasma mycoides* subsp *mycoides* small colony (contagious bovine pleuropneumonia). Fibrinous bronchopneumonia can also be the result of bronchoaspiration of irritant materials, such as gastric contents.

Interstitial Pneumonia

Interstitial pneumonia refers to a particular type of pneumonia in which injury and the inflammatory process take place primarily in any of the three layers of the alveolar walls (endothelium, basement membrane, and alveolar epithelium) and the contiguous bronchiolar interstitium. This type of pneumonia is perhaps the most difficult to diagnose at necropsy and generally requires microscopic confirmation. The pathogenesis of interstitial pneumonia is complex and can result from aerogenous injury to the alveolar epithelium (pneumonocytes I and II) or from hematogenous injury to the alveolar capillary endothelium or alveolar basement membrane. Inhalation of toxic gases, toxic fumes such as smoke, local generation of toxic metabolites by Clara cells, release of free radicals, and infection with pneumotropic viruses are just a few of the different agents that can damage alveolar epithelium. Injury to the vascular endothelium occurs in septicemias, in disseminated intravascular coagulation, from microembolism, from circulating larva migrans, from toxins absorbed in the alimentary tract or toxic metabolites locally generated in the lungs, and from infections with endotheliotropic viruses. Damage to the alveolar wall can also occur when inhaled antigens such as fungal spores combine with circulating antibodies and form deposits of antigen-antibody complexes in the alveolar wall, which initiate a cascade of inflammatory responses and injury (allergic alveolitis). As are interstitial pneumonias in human beings, those of the domestic animals are also subdivided, based on some morphologic features, into acute and chronic. It should be kept in mind, however, that not all acute interstitial pneumonias are fatal and that they do not necessarily progress into the chronic form.

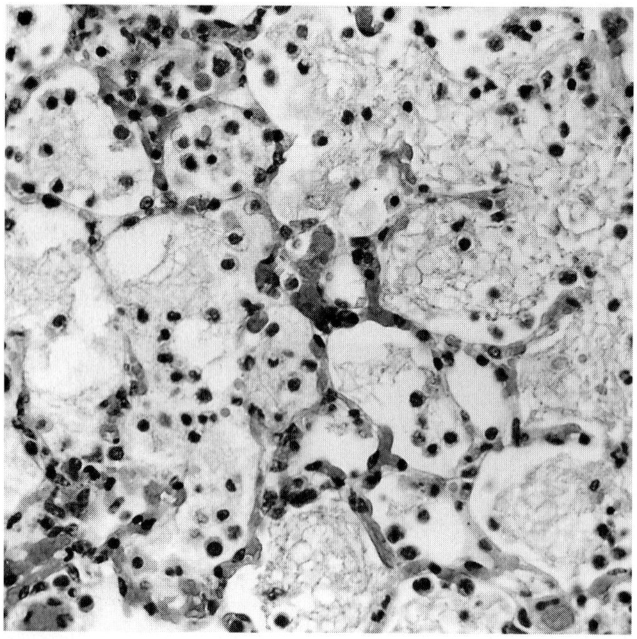

Figure 3-30 Lung; calf. Pneumonic pasteurellosis *(P. haemolytica)*. Alveoli contain abundant fibrin mixed with neutrophils and macrophages. H & E stain.

Acute interstitial pneumonias begin with injury to either type I pneumonocytes or alveolar capillary endothelium, which provokes a disruption of the air-blood barrier and a subsequent exudation of plasma proteins into the alveolar space. This spillage of proteinaceous fluid into the alveolar lumen constitutes the **exudative phase** of acute interstitial pneumonia. In some cases of diffuse alveolar damage, exuded plasma proteins mix with lipids and other components of pulmonary surfactant and form elongate membranes that become partially attached to the alveolar and bronchiolar walls. These membranes are referred to as **hyaline membranes** because they have a hyaline appearance (eosinophilic, homogenous, amorphous) on microscopic examination. In addition to intraalveolar exudation of fluid, inflammatory edema and neutrophils accumulate in the alveolar interstitium and cause thickening of the alveolar walls. This acute exudative phase is generally followed a few days later by the **proliferative phase** of acute interstitial pneumonias characterized by hyperplasia of type II pneumonocytes to replace the lost type I alveolar cells. Type II pneumonocytes are, in fact, progenitor cells that differentiate and replace necrotic type I pneumonocytes (see General Aspects of Lung Inflammation). As a consequence, the alveolar walls become increasingly thickened. This process is, in part, the reason why lungs become rubbery on palpation, what prevents their normal collapse after the thorax is opened and why the cut surface of the lung has a "meaty appearance."

Acute interstitial pneumonias are often mild and transient, especially those caused by some respiratory viruses. These mild forms of pneumonia are rarely seen in the postmortem room since they are not fatal and do not leave significant sequelae (see Defense Mechanisms of the Exchange System [Alveoli]). In severe cases of acute interstitial pneumonias, animals may die of respiratory failure, usually as a result of diffuse alveolar damage, a profuse exudative phase (leakage of proteinaceous fluid) leading to a fatal pulmonary edema. Examples of this type of fatal acute interstitial pneumonia are bovine pulmonary edema and emphysema in cattle, ARDS in all species, and massive pulmonary migration of ascaris larvae in pigs.

When the source of alveolar injury persists, the proliferative and infiltrative lesions of acute interstitial pneumonia can progress into a different morphologic stage referred to as **chronic interstitial pneumonia.** The hallmark of chronic interstitial pneumonias is alveolar fibrosis and, in some cases, accumulation of mononuclear inflammatory cells in the interstitium and persistence of hyperplastic type II pneumonocytes. It should be emphasized again that, although the lesions in interstitial pneumonia are centered in the alveolar walls and interstitium, a mixture of desquamated epithelial cells, macrophages, and mononuclear cells are usually present in the lumen of bronchioles and alveoli. Other concurrent changes that can accompany some forms of chronic interstitial pneumonia are formation of microscopic granulomas and hyperplasia of smooth muscle in airways or pulmonary vasculature. Ovine progressive pneumonia, hypersensitivity pneumonitis in cattle and dogs, and silicosis in horses are good veterinary examples of chronic interstitial pneumonia. Pneumoconioses (silicosis, asbestosis), paraquat toxicity, pneumotoxic antineoplastic drugs (bleomycin), and extrinsic allergic alveolitis (farmer's lung) are well-known examples of diseases that lead to chronic interstitial pneumonias in human beings.

In contrast to bronchopneumonias, where distribution of lesions is generally cranioventral, in acute or chronic interstitial pneumonias, lesions are more diffusely distributed and generally involve all pulmonary lobes, or, in some cases, they appear to be more pronounced in the dorsocaudal aspects of the lungs. Three important gross features of interstitial pneumonia are the failure of lungs to collapse when the thoracic cavity is opened, the occasional presence of rib impressions on the lung's pleural surface, and the lack of visible exudate in airways unless complicated with secondary bacterial pneumonia. The color of affected lungs varies from diffusely red to diffusely pale gray to a mottled red, pale appearance. Pale lungs are due to severe obliteration of alveolar capillaries (reduced blood/tissue ratio), especially when there is fibrosis. The texture of lungs with uncomplicated interstitial pneumonia is typically elastic or rubbery, but definitive diagnosis based on texture alone is difficult due to the intrinsic subjectivity of palpation. On cut surface, the lungs may appear more "meaty" and have no evidence of exudate. It should be remembered, however, that acute interstitial pneumonias, particularly in cattle, are frequently accompanied by pulmonary edema (exudative phase) and interstitial emphysema secondary to partial obstruction of bronchioles and strenuous air gasping before death. Since edema tends to gravitate into the cranioventral portions of the lungs and emphysema is often more obvious in the dorsocaudal aspects, acute interstitial pneumonias in cattle occasionally have a gross cranioventral-like pattern that may resemble that of bronchopneumonia generally. Lungs are notably heavy due to infiltrative and proliferative changes.

The term **"bronchointerstitial pneumonia"** has been introduced into veterinary pathology to describe cases in which pulmonary lesions share some histologic features of both bronchopneumonia and interstitial pneumonia. This combined type pneumonia is, in fact, frequently seen in many viral infections in which viruses replicate and cause injury in bronchial, bronchiolar, and alveolar cells. Damage to the bronchial and bronchiolar epithelium causes influx of neutrophils similar to that of bronchopneumonias, and damage to alveolar walls causes proliferation of type II pneumonocytes, similar to that which takes place in the proliferative phase of acute interstitial pneumonias. Examples of bronchointerstitial pneumonia include uncomplicated cases of respiratory syncytial virus infections in cattle and lambs, canine distemper, and influenza in pigs and horses (Fig. 3-31).

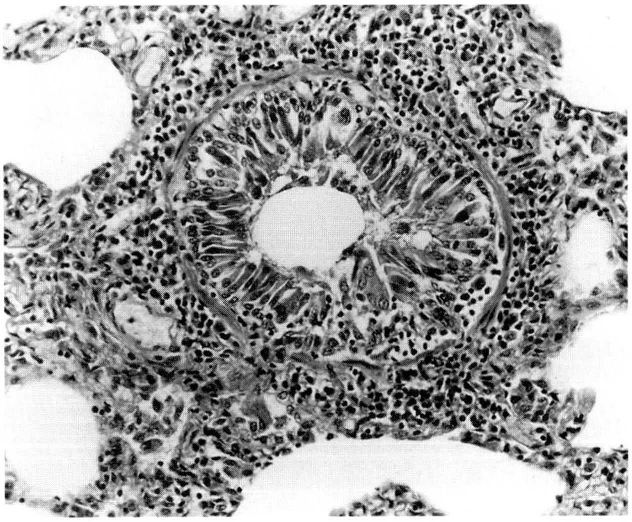

Figure 3-31 Lung; horse. Bronchointerstitial pneumonia (unknown etiology). The bronchiolar epithelium is intact, but an inflammatory cell infiltrate in the mucosa has extended peribronchially into the alveolar interstitium. H & E stain. *Courtesy of Western College of Veterinary Medicine.*

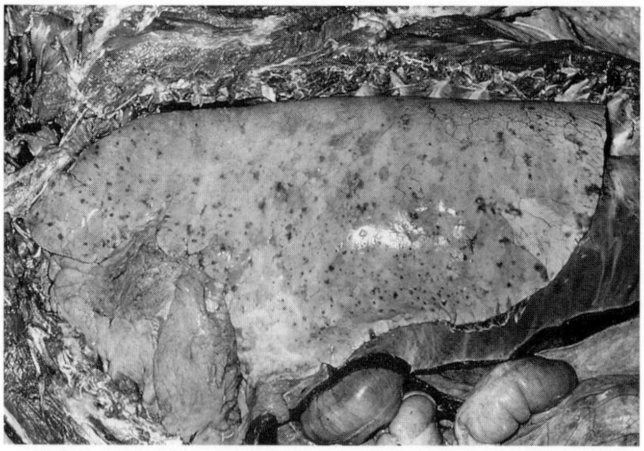

Figure 3-32 Left lung; foal. Acute embolic pneumonia. Note numerous small, dark foci of hermorrhage and inflammatory exudate randomly distributed in the pulmonary parenchyma.

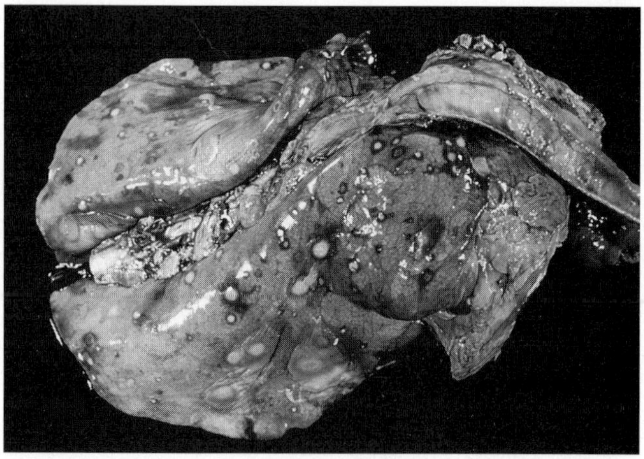

Figure 3-33 Lungs; 3-week-old lamb. Embolic pneumonia *(Staphylococcus aureus).* The lesions are spherical abscesses surrounded by a hyperemic border caused by septic emboli (pyemia). Heart, kidney, meninges, and joints were similarly affected. *Courtesy of Western College of Veterinary Medicine.*

Embolic Pneumonia

Embolic pneumonia is characterized by multifocal lesions randomly distributed in all pulmonary lobes, caused by entrapment of septic emboli. Lungs act as a biologic filter for circulating particulate matter. Sterile thrombi, unless extremely large, are rapidly dissolved and removed from the pulmonary vasculature by fibrinolysis, causing little if any ill effects. Experimental studies have confirmed that most types of bacteria when injected intravenously (bacteremia) generally bypass the lungs and are finally trapped in the liver, spleen, joints, or other organs. To cause pulmonary infection, circulating bacteria must first attach to the pulmonary endothelium and then evade phagocytosis by intravascular macrophages or leukocytes. Infected thrombi facilitate entrapment of bacteria in the pulmonary vessels and provide a favorable environment to escape phagocytosis. Once trapped in the pulmonary vasculature, usually in alveolar capillaries, offending bacteria spread from the vessels to the interstitium and then to surrounding lung, forming finally a nidus of infection. Early lesions in embolic pneumonia are characterized grossly by the presence of very small (1 mm), white foci in the lungs surrounded by a discrete, red, hemorrhagic halo (Fig. 3-32). Unless emboli arrive in massive numbers, causing fatal pulmonary edema, embolic pneumonia is seldom fatal; therefore, these acute lesions are rarely seen at postmortem examination. In most instances, acute lesions if unresolved rapidly progress into the formation of pulmonary abscesses (Fig. 3-33) that are randomly distributed in all pulmonary lobes and are not restricted to the cranioventral aspects of the lungs, as is the case of abscesses developing from suppurative bronchopneumonia. The early inflammatory lesions in embolic pneumonias are always focal; thus, they differ from those of endotoxemia or septicemia, in which endothelial damage and interstitial reactions (interstitial pneumonia) are diffusely distributed in the lungs.

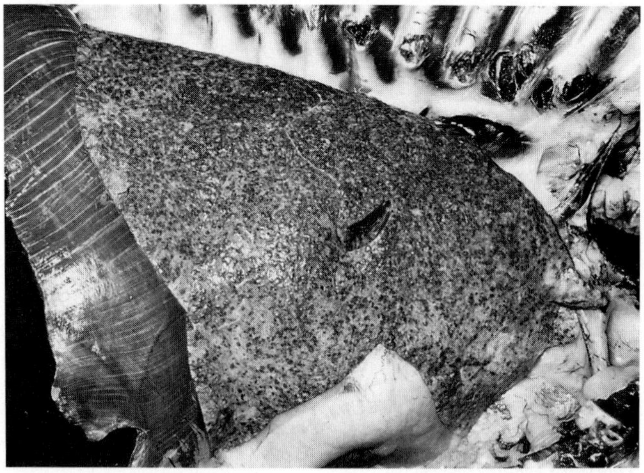

Figure 3-34 Right lung; dog. Granulomatous pneumonia. Blastomycosis *(Blastomyces dermatitidis).* The lung contains large numbers of small granulomas distributed throughout all pulmonary lobes.

When embolic pneumonia or its sequelae (abscesses) are encountered, careful postmortem examination is required to locate the source of septic emboli. Most common causes include rupture of hepatic abscesses into the caudal vena cava in cattle, omphalophlebitis in farm animals, chronic bacterial skin or hoof infections, and infected jugular catheter in all species (Fig. 3-20). Valvular or mural endocarditis in the right side of the heart is also a usual source of septic emboli and embolic pneumonia in all species. Most frequently, bacterial isolates from septic pulmonary emboli in domestic animals are *Arcanobacterium (Actinomyces) pyogenes, Fusobacterium necrophorum, Erysipelothrix rhusiopathiae, Streptococcus suis* type II, *Staphylococcus aureus,* and *Streptococcus equi.*

Granulomatous Pneumonia

The term "granulomatous" is used here to describe an anatomic pattern of pneumonia typically characterized by the presence of pulmonary granulomas. It does not presuppose that all granulomatous inflammation, as seen in other organs, necessarily results in the formation of granulomas.

Granulomatous pneumonia is characterized by the presence of variable numbers of caseous or noncaseous granulomas randomly distributed in the lungs (Fig. 3-34). On palpation, lungs have a typical nodular character given by well-circumscribed, variably sized nodules that, generally, have a firm texture, especially if calcification has occurred. During postmortem examination, granulomas in the lungs occasionally can be mistaken for neoplasms.

The pathogenesis of granulomatous pneumonia shares some similarities with those of interstitial and embolic pneumonias. Not surprisingly, some pathologists group granulomatous pneumonias within one of these types of pneumonias (e.g., granulomatous interstitial pneumonia). What makes granulomatous pneumonia a distinctive type is not so much the portal of entry or site of initial injury in the lungs, but the unique type of inflammatory response that results in the formation of granulomas, which can be easily recognized at gross and microscopic examination. The portal of agent entry into lungs can be aerogenous or hematogenous. As a rule, agents causing granulomatous pneumonia are resistant to intracellular killing by phagocytic cells and to the acute inflammatory response and persist in affected tissues for a long time.

The most common causes of granulomatous pneumonia in animals include systemic fungal diseases such as cryptococcosis *(Cryptococcus neoformans),* coccidioidomycosis *(Coccidioides immitis),* histoplasmosis *(Histoplasma capsulatum),* and blastomycosis *(Blastomyces dermatitidis)* (Fig. 3-35). In most of these fungal diseases, the port of entry is aerogenous and from the lungs the fungi disseminate systemically to other organs, particularly lymph nodes, liver, and spleen. Granulomatous pneumonia is also caused by some bacterial diseases such as tuberculosis *(Mycobacterium bovis)* in all species (Fig. 3-36), *Rhodococcus equi* in foals, and inhaled foreign material (starch). Sporadically, aberrant parasites such as *Fasciola hepatica* in cattle and aspiration of foreign bodies can also cause granulomatous pneumonia. Feline infectious peritonitis is one of a few viral infections of domestic animals that result in granulomatous pneumonia. Lesions are caused by the deposition of antigen-antibody complexes in the vasculature of many organs and subsequent vasculitis, including the lungs.

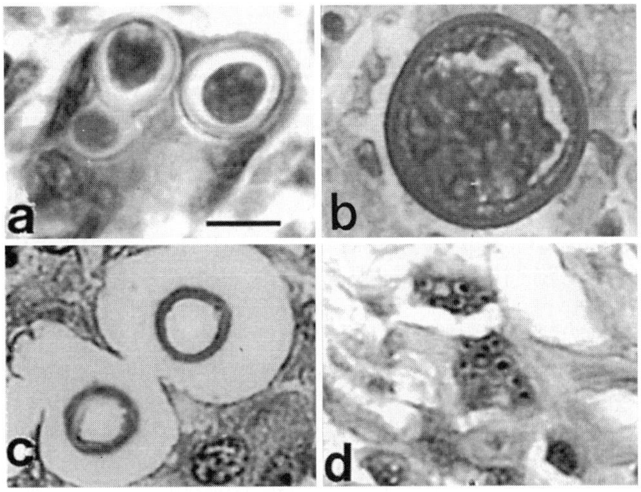

Figure 3-35 Systemic (deep) mycoses. **A,** *Blastomyces dermatitides.* Bar = 10 μm. **B,** *Coccidioides immitis.* **C,** *Cryptococcus neoformans.* **D,** *Histoplasma capsulatum.* All photographs were taken at the same magnification to preserve relative sizes.

A

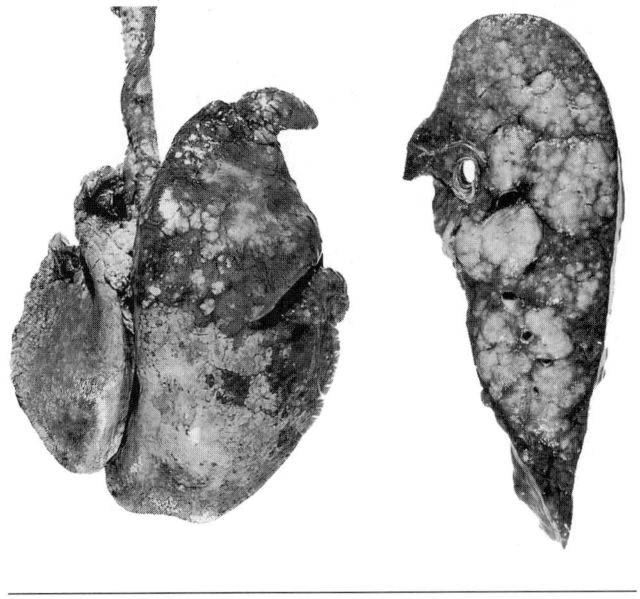

B

Figure 3-36 Lungs; foal. Granulomatous pneumonia *(Rhodococcus equi).* **A,** Cranioventral consolidation of the lungs with subpleural granulomas. **B,** Cut surface. Note the large, often confluent, caseated granulomas. *Johnson et al. Vet Pathol 1983; 20:440-449.*

Microscopically, pulmonary granulomas are composed of a center of necrotic tissue, surrounded by a rim of macrophages (epitheliod cells) and giant cells and an outer delineated layer of connective tissue commonly infiltrated by lymphocytes and plasma cells. Unlike other types of pneumonias, the causative agent in granulomatous pneumonia can, in many cases, be identified microscopically in sections stained by periodic acid–Schiff stain (PAS) or by

Grocott-Gomori methenamine silver (GMS) stains for fungi or the acid-fast stain for mycobacteria.

Pneumonias of Horses

Viral infections of the respiratory tract, particularly equine viral rhinopneumonitis and equine influenza, are important diseases of horses around the world. The effects of these and other respiratory viruses on the horse can be manifested in three distinct ways. First, as pure viral infections, their severity may range from mild to severe, making them a frequent interfering factor in training and athletic performance. Second, superimposed infections by opportunistic bacteria such as *Streptococcus* spp., *Escherichia coli, Klebsiella pneumoniae, Rhodococcus equi* and various anaerobes can cause fibrinous or suppurative bronchopneumonias. Third, it is possible, but yet unproven, that viral infections may also predispose horses to "airway hyperresponsivness" and "chronic obstructive pulmonary disease."

Equine Influenza

This contagious respiratory disease of horses has high morbidity and low mortality, and severe outbreaks occur in susceptible populations of horses. Two antigenically unrelated subtypes of equine influenza viruses have been identified (A/equine-1 and A/equine-2). The course of the disease is generally mild and transient, and its importance is primarily due to its economic impact on horse racing. The types of injury and host response in the conductive system are described under Specific Diseases of Nasal Cavity and Sinuses (Equine Nasal Diseases). Uncomplicated lesions in the lungs are those of a mild and self-limiting bronchointerstitial pneumonia. The influenza virus antigen can be readily demonstrated in ciliated cells and alveolar macrophages. Secondary infection is a common complication of equine influenza.

Equine Viral Rhinopneumonitis (EVR)

This respiratory disease of young horses is particularly important in weanlings between 4 and 8 months of age and, to a much lesser extent, in young foals and adult horses. The causative agent is an equine herpesvirus that, in addition to respiratory disease, can cause abortion in pregnant mares and neurologic diseases in horses of all ages (see also EVR under Equine Nasal Diseases).

The respiratory form of EVR in adult horses is a mild and a transient bronchointerstitial pneumonia and is seen only by pathologists when complications with secondary bacterial infections cause a fatal bronchopneumonia. Uncomplicated lesions in EVR are seen only in aborted fetuses or in foals that die within the first few days of life. They consist of focal areas of necrosis (0.5 to 2 mm) in various organs, including liver, adrenal glands, and lungs.

Equine Viral Arteritis (EVA)

This pansystemic disease of foals and horses, caused by Arterivirus, occurs sporadically throughout the world, sometimes as an outbreak. Clinical signs are respiratory distress, fever, abortion, diarrhea, colic, and edema of the limbs and ventral abdomen. Respiratory signs are frequently seen and consist of serous or mucopurulent rhinitis and conjunctivitis with palpebral edema. Like most viral respiratory infections, EVA can also predispose horses to opportunistic secondary bacterial pneumonias. Gross lesions consist of hemorrhage in most tissues, pulmonary edema, voluminous hydrothorax and hydroperitoneum, enteritis, and edema of the intestinal wall. Fibrinoid de generation and inflammation of the vessel walls (vasculitis), particularly the small muscular arteries (arteritis), are the underlying microscopic lesions that explain most of the clinical and pathologic features. Pulmonary lesions are those of the interstitial pneumonia with hyperplasia of type II pneumonocytes and vasculitis with distended pulmonary lymphatic vessels and abundant fluid in the bronchoalveolar spaces. Viral antigen can be detected in affected pulmonary vessels by immunoperoxidase techniques.

African Horse Sickness

This vector-borne disease of horses and, to a lesser extent, other equidae is caused by an orbivirus (family Reoviridae) and is characterized by respiratory distress or cardiovascular failure. It has a high mortality rate—up to 95% in the native population of horses in Africa, the Middle East, India, Pakistan, and, most recently, in Spain. Although the virus is transmitted primarily by insects *(Culicoides)* to horses, other animals such as dogs can be infected by eating infected equine flesh. Based on clinical signs (not pathogenesis), African horse sickness is arbitrarily divided into four different forms, namely: pulmonary, cardiac, mixed, and mild. The pulmonary form is characterized by severe respiratory distress and rapid death due to massive pulmonary edema. Grossly, large amounts of froth are present in the airways, lungs fail to collapse, subpleural lymph vessels are distended, and the ventral parts of the lungs are notably edematous. In the cardiac form, recurrent fever is detected, and heart failure results in subcutaneous and interfascial edema, most notably in the neck and supraorbital region. The mixed form is a combination of the respiratory and cardiac forms. Finally, the mild form is characterized by fever and clinical signs resembling those of equine influenza; it is in most cases, transient and followed by a complete recovery. This mild form is most frequently seen in donkeys, mules, and zebras and in horses with some degree of immunity. The pathogenesis remains unclear, but this equine orbivirus has an obvious tropism for pulmonary and cardiac endothelial cells, and to some lesser extent mononuclear cells; detection of viral antigen for diagnostic purposes could be done by immunohistochemistry in paraffin-embedded tissues.

Hendra Virus (Equine Morbillivirus)

Fatal cases of a novel respiratory disease in horses and human beings suddenly appeared around 1994 in Hendra, Australia. This outbreak was attributed to a newly recognized virus that was tentatively classified as **equine morbillivirus** and is currently referred to as **Hendra virus,** a new member of the subfamily Paramyxoviridae. The lungs of affected horses are severely edematous with gelatinous distension of pleura and subpleural lymph vessels. Microscopically, the lungs have diffuse alveolar edema associated with vasculitis, capillary thrombosis, distension of lymphatic vessels, and presence of multinucleated syncytial cells typical of morbillivirus infections in the endothelium of small pulmonary blood vessels and along the alveolar septa. The characteristic inclusion bodies seen in other morbillivirus infections are not seen in horses; however, the virus can be easily detected by immunohistochemistry in pulmonary endothelial cells and alveolar epithelial cells.

Rhodococcosis

Rhodococcus equi, formerly known as *Corynebacterium equi,* is an important cause of morbidity and mortality in foals around the world. It is a facultative intracellular bacterium that causes two major forms of disease—one involves the intestine, causing ulcerative enterocolitis, and the other affects the respiratory tract, resulting in a severe and often fatal bronchopneumonia. Although half of foals with pneumonia have enterocolitis, it is rare to find animals with enterocolitis alone. Occasionally, infection is disseminated to lymph nodes, joints, bones, genital tract, and other organs. Because *R. equi* is present in soil and feces of herbivores (particularly foals), it is not unusual for the disease to become enzootic on farms where the organism has been shed earlier by infected foals. Serologic evidence of infection in horses is widespread, yet clinical disease is sporadic and largely restricted to young foals or to adult horses with severe immunosuppression. Virulence factors encoded by plasmids appear to be responsible for the survival or *R. equi* in macrophages and thus determining the evolution of the disease. This bacterium also has been incriminated in cases of cervical lymphadenitis in cattle, goats, and pigs and quite often in immunocompromised human beings, for example, those infected with the AIDS virus, after organ transplantation, or undergoing chemotherapy.

Clinically, *R. equi* infection can be acute, with rapid death due to severe bronchopneumonia, or chronic, with depression, cough, weight loss, and respiratory distress. In either form, there may be diarrhea, arthritis, or subcutaneous abscess formation.

It is still debatable whether natural infection starts as a bronchopneumonia (aerogenous route) from which *R. equi* reaches the intestine via swallowed sputum, or whether infection starts as an enteritis (oral route) with subsequent bacteremia into the lungs. The results of experimental studies suggest that natural infection with this organism likely starts from inhalation of infected dust or aerosols. Once in the lung, *R. equi* undergoes rapid phagocytosis by alveolar macrophages, but defective phagosome-lysosome fusion and premature lysosomal degranulation result in bacteria survival and multiplication, eventually leading to the destruction of the macrophage. Interestingly, *R. equi* appears to be easily killed by neutrophils but not macrophages. Released cytokines and lysosomal enzymes and bacterial toxins are responsible for extensive caseous necrosis of the lungs and the recruitment of large numbers of neutrophils, macrophages, and giant cells containing intracellular gram-positive organisms in their cytoplasm. These changes eventually lead to a pyogranulomatous pneumonia (Fig. 3-36) with abscesses and tracheobronchial pyogranulomatous lymphadenitis, the hallmark lesions of *R. equi* disease. PCR analysis of tracheal aspirates has successfully been used as an alternative to bacteriologic culture in the diagnosis of *R. equi* infection in live foals.

Other Pneumonias of Horses

Chlamydia psittaci, an obligatory intracellular pathogen, can cause systemic infection in many mammalian and avian species; in horses, it has been associated with keratoconjunctivitis, rhinitis, pneumonia, abortion, polyarthritis, enteritis, hepatitis, and encephalitis. Serologic studies suggest that infection without apparent disease is common in horses. Horses experimentally infected with *C. psittaci* develop a mild and transient bronchointerstitial pneumonia. Detection of chlamydial organisms in affected tissue is not easy and requires special laboratory techniques.

Horses are susceptible to *Mycobacterium avium, Mycobacterium tuberculosis,* and *Mycobacterium bovis.* The intestinal tract and associated lymph nodes are usually affected, but with hematogenous dissemination, the lungs are involved (Fig. 3-37). The tubercles (granulomas) definitely differ from those in ruminants and pigs, being smooth, gray, solid nodules without grossly visible caseous necrosis or calcification; they typically appear more like sarcomas. Microscopically, the tubercles are composed of macrophages, epithelioid cells, and multinucleated giant cells. Fibrosis increases with time, accounting in part for the sarcomatous appearance.

Adenovirus and *Pneumocystis carinii* infections occur commonly in Arabian foals with **combined immunodeficiency,** a hereditary lack of B and T lymphocytes. In cases of viral infection, large basophilic or amphophilic

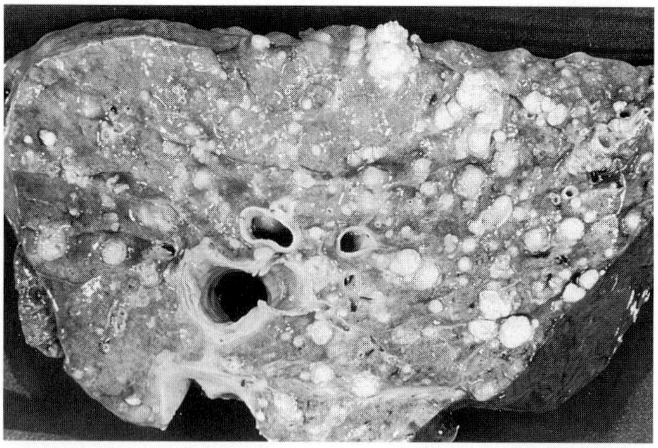

Figure 3-37 Lung, cut surface; aged horse. Tuberculosis *(Mycobacterium avium-intracellulare)*. Multifocal, granulomatous pneumonia. *Courtesy of Western College of Veterinary Medicine.*

adenoviral inclusion are present in the nuclei of tracheal, bronchial, bronchiolar, alveolar, renal, and intestinal epithelial cells. In infections with *P. carinii,* the pulmonary lesion is an interstitial pneumonia. Characteristically, alveoli are filled with a distinctive foamy exudate that contains the organism (not visible in H & E stain), which is easily demonstrated with Gomori's methenamine silver stain. In human beings, *P. carinii* pneumonia (pneumocystosis) is one of the most common and often fatal complications in AIDS patients. As in AIDS patients, in foals, abnormal populations of CD4 and CD8 lymphocytes have been incriminated as the underlying mechanism leading to pneumocystosis.

Diffuse proliferative interstitial pneumonias of undetermined etiology have been repeatedly reported in North American horses. The gross and microscopic lesions are reminiscent of those of bovine pulmonary edema and emphysema in cattle with hyperplasia of type II pneumonocytes. The etiology of this form of equine interstitial pneumonia is not known, but toxic and viral etiologies already have been proposed.

Aspiration pneumonia is often a devastating sequela to improper gastric tubing of horses, particularly exogenous lipid pneumonia from mineral oil delivered into the trachea in treatment of colic. Gross and microscopic lesions are described in detail in the section *Aspiration Pneumonias of Cattle.*

Parasitic Pneumonias of Horses

Parascaris equorum is a large nematode (roundworm) of the small intestine of horses; the larval stages migrate through the lungs as ascarid larvae do in pigs. It is still unclear whether migration of *P. equorum* larvae can cause significant pulmonary lesions under natural conditions. Experimentally, migration of larvae results in coughing, anorexia, and weight loss. Small necrotic foci and petechiae occur in the liver, hepatic and tracheobronchial lymph nodes, and lungs. These changes are also apparent microscopically, but eosinophils are also prominent as part of the focal, granulomatous, interstitial pneumonia associated with larvae. Eosinophilic bronchitis and bronchiolitis also occur.

Dictyocaulus arnfieldi is not a very pathogenic nematode, but should be considered if there are signs of coughing in horses that are pastured together with donkeys. Donkeys are considered the natural hosts and can tolerate large numbers of parasites without ill effects. *D. arnfieldi* does not usually become patent in horses, so examination of fecal samples is not useful; BALs are only occasionally diagnostic as eosinophils but not parasites are typically found in the lavage fluid. Mature parasites cause obstructive bronchitis, edema, and atelectasis particularly along the dorsocaudal lung. The microscopic lesion is an eosinophilic bronchitis similar to the less acute infestations seen in cattle and sheep with their *Dictyocaulus* species.

Pneumonias of Cattle

Bovine Respiratory Disease (BRD) Complex

This general term is often used by clinicians to describe acute and severe bovine respiratory illness of clinically undetermined etiology. The BRD complex includes enzootic pneumonia of calves (multifactorial etiology), bovine pneumonic pasteurellosis *(Pasteurella haemolytica),* respiratory hemophilosis *(Haemophilus somnus),* respiratory viral infections such as infectious bovine rhinothracheitis (IBR/BHV-1), parainfluenza-3 (PI-3 virus), bovine respiratory syncytial virus (BRSV), and noninfectious interstitial pneumonias such as bovine pulmonary edema and emphysema, reinfection syndrome, and many others.

Enzootic pneumonia, sometimes simply referred to as "calf pneumonia," is a disease caused by a variety of etiologic agents and with a variety of lesions in young, intensively housed calves. Morbidity is often high (up to 90%), but fatalities are uncommon (less than 5%) unless management is poor or unless new, virulent pathogens are introduced by additions to the herd. Clinically, enzootic pneumonia is usually mild, but fatal cases are occasionally seen even in farms with optimal health management.

Enzootic pneumonia is also called **viral pneumonia** because it often begins with an acute respiratory infection with PI-3 virus, BRSV, or possibly with one or more of several others viruses (adenoviruses, BHV-1, reoviruses, rhinoviruses). Mycoplasmas, notably *M. dispar, M. bovis, Ureaplasma,* and possibly *Chlamydia,* may also be primary agents. Following infection with any of these agents, opportunistic bacteria such as *Pasteurella multocida, Arcanobacterium (Actinomyces) pyogenes, H. somnus,* and *Escherichia coli* cause a secondary suppurative bronchopneumonia, the most serious stage of enzootic pneumonia. The pathogenesis of the primary invasion and how it predisposes the host to invasion by the opportunists are poorly understood, but it is likely that there is impairment of pulmonary defense mechanisms. Environmental factors, including air quality (poor ventilation), relative humidity, and animal crowding have been strongly incriminated. The immune status of the calf also plays an important role in the development and severity of enzootic pneumonia. Calves with **bovine leukocyte adhesion deficiency (BLAD)** are highly susceptible to bronchopneumonia.

Lesions are variable and depend largely on the agents involved as well as on the duration of the inflammatory process. In the acute phases, lesions caused by viruses are those of bronchointerstitial pneumonia, which are generally mild and transient and, therefore, are seen only sporadically at necropsy. Microscopically, the lesions are necrotizing bronchiolitis, necrosis of type I pneumonocytes with hyperplasia of type II pneumonocytes, and mild interstitial and alveolar edema. In the case of PI-3 and BRSV infection, intracytoplasmic inclusion bodies and the formation of large multinucleated syncytia resulting from the fusion of infected bronchiolar epithelial cells can also be observed in the lungs. The mycoplasmas, too, can cause bronchiolitis, necrosis, and an interstitial reaction, but, in contrast to viral-induced pneumonias, mycoplasmal lesions tend to progress to a chronic stage characterized by striking peribronchiolar lymphoid hyperplasia (cuffing pneumonia). When complicated by secondary bacterial infections, viral or mycoplasmal lesions change from a pure bronchointerstitial to a suppurative bronchopneumonia (Fig. 3-26). In late stages of bronchopneumonia, the lungs contain a creamy-mucoid exudate in the airways and, often, have pulmonary abscesses or bronchiectasis (Fig. 3-22). Airway hyperreactivity has been recently described in neonatal calves following BRSV infection; however, the significance of this syndrome in relation to enzootic pneumonia of calves is still under investigation.

It should be noted that the same viruses and mycoplasmas involved with the enzootic pneumonia complex can also predispose cattle to other diseases such as pneumonic pasteurellosis (shipping fever).

"Shipping fever" (transit fever) is a vague clinical term used in the past to denote acute respiratory diseases that occurred in cattle several days or weeks after shipment. The disease is characterized by a severe fibrinous bronchopneumonia. Because *P. haemolytica* and *P. multocida* are generally isolated from affected lungs, the name pneumonic pasteurellosis has been used synonymously. Currently, it is known that shipping fever can occur in animals that have not been shipped and that organisms other than *Pasteurella* spp. can cause similar lesions. Therefore, the term "shipping fever" should be relinquished in favor of more specific names such as pneumonic pasteurellosis, respiratory hemophilosis, and others.

Pneumonic pasteurellosis (shipping fever) is the most important respiratory disease of cattle in North America, particularly in feedlot animals that have been through the stressful marketing and assembly processes. It is clinically characterized by acute fibrinous bronchopneumonia with toxemia.

P. haemolytica biotype A, serotype 1 is the etiologic agent responsible for the severe pulmonary lesions. A few investigators still consider that *P. multocida* and other serotypes of *P. haemolytica* are also causes of this disease.

Even after many years of intense investigation, the pathogenesis of pneumonic pasteurellosis still remains incompletely understood. Experiments have established that *P. haemolytica* A1 alone is usually incapable of causing disease, since it is rapidly cleared by pulmonary defense mechanisms. These findings may explain why *P. haemolytica* A1, in spite of being present in the nasal cavity of healthy animals, only sporadically causes disease. For *P. haemolytica* to be established as a pulmonary infection, it is first required that stressors impair the defense mechanisms. These stressors include weaning, transport, fatigue, crowding, mixing of cattle from various sources, inclement weather, temporary starvation, and viral infections. Horizontal transmission of viruses and *P. haemolytica* occurs during crowding and transportation of cattle. Viruses that most commonly predispose cattle to pneumonic pasteurellosis include BHV-1, PI-3, BRSV, and several others. Once established in the lungs, *P. haemolytica* causes lesions by means of different virulence factors that include endotoxin and outer membrane proteins, but the most important is probably the production of a leukotoxin (exotoxin) that binds and kills bovine macrophages and neutrophils. The fact that this toxin exclusively affects ruminant leukocytes probably explains why *P. haemolytica* is a respiratory pathogen in cattle and sheep but not in other species. During *P. haemolytica* infection, alveolar macrophages release maximum amounts of proinflammatory cytokines, particularly TNF-α, IL-8, and leukotrienes, and bacterial toxins further amplify the inflammatory response.

Clinically, pneumonic pasteurellosis is characterized by a severe toxemia that can kill animals even when considerable parts of the lungs remain functional and structurally normal. Cattle usually become depressed, febrile, and anorexic and have a productive cough, encrusted nose, mucopurulent nasal exudate, shallow respiration, or an expiratory grunt.

The gross lesions of pneumonic pasteurellosis are the prototype of fibrinous (lobar) bronchopneumonia with prominent fibrinous pleuritis (Fig. 3-28) and pleural effusion. Lesions are always cranioventral and usually ventral to a horizontal line through the tracheal bifurcation. The interlobular septa are distended by yellow, gelatinous edema and fibrin. The "marbling" of lobules is the result of areas of coagulation necrosis, interlobular interstitial edema, and congestion (Fig. 3-29). The necrotic areas are typically bordered by a rim of elongated cells often referred to as "swirling macrophages" or "oat-shaped cells," now known to be degenerating neutrophils mixed with a few alveolar macrophages. Edema and fibrin are the major components of the exudate in alveoli and interlobular septa (Fig. 3-30). The extensive deposition of fibrin is the result of altered platelet function, increased procoagulant activity, and diminished profibrinolytic activity in the lungs. The conducting airways also have considerable amounts of exudate from deep within the lungs, but their walls are not particularly involved. Because of the necrotizing process, sequelae to pneumonic pasteurellosis can be serious and can include abscesses, sequestra, chronic pleuritis, fibrous pleural adhesions, and bronchiectasis.

Pneumonic pasteurellosis should not be confused with other forms of bovine pasteurellosis, such as **hemorrhagic septicemia** of ruminants caused by serotypes B and E of *P. multocida.* This disease does not occur in North America and currently is reported only from some countries in Asia and Africa. In contrast to pneumonic pasteurellosis, in which lesions are always confined to the lower respiratory tract, the bacteria in hemorrhagic septicemia are always disseminated hematogenously to many organs. The disease is clinically characterized by a severe, acute septicemia, high fever, and rapid death. At necropsy, typically, generalized petechiae are present on the serosal surfaces of intestine, heart, lungs, and in skeletal muscles. Superficial and visceral lymph nodes are swollen and hemorrhagic. Variable lesions include fibrinohemorrhagic interstitial pneumonia, hemorrhagic enteritis, blood-tinged fluid in the thorax and abdomen, and subcutaneous edema.

Respiratory hemophilosis is part of the **"*Haemophilus somnus* disease complex"** caused by *H. somnus,* which has different clinicopathologic forms, each one involving different organs. This complex includes septicemia, encephalitis known as thrombotic meningoencephalitis (TME), pneumonia (respiratory hemophilosis), pleuritis, myocarditis, arthritis, ophthalmitis, conjunctivitis, otitis, and abortion.

The respiratory form of bovine hemophilosis is the result of the bacterium's capacity to produce both suppurative and fibrinous bronchopneumonia. The latter is, in some cases, indistinguishable from that of pneumonic pasteurellosis. The pathogenesis of respiratory hemophilosis is still poorly understood, and the disease cannot be reproduced consistently by administration of *H. somnus* alone. Like *P. haemolytica,* it requires predisposing factors such as stress or a preceding viral infection. The capacity of *H. somnus* to cause septicemia, as well as localized infections in the lungs, brain, eyes, ear, heart, mammary gland, male and female genital organs, or placenta, is perhaps attributable to specific virulence factors. It has been shown that *H. somnus* has the ability to undergo structural and antigenic variation, evade phagocytosis by promoting leukocytic apoptosis, inhibit intracellular killing, and reduce transferrin concentrations in affected calves. Mixed infections of *H. somnus,* pasteurellae, and mycoplasmas are fairly common.

Contagious bovine pleuropneumonia is of historical interest in veterinary medicine, as the object of early national control programs for infectious disease. It was eradicated from North America in 1892 and from Australia in the 1970s, but it is still enzootic in large areas of Africa, Asia, and Eastern Europe. The etiologic agent, *Mycoplasma mycoides* subsp. *mycoides* small colony, was the first *Mycoplasma* isolated and is the most pathogenic of any that infect domestic animals. Pathogenetic mechanisms are still inadequately understood, but are suspected to involve toxin production, unregulated production of TNF-α, ciliary dysfunction, immunosuppression, and immune-mediated vasculitis. Vasculitis and thrombosis of blood vessels lead to lobular infarction.

The name of the disease is a good indication of the gross lesions. It is a severe, fibrinous bronchopneumonia (pleuropneumonia) similar to that of pneumonic pasteurellosis but having a more pronounced "marbling" of the lobules (different stages of inflammation), 60% to 79% of lesions in the caudal lobes (not cranioventrally), and more frequent and larger pulmonary sequestra (necrotic lung encapsulated by connective tissue). Microscopically, the appearance again is like that of pneumonic pasteurellosis, except that vasculitis and thrombosis of pulmonary arterioles and capillaries are much more obvious and are clearly the major cause of the infarction. *M. mycoides* remains viable in the sequestra for many years, and under stress the fibrous capsule may break down and the mycoplasma are released into the airways and become a source of infection for other animals. Vaccination is highly effective in preventing the disease.

Tuberculosis is an ancient, communicable, worldwide, chronic disease of human beings and domestic animals. It continues to be a major problem in human beings in underdeveloped countries, and it is on the rise in some industrialized nations, largely due to the immunosuppressive effects of AIDS, immigration, and movement of infected animals across borders. The World Health Organization (WHO) estimated that 30 million people, mostly in developing countries, died of tuberculosis between 1990 and 1999. *Mycobacterium tuberculosis* is transmitted between human beings, but, where unpasteurized cow's milk is consumed, *M. bovis* from the milk of cattle with mammary tuberculosis is also important. Cattle can be infected with *M. bovis, M. tuberculosis,* and *M. avium-intracellulare* by several routes, but infection of the lungs by inhalation of *M. bovis* is the most common in adult animals, whereas ingestion of infected milk is more predominant in young animals. Respiratory infection usually starts when inhaled bacilli reach the alveoli and are phagocytosed by pulmonary alveolar macrophages. If these cells are successful in destroying the bacteria, infection is averted. However, *M. bovis* may multiply intracellularly, kill the macrophage, and initiate infection. From this first nidus of infection, bacilli spread via airways within the lungs and eventually to tracheobronchial and mediastinal lymph nodes via the lymph vessels. The initial focus of infection at the portal of entry (lungs) plus the involvement of regional lymph nodes is termed the *primary (Ghon's) complex* of tuberculosis. If the infection is not contained within this primary complex, bacilli disseminate via the lymph vessels to distant organs and other lymph nodes. Hematogenous dissemination occurs sporadically when the inflammatory process containing the mycobacteria erodes the walls of blood vessels. If bacterial dissemination is sudden and massive, numerous small foci of infection develop in many tissues and organs and is referred to as **miliary tuberculosis** (like millet seeds). The host becomes hypersensitive to the mycobacterium, which enhances the cell-mediated immune defenses in early or mild infections, but can result in host-tissue destruction in the form of caseous necrosis. The evolution and dissemination of the pulmonary infection are closely regulated by cytokines and TNF-α production by alveolar macrophages.

Clinically, the signs relate to the dysfunction of a particular organ system or to general debilitation, reduced milk production, and emaciation. In the pulmonary form, which is more than 90% of bovine cases, a chronic, moist cough can progress to dyspnea. Enlarged tracheobronchial lymph nodes can contribute to the dyspnea by impinging on airways, and the enlargement of caudal mediastinal nodes can compress the caudal thoracic esophagus and cause bloating.

Tuberculosis, the prototype for granulomatous pneumonia, is characterized by the presence of a few or many caseated granulomas (Fig. 3-38). The early gross changes are small foci *(tubercles)* most frequently seen in the dorsocaudal, subpleural areas. With progression, the lesions enlarge and become confluent with the formation of large areas of caseous necrosis. Single nodules or clusters occur on the pleura and peritoneum, and this presentation has been termed *pearl disease*. Microscopically, the tubercle is composed of mononuclear cells of various types. In young tubercles, which are noncaseous, epithelioid and Langhans' giant cells are at the center, surrounded by lymphocytes, plasma cells, and macrophages. Later, caseous necrosis is at the center, secondary to the effects of cell-mediated hypersensitivity, enclosed by other cell types and fibrosis at the periphery. Acid-fast organisms may be numerous but, more often, are difficult to find in histologic section or smears.

Atypical interstitial pneumonia (AIP) is a vague clinical term well entrenched in veterinary literature, but one that has led to enormous confusion among veterinarians. It was first used to describe acute or chronic forms of bovine pneumonia that did not fit in any of the "classical" forms because of the lack of exudate and lack of productive cough. Microscopically, the criteria for diagnosis of AIP in cattle were based on the absence of obvious exudate and the presence of edema, interstitial emphysema (see Pulmonary Emphysema), hyaline membranes, hyperplasia of type II pneumonocytes, and fibrosis of cellular infiltrates in the interstitium. At that time, any pulmonary disease or pulmonary syndrome that had a few of the above lesions was traditionally diagnosed as AIP, and grouping all these different syndromes together was inconsequential since their etiopathogenesis were then unknown.

Field and laboratory investigations have demonstrated that most of the syndromes previously grouped under AIP have rather different etiologies and pathogeneses (Fig. 3-39). Further, what was "atypical" in the past has become

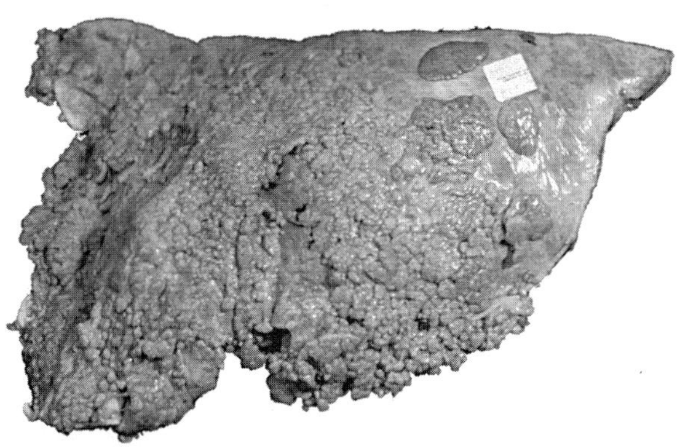

Figure 3-38 Lung; aged cow. Pulmonary tuberculosis. Multifocal, granulomatous pneumonia.

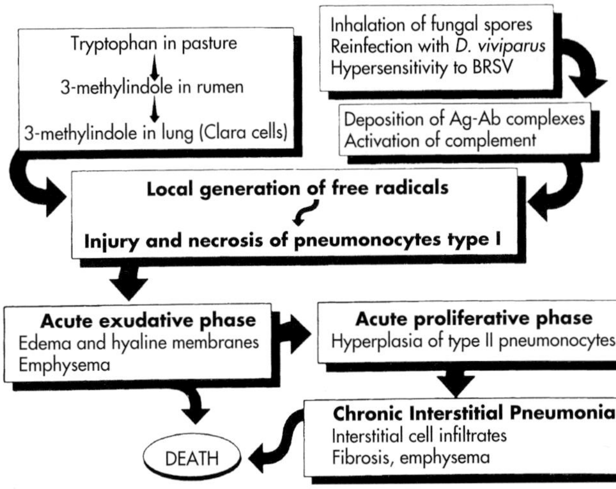

Figure 3-39 Pathogenesis of toxic and allergic pneumonias ("atypical interstitial pneumonia") in cattle.

so routine that it is fairly common nowadays to find "typical cases" of AIP. For all these reasons, investigators, largely from Britain, proposed that all these syndromes previously clustered into AIP should be named according to their specific etiology or pathogenesis. The most common bovine syndromes characterized by edema, emphysema, hyaline membranes, and hyperplasia of type II pneumonocytes include **bovine pulmonary edema and emphysema ("fog fever"), "extrinsic allergic alveolitis" (hypersensitivity pneumonitis), "reinfection syndrome" (hypersensitivity to *Dictyocaulus* sp.), milk allergy,** and others.

Acute bovine pulmonary edema and emphysema (ABPE), known in Britain as "fog fever" (no association with atmospheric conditions), occurs in cattle usually grazing "fog" pastures (that is, aftermath or foggage, regrowth after a hay or silage has been cut). Epidemiologically, ABPE usually occurs in adult beef cattle in the fall when there is a change in pasture, from a short, dry grass to a lush, green grass. It is generally accepted that L-tryptophan present in the pasture is metabolized in the rumen to 3-methylindole, which in turn is absorbed into the bloodstream and carried to the lungs. Mixed function oxidases present in the nonciliated bronchiolar epithelial (Clara) cells metabolize 3-methylindole into a highly pneumotoxic compound that causes extensive necrosis of bronchiolar cells and type I pneumonocytes (Fig. 3-39), and increases alveolar permeability leading to edema, interstitial pneumonia, and alveolar and interstitial emphysema. Clinically, severe respiratory distress develops within 2 weeks of the pasture change, and cattle develop expiratory dyspnea, oral breathing, and evidence of emphysema within the lungs and even subcutaneously along the back. Experimentally, reducing ruminal conversion of L-tryptophan to 3-methylindole prevents the development of ABPE. The gross lesions are those of a diffuse interstitial pneumonia with severe alveolar and interstitial edema and interlobular emphysema (Figs. 3-15 and 3-40). The lungs are enlarged, pale, and rubbery in texture, and the lesions are most notable in the caudal lobes. Microscopically, the lesions are alveolar and interstitial edema and emphysema, formation of hyaline membranes within alveoli, and, in those animals that survive for several days, hyperplasia of type II alveolar epithelial cells.

A number of other agents cause virtually the same clinical and pathologic syndrome as is seen in ABPE. The pathogenesis is assumed to be similar, although presumably other toxic factors will be specific for each syndrome. One of these pneumotoxic factors is 4-ipomeanol, which is found in moldy sweet potatoes contaminated with the fungus *Fusarium solani*. Mixed-function oxidases in the lungs activate 4-ipomeanol into a potent pneumotoxicant capable of producing irreversible injury to type I pneumonocytes and bronchiolar epithelial cells. Similarly, purple mint *(Perilla frutescens),* stinkwood *(Zieria arborescens),* and rapeseed and kale (*Brassica* species) also cause pulmonary edema, emphysema, and interstitial pneumonia.

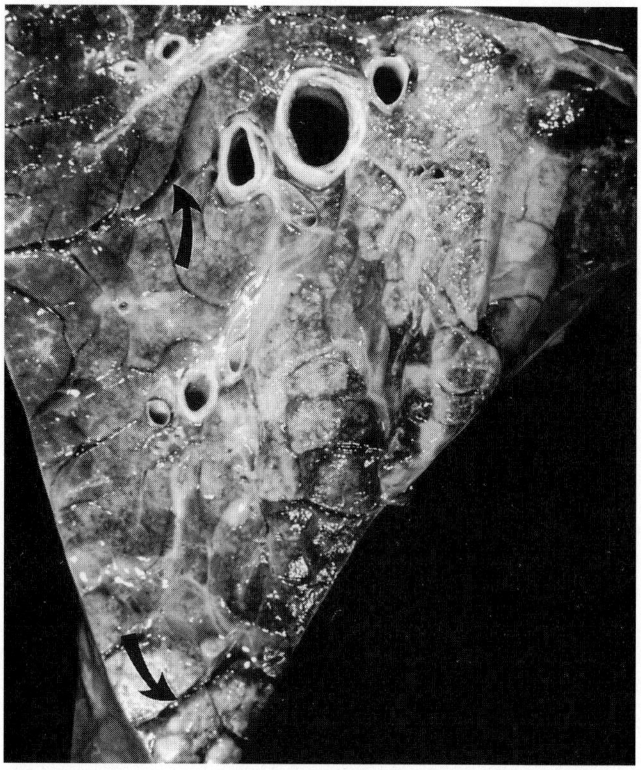

Figure 3-40 Lung, cut surface; yearling calf. Interstitial pneumonia (unknown etiology). The lung is heavy, rubbery in texture, dark red-blue cranioventrally, and pale caudally. Interstitial emphysema and edema, both lesions characteristic of those of bovine pulmonary edema and emphysema, are evident in the interlobular septa *(arrows)* of the caudal lobes. *Courtesy of Western College of Veterinary Medicine.*

Extrinsic allergic alveolitis (hypersensitivity pneumonitis), one of the most common allergic diseases in cattle, is seen mainly in housed, adult dairy cows in the winter. This disease shares many similarities with its human counterpart known as **farmer's lung,** which results from a type III hypersensitivity reaction to inhaled organic antigens and local deposition of antigen-antibody complexes (Arthus reaction) in the lungs. The most common type of inhaled antigens triggering this disease are fungal spores, mainly of the thermophilic actinomycete, *Saccharopolyspora rectivirgula (Micropolyspora faeni),* commonly found in moldy hay. Since it occurs only in a few animals of the herd or sporadic farmer, it is presumed that intrinsic host factors such as dysregulation of IgG, interleukines, IFN-γ and T lymphocytes are involved in the pathogenesis of the disease. Clinically, it can be acute or chronic; the latter has a cyclical pattern of exacerbation during winter months. Weight loss, coughing, and poor exercise tolerance are clinical features. Grossly, the postmortem lesions vary from subtle, gray, subpleural foci (granulomatous inflammation) to severe, in which the lungs are firm and heavy and have a "meaty appearance" due to alveolar epithelial hyperplasia, lymphocytic infiltration, and fibrosis (Fig. 3-39). Characteristically, discrete noncaseous granulomas formed in response to the deposition of antigen-antibody complexes are scattered throughout the lungs. Chronic cases of extrinsic allergic alveolitis can eventually progress into diffuse fibrosing alveolitis. Full recovery can occur if it is recognized and treated at the early stages of the disease.

Other allergic syndromes manifested in the lungs include hypersensitivity to reinfection with larvae of *Dictyocaulus viviparus,* which cause signs and lesions indistinguishable from ABPE, with the exception of a component of eosinophils and possibly larvae seen microscopically in the alveolar exudate. It has been suggested that emphysema with diffuse proliferative alveolitis and formation of hyaline membranes can also occur in the late stages of BRSV infection in cattle. Presumably, this disease shares many similarities with severe infections occasionally seen in children with respiratory syncytial virus (RSV human strain), in which a hypersensitivity to the virus has been implicated as primary cause of disease (Fig. 3-39).

A type of systemic anaphylaxis (type I hypersensitivity) known as milk allergy can cause acute pulmonary congestion, edema, and even hemorrhage and emphysema in cows sensitized to their own milk casein and lactalbumin. Occasionally, adverse drug reactions can induce a similar allergic response in the lung.

Inhalation of manure ("pit") gases, such as hydrogen sulfide (H_2S) and ammonia (NH_3), and nitrogen dioxide (NO_2) from silos, can be a serious hazard to animals and human beings. At toxic concentrations, these gases cause necrosis of bronchiolar cells and type I pneumonocytes, fulminating pulmonary edema that causes asphyxiation, and rapid death. In addition, NO_2, like other oxidant gases, also causes bronchiolitis, edema, and interstitial pneumonia and in survivors fibrosis ("silo filler's disease").

Parasitic Pneumonias of Cattle

Pulmonary lesions in parasitic pneumonias (the word is used here in its restricted sense to mean helminth infestations of the lungs) vary from interstitial in larvae migration to chronic bronchitis caused by some intrabronchial adult parasites to granulomatous pneumonia caused by dead larvae, aberrant parasites, or eggs of parasites. In many cases, an "eosinophilic syndrome" in the lungs is characterized by infiltrates of eosinophils in the pulmonary interstitium and bronchoalveolar spaces and blood eosinophilia. Atelectasis and emphysema secondary to the obstruction of airways are also common findings in many parasitic pneumonias. The adult parasites are often visible grossly (Fig. 3-16). The severity of the lesions relates to the numbers and size of the parasites and the nature of the host reaction, which sometimes includes hypersensitivity reactions. A common general term for all of these diseases is **verminous pneumonia.**

Dyctiocaulus viviparus is an important pulmonary nematode (lungworm) responsible for a disease in cattle referred to as verminous pneumonia or **verminous bronchitis.** Adult parasites live in the intrapulmonary bronchi of cattle, mainly in those of the caudal lobes of the lungs. Adult parasites cause severe bronchial irritation, bronchitis, and pulmonary edema, which in turn induce lobular atelectasis and interstitial emphysema. Atelectasis is clearly confined to the lobules of the lungs ventilated by the obstructed bronchi (dorsocaudal); interstitial emphysema (interlobular) is caused by forced expiratory movements due to obstruction of the small bronchi. In addition to the inflammation of bronchial mucosa, bronchoaspiration of larvae and eggs also causes an influx of leukocytes into the bronchoalveolar space (alveolitis). Verminous pneumonia is most commonly seen in calves during their first summer grazing pastures used repeatedly from year to year, particularly in regions of Europe with a moist, cool climate. The parasite can overwinter in pastures even in climates as cold as Canada's, and older animals may be carriers for a considerable length of time.

The clinical signs (coughing) vary with the severity of infection, and severe cases can be confused clinically with interstitial pneumonias. Expiratory dyspnea and death can occur with heavy infestations when there is massive obstruction of airways.

At necropsy, lesions appear as large, dark or gray, depressed, wedge-shaped areas of atelectasis present usually along the dorsocaudal aspect of the lungs. On cut surface, edematous foam and mucus mixed with white, slender (up to 80 mm long) nematodes are visible in the bronchi (see Fig. 3-16). In most severe cases, massive numbers of nematodes fill the entire bronchial tree. Microscopically, the bronchial lumen is filled with parasites admixed with mucus due to goblet cell hyperplasia and metaplasia of bronchial and bronchiolar epithelium (chronic irritation). There is also alveolar edema, hyperplasia of BALT due to persistent immunologic stimulus, hypertrophy and hyperplasia of bronchiolar smooth muscle due to increased contraction and decreased muscle relaxation, and a few eosinophilic granulomas around the eggs and dead larvae. These granulomas, grossly, are gray nodules (2 to 4 mm) and may be confused with those caused by tuberculosis.

A different form of bovine pneumonia, an acute allergic reaction known as **reinfection syndrome,** occurs when previously sensitized adult cattle are exposed to large numbers of larvae *(D. viviparus).* Lesions in this syndrome are those of a hypersensitivity pneumonia as previously described.

Ascaris suum is the common intestinal roundworm of pigs; larvae cannot complete their life cycle in calves, but, the larvae can cause severe pneumonia and death within 2 weeks if calves are housed in places where infested pigs were previously kept. Pigs, the natural host, also can be killed if exposed to an overwhelming larval migration. Clinical signs due to migration of larvae through the lungs include cough and expiratory dyspnea to the point of oral breathing. The lesions are of a diffuse interstitial pneumonia with hemorrhagic foci, atelectasis, and interlobular edema and emphysema. Microscopically, larvae are present in bronchioles and alveoli; the latter have thickened walls and contain edema fluid and cellular exudate (including eosinophils) in the lumens.

Hydatid cysts, the intermediate stage of *Echinococcus granulosus,* can be found in the lungs and other viscera of sheep and to a lesser extent in cattle, pigs, goats, horses, and human beings. The adult stage is a tapeworm that parasitizes the intestine of canidae. Hydatidosis is still an important zoonosis in some countries and perpetuation of the parasite life cycle results from close association of sheep, dogs, and consumption of uninspected meat from privately slaughtered sheep. Hydatid cysts are generally 5 to 15 cm in diameter; they have little clinical significance in animals, but are of economic importance due to carcass condemnation.

Aspiration Pneumonias of Cattle

The inhalation of regurgitated ruminal contents or iatrogenic deposition of medicines or milk into the trachea can cause a severe and often fatal **aspiration pneumonia.** Bland substances such as mineral oil may incite only a mild or suppurative or histiocytic bronchopneumonia, whereas some "home remedies" or ruminal contents may be highly irritating and cause a fibrinous, necrotizing bronchopneumonia. The right lung tends to be more severely affected since the right cranial bronchus is closest to the trachea. However, the distribution may vary when animals aspirate during prostration. In some severe cases, pulmonary necrosis can be complicated by infection with saprophytic organisms present in ruminal contents, causing fatal gangrenous pneumonia. Aspiration pneumonia should always be considered in animals with cleft palate or in those whose swallowing has been compromised because of disorders such as hypocalcemia (milk fever). On the other hand, neurologic diseases such encephalitis (e.g., rabies) or encephalopathy (e.g., lead poisoning) should be investigated in animals where the cause of aspiration pneumonia could not be explained otherwise.

Pneumonias of Sheep and Goats

Four major forms of *Pasteurella haemolytica* infection occur in sheep. Two are acute or chronic pulmonary infections and are referred to as **ovine pneumonic pasteurellosis** and **chronic enzootic pneumonia,** respectively; the third form is a systemic and often fulminating infection known as **septicemic pasteurellosis;** the fourth form affects the mammary gland causing severe **mastitis** in ewes (blue bag). These forms of pasteurellosis are generally associated with particular biotypes and serotypes of *P. haemolytica* that are usually carried in the tonsils and upper respiratory tract of normal sheep.

Ovine Pneumonic Pasteurellosis

Ovine pneumonic pasteurellosis is one of the most common and economically significant diseases in most areas where sheep are raised. It is caused by *P. haemolytica* biotype A and has pathogenetic features and lesions similar to those of pneumonic pasteurellosis of cattle. Colonization and infection of lungs are facilitated by stressors such as changes in weather, handling, deworming, dipping, and by viral infections such as PI-3 virus, RSV, adenovirus, and probably chlamydias and *Bordetella parapertussis.* Lesions are characterized by a severe fibrinous bronchopneumonia (lobar, cranioventral) (Fig. 3-41) with pleuritis. Subacute to chronic cases appear as a fibrinopurulent bronchopneumonia, and sequelae include abscesses and fibrous pleural adhesions.

Chronic Enzootic Pneumonia

In sheep, this entity is a multifactorial disease complex that, in contrast to ovine pneumonic pasteurellosis, causes only a mild to moderate pneumonia, and it is rarely fatal. It generally affects animals younger than 1 year of age. Significant costs associated with chronic enzootic pneumonia include reduction of weight gain, labor costs, veterinary fees, and slaughterhouse waste. The modifier "chronic" is used here to avoid any confusion with pneumonic pasteurellosis ("acute enzootic pneumonia").

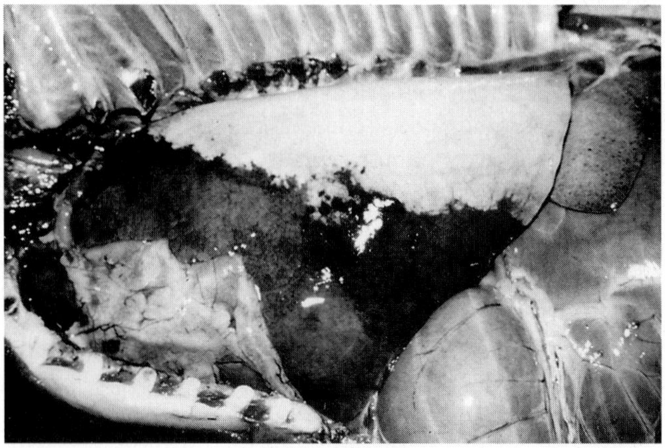

Figure 3-41 Thoracic cavity, left lung; 3-week-old lamb. Fibrinous bronchopneumonia. Pneumonic pasteurellosis *(P. haemolytica).* The cranioventral aspects of the lungs were red, swollen, and very firm with some fibrin on the pleural surface. *Courtesy of Western College of Veterinary Medicine.*

It is also sometimes called *atypical pneumonia, chronic nonprogressive pneumonia, proliferative pneumonia,* or other names.

Chronic enzootic pneumonia is a clinicoepidemiologic term and does not imply a single causal agent, but a combination of infectious, environmental, and managerial factors. The list of infectious agents involved in ovine enzootic pneumonia includes PI-3, adenovirus, reovirus, and RSV, as well as chlamydias, pasteurellae, and mycoplasmas *(M. ovipneumoniae).*

In the early stages of the disease, a cranioventral bronchointerstitial pneumonia is characterized by moderate thickening of alveolar walls due to hyperplasia of type II pneumonocytes. In some cases, it may progress to suppurative bronchopneumonia when further colonization of the lungs with secondary pathogens such as *P. multocida* takes place. One might expect some specific evidence pointing to the infectious agents (for example, large intranuclear inclusion bodies in epithelial cells with adenoviral infection), but such is often not the case, either because examination is seldom done at acute stages when the lesions are still present or because secondary bacterial infections mask the primary lesions. In the late stages, chronic enzootic pneumonia is characterized by hyperplastic bronchitis, atelectasis, alveolar and bronchiolar fibrosis, and severe peribronchial lymphoid hyperplasia (cuffing pneumonia).

Septicemic Pasteurellosis

This condition is a common ovine disease caused by *Pasteurella haemolytica* biotype T in animals 5 months or older, or by the biotype A in lambs younger than 2 months of age. Both biotypes of *P. haemolytica* are carried in the tonsils and oropharynx of normal sheep; but, under abnormal circumstances, bacteria can invade adjacent tissues, enter the bloodstream, and cause septicemia particularly in association with stresses, such as dietary or environmental changes. Affected animals die after short illness and only rarely have clinical signs such as dullness, recumbency, and dyspnea. Gross lesions include a distinctive necrotizing pharyngitis and tonsillitis, severe congestion and edema of the lungs, focal hepatic necrosis, infarcts and petechiae in tongue, esophagus, and intestine, but particularly of the lungs. Microscopically, the hallmark lesion is a disseminated intravascular thrombosis often associated with the presence of bacterial colonies in affected tissues. *P. haemolytica* is readily isolated from many organs.

Contagious Caprine Pleuropneumonia

This disease in goats is the counterpart of contagious bovine pleuropneumonia in cattle; sheep do not have a corresponding disease. The etiopathogenesis and geographic distribution of contagious caprine pleuropneumonia are yet to be determined. Three mycoplasmas, namely *M. mycoides* spp. *mycoides* large colony, *M. mycoides* spp. *capri,* and *Mycoplasma* strain F38, have all been associated with respiratory infections in goats; however, the classification of these mycoplasmas and their relation to specific diseases remain unsettled.

Caprine pleuropneumonia is important in Africa, the Middle East, and parts of Asia but is also seen elsewhere; one of the etiologic agents, *M. mycoides* spp. *mycoides* large colony, is widespread in North America, yet the actual importance of this organism as a cause of disease is unclear. Although it is unwise to speak in absolute terms when dealing with many aspects of biology, transmission from goats to sheep or cattle does not occur to any significant degree.

Clinically, the disease is similar to contagious bovine pleuropneumonia, with high morbidity and mortality, fever, cough, dyspnea, and increasing distress and debility. The gross lesions, particularly those caused by the F38 strain, are similar to the bovine disease and consist of a severe fibrinous bronchopneumonia and pleuritis; however, sequestra formation in the lungs and interlobular septal distension are less obvious than in the bovine disease. Fibrinous polyarthritis, septicemia, meningitis, mastitis, peritonitis, and abortion are other manifestations of this disease.

Other Mycoplasma Infections

The pathogenicity of other mycoplasmas such as *M. ovipneumoniae* and *M. capricolum* in sheep and goats is still being defined, and specific description of the lesions would be premature. These organisms probably cause disease only in circumstances similar to those for enzootic pneumonia, where host, infectious, and environmental factors play a complex interaction in the pathogenesis of the disease. Most recently, it has been suggested that IgG antibodies directed against unknown ovine antigens cross-react with ciliary proteins causing a condition in lambs referred to as "coughing syndrome."

Maedi (Maedi-Visna)

This entity is an important, lifelong, persistent viral disease of sheep and occurs in most countries, except Australia and New Zealand. Maedi means "shortness of breath" in the Icelandic language, and it is known locally as **Graaff-Reinet disease** in South Africa, **Zwoegerziekte** in The Netherlands, **la bouhite** in France, and **ovine (Montana** or **Marsh's) progressive pneumonia (OPP)** in the United States. More recently, the disease has also been referred to as ovine lentivirus-induced lymphoid interstitial pneumonia or simply, **lymphoid interstitial pneumonia (LIP).**

Maedi is caused by a nononcogenic retrovirus of the lentivirus subfamily (ovine lentivirus) antigenically related to the retrovirus causing caprine arthritis-encephalitis. Seroepidemiologic studies indicate that infection is widespread in the sheep population, yet the clinical disease seems to be rare. The pathogenesis is incompletely understood, but it is known that transmission occurs largely through ingestion of infected colostrum and to a lesser extent by close contact between infected and susceptible sheep. Once in the body, the ovine lentivirus remains for long periods of time within monocytes and macrophages, including alveolar and pulmonary intravascular macrophages; clinical signs do not develop until after a long incubation period of 2 years or more (slow virus infection).

Maedi is clinically characterized by dyspnea and an insidious, slowly progressive emaciation despite good appetite. Death is inevitable once clinical signs are present, but may take many months.

Pulmonary lesions are a severe interstitial pneumonia, and the lungs fail to collapse when the thorax is opened. Notable rib imprints, indicators of expanded lungs, are often present on the pleural surface. The lungs are pale and mottled (Fig. 3-42) and typically heavy (2 to 3 times normal weight), and the tracheobronchial lymph nodes are enlarged. Microscopically, the interstitial pneumonia is characterized by alveolar walls, BALT, and bronchointerstitial tissue markedly thickened due to a heavy infiltration of lymphocytes, largely T cells (Fig. 3-43). Recruitment of mononuclear cells into the pulmonary interstitium is presumably the result of sustainable production of cytokines by retrovirus-infected pulmonary macrophages and lymphocytes. Hyperplasia of type II pneumonocytes is not a prominent feature of maedi, but there is some fibrosis and smooth muscle hypertrophy in bronchioles. Secondary bacterial infections often confound the microscopic lesions of the disease. Enlargement of regional lymph nodes is due to severe lymphoid hyperplasia, primarily of B lymphocytes. The virus also can infect many other tissues, causing nonsuppurative encephalitis (visna), lymphocytic arthritis, lymphofollicular mastitis, or vasculitis.

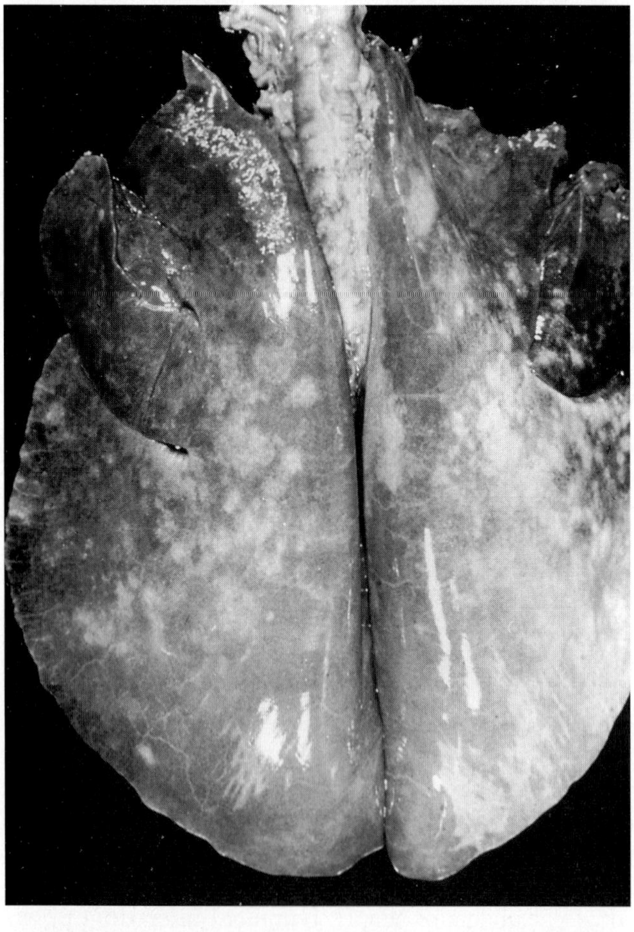

Figure 3-42 Lungs; 7-year-old ewe. Maedi (lymphoid interstitial pneumonia, lentivirus). The lungs are extremely heavy and firm. The interstitial pneumonia has a mottled pattern in all but the dorsocaudal areas, where it is diffuse. *Courtesy of Western College of Veterinary Medicine.*

Caprine Arthritis-Encephalitis (CAE)

This retroviral disease of goats (lentivirus) has a pathogenesis remarkably similar to that of maedi-visna in sheep. It was first described in the United States in the 1970s, but also occurs in Canada, Europe, Australia, and probably elsewhere. This disease has two major clinicopathologic forms: one involves the central nervous system of goat kids and young goats and is characterized by a nonsuppurative leukoencephalomyelitis; the other involves the joints of adults goats and is characterized by a chronic, nonsuppurative arthritis-synovitis. In addition, infection with CAE virus can also cause chronic lymphocytic interstitial pneumonia.

The lentivirus of CAE is closely related to the maedi-visna virus, and, in fact, cross-infection with CAE virus in sheep has been achieved experimentally. Similar

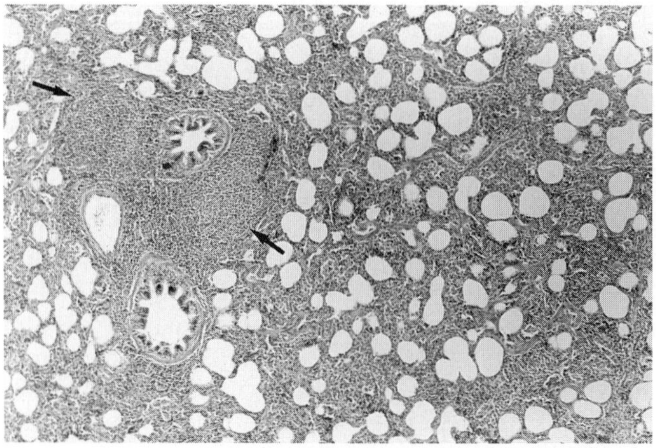

Figure 3-43 Lung; aged ewe. Maedi (lymphoid interstitial pneumonia, lentivirus). Peribronchiolar lymphoid nodules *(arrows)* are hyperplastic, and interalveolar septa are thickened by lymphocytes and other mononuclear leukocytes. H & E stain. *Courtesy of Western College of Veterinary Medicine.*

to what occurs with maedi, CAE infection presumably occurs during the first weeks of life when the doe transmits the virus to her offspring through infected colostrum or milk. Horizontal transmission between infected and susceptible goats has also been described. After coming into contact with mucosal cells at the portal of entry, the virus initially replicates in monocytes-macrophages. Infected macrophages are disseminated to the central nervous system, joints, lungs, and mammary glands. Like maedi, there is some evidence that recruitment of lymphocytic cells results from dysregulation of cytokine production by infected macrophages and lymphocytes in affected tissues. It can take several months before serum antibodies can be detected in infected goats.

Clinically, goats are active and afebrile, but progressively lose weight in spite of normal appetite. The encephalitic or arthritic signs tend to obscure the respiratory signs, which are only evident on exertion. Secondary bacterial infections are common in affected animals.

Grossly, a diffuse interstitial pneumonia tends to be most severe in the caudal lobes. The lungs are gray-pink and firm in texture with numerous, 1- to 2-mm, gray-white foci on the cut surface. The tracheobronchial lymph nodes are consistently enlarged. Microscopically, thickening of the alveolar wall is due to infiltration of lymphocytes and conspicuous hyperplasia of type II pneumonocytes. One important difference between CAE pneumonia and maedi is that pulmonary lesions in goats may be accompanied by accumulation of proteinaceous eosinophilic material in the alveoli, which in electron micrographs has structural features of pulmonary surfactant. The pulmonary form of CAE can be mistaken for parasitic pneumonia, as these two diseases share some macroscopic similarities, and the two diseases can coexist in the same goat.

Tuberculosis

This disease is uncommon in sheep and goats, but infection with *Mycobacterium bovis* or *Mycobacterium avium* does occur when the disease is prevalent in other species in the locality. The pulmonary form, similar to that seen in cattle, is characterized by a granulomatous pneumonia with multiple, large, caseous, calcified, and well-encapsulated granulomas scattered throughout the lungs. Intralesional acid-fast organisms within macrophages are not as abundant as in bovine tuberculosis.

Parasitic Pneumonias of Sheep and Goats

Dictyocaulus filaria is a serious, worldwide, parasitic disease of the lungs, most commonly of lambs and goat kids, but occurring in adults as well. The life cycle and lesions are similar to those of *Dictyocaulus viviparus* of cattle. The clinical signs (cough, moderate dyspnea, and loss of condition) and lesions relate mainly to obstruction of the small bronchi by adult worms and exudate. As seen in cattle with *D. viviparus,* areas of atelectasis and pneumonia are microscopically characterized by a catarrhal, eosinophilic bronchitis with peribronchial lymphoid hyperplasia, thickening of alveolar interstitium due to hyperplasia of type II pneumonocytes and focal infiltration of lymphocytes, and an alveolar exudation. Anemia of undetermined pathogenesis and secondary bacterial pneumonia are common in small ruminants with this parasitic disease.

Muellerius capillaris, also called the nodular lungworm, occurs in sheep and goats in most areas of the world and is the most common lung parasite of sheep in Europe and Northern Africa. It requires slugs or snails as intermediate hosts. Clinical signs are usually not apparent. The lesions in sheep are typically multifocal, subpleural nodules that tend to be most numerous in the dorsal areas of the caudal lung lobes. These nodules are soft and hemorrhagic in the early stages but, later, become gray-green and hard or even calcified. Microscopically, a focal, eosinophilic, and granulomatous reaction occurs in the subpleural alveoli where the adults, eggs, and larvae reside (Fig. 3-44).

Goats differ from sheep by having diffuse interstitial rather than focal lesions, and the reaction to the parasites seen microscopically varies from almost no lesions to a severe pneumonia with some eosinophils. Secondary effects include decreased weight gain and, possibly, secondary bacterial infections.

Protostrongylus rufescens is a worldwide parasite of sheep and goats. It requires an intermediate snail as a host. Infection is usually subclinical, but *P. rufescens* can be pathogenic for lambs and goat kids and cause anorexia, diarrhea, weight loss, and mucopurulent nasal discharge.

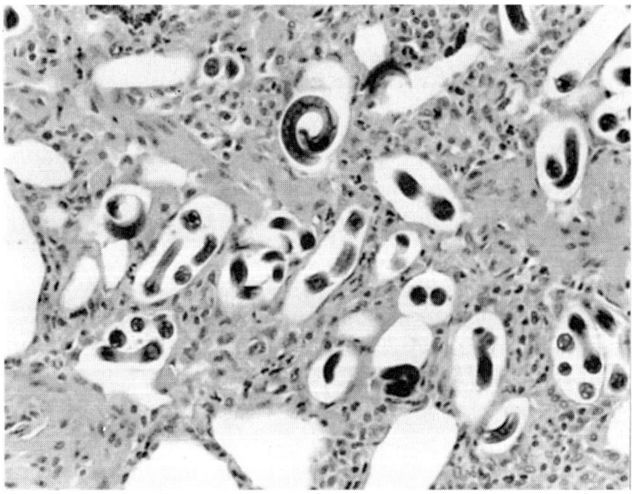

Figure 3-44 Lung; adult ewe. Granulomaotus (parasitic) pneumonia *(Mullerius capillaris).* There is notable thickening of the alveolar walls due to fibrosis, lymphoplasmacytic infiltration and smooth muscle hypertrophy. Cross-section of adults and larvae. H & E stain.

The adult parasite lives in bronchioles as *Dictyocaulus* spp. but causes pulmonary nodules similar to *Muellerius capillaris*.

Pneumonias of Pigs

Porcine pneumonias are unequivocally a major component of the problems facing the contemporary swine industry. The incidence, prevalence, and mortality rates of pneumonias in pigs are dependent on a series of complex, multifactorial interactions. Among the most commonly recognized elements linked to porcine pneumonias are host (age, genetic makeup, immune status), infectious agents (viruses, bacteria, mycoplasmas), environmental determinants (humidity, temperature, ammonia concentrations), and management practices (crowding, mixing of animals, air quality, nutrition, stress). Because of the nature of these multifactorial interactions, it will become obvious in the following paragraphs that, more often than not, a specific type of pneumonia frequently progresses to or coexists with another one.

Swine Influenza

It is generally accepted that the swine disease resulted from adaptation of the **type A influenza virus,** the cause of the human influenza pandemic during World War I. Swine influenza is enzootic worldwide and is known to infect human beings who are in close contact with sick pigs. Infection between pigs occurs mainly by aerosols or oral route; however, the virus can also be transmitted by lungworms and the common earthworm (when ingested). The infection of epithelial cells spreads throughout the respiratory tract, with the more severe outbreaks reflecting more involvement of intrapulmonary airways and secondary infection with *Pasteurella multocida, Arcanobacterium pyogenes,* or *Haemophilus* spp.

Clinically, a sudden onset of painful and often paroxysmal coughing is followed by respiratory distress, nasal discharge, high fever, stiffness, and weakness or even prostration in most or all of the herd, including animals of all age groups. The outbreak subsides virtually without mortality within a week; the clinical appearance is much more alarming than the pathologic changes, unless the pigs have secondary infection with bacteria. Infection can be confirmed using PCR in secretion collected with nasal swabs. The most important effect of most outbreaks of influenza is severe weight loss, but pregnant sows also abort or give birth to weak piglets.

Pulmonary lesions caused by influenza virus alone are rarely seen in the postmortem room since this disease has very low mortality unless complicated with secondary bacterial infections. Grossly, a copious catarrhal to mucopurulent inflammation extends from the nasal passages to the bronchioles, the volume of mucus being sufficient to plug small airways and cause a lobular or multilobular atelectasis in the cranioventral regions of the lungs. The appearance can be quite similar grossly, though not microscopically, to that of *Mycoplasma* pneumonia. Fatal cases have severe alveolar and interstitial pulmonary edema. Microscopically, the lesions in uncomplicated cases are typical of a virus-induced, necrotizing bronchitis-bronchiolitis that in severe cases extends into the alveoli as a bronchointerstitial pneumonia. It is characterized by thickening and infiltration of the alveolar wall with mononuclear cells, and aggregates of macrophages, neutrophils, mucus, and some necrotic cells within the alveolar lumen (Fig. 3-45). If these changes are extensive enough, the lumen of bronchioles can be occluded by exudate causing lobular atelectasis. Viral antigen can be demonstrated in infected epithelial cells by immunoperoxidase techniques. In the later stages of alveolar inflammation, neutrophils are progressively replaced by intraalveolar macrophages, unless the pneumonia is complicated by secondary bacterial infections. Recent serologic survey indicates that infection is also prevalent in wild pigs.

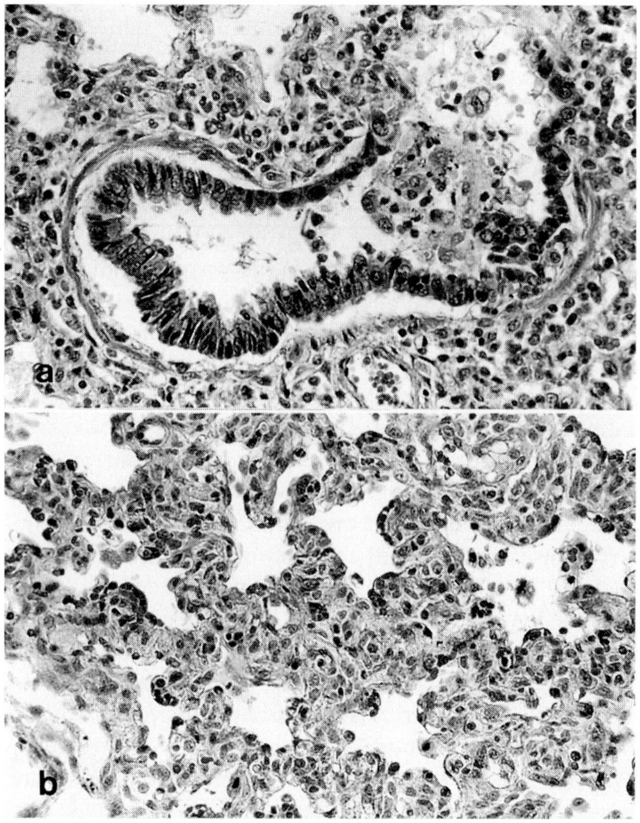

Figure 3-45 Lung; pig. Bronchointerstitial pneumonia (unidentified virus). **A,** Focal necrosis and exfoliation of bronchiolar epithelium with discrete infiltrates of mononuclear cells in the peribronchiolar interstitium. **B,** Thickening of alveolar walls by mononuclear cells and proliferating type II pneumonocytes. H & E stain. *From López et al. Can Vet J 1993; 34:622-623.*

Porcine Reproductive and Respiratory Syndrome (PRRS)

A novel disease named "mystery disease of swine" was first recognized in the United States in 1987, in 1990 it was also seen in Europe, and since then the disease has been reported in many Latin American and Asian countries. In 1991, Dutch investigators isolated a virus as the etiologic agent that is currently classified under the Arterivirus group.

As its name implies, porcine reproductive and respiratory syndrome is characterized by late-term abortions and stillbirths and respiratory problems in young pigs. The respiratory form generally seen in nursing or young pigs is clinically characterized by anorexia, dyspnea, cough, and occasional death. Some piglets develop severe cyanosis of the abdomen and ears, which explains why this syndrome when first described in Europe was named "blue ear disease." The pathogenesis has not been completely elucidated, but it is presumed there is a mucosal portal of entry with virus replication in local macrophages followed by transient viremia and finally dissemination to phagocytic cells in the lungs and other organs such as thymus, liver (Kupffer cells), spleen, all lymph nodes, and intestine. Recently, PRRS virus was added to the list of viruses known to induce apoptosis as a mechanism of cell destruction. Although clinical evidence suggests that PRRS virus also compromises the pulmonary defense mechanism, experimental studies have been inconsistent in producing dual infections with other secondary pathogens. Detection of porcine parvovirus and circovirus in pigs with PRRS has created controversy regarding the pathogenesis of this disease (see Postweaning Multisystemic Wasting Syndrome).

On postmortem examination, pulmonary lesions vary from very mild changes to failure of the lung to collapse when the thorax is opened, to consolidation in cases complicated with bacterial pneumonia. Tracheobronchial and mediastinal lymph nodes are enlarged. Microscopically, pulmonary changes are those of interstitial pneumonia characterized by thickening of alveolar walls by infiltrating of macrophages, lymphocytes, and mild hyperplasia of pneumonocytes type II. Necrotic cells are scattered in the alveolar lumens. Unlike some other viral infections, bronchiolar epithelium appears not to be affected. Diagnosis of PRRS in tissues collected at the postmortem room can be confirmed by immunohistochemistry and PCR techniques. Infected pigs may become carriers and transmit the infection through body fluids and semen.

Postweaning Multisystemic Wasting Syndrome (PMWS)

Another newly recognized porcine syndrome, clinically characterized by progressive emaciation in weaned pigs, has been recently described in Canada, United States, and Europe. Because of the clinical signs and lesions in many organs, this syndrome was named postweaning multisystemic wasting syndrome (PMWS); a porcine circovirus, alone or in combination with porcine parvovirus, has been incriminated as the etiologic agent. At necropsy, affected pigs are in poor body condition, and the most remarkable changes, not considering other possible secondary infections, are enlargement of the superficial and visceral lymph nodes and a mild interstitial pneumonia characterized by failure of the lungs to collapse when the thorax is opened. Microscopically, there is granulomatous lymphadenitis with syncytial cells and large basophilic inclusion bodies in the cytoplasm of macrophages. The lungs show thickening of the alveolar walls due to hyperplasia of type II pneumonocytes and interstitial infiltrates of mononuclear cells, some of which contain intracytoplasmic inclusion bodies. Circovirus antigen can be confirmed in affected tissues by immunohistochemical or PCR techniques.

Porcine Enzootic Pneumonia (Mycoplasmal Pneumonia of Swine)

This highly contagious disease of pigs caused by *Mycoplasma hyopneumoniae* is characterized by suppurative bronchopneumonia (see Fig. 3-25). When its worldwide prevalence and deleterious effect on feed conversion are taken into account, this disease is probably the most economically significant respiratory disease of pigs. Although an infectious disease, it is very much influenced by immune status and management factors such as crowding (airspace and floor space), ventilation (air exchange rate), concentrations of noxious gases in the air (ammonia, hydrogen sulfide), relative humidity, temperature fluctuations, and mixing of stock from various sources. It has been recently demonstrated with PCR technique that *M. hyopneumoniae* is present in the air of infected farms.

The etiology of porcine enzootic pneumonia remained unclear for many years, and so the disease was mistakenly known as "virus pneumonia of pigs" on the assumption that if the agent was hard to find it must be a virus. The causative agent, *M. hyopneumoniae,* is a fastidious organism and very difficult to grow; thus, the final diagnosis is frequently based on interpretation of lesions alone, or supported by ancillary tests directed at the detection of this mycoplasma in affected lungs by immunohistochemical, immunofluorescence, enzyme-linked immunosorbent assay (ELISA), or PCR techniques. The bronchopneumonic lesions of porcine enzootic pneumonia are, in most cases, mild to moderate, and, thus, mortality is low unless complicated with secondary pathogens such as *Pasteurella multocida, Arcanobacterium pyogenes, Bordetella bronchiseptica, Haemophilus* spp., *Mycoplasma hyorhinis,* and other mycoplasmas and ureaplasmas. Although the pathogenesis of porcine enzootic pneumonia is not completely elucidated, it is known that *M. hyopneumoniae* first adheres to the cilia of the bronchi by means of a unique adhesive protein, produces ciliostasis, and finally colonizes the respiratory system by firmly attaching to the ciliated epithelial cells of the trachea and the bronchi of the cranioventral regions of the lungs. Once attached to the respiratory epithelium, it provokes an influx of neutrophils into the tracheobronchial mucosa, causes extensive loss of cilia, stimulates an intense hyperplasia of lymphocytes in the BALT, and attracts mononuclear cells into the bronchoalveolar interstitium. Additional virulence factors include the ability of *M. hyopneumoniae* to reduce the phagocytic activity of neutrophils in the lung and change the chemical composition of mucus predisposing the lung to secondary bacterial infections.

Clinically, enzootic pneumonia occurs as a herd problem in two disease forms. A newly acquired infection of a previously clean herd causes disease in all age groups, resulting in acute respiratory distress and low mortality. In a chronically infected herd, the mature animals are immune, and clinical signs are usually apparent only in growing pigs at times of particular stress, such as at weaning. In such herds, coughing and reduced rate of gain are the most notable signs unless secondary bacterial infection causes severe bronchopneumonia.

The lesions caused by *M. hyopneumoniae* are characterized initially by a bronchointerstitial pneumonia (rarely seen at necropsy) that rapidly progresses to suppurative bronchopneumonia once secondary pathogens such as *P. multocida, B. bronchiseptica,* or *A. pyogenes* are involved (commonly seen at necropsy). In most pigs, gross lesions affect only portions of the cranial and accessory lobes, but, in more severely affected pigs, lesions involve 50% or more of the cranioventral portions of the lungs. The affected lungs are dark red in the early stages and have a homogeneous pale-gray ("fish flesh") appearance in the more chronic stages of the disease. On cut surface, exudate can easily be expressed from airways, and, depending on the stage of the lesions and secondary infections, the exudate varies from purulent to mucopurulent to mucoid. Microscopic lesions are characterized by an influx of macrophages and neutrophils into the bronchoalveolar spaces with marked peribronchial and BALT hyperplasia. In some cases, accumulation of exudate can be severe enough to cause occlusion of airways and atelectasis of neighboring lobules. The suppurative bronchopneumonia may be accompanied by a mild fibrinous pleuritis, which is often more severe if *M. hyorhinis, P. multocida,* or *Actinobacillus pleuropneumoniae* is involved concurrently. Abscesses and pleural fibrous adhesions can be long-term sequelae to chronic complicated infections.

Porcine Pasteurellosis

This infectious disease complex with unclear pathogenesis includes primary infections caused by *Pasteurella multocida* alone, or more frequently, as a secondary infection when the bacterium colonizes the lung only after the defense mechanisms are impaired (porcine pneumonic pasteurellosis). In some rare cases, *P. multocida* causes acutely fatal septicemias in pigs. Although *P. multocida* is part of the normal nasal flora, it is also an important secondary pathogen for porcine lungs, especially when defense mechanisms have been impaired by viral or mycoplasmal infections or following stress associated with poor management practices. In contrast to responses in cows, *P. haemolytica* can cause abortion in sows, but has no important role in respiratory diseases of swine.

The most common role of *P. multocida* in porcine pneumonias is its secondary involvement in porcine influenza, pseudorabies, hog cholera, enzootic pneumonia, and porcine pleuropneumonia. Secondary infections with *P. multocida* notably modify the early and mild bronchointerstitial reaction of enzootic pneumonia into a severe suppurative bronchopneumonia with multiple abscesses and sometimes pleuritis. The other important role for *P. multocida* in porcine pneumonias is as a cause of a fulminating, cranioventral, fibrinous bronchopneumonia (pleuropneumonia) without a previous mycoplasmal infection. The nature of the lesion and the predisposing factors of poor management and concurrent viral infections suggest that porcine pasteurellosis has a pathogenesis similar to that of pneumonic pasteurellosis of cattle. Pharyngitis with cervical subcutaneous edema, fibrinohemorrhagic polyarthritis, and focal nephritis are associated with porcine pneumonic pasteurellosis. Whether this disease is a separate form of pasteurellosis (septicemic) or a change to bronchopneumonia needs to be elucidated. Sequelae to porcine pneumonic pasteurellosis include fibrous pleuritis and pericarditis, pulmonary abscesses, the formation of the so-called sequestra, and, usually, death.

Porcine Pleuropneumonia

This entity is a highly contagious, worldwide disease of pigs, caused by *Actinobacillus pleuropneumoniae (Haemophilus pleuropneumoniae),* that is characterized by a severe, often fatal, fibrinous bronchopneumonia with extensive pleuritis (pleuropneumonia). Survivors generally develop notable residual lesions and become carriers of the organisms. Porcine pleuropneumonia is an increasingly important cause of acute and chronic pneumonias, particularly in intensively raised pigs (2 to 5 months old). Transmission of *A. pleuropneumoniae* occurs by the respiratory route, and the disease can be reproduced experimentally by intranasal inoculation of the bacterium. Considered as a primary pathogen, *A. pleuropneumoniae* can sporadically produce septicemia in young pigs and otitis media and interna with vestibular syndrome in weaned pigs. Twelve serotypes of the organism, most of which can cause the disease, have been identified. The pathogenesis is not yet well understood, but specific virulence factors such as capsular factors, lipopolysaccharide, hemolysins, cytotoxins, and permeability factors can damage capillaries, alveolar cells, and impair phagocytic function, resulting in vascular leakage or thrombosis and failure of clearance mechanisms.

Clinically, **porcine pleuropneumonia** can vary from an acute form with unexpected death and blood-stained froth at the nostrils and mouth to a subacute form characterized by coughing and dyspnea accompanied with clinical signs of sepsis such as high fever, hypoxemia, anorexia, and lethargy. A chronic form is characterized by decreased growth rate and persistent cough. Animals that survive often carry the organism in the tonsils, shed the organism, and infect susceptible pigs.

The gross lesions in the acute and subacute forms consist of a fibrinous bronchopneumonia characterized by severe consolidation and a fibrinous exudate on the pleural surface. Although all lobes can be affected, a common site is the dorsal area of the caudal lobes (Fig. 3-46). In fact, a large area of fibrinous pleuropneumonia involving the caudal lobe of a pig's lung is considered almost pathognomonic for this disease. On the cut surface, consolidated lungs have markedly dilated interlobular septa and irregular, but well-circumscribed areas of coagulative necrosis caused by potent cytotoxins produced by *A. pleuropneumoniae.* Except for the distribution, pulmonary lesions of porcine pleuropneumonia are identical to those of pneumonic pasteurellosis of cattle. The microscopic lesions are also very similar to those of bovine pneumonic pasteurellosis and include areas of necrosis surrounded by a thick cluster of "streaming (oat-shaped) leukocytes," and a notable distension of the interlobular septa due to severe edema and lymph vessel thrombosis. Pigs with the chronic form have multiple pulmonary abscesses and large pieces of necrotic lung encapsulated by connective tissue (sequestra). These sequestra and abscesses result in an occasional abortion, and a high incidence of pleural fibrous adhesions at slaughter.

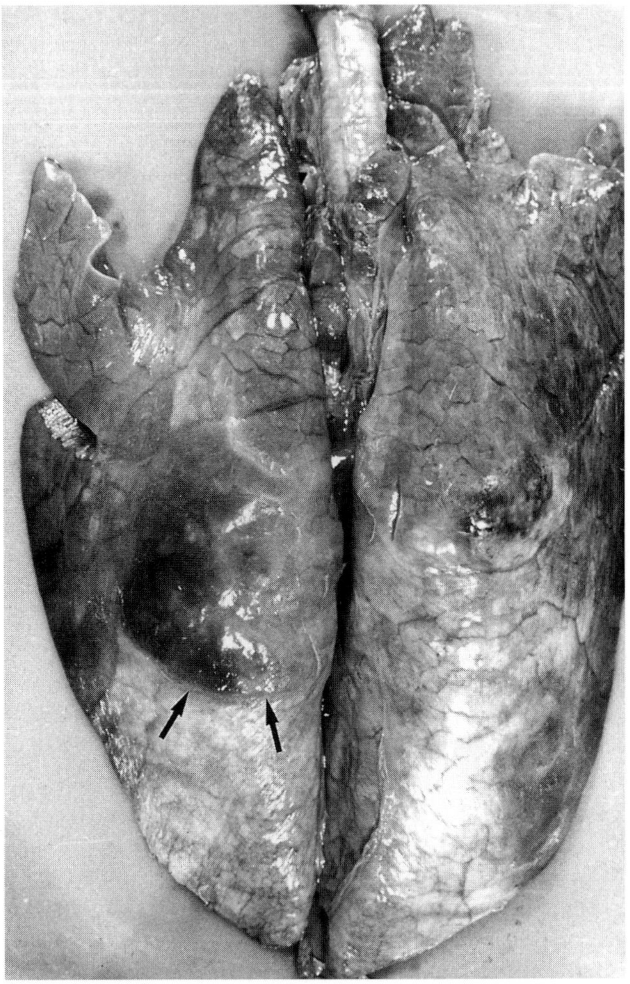

Figure 3-46 Lungs; 4-month-old pig. Porcine pleuropneumonia *(Actinobacillus pleuropneumoniae).* Note the large focus of hemorrhagic necrotizing fibrinous bronchopneumonia involving the dorsal aspect of the left caudal lobe *(arrows).* This dorsocaudal location is typical of porcine pleuropneumonia. *Courtesy of Western College of Veterinary Medicine.*

Haemophilus Pneumonia

In addition to **polyserositis and polyarthritis (Glasser's disease),** some serotypes of *Haemophilus parasuis* (originally, *H. suis*) can also cause pulmonary infections characterized by a suppurative bronchopneumonia that, in some severe cases, can be fatal. The causal organism, *H. parasuis,* is usually carried in the nasopharynx of normal pigs and requires abnormal circumstances such as those following stress (weaning, cold weather) or viral infections (e.g., swine influenza) to cause pulmonary infection. Specific pathogen–free (SPF) pigs seem to be particularly susceptible to Glasser's disease (arthritis and serositis) but not to pulmonary infection (bronchopneumonia).

Streptococcal Pneumonia

***Streptococcus suis* type II,** a pathogen that produces lesions in several body systems, has been a problem in Europe for two decades, and is of increasing concern in North America. It is a serious zoonosis capable of causing death by septic shock or meningitis and residual deafness in survivors; butchers and pig farmers are particularly at risk. In pigs, *S. suis* type II may be carried in the nasal cavity, tonsils, and mandibular lymph nodes of healthy animals, particularly in survivors in the aftermath of an outbreak, while sows can vertically transmit the infections to their offspring. Some serotypes of *S. suis* (type I) are associated with neonatal septicemia, and this can result in meningitis, arthritis, polyserositis, myocarditis, abortion, valvular endocarditis, and embolic pneumonia. Other serotypes may reach the lung by the aerogenous route and cause suppurative bronchopneumonia, generally in combination with *Pasteurella multocida* and *Escherichia coli.* It can also produce fibrinous bronchopneumonia when *S.*

suis infection occurs in combination with *Actinobacillus pleuropneumonia*.

Tuberculosis

Tuberculosis is an important disease in pigs, which, in many countries, including those in North America, has a much greater prevalence in pigs than in cattle or other domestic mammals. Because pigs are susceptible to *Mycobacterium avium, Mycobacterium bovis,* and *Mycobacterium tuberculosis,* the incidence of porcine tuberculosis in a geographic region reflects what is occurring in the poultry, cattle, and human populations. A common scenario in small mixed-farming operations is the diagnosis of avian tuberculosis at the time that pigs are slaughtered, the source being ingestion of tuberculous chickens or contaminated litter. Tuberculous granulomas generally involve the mandibular and mesenteric lymph nodes, to a lesser extent the intestine, liver, and spleen, and only in rare cases the lung. The route of infection in pulmonary tuberculosis of pigs is most often hematogenous after oral exposure and intestinal infection. The microscopic lesions are basically those of tubercles, but the degree of encapsulation, caseation, and calcification vary with the type of mycobacterium, age of the lesion, and host immune response.

Other Infectious Pneumonias of Pigs

Porcine respiratory coronavirus (PRCV) is sporadically incriminated in pneumonia in pigs. This viral pneumonia is generally mild, and most pigs fully recover if the pneumonia is not complicated with other infections. **Septicemias** often cause petechiae and pulmonary edema, and these features may be a part of African swine fever, hog cholera, pseudorabies, and other diseases. Salmonellae, *Escherichia coli,* and *Listeria monocytogenes* can cause severe interstitial pneumonia as part of a septicemic process in very young animals. *Salmonella choleraesuis* causes a necrotizing fibrinous pneumonia, and *Salmonella typhisuis,* a chronic suppurative bronchopneumonia.

Foreign body granulomatous pneumonia occurs frequently in pigs following inhalation of vegetable material (starch pneumonia), presumably from dusty (nonpelleted) feed. Lesions are clinically silent but are often mistaken for other pneumonic processes during inspection at slaughter houses. Microscopically, pulmonary changes are typical of foreign body granulomatous inflammation in which variably sized feed particles are surrounded by macrophages and neutrophils, and often are found in multinucleated giant cells.

Parasitic Pneumonias of Pigs

Metastrongylus apri (elongatus), M. salmi, and *M. pudendotectus* (lungworms) of domestic and feral pigs occur throughout most of the world and require earthworms as intermediate hosts for transmission. Lungworms may transmit the virus of swine influenza. The importance of swine lungworms is mainly due to growth retardation of the host. Clinical signs include coughing due to parasitic bronchitis.

The gross lesions, when noticeable, consist of small gray nodules, particularly along the ventral borders of the caudal lobes. The adult worms are grossly visible in bronchioles and small bronchi and cause a catarrhal inflammation with infiltration of eosinophils and lobular atelectasis (Fig. 3-47).

During migration through the lungs of pigs, larvae of *Ascaris suum* can cause edema, focal subpleural hemorrhages, and interstitial inflammation (Fig. 3-48). Hemorrhages also occur in the liver, and after fibrosis they become the large, white "milk spots" seen so frequently as

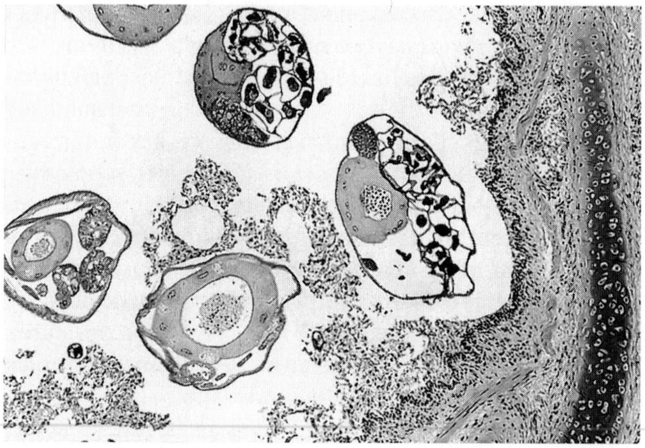

Figure 3-47 Lung; pig. Verminous pneumonia. Cross-section of bronchus with nematode parasites *(Metastrongylus apri)* admixed with mucus, neutrophils and eosinophils. H & E stain.

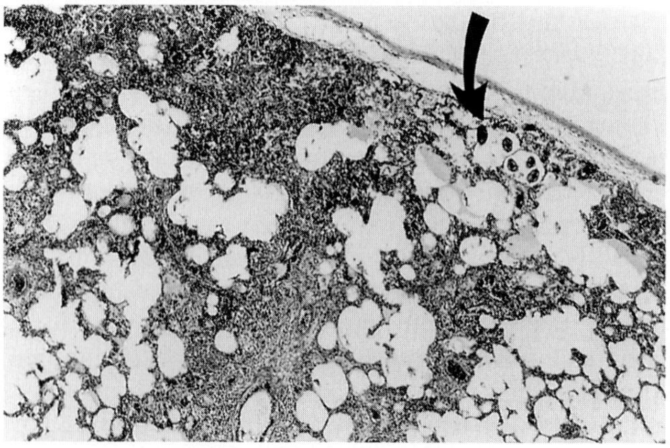

Figure 3-48 Lung; pig. Larva migrans. Cross sections of *Ascaris suum* larvae *(arrows)* are located subpleurally and have caused focal hemorrhage and interstitial inflammation. H & E stain. *Courtesy of Western College of Veterinary Medicine.*

incidental findings at necropsy. It has recently been reported that *A. suum* may cause immunosuppression in severely affected pigs.

Pneumonias of Dogs

In general, inflammatory diseases of the lungs are less of a problem in dogs than in food-producing species and could be subdivided in two major groups, infectious and noninfectious pneumonias. Of the infectious causes, two account for most cases: infectious tracheobronchitis (kennel cough), which was discussed previously, and canine distemper. Uremia and paraquat toxicity are perhaps the two most notable noninfectious causes of pulmonary disease in dogs.

Canine Distemper

Canine distemper is an important and ubiquitous infectious disease of dogs, other canidae, wild felidae, mustelidae, and marine mammals around the world. It is caused by a morbillivirus that is antigenically related to the human measles, rinderpest, and "peste de petit ruminants" viruses. Distemper virus invades through the upper respiratory tract, proliferates in all lymphoid tissues, becomes viremic, and, in dogs with an inadequate antibody response, infects nearly all body tissues (pantropic), particularly the epithelial cells. During viremia, distemper virus hampers the immune response and appears to down-regulate cytokine production. This virus can target the lungs either directly as a viral pneumonia or by its immunosuppressive effects rendering the lungs susceptible to secondary bacterial infections. Clinical signs consist of biphasic fever, diarrhea, vomiting, weight loss, mucopurulent oculonasal discharge, coughing, respiratory distress, and possible loss of vision. Weeks later, hyperkeratosis of foot pads ("hard pad") and nose are observed, along with nervous signs including ataxia, paralysis, convulsions, or residual myoclonus (muscle twitches, tremors, "tics").

Gross lesions in the acute stages include serous to catarrhal to mucopurulent nasopharyngitis and conjunctivitis. The lungs are edematous and have a diffuse interstitial pneumonia microscopically characterized by necrotizing bronchiolitis, necrosis and exfoliation of pneumonocytes, mild alveolar edema, and several hours later, thickening of the alveolar walls due to interstitial mononuclear cells infiltrates and hyperplasia of type II pneumonocytes. Secondary infections with *Bordetella bronchiseptica* and mycoplasmas are common and induce life-threatening suppurative bronchopneumonia. The thymus may be small relative to the age of the animal due to viral-induced lympholysis. Microscopically, eosinophilic inclusions are present in the epithelial cells of many tissues, in the nuclei or cytoplasm, or in both. They appear early in the bronchiolar epithelium, but are most prominent in the epithelium of the stomach, renal pelvis, and urinary bladder, making these tissues good choices for diagnostic examination. The suppurative secondary bronchopneumonias often hinder the detection of viral lesions in the lung, particularly bronchiolar necrosis and inclusion bodies. Distemper virus antigens can be readily demonstrated in infected cells by the immunoperoxidase technique.

Distemper virus also has a tendency to affect developing tooth buds and ameloblasts, causing enamel hypoplasia in dogs that recover from infection. Of all distemper lesions, demyelinating encephalomyelitis, which develops late, is the most devastating (see Diseases of the Nervous System). Sequelae to distemper include the nervous and pneumonic complications mentioned previously and such various systemic infections as toxoplasmosis. Persistent viral infection occurs in some animals that survive the disease.

Canine Adenovirus Type 2 (CAV-2) Infection

This entity is a common and contagious disease of the respiratory tract of dogs, causing mild fever, oculonasal discharge, coughing, and poor weight gain. Pulmonary lesions are initially those of a bronchointerstitial pneumonia, with necrosis and exfoliation of bronchiolar and alveolar epithelium and edema, and a few days later, proliferation of type II pneumonocytes, mild infiltration of neutrophils and lymphocytes in alveolar interstitium, and hyperplastic bronchitis and bronchiolitis. Large basophilic intranuclear viral inclusions are typically seen in bronchiolar and alveolar epithelial cells. The disease is sometimes associated with the infectious tracheobronchitis complex (kennel cough) and occasionally can coexist with distemper. It is clinically mild unless complicated with a secondary bacterial infection. Experimental work suggests CAV-2 reinfection may lead to hyperreactive airways. However, it is not clear if this outcome is true in natural infections.

Canine Herpesvirus 1 (CH-1)

This viral infection can cause fatal generalized disease in newborn puppies, and it is probably part of the variety of factors that result in the "fading puppy syndrome." Hypothermia has been suggested as a pivotal component in the pathogenesis of fatal infections in puppies. CH-1 also causes necrotizing rhinotracheitis and secondary bronchopneumonia in older animals. Many dogs are seropositive, suggesting that transient or subclinical infections are more common than realized; the virus remains latent and can be reactivated following stress, resulting in asymptomatic transmission of CH-1 virus to offspring via the placenta resulting in abortion or stillbirths. Distemper virus is also transmitted to susceptible puppies through infective body fluids.

Bacterial Pneumonias of Dogs

Dogs generally have bacterial pneumonias when the pulmonary defense mechanisms have been impaired.

Pasteurella multocida, Streptococcus spp., *Escherichia coli, Klebsiella pneumoniae,* and *Bordetella bronchiseptica* can be involved in pneumonia secondary to distemper or after aspiration of gastric contents. *Streptococcus zooepidemicus* also causes acute and fatal hemorrhagic pleuropneumonia with hemorrhagic pleural effusion in dogs. Death is generally a consequence of generalized septic embolism and affects the lungs, liver, brain, and lymph nodes, but, often, the primary source of the infection cannot be determined. Dental disease in dogs may be a source of systemic and pulmonary infection, which is not a new concept as human medicine has recognized it for many years. The role of **mycoplasmas** in canine pneumonia is still unclear as generally these organisms are isolated along with other bacterial pathogens or are part of the normal nasopharyngeal flora.

Tuberculosis is uncommon in dogs. Dogs appear to be quite resistant to infection; most cases occur in immunocompromised dogs or dogs with a familial defect in cell-mediated immunity (e.g., basset hounds). Dogs are susceptible to the *M. tuberculosis, M. bovis,* and *M. avium* strains, and therefore canine infection presupposes contact with human or animal tuberculosis. The clinicopathologic manifestation is pulmonary after inhalation or alimentary after oral exposure, but in most cases infection is disseminated to lymph nodes and visceral organs. The gross pulmonary lesions are multifocal, firm, usually calcified nodules with necrotic centers, most often in the caudal lung lobes. Diffuse granulomatous pleuritis and pericarditis with copious serofibrinous or sanguineous effusion are common.

Mycotic Pneumonias of Dogs

These are serious diseases seen commonly in animals in some areas. There are two main types: those caused by opportunistic fungi and those caused by a group of fungi associated with systemic "deep" mycoses. All these fungi affect human beings and most domestic animals but are probably not transmitted between species.

Opportunistic fungi, such as *Aspergillus fumigatus,* are important in birds, but in domestic animals they mainly affect immunosuppressed animals or those animals on prolonged antibiotic therapy. The pulmonary lesion is a focal, nodular, pyogranulomatous, or granulomatous pneumonia. Microscopically, the fungal hyphae are present, and there is usually necrosis, vasculitis, infiltrations of neutrophils, macrophages, lymphocytes, and fibroblasts, eventually leading to the formation of granulomas.

Systemic (deep) mycoses are caused by *Blastomyces dermatitidis, Histoplasma capsulatum, Coccidioides immitis,* and *Cryptococcus neoformans* (Fig. 3-35). Blastomycosis mainly affects dogs and is discussed here, whereas cryptococcosis is discussed in the section Pneumonias of Cats. In contrast to other fungi such as *Aspergillus* sp., organisms of the systemic mycosis group are all primary pathogens of human beings and animals and, thus, do not necessarily require a preceding immunosuppression in order to cause disease. These fungi posses virulence factors that favor hematogenous dissemination and evasion of immune and phagocytic responses. In general, cytologic examination of affected tissues is very rewarding in the antemortem diagnosis of all systemic mycoses.

Blastomycosis occurs in many countries of the American continent, Africa, and the Middle East and occasionally in Europe. In the United States, it is most prevalent in the Atlantic, St. Lawrence, and Ohio-Mississippi River Valley states as compared with the Mountain-Pacific region. *B. dermatitidis* is a dimorphic fungus (mycelia-yeast) seen mainly in young dogs and occasionally in cats (Fig. 3-35). This fungus is present in the soil, and inhalation of spores is considered the principal route of infection, thus most frequently affects outdoor and hunting dogs. From the lung, infection is disseminated hematogenously to other organs. Clinical signs can reflect involvement of virtually any body tissue; pulmonary effects include cough, decreased exercise tolerance, and terminal respiratory distress. Pulmonary lesions are characterized by a granulomatous pneumonia, generally with multiple firm nodules (pyogranulomas) scattered throughout the lungs (Fig. 3-34). Microscopically, nodules are granulomas with numerous macrophages (epitheliod cells), some neutrophils, multinucleated giant cells, and thick-walled yeasts (Fig. 3-35). Yeasts are 5 to 25 μm in diameter and are much better visualized when tissue sections are stained with PAS or Gomori's methenamine silver stain. Nodules can also be present in other tissues, chiefly lymph nodes, skin, spleen, liver, kidneys, bones, testes, prostate, and eyes. This fungus can be easily identified in properly prepared and stained transtracheal washes or aspirates of affected lymph nodes.

Coccidioidomycosis (San Joaquin Valley Fever), caused by the dimorphic fungus *Coccidioides immitis,* occurs mainly in animals living in arid regions of the southwestern United States and Central and South America (Fig. 3-35). It is a primary respiratory tract (aerogenous) infection seen commonly at slaughter in clinically normal feedlot cattle. In dogs, coccidioidomycosis is generally systemic and clinical signs relate to the location of lesions, so there can be respiratory distress, lameness, generalized lymphadenopathy, or cutaneous lesions, among others. Again, the lesions are focal granulomas or pyogranulomas that can have suppurative or caseated centers. The fungal organisms are readily seen in histologic or cytologic preparation as small spores or large spherules from 10 to 80 μm in diameter (Fig. 3-35).

Histoplasmosis is a systemic infection that results from inhalation of another dimorphic fungus, *Histoplasma capsulatum* (Fig. 3-35). Histoplasmosis occurs sporadically in dogs and human beings, and to a lesser extent, in cats and horses. Bat and bird droppings appear to promote its growth and survival in the soil of enzootic areas. Pulmonary lesions are grossly characterized by variably sized, firm, well-encapsulated granulomas, and, sometimes, more diffuse involvement of the lungs. Microscopically, granulomatous tissue typically has many macrophages filled with small (1 to 3 μm), punctiform, intracytoplasmic dark bodies (yeasts), best demonstrated with PAS or Gomori methenamine silver stains (Fig. 3-35) Similar nodules can be present in other tissues, chiefly lymph nodes, spleen, intestines, and liver.

Aspiration Pneumonia

This disease is an important form of pneumonia in dogs when vomited, or regurgitated materials are aspirated into the lungs or when drugs or radiographic contrast media is accidentally introduced into the airways. As in other animal species, aspiration pneumonia may be unilateral or affecting more severely the right cranial lobe. The severity of lesions depends very much on the chemical and microbiologic composition of the aspirated material. In general, aspiration in monogastric animals, particularly in dogs and cats, is more severe because of the low pH of the gastric contents (chemical pneumonitis). In severe cases, dogs die acutely from septic shock (ARDS), whereas in chronic cases lesions progress into bronchopneumonia. Aspiration pneumonia is a common sequela to cleft palate, and megaesophagus in dogs with myasthenia gravis and persistent right aortic arch. It is also an important anesthetic complication.

Toxic Pneumonias

Paraquat, a broad-spectrum herbicide widely used in gardening and agriculture, can cause severe and often fatal toxic interstitial pneumonia (pneumonitis) in dogs, cats, human beings, and other species. Following ingestion or inhalation, paraquat metabolites promote local release of free radicals, which cause extensive injury to the air-blood barrier, presumably through lipid peroxidation of type I and II pneumonocytes and alveolar endothelial cells. Paraquat toxicity has been used experimentally as a model of oxidant-induced alveolar injury and pulmonary fibrosis. Soon after poisoning, the lungs are heavy, edematous, and hemorrhagic due to extensive necrosis of alveolar epithelial and endothelial cells. The lungs of animals that survive acute paraquat toxicosis become pale, fail to collapse when the thorax is opened, and have interstitial emphysema, bullous emphysema, and pneumomediastinum. Microscopic findings in the acute and subacute phases include necrosis of type I pneumonocytes, interstitial and alveolar edema, intraalveolar hemorrhages, and proliferation of type II pneumonocytes. In the chronic stages (4 to 8 weeks later), the lesions are typically characterized by severe interstitial and intraalveolar fibrosis.

Uremic pneumonopathy (pneumonitis) is one of the many nonrenal lesions seen in dogs with chronic uremia.

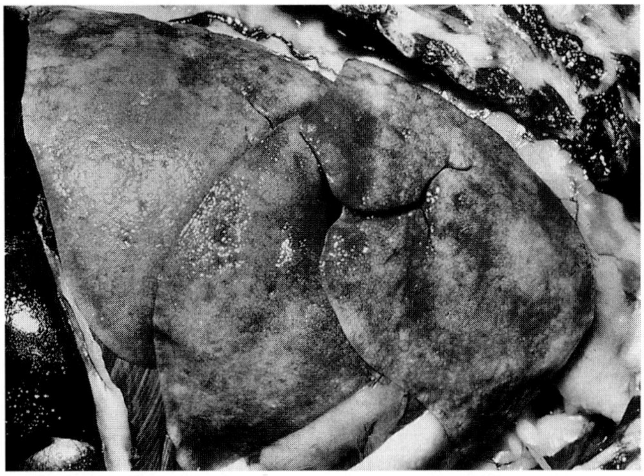

Figure 3-49 Lung; dog. Uremic pneumopathy from chronic renal failure. The lungs of this dog failed to collapse when the thorax was opened due to extensive calcification of alveolar walls.

Lesions are characterized by a combination of pulmonary alveolar edema and calcification of vascular smooth muscle. In severe cases, calcification involving the alveolar walls prevents lung collapse when the thorax is opened. Grossly, the lungs appear diffusely distended, pink or red in color, and show a rough pleural surface with rib imprints (Fig. 3-49). On palpation, the pulmonary parenchyma has a typical "gritty" texture due to mineralization of the alveolar and vascular walls. Since this is not primarily an inflammatory lesion, the term pneumonitis should be avoided.

Parasitic Pneumonias of Dogs

Toxoplasmosis is a worldwide disease caused by an obligate intracellular, protozoal parasite *Toxoplasma gondii.* Cats and other felidae are the definitive host where the mature parasite divides sexually in the intestinal mucosa. Human beings, dogs, cats, and many wild mammals can become intermediate hosts following accidental ingestion of fertile oocysts shed in cat feces, or fetuses can be infected transplacentally. In most instances, the parasite infects many cells of different tissues, induces an antibody response (seropositive animals), but does not cause clinical disease. Toxoplasmosis is often triggered by immunosuppression, such as that caused by canine distemper virus. Toxoplasmosis is characterized by necrosis. Pulmonary lesions are severe, multifocal necrotizing interstitial pneumonia with notable proliferation of type II pneumonocytes and infiltrates of macrophages and neutrophils. Other lesions in disseminated toxoplasmosis include focal necrotizing hepatitis, myocarditis, splenitis, myositis, encephalitis, and ophthalmitis. The parasites appear microscopically as small (3 to 6 μm) basophilic cysts that can be found free in affected tissues or within the cytoplasm of many epithelial cells and macrophages.

Pneumocystis carinii has also been reported as a sporadic cause of chronic interstitial pneumonia in dogs with a compromised immune system (see Equine Pneumonias).

Filaroides hirthi, a lungworm of the alveoli and bronchioles of dogs, has long been known as a cause of mild subclinical infection in large colonies of beagle dogs in the United States. However, it can on occasion cause severe and even fatal disease in individual pets, presumably as result of immunosuppression. Clinical signs may include coughing and terminal respiratory distress. Grossly, the lesions are multifocal subpleural nodules, often with a green hue due to eosinophils, scattered throughout the lungs. Microscopically, these nodules are eosinophilic granulomas associated with larvae or dead worms, as little reaction develops to the live adults.

Crenosoma vulpis is a lungworm seen in dogs and foxes with access to the intermediate hosts, slugs and snails. The adults live in small bronchi and bronchioles, causing eosinophilic, catarrhal bronchitis-bronchiolitis manifested grossly as gray areas of inflammation and atelectasis in the caudal lobes.

Paragonimus kellicotti in North America and *P. westermanii* in Asia are generally asymptomatic fluke infections in fish-eating species; cats and dogs acquire it in North America by eating crayfish. Gross lesions include pleural hemorrhages when the metacercariae migrate into the lungs. Later, multifocal eosinophilic pleuritis and cysts up to 7 mm long, containing pairs of adult flukes, are found along with eosinophilic granulomas around clusters of eggs. Like many other parasitic pneumonias, lesions and scars are more frequent in the caudal lubes. Pneumothorax can occur if a cyst that communicates with an airway ruptures to the pleural surface.

Angiostrongylus vasorum and *Dirofilaria immitis* are parasites of the vascular system and depending on the stage, can produce different forms of pulmonary lesions. Adult parasites can cause chronic arteritis that leads to pulmonary hypertension, pulmonary eosinophilia, congestive right cardiac failure, and eventually caudal vena caval syndrome. Other lesions include pleural petechiae, interstitial fibrosis, diffuse hemosiderosis, and multifocal pulmonary infarcts. Larvae cause alveolar injury, which leads to thickening of the alveolar walls with eosinophils and lymphocytes (interstitial pneumonia), and alveolar rupture and release of eggs into the alveoli producing multifocal granulomatous pneumonia.

Pneumonias of Cats

Although upper respiratory tract infections are common and important in cats, pneumonias are uncommon except when there is immunosuppression. Viral infections such as *feline rhinotracheitis* and *calicivirus* may cause lesions in the lungs, but, unless there is secondary invasion by bacteria, they do not usually pose a problem (see Specific Diseases of the Nasal Cavity, Feline Diseases).

Feline Pneumonitis

This mild, subclinical bronchointerstitial pneumonia is caused by *Chlamydia psittaci (felis).* The term "feline pneumonitis" is a misnomer since the major lesions from chlamydial infections are a severe conjunctivitis and rhinitis (see Nasal Cavity and Sinuses), but pneumonia is mild. The elucidation of the importance of feline viral rhinotracheitis and feline calicivirus has removed *Chlamydia* from its previously overstated importance.

Bacterial Pneumonias

Bacteria from the nasal flora such as *Pasteurella multocida* and *Pasteurella*-like organisms are occasionally associated with secondary bronchopneumonias in cats (Fig. 3-50). *P. multocida* also causes otitis media and meningitis, but its role as a respiratory pathogen is mainly associated with pyothorax. Interestingly, there are reports of *P. multocida* pneumonia in older or immunosuppressed human beings acquired through contact with domestic cats. Mycoplasmas are often isolated from the lungs of cats with

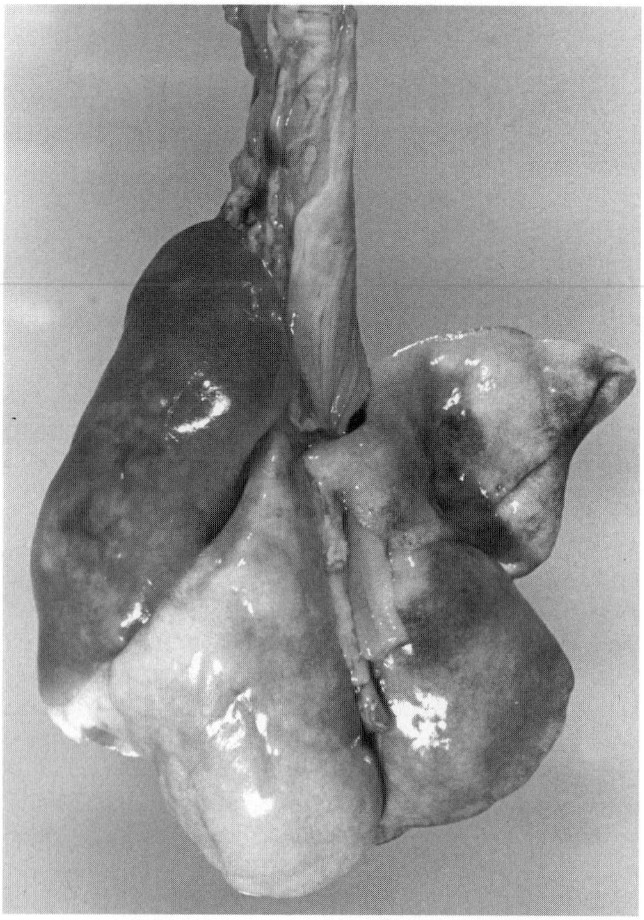

Figure 3-50 Lungs; 5-month-old kitten with history of conjunctivitis, rhinitis, and bacterial pneumonia. Fibrinopurulent bronchopneumonia. Cranioventral consolidation of the lungs involves around 40% of lung parenchyma.

pulmonary diseases, but are not definitively established as primary pathogens in feline pneumonias.

Cats are susceptible to three types of mycobacterial infections: classical tuberculosis, feline leprosy, and atypical mycobacteriosis. Classical tuberculosis in cats is generally caused by *M. bovis,* but *M. tuberculosis* and *M. avium* are sporadically involved. The usual route of infection for feline tuberculosis is oral, through infected milk, so the lesions are mainly in the alimentary tract from where they may disseminate to other organs. The gross appearance of tuberculous nodules is similar to that of neoplasms, so they must be differentiated from pulmonary neoplasms (e.g., lymphosarcoma). Classic tuberculosis with dermal lesions in cats should be differentiated from feline leprosy (localized skin granulomas) caused by *M. lepraemurium* and other nonculturable species of acid-fast bacilli and from atypical mycobacteriosis caused by contamination of a skin wound with saprophytic mycobacteria. Advances in PCR techniques have notably reduced the time required for diagnosis of mycobacteriosis in veterinary diagnostic laboratories.

Mycotic Pneumonias

Cryptococcosis (pulmonary *Cryptococcus neoformans*) is the most frequent systemic mycosis in cats, and lesions are akin to those discussed under Pneumonias of Dogs, Mycotic Pneumonias. It occurs worldwide in all species but is diagnosed most frequently in cats, horses, dogs, and human beings. Some dogs and cats are asymptomatic carriers of *C. neoformans*. Animals that are compromised immunologically, such as by feline leukemia virus infection, malnutrition, or corticosteroid treatment, are most susceptible to clinical infection.

Lesions can occur in nearly any tissue, resulting in a wide variety of clinical signs. However, granulomatous rhinitis, sinusitis, pneumonia, ulcerative dermatitis, and meningoencephalitis are common. The pulmonary lesion is a multifocal granulomatous pneumonia and, as with those occurring in other internal organs, has the appearance of small, gelatinous, white foci. The gelatinous appearance is due to the wide mucous capsule around the yeast (4 to 10 μm). Lesions caused by *C. neoformans* contain great numbers of fungi and only a few macrophages, lymphocytes, and multinucleated giant cells. This fungus has a typical thick polysaccharides capsule, which does not stain well on routine histological preparations, leaving a large empty space or halo around the yeast (Fig. 3-35).

Other Pneumonias of Cats

Endogenous Lipid (Lipoid) Pneumonia. This condition is an obscure, subclinical pulmonary disease of cats and occasionally of dogs, which is unrelated to aspiration of foreign material. Although the pathogenesis is not understood, it is presumed that lipids from pulmonary surfactant and from degenerated cells accumulate within alveolar macrophages. The gross lesions are multifocal, white, firm nodules scattered throughout the lungs. Microscopically, the alveoli are filled with foamy, lipid-laden macrophages accompanied by interstitial infiltration of lymphocytes and plasma cells, fibrosis, and alveolar epithelialization.

Lipid (lipoid) pneumonia occurs frequently in the vicinity of cancerous lung lesions in human beings, cats, and dogs. The reason for this association remains enigmatic and frequently unrecognized by pathologists. Recent investigations suggest that lipids are the breakdown products of neoplastic cells.

Exogenous Lipid Pneumonia. Another form of lipid pneumonia occurs accidentally in cats given mineral oil by their owners in attempts to remove hairballs.

Aspiration Pneumonias. This condition is common in cats as a result of vomiting, regurgitation, dysphagia, anesthetic complication, or following accidental administration of food, oral medicaments, or contrast media into the trachea (iatrogenic); pulmonary lesions are similar to those described for dogs (see Aspiration Pneumonia of Dogs).

Parasitic Pneumonias. *Aelurostrongylus abstrusus,* known as "feline lungworm," is a parasite that occurs in cats wherever the necessary slug and snail intermediate hosts are found. It can cause chronic respiratory disease with coughing and weight loss and, sometimes, severe dyspnea and death, particularly if there are secondary bacterial infections. The gross lesions are multifocal, amber, subpleural nodules up to 1 cm in diameter throughout the lungs. On incision, these granulomatous nodules typically contain eggs, larvae, and turbid, viscous exudate. Microscopically, the parasites and their eggs and larvae are in the bronchioles and alveoli where they cause catarrhal bronchiolitis, hyperplasia of submucosal glands, granulomatous alveolitis, alveolar fibrosis, and fibromuscular hyperplasia. During routine examination of feline lungs, it is quite common to find fibromuscular hyperplasia of bronchioles, alveoli, and arterioles, presumably the long-term sequela of this pulmonary nematode in otherwise normal cats.

Toxoplasma gondii, Paragonimus kellicotti, and *Dirofilaria immitis* can also affect cats (see Parasitic Pneumonias under Pneumonias of Dogs).

Fetal and Perinatal Pneumonias

Fetal Pneumonias

Pneumonia is one of the most frequent lesions found in fetuses submitted for postmortem examination, particularly in foals and food-producing animals. Because of autolysis, lack of inflation, and the lungs being at various stages of development, lesions are often missed or misdiagnosed. In the nonaerated fetal lung, the bronchoalveolar spaces are filled with a viscous, locally produced fluid known as "lung fluid" or "lung liquid." It has been estimated that each hour an ovine fetus produces about 2.5 ml of "lung fluid" per kilogram of body weight. In the fetus, this fluid normally moves along the tracheobronchial tree, reaching the oropharynx, and is swallowed or discharged into the amniotic fluid. At the time of birth the "lung fluid" is rapidly reabsorbed from the lungs by the pulmonary lymph vessels and by alveolar absorption.

Aspiration of amniotic fluid contaminated with meconium and bacteria is the most common route by which microbial pathogens reach the fetal lungs. This form of pneumonia is secondary to fetal hypoxia and acidosis ("fetal distress") that cause the fetus to relax the anal sphincter, release meconium into amniotic fluid, and, in the terminal stages, inspire deeply with open glottis, resulting in the aspiration of contaminated fluid. Gross lesions are only occasionally recognized, but microscopic changes are similar to those of a bronchopneumonia. Microscopically, bronchoalveolar spaces contain variable numbers of neutrophils, macrophages, and pieces of meconium that appear as bright yellow material because of its bile content. In contrast to postnatal bronchopneumonia, lesions in fetuses are not restricted to the cranioventral aspects of the lungs, but involve all pulmonary lobes.

In cattle, *Brucella abortus* and *Arcanobacterium (Actinomyces) pyogenes* are two of the most common bacteria isolated from the lungs of aborted fetuses. These bacteria are usually present in large numbers in the amniotic fluid of cows with bacterial placentitis. Inflammation of the placenta interferes with oxygen exchange between fetal and maternal tissues, inducing fetal hypoxia and predisposing the fetus to "breathe" with an open glottis inside the amniotic sac. Aspiration of amniotic fluid carries the organisms into the fetal lungs, causing a suppurative bronchopneumonia characterized by severe necrosis and cellular exudate in bronchi, bronchioles, and alveoli. Microscopically, leukocytes, bacteria, necrotic debris, and occasional pieces of meconium are present in the bronchoalveolar spaces. *Aspergillus* spp. (mycotic abortion) and *Ureaplasma diversum* cause sporadic cases of placentitis, which result in fetal pneumonia and abortion.

In addition to aspiration of bacteria, pathogens can also reach the lungs via fetal blood and cause interstitial pneumonia. Listeriosis (*Listeria monocytogenes*), salmonellosis (*Salmonella* spp.), and chlamydiosis (*Chlamydia psittaci*) are the best known examples of blood-borne diseases causing fetal pneumonia in farm animals. Gross lesions in the lungs are generally undetected, but microscopic lesions include focal necrotizing interstitial pneumonia, as well as focal necrosis in liver, spleen, or brain. Fetal bronchointerstitial pneumonia occurs also in some viral abortions, such as those caused by infectious bovine rhinotracheitis virus and PI-3 virus in cattle and equine viral rhinopneumonitis in horses. Fetal pneumonias in dogs and cats are infrequently described, perhaps because aborted puppies and kittens are rarely submitted for postmortem examination. With advancements in molecular biology techniques, the etiological diagnosis of abortions and their association with pulmonary fetal lesions are rapidly improving.

Neonatal Pneumonias and Septicemias

These entities are rather common in newborn animals lacking passive immunity from hypogammaglobulinemia because of lack of either ingestion or absorption of maternal colostrum (failure of passive transfer). In addition to septicemic states causing interstitial pneumonia, farm animals with hypogammaglobulinemia can also develop bronchopneumonia by inhalation of bacterial pathogens such as *Haemophilus somnus* and *Pasteurella multocida* in calves, *Streptococcus* spp. in foals, and *Escherichia coli* and streptococci in pigs.

Meconium Aspiration Syndrome (MAS). This is an important but preventable condition in human babies that originates when amniotic fluid contaminated with meconium is aspirated during labor or immediately after birth. The pathogenesis of MAS is basically the same as in fetal bronchopneumonia and abortion. Fetal hypoxia, a common event during parturition, causes the fetus to expel meconium into the amniotic fluid. Aspiration can occur directly from aspirating contaminated amniotic fluid before delivery (respiratory movements with an open glottis), or immediately after delivery when the meconium lodged in the nasopharynx is carried into the lung with the first breath of air. This later form of aspiration is prevented in delivery rooms by routine suction of the nasopharynx in meconium-stained babies. MAS is well known in human babies, but the occurrence and significance in animals remains largely unknown. Although pulmonary lesions due to meconium are generally mild and transient, MAS can be life threatening for newborn babies since it is accompanied by neonatal hypoxia and acidosis. There is a great deal of evidence that pulmonary hypertension and possibly airway hyperreactivity can be sequelae to this syndrome. In the most severe cases, focal (patchy) atelectasis can be observed grossly (see Fig. 3-14). Microscopically, keratin exfoliated from skin into the amniotic fluid and meconium are present in bronchoalveolar spaces accompanied by mild alveolitis characterized by infiltration of leukocytes followed by alveolar macrophages and occasional giant cells.

NEOPLASMS OF THE LUNGS

General Considerations

Lung cancer in animals is rare, unlike in human beings where the incidence is alarmingly on the rise. Recent estimates in Canada and United States show that 32% and 25% of cancer deaths in human beings are attributed to lung cancer for male and females, respectively. Interestingly, prostatic and breast cancers, so much feared by men and women, are distant second places with estimated cancer deaths of 14% and 17%, respectively. To say that

Table 3-6 Classification of Pulmonary Neoplasms

Primary
Epithelial origin
Benign
- Bronchial papilloma
- Bronchial gland adenoma
- Bronchiolar-alveolar adenoma

Malignant
- Carcinomas
  - Squamous cell (epidermoid) carcinoma
  - Adenocarcinoma
  - Adenosquamous carcinoma
  - Anaplastic (undifferentiated) carcinoma
    - Small cell type
    - Large cell type
- Bronchiolar-alveolar carcinoma
- Alveolar carcinoma
- Bronchial gland carcinoma
- Carcinoid tumor (neuroendocrine)

Mesenchymal origin
Benign, e.g., hemangioma; granular cell tumor (myoblastoma) of horses
Malignant, e.g., hemangiosarcoma

Secondary (metastatic)
Any malignant tumor metastatic from another body location, e.g., osteogenic sarcoma in dogs, uterine carcinoma in cows, malignant melanoma in horses

cigarette smoking is responsible for this epidemic is redundant. A recent study suggests that dogs are valuable "sentinels" for environmental hazards such as exposure to passive smoking, asbestos, dyes, and insecticides.

As with many other forms of cancer, epidemiologic studies indicate that the incidence of pulmonary neoplasms increases with age, but there are still insufficient data to confirm that particular canine or feline breeds have a higher predisposition to spontaneous lung neoplasms.

A standard nomenclature of pulmonary neoplasms in domestic animals is not universally accepted, and, as a consequence, multiplicity of names and synonyms occur in the veterinary literature. The most common types of benign and malignant pulmonary neoplasms in domestic mammals are listed in Table 3-6.

Clinically, the signs vary with the degree of invasiveness, the amount of parenchyma involved, and locations of metastases. Signs may be vague, such as cough, lethargy, anorexia, weight loss, and, perhaps, dyspnea. In addition, paraneoplastic syndromes such as hypercalcemia, endocrinopathies, and pulmonary hypertrophic osteoarthropathy (see Chapter 10, Diseases of Bones and Joints) have been associated with pulmonary neoplasms.

Primary Neoplasms of the Lungs

Primary neoplasms of the lungs arise from cells normally present in the pulmonary tissue and can be epithelial or mesenchymal, although the latter are rare. Primary benign neoplasms of the lungs, such as **pulmonary adenomas,** are highly unusual in domestic animals. Most primary neoplasms are malignant and appear as solitary masses of variable size that, with time, can metastasize to other areas of the lungs and to distant organs. Without a diligent necropsy, it is sometimes difficult to differentiate primary lung cancer from pulmonary metastasis resulting from malignant neoplasms elsewhere in the body.

It is often difficult to determine the precise topographic origin of a neoplasm within the lungs, for instance, whether it originates in the conductive system **(bronchogenic carcinoma),** transitional system **(bronchiolar carcinoma),** exchange system **(alveolar carcinoma),** or bronchial glands **(bronchial gland carcinoma).** However, according to the literature, pulmonary carcinomas in animals seem to arise generally from the bronchioloalveolar region (Clara cells or type II pneumonocytes), in contrast to those in human beings, which are mostly bronchogenic. Because of histologic architecture, many malignant epithelial neoplasms are frequently classified as **pulmonary adenocarcinomas** irrespective of their cell of origin.

Dogs and cats are the species most frequently affected with primary pulmonary neoplasms, largely carcinomas and generally in animals 6 years of age or older (Figs. 3-51 and 3-52). Pulmonary carcinomas in other domestic animals are less common, possibly because fewer are allowed to live a natural life span. These neoplasms can be invasive or expansive, have varying color (white, tan, or grey) and texture (soft or firm), and often have areas of necrosis and hemorrhage, which result in a "craterous" or "umbilicate" appearance. Some lung neoplasms mimic pulmonary consolidation. In cats, moderately differentiated neoplasms have significantly longer survival time (median, 698 days) than cats with poorly differentiated neoplasms (median, 75 days). In a study with dogs, primary lung neoplasms with grades I, II, and III had 790, 251, and 5 days of survival time, respectively.

Ovine Pulmonary Carcinoma (Pulmonary Adenomatosis)

This disease, also known as ***pulmonary adenomatosis*** and **jaagsiekte** (from the South African Afrikaans word for "driving sickness"), is a transmissible, retrovirus-induced neoplasia of ovine lungs. It occurs in sheep around the world with the notable exception of Australia and New Zealand; its incidence is great in Scotland, South Africa, and Peru and unknown, but probably low, in North America. This pulmonary carcinoma behaves very much like a chronic pneumonia, and the putative etiology shares many epidemiologic similarities with the ovine lentivirus responsible for maedi. Pulmonary adenomatosis has been transmitted to goats experimentally but is not known to be a spontaneous disease in that species.

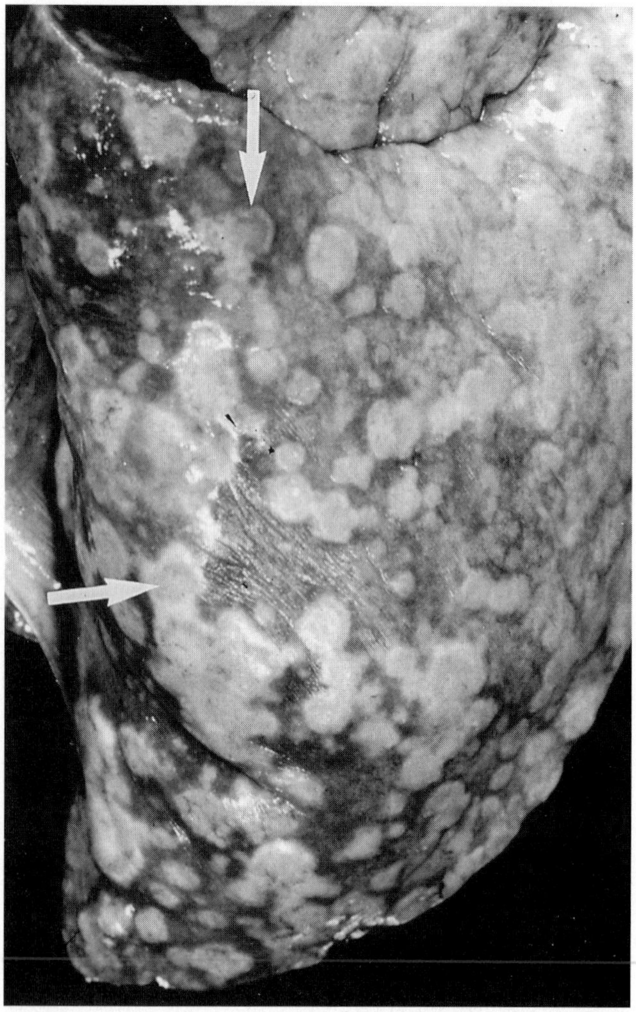

Figure 3-51 Lungs, right caudal lobe; 12-year-old dog. Pulmonary adenocarcinoma. Metastases are present widely within the lung but not beyond. Some of the tumorous nodules are "umbilicated" *(arrows)* due to central necrosis. *Courtesy of Western College of Veterinary Medicine.*

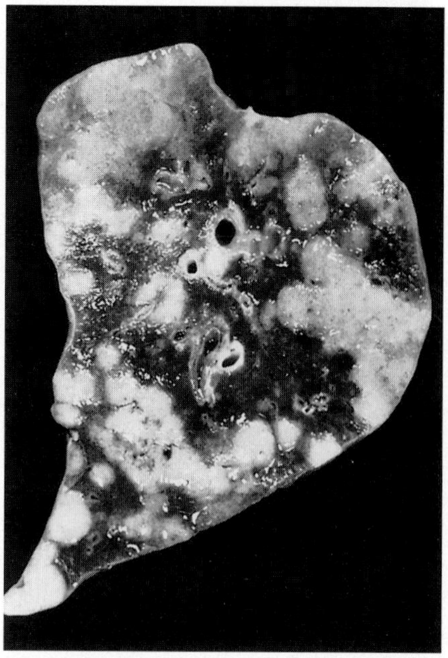

Figure 3-52 Lungs, cross-section of the primary pulmonary carcinoma shown in Figure 3-51. Multiple, pale, often coalescing tumoral nodules scattered throughout the pulmonary parenchyma.

This disease affects mainly mature sheep but can occasionally affect young stock. Clinical signs are a gradual loss of condition, sometimes coughing, and respiratory distress, especially after exercise (such as herding or "driving"). Appetite and temperature are normal, unless there are secondary bacterial infections. An important differentiating feature from maedi can be observed if the animals are raised by the hind limbs: copious, thin, mucoid fluid, produced by neoplastic cells in the lungs, pours from the nostrils of some animals with pulmonary adenomatosis. Intensive husbandry probably facilitates horizontal transmission by this copious nasal discharge and explains why the disease occurs in Iceland as a devastating epizootic disease with 5% to 80% mortality.

During the early stages of the disease, the lungs are enlarged, heavy, and wet and have several firm, gray, variably sized nodules. In the later stages, the nodules become confluent, and large segments of both lungs are diffusely, but not symmetrically, infiltrated by neoplastic cells. On cross section, a copious mucoid secretion is present in the airways. Microscopically, the nodules are composed of cuboidal or columnar epithelial cells lining airways and alveoli and forming papillary structures in adenomatous (glandlike) patterns (Fig. 3-53). Because the cells have been identified ultrastructurally as originating from both the type II alveolar epithelial cells and the nonciliated bronchiolar epithelial (Clara) cells, the neoplasm is considered a "bronchioloalveolar" carcinoma. Sequelae often include secondary bronchopneumonia, abscesses, and fibrous pleural adhesions. Metastases occur to tracheobronchial and mediastinal lymph nodes and to a lesser extent to other tissues such as pleura, muscle, liver, and kidneys. Death is inevitable after several months of the initial onset of respiratory signs. Differential diagnosis between maedi and pulmonary adenomatosis often proves difficult, since both diseases often co-exist in the same flock or in the same animal.

Carcinoid of the Lungs

This neoplasm, presumably arising from neuroendocrine cells, is sporadically seen in the respiratory tract of dogs as multiple, large, firm masses close to the main stem bronchi. It has also been reported in the nasal cavity of horses.

Lymphomatoid Granulomatosis

This is a rare but interesting disease of human beings and dogs characterized by nodules or large solid masses in one or more lung lobes that metastasize frequently to

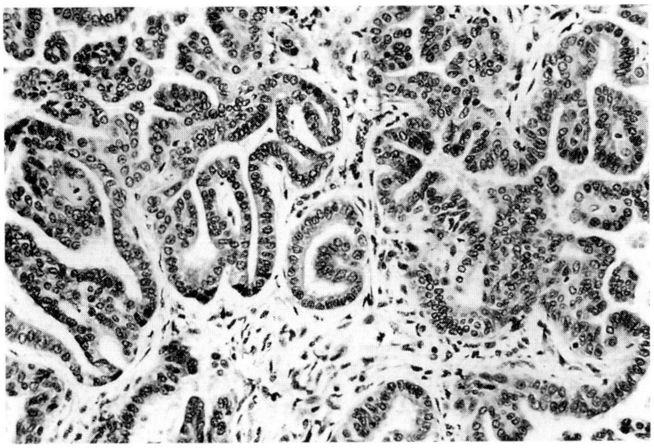

Figure 3-53 Lung; sheep. Ovine pulmonary carcinoma (pulmonary adenomatosis, jaagsiekle). Papillary proliferation of cuboidal epithelial cells (presumed type II pneumonocytes) in a pulmonary nodule of a lamb with experimentally induced ovine pulmonary carcinoma. H & E stain. *Rosadio et al. Vet Pathol 1988; 25:475-483.*

lymph nodes, kidneys, and liver. Microscopically, these masses are formed by large pleomorphic mononuclear cells with high mitotic rate and frequent formation of binucleated or multinucleated cells. Lymphomatoid granulomatosis shares some resemblance with lymphomas, and phenotypic marking confirmed that neoplastic cells are a mixed population of plasma cells, B and T lymphocytes, and histiocytes. Tumor cells have a distinct tendency to grow around blood vessels and destroy the vascular walls.

Secondary Neoplasms of the Lungs

These are all malignant by definition because they are the result of metastasis to the lungs from malignant neoplasms elsewhere. They too can be of epithelial or mesenchymal origin. Common sources include **mammary** and **thyroid carcinomas,** and recently **vaccination-site fibrosarcoma** in cats, **uterine carcinoma** in cows, **hemangiosarcoma** (Fig. 3-54), **osteogenic sarcoma, malignant melanoma** in dogs, and **malignant lymphoma** in dogs and pigs. Secondary neoplasms are relatively common in comparison to primary ones. Usually, secondary pulmonary neoplasms are multiple and scattered throughout all pulmonary lobes (hematogenous dissemination), of variable size, and, according to the growth pattern, can be nodular, diffuse, or radiating. The appearance of metastatic neoplasms differs according to the type of neoplasm. For instance, dark cystic nodules containing blood are indicative of hemangiosarcoma; dark solid nodules, of melanoma; and hard solid nodules with bone spicules, of osteogenic sarcoma. The gross appearance of metastatic carcinomas is generally similar to the primary neoplasm and sometimes have umbilicated centers.

Proper diagnoses of pulmonary neoplasms in live animals require history, clinical signs, radiographs, cytologic analysis of BAL fluid, and when necessary a lung biopsy. Identification of a specific lineage of neoplastic cells in biopsy or postmortem specimens is often difficult and requires electron microscopy or immunohistochemical techniques. Electron microscopy allows identification of distinctive cellular components such as lamellar phospholipid bodies in alveolar type II epithelial cells or melanosomes in melanomas. Immunohistochemical staining of intermediate filaments is also helpful in identifying tumor cells, for instance, a metastatic neurofibrosarcoma can be distinguished from an anaplastic hemangiosarcoma by the presence of S-100 protein and factor VIII–related markers.

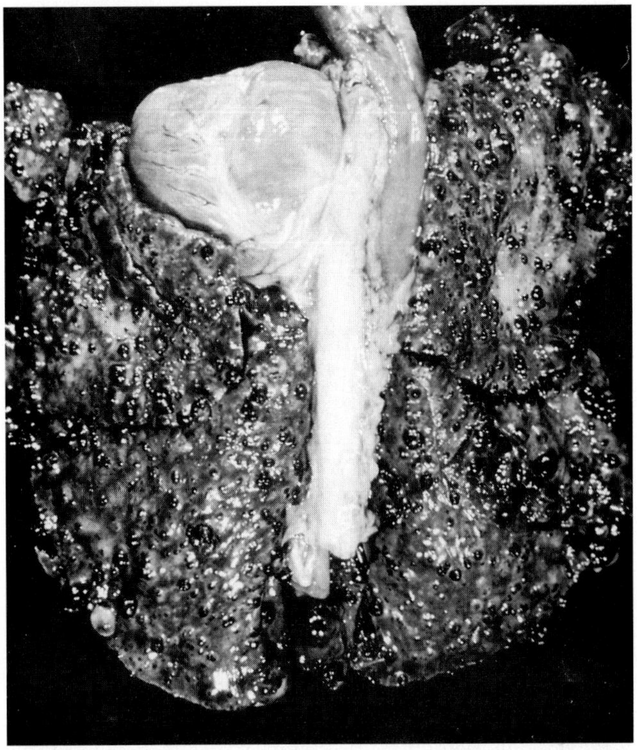

Figure 3-54 Lungs; 9-year-old boxer dog. The animal collapsed suddenly and died of hemothorax. Metastatic hemangiosarcoma. Note the numerous, blood-filled, cystic nodules. The primary site was the right atrium. *Courtesy of Western College of Veterinary Medicine.*

DISEASES OF THE PLEURA AND THORACIC CAVITY

The thoracic wall, diaphragm, and mediastinum are lined by the parietal pleura, which reflects onto the lungs at the hilum and continues as the visceral pleura, covering the entire surface of the lungs. The space between these two pleurae (pleural space) is only minimal and, under normal conditions, contains only traces of clear fluid with a few exfoliated cells. Samples of this fluid are obtained by thoracocentesis, a simple procedure in which a needle is passed into the pleural cavity. Volumetric, biochemical, and cytologic changes in this fluid are routinely used in veterinary diagnostics.

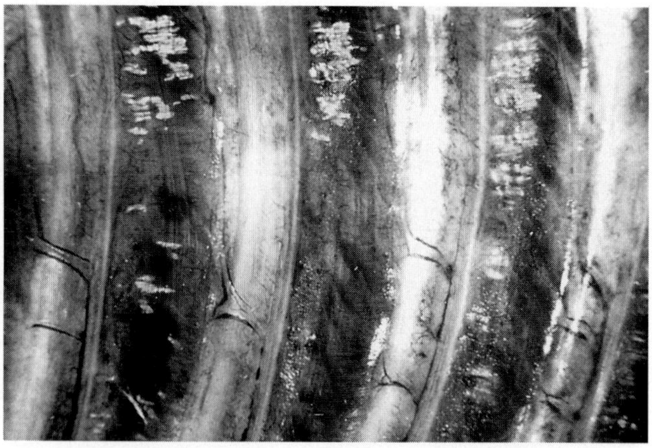

Figure 3-55 Rib cage; 5-year-old male dog. Hypervitaminosis D. Foci of mineralization in the intercostal pleura caused by excessive vitamin D in the diet. Identical lesion occurs in dogs with uremia. *Courtesy of Western College of Veterinary Medicine.*

Anomalies

Congenital defects are rare and generally of little clinical significance. **Cysts** within the mediastinum of dogs can be large enough to compromise pulmonary function or mimic neoplasia in thoracic radiographs. These cysts may arise from the thymus (thymic branchial cysts), perinephric tissue (perinephric pseudocyst), bronchi, or from remnants of the branchial pouches and are generally lined by epithelium and surrounded by a capsule of stromal tissue. Anomalies of the thoracic duct cause some cases of chylothorax.

Degenerative Disturbances

Pleural Calcification

This disorder is commonly found in dogs with chronic uremia. Lesions appear as linear white streaks in parietal pleura, mainly over the intercostal muscles of the cranial part of the thoracic cavity. The lesions are not functionally significant but indicate a severe underlying renal problem. **Vitamin D toxicity (hypervitaminosis D)** can cause a similar pleural lesion (Fig. 3-55).

Pneumothorax

This disorder is the presence of air in the thoracic cavity where there should normally be negative pressure to facilitate inspiration. Human beings have a complete and strong mediastinum so that pneumothorax is generally unilateral and, thus, not a serious problem. In dogs the barrier is variable but, in general, less complete, so often some communication exists between left and right sides.

Causes of pneumothorax include accidental (penetrating wound) or iatrogenic trauma (biopsy of the lung) and spontaneous rupture of emphysematous bullae or parasitic cysts that communicate with airways (*Paragonimus* spp.). Pneumothorax and pneumomediastinum due to barotrauma are well documented in cats after equipment failure during anesthesia. Clinical signs of pneumothorax include respiratory distress, and the lesion is simply a collapsed, atelectatic lung. The air is readily reabsorbed from the cavity if the site of entry is sealed.

Circulatory Disturbances

Pleural Effusion

This general term is used to describe accumulation of any fluid (transudate, modifies transudate, exudate, blood, lymph, or chyle) in the thoracic cavity. Cytologic evaluations of pleural effusions are sometimes helpful in suggesting a possible pathogenesis. According to protein concentration and total numbers of nucleated cells, pleural effusions are cytologically divided into transudates, modified transudates, and exudates.

Hydrothorax

When this fluid is serous, clear, and odorless, and fails to coagulate when exposed to air, the condition is referred to as hydrothorax (transudate). Causes of hydrothorax are the same as those involved in edema formation in other organs: increased hydrostatic pressure (heart failure), decreased oncotic pressure (hypoproteinemia, as in liver disease), alterations in vascular permeability (ANTU toxicity), or obstruction of lymph drainage (neoplasia). In cases where the leakage is corrected, if the fluid is a transudate, it is rapidly reabsorbed. If the fluid persists, it irritates the pleura and causes mesothelial hyperplasia and fibrosis, which thickens the pleura.

In severe cases, the amount of fluid present in the thoracic cavity can be considerable. For instance, a medium size dog can have 2 L of fluid, and a cow may accumulate 25 L or more. Excessive fluid in the thorax causes compressive atelectasis of the ventral portions of the lungs and respiratory distress. Hydrothorax is most commonly seen in cattle with right heart failure or cor pulmonale, dogs with congestive heart failure or nephrotic syndrome, pigs with mulberry heart disease, and horses with African horse sickness.

Hemothorax

Blood in the thoracic cavity is called hemothorax, but the term has been used for exudates with a sanguineous component. Causes include rupture of a major blood vessel as a result of severe trauma (e.g., hit by car), erosion of a vascular wall by malignant cells or inflammation (e.g., aortitis caused by *Spirocerca lupi*), or ruptured aortic aneurysms, clotting defects (coagulopathies as in warfarin toxicity), disseminated intravascular coagulation (consumption coagulopathy), and bone marrow suppression. Hemothorax is generally acute and fatal. On gross examination, the thoracic cavity is filled with blood, and the lungs are partially or completely atelectatic (Fig. 3-56).

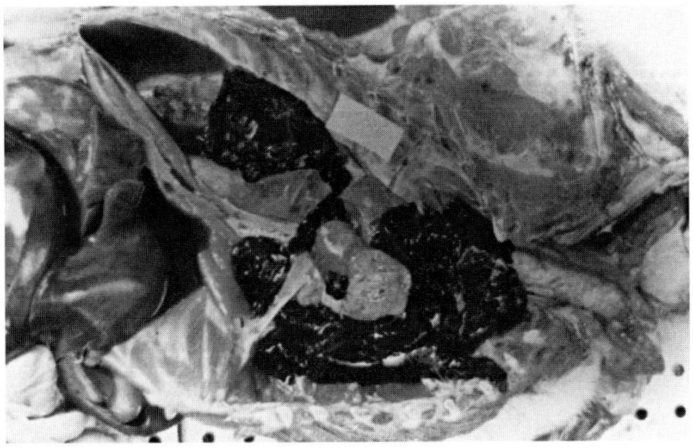

Figure 3-56 Thoracic cavity; dog. Hemothorax. A large ruptured aneurysm of the thoracic aorta caused sudden death. Aortic aneurysms are associated with migration of *Spirocerca lupi* larvae.

Chylothorax

The accumulation of chyle (lymph rich in triglycerides) in the thoracic cavity (Fig. 3-57) is due to rupture of major lymph vessels, usually the thoracic duct or the right lymph duct. The clinical and pathologic effects of chylothorax are similar to those of the other pleural effusions. Causes include neoplasia (the most common cause in human beings but a distant second to idiopathic cases in dogs), trauma, congenital lymph vessel anomalies, and iatrogenic rupture of thoracic duct during surgery. The source of the leakage of chyle is rarely found at necropsy.

Inflammation of the Pleura

Pleuritis or Pleurisy

Inflammation of the visceral or parietal pleurae is called pleuritis and, according to the type of exudate, can be fibrinous, suppurative, granulomatous, hemorrhagic, or a combination of exudates. When suppurative pleuritis results in accumulation of purulent exudate in the cavity, the lesion is called **pyothorax** or **thoracic empyema** (Fig. 3-58). Clinically, pleuritis causes considerable pain, and, in addition, empyema can result in severe toxemia. **Pleural adhesions** and **fibrosis** are the most common sequelae to chronic pleuritis and can notably interfere with inflation of the lungs.

Pleuritis can occur as part of pneumonia, particularly in fibrinous bronchopneumonias (pleuropneumonia), or it can occur alone, without notable pulmonary involvement. Bovine and ovine pneumonic pasteurellosis and porcine and bovine pleuropneumonia are good examples of pleuritis associated with fibrinous bronchopneumonias. Polyserositis in pigs and pleural empyema, particularly in cats and horses, are examples of pleural inflammation in which involvement of the lungs may not accompany the pleurisy. Pleuritis is most frequently caused by bacteria, which can reach the pleural surface hematogenously, as in bacteremias causing polyserositis. This type of polyserositis is caused by *Haemophilus parasuis* (Glasser's disease) *Streptococcus suis* type II, and some strains of *Pasteurella multocida* in pigs, *Streptococcus equi* and *Steptococcus zooepidemicus* in horses, *Escherichia coli* in calves, and *Mycoplasma* spp. and *Haemophilus* spp. in sheep and goats. Implantation of bacterial pathogens onto the pleural surface can be the result of extension of a septic process. Examples are puncture wounds of the thoracic wall, traumatic reticulopericarditis, and ruptured pulmonary

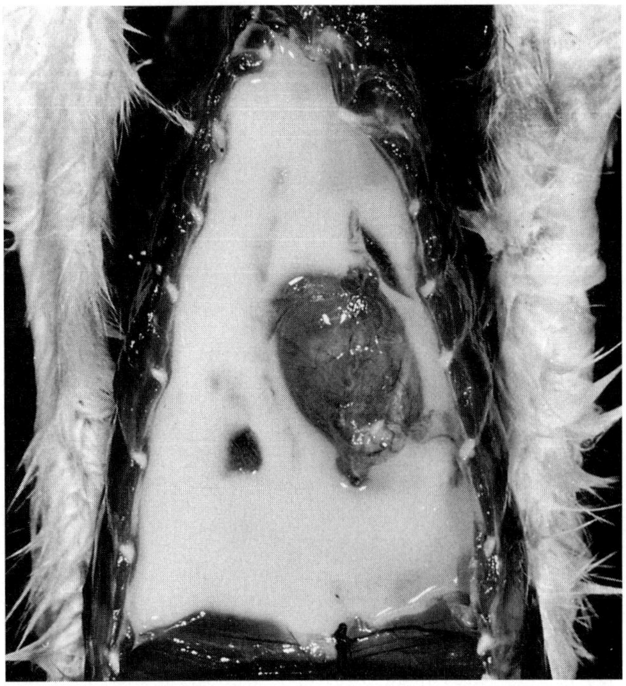

Figure 3-57 Thoracic cavity; cat. Chylothorax (etiology unknown). Lymph (chyle) fills the thoracic cavity. *Courtesy of Western College of Veterinary Medicine.*

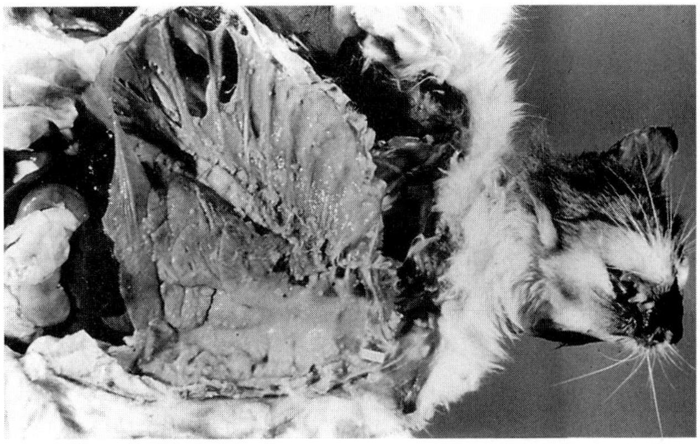

Figure 3-58 Right thoracic cavity; cat. Pyothorax *(Pasteurella multocida).* Large amounts of purulent exudate have caused thickening of visceral and parietal pleurae.

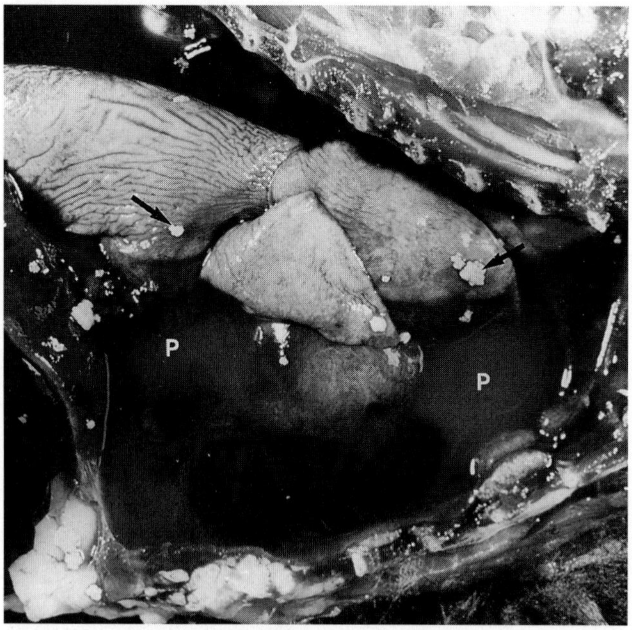

Figure 3-59 Right thorax and lung; cat. Nocardiosis *(Nocardia asteroides).* Note flecks of exudate ("sulfur granules") *(arrows),* fibrinopurulent pleuritis, and mild pyothorax *(P). Courtesy Dr. M.D. McGavin.*

abscesses (e.g., *Arcanobacterium [Actinomyces] pyogenes*) in cattle.

In dogs and cats, bacteria (such as *Nocardia, Actinomyces,* and *Bacteroides*) can cause **pyogranulomatous pleuritis** characterized by accumulation of blood-stained pus ("tomato soup") in the thoracic cavity. This exudate usually contains yellowish flecks called "sulfur granules" (Fig. 3-59), although these do not occur in nocardial empyema in cats. Many species of bacteria such as *E. coli, A. pyogenes, P. multocida,* and *Fusobacterium necrophorum* can be present in pyothorax of dogs and cats. These bacteria occur alone or in mixed infections. The pathogenesis of pleural empyema in cats is still debatable, but bite wounds or penetration of foreign material (migrating grass awns) are likely. Pyogranulomatous pleuritis with empyema occur occasionally in dogs, presumably associated with inhaled small plant material (grass awns) and nasal flora microorganisms.

Cats with the noneffusive ("dry") form of **feline infectious peritonitis** frequently have focal, pyogranulomatous pleuritis, in contrast to those with the "wet" or "effusive" form, in which thoracic involvement is primarily that of a pleural effusion. Cytologic evaluation of the effusion typically shows a high cellularity with many degenerated leukocytes, lymphocytes, macrophages and mesothelial cells, and a pink granular background due to the high protein content.

Pleuritis is also an important problem in horses. *Nocardia asteroides* and *Nocardia brasiliensis* can cause fibrinopurulent pneumonia and pyothorax with characteristic sulfur granules. Although *Mycoplasma felis* can be isolated from the respiratory tract of normal horses, it is also isolated from horses with pleuritis and pleural effusion, particularly during the early stages of infection.

Neoplasms

The pleural surface of the lung is often involved in neoplasms that have metastasized from other organs to the pulmonary parenchyma. Mesothelioma is the only primary neoplasm of the pleura.

Mesothelioma

This rare neoplasm of the thoracic, pericardial, and peritoneal mesothelium of human beings and most domestic animals is seen most commonly in calves, in which it can be congenital. In human beings, it has long been associated with inhalation of certain types of asbestos fibers (asbestos mining, ship building) alone or with cigarette smoking as a probable cocarcinogen; no association between mesothelioma and asbestos has been made convincingly in domestic animals. In animals there may be pleural effusion with resulting respiratory distress, cough, and weight loss.

Grossly, mesothelioma appears as multiple, discrete nodules or arborescent, spreading growths on the pleural surface. Microscopically, either the mesothelial covering cells or the supporting tissues can be the predominant malignant component, so the neoplasm can appear microscopically as a carcinoma or as a fibrosarcoma. Although considered malignant, mesotheliomas rarely metastasize.

Suggested Readings

Allan GM, McNeilly F, Kennedy S, Daft B, Clarke EG, Ellis JA, Haines DM, Meehan BM, Adair BM. Isolation of porcine circovirus-like viruses from pigs with a wasting disease in the USA and Europe. J Vet Diagn Invest 1998; 10:3-10.

Arceneaux KA, Taboada J, Hosgood G. Blastomycosis in dogs: 115 cases (1980-1995). J Am Vet Med Assoc 1998; 213:658-664.

Beech J. Equine Respiratory Disorders. Philadelphia: Lea & Febiger, 1991.

Blood DC, Radostits OM. Veterinary Medicine: A Textbook of the Diseases of Cattle, Sheep, Pigs, Goats and Horses. 8th ed. London: Balliere Tindall, 1994.

Brogden KA, Lehmkuhl HD, Cutlip RC. *Pasteurella haemolytica* complicated respiratory infections in sheep and goats. Vet Res 1998; 29:233-254.

Castleman WL, Sorkness RL, Lemanske RF, McAllister PK. Viral bronchiolitis during early life induces increased numbers of bronchiolar mast cells and airway hyperresponsiveness. Am J Pathol 1990; 137:821-831.

Carman S, Rosendal S, Huber L, Gyles C, McKee S, Willoughby RA, Dubovi E, Thorsen J, Lein D. Infectious agents in acute respiratory disease in horses in Ontario. J Vet Diagn Invest 1997; 9:17-23.

Davies C, Troy GC. Deep mycotic infections in cats. J Am Anim Hosp Assoc 1996; 32:380-391.

De la Concha-Bermejillo A. Maedi-visna and ovine progressive pneumonia. Vet Clin North Am Food Anim Pract 1997; 13:13-33.

DeMartini JC, York DF. Retrovirus-associated neoplasms of the respiratory system of sheep and goats. Ovine pulmonary carcinoma and enzootic nasal tumor. Vet Clin North Am Food Anim Pract 1997; 13:55-70.

Dungworth DL. The respiratory system. In: Jubb KVF, Kennedy PC, Palmer N, eds. Pathology of Domestic Animals. 3rd ed. Vol 2. Toronto: Academic Press, 1993:539.

Dungworth DL, Schwartz LW. The reaction of lung to injury. In: Philippson AT, Hall LW, eds. Pritchard WR, Scientific Foundations of Veterinary Medicine. London: William Heinemann Medical Book Ltd, 1980.

Fossum TW, Jacobs RM. Chylothorax in 34 dogs. J Am Vet Med Assoc 1986; 188:1315-1318.

Gail DB, Lenfant CJM. Cells of the lung: Biology and clinical implications. Am Rev Respir Dis 1983; 127:366-387.

Griffiths IR. The pathogenesis of equine laryngeal hemiplegia. Equine Vet J 1991; 23:75-76.

Gunn-Moore DA, Jenkins PA, Lucke VM. Feline tuberculosis: A literature review and discussion of 19 cases caused by an unusual mycobacterial variant. Vet Rec 1996;138:53-58.

Hahn KA, McEntee MF. Prognosis factors for survival in cats after removal of a primary lung tumor: 21 cases (1979-1994). Vet Surg 1998; 27:307-311.

Hondalus MK. Pathogenesis and virulence of *Rhodococcus equi*. Vet Microbiol 1997; 56:257-268.

Johnson LR, Lappin MR, Baker DC. Pulmonary thromboembolism in 29 dogs: 1985-1995. J Vet Intern Med 1999; 13:338-345.

Jones GE. Mycoplasmas of sheep and goats: A synopsis. Vet Rec 1983; 113:619-620.

Maus U, Rosseau S, Knies U, Seeger W, Lohmeyer J. Expression of pro-inflammatory cytokines by flow-sorted alveolar macrophages in severe pneumonia. Eur J Resp Dis 1998; 111:534-541.

McNiel EA, Ogilvie GK, Powers BE, Hutchison JM, Salman MD, Withrow SJ. Evaluation of prognostic factors for dogs with primary lung tumors: 67 cases (1985-1992). J Am Vet Med Assoc 1997; 211:1422-1427.

Moulton JE. Tumours of the respiratory system. In: Mouton JE, ed. Tumours in Domestic Animals. 3rd ed. Berkeley: University of California Press, 1990:308.

Norris AM, Laang EA. Diseases of the nose and sinuses. Vet Clin North Am Small Anim Pract 1985; 15:865-890.

Robinson NE. Some functional sequences of species differences in lung anatomy. Adv Vet Sci Comp Med 1982; 26:1-33.

Rossow KD. Porcine reproductive and respiratory syndrome. Vet Pathol 1998; 35:1-20.

Sibille Y, Reynolds HY. Macrophages and polymorphonuclear neutrophils in lung defense and injury. Am Rev Respir Dis 1990; 141:471-501.

Slauson DO. The mediation of pulmonary inflammatory injury. Adv Vet Sci Comp Med 1982; 26:99-153.

Slauson DO, Cooper BJ. Mechanisms of Disease: A Textbook of Comparative General Pathology. 2nd ed. Baltimore: Williams & Wilkins, 1990.

Sweeney CR. Exercise-induced pulmonary hemorrhage. Vet Clin North Am Equine Pract 1991; 7:93-103.

Standiford TJ, Huffnagle GB. Cytokines in host defense against pneumonia. J Invest Med 1997; 45:335-345.

Staats JJ, Feder I, Okowumabuao, Chengappa MM. *Streptococcus suis:* Past and present. Vet Res Commun 1997; 21:381-407.

Toews G. Pulmonary defense mechanisms. Semin Respir Infect 1993; 8:160-176.

Yates WDG. A review of infectious bovine rhinotracheitis, shipping fever pneumonia, and viral-bacterial synergism in respiratory disease of cattle. Can J Comp Med 1982; 46:225-263.

Zink MC, Yager JA, Myers JD. Pathogenesis of caprine arthritis encephalitis virus. Am J Pathol 1990; 136:843-954.

Acknowledgments

I credit Dr. William Yates (Canadian Food Inspection Agency) for having provided the basis of this chapter and Dr. Donald McGavin, University of Tennessee, for critically reviewing the text. I thank Shelley Ebbett and Tom MacDonald for photographic assistance and Glenda Clements for illustrations; Tracy O'Flaherty for preparation of the manuscript; all pathologists at the Atlantic Veterinary College for providing case material; Dr. Julio Martínez, University of Tamaulipas, Mexico, for his suggestions. Finally, I acknowledge Dr. Reginald G. Thomson, former Dean of the Atlantic Veterinary College, for years of advice, and Rosalie and Adriana for their support.

CHAPTER 4

Cardiovascular System

John F. Van Vleet
Victor J. Ferrans

HEART

Introduction

Normal Morphology

The heart is a conical, muscular organ that in mammals and birds has evolved to form a four-chambered pump with four valves. During early fetal development, the heart is converted from an elongated muscular tube into a C-shaped structure by a process termed looping. Subsequently, septation to produce right and left atrial and ventricular chambers and separation of the common truncus arteriosus into the aorta and pulmonary artery occurs. The heart lies within a fibroelastic sac, the pericardium, that normally contains a small amount of clear, serous fluid. The heart is interposed as a pump into the vascular system, with the right side supplying the pulmonary circulation and the left side the systemic circulation.

The wall of the heart is composed of three layers: the epicardium, the myocardium, and the endocardium. The epicardium, the outermost layer of the heart, is the visceral pericardium, which is continuous at the cardiac base with the parietal pericardium, the fibrous pericardium. The entire inner surface of the pericardial cavity is covered by mesothelium. The subepicardial layer is attached to the myocardium and consists of a thin layer of fibrous connective tissue, variable but generally abundant amounts (in well-nourished animals) of adipose tissue, and numerous blood vessels, lymph vessels, and nerves (Fig. 4-1).

The myocardium is the muscular layer of the heart. It is composed of cardiac muscle cells (myocytes) arranged in overlapping spiral patterns. These sheets of cells are anchored to the fibrous skeleton of the heart that surrounds the atrioventricular valves and the origins of the aorta and pulmonary artery. The myocardial thickness is related to the pressures present in each chamber; the atria are thin walled and the ventricles are thicker. The thickness of the left ventricular free wall is approximately threefold that of the right ventricle, measured in a transverse section across the middle of the ventricles, because the pressures are greater in the systemic circulation than in the pulmonary circuit.

The endocardium is the innermost layer of the heart and lines the chambers and extends over projecting structures such as the valves, chordae tendineae, and papillary muscles. The endocardium of the atria is thicker than that of the ventricles and normally appears white at gross examination. The surface of the endocardium is formed by endothelium that lies on a thin layer of connective tissue; the subendocardial layer contains blood vessels, nerves, and connective tissue. Purkinje fibers are distributed in the subendocardium throughout the ventricles.

The arterial supply to the heart is the left and right coronary arteries, which arise from the aorta at the sinuses of Valsalva behind the left and right cusps of the aortic valves. The arteries radiate over the heart in the subepicardium and give off perforating intramyocardial arteries that supply a rich capillary bed throughout the myocardium. Extensive anastomoses occur between the capillaries that tend to run parallel to the elongated cardiac muscle cells. The ratio of the area of capillaries to muscle cells is approximately 1:1, a fact evident when myocardium is viewed in cross section.

The cardiac conduction system is infrequently examined in animals. Components include (1) the sinoatrial node at the junction of the cranial vena cava and the right atrium, (2) the atrioventricular node and bundle located beneath the septal leaflet of the tricuspid valve and traversing the lower atrial septum onto the dorsal portion of the muscular interventricular septum, and (3) the right and left bundle branches that descend on each side of the muscular interventricular septum and eventually ramify over the ventricles as the Purkinje fiber network.

Occasionally, normal features in animal hearts can be misinterpreted as lesions. The epicardial lymph vessels, especially in cattle, can appear as prominent white streaks that could be interpreted as areas of necrosis. The septal cusp of the tricuspid valve in dogs is normally rather tightly attached to the ventricular septum. In young ruminants, the ductus arteriosus and foramen ovale can be probe patent, but unless the openings are large, no significant shunting of blood is likely to occur during life.

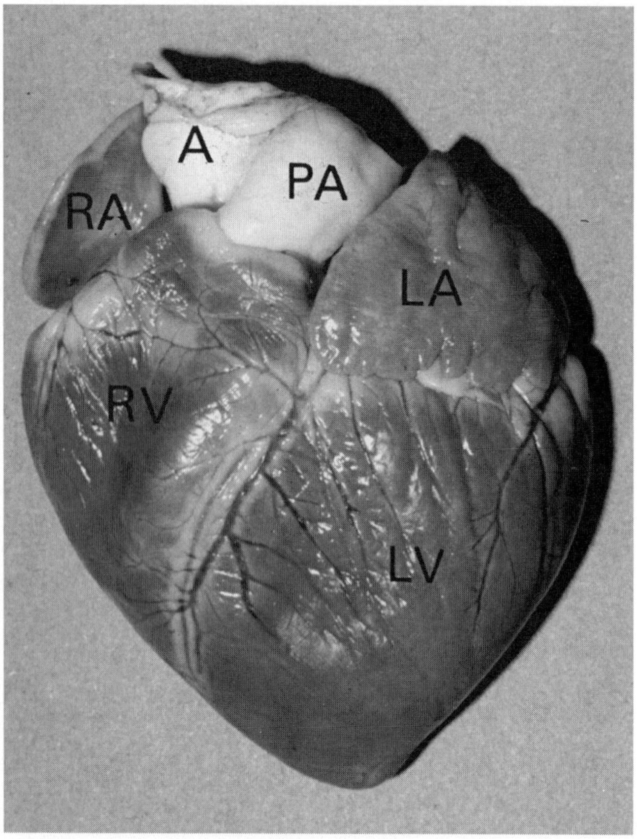

Figure 4-1 Normal heart; pig. *LV,* left ventricle; *RV,* right ventricle; *LA,* left atrium; *RA,* right atrium; *PA,* pulmonary artery; *A,* aorta.

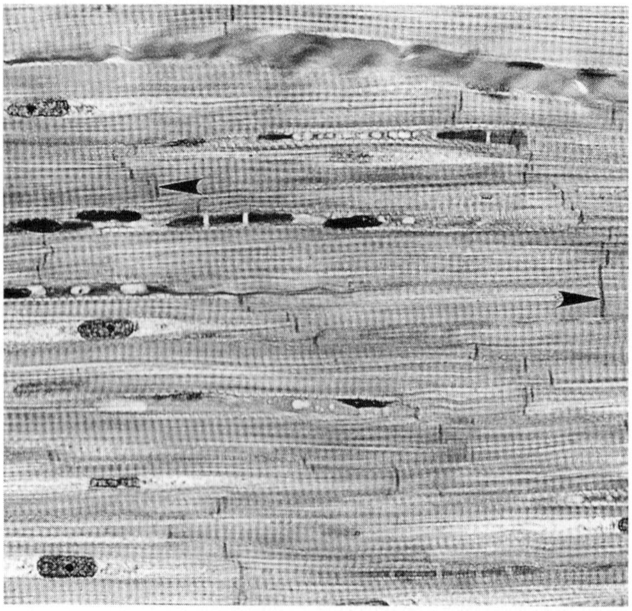

Figure 4-2 Normal left ventricular myocardium; dog. The longitudinally sectioned myocytes show prominent cross-striations and several intercalated discs *(arrowheads).* Toluidine blue–stained, plastic-embedded section. ×425.

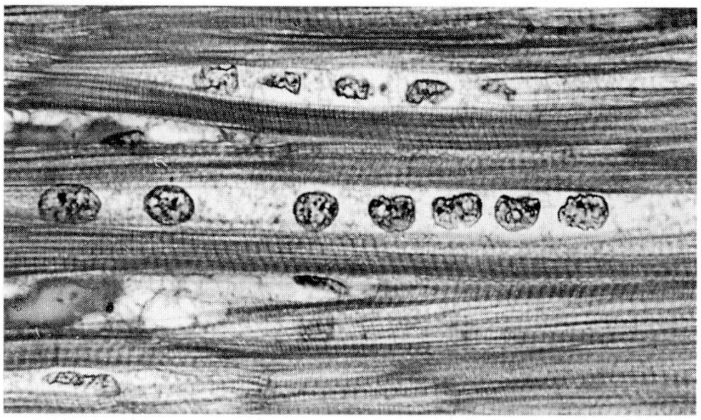

Figure 4-3 Left ventricular myocardium; normal young pig. Multinucleated myocytes are present. Toluidine blue–stained, plastic-embedded section. ×375.

The overall shape of normal hearts can vary from the elongated conical profile in the horse to the somewhat rounded shape in the dog. Cardiac weights vary greatly among species; pigs have relatively small hearts (approximately 0.3% of body weight) and dogs have relatively large hearts (from 0.75% of body weight in nonathletic breeds to 1.25% in athletic breeds).

Postmortem alterations in hearts must be recognized and correctly interpreted. Rigor mortis occurs in myocardium much as in skeletal muscles and produces contracted, rigid ventricular walls, which empties the more powerful left ventricle. Postmortem blood clotting produces red ("currant jelly") clots in the atria, right ventricle, and large vessels at the base of the heart. Occasionally, pale "chicken fat" clots that are poor in erythrocytes form in animals with severe anemia or after prolonged agonal periods. Horses more often have pale clots due to a rapid erythrocyte sedimentation rate. Postmortem lysis of erythrocytes followed by imbibition of hemoglobin produces diffuse red staining of the endocardium and epicardium and simulates the appearance of hemorrhage.

Other potentially misleading findings at necropsy of young dogs and horses include diffuse or patchy myocardial pallor that subsequently fails to correlate with any detectable microscopic alterations. Also, the intracardiac injection of euthanasia solution and other substances can cause hemopericardium and myocardial pallor and crystalline deposits at the site of solution deposition.

Cardiac muscle cells are surrounded by interstitial components, which include blood and lymph vessels, nerves, connective tissue cells such as fibroblasts, histiocytes, mast cells, pericytes, primitive mesenchymal cells, and extracellular elements of connective tissue, including collagen fibrils, elastic fibers, and acid mucopolysaccharides. Cardiac muscle cells can be divided into two populations: the working myocytes and the specialized fibers of the conduction system. The working

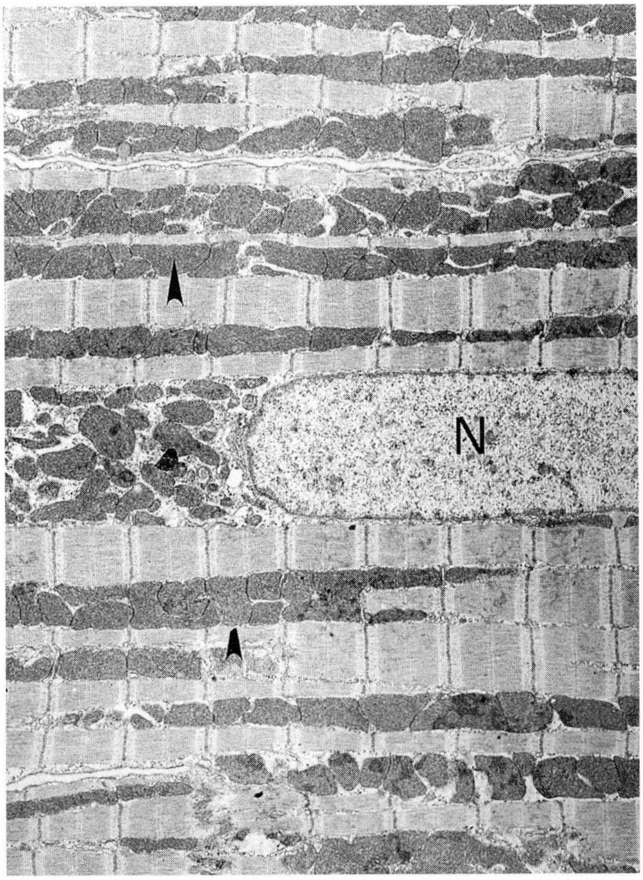

Figure 4-4 Transmission electron micrograph. Heart, longitudinally sectioned left ventricular myocytes; normal rat. Numerous dense mitochondria *(arrowheads)* lie between myofibrils which have prominent bands. *N*, nucleus. ×8250.

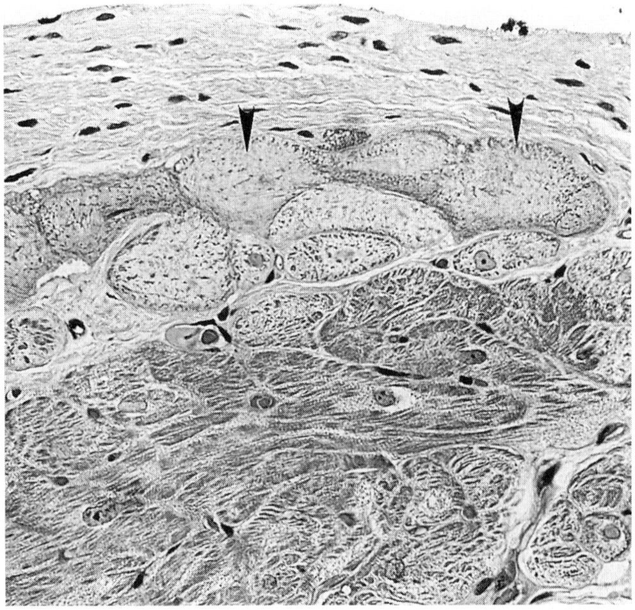

Figure 4-5 Inner left ventricular wall; normal pig. Note fibrous endocardium *(top)*, several large pale Purkinje fibers *(arrowheads)*, and underlying contractile myocytes. Toluidine blue–stained, plastic-embedded section. ×530.

myocyte is a cross-striated branching fiber of an irregular cylindrical shape that measures 60 to 100 μm in length and 10 to 20 μm in diameter with centrally located, elongated nuclei (Fig. 4-2). Myocytes in young animals are smaller and have small amounts of sarcoplasm. Atrial myocytes are smaller than ventricular myocytes. Adjacent myocytes are joined end-to-end by specialized junctions known as intercalated discs and, less frequently, by side-to-side connections termed lateral junctions. Multinucleated fibers with nuclei arranged in central rows are frequently seen in hearts of growing swine (Fig. 4-3). The hearts of old animals commonly have large polyploid nuclei. The cytoplasm (sarcoplasm) of myocytes is largely occupied by the contractile proteins that are highly organized into sarcomeres. Myofibrils are formed by end-to-end attachment of many sarcomeres. The cross-striated or banded appearance of myocytes is the result of sarcomeric organization into A bands composed of myosin in the form of "thick" filaments (12 to 16 nm in diameter), I bands composed of actin in the form of "thin" filaments (5 to 8 nm in diameter), and dense Z bands at the end of each sarcomere. Thick and thin filaments interdigitate and provide the basis for the sliding mechanism of muscle contraction. Myocytes are enclosed by the sarcolemma, which consists of the plasma membrane and the covering basal lamina (external lamina). Other important components of cardiac muscle cells are generally only apparent in electron micrographs and include abundant mitochondria, a highly organized network of intracellular tubules termed the sarcoplasmic reticulum, cylindrical invaginations of the plasma membrane called T tubules, ribosomes, cytoskeletal filaments, glycogen particles, lipid droplets, Golgi complexes, atrial granules (contain atrial natriuretic factor), lysosomes, and residual bodies (Fig. 4-4).

The morphologic features of the cardiac muscle cells of the specialized conduction tissues, including the sinoatrial node, atrioventricular node, atrioventricular bundle (bundle of His), and bundle branches vary greatly at different sites and among animal species, but generally are thin fibers surrounded by abundant fibrous connective tissue and have only small amounts of contractile material. The Purkinje fibers are distinguished by their large diameters (in horse, ox) and abundant pale eosinophilic sarcoplasm rich in glycogen and poor in myofibrils (Fig. 4-5).

Reaction to Injury

Cardiac muscle cells respond to injury by a limited spectrum of reactions. Reversible morphologic alterations include cellular growth disturbances that lead to atrophy or hypertrophy (Fig. 4-6). Various sublethal injuries or

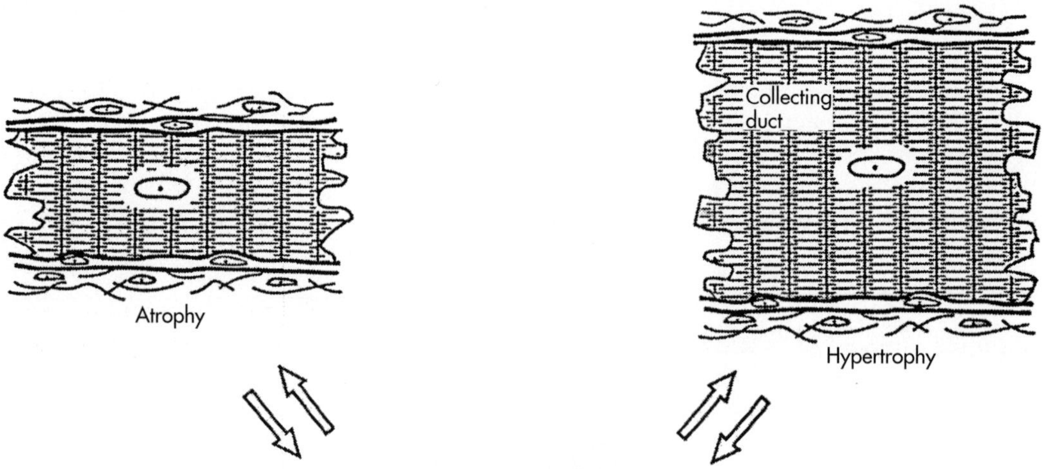

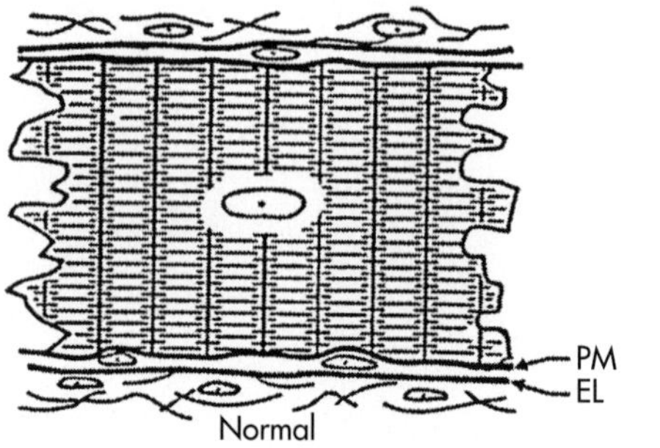

Figure 4-6 Schematic of cardiac muscle cells. Growth disturbances of atrophy and hypertrophy are illustrated. *EL,* external lamina; *PM,* plasma membrane.

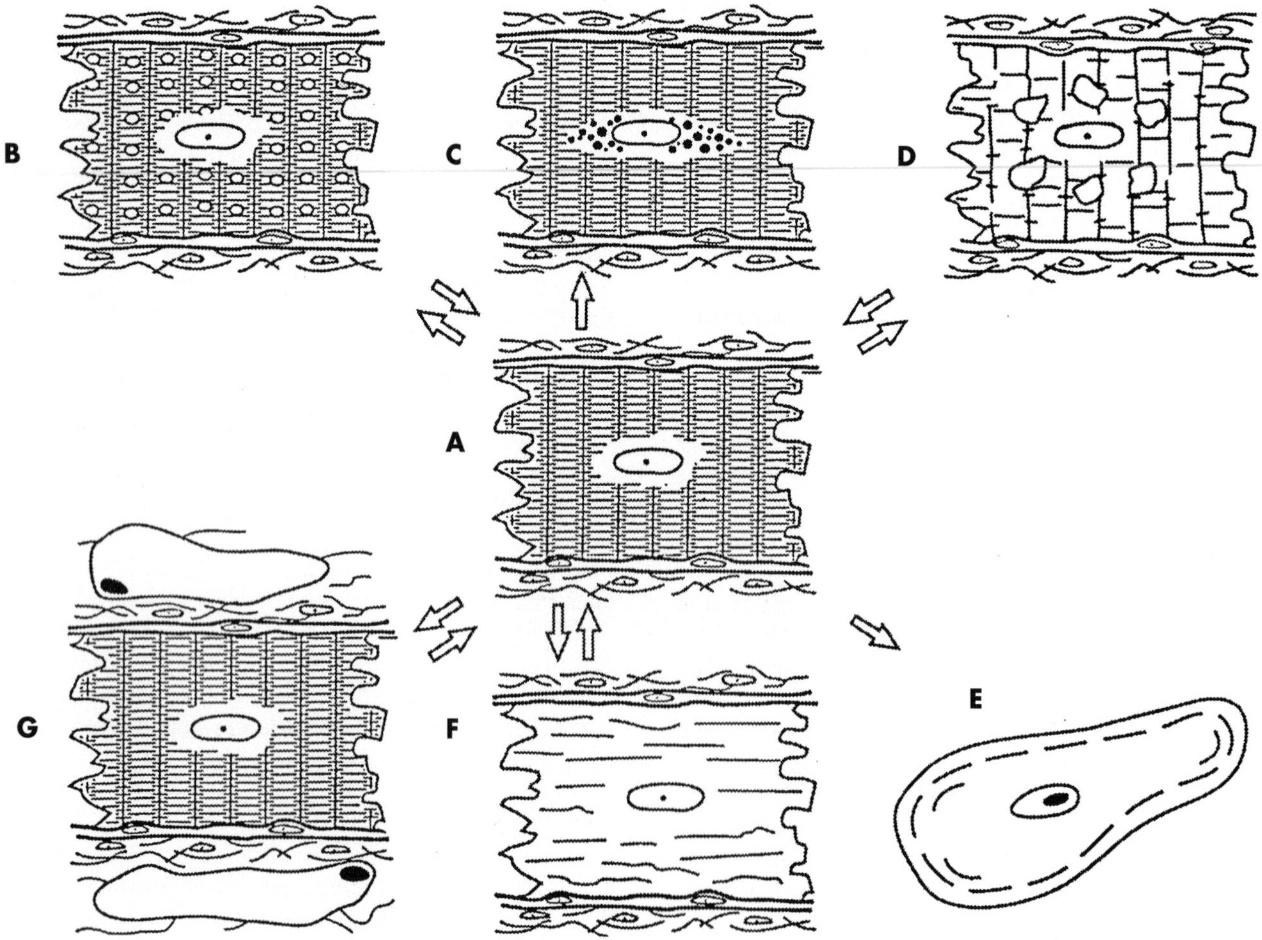

Figure 4-7 Schematic of various cardiac muscle cell sublethal injuries. **A,** Normal muscle cell. **B,** Fatty degeneration. **C,** Lipofuscinosis. **D,** Vacuolar degeneration. **F,** Myocytolysis. Also illustrated is fatty infiltration of interstitium, **G,** and neoplastic transformation of myocytes, **E.**

degenerations such as fatty degeneration, lipofuscinosis, vacuolar degeneration, and myocytolysis result in distinctive myocyte alterations (Fig. 4-7). Lethal injury to myocytes results in necrosis or apoptosis (Fig. 4-8).

Necrosis of cardiac muscle cells is generally followed by leukocytic invasion and phagocytosis of sarcoplasmic debris. The end result is persistence of collapsed sarcolemmal "tubes" of basal lamina surrounded by condensed interstitial stroma and vessels. Lesions with severe disruption of the myocardium have residual changes of fibroblastic proliferation and collagen deposition to form scar tissue. Regeneration of cardiac muscle cells generally does not occur; the continual contraction of intact cardiac muscle cells impairs the mechanisms for regeneration. Rarely, in hearts of neonatal animals and, more often, in avian hearts, a limited amount of myocyte regeneration has been reported. Hyperplasia of myocytes is a normal component of cardiac growth in the first several months of life. Then, proliferation ceases. Growth then is the result of hypertrophy of myocytes until cell sizes normal for the species are reached.

Apoptosis (programmed cell death of myocytes) is increasingly recognized for its role in the development of various myocardial lesions and cardiac diseases. These conditions include cardiac development, ischemic injury, several types of heart failure, and cardiotoxicity. In some cell systems, apoptosis can be triggered by the presence of excessive amounts of oxygen free radicals. Cells dying by apoptosis shrink and form apoptotic bodies. In contrast to cell death by necrosis, apoptosis is not accompanied by an inflammatory reaction and fibrosis.

Histopathologic study of sections of the myocardium is substantially limited in respect to specific diagnoses and only rarely can an etiologic diagnosis be made from the morphologic alterations. This limitation exists because the spectrum of pathologic reactions is a limited one and many agents that damage the heart produce similar lesions. Myocardial necrosis can be confused with myocardial inflammation with secondary necrosis as both lesions have substantial leukocytic infiltration. Some animals that die peracutely from cardiac failure lack detectable microscopic alterations. Hearts with long-standing myocardial

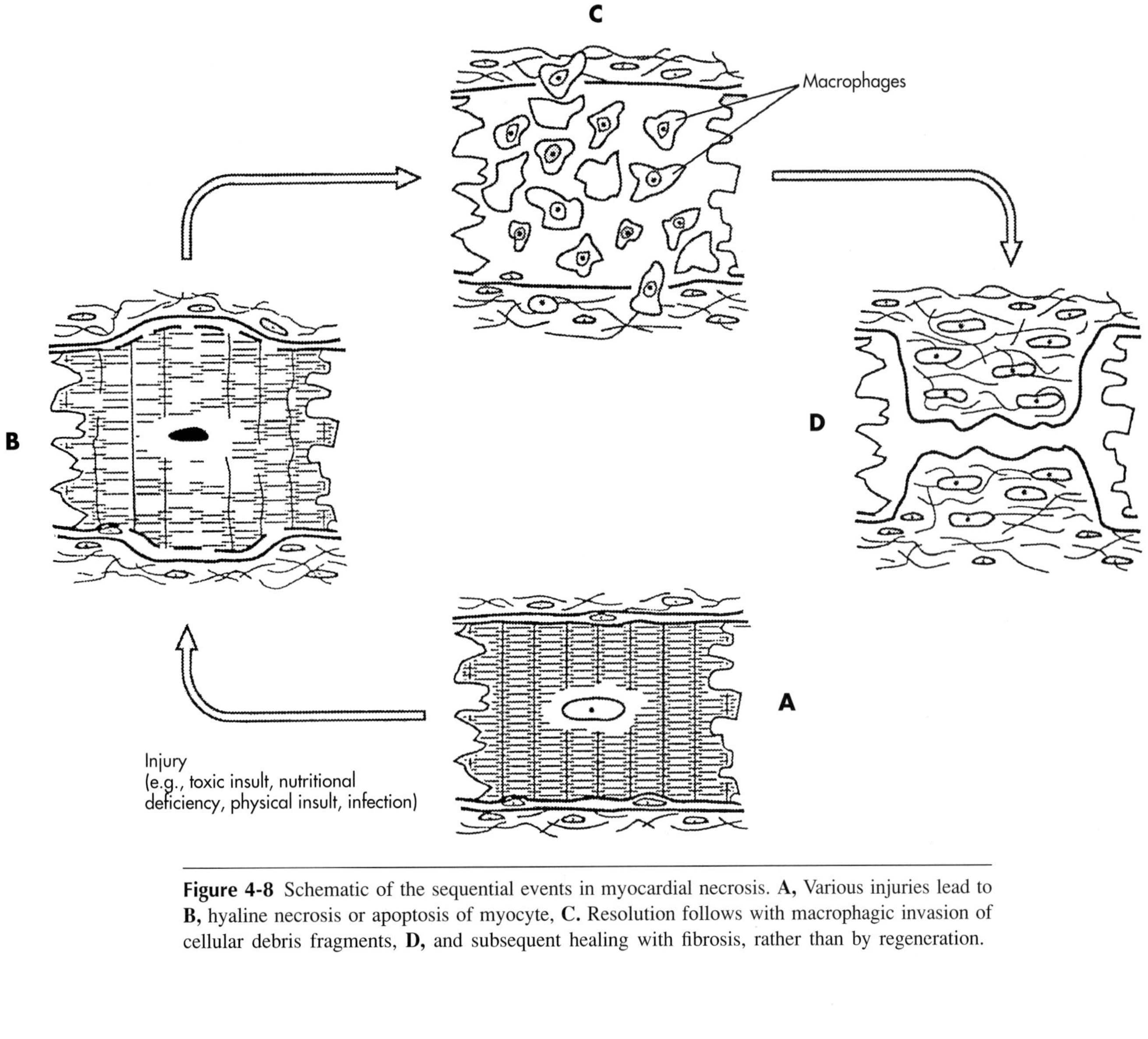

Figure 4-8 Schematic of the sequential events in myocardial necrosis. **A,** Various injuries lead to **B,** hyaline necrosis or apoptosis of myocyte, **C.** Resolution follows with macrophagic invasion of cellular debris fragments, **D,** and subsequent healing with fibrosis, rather than by regeneration.

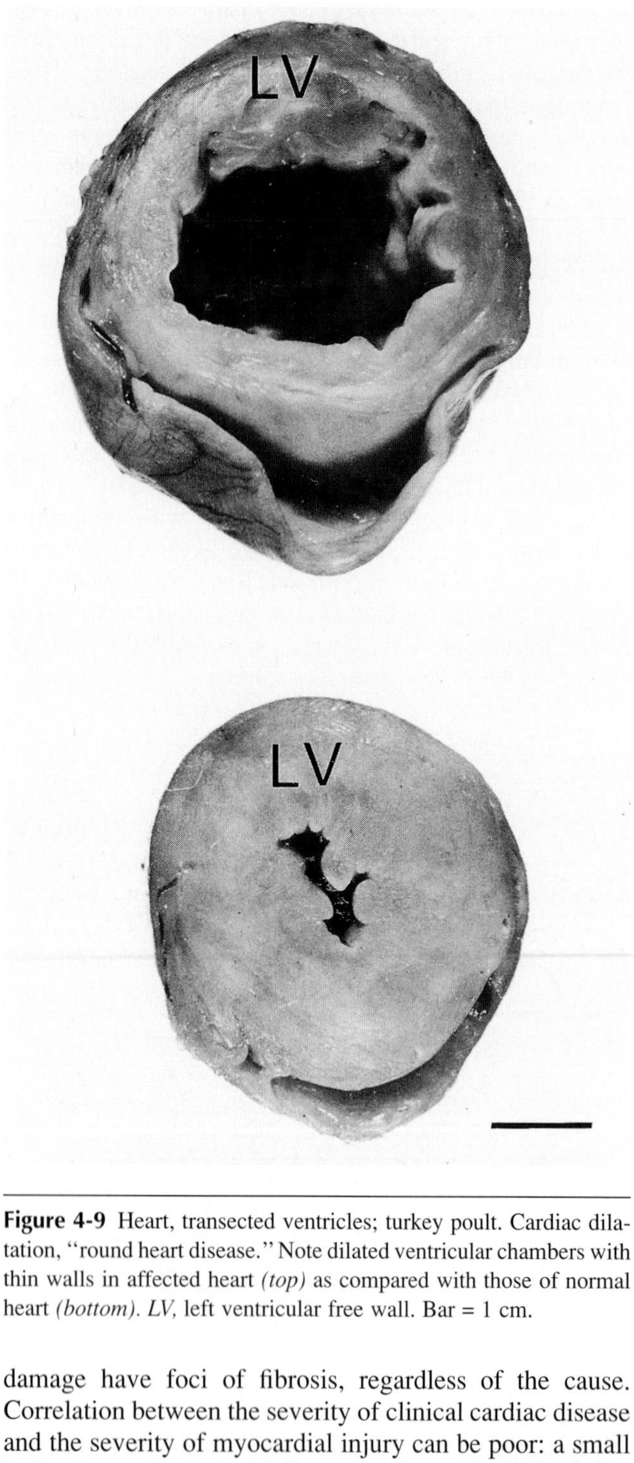

Figure 4-9 Heart, transected ventricles; turkey poult. Cardiac dilatation, "round heart disease." Note dilated ventricular chambers with thin walls in affected heart *(top)* as compared with those of normal heart *(bottom)*. *LV,* left ventricular free wall. Bar = 1 cm.

damage have foci of fibrosis, regardless of the cause. Correlation between the severity of clinical cardiac disease and the severity of myocardial injury can be poor: a small lesion in a critical site such as a portion of the conduction system can be fatal, whereas a widespread myocardial lesion, such as myocarditis, can be asymptomatic.

Cardiac Pathophysiology

The results of normal cardiac function include the maintenance of adequate blood flow to peripheral tissues that provide delivery of oxygen and nutrients, the removal of carbon dioxide and other metabolic products, the

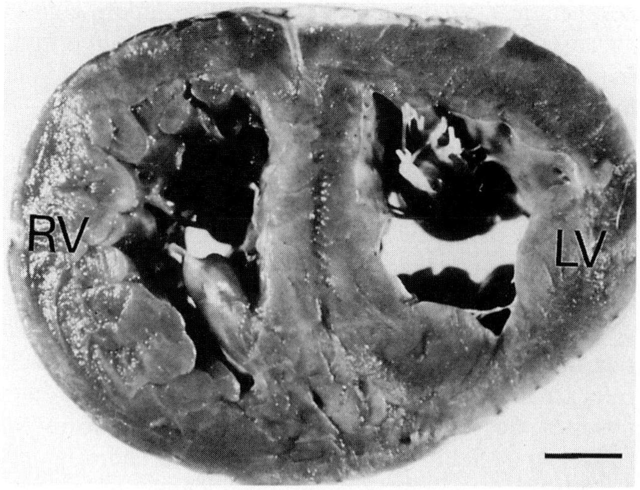

Figure 4-10 Heart, right ventricular myocardium; dog. Hypertrophy, tetralogy of Fallot. Note similar thickness of the right *(RV)* and left *(LV)* ventricular walls. Bar = 1 cm.

distribution of hormones and other cellular regulators, and the maintenance of adequate thermoregulation and urine output. The normal heart has a three- to fivefold functional reserve capacity, but this capacity can eventually be lost in cardiac disease and the result is impaired function. Compensatory mechanisms operate in both normal and diseased hearts in an attempt to meet both the short-term and long-term demands for adequate cardiac output. These mechanisms include cardiac dilatation, myocardial hypertrophy, increase in heart rate, increase in peripheral resistance, increase in blood volume, and redistribution of blood flow. These compensatory mechanisms can maintain cardiac output, adequate for some time even in animals with rather severe cardiac disease that could compromise cardiac function from loss of myocardial contractility, sustained pressure overload, or sustained volume overload.

Cardiac dilatation can occur as a terminal lesion in many cardiac diseases (Fig. 4-9). As a compensatory response to achieve increased cardiac output, dilatation allows stretching of cardiac muscle cells to increase contractile force according to the Frank-Starling phenomenon, and increased stroke volume is the result. However, stretching beyond certain limits decreases contractile strength.

Myocardial hypertrophy is an important long-term compensatory response of the heart to maintain adequate cardiac output in the face of increased pressure or volume overload (see Myocardial Diseases) (Fig. 4-10).

Circulatory Disturbances

Hemorrhage is a frequent lesion of the epicardium, endocardium, and myocardium. Hemorrhages vary in size from petechiae to ecchymoses to suffusion in size. Animals

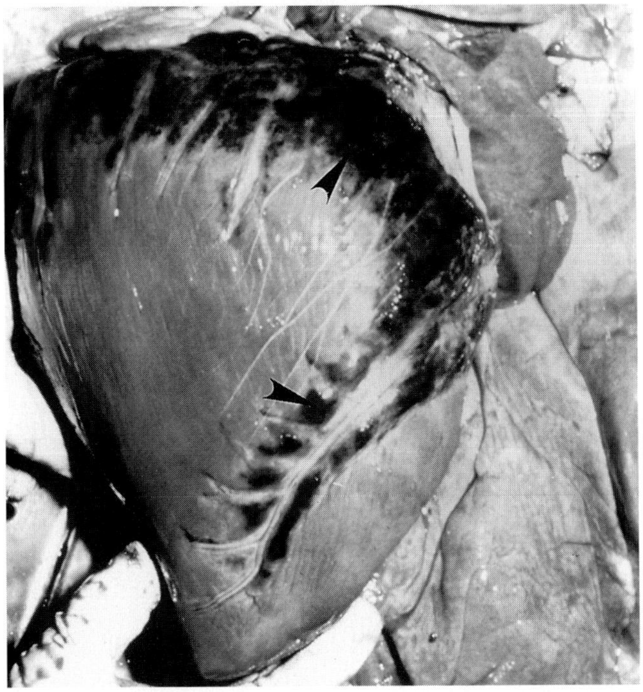

Figure 4-11 Heart, epicardial surface; horse. Epicardial hemorrhage. A dark sheet of suffusive hemorrhage *(arrowheads)* extends along coronary vessels and atrioventricular groove.

dying from septicemia, endotoxemia, anoxia, or electrocution often have prominent epicardial and endocardial hemorrhages (Fig. 4-11). Horses dying of any cause usually have agonal hemorrhages on the epicardial and endocardial surfaces. A distinctive example of a specific disease with cardiac hemorrhage is so-called mulberry heart disease, associated with selenium–vitamin E deficiency in growing swine. In these pigs, hydropericardium accompanies severe myocardial hemorrhage that results in a red, mottled (mulberrylike) appearance of the heart.

Syndromes of Cardiac Failure or Decompensation (Table 4-1)

Cardiac syncope, an acute expression of cardiac disease, is characterized clinically by collapse, loss of consciousness, and extreme changes in heart rate and blood pressure, and with or without demonstrable lesions. Syncope can be caused by massive myocardial necrosis, ventricular fibrillation, heart block, arrhythmias, and reflex cardiac inhibition (e.g., that associated with high intestinal blockage).

Congestive heart failure usually develops slowly from gradual loss of cardiac pumping efficiency associated with either pressure or volume overload or myocardial damage (Fig. 4-12). Pathogenetically, congestive heart failure is initiated by development of cardiac disease (myocardial, valvular, congenital, etc.) or increased workload associated with pulmonary, renal, or vascular disease leading to

Table 4-1 Experimental Models of Heart Failure[a]

Experimental Technique	Species
Pressure loading	
Pulmonary artery banding	Rat, dog, pig, sheep, pony
Aortic constriction	Rat, rabbit, dog, sheep
Supravalvular aortic constriction	Dog
Aortic valve stenosis	Rabbit, dog
Pulmonary valve stenosis	Dog
Experimental hypertension	Rat, dog
Volume loading	
Fluid overload	Baboon
Aorta-to-vena cava fistula	Rat, dog
Aortic valve incompetence	Rat, rabbit
Atrial septal defect	Cat
Myocardial infarction	
Sustained atrial pacing	Dog
Coronary ligation	Dog, pig
Controlled occlusion—subclavian-to-carotid shunt	Dog
Coronary embolism	Dog, calf, pig
Thrombus generation	Dog
Chronic hypoxia	Rat
Cardiomyopathy and other conditions	
Left ventricular dacron patch	Dog
Spontaneous cardiomyopathy	Hamster, mice, cattle, rat, turkey, cat, dog
Barbiturate overdosage	Dog
Furazolidone cardiomyopathy	Turkey, duckling
Adriamycin cardiomyopathy	Rat, dog, mouse, pig
Isoprenaline	Rat
Noradrenaline	Dog
Amphetamine	Rat
Cobalt chloride	Rat, pig
Vitamin E deficiency	Rat, mouse, calf, lamb
Alcohol intoxication	Rat
Coxsackie viral myocarditis	Mouse
Viral encephalomyocarditis	Mouse
Altered cardiac development and/or function	Transgenic mice

[a]Modified from Smith and Nuttal, Cardiovasc Res 1985; 19:181.

loss of cardiac reserve and development of decreased blood flow to peripheral tissues (forward failure) and accumulation of blood behind the failing chamber (backward failure). Reduced renal blood flow creates hypoxia in the kidneys and increases renin release from the juxtaglomerular apparatus, resulting in stimulation of aldosterone release from the zona glomerulosa of the adrenal cortex. Sodium and water retention are the results of the action of aldosterone on the renal tubules; increased plasma volume follows, as does accumulation of edema fluid (mainly in body cavities). Hypoxia also stimulates increased erythropoiesis in bone marrow, causing polycy-

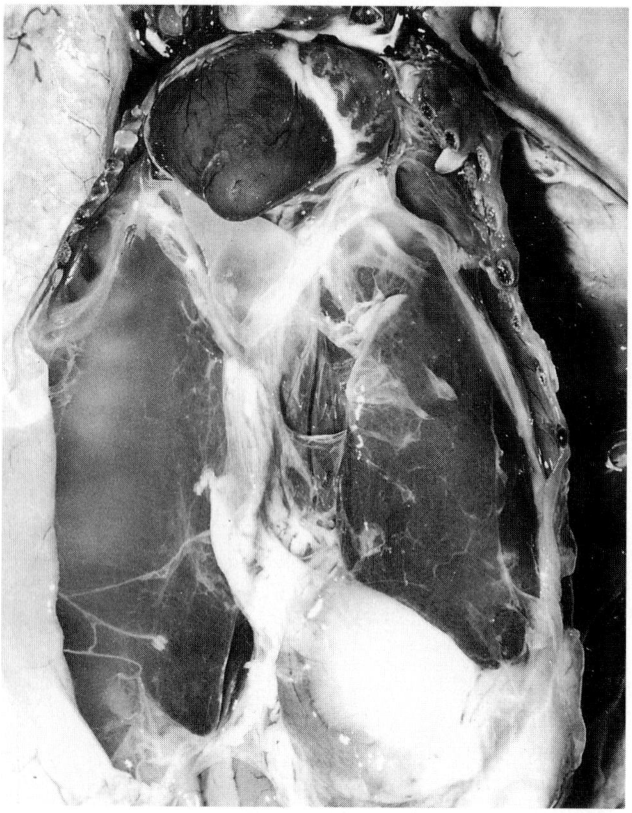

Figure 4-12 Heart, liver; duckling. Congestive heart failure, furazolidone cardiotoxicity. Note prominent accumulations of serous fluid in the abdomen and fibrin deposits over the liver. The heart *(top)* is dilated.

themia and thus increased viscosity of the blood. The hypervolemia from aldosterone-induced water retention increases the workload on the already failing heart. Thus a vicious cycle of cardiac decompensation is initiated that will lead to death from cardiac failure unless therapeutic intervention occurs. Cardiac dilatation, hypertrophy, and increased heart rate can provide some compensation for the increased workload.

Left heart failure is manifested by pulmonary congestion and edema. The most common causes are (1) myocardial contractility loss associated with myocarditis, myocardial necrosis, or cardiomyopathy; (2) dysfunction of the mitral or aortic valves; and (3) several congenital heart diseases.

Chronic right heart failure results in hepatic congestion ("nutmeg liver") and more severe sodium and water retention than in left heart failure. Edema is evident predominantly as ventral subcutaneous edema in horses and ruminants, ascites in dogs, and hydrothorax in cats. Causes of right-sided failure include (1) pulmonary hypertension, (2) cardiomyopathy, and (3) disease of the tricuspid and pulmonary valves. See Chapters 2 and 3 for further details on pulmonary and hepatic lesions associated with congestive heart failure.

A wide variety of experimental animal models of heart failure exist (Table 4-1). The models have been used to develop an understanding of human cardiac diseases.

Diagnostic Procedures

The array of diagnostic tools available to the veterinarian to evaluate changes in cases of cardiac disease has grown dramatically in the past decade as many procedures have been adapted from use in human patients. Procedures include physical examination, radiography, electrocardiology, echocardiography, angiocardiography, and cardiac catheterization. Cardiac damage can be detected by increased activity of serum enzymes and isoenzymes such as creatine phosphokinase, lactate dehydrogenase, troponin T, and aspartate aminotransferase, which are specifically released from injured cardiac muscle cells. In research studies of cardiac diseases in animals, endomyocardial biopsies have been used to assess the light microscopic and ultrastructural alterations during the course of the disease.

Examination of the Heart at Necropsy and Tissue Sampling for Histopathologic Evaluation

Following exposure of the thoracic organs, the pericardial sac should be incised and observations made on the presence of pericardial thickening and adhesions and the nature and amount of pericardial fluid present. The heart and lungs should be removed together. The great vessels are transected, and the entire heart is examined to determine the overall shape, size, and color.

The hearts of most animals are dissected to expose the endocardium and the four valves. A systematic approach should be followed; usually the heart is opened in the direction of blood flow with incisions through the right atrium and right ventricle to the apex and then along the interventricular septum into the pulmonary outflow tract. The left side is incised from the atrium to the left ventricular apex to expose the endocardial surfaces and mitral valve; subsequently, the mitral valve leaflet is incised to expose the outflow tract into the aorta. After all observed lesions and the weight of the heart are recorded in the written record, the heart is placed in fixative solution.

The hearts of small-sized animals such as rodents, birds, puppies, and kittens are often collected and placed intact into the fixative solution.

Other procedures that can be performed on hearts before fixation to quantitate hypertrophy and dilatation include measurements of ventricular wall thicknesses, determination of weights of individual cardiac chambers and septum, and measurements of atrioventricular valve ring circumferences.

After fixation for at least 24 hours, tissue samples should be removed from standard sites for histopathologic evaluation (Fig. 4-13). If gross lesions are apparent,

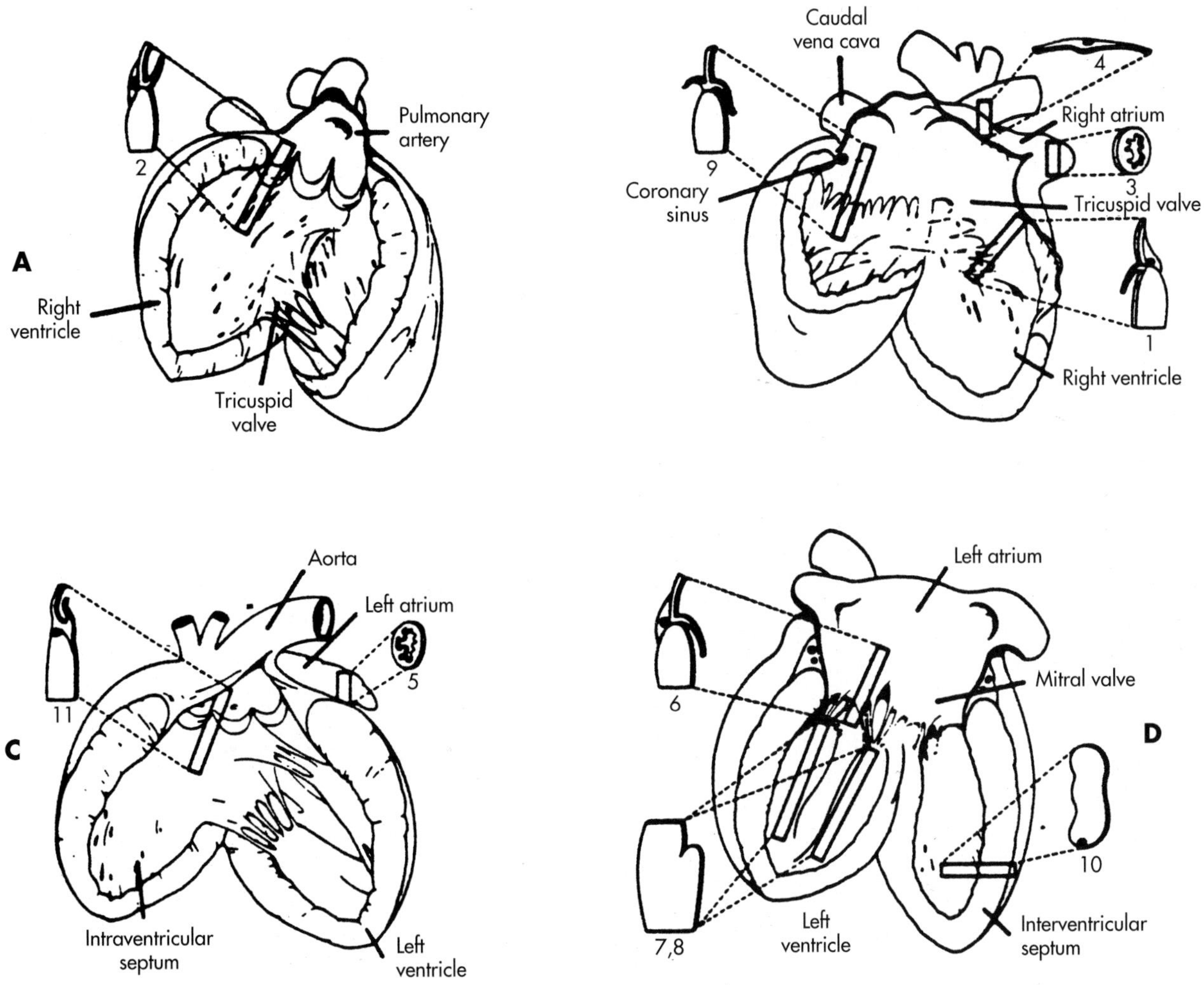

Figure 4-13 Gross and microscopic examination of the heart. Diagrams **A** to **D** illustrate the heart opened. The numbers indicate the area and the shape of the blocks of tissue removed for histopathology. **A,** Right ventricular cavity and pulmonary outflow tract. **B,** Right ventricle and right atrium. **C,** Left ventricle and aortic outflow tract. **D,** Left ventricle and left atrium. Block *1*. Right ventricular free wall, atrioventricular valve, and atrium. *2*. Pulmonic valve, right ventricular outflow tract, and pulmonary artery. *3*. Right auricular appendage. *4*. Sinoatrial node. *5*. Left auricular appendage. *6*. Left atrioventricular valve, ventricle, and atrium. *7, 8*. Left ventricular free wall and papillary muscles. *9*. Atrioventricular node, right atrioventricular valve, and atrium. *10*. Interventricular septum. *11*. Aortic valve, left aortic outflow tract and aorta. *From Canine and Feline Cardiology, Philip R. Fox (ed.) and Sanford P. Bishop, Churchill Livingstone, 1988, with permission.*

representative samples should be taken of these lesions. In small-sized hearts the fixed specimen is bisected perpendicular to the septum to provide a sample for histopathologic study that includes sections of all four chambers and interventricular and interatrial septa.

Special sampling procedures are available for comprehensive evaluation of the cardiac conduction tissues.

Congenital Anomalies

The complex events involved in the embryologic development of the heart and great vessels allow substantial opportunities for congenital anomalies to develop. The functional significance of these anomalies varies widely. Animals with the most extreme defects will be unable to survive in utero, and those with the mildest lesions could have no clinical signs of disease during life. However, animals with defects of intermediate severity are most likely to be presented to a veterinarian because of gradually developing signs of cardiac failure, including poor exercise tolerance, cyanosis, and stunted body growth. The most frequently observed cardiovascular anomalies in domestic animals are listed in Box 4-1.

The etiologies of congenital cardiovascular anomalies are varied. Most animal species have a low background frequency of spontaneous cardiac malformations. In many species, especially in dogs, these defects are heritable and can be attributed to either single or multiple gene effects. Under experimental conditions, at least, cardiovascular congenital defects can be elicited by exposure of pregnant dams to various chemicals and drugs, physical agents, toxins, or nutritional deficiencies. Chemical compounds implicated include thalidomide, ethanol, salicylates, griseofulvin, and cortisone. Prenatal exposure to x-irradiation or fetal hypoxia can induce defects. Maternal nutritional deficiencies of vitamin A, pantothenic acid, riboflavin, or zinc and excess intake of vitamin A, retinoic acid, or copper can result in cardiovascular anomalies in newborn.

BOX 4-1 MOST COMMON CARDIOVASCULAR ANOMALIES IN SEVERAL DOMESTIC ANIMAL SPECIES

Dog	**Cow**
Patent ductus arteriosus	Atrial septal defect
Pulmonic stenosis	Ventricular septal defect
Subaortic stenosis	Transposition of aorta
Persistent right aortic arch	Pulmonary artery valvular hematomas
Cat	
Endocardial cushion defects	**Pig**
Mitral malformation	Subaortic stenosis
	Endocardial cushion defect

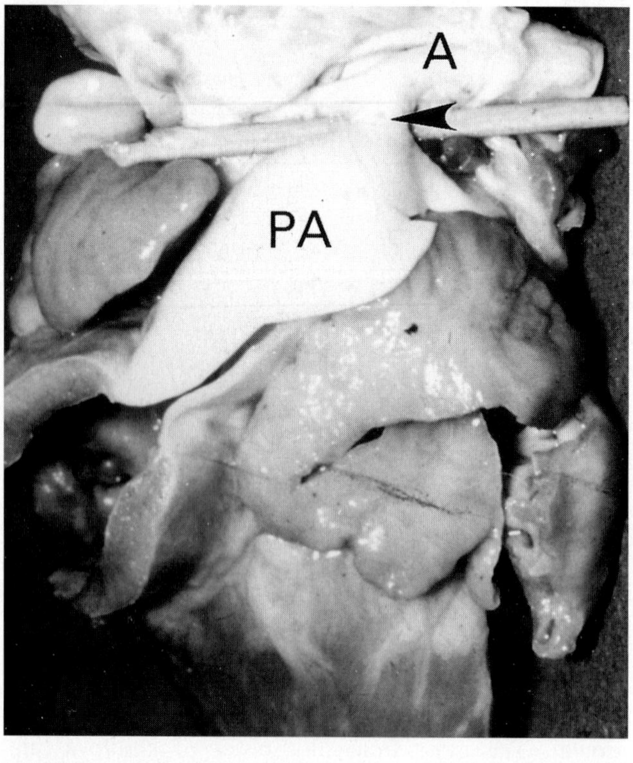

Figure 4-14 Heart; pig. Patent ductus arteriosus. Note the prominent ductus *(arrowhead)* between the unopened pulmonary artery *(PA)* and aorta *(A)*.

Anomalies from Failure of Closure of Fetal Cardiovascular Shunts

Patent ductus arteriosus is a frequent anomaly in poodle, collie, Pomeranian, Chihuahua, Maltese, English springer spaniel, keeshond, bichon frise, and Shetland sheepdog breeds (Fig. 4-14). In poodles, it is an inherited lesion. Female dogs have a greater incidence. This vascular channel between the pulmonary artery and aorta allows blood to bypass the lungs during fetal life and normally is converted to the solid ligamentum arteriosum postnatally. It remains patent in dogs with this anomaly. Generally, blood is shunted from the left to the right ventricle resulting in pulmonary hypertension.

An **atrial septal defect** could represent the failure of closure of the foramen ovale, which is an interatrial septal shunt that allows blood to bypass the lungs of the fetus, or it can be the result of true septal defects because of faulty development of the interatrial septum (Fig. 4-15). Dog breeds with greatest frequency of this defect are the boxer, Doberman pinscher, and Samoyed.

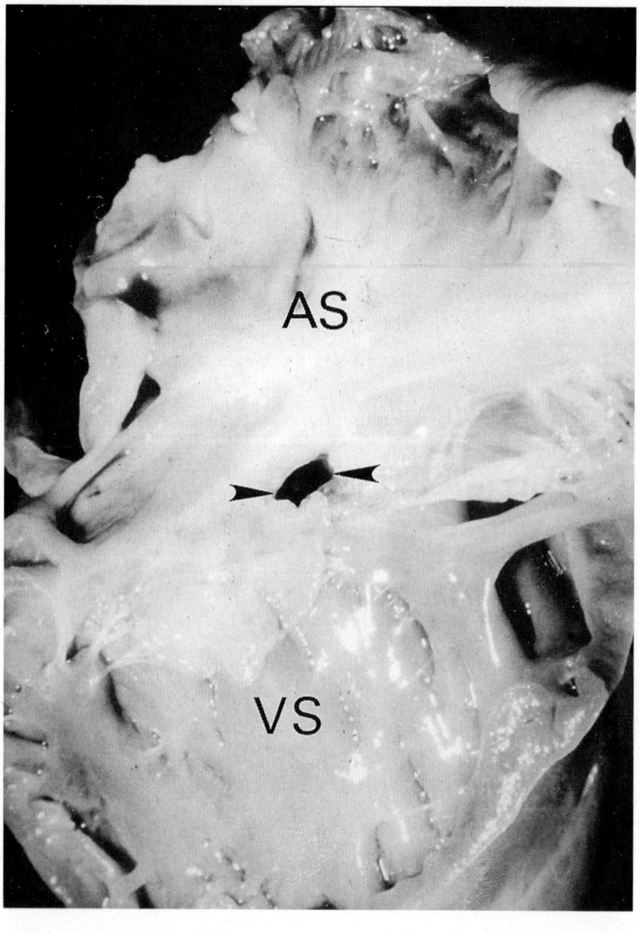

Figure 4-15 Heart, opened right side; pig. Atrial septal defect. There is a prominent opening *(arrowheads)* low in the atrial septum *(AS)*. *VS*, ventricular septum.

A **ventricular septal defect** indicates failure of complete development of the interventricular septum and allows the shunting of blood between the ventricles (Fig. 4-16). The defect occurs in many species and more commonly in the upper, membranous portion of the interventricular septum rather than in the lower, muscular septum. Among breeds of dogs, the greatest frequency has been observed in the English bulldog, English springer spaniel, and West Highland white terrier.

The **tetralogy of Fallot** is a complicated cardiac anomaly with four lesions (Fig. 4-17). The three primary defects are a ventricular septal defect located high in the septum, pulmonic stenosis (see below), and dextroposition of the aorta (see below). The fourth defect, which develops secondarily, is hypertrophy of the right ventricular myocardium. This complex anomaly is inherited in keeshond dogs and is frequent in English bulldogs. Cyanosis is often an associated clinical sign. The anomaly is one of the most common cardiac abnormalities seen in hearts of human beings (so-called blue babies). By genetic and pathologic studies of keeshond dogs, the basic defect has been determined to be hypoplasia and malpositioning of the conotruncal septum. Wide variability in the severity of the lesions has been observed.

Anomalies from Failure of Normal Valvular Development

Pulmonic stenosis has been recognized as a frequently occurring anomaly in dogs and is inherited in such breeds as beagle, English bulldog, and Chihuahua (Fig. 4-18).

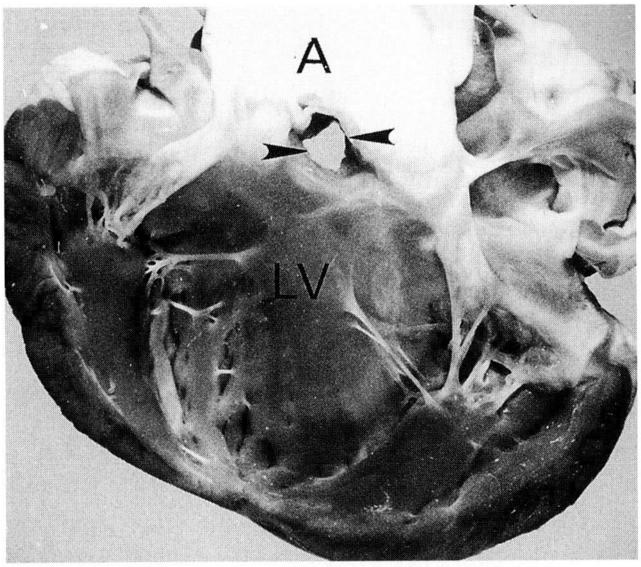

Figure 4-16 Heart, left side; dog. Ventricular septal defect. Note the large opening in the basal portion of the septum *(arrowheads)*. *LV,* left ventricle; *A,* aorta.

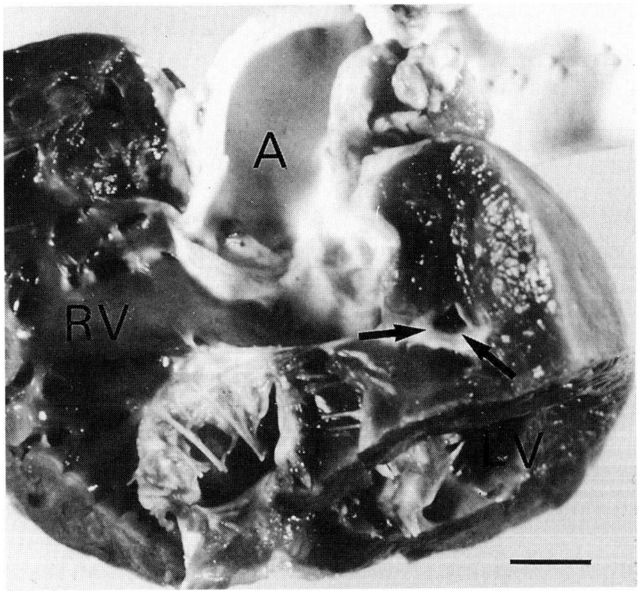

Figure 4-17 Heart, dissected; dog. Tetralogy of Fallot. This large basal ventricular septal defect has an overlying, straddling aorta *(A)* and severe pulmonic stenosis *(arrows)* with massive right ventricular hypertrophy. *RV,* right ventricle; *LV,* left ventricle. Bar = 1 cm.

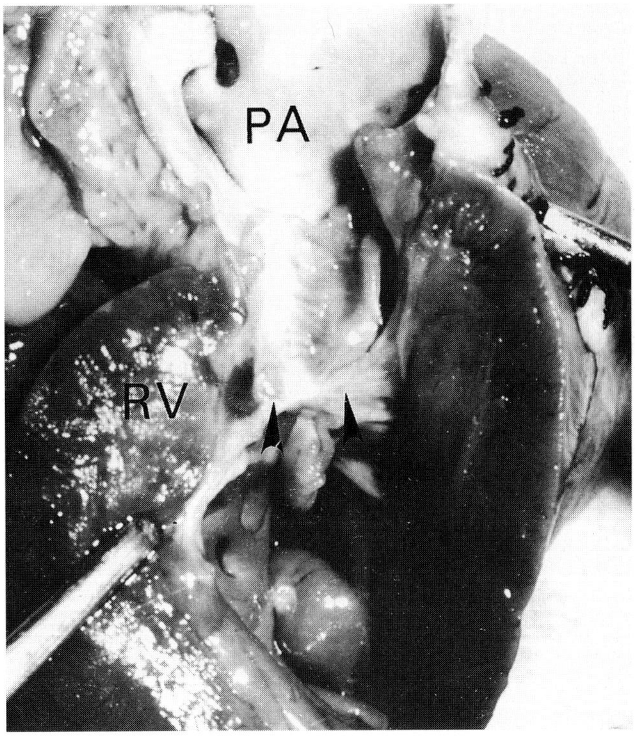

Figure 4-18 Heart; dog. Pulmonic stenosis. Note the prominent right ventricular *(RV)* hypertrophy and white, thick mass of fibrous connective tissue *(arrowheads)* lining the outflow tract beneath the pulmonary valve. The pulmonary artery *(PA)* is dilated above the stenotic valve.

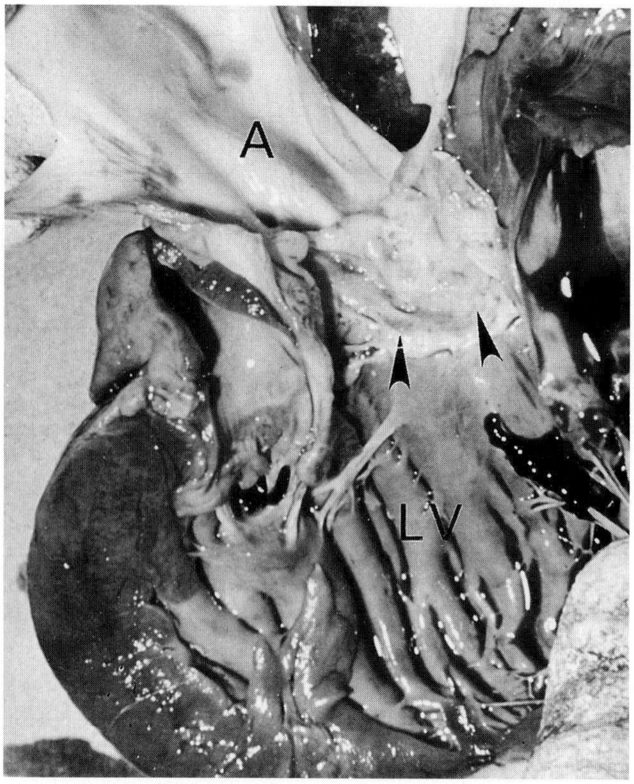

Figure 4-19 Heart, opened left side; dog. Subaortic stenosis. A thick, white, broad band of fibrous connective tissue *(arrowheads)* lies along the left ventricular outflow tract below the aortic valve (*A*, aorta). Left ventricular hypertrophy is evident by the thick wall and prominent muscular trabeculae. *LV,* left ventricle.

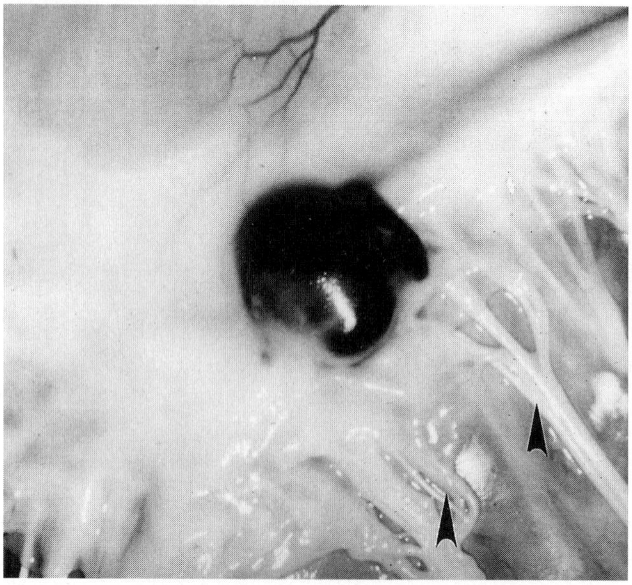

Figure 4-20 Heart, opened left side; calf. Valvular hematoma. A dark, blood-filled cyst is on a cusp of the mitral valve. Chordae tendinae *(arrowheads)* are present.

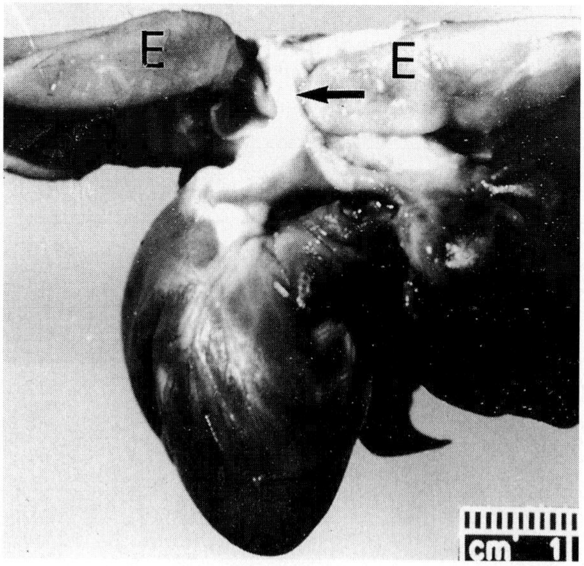

Figure 4-21 Heart, esophagus; dog. Persistent right aortic arch. Vascular ring *(arrow)* and the trachea overlie the esophagus *(E),* which is dilated proximally.

Other breeds in which this lesion is frequent are basset hound, boxer, chow chow, cocker spaniel, Labrador retriever, mastiff, Newfoundland, Samoyed, schnauzer, and terriers. Several types of valvular lesions have been described and include formation of a band of fibrous or muscular tissue beneath the valve (subvalvular stenosis) or malformation of the valve (valvular stenosis), with a small central orifice in a dome of thickened valvular tissue. Marked concentric hypertrophy of the right ventricle will develop from the resulting pressure overload.

Subaortic stenosis is a cardiac anomaly frequently observed in pigs and dogs. It apparently is inherited in Newfoundland, boxer, and German shepherd dogs (Fig. 4-19). The lesion is also observed in the German shorthair pointer, golden retriever, Great Dane, rottweiler, Samoyed, and bull terrier breeds. The stenosis is produced by the presence of a thick zone of endocardial fibrous tissue that encircles the left ventricular outflow tract below the valve. Microscopically, the altered endocardial tissue can contain proliferated mesenchymal cells, mucinous ground substance, and foci of metaplastic cartilage. Other cardiac lesions develop as a result of the altered left ventricular outflow; these include left ventricular concentric hypertrophy, disseminated foci of myocardial necrosis, fibrosis in the inner left ventricular wall, and thickening of the walls of intramyocardial arteries.

Valvular hematomas (hematocysts) frequently are observed on the atrioventricular valves of young ruminants (Fig. 4-20). These lesions, which generally regress spontaneously when animals are several months of age, do not produce any functional abnormalities. Lesions are bulging, blood-filled cysts, several millimeters in diameter, on the edges of the atrioventricular valves.

Other valvular developmental anomalies include **endocardial cushion defects** (persistent atrioventricular canal) in pigs and cats, **mitral dysplasia** in cats and dogs, and **tricuspid dysplasia** in cats and dogs.

Anomalies from Malpositioning of Great Vessels

Persistent right aortic arch occurs in dogs; German shepherd, Irish setter, and Great Dane dogs are predisposed (Fig. 4-21). This defect arises because the right fourth aortic arch, rather than the left, develops and ascends on the right side of the midline so that the ligamentum arteriosum forms a vascular ring over the esophagus and trachea. This arrangement eventually results in esophageal obstruction and proximal dilatation (megaesophagus) as the animal matures and consumes solid feed.

Transposition of the aorta and pulmonary artery are severe anomalies, of which there are several types.

Other Cardiac Anomalies

Ectopia cordis is the congenital development of the heart at an abnormal site outside of the thoracic cavity. In cattle, cases in healthy adult animals have been described where the heart was located subcutaneously in the caudoventral neck area.

Endocardial fibroelastosis in animals has been most recognized as a primary cardiac defect in Burmese cats. In this heritable disease, the heart has prominent, white, thickened endocardium, especially of the left ventricle, due to proliferation of fibroelastic tissue.

Peritoneopericardial diaphragmatic hernias occur in dogs with incomplete development of the diaphragm. Abdominal viscera can be located in the pericardial sac.

Pericardial Diseases

Fluid Accumulations in the Pericardial Sac

Hydropericardium is the accumulation of clear to light yellow, watery, serous fluid in the pericardial sac, which becomes distended. In cases associated with vascular injury, such as "mulberry heart disease" (dietary microangiopathy of swine), a few fibrin strands are present, and the fluid could clot following exposure to air (Fig. 4-22). The pericardial surfaces are smooth and glistening in acute cases, but, in chronic cases, the epicardium becomes opaque because of mild fibrous thickening and can appear roughened and granular when there is villous proliferation of fibrous tissue, especially over the atria.

Hydropericardium occurs in those diseases that have generalized edema. Thus, ascites and hydrothorax often occur concurrently with hydropericardium. Congestive heart failure is an important mechanism of hydropericardium and is usually due to primary myocardial, valvular, congenital, or neoplastic diseases. Common specific diseases include dilated cardiomyopathy of dogs and cats

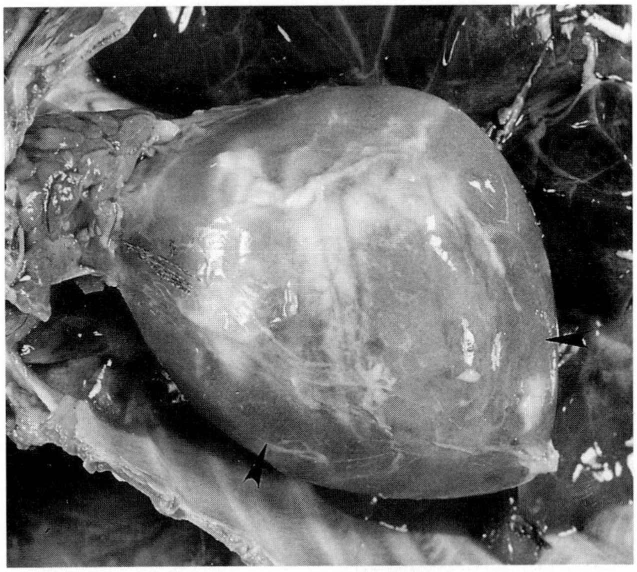

Figure 4-22 Pericardial sac hydropericardium; pig. "Mulberry heart disease." The thin-walled pericardial sac *(arrowheads)* is distended by serous fluid that has a few clumps of fibrin.

and "ascites syndrome" of poultry. Hydropericardium can also accompany pulmonary hypertension (e.g., "brisket disease" or "high-altitude disease" of cattle), renal failure, and hypoproteinemia from various chronic debilitating diseases. Hydropericardium can also occur in various systemic diseases with vascular injury such as septicemia in swine, "heartwater" (*Cowdria ruminantium* infection) in small ruminants, African horse sickness, and bovine ephemeral fever.

Hydropericardium of rapid onset and of sufficient volume leads to development of cardiac tamponade or compression, which interfere with cardiac filling (especially of the atria) and venous return to the heart. In cases with slow development, stretching of the pericardium allows accumulation of a large volume of fluid without tamponade. Hydropericardium can be reversed if the underlying cause is removed. However, many cases are associated with progressive cardiac diseases and death is the outcome.

Hemorrhagic pericardial effusion of unknown etiology is seen in dogs. Large breeds such as great Dane, Saint Bernard, great Pyrenees, German shepherd, and golden retriever are most often affected. Similar effusions have occurred in dogs with cardiac hemangiosarcomas and heart base tumors, common cardiac neoplasms in this species.

Hemopericardium is accumulation of whole blood in the pericardial sac. Death often occurs suddenly from cardiac tamponade. Bleeding into the pericardial sac can result from spontaneous atrial rupture in dogs, rupture of the intrapericardial aorta in horses, or as a complication of intracardiac injections.

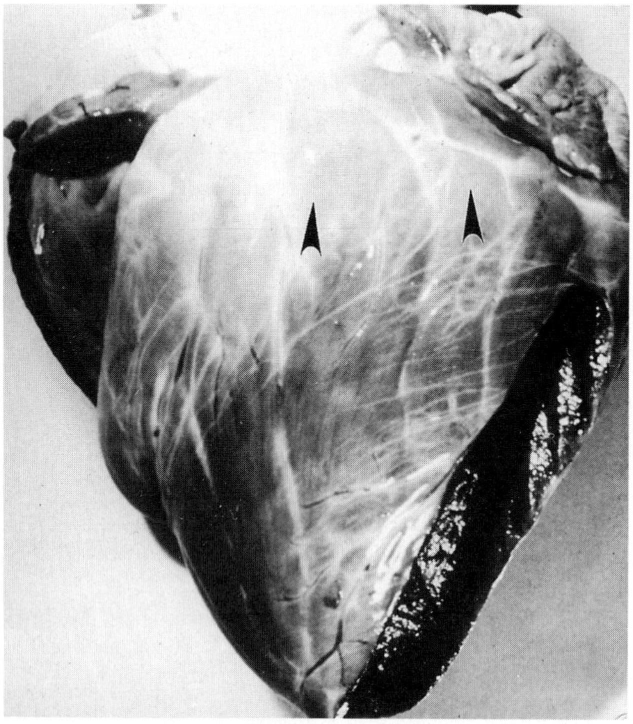

Figure 4-23 Heart, myocardium; cow. Serous atrophy of fat and brown atrophy of myocardium. The epicardial fat deposits are gray and gelatinous *(arrowheads),* and the incised myocardium is dark brown due to deposits of lipofuscin in myocytes.

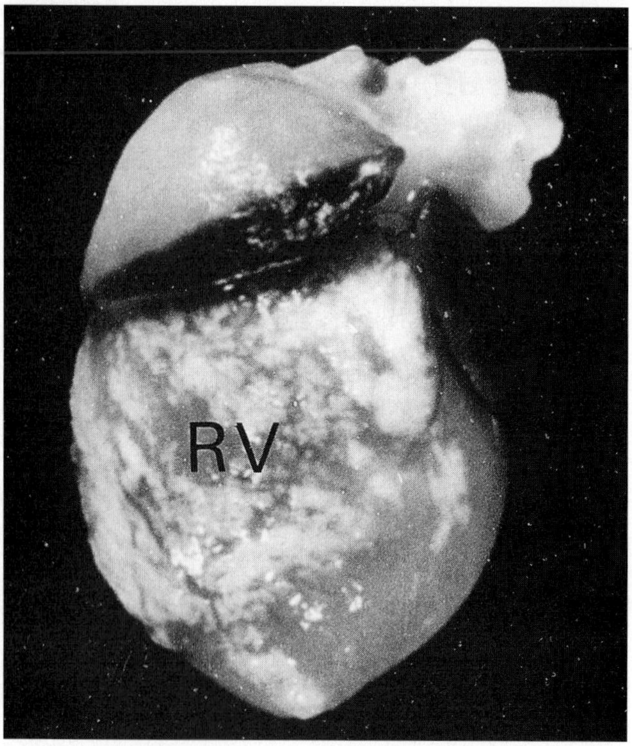

Figure 4-24 Heart, right ventricle; mouse. Epicardial calcification. Note the prominent white mineralized deposits over the right ventricle *(RV).*

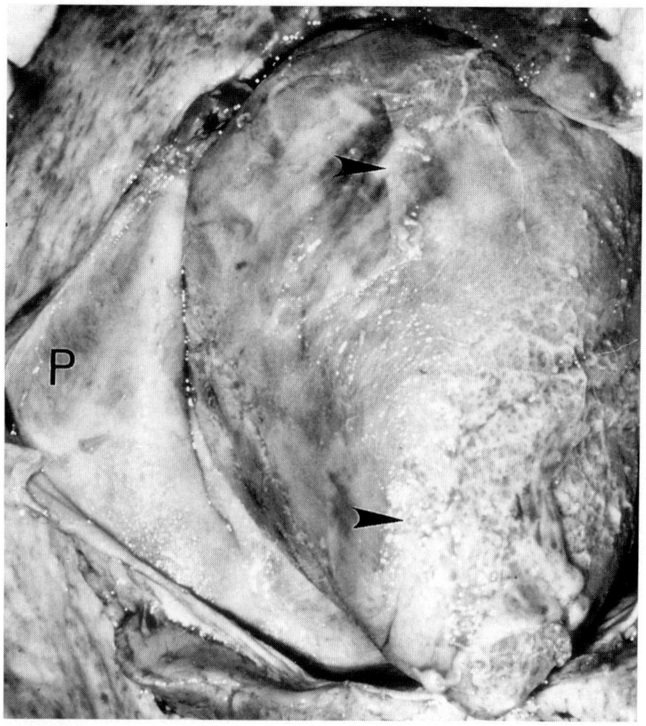

Figure 4-25 Heart, epicardium; horse. Fibrinous pericarditis. The epicardium is covered by a thick, yellow layer of fibrin *(arrowheads). P,* reflected pericardium.

Metabolic Alterations

Serous atrophy of fat is readily identified by the gray gelatinous appearance of epicardial fat deposits (Fig. 4-23). Healthy animals normally have abundant white or yellow epicardial fat deposits, especially along the atrioventricular junction. Microscopically, lipocytes are atrophic and edema fluid is present in interstitial tissues. Serous atrophy of epicardial fat occurs rapidly during anorexia, starvation, or cachexia.

Epicardial mineralization (cardiac calcinosis) is a striking lesion of certain inbred strains of mice (Fig. 4-24). In this inherited disorder, white, firm, mineralized plaques are present, especially over the right ventricular epicardium. The lesion, arising by dystrophic calcification, does not tend to cause cardiac dysfunction.

Urate deposits on the pericardium occur in birds and snakes with visceral gout. The affected serosal surface appears thickened and white.

Inflammation

Fibrinous pericarditis, the most common type of pericardial inflammation in animals, is usually the result of hematogenously spread infection. Specific diseases with this lesion include cattle (pasteurellosis, blackleg, coliform septicemias, and sporadic bovine encephalomyelitis), swine (Glasser's disease, streptococcal infections, pasteurellosis, enzootic mycoplasmal pneumonia, and salmonellosis), horses (streptococcal infections), and birds (psittacosis). Grossly, both the visceral and parietal pericardial surfaces are covered by variable amounts of yellow fibrin deposits that can result in adherence between the parietal and visceral layers. When the pericardial sac is opened at necropsy, these attachments are torn away (so-called bread-and-butter heart) (Fig. 4-25). Microscopically, an eosinophilic layer of fibrin with admixed neutrophils lies over a congested pericardium.

The outcome of fibrinous pericarditis varies. Early death is frequent because many of these lesions result from infection by highly virulent bacteria and concurrent septicemia. When survival is prolonged, fibrous adhesions form between the pericardial surfaces after fibrous organization of the exudate.

Suppurative pericarditis is seen mainly in cattle as a complication of traumatic reticuloperitonitis ("hardware disease"). Foreign bodies, such as nails or pieces of wire that accumulate in the reticulum, occasionally penetrate the reticular wall and diaphragm, and enter the adjacent pericardial sac and introduce infection. Some affected cattle survive for weeks to months until death ensues from congestive heart failure and septicemia. Grossly, the pericardial surfaces are markedly thickened by white, often rough, shaggy-appearing masses of fibrous connective tissue that enclose an accumulation of white to gray, thick, foul-smelling, purulent exudate (Fig. 4-26).

Constrictive pericarditis is a chronic inflammatory lesion of the pericardium accompanied by extensive fibrous proliferation and eventual formation of fibrous adhesions between the surfaces of the visceral and parietal pericardium. Severe lesions obliterate the pericardial sac and constrict the heart by fibrous tissue and can interfere with cardiac filling. Compensatory myocardial hypertrophy can result in diminished ventricular chamber volumes and contribute to the eventual development of congestive cardiac failure.

Endocardial Diseases

Degeneration

Endocardial mineralization and **endocardial fibrosis** can occur singly or together. Mineralization occurs from intake of excessive amounts of vitamin D and from intoxication by calcinogenic plants *(Cestrum diurnum, Tristetum flavescens, Solanum malacoxylon, Solanum torvum)* that contain vitamin D analogs. These plant-induced syndromes of cattle have been called by different names in various areas of the world, such as "Manchester wasting disease" in Jamaica, "enzootic calcinosis" in Europe, "naahelu disease" in Hawaii, "enteque seco" in Argentina, and "espichamento" in Brazil. Multiple, large, white, rough, firm plaques of mineralized fibroelastic tissue are present in the endocardium and intima of large elastic arteries. Fibrosis, with or without mineralization, occurs in chronically dilated hearts, in hearts of debilitated cattle with Johne's disease (Fig. 4-27), in dogs with healed lesions of left atrial ulcerative endocarditis associated with a prior uremic episode, and in the so-called jet lesions produced by the trauma by refluxed blood in valvular insufficiencies.

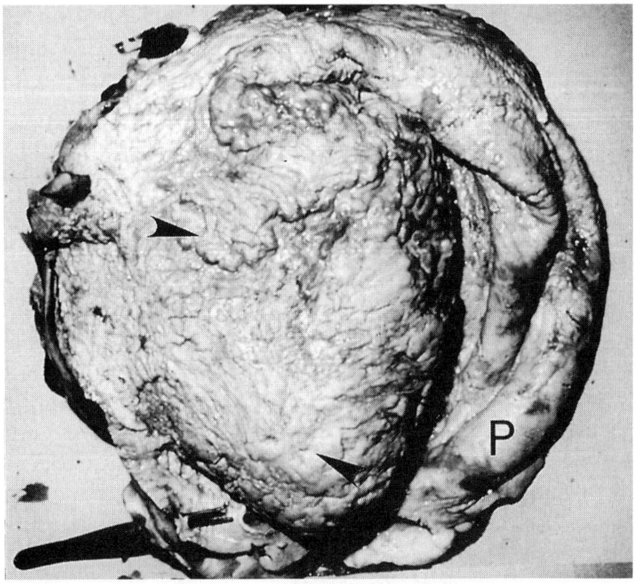

Figure 4-26 Heart, pericardium; cow. Suppurative pericarditis, traumatic reticuloperitonitis ("hardware disease"). The exposed pericardial surface is markedly thickened by fibrous connective tissue and is covered by shaggy, white masses of fibrinopurulent exudate *(arrowheads)*. *P,* reflected pericardium.

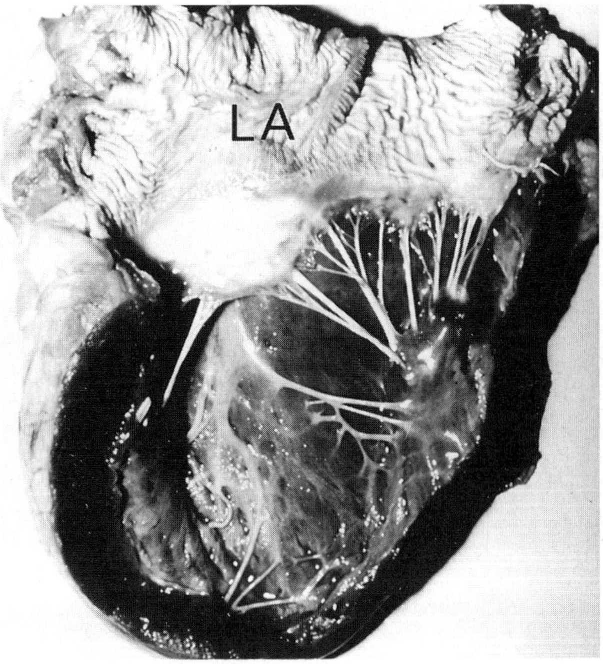

Figure 4-27 Heart, left atrial endocardium; cow. Endocardial mineralization, Johne's disease. The left atrial *(LA)* endocardium is white, thick, and wrinkled.

Valvular endocardiosis is an important age-related cardiac disease of old dogs associated with degeneration of valvular collagen. Other names used for this disease include valvular fibrosis and myxomatous or mucoid valvular degeneration. This disease, the most common cause of congestive heart failure in old dogs, could have a genetic basis as males of certain breeds are most frequently affected. The cavalier King Charles spaniel breed has a unique susceptibility with more than 50% prevalence by 4 years of age and 100% prevalence by 10 years of age. Other breeds with high incidence include cocker spaniel, beagle, dachshund, poodle, schnauzer, Chihuahua, Doberman pinscher, fox terrier, Boston terrier, Pekinese, deerhound, and wolfhound. Lesions occur most frequently on the mitral valve, less commonly on the tricuspid, and infrequently on the aortic and pulmonary valves. Affected valves are shortened and thickened, either diffusely or nodular, and appear smooth rather than roughened, as is usual in cases of valvular endocarditis (Fig. 4-28). These lesions result in valvular insufficiency with subsequent atrial dilatation and development of atrial "jet lesions." Other complications of valvular endocardiosis include occasional rupture of the chordae tendineae and occasional splitting or rupture of the left atrial wall. Microscopically, the thickened valves have markedly increased fibroblastic proliferation and deposition of acid mucopolysaccharides. Frequent accompanying myocardial alterations include arteriosclerosis of intramyocardial arteries and multifocal myocardial necrosis and fibrosis.

Circulatory Disturbances

Atrial thrombosis is a frequent lesion in aged Syrian hamsters and in certain strains of mice and has been found in the failing hearts of dogs and cats with idiopathic cardiomyopathies. In affected hamsters and mice, the atria are swollen, firm, mottled and have gray to tan, laminated masses of fibrin. Fibroblastic organization occurs rapidly in the thrombi. Etiologic factors include aging and genetic and dietary influences. Susceptible strains fed a thrombogenic diet (high-fat, low-protein, and hypolipotropic) have a high incidence of atrial thrombosis.

Inflammation

Endocarditis is usually the result of bacterial infections, except for lesions produced by migrating *Strongylus vulgaris* larvae in horses and an occasional case of mycotic infection. The lesions are often very large by the time of death and are present on the valves (valvular endocarditis), although some lesions extend to the adjacent wall (mural endocarditis). Grossly, the affected valves have large, adhering, friable, yellow to gray masses of fibrin termed "vegetations" that can largely occlude the valvular orifice (Fig. 4-29). In chronic lesions, the fibrin deposits are organized by fibrous connective tissue to produce irregular nodular masses termed "verrucae" (wartlike lesions). Microscopically, the lesion consists of accumulated layers of fibrin and numerous embedded bacterial colonies

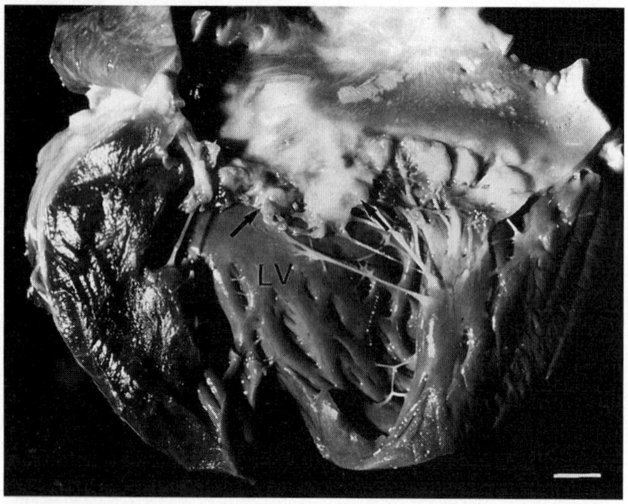

Figure 4-28 Heart, left ventricle; dog. Valvular endocardiosis. The affected cusps of the mitral valve are thickened by white, smooth, fibrotic nodules *(arrows)*. *LV,* left ventricle. Bar = 1 cm. *Courtesy Dr. M.D. McGavin.*

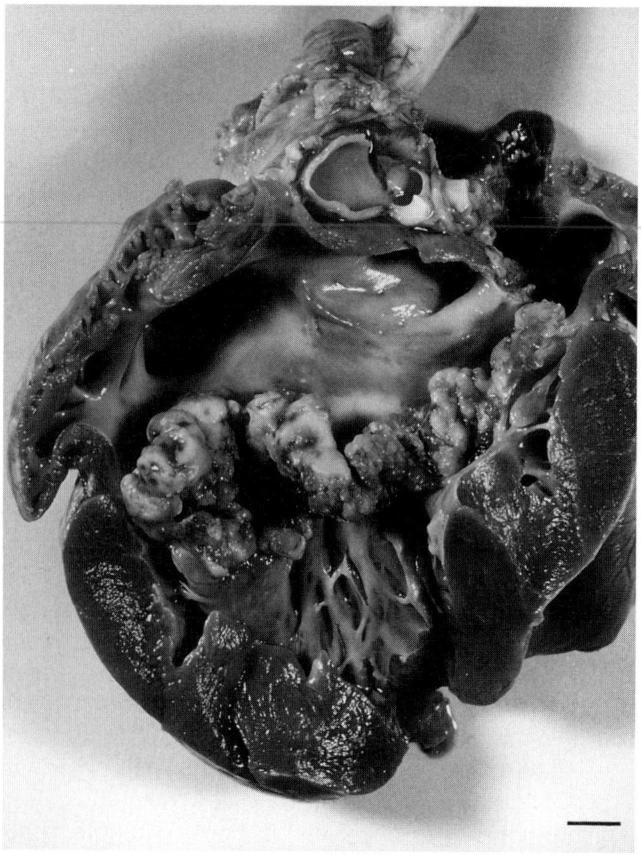

Figure 4-29 Heart, mitral valve; pig. Vegetative valvular endocarditis, streptococcal infection. Multiple, large, raised, friable, yellow-red thrombotic masses are attached to the affected mitral valve. Bar = 1 cm. *Courtesy Dr. M.D. McGavin.*

underlain by a zone of infiltrated leukocytes and granulation tissue (Fig. 4-30). Relative frequency of valvular involvement with endocarditis in animals is mitral > aortic > tricuspid > pulmonary.

The pathogenesis of endocarditis is complicated and frequently incompletely understood. Affected animals often have preexisting extracardiac infections that have resulted in one or more bouts of bacteremia. Focal endothelial disruption on the surface of the normally avascular valves allows bacteria to adhere, proliferate, and initiate an inflammatory reaction that results in subsequent deposition of masses of fibrin. Bacteria frequently recovered from the vegetative lesions are *Actinomyces pyogenes* in cattle, *Streptococcus* spp. and *Erysipelothrix rhusiopathiae* in pigs, and *Streptococcus* spp. and *E. coli* in dogs and cats. Death is the result of cardiac failure from valvular dysfunction or the effects of bacteremia. In some animals, septic emboli lodge in organs such as the heart and kidneys leading to infarction.

Ulcerative endocarditis of the left atrium is a distinctive lesion associated with acute renal insufficiency

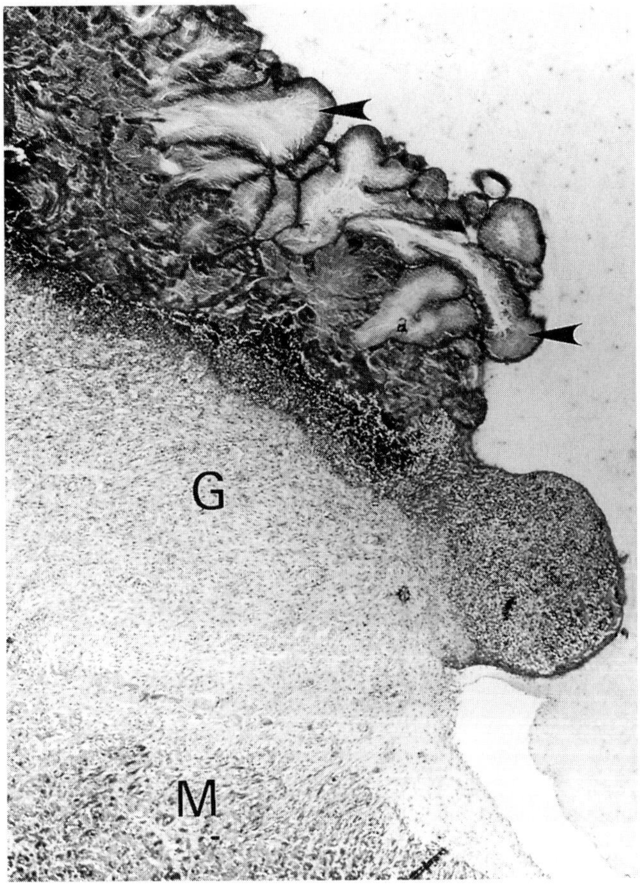

Figure 4-30 Heart, endocardium and myocardium from the affected valve cusp; pig. Vegetative valvular endocarditis. Note abundant masses of bacterial colonies *(arrowheads)* overlying a zone of inflammatory cells and granulation tissue *(G)*. *M*, myocardium. H & E stain. ×105.

in dogs. Grossly, after the initial ulcer heals, the area is replaced by raised, white plaques of fibrous and mineralized tissue.

Myocardial Diseases

Growth Disturbances

Hypertrophy of the myocardium represents an increase in muscle mass, the result of an increase in size of cardiac muscle cells. Hypertrophy is generally secondary and is the result of a compensatory response to increased workload; it is usually reversible on removal of the cause. However, primary hypertrophy also occurs, as in cats and dogs with idiopathic hypertrophic cardiomyopathy (see below), and is not reversible. Two anatomic forms of hypertrophy are recognized. **Eccentric hypertrophy** results in a heart with enlarged ventricular chambers and walls of normal to somewhat decreased thickness; it is produced by lesions that increase blood volume load, such as valvular insufficiencies and septal defects. In **concentric hypertrophy** the heart is characterized by small ventricular chambers that have thick walls; it results from lesions that increase pressure load, such as valvular stenosis, systemic hypertension, and pulmonary disease. Some cats with hyperthyroidism have a cardiac hypertrophy that is mediated by enhanced production of myocardial contractile proteins under the influence of increased concentration of circulating thyroid hormones. The hypertrophy is reversible on return to euthyroidism.

Three stages of myocardial hypertrophy are recognizable: (1) initiation, (2) stable hyperfunction, and (3) deterioration of function associated with degeneration of hypertrophied myocytes. Microscopically, in myocardial hypertrophy the myocytes are enlarged and have large nuclei.

Diseases that can result in right ventricular hypertrophy include dirofilariasis (Fig. 4-31) and congenital pulmonic stenosis in dogs, "brisket disease" ("high-altitude disease") in cattle, and chronic alveolar emphysema ("heaves") in horses. Cattle maintained under the hypoxic conditions that exist at altitudes above 7000 feet above sea level develop pulmonary hypertension and subsequent right heart failure with subcutaneous edema, chronic passive congestion of the liver ("nutmeg liver"), and right ventricular hypertrophy. Exposure to certain poisonous plants (*Oxytropis* spp. and *Astragalus* spp.) increases the severity of the disease.

Left ventricular hypertrophy occurs in dogs with congenital subaortic stenosis. Biventricular hypertrophy can occur with hypertrophic cardiomyopathy and various congenital cardiac anomalies. Eccentric hypertrophy develops in the late stages of diseases that initially cause concentric hypertrophy.

Infiltration

Fatty infiltration is the presence of increased numbers of lipocytes interposed between myocardial fibers. The lesion

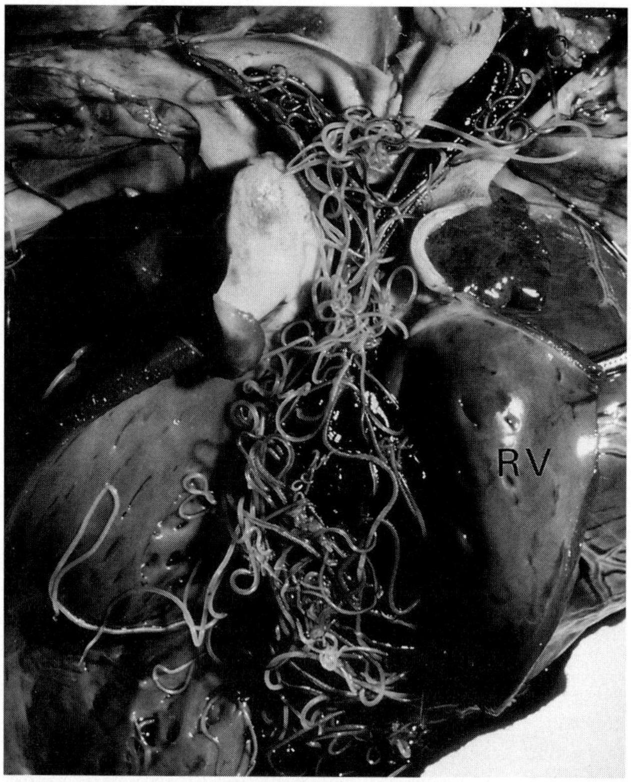

Figure 4-31 Heart, opened; dog. Dirofilariasis. Numerous adult *Dirofilaria immitis* are surrounded in clotted blood in the right ventricle *(RV),* and pulmonary artery. *Courtesy Dr. M.D. McCracken.*

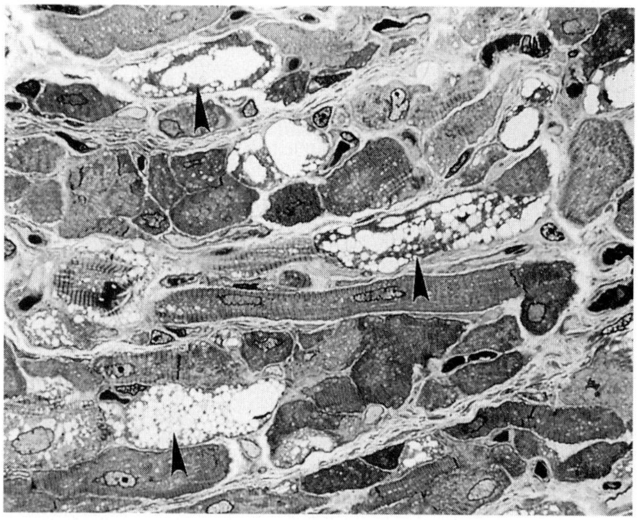

Figure 4-32 Heart, section of myocardium; dog. Myocardial vacuolar degeneration, chronic doxorubicin cardiotoxicity. The affected myocytes have prominent sarcoplasmic vacuolation *(arrowheads).* Plastic-embedded, toluidine blue–stained section. ×425.

is associated with obesity and appears as abundant epicardial and myocardial deposits of adipose tissue.

Degeneration

Fatty degeneration (fatty change) is the accumulation of abundant lipid droplets in the sarcoplasm of myocytes. Grossly, the myocardium is pale and flabby. Microscopically, affected myocytes have numerous variably sized spherical droplets that appear as empty vacuoles in paraffin sections but stain positively for lipids with lipid-soluble stains in frozen sections. This lesion occurs with systemic disorders such as severe anemia, toxemia, and copper deficiency but is seen much less often in the heart than in the liver and kidneys.

Hydropic degeneration, a distinctive microscopic alteration in cardiac muscle cells, is associated with chronic administration of anthracyclines, a group of antineoplastic drugs. Affected fibers have extensive vacuolization of sarcoplasm that is initiated by distension of elements of sarcoplasmic reticulum and, eventually, ends in lysis of contractile material (Figs. 4-32 and 4-33).

Lipofuscinosis (brown atrophy) of the myocardium occurs in aged animals and in animals with severe cachexia, but it also has been described as a hereditary lesion in healthy Ayrshire cattle (see Fig. 4-23). Severely affected hearts appear brown and microscopically have clusters of yellow-brown granules at the nuclear poles of myocytes. These granules represent intralysosomal accumulation of membranous and amorphous debris (residual bodies).

BOX 4-2 CAUSES OF MYOCARDIAL NECROSIS IN ANIMALS

Nutritional Deficiencies

Selenium–vitamin E, potassium, copper, thiamine, magnesium

Toxicities

Cobalt, catecholamines, vasodilator antihypertensives, methylxanthines (theobromine, theophylline, caffeine), ionophores (monensin, lasalocid, salinomycin, narasin), vitamin D and calcinogenic plants *(Cestrum diurnum, Trisetum flavescens, Solanum malacoxylon, Solanum torvum),* other poisonous plants *(Acacia georginae, Gastrolobium* spp., *Oxylobium* spp., *Dichapetalum cymosum, Persea americana, Cassia occidentalis, Cassia obtusifolia, Karwinskia humboldtiana),* blister beetles (Epicauta), high-erucic-acid rapeseed oil, brominated vegetable oils, gossypol, T-2 mycotoxin, uremia

Physical Injuries and Shock

Central nervous system lesions and trauma ("heart-brain syndrome"), stress, overexertion, electrical defibrillation, hemorrhagic shock

Myofibrillar degeneration (myocytolysis) represents a distinctive sublethal injury of cardiac muscle cells. Affected fibers have pale eosinophilic sarcoplasm and lack cross-striations. Ultrastructurally, myofibrils have variable

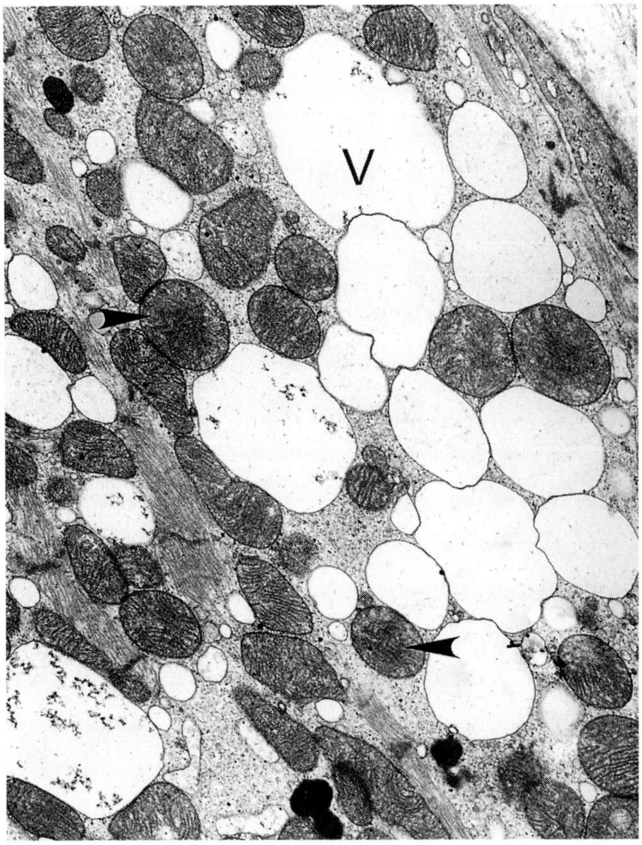

Figure 4-33 Transmission electron micrograph. Heart, section of myocardium; dog. Chronic doxorubicin cardiotoxicity. The prominent sarcoplasmic vacuolation *(V)* is produced by distension of elements of sarcoplasmic reticulum. Even though the myofibrils have extensive lysis, mitochondria *(arrowheads)* are intact. ×14,400.

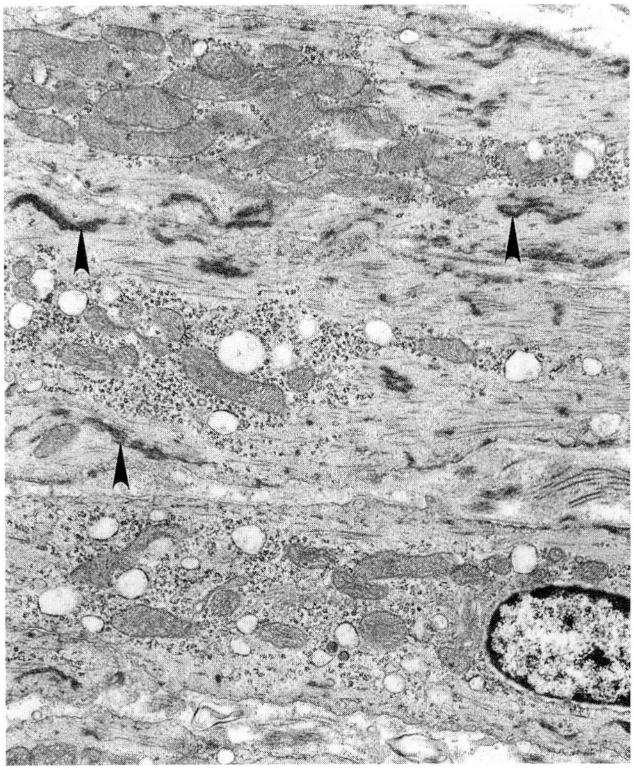

Figure 4-34 Transmission electron micrograph. Heart, ventricular myocardium; duckling. Myofibrillar lysis, furazolidone cardiotoxicity. Affected myocytes have extensive dissolution of myofibrils with scattered free myofilaments and dense clumps of Z-band material *(arrowheads)*. Other organelles appear normal. ×12,350.

extent of dissolution (myofibrillar lysis). This lesion has been described in furazolidone cardiotoxicity in birds (Fig. 4-34) and potassium deficiency in rats.

Necrosis and Mineralization

Myocardial necrosis can result from a number of causes, including nutritional deficiencies, chemical and plant toxins, ischemia, metabolic disorders, and physical injuries (Box 4-2). From this large list of causes of myocardial injury, some of the most frequently observed current examples are ionophore toxicity in horses and ruminants, vitamin E–selenium deficiency in the young of all species, "brain-heart syndrome" of dogs, anthracycline toxicity in dogs, and gossypol toxicosis in swine. In various localized areas throughout the world, numerous deaths in ruminants have resulted from consumption of poisonous plants such as *Acacia georginae* and *Dichapetalum cymosum*.

Cardiotoxicity has emerged as a significant clinical entity in veterinary medicine in recent years with the growing use of antineoplastic drugs in small animal practice and the widespread use of growth promotants in ruminants. The mechanisms of cardiotoxicities include (1) exaggerated pharmacologic action of drugs acting on cardiovascular tissues, (2) exposure to substances that depress myocardial function, (3) direct injury of cardiac muscle cells by chemicals, and (4) hypersensitivity reactions.

Grossly, affected areas appear pale initially, and some progress to prominent yellow to white, dry areas made gritty by dystrophic mineralization (Figs. 4-35 to 4-37). The lesions are focal, multifocal, or diffuse. The most frequent sites of focal lesions are the left ventricular papillary muscles and the subendocardial myocardium, especially when such lesions are related to transient reduction of vascular perfusion. These lesions can be overlooked at necropsy unless multiple incisions are made in the ventricular myocardium. In diseases with diffuse cardiac necrosis, such as so-called white muscle disease of calves and lambs due to selenium–vitamin E deficiency, the pale lesions can be readily observed on the epicardial and endocardial surfaces.

Microscopically, fibers in areas of recent necrosis often appear swollen and hypereosinophilic (hyaline necrosis).

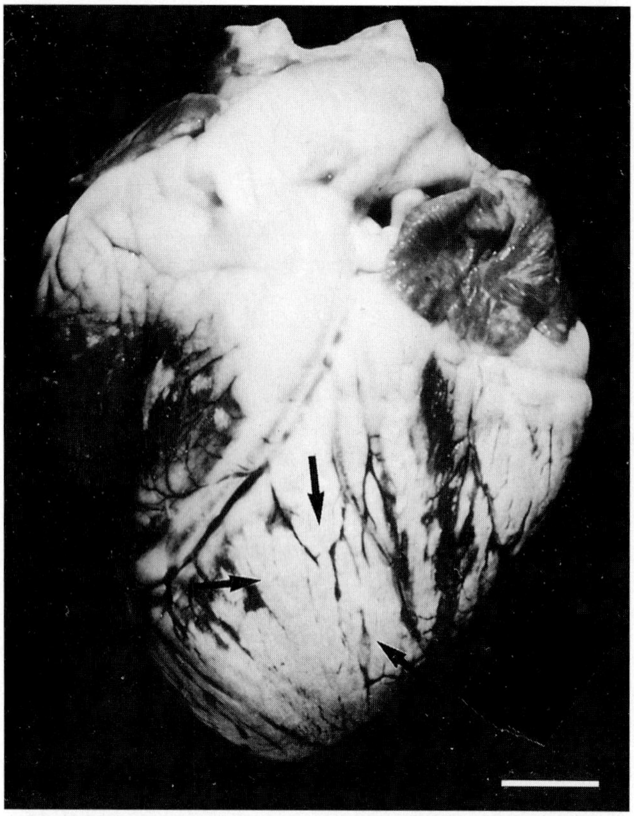

Figure 4-35 Heart, left ventricular myocardium; calf. Myocardial necrosis, selenium–vitamin E deficiency. Note prominent white chalky areas of necrosis with mineralization *(arrows)*. Bar = 2 cm.

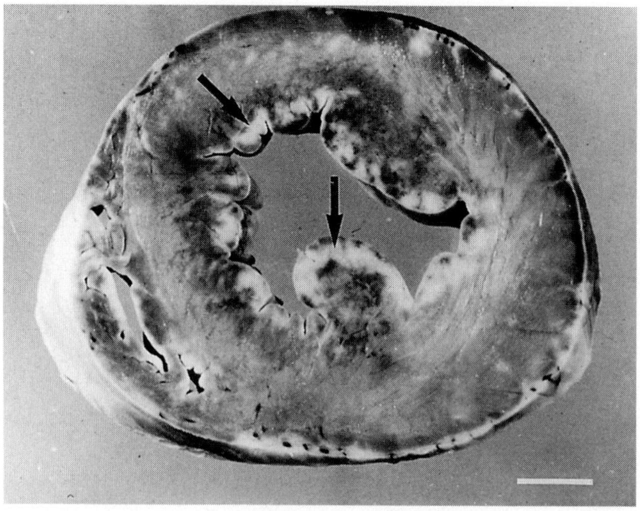

Figure 4-36 Heart, transected ventricles; dog. Myocardial necrosis and hemorrhage. Prominent pale and red affected areas are concentrated in the subendocardium *(arrows)* and subepicardium. Bar = 1 cm.

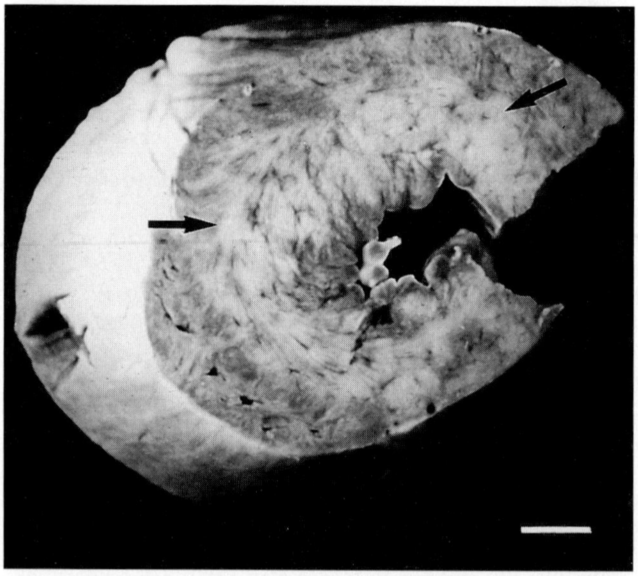

Figure 4-37 Heart, ventricular myocardium; calf. Myocardial necrosis, acute monensin toxicosis. Note the pale, mottled, necrotic areas *(arrows)* distributed throughout the cross-sectioned ventricular myocardium. Bar = 1 cm.

Striations are indistinct, and nuclei are pyknotic. Necrotic fibers often have scattered basophilic granules that represent calcified mitochondria and can be confirmed by electron microscopy (Fig. 4-38). In a second pattern of necrosis, affected myocytes have a "shredded" appearance due to hypercontraction and the formation of multiple transversely oriented bars of disrupted contractile material (often termed contraction band necrosis). A third pattern is seen in necrotic myocytes in large areas of ischemic necrosis (infarcts). These myocytes have features of coagulation necrosis and have relaxed rather than hypercontracted contractile elements.

Within 24 to 48 hours after injury, necrotic areas are infiltrated by inflammatory cells, mainly macrophages and a few neutrophils; these phagocytose and lyse the necrotic cellular debris (Fig. 4-39). In early stages of healing of necrosis, it is often difficult to distinguish the lesions from those found in some types of myocarditis (see below). Later, when necrosis has progressed somewhat, lesions consist of persistent stromal tissues (interstitial fibroblasts and collagen and capillaries) and empty "tubes" of basal laminae formally occupied by necrotic myocytes (Fig. 4-40). The healing phase is characterized by proliferation of connective tissue cells (fibroblasts and capillary endothelial cells) and by deposition of connective tissue (collagen and elastic tissue and acid mucopolysaccharides). Grossly, these areas with healing of myocardial necrosis appear as white, firm, contracted scars.

The outcome of myocardial necrosis varies depending on the extent of the damage. First, many animals die unexpectedly of acute cardiac failure if the myocardial damage is extensive. Second, early deaths from necrosis-related arrhythmias also occur when cardiac conduction is disrupted. Third, some cases eventually develop cardiac

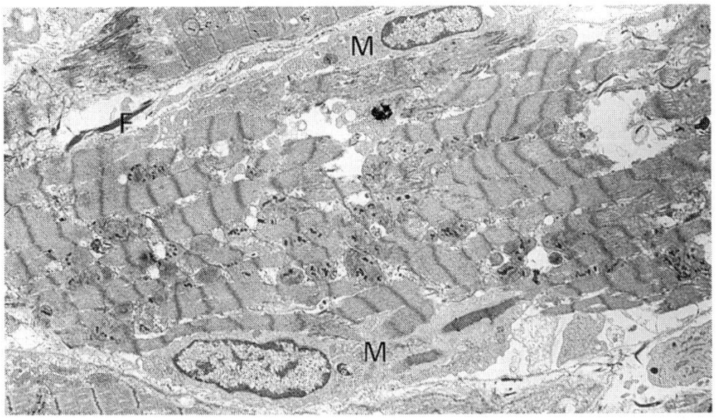

Figure 4-38 Transmission electron micrograph. Heart, necrotic myocyte, longitudinal section; calf. Myocardial necrosis, monensin toxicosis. The necrotic myocyte *(center)* has disrupted myofibrils, damaged mitochondria with matrical densities, and several invading macrophages *(M)*. *F*, fibrin. ×6000.

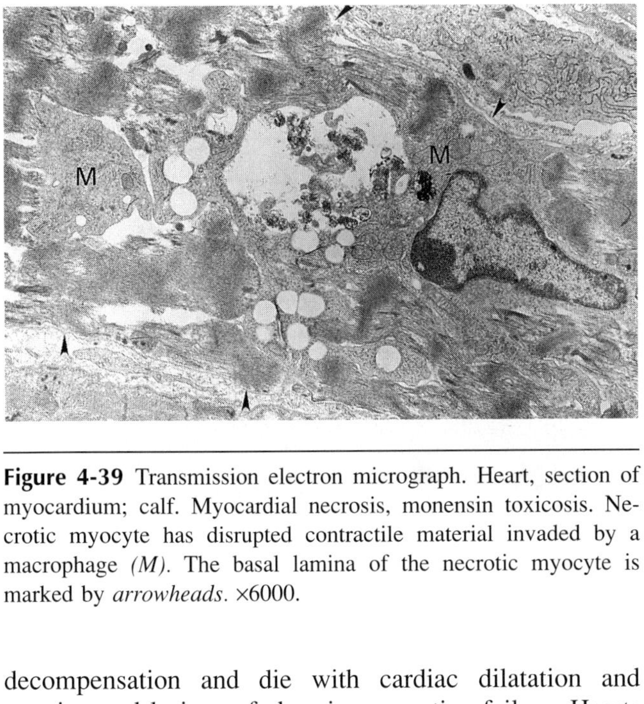

Figure 4-39 Transmission electron micrograph. Heart, section of myocardium; calf. Myocardial necrosis, monensin toxicosis. Necrotic myocyte has disrupted contractile material invaded by a macrophage *(M)*. The basal lamina of the necrotic myocyte is marked by *arrowheads*. ×6000.

decompensation and die with cardiac dilatation and scarring and lesions of chronic congestive failure. Hearts with minimal damage have only microscopically detectable myocardial fibrosis when death eventually occurs from other diseases.

Myocardial mineralization is a prominent feature in several diseases, such as hereditary calcinosis in mice, cardiomyopathy in hamsters, vitamin E–selenium deficiency in sheep and cattle, vitamin D toxicity in several species, calcinogenic plant toxicosis in cattle ("Manchester wasting disease"), and spontaneous myocardial calcification in aged rats and guinea pigs.

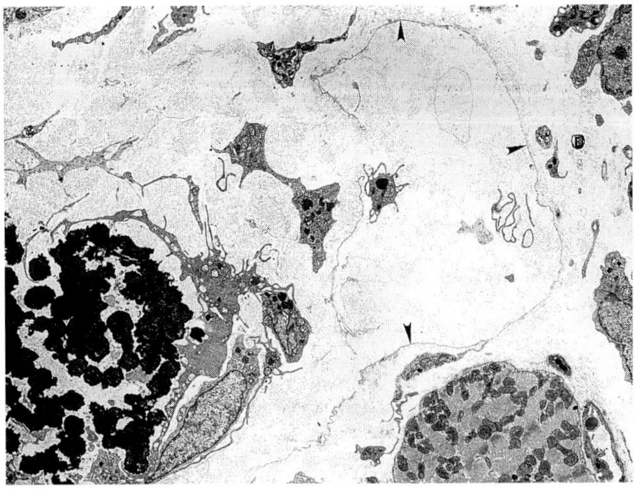

Figure 4-40 Transmission electron micrograph. Heart, section of myocardium; mouse. Myocardial necrosis and calcification, cardiac calcinosis. Necrotic myocyte *(lower left)* has dark granular masses of calcified debris and several invading macrophages. Another necrotic myocyte *(right center)* is outlined by a shell of external lamina *(arrowheads)*. Numerous macrophages are scattered in the interstitium. ×3000.

BOX 4-3 CARDIOMYOPATHIES IN ANIMALS

PRIMARY CARDIOMYOPATHIES (IDIOPATHIC)
Hypertrophic: cat, dog, rat, pig
Dilated (congestive): cat, dog, hamster, turkey, pig, cow
Restrictive: cat

SECONDARY CARDIOMYOPATHIES (SPECIFIC HEART MUSCLE DISEASES)
Heritable (known or suspected): hereditary cardiomyopathy of hamsters, mice, rats, turkeys and cattle; Duchenne-type muscular dystrophy of golden retriever dogs; glycogenoses
Nutritional deficiencies: see list in Box 4-2; other examples include taurine deficiency in cats and foxes
Toxic: see list in Box 4-2; other examples include anthracycline toxicity, furazolidone toxicity, NaCl toxicity
Physical injuries and shock: see list in Box 4-2
Endocrine disorders: hyperthyroidism, acromegaly (hypersomatotropism), hypothyroidism, glucocorticoid excess, functional pheochromocytoma, diabetes mellitus
Infections: see list in Box 4-4
Neoplastic infiltration: malignant lymphoma
Systemic hypertension in cats: spontaneous or associated with chronic renal disease, hyperthyroidism, diabetes mellitus, acromegaly, primary aldosteronism

Cardiomyopathies

Primary and **secondary cardiomyopathies** (Box 4-3) represent important generalized myocardial diseases of either idiopathic or known causation. The primary or idiopathic cardiomyopathies are progressive cardiac diseases. These diseases affect cats and dogs and resemble some diseases of human beings. These diseases are divided into three morphologic types: hypertrophic, dilated, and restrictive cardiomyopathies.

Hypertrophic cardiomyopathy occurs frequently in cats, especially in middle-aged males, and is seen infrequently in dogs, usually affecting males of large breeds. Cats usually present with congestive heart failure, and approximately 10% to 20% have posterior paresis from concurrent thromboembolism of the caudal abdominal aorta ("saddle thrombosis") due to left atrial thrombosis. The occurrence of clusters of cases in Persians and Maine coon cat breeds suggests heritability of the disease in some cases. Some dogs die unexpectedly as the first clinical expression of the disease. In both cats and dogs, the hearts are enlarged and have prominent hypertrophy of the left ventricle and interventricular septum. The left ventricular cavity is small and the left atrium is dilated. In a few cases, the interventricular septum is disproportionately hypertrophied in relation to the remainder of the myocardium. Microscopically, the lesions of the myocardium are prominent disarray or disorganization of myocytes with interweaving rather than parallel arrangement of fibers (Fig. 4-41). Interstitial fibrosis and various degenerative alterations in myocytes also are present.

Dilated or **congestive cardiomyopathy** is an important cause of congestive heart failure in cats and dogs. Many affected cats have low tissue concentrations of taurine, and supplementation with taurine has reversed the clinical signs of cardiac failure. Taurine-deficient foxes also develop cardiac failure.

Affected cats often are middle-aged males and affected dogs often are males of large breeds, such as Doberman pinschers, Scottish deerhounds, Irish wolfhounds, Saint Bernards, Afghan hounds, Newfoundlands, Old English sheepdogs, English cocker spaniels, Great Danes, and boxers. Some cats develop aortic thromboembolism. At necropsy, lesions of congestive heart failure are present and the hearts are rounded because of biventricular dilatation (Fig. 4-42). The dilated cardiac chambers often have a diffusely white, thickened endocardium. Microscopic and ultrastructural alterations are nonspecific, can be either mild or absent, and include interstitial fibrosis and changes of myocyte degeneration.

Restrictive cardiomyopathy occurs infrequently. It occurs in cats as one of two types of endocardial lesions that result in impaired ventricular filling. In one type, the left ventricular endocardium has diffuse marked fibrosis. Available evidence suggests that the fibrotic lesion is preceded by endomyocarditis. The second type results from numerous moderator bands that traverse the left ventricular cavity. Other examples of restrictive cardiomyopathy in animals include endocardial fibrosis in certain strains of aged rats and congenital endocardial fibroelastosis in Burmese cats.

Secondary cardiomyopathies (also termed specific heart muscle diseases) are those generalized myocardial diseases of known cause. Box 4-3 lists examples (many

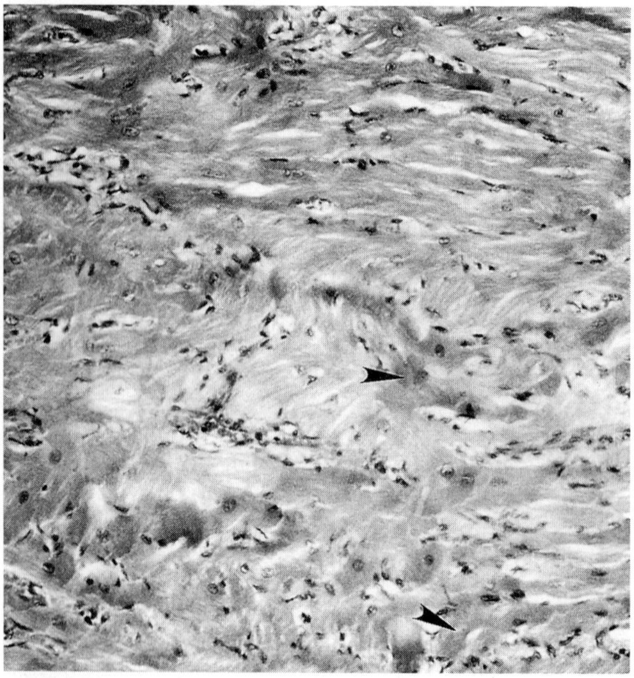

Figure 4-41 Heart, section of the ventricular myocardium; cat. Hypertrophic cardiomyopathy. Large hypertrophied myocytes with interweaving patterns are indicated by the arrowheads. H & E stain. ×105.

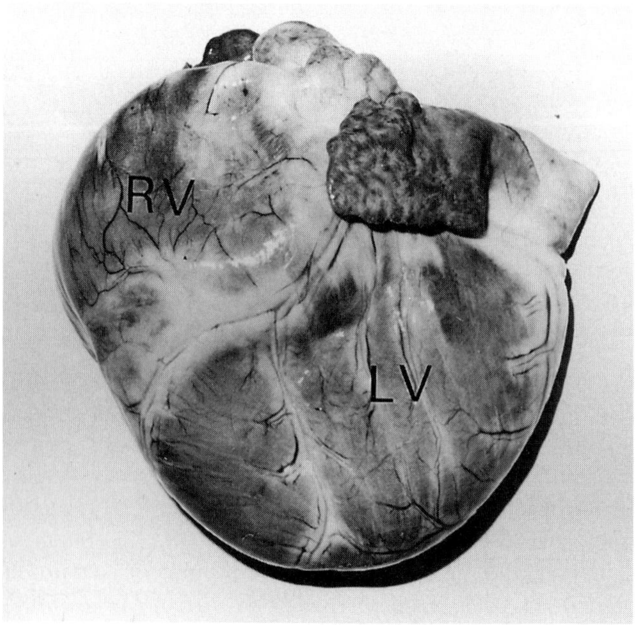

Figure 4-42 Heart, left ventricle *(LV)* and right ventricle *(RV)*; dog. Dilated (congestive) cardiomyopathy. Biventricular dilatation has given the heart a rounded profile.

are discussed either previously under Degeneration and Necrosis of the Myocardium or below under Myocarditis).

Our understanding of the molecular mechanisms of the hereditary cardiomyopathies is developing rapidly. In human patients with familial hypertrophic cardiomyopathy, inherited in an autosomal dominant manner, a variety of single-gene mutations have been documented. The mutations affect genes that encode sarcomeric proteins of cardiac myocytes. Altered cardiac proteins include cardiac β-myosin heavy chain, cardiac troponin T, cardiac troponin I, α-tropomyosin, ventricular myosin essential light chain, ventricular myosin regulatory light chain, and cardiac myosin-binding protein C. It remains unclear how these mutant proteins result in functional and structural alterations of cardiac muscle cells. It is expected that similar gene mutations and altered proteins will be discovered in the various heritable cardiomyopathies of animals.

Also, a portion of cases of dilated cardiomyopathy in human patients appears to be inherited. In these patients, alterations in several myocytic proteins including dystrophin and actin have been documented.

Inflammation

Myocarditis generally is the result of infections spread hematogenously to the myocardium and occurs in various systemic diseases. Infrequently, myocarditis is the primary lesion in affected animals and responsible for their death. Types of inflammation provoked by infectious agents that produce myocarditis include suppurative, necrotizing, hemorrhagic, lymphocytic, and eosinophilic. **Suppurative myocarditis** results from localization of pyogenic bacteria in the myocardium. These often originate from the vegetations of vegetative valvular endocarditis on the mitral and aortic valves. Pale, disseminated lesions are present grossly in the myocardium. These foci consist of neutrophils and necrotic myocytes that form abscesses. **Necrotizing myocarditis** is a frequent lesion of toxoplasmosis, a common disease of cats and dogs. **Hemorrhagic myocarditis** occurs together with the hemorrhagic inflammation typically found in skeletal muscle of cattle with blackleg *(Clostridium chauvoei)*. **Lymphocytic myocarditis** is usually a lesion of viral infections and is well illustrated by the lesions of parvoviral myocarditis of puppies. Dogs with parvoviral myocarditis die unexpectedly and have generalized lesions of acute congestive heart failure, but lack lesions in the intestine, the primary site of viral damage in approximately 95% of clinical cases. The heart is pale and flabby and has disseminated interstitial lymphocytic infiltrations, scattered myocytes with large, basophilic, intranuclear viral inclusion bodies, and, in dogs that survive, fibrosis (Fig. 4-43). **Eosinophilic myocarditis** is the result of some parasitic infections, such as sarcocystosis. The various infectious diseases that cause myocarditis in animals are summarized in Box 4-4.

The pathogenesis and expected outcome of cases of myocarditis remain an important area of research because

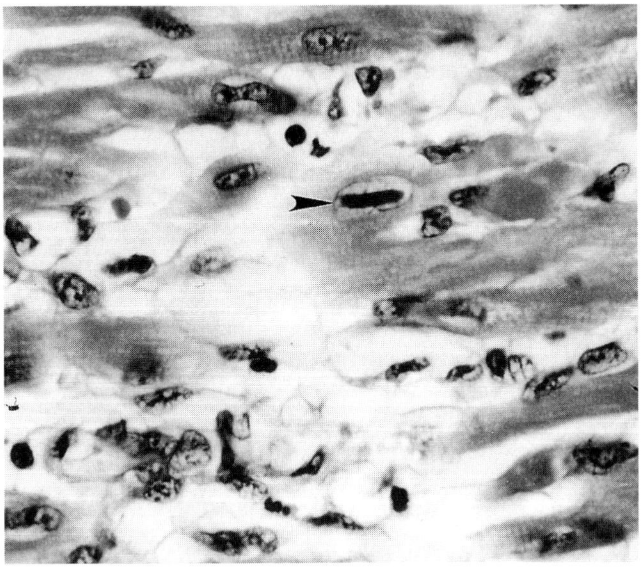

Figure 4-43 Heart, section of myocardium; dog. Myocarditis, parvovirus infection. Note intranuclear inclusion body in a myocyte *(arrowhead)*. H & E stain. ×425.

BOX 4-4 DISEASES THAT CAUSE MYOCARDITIS IN ANIMALS

Viral

Canine parvovirus, encephalomyocarditis, foot-and-mouth disease, pseudorabies, canine distemper, cytomegalovirus, Newcastle disease, avian encephalomyelitis, Eastern and Western equine encephalomyelitis

Bacterial

Blackleg *(Clostridium chauvoei)*, listeriosis *(Listeria monocytogenes)*, Tyzzer's disease *(Bacillus piliformis)*, necrobacillosis *(Fusobacterium necrophorum)*, tuberculosis (*Mycobacterium* spp.), caseous lymphadenitis *(Corynebacterium pseudotuberculosis)*, disseminated infections by *Actinobacillus equuli, Staphylococcus* sp., *Corynebacterium kutscheri, Pseudomonas aeruginosa,* and *Streptococcus pneumoniae*

Protozoan

Toxoplasmosis *(Toxoplasma gondii)*, sarcocystosis (*Sarcocystis* sp.), encephalitozoonosis *(Encephalitozoon cuniculi)*, trypanosomiasis (Chagas' disease [*Trypanosoma cruzi*])

Parasitic

Cysticercosis *(Cysticercus cellulosae)*, trichinosis (*Trichinella* sp.)

Idiopathic

Eosinophilic myocarditis

of the importance of this lesion in cardiac failure in human beings. The sequellae to myocarditis include (1) complete resolution of lesions, (2) scattered residual myocardial scars, or (3) progressive myocardial damage with acute or, in some cases, chronic cardiac failure as secondary dilated (congestive) cardiomyopathy. In experimental studies of myocarditis induced in mice by coxsackie B virus, the severity of myocarditis was influenced by the virulence of the virus and mouse strain and was enhanced by host factors such as young age, male sex, pregnancy, poor nutrition, whole-body ionizing radiation, cold environmental temperatures, alcohol ingestion, exercise, and cortisone administration. Much of the myocardial damage in coxsackie B virus infection is induced by immunologic reactions (with T lymphocyte involvement) rather than by direct viral injury.

Conduction System Diseases

Conduction system disorders have been described mainly in dogs and horses, probably because clinical cardiologic evaluations are done most frequently in these species. Few pathologic evaluations of the tissues of the conduction system have been reported. Specific presumably inherited diseases in dogs include (1) unexpected death in Doberman pinscher dogs associated with focal degeneration of the bundle of His, (2) syncope in pug dogs with lesions of the bundle of His, (3) intermittent sinus arrest in deaf dalmatian dogs, presumably associated with lesions in the sinus node, and (4) sinoatrial syncope (sick sinus syndrome) in miniature schnauzers and springer spaniels. Other arrhythmias in dogs and horses are atrial fibrillation and heart block. Dogs with atrial fibrillation usually have short survival times and have atrial dilatation with mitral insufficiency, but some horses survive longer and at necropsy have atrial fibrosis. Heart block of first degree (incomplete), second degree (incomplete with dropped beats), and third degree (complete) have been associated with myocardial lesions, such as areas of scarring in horses and dogs. However, some investigators consider second-degree heart block in horses a normal phenomenon.

Neoplastic Diseases

Various primary and secondary neoplasms develop either in or near the heart. The primary neoplasms include rhabdomyoma, rhabdomyosarcoma, schwannoma, and hemangiosarcoma. **Rhabdomyomas** and **rhabdomyosarcomas** are rare in animals and form gray nodules in the myocardium that often project into the cardiac chambers. **Congenital rhabdomyomatosis** in swine and guinea pigs is really a nonneoplastic hamartoma. Multiple, pale, poorly circumscribed areas are scattered in the myocardium and are composed of large glycogen-laden myocytes. **Schwannomas** involve cardiac nerves in cattle and appear as single or multiple white nodules detected as incidental findings at slaughter.

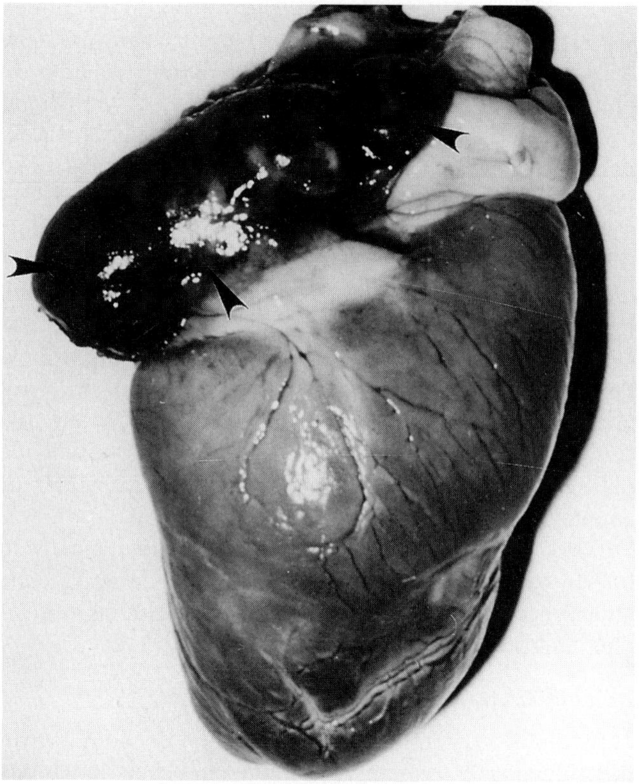

Figure 4-44 Heart, right atrium; dog. Hemangiosarcoma. The atrium is enlarged by the dark red neoplastic mass *(arrowheads)*.

Cardiac **hemangiosarcoma** is an important neoplasm of dogs and can arise either in the heart (primary) or by metastasis (secondary) from sites such as the spleen. This neoplasm is usually seen in the right atrium and only occasionally involves the right ventricle. Grossly, protruding red to red-black blood-containing masses are located on the epicardial surface. Rupture produces fatal hemopericardium and cardiac tamponade (Fig. 4-44). Microscopically, the neoplasms are composed of scattered, elongated, plump neoplastic endothelial cells that may or may not form vascular spaces containing blood. Pulmonary metastases are frequent.

Malignant lymphoma (lymphosarcoma) often causes lesions in the hearts of cattle, and these can be severe enough to cause death from cardiac failure. Cardiac lesions may also be present in dogs and cats with malignant lymphoma. The neoplastic cell infiltration can be diffuse or nodular and involve the myocardium and pericardium. Lymphomatous tissue appears as white masses that resemble deposits of fat (Fig. 4-45). Microscopically, extensive infiltrations of neoplastic lymphocytes are present between myocytes (Fig. 4-46). Other generalized neoplasms occasionally have metastatic lesions in the heart.

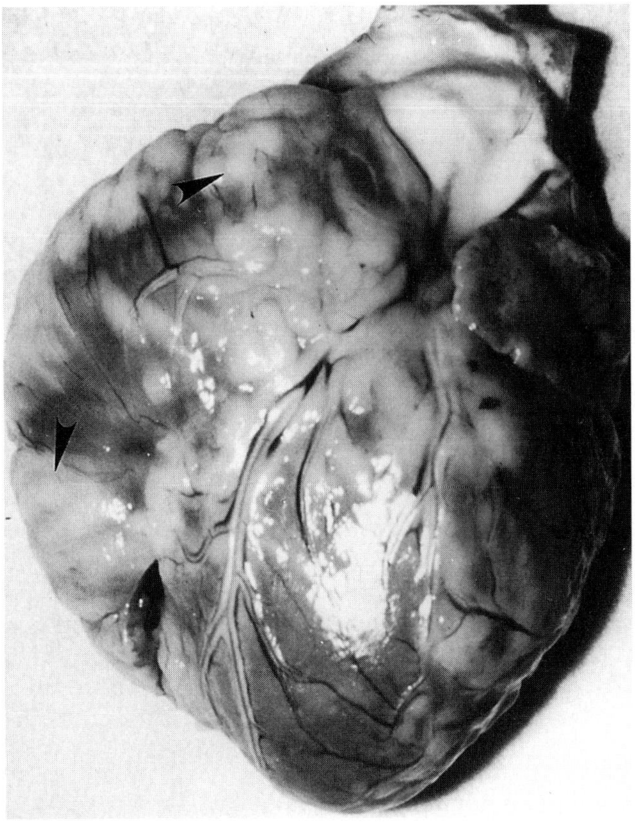

Figure 4-45 Heart, myocardium; dog. Lymphosarcoma. Neoplastic infiltration of the ventricular myocardium is evident as numerous white areas *(arrowheads)*.

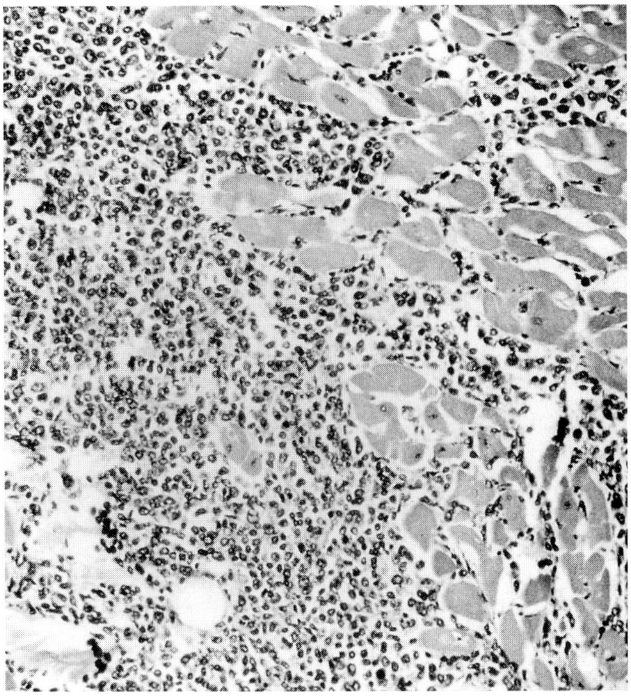

Figure 4-46 Heart, section of myocardium; cow. Lymphosarcoma. Neoplastic lymphocytes have extensively infiltrated the ventricular myocardium. H & E stain. ×265.

Heart base tumors are primary neoplasms of extracardiac tissues in dogs but arise at the base of the heart and can produce vascular obstruction and cardiac failure. The most common neoplasm arising at this location is the **aortic body tumor** or **chemodectoma** (paraganglioma), but, occasionally, ectopic thyroid or parathyroid tissue gives origin to neoplasms in this area. The aortic body is a chemoreceptor organ. In some cases, aortic body tumors become large, white, firm masses that surround and compress the great vessels and atria (Fig. 4-47). Brachycephalic dog breeds are most frequently affected. Microscopically, the neoplastic cells are polyhedral with vacuolated cytoplasm and are supported by an abundant, fine connective tissue stroma.

VASCULAR SYSTEM

Introduction

Normal Morphology

The vascular system is subdivided into **arterial, capillary, venous,** and **lymph segments.** The arteries are classified into three types: elastic arteries, muscular arteries, and arterioles. The venous vessels are termed venules and veins. The lymph vasculature includes lymph capillaries and lymph vessels. Interposed between the arterial and venous segments are the capillary beds. A vascular segment termed the **microcirculation** includes arterioles, capillaries, and venules and is the major area of exchange between the circulating blood and the peripheral tissues.

The overall design of the blood and lymph vessels is similar, except that luminal diameter, wall thickness, and the presence of other anatomic features such as valves vary between the different segments. The luminal surface of all vessels is lined by longitudinally aligned endothelial cells lying over a basal lamina. Vessel walls are divided into three layers or tunics: intima, media, and adventitia. However, some of the layers can be deleted or all of the layers can be thinned in some segments of the vascular system, depending on the intravascular pressures. The large **elastic arteries,** such as the aorta, have (1) an intima composed of endothelium and subendothelial connective tissue, (2) a very thick tunica media composed of fenestrated elastic laminae with interposed smooth muscle cells and ground substance and bordered internally by the internal elastic lamina and externally by the external elastic lamina, and (3) an outer tunica adventitia layer composed of collagen and elastic fibers and connective tissue cells with penetrating blood vessels, termed the vasa vasorum, supplying nutrients to the adventitia and the

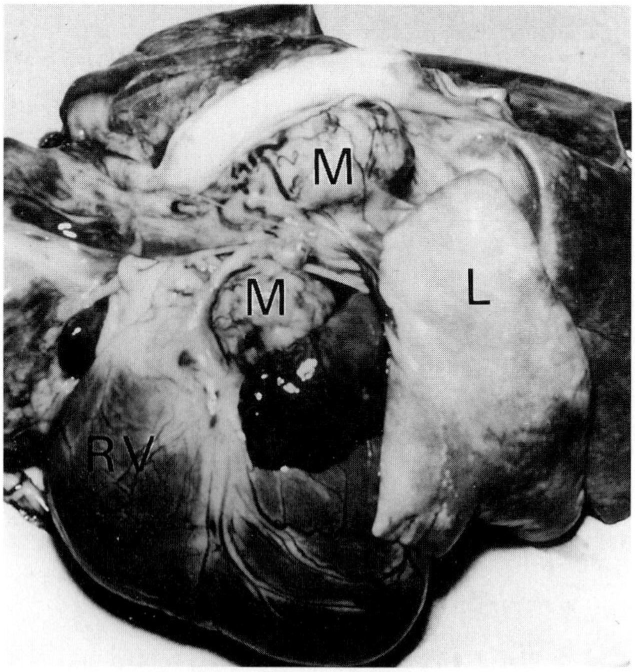

Figure 4-47 Heart, right ventricle *(RV)*; lung *(L)*; dog. Heart base tumor (aortic body tumor, chemodectoma). Multiple tumor masses *(M)* surround the large vessels at the base of the heart.

outer half of the media. In **muscular arteries** and **arterioles,** the tunica media is composed largely of smooth muscle cells arranged in a circumferential pattern. Arterioles are the smallest arterial channels and are generally less than 100 μm in diameter and with one to three layers of smooth muscle cells in the tunica media.

Capillaries are 5 to 10 μm in diameter and their endothelium is one of three types: (1) continuous, (2) fenestrated (as in the endocrine glands), and (3) porous (as in renal glomeruli). The endothelium rests on an external lamina surrounded by pericytes. Lesions of the endothelium might not be evident by light microscopy and electron microscopy is required for characterization.

Veins have thin walls in relation to their luminal size when compared with those of arteries, in which blood pressures are greater. The adventitia is the thickest layer. Valves are present to prevent retrograde blood flow (i.e., away from the heart).

Lymph capillaries lack a basal lamina. **Large lymph vessels** are similar in structure to veins and generally have large lumina, thin walls, and intimal valves, but contain lymph.

Reactions to Injury

The response of vessels to injury involves a complex interaction among the cellular and noncellular elements of the vessel wall and the cellular and noncellular elements of the blood. The key cells of vessels in these reactions are endothelial cells and smooth muscle cells. Endothelial cells are metabolically active and provide a thromboresistant monolayer at the interface of blood and the vessel wall. Key functions of endothelial cells include prostacyclin production, macromolecular transport, and recruitment of inflammatory cells. Injury of endothelial cells is followed by movement of plasma proteins into the subendothelium. Necrosis of endothelium will expose subendothelial collagen and elicit thrombus formation. Endothelial cells at the margin of denuded areas proliferate and reendothelialize the damaged area. The arterial intima has regional differences in the uptake of macromolecules, as well as other unique structural and functional features that result in lesion-prone areas of the vasculature.

The other major cellular component of vessels involved in reaction to injury is the smooth muscle cell. These cells have important functions, including production of extracellular components such as collagen, elastin, and proteoglycans; maintenance of vascular tone; blood monocyte recruitment; lipoprotein metabolism; production of bioactive lipids such as prostaglandins; and formation of oxygen free radicals. These functions are regulated by a wide variety of biochemical mediators, such as various growth factors, cytokines, and inflammatory mediators.

Postmortem Alterations

Usually 12 to 24 hours after death, erythrocytes lyse, and the resultant **imbibition of hemoglobin** produces red discoloration of the normally white intima of blood vessels. Postmortem clotting must be differentiated from thrombosis. **Postmortem clots,** found in veins and large elastic arteries as red "currant jelly" type or, occasionally, as pale "chicken fat" type, are readily removed by traction or gentle flushing at necropsy in contrast to thrombi, which are adherent. **Postmortem contraction** of muscular arteries due to rigor mortis extrudes blood. Microscopically, these muscular arteries are devoid of blood, and their internal elastic lamina is wavy in cross sections of the vessel.

Arterial Diseases

Aneurysms and Ruptures

An **aneurysm** is a localized dilatation or outpouching of a thinned and weakened portion of a vessel. Usually arteries are affected, especially large elastic arteries, but the lesion can also occur in veins. Known causes include copper deficiency in pigs, as copper is needed for normal development of elastic tissue, and infection with *Spirocera lupi* in dogs or *Strongylus vulgaris* in horses. Most cases are idiopathic. **Dissecting aneurysms** are infrequent but have been seen in birds. They result from disruption of the intima, which allows entry of blood into the media, and this dissects along the wall (Fig. 4-48). Aneurysms can rupture. Usually the consequences are rapidly fatal, as rather large arteries typically are involved.

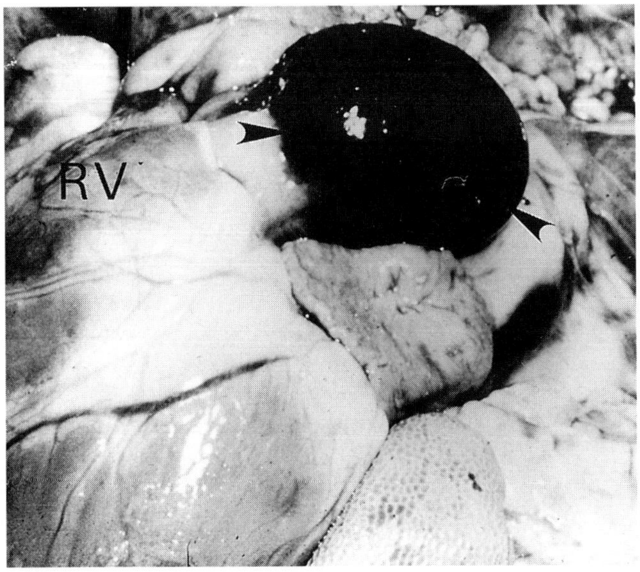

Figure 4-48 Heart, pulmonary artery, right ventricle *(RV);* pig. Dissecting aneurysm, copper deficiency. The dark, blood-filled, bulging segment of the artery wall *(arrowheads)* has resulted from disruption of elastic fibers.

Aortic rupture and rupture of large arteries can be the sequela of severe trauma or occur spontaneously. Sudden rupture of the ascending aorta in horses is associated with marked exertion. Death ensues rapidly from cardiac tamponade as the tear is in that portion of the aorta within the pericardial sac. In horses, the internal carotid artery can rupture into the adjacent guttural pouch, with subsequent epistaxis. This is a consequence of deep mycotic infection of the guttural pouch. Aortic rupture, with or without dissection, is an important cause of death in male turkeys.

Growth Disturbances

Arterial hypertrophy is a response to sustained increases in pressure or volume loads. Affected vessels are generally muscular arteries, and the increase in wall thickness is predominantly due to hypertrophy (and, to some degree, hyperplasia) of smooth muscle cells of the tunica media. Muscular pulmonary arteries of cats are frequently affected, and the lesion has been associated with infection by several parasites, including *Aelurostrongylus abstrusus* (the lungworm of cats), *Toxocara* sp., and *Dirofilaria immitis* (Fig. 4-49). However, the lesions often occur in the absence of parasitic infections. Often, no clinical disease is associated with the lesion in cats, but asthmatic signs have been seen in cats with these parasitic infections. Similar hypertrophy of muscular pulmonary arteries occurs in cattle with hypoxia-induced pulmonary arterial vasoconstriction and subsequent pulmonary hypertension associated with exposure to high altitudes (so-called high-altitude disease or "brisket disease"). (See Myocardial Hypertrophy and Myocardial Diseases). Also, animals with cardiovascular anomalies that shunt blood left to right result in pulmonary hypertension and have hypertrophy of the muscular pulmonary arteries. Uterine arteries in pregnant animals also are hypertrophic.

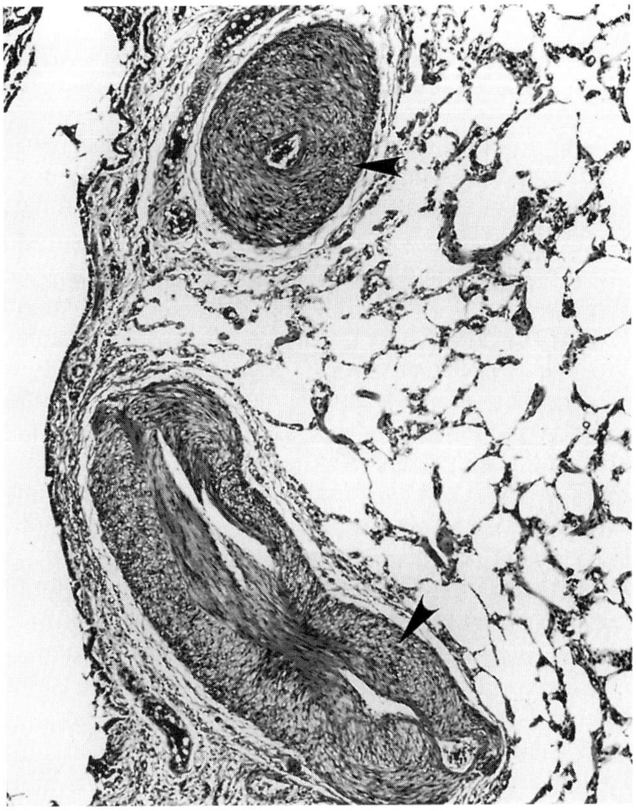

Figure 4-49 Lung, small pulmonary arteries; cat. Medial hypertrophy. Proliferation of smooth muscle cells *(arrowheads)* has resulted in marked thickening of the tunica media. Note luminal narrowing. H & E stain. ×50.

Degeneration and Necrosis

Generalized vascular degenerative diseases in animals are classified into three principal groups. Arteriosclerosis is characterized by intimal fibrosis of large elastic arteries, atherosclerosis by intimal and medial lipid deposits in elastic and muscular arteries, and medial calcification has characteristic mineralization of the walls of elastic and muscular arteries.

Arteriosclerosis is an age-related disease that is frequent in many animal species but rarely causes clinical signs. The disease develops as chronic degenerative and proliferative responses in the arterial wall and results in loss of elasticity ("hardening of the arteries") and luminal narrowing. The abdominal aorta is most frequently affected but other elastic arteries and peripheral large muscular vessels may be involved. Lesions are often localized around the orifices of arterial branches. Etiologic factors in the development of arteriosclerosis are not well defined, but the significant role of hemodynamic influences is suggested by the frequent involvement at arterial branching sites, where blood flow is turbulent. Grossly, the lesions are seen as slightly raised, firm, white plaques. Microscopically, initially the intima is thickened by accumulation of mucopolysaccharides and later by the proliferation of smooth muscle cells in the tunica media and fibrous tissue infiltration into the intima. Splitting and fragmentation of the internal elastic lamina are common.

Atherosclerosis, the vascular disease of greatest importance in human beings, occurs only infrequently in animals and rarely leads to clinical disease, such as resulting in infarction of the heart or brain. The principal alteration is accumulation of deposits (atheroma) of lipid, fibrous tissue, and calcium in vessel walls, which eventually results in luminal narrowing. Many studies have established that the pig, rabbit, and chicken are susceptible to the experimental disease produced by the feeding of a high-cholesterol diet; the dog, cat, cow, goat, and rat are resistant. Lesions of the naturally occurring disease have been detected in aged pigs and birds, and in dogs with hypothyroidism that develop an accompanying hypercholesterolemia. Arteries of the heart, mesentery, and kidneys are prominently thickened, firm, and yellow-white (Fig. 4-50). Microscopically, lipid globules accumulate in the cytoplasm of smooth muscle cells and macrophages, often termed "foam cells," in the media and intima (Fig. 4-51). Necrosis and fibrosis develop in some arterial lesions.

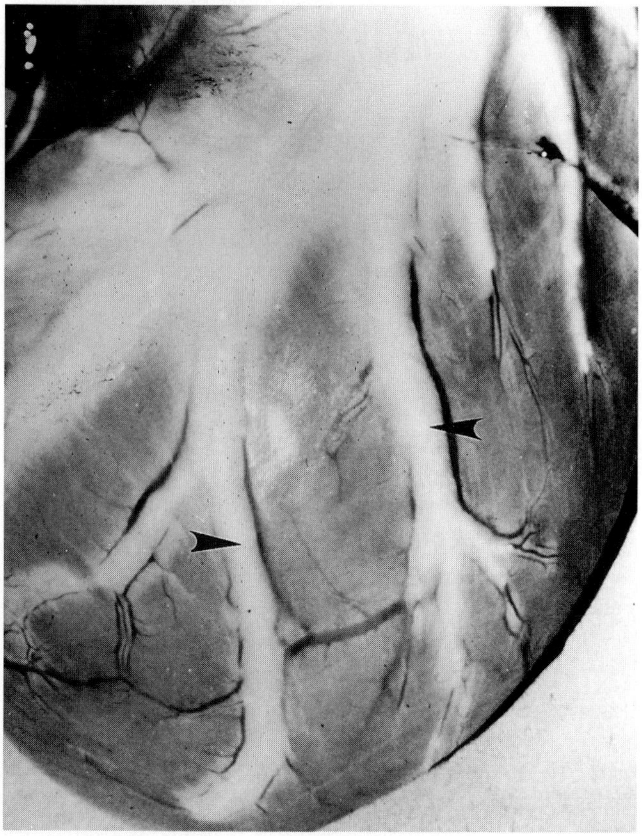

Figure 4-50 Heart, left ventricle; dog. Coronary atherosclerosis, hypothyroidism. The affected epicardial arteries appear as prominent, white, cordlike structures *(arrowheads).*

Arterial medial calcification is a frequent lesion in animals that often have concurrent endocardial mineralization and involves both elastic and muscular arteries. The etiologies of arterial calcification include calcinogenic plant toxicosis, vitamin D toxicosis, renal insufficiency, and severe debilitation, as seen in cattle with Johne's disease. Medial calcification occurs spontaneously in rabbits and in aged guinea pigs and rats with chronic renal disease. Affected arteries such as the aorta have a unique gross appearance; they appear as solid, dense, pipelike structures with raised, white, solid intimal plaques. Microscopically, in elastic arteries prominent basophilic granular mineral deposits are present on elastic fibers of the media but in muscular arteries form a complete ring of mineralization in the tunica media (Fig. 4-52). **Siderocalcinosis** (so-called iron rings), the result of deposition of both iron and calcium salts, occurs in the cerebral arteries of aged horses. Lesions in the surrounding brain tissue are generally absent. Siderocalcinosis lesions are considered incidental.

Arterial intimal calcification (intimal bodies) are distinctive small, mineralized masses within the subendothelium in small muscular arteries and arterioles of horses. They have no deleterious effect.

Hyaline degeneration, fibrinoid necrosis, and **amyloidosis** are vascular lesions of small muscular arteries and arterioles and occur in all animal species. These lesions are generally not detected grossly, but, in some diseases with fibrinoid necrosis of vessels, hemorrhages and edema are seen in affected organs at necropsy. The microscopic feature shared by these lesions is the formation of a homogeneous eosinophilic zone in the vessel wall. Special stains allow differentiation into three types: (1) amyloid confirmed by Congo red and methyl violet; (2) fibrinoid deposits, positive by the periodic acid–Schiff method; and (3) negative staining of hyaline deposits by these stains. Amyloidosis and hyaline degeneration are often observed in small muscular arteries of the myocardium, lungs, and spleen of old dogs. Lesions in the intramyocardial arteries can cause small foci of myocardial infarction.

Fibrinoid necrosis of arteries is associated with endothelial damage and is characterized by entry and accumulation of serum proteins followed by fibrin polymerization in the vessel wall. These materials form an intensely eosinophilic collar that obliterates cellular detail. This lesion is frequent in many acute degenerative and inflammatory diseases of small arteries and arterioles. It is particularly frequent in swine and is an important

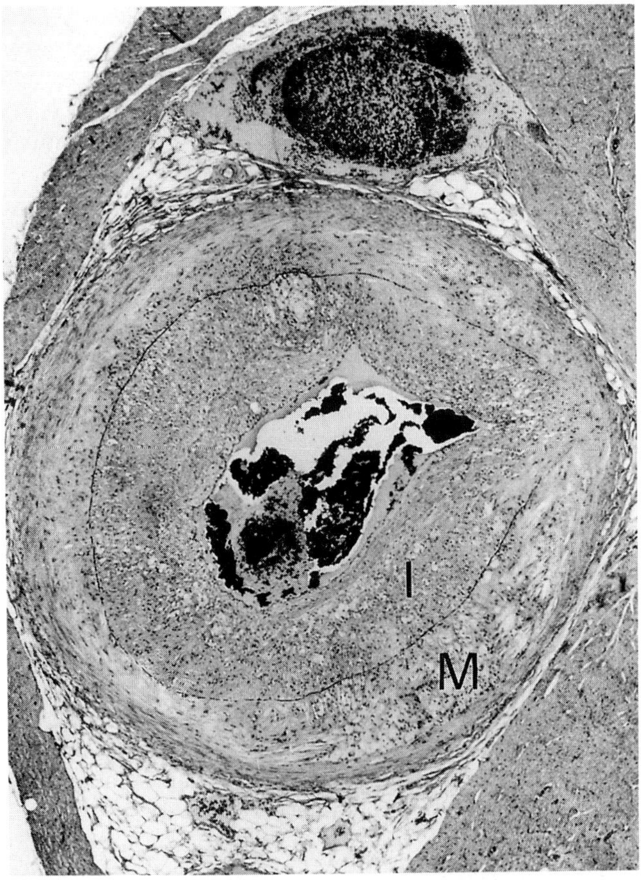

Figure 4-51 Heart, cross section of affected coronary artery; dog. Coronary atherosclerosis. Note extensive accumulation of lipid in "foam cells" throughout the thickened intima *(I)* and media *(M)*. H & E stain. ×25.

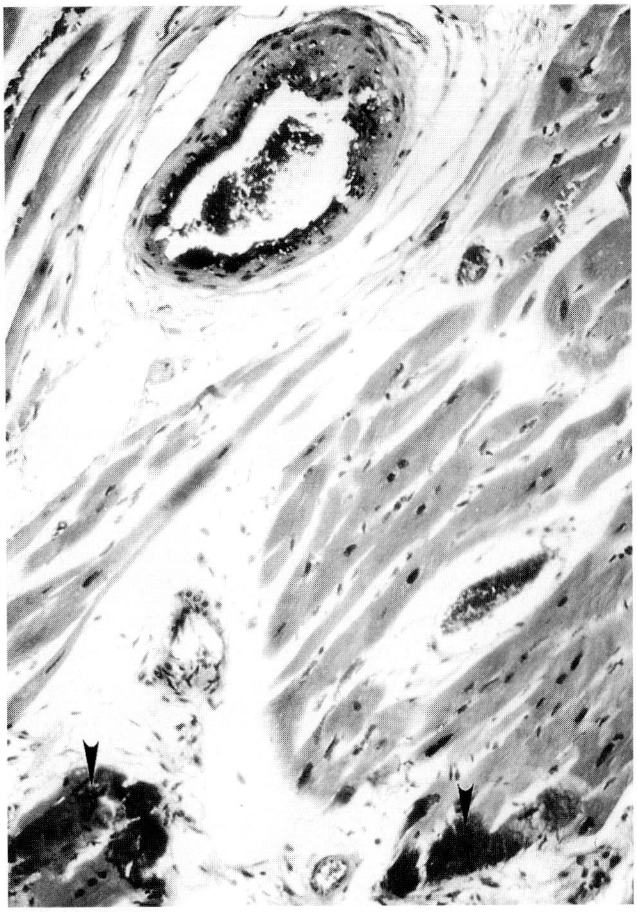

Figure 4-52 Heart, section of myocardium; pig. Arterial and myocardial calcification, vitamin D toxicosis. Dark, basophilic masses of calcium deposits are present in the arterial intima and media *(top)* and in scattered necrotic myocytes *(arrowheads at bottom)*. H & E stain. ×105.

diagnostic feature in cases of selenium–vitamin E deficiency (heart), edema disease (gastric submucosa), cerebrospinal angiopathy, and organic mercury toxicosis (meninges). Fibrinoid necrosis is seen frequently in dogs with uremia and in dogs with hypertension, although hypertension is an uncommon finding in animals compared with human beings.

In pigs with selenium–vitamin E deficiency the vascular lesions produce gross lesions of cardiac hemorrhage ("mulberry heart disease") and massive hemorrhagic hepatic necrosis (hepatosis dietetica). With either form of the disease, fibrinoid necrosis of small muscular arteries and arterioles is widespread and is accompanied by fibrin thrombi in capillaries, especially capillaries of the myocardium (Fig. 4-53). This complex of vascular lesions has been termed dietary microangiopathy. Similar capillary lesions of endothelial damage and occlusion by fibrin thrombi are seen in the cerebellum of vitamin E–deficient chicks with ischemia-induced encephalomalacia and in the skin and skeletal muscles of selenium–vitamin E-deficient chicks with exudative diathesis.

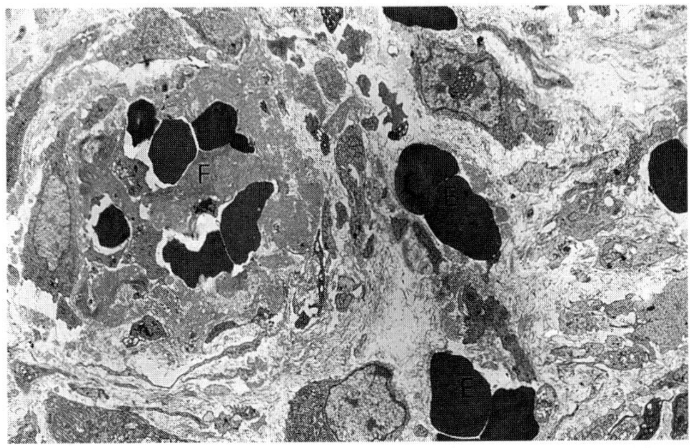

Figure 4-53 Transmission electron micrograph. Heart, section of myocardium; pig. Fibrinoid necrosis, "mulberry heart disease," selenium–vitamin E deficiency. The affected arteriole *(left)* has intraluminal masses of fibrin *(F)* and entrapped erythrocytes. Fibrin masses are also present in the vessel wall, and the adjacent interstitium has edema and hemorrhage. Note scattered erythrocytes *(E)*. ×3500.

Cerebrospinal angiopathy in swine is characteristically sporadic in pigs with signs of nervous system disease. Vascular lesions, with fibrinoid necrosis, are present consistently in arteries of the central nervous system. Similar lesions occur in the arteries of the gastric submucosa of pigs with edema disease, a form of colibacillosis, and many researchers believe that cerebrospinal angiopathy represents a subacute form of edema disease.

Thrombosis and Embolism

Thrombosis represents the product of intravascular coagulation during life. Predisposing factors to thrombosis include (1) endothelial damage, (2) turbulence or stasis of blood flow, and (3) hypercoagulative states. Endothelial damage can be a feature of many arterial diseases. It is frequently present in arteritis, but is uncommon with most of the degenerative arterial diseases other than fibrinoid necrosis and atherosclerosis. Alterations in blood flow occur with vascular or cardiac valvular lesions that cause turbulence; stasis of blood flow can accompany congestive cardiac failure and cardiovascular collapse, as occurs in systemic shock. Hypercoagulative states have occurred in dogs with amyloidosis and some types of renal disease.

Examples of arterial thrombosis frequently observed in animals include caudal aortic thromboembolism in cats and dogs with primary cardiomyopathy (Fig. 4-54), thrombosis of mesenteric and intestinal arteries in horses with verminous arteritis from strongylosis, thrombosis of the pulmonary arteries in dogs with dirofilariasis, and aortoiliac thrombosis in horses. In these diseases, because large arteries can be affected, ischemia in the peripheral tissues results unless adequate collateral circulation exists. Recently formed mural thrombi appear as yellow, firm masses of fibrin adhered focally to the arterial intima. Fibroblastic proliferation and organization develop within days in the thrombi.

Thrombosis or **embolism** of the coronary arteries can result in **myocardial infarction** (Fig. 4-55) and cardiac failure. These lesions are much less common in animals than in human beings. Affected animals generally have one of several types of coronary arterial disease, including atherosclerosis, arteriosclerosis, or periarteritis. In atherosclerosis associated with hypothyroidism (discussed above), severe lesions are present in the extramural (epicardial) coronary arteries of dogs, but this only rarely leads to thrombosis and myocardial infarction. In contrast, severe arteriosclerosis of intramural cardiac arteries in aged dogs can cause small multifocal myocardial infarcts. Affected dogs often also have valvular endocardiosis.

Disseminated intravascular coagulation, initiated by a variety of causes, results in formation of widespread clotting within arterioles and blood capillaries. This clotting phenomenon is due largely to (1) endothelial damage with exposure of subendothelial collagen and subsequent platelet aggregation and (2) intravascular

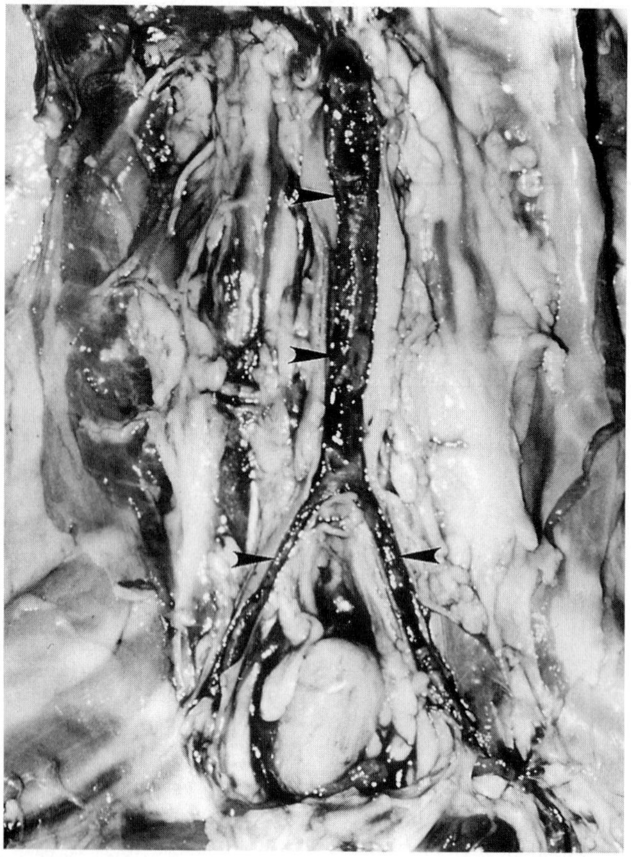

Figure 4-54 Aorta and iliac arteries; dog. Aortic thrombosis. A dark-red, friable thrombus occludes the caudal abdominal aorta and iliac arteries *(arrowheads)*.

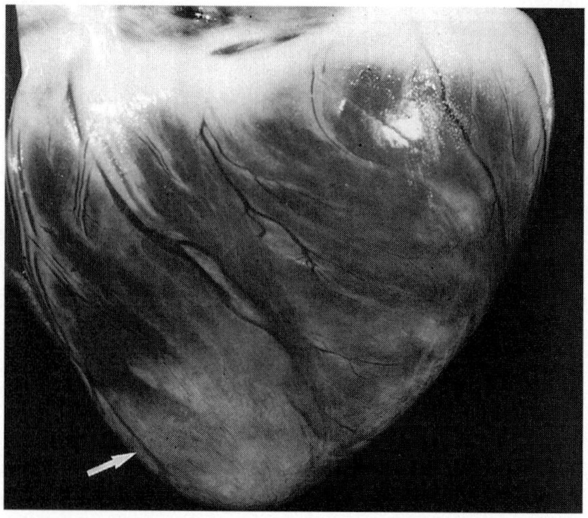

Figure 4-55 Heart, left and right ventricles; dog. Myocardial infarction. Pale, necrotic, circumscribed areas *(arrow)* are present in the ventricular wall. *Courtesy Dr. C.S. Patton.*

activation of the coagulation process. Diseases that can be accompanied by disseminated intravascular coagulation include bacterial endotoxemias, certain viral infections such as feline infectious peritonitis and infectious canine hepatitis, dirofilariasis, certain neoplastic diseases, shock, hemolysis, and extensive tissue necrosis, such as occurs in animals with burns. Extensive clotting depletes coagulation factors (termed consumption coagulopathy), which results in widespread hemorrhages. Hemorrhagic lesions produced by this mechanism include hemorrhagic renal cortical necrosis (Shwartzman-like reaction) or hemorrhagic adrenal gland necrosis in cases of septicemia. Microscopically, organs in cases of disseminated intravascular coagulation have numerous fibrin thrombi in arterioles and capillaries (Fig. 4-56). Fibrinolysis, an intravascular enzymatic process to lyse clots, can continue to be active following the death of the animal and could lead to failure to observe fibrin thrombi in autolyzed tissue.

Embolism is the occlusion of arteries by lodgment of foreign materials, such as disrupted fragments of thrombi (thromboemboli), neoplastic cells, and bacteria. Thromboemboli originating from thrombotic lesions are either bland (sterile) or septic. Septic emboli most often originate from lesions of vegetative endocarditis. Right-sided lesions are disseminated into the lungs and left-sided

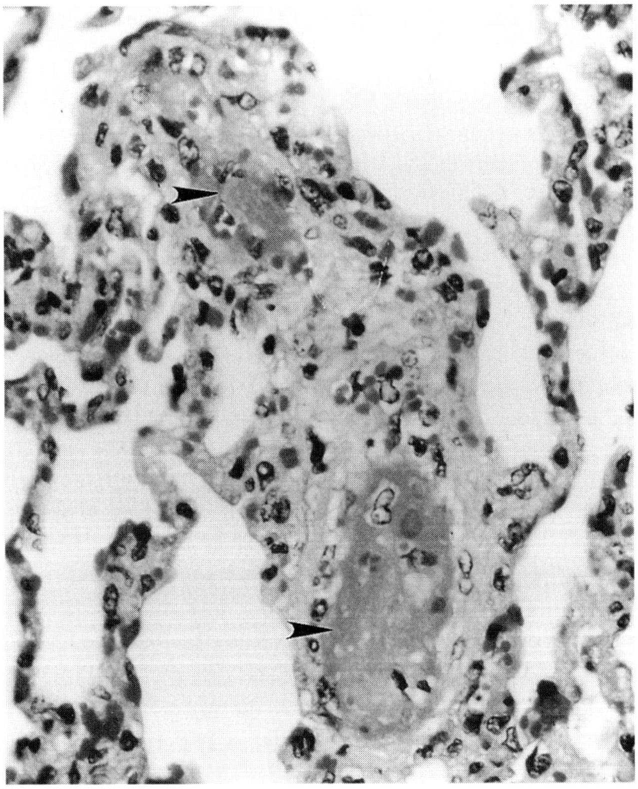

Figure 4-56 Lung; horse. Fibrin thrombi, disseminated intravascular coagulation. Multiple fibrin thrombi *(arrowheads)* occlude pulmonary vessels. H & E stain. ×265.

lesions to the myocardium, kidneys, spleen, joints, and leptomeninges. Other types of emboli include air bubbles or hair fragments forced into the circulation during intravenous injections, release of fat into the vasculature from fractures, release of fragments of dead intravascular parasites such as *Dirofilaria immitis* into the pulmonary circulation of carnivores following administration of adulticidal drugs, and introduction of fragments of fibrocartilage into spinal arteries of dogs and less frequently in other species from disruption of degenerated intervertebral disc material.

Inflammation

Arteritis occurs as a feature of many infections and immune-mediated diseases (Box 4-5). Often, all types of vessels are affected rather than only arteries, and then vasculitis or angiitis is the term applied to the lesions. In inflamed vessels, leukocytes will be present within and surrounding the walls, and damage to the vessel wall will be evident as fibrin deposits or necrotic endothelial and smooth muscle cells. These vascular alterations are accompanied by thrombosis which can result in ischemic injury or infarction in the circulatory field. The "diamond skin" lesions of porcine erysipelas caused by *Erysipelothrix rhusiopathiae* (Fig. 4-57) is an example of cutaneous infarction.

Arteritis and vasculitis can develop from endothelial injury caused by either infectious agents or immune-mediated mechanisms or may be caused by local extension

BOX 4-5 DISEASES THAT CAUSE VASCULITIS IN ANIMALS

Viral

Equine viral arteritis, malignant catarrhal fever, hog cholera, feline infectious peritonitis, bluetongue, African swine fever, equine infectious anemia, bovine virus diarrhea

Bacterial

Salmonellosis, erysipelas *(Erysipelothrix rhusiopathiae)*, *Hemophilus* spp. infections *(H. suis, H. somnus, H. parasuis)*

Mycotic

Phycomycosis, aspergillosis

Parasitic

Equine strongylosis *(Strongylus vulgaris)*, dirofilariasis *(Dirofilaria immitis)*, spirocercosis *(Spirocerca lupi)*, onchocerciasis, elaeophoriasis *(Elaphora schneideri)*, filariasis in primates, aelurostrongylosis, angiostrongylosis

Immune-Mediated

Canine systemic lupus erythematosus, rheumatoid arthritis, Aleutian disease, polyarteritis nodosa, lymphocytic choriomeningitis, drug-induced hypersensitivity

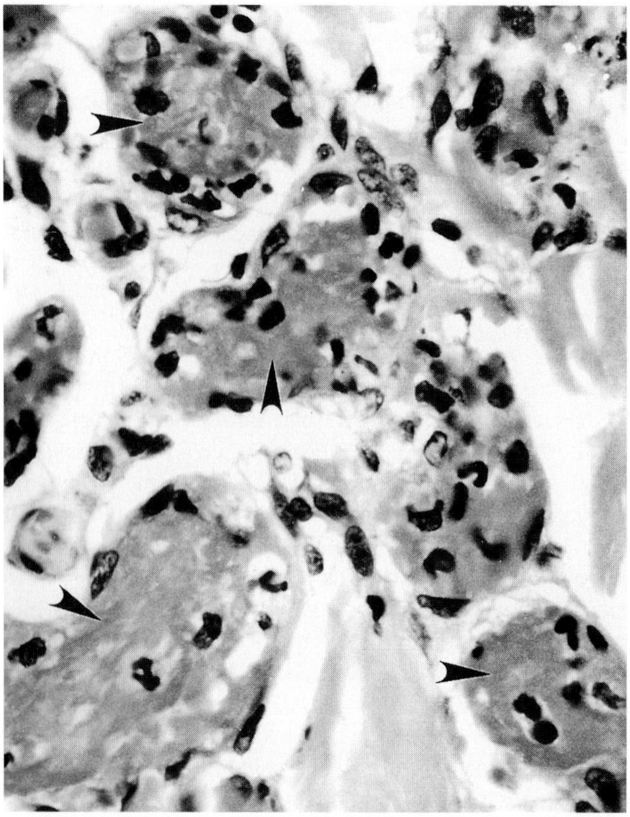

Figure 4-57 Skin; pig. Vasculitis, erysipelas. The dermal vessels *(arrowheads)* contain masses of fibrin. Numerous scattered leukocytes invade their walls. H & E stain. ×425.

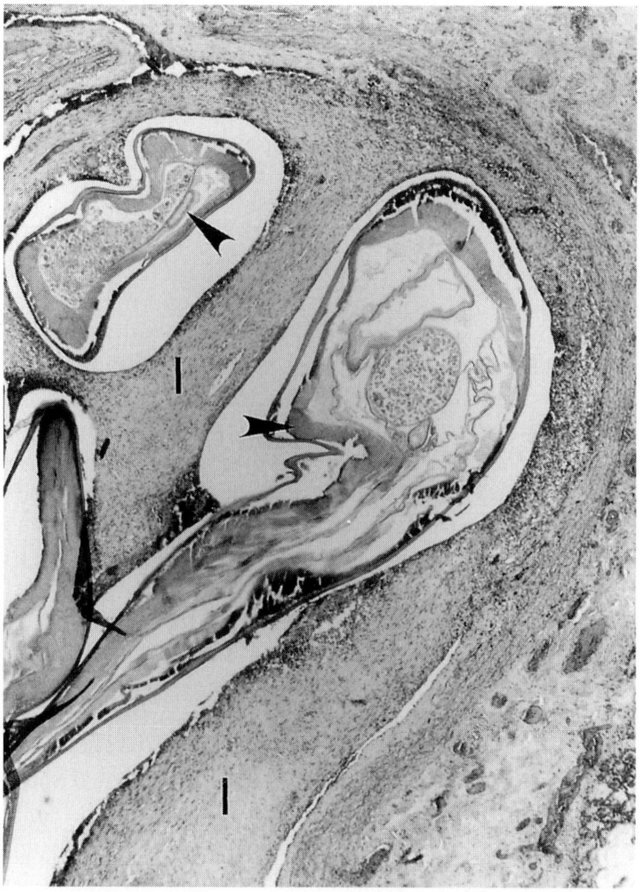

Figure 4-58 Pulmonary artery; dog. Chronic proliferative verminous arteritis, dirofilariasis. Multiple, dead adult *Dirofilaria immitis (arrowheads)* are in the lumen and are surrounded by fibrous proliferation of the intima *(I)*. H & E stain. ×25.

of suppurative and necrotizing inflammatory processes. Equine viral arteritis is a systemic viral infection with a tropism for vascular endothelial cells. In this disease, affected small muscular arteries have lesions of fibrinoid necrosis, extensive edema, and leukocytic infiltration. Grossly, the vascular injury is reflected by severe edema of the intestinal wall and mesentery accompanied by marked accumulation of serous fluids in body cavities.

Arteritis is a prominent feature of several parasitic diseases. In canine dirofilariasis (heartworm infection), maturation of adult parasites occurs in the pulmonary arteries and right atrium and ventricle. The pulmonary arteries containing parasites initially have an eosinophilic infiltration of the intima (termed endoarteritis), with subsequent development of an irregular fibromuscular proliferation of the intima visible grossly as a rough granular or shaggy appearance of the luminal surface (Fig. 4-58). Live or dead parasites can be present within these vascular lesions and be accompanied by thromboembolism and pulmonary infarction. Infection of horses by *Strongylus vulgaris* is very common. During its larval development, the parasite migrates through the intestinal arteries, and the most severe lesions are generally found in the cranial mesenteric artery. The affected vessel is enlarged and its wall is firm and fibrotic. The intimal surface often has an adhering thrombus admixed with larvae. Microscopically, the affected vessel has extensive infiltration of inflammatory cells and proliferation of fibroblasts throughout the wall. Thromboembolism of the intestinal arteries frequently occurs and can produce colic, but the abundant collateral circulation to the equine intestinal tract makes intestinal infarction an unusual event.

Polyarteritis is a disease that occurs sporadically in many animal species and is an important disease of aged rats. Several reports have described the occurrence of polyarteritis (idiopathic necrotizing arteritis) involving the coronary and meningeal arteries in colonies of beagle dogs ("canine pain syndrome"). The lesions are usually attributed to an immune-mediated vascular injury. Medium-sized muscular arteries are selectively involved and grossly appear thick and tortuous, have associated focal hemorrhage, and develop aneurysms and thrombosis (Fig. 4-59). Microscopically, the early lesions include fibrinoid necrosis and leukocytic invasion of the intima

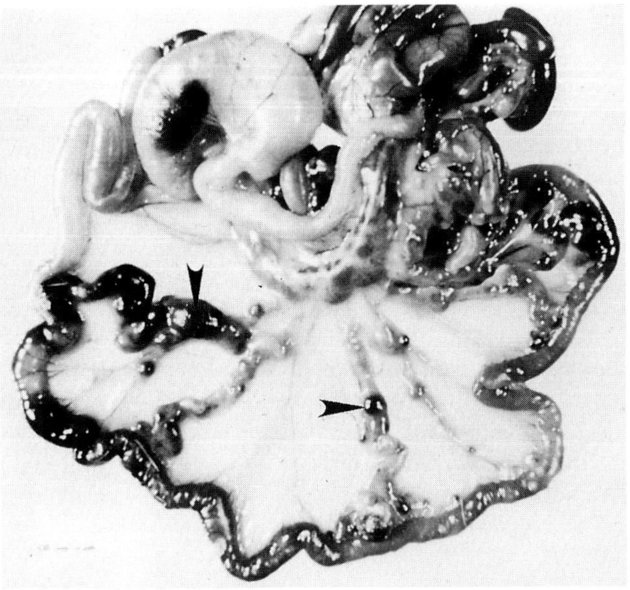

Figure 4-59 Mesenteric arteries; rat. Polyarteritis nodosa. The affected segments of the arteries are thick, red, hemorrhagic, tortuous structures *(arrowheads)*.

and media. In chronic lesions, inflammatory cells and fibrosis involve all layers of the vascular wall.

Neoplastic Diseases

Neoplasms arising from vascular endothelial cells develop in many different organs. **Hemangiomas** are benign neoplasms often found in the skin of dogs. These red, blood-filled masses are well circumscribed. The malignant neoplasm, the **hemangiosarcoma,** occurs frequently in the spleen and the right atrium of dogs. This neoplasm is also generally a red mass, but, microscopically, the neoplastic cells are pleomorphic and do not form distinct vascular spaces. Another neoplasm of vascular origin is the **hemangiopericytoma** of the canine skin. The distinctive microscopic feature is a laminated arrangement of elongated, plump neoplastic pericytes around small blood vessels.

Metastasis of primary sarcomas to distant sites often occurs after invasion of blood vessels.

Venous Diseases

Congenital Anomalies

Portocaval shunts occur in dogs and, because blood bypasses the liver, can result in signs of nervous system disease associated with failure of hepatic degradation of nitrogenous products such as ammonia (hyperammonemia). The resulting nervous system syndrome is termed hepatic encephalopathy. Specifically, the shunts represent retained fetal vascular structures, as in persistent ductus venosus, or arise from prominent dilatation of various portosystemic shunts that normally are quite small vessels. See Chapter 2 on diseases of the liver for further details.

Dilatation

A venous dilatation from weakened vascular walls is termed a **varicosity** (localized involvement) or **phlebectasia** (generalized alteration). Although a frequent lesion in the superficial veins of the legs in women, it is rather uncommon in animals. The pampiniform plexus in the spermatic cord in aged rams and bulls has been affected.

Inflammation

Phlebitis is a common vascular lesion and is often complicated by thrombosis. The vascular lesion arises from (1) systemic infections, (2) local extension of infection, and (3) faulty intravenous injection procedure. Systemic infections with phlebitis as a lesion include salmonellosis in several species and feline infectious peritonitis. In pigs with various septicemias, the gastric fundic mucosa is often severely congested and hemorrhagic because of venous endothelial damage and thrombosis. In severe local infections, such as in metritis or hepatic abscesses, inflammation extends into the walls of adjacent veins and produce phlebitis, with or without thrombosis. Intravenous injections of irritant solutions, injecting solutions into the vascular wall, or intimal trauma produced by indwelling venous catheters result in vascular damage and create an opportunity for localization and proliferation of infectious agents and development of phlebitis. Animals with phlebitis complicated by thrombosis have the additional risk of septic embolism and development of endocarditis and pulmonary abscesses.

Omphalophlebitis ("navel ill") is inflammation of the umbilical vein and often occurs in neonatal farm animals due to bacterial contamination of the umbilicus immediately following parturition. Bacteria from this site can cause septicemia, suppurative polyarthritis, hepatic abscesses (the umbilical vein drains into the liver), and umbilical abscesses.

Cats with feline infectious peritonitis often develop phlebitis in various abdominal organs. This lesion appears to result from deposition of immune complexes that subsequently induce an inflammatory reaction in affected vessels. Occasionally, in some cattle with hepatic abscesses, infection extends into the adjacent large hepatic veins and results in formation of a septic thrombus in the caudal vena cava. Release of the contents of the abscess into the lumen can cause unexpected death of the affected animal.

Several parasitic diseases important in tropical regions of the world are characterized by presence of parasites in the lumens of veins. These diseases include schistosomiasis (blood fluke infection) and infection of cats in South America by *Gurltia paralysans*. Affected cats have spinal cord damage from thrombophlebitis in the lumbar veins, associated with the presence of adult parasites in affected vessels. In schistosomiasis, adult parasites are present in the mesenteric and portal veins, and the resulting phlebitis is characterized by intimal proliferation and thrombosis.

Lymph Vessel Diseases

Congenital Anomalies

Hereditary lymphedema has been described in dogs, Ayrshire calves, and pigs. Affected animals have prominent subcutaneous edema that, in calves, often causes severe swelling of the tips of the ears. Interference with lymph drainage results from defective development of the lymph vessels that are aplastic or hypoplastic.

Dilatation and Rupture

Lymphangiectasis is dilatation of lymph vessels. One cause is obstruction of lymph drainage by invading masses of malignant neoplasms. Another example is intestinal lymphangiectasis, an important disease of dogs in which there is a protein-losing enteropathy. Lacteals in the intestinal villi are prominently dilated, and lymph vessels throughout the wall of the bowel and the mesentery are distended. The role of obstruction of lymph vessels in the pathogenesis of this disease is still unclear. Many diseases with severe acute inflammatory alterations accompanied by vascular damage, as with the pulmonary lesions of bovine pasteurellosis, have prominently dilated lymph vessels.

Rupture of the thoracic duct, either as a result of trauma or from spontaneous disruption, causes chylothorax in dogs and cats. However, many cases of chylothorax occur without injury to the thoracic duct and have been attributed either to lesions that interfere with central venous return or produce obstruction of the thoracic duct (right-sided heart failure, neoplasms, granulomas, cranial vena cava thrombosis, dirofilariasis) or are idiopathic.

Inflammation

Lymphangitis is a feature of many diseases (Box 4-6). The affected vessels are often located in the distal limbs and are thick, cordlike structures. Lymphedema also can be present. Nodular suppurative lesions of lymphangitis often ulcerate and discharge pus onto the surface of the skin. In Johne's disease, the mesenteric lymph vessels are often prominent due to granulomatous lymphangitis, an extension of the enteric infection producing a granulomatous enteritis and lymphangitis (Fig. 4-60).

BOX 4-6 DISEASES THAT CAUSE LYMPHANGITIS IN ANIMALS

BACTERIAL

Porcine anthrax *(Bacillus anthracis),* Johne's disease *(Mycobacterium paratuberculosis),* tuberculosis (*Mycobacterium* spp.), actinobacillosis *(Actinobacillus lignieresii),* glanders ("farcy") *(Pseudomonas mallei),* cutaneous streptothricosis *(Dermatophilus congolensis),* bovine farcy, ulcerative lymphangitis of horses, sporadic lymphangitis of horses

MYCOTIC

Epizootic lymphangitis of horses *(Histoplasma farciminosum),* sporotrichosis *(Sporothrix schenckii)*

PARASITIC

Brugia spp. infection of dogs and cats

Neoplastic Diseases

Lymphangioma represents a rare benign neoplasm composed of lymph channels. The lymphangiosarcoma occurs more often than the benign neoplasm. Vascular spaces contain lymph rather than the blood. Lymph vessels are frequently invaded by primary carcinomas and are a common route of metastasis.

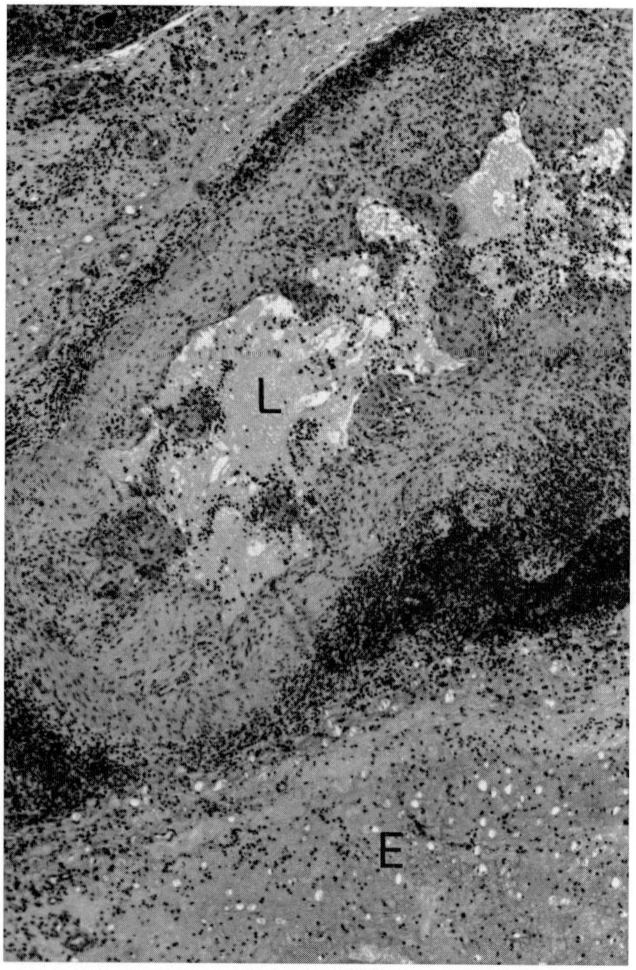

Figure 4-60 Mesenteric lymph vessel; cow. Granulomatous lymphangitis, Johne's disease. The vessel wall is markedly thickened by infiltration of mononuclear leukocytes and proliferation of fibrous connective tissue. Extensive edema *(E)* surrounds the lymph vessel. *L,* lumen. H & E stain. ×56.

Suggested Readings

Allen A. The cardiotoxicity of chemotherapeutic drugs. Semin Oncol 1992; 19:529-542.

Anversa P, Leri A, Beltrami C, Guerra S, Kajstura J. Myocyte death and growth in the failing heart. Lab Invest 1998; 78:767-786.

Ayers KM, Jones SR. The cardiovascular system. In: Benirschke K, Garner FM, Jones TC, eds. Pathology of Laboratory Animals. Vol I. New York: Springer-Verlag, 1978:1-69.

Balazs T, ed. Cardiac Toxicology. Vols I, II, III. Boca Raton, Fl: CRC Press, 1981.

Bastianello SS, Fourie N, Prozesky L, Nel PW, Kellerman TS. Cardiomyopathy of ruminants induced by the litter of poultry fed on rations containing the ionophore antibiotic, maduramicin. II. Macropathology and histopathology. Onderstepoort J Vet Res 1995; 62:5-18.

Beardow AW, Buchanan JW. Chronic mitral valve disease in cavalier King Charles spaniels: 95 cases (1987-1991). J Am Vet Med Assoc 1993; 203:1023-1029.

Bennett D, Taylor DJ. Bacterial endocarditis and inflammatory joint disease in the dog. J Small Anim Pract 1987; 29:347-365.

Birchard SJ, Fossum TW. Chylothorax in the dog and cat. Vet Clin North Am Small Anim Pract 1987; 17:271-283.

Birchard SJ, Smeak DD, McLaughlin MA. Treatment of idiopathic chylothorax in dogs and cats. J Am Vet Med Assoc 1998; 212:652-657.

Bishop SP. Cardiovascular system. In: Andrews ET, Ward BC, Altman NH, eds. Spontaneous Animal Models of Human Disease. Vol. I. New York: Academic Press, 1979:39-79.

Bishop SP. Necropsy techniques for the heart and great vessels. In: Fox PR, ed. Canine and Feline Cardiology. New York: Churchill Livingstone, 1988:637-640.

Bishop SP, Louden C. Morphologic evaluation of the heart and blood vessels. In: Bishop SP, Kerns WD, eds. Comprehensive Toxicology. Vol. 6. Cardiovascular Toxicology. New York: Elsevier Science, 1997:73-93.

Bonagura JD, Darke PGG. Congenital heart disease. In: Ettinger SJ, Feldman EC, eds. Textbook of Veterinary Internal Medicine. Vol. I. Philadelphia: WB Saunders, 1995:892-943.

Bristow MR. Drug-Induced Heart Disease. New York: Elsevier/North Holland Biomedical Press, 1980.

Buchanan JW. Causes and prevalence of cardiovascular disease. In: Kirk RW, Bonagura JD, eds. Current Veterinary Therapy XI. Small Animal Practice. Philadelphia: WB Saunders, 1992:647-655.

Buchanan JW. Chronic valvular disease (endocardiosis) in dogs. Adv Vet Sci Comp Med 1977; 21:75-104.

Calvert CA, Hall G, Jacobs G, Pickus C. Clinical and pathologic findings in Doberman pinschers with occult cardiomyopathy that died suddenly or developed congestive heart failure: 54 cases (1984-1991). J Am Vet Med Assoc 1997; 210:505-511.

Chiu YT, Liu SK, Tsau HL, Shyu JJ, Yang PC, Huang SY. Pathological studies on hypertrophic cardiomyopathy in pigs. J Chin Soc Vet Sci 1994; 20:126-133.

Combs AG, Acosta D. Toxic mechanisms of the heart: A review. Toxicol Pathol 1990; 18:583-596.

Czarnecki CM. Animal models of drug-induced cardiomyopathy. Comp Biochem Physiol 1984; 79C:9-14.

Easley JR. Necrotizing vasculitis: An overview. J Am Anim Hosp Assoc 1979; 15:207-211.

Eschenhagen T, Diederich M, Kluge SH, et al. Bovine hereditary cardiomyopathy: An animal model of human dilated cardiomyopathy. J Mol Cell Cardiol 1995; 27:357-370.

Ferrans VJ. Overview of morphologic reactions of the heart to toxic injury. In: Balazs T, ed. Cardiac Toxicology. Boca Raton, Fla: CRC Press, 1981:83-109.

Feuerstein G, Ruffolo RR, Yue TL. Apoptosis and congestive heart failure. Trends Cardiovasc Med 1997; 7:249-255.

Franklin MT, Field LJ. Use of transgenic animals in cardiovascular toxicology testing. In: Bishop SP, Kerns WD, eds. Comprehensive Toxicology, Vol 6. Cardiovascular Toxicology. New York: Elsevier Science, 1997:201-212.

Freeman LM, Michel KE, Brown DJ, Kaplan PM, Stamoulis ME, Rosenthal SL, Keene BW, Rush JE: Idiopathic dilated cardiomyopathy in Dalmations: nine cases (1990-1995). J Am Vet Med Assoc 1996, 209:1592-1596.

Gibbs C, Gaskell CJ, Darke PGG, Wotton PR. Idiopathic pericardial hemorrhage in dogs: A review of fourteen cases. J Small Anim Pract 1982; 23:483-500.

Granville DJ, Carthy CM, Hunt DWC, McManus BM. Apoptosis: molecular aspects of cell death and disease. Lab Invest 1998, 78:893-913.

Haggstrom J, Hansson K, Kvart C, Swenson L. Chronic valvular disease in the cavalier King Charles spaniel in Sweden. Vet Rec 1992; 131:549-553.

Harpster NK. Cardiovascular diseases of the domestic cat. Adv Vet Sci Comp Med 1977; 21:39-74.

Hayes TJ, Roberts GKS, Halliwell WH. An idiopathic febrile necrotizing arteritis syndrome in the dog: Beagle pain syndrome. Toxicol Pathol 1989; 17:129-137.

Herman EH, Ferrans VJ. Animal models of anthracycline cardiotoxicity-basic mechanisms and cardioprotective activity. Prog Pediatr Cardiol 1997; 8:49-58.

Hongo M, Ryoke T, Ross J. Animal models of heart failure—recent developments and perspectives. Trends Cardiovasc Med 1997; 7:161-167.

Holman RL. Acute necrotizing arteritis, aortitis, and auriculitis following uranium nitrate injury in dogs with altered plasma proteins. Am J Pathol 1941; 17:359-381.

Isaacs KR. The cardiovascular system. In: Turton J, Hooson J, eds. Target Organ Pathology. London: Taylor & Francis, 1998:141-176.

James TN. Normal and abnormal consequences of apoptosis in the human heart. From postnatal morphogenesis to paroxysmal arrhythmias. Circulation 1994; 90:556-573.

Jones JET. Experimental streptococcal endocarditis in the pig: The development of lesions 3 to 14 days after inoculation. J Comp Pathol 1981; 91:51-62.

Jones TC, Gleiser CA. Veterinary Necropsy Procedures. Philadelphia: Lippincott JB, 1954:21-23, 29-31, 52-53.

Jonsson L. Coronary arterial lesions and myocardial infarcts in the dog: A pathologic and microangiographic study. Acta Vet Scand 1972; 38(Suppl):1-80.

Kajstura J, Cheng W, Reiss K, Clark W, Sonnerblick E, Krajewski S, Reed J, Olivetti G, Anversa P. Apoptotic and necrotic myocyte cell deaths are independent contributing variables of infarct size in rats. Lab Invest 1996; 74:86-107.

Karmazyn M, Bend JR. Biochemical and molecular mechanisms of myocardial injury. In: Bishop SP, Kerns WD, eds. Comprehensive Toxicology. Vol. 6. Cardiovascular Toxicology. New York: Elsevier Science, 1997:255-278.

Kellerman TS, Coetzer JAW, Naude' TW. Heart. In: Plant Poisonings and Mycotoxicoses of Livestock in Southern Africa. Capetown, South Africa: Oxford University Press, 1988:83-130.

Kienle RD, Bruyette D, Pion PD. Effects of thyroid hormone and thyroid dysfunction on the cardiovascular system. Vet Clin North Am Small Animal Pract 1994; 24:495-507.

King JM, Roth L, Haschek WM. Myocardial necrosis secondary to neural lesions in domestic animals. J Am Vet Med Assoc 1982; 180:144-148.

Kittleson MD. Feline hypertrophic cardiomyopathy. In: Kirk RW, ed. Kirk's Current Veterinary Therapy XII. Small Animal Practice Philadelphia: WB Saunders. 1995; 854-862.

Kittleson MD, Kienle RD: Small Animal Cardiovascular Medicine. St. Louis: Mosby, 1998:297-318, 319-346, 347-362, 363-369, 370-401, 413-432.

Lamb CR, White RN. Morphology of congenital intrahepatic portacaval shunts in dogs and cats. Vet Rec 1998; 142:55-60.

Laste NJ, Harpster NK. A retrospective study of 100 cases of feline distal aortic thromboembolism: 1977-1993. J Am Anim Hosp Assoc 1995; 31:492-500.

Littman MP. Spontaneous systemic hypertension in 24 cats. J Vet Intern Med 1994; 8:79-86.

Liu SK. Cardiovascular pathology. In: Fox PR, ed. Canine and Feline Cardiology. New York: Churchill Livingstone. 1988:641-660.

Liu SK. Postmortem examination of the heart. Vet Clin North Am Small Anim Pract 1983; 13:379-394.

Liu SK, Peterson ME, Fox PR. Hypertrophic cardiomyopathy and hyperthyroidism in the cat. J Am Vet Med Assoc 1984; 185:52-57.

Liu SK, Roberts WC, Maron BJ. Comparison of morphologic findings in spontaneously occurring hypertrophic cardiomyopathy in humans, cats, and dogs. Am J Cardiol 1993; 72:944-951.

Luginbuhl H, Detweiler D. Cardiovascular lesions in dogs. Ann N Y Acad Sci 1965; 127:517-540.

Luginbuhl H, Rossi GL, Ratcliffe HL, Muller R. Comparative atherosclerosis. Adv Vet Sci Comp Med 1977; 21:421-448.

Markwell PJ, Earle KE. Taurine: An essential nutrition for the cat. A brief review of the biochemistry of its requirement and the clinical consequences of deficiency. Nutr Res 1995; 15:53-58.

Martin RA. Congenital portosystemic shunts in the dog and cat. Vet Clin North Am 1993; 23:605-623.

Maxson AD, Reef VB. Bacterial endocarditis in horses: ten cases (1984-1995). Eq Vet J 1997; 29:394-399.

Mayer NJ, Rubin SA. The molecular and cellular biology of heart failure. Current Opin Cardiol 1995; 10:238-245.

Miller MW, Sisson DD. Pericardial disorders. In: Ettinger SJ, Feldman EC, eds. Textbook of Veterinary Internal Medicine. Vol. I. Philadelphia: WB Saunders, 1995; 1032-1045.

Moise NS, Gilmour RF, Riccio ML. An animal model of spontaneous arrhythmic death. J Cardiovas Electrophys 1997, 8:98-103.

Murdoch DB, Baker JR. Bacterial endocarditis in the dog. J Small Anim Pract 1977; 18:687-699.

Newsholme SJ. Reaction patterns in myocardium in response to injury. J S Afr Vet Assoc 1982; 53:52-59.

Niimura H, Bachinski LL, Sangwatanaroj S, Watkins H, Chudley AE, McKenna W, Kristinsson A, Roberts R, Sole M, Maron BJ, Seidman JG, Seidman CE. Mutations in the gene for cardiac myosin-binding protein C and late-onset familial hypertrophic cardiomyopathy. N Engl J Med 1998; 338:1248-1257.

O'Toole D, Li H, Roberts S, Rovnak J, DeMartini J, Cavender J, Williams B, Crawford T. Chronic generalized obliterative arteriopathy in cattle: A sequel to sheep-associated malignant catarrhal fever. J Vet Diag Invest 1995; 7:108-121.

Palate BM, Denoel SR, Roba JL. A simple method for performing routine histopathological examination of the cardiac conduction tissue in the dog. Toxicol Pathol 1995; 23:56-62.

Patterson DF. Congenital defects of the cardiovascular system of dogs: Studies in comparative cardiology. Adv Vet Sci Comp Med 1976; 20:1-35.

Piper RC. Morphologic evaluation of the heart in toxicology studies. In: Balazs T, ed. Cardiac Toxicology. Vol III. Boca Raton, Fla: CRC Press, 1981:111-136.

Pion PD, Kittleson MD, Rogers QR, Morris JG. Myocardial failure in cats associated with low plasma taurine: A reversible cardiomyopathy. Science 1987; 237:764-768.

Reichenbach DD, Benditt EP. Myofibrillar degeneration: A response of the myocardial cell to injury. Arch Pathol 1968; 85:189-199.

Riddell C. Cardiovascular system. In: Avian Histopathology. Lawrence, Kansas: Allen Press, 1987; 31-36.

Robinson WF, Huxtable CR, Pass DA. Canine parvoviral myocarditis: A morphologic description of the natural disease. Vet Pathol 1980; 17:282-293.

Robinson WF, Maxie MG. The cardiovascular system. In: Jubb KVF, Kennedy PC, Palmer N, eds. Pathology of Domestic Animals. Vol. 3. 4th ed. New York: Academic Press, 1993:1-100.

Rush JE, Freeman LM. The cardiovascular system. In: Goldston RT, Hoskins JD, eds. Geriatrics and Gerontology of the Dog and Cat. Philadelphia: WB Saunders, 1995:89-115.

Schwartz CJ, Sprague EA, Valente AJ, Kelley JL, Edwards EH. Cellular mechanisms in the response of the arterial wall to injury and repair. Toxicol Pathol 1989; 17:66-71.

Sharov UG, Sabbah HN, Shimoyama H, Goussev A, Lesch M, Goldstein S. Evidence of cardiocyte apoptosis in myocardium of dogs with chronic heart failure. Am J Pathol 1996; 148:141-149.

Sisson DD. Acquired valvular heart disease in dogs and cats. In Bonagura JD, ed. Cardiology. New York: Churchill Livingstone, 1987:59-116.

Sisson DD, Thomas WP. Myocardial diseases. In: Ettinger SJ, Feldman EC, eds. Textbook of Veterinary Internal Medicine. Vol. 1. Philadelphia: WB Saunders, 1995:995-1032.

Smith HJ, Nuttall A. Experimental models of heart failure. Cardiovasc Res 1985; 19:181-186.

Snyder PW, Kazacos EA, Scott-Moncrieff JC, HogenEsch H, Carlton WW, Glickman LT, Felsburg PJ. Pathologic features of naturally occurring juvenile polyarteritis in beagle dogs. Vet Pathol 1995; 32:337-345.

Stalis IH, Bossbaly MJ, VanWinkle TJ. Feline endomyocarditis and left ventricular endocardial fibrosis. Vet Pathol 1995; 32:122-126.

Suter PF, Fox PR. Peripheral vascular disease. In: Ettinger SJ, Feldman EC, eds. Textbook of Veterinary Internal Medicine. Vol. I. Philadelphia: WB Saunders, 1995:1068-1081.

Swenson L, Haggstrom J, Kvart C, Juneja RK. Relationship between parental cardiac status in cavalier King Charles spaniels and prevalence and severity of chronic valvular disease in offspring. J Am Vet Med Assoc 1996; 208:2009-2012.

Szabo KT. Heart and cardiovascular system. In: Szabo KT, ed. Congenital Malformations in Laboratory and Farm Animals. New York: Academic Press, 1989:216-226.

Tanigawa G, Jarcho JA, Kass S, Solomon SD, Vosberg H, Seidman JG, Seidman CE. A molecular basis for familial hypertrophic cardiomyopathy: An alpha/beta cardiac myosin heavy chain hybrid gene. Cell 1990; 62:991-998.

Tidholm A. Retrospective study of congenital heart defects in 151 dogs. J Small Anim Pract 1997; 38:94-98.

Tidholm A, Jonsson L. A retrospective study of canine dilated cardiomyopathy (189 cases). J Am Anim Hosp Assoc 1997; 33:544-550.

Tidholm A, Jonsson L. Dilated cardiomyopathy in the Newfoundland: A study of 37 cases (1983-1994). J Am Anim Hosp Assoc 1996; 32:465-470.

Tontis A, Zwahlen R, Lobsiger C, Luginbuhl H: Pathology of bovine cardiomyopathy. Schweiz Arch Tierheilkd 1990; 132:105-116.

Turk JR. Necropsy of the canine heart: A simple technique for quantifying ventricular hypertrophy and valvular alterations. Comp Contin Ed Pract Vet 1983; 5:905-910.

Van Stee EW, ed. Cardiovascular Toxicology. New York: Raven Press, 1982.

Van Vleet JF, Amstutz HE, Weirich WE, Rebar AH, Ferrans VJ. Clinical, clinicopathologic and pathologic alterations in acute monensin toxicosis in cattle. Am J Vet Res 1983; 44:2133-2144.

Van Vleet JF, Ferrans VJ. Characterization of myocardial toxicity caused by agents that affect the myocytes. In: Bishop SP, Kerns WD, eds. Comprehensive Toxicology. Vol. 6. Cardiovascular Toxicology. New York: Elsevier Science, 1997:333-367.

Van Vleet JF, Ferrans VJ. Clinical and pathologic features of chronic adriamycin toxicosis in rabbits. Am J Vet Res 1980; 41:1462-1469.

Van Vleet JF, Ferrans VJ. Congestive cardiomyopathy induced in ducklings fed graded amounts of furazolidone. Am J Vet Res 1983; 44:76-85.

Van Vleet JF, Ferrans VJ. Myocardial disease of animals. Am J Pathol 1986; 124:98-178.

Van Vleet JF, Ferrans VJ, Herman E. Cardiovascular and skeletal muscular systems. In: Haschek WM, Rousseaux CG, eds. Handbook of Toxicologic Pathology. New York: Academic Press, 1991:539-624.

Van Vleet, JF, Ferrans VJ, Weirich WE. Cardiac disease induced by chronic adriamycin administration in dogs and an evaluation of vitamin E and selenium as cardioprotectants. Am J Pathol 1980; 99:13-42.

Van Vleet JF, Ferrans VJ, Weirich WE. Pathologic alterations in congestive cardiomyopathy of dogs. Am J Vet Res 1981; 42:416-424.

Van Vleet JF, Ferrans VJ, Weirich WE. Pathologic alterations in hypertrophic and congestive cardiomyopathy of cats. Am J Vet Res 1980; 41:2037-2048.

Van Vleet JF, Rebar AH, Ferrans VJ. Acute cobalt and isoproterenol cardiotoxicity in swine: Protection by selenium-vitamin E supplementation and potentiation by stress-susceptible phenotype. Am J Vet Res 1977; 38:991-1002.

Vracko R, Cunningham D, Frederickson RG, Thorning D. Basal lamina of rat myocardium: Its fate after death of cardiac myocytes. Lab Invest 1988; 58:77-87.

Vracko R, Throning D, Frederickson RG, Cunningham D. Myocytic reactions at the borders of injured and healing rat myocardium. Lab Invest 1988; 59:104-114.

Walter JH, Rudolph R. Systemic, metastatic eu- and heterotope tumours of the heart in necropsied dogs. Zentralbl Fur Veterinarmed A 1996; 43:31-45.

Woodruff JF. Viral myocarditis. Am J Pathol 1980; 101:427-484.

CHAPTER 5

The Urinary System

ANTHONY W. CONFER
ROGER J. PANCIERA

GENERAL RESPONSE TO INJURY

The urinary system is composed of kidneys, ureters, urinary bladder, and urethra. Injury to or obstruction of any component that significantly decreases or blocks renal function can result in major systemic effects, including azotemia; uremia; plasma protein loss; water, electrolyte, and acid-base imbalances; retention of drugs; and hyperparathyroidism and osteodystrophy. The functional unit of the kidney is the nephron. Each nephron has a glomerulus, proximal convoluted tubule, loop of Henle, distal convoluted tubule, collecting duct, and a closely associated portion of the blood-vascular system. Because the nephron is a functional unit, damage to any component of that unit results first in diminished function of the entire nephron and subsequently damage to other components.

Primary glomerular damage often occurs as a result of deposition of immune complexes, thrombosis, embolism, or direct viral or bacterial infection of glomerular components. Such insults are reflected morphologically in necrosis, or proliferation of cells or membranes of the glomerulus, or by infiltration of leukocytes, and, functionally by reduced vascular perfusion or increased vascular permeability characterized by leakage of large quantities of plasma proteins and other plasma macromolecules into the glomerular filtrate. Continued or severe injury can result in chronic changes characterized by atrophy and fibrosis of the glomerular tuft and secondary atrophy of renal tubules. Similar chronic glomerular changes can result from the chronic loss of tubular function or reduced blood flow to the glomerulus.

Renal tubules consist of epithelial cells whose basilar surfaces rest on basement membrane. Cells respond to injury by degeneration, necrosis, apoptosis, and atrophy. The basement membrane can respond by rupture or thickening. Tubular disease occurs as a result of tubular epithelial damage from blood-borne or ascending infection, direct damage from toxins, or ischemia. When nephrons are lost because of injury, remaining tubules can undergo compensatory hypertrophy that can maintain overall renal function. In many instances of tubular epithelial cell necrosis, particularly as a response to toxins, tubular epithelium can regenerate and restore function. Severe damage to or loss of tubular basement membranes results in loss of tubular segments, failure of functional repair, and permanent loss of function of the entire nephron. Tubular atrophy is due to reduced oxygen tension, interstitial fibrosis, tubular obstruction, or to diminished glomerular perfusion and filtration.

The renal interstitium is the fibrovascular stroma that surrounds the nephron and is significantly involved in renal disease. Interstitial inflammation occurs as the result of ascending urinary tract infections (pyelonephritis), systemically derived infections of tubules and interstitium, and secondary to injury of tubules or glomeruli. Common acute lesions of the interstitium include edema, hemorrhage, and inflammation characterized by infiltration of neutrophils. As lesions become subacute to chronic, neutrophils become less prominent, and in several diseases, infiltrates of macrophages, lymphocytes, and plasma cells predominate. With chronic injury to or atrophy of nephrons, fibrosis of the interstitium can be severe, resulting in marked reduction in nephron function.

Diseases of the lower urinary tract (urinary bladder and urethra) result from infection, obstruction, intoxication, congenital defects, physical trauma, or neoplasia. The initial sequence of events after damage to the lower urinary tract is erosion or ulceration of the transitional epithelium, neutrophilic infiltrates in the lamina propria, hemorrhage, and edema. With time, healing can be complete. Chronic damage results in hyperplasia or metaplasia of transitional epithelium, lymphocyte and plasma cell infiltrates, fibrosis of the lamina propria, and hypertrophy of smooth muscle.

THE KIDNEY

Normal Structure and Function

Gross Anatomy

Mammalian kidneys are complex, paired organs that lie in the retroperitoneum ventral and adjacent to the lumbar vertebrae. Kidneys are organized functionally and anatomically into lobules. Each lobule represents those nephrons separated by the medullary rays. Renal lobules should not be confused with renal lobes. Each lobe is represented by a renal pyramid. Among domestic animals, carnivores and horses have unilobar (or unipyramidal) kidneys. Kidneys from pigs and cattle are multilobar (or multipyramidal); however, only bovine kidneys have external lobation. Kidneys are covered by a fibrous capsule that normally can be easily removed from the renal surface. The renal parenchyma is divided into a cortex and medulla. The corticomedullary ratio is usually approximately 1:2 or 1:3 in domestic animals. The ratio varies among species; for example, those adapted to the desert have a far larger medulla and thus a smaller corticomedullary ratio. The ratio also is altered in certain disease states. The medulla generally can be subdivided into an outer zone, that portion of the medulla close to the cortex, and an inner zone, that portion closer to the pelvis. Normally, the cortex is radially striated and dark red-brown except in mature cats, in which the cortex is often yellow because of the large lipid content of tubular epithelial cells. The renal medulla is pale gray and has either a single renal papilla in cats, a fused, crestlike papilla (renal medullary crest) in dogs, sheep, and horses, or multiple renal papillae in pigs and cattle.

Organization and Functions of the Kidney

The functional unit of the kidney is the nephron, which includes the glomerulus, and a tubular system that includes convoluted and straight tubules that become collecting ducts (Fig. 5-1). The glomerulus is a complex, convoluted tuft of capillaries held together by a supporting structure of cells in a glycoprotein matrix, the mesangium. The capillary tuft is covered by the visceral epithelial cells and contained within a membranous "cap," called Bowman's capsule, which is lined by parietal epithelial cells. Blood perfusing the glomerulus is the source of the glomerular filtrate. This ultrafiltrate of plasma, which contains water, salts, ions, glucose, and albumin, passes between visceral epithelial cells into Bowman's (urinary) space and then into the proximal convoluted tubule. This tubule is lined by columnar epithelial cells that have a microvillous (brush) border that greatly increases their absorptive surface.

A major function of the proximal tubules is to reabsorb sodium, albumin, glucose, water, and bicarbonate. The proximal tubule is continuous with the loop of Henle that is in close physiologic and anatomic association with the capillary network referred to as the vasa recta. The loop of Henle, via a countercurrent mechanism, absorbs Na^+ and Cl^- ions, producing a hypotonic filtrate that flows into the next portion of the nephron, the distal convoluted tubule. In the distal convoluted tubule, water is reabsorbed from the tubule into the interstitium because of a solute concentration gradient and by the effects of antidiuretic hormone. The filtrate is further concentrated in the collecting ducts by water reabsorption into the medullary interstitium by a urea gradient. Thus, the final excretory product, urine, is formed.

Renal function can be summarized into five basic components:

1. Formation of urine for the purpose of elimination of metabolic wastes.
2. Acid-base regulation, predominantly through reclamation of bicarbonate from the glomerular filtrate.
3. The conservation of water through reabsorption by the proximal convoluted tubules, the countercurrent mechanism of the loop of Henle, antidiuretic hormone activity in the distal tubules, and the urea

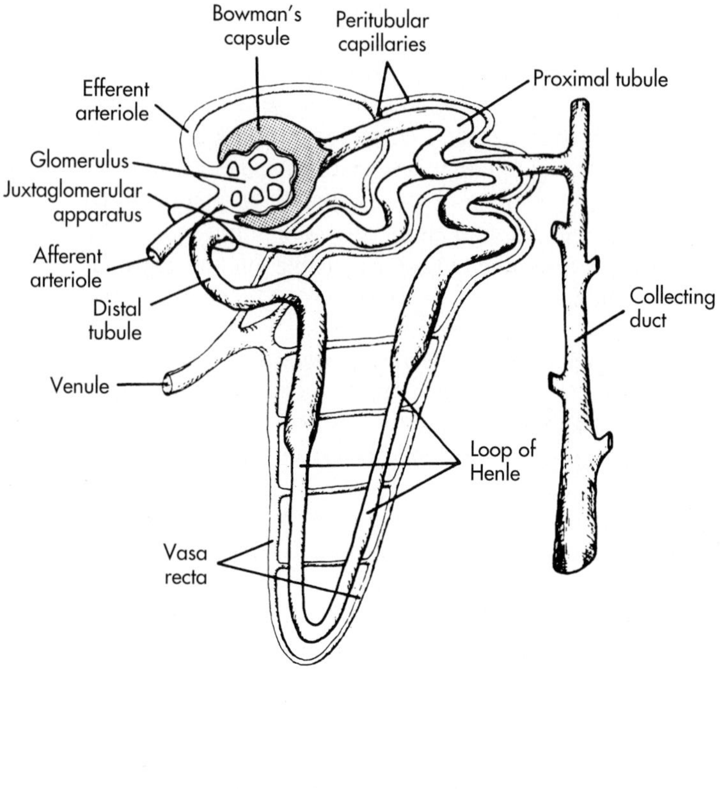

Figure 5-1 Kidney, normal. The diagram depicts the organization of the normal nephron.

gradient in the medulla. The tubular system is capable of absorbing up to 99% of the water of the glomerular filtrate.

4. The maintenance of normal extracellular potassium ion concentration through passive reabsorption in the proximal tubules and tubular secretion in the distal tubules under the influence of aldosterone.
5. Endocrine function through three hormonal axes: erythropoietin, renin-angiotensin, and vitamin D.

   Erythropoietin, produced in the kidneys in response to reduced oxygen tension, is released into the blood and stimulates bone marrow to produce erythrocytes.

   Renin, produced by cells of the juxtaglomerular apparatus, stimulates the production of the angiotensins that constrict afferent renal arterioles, maintain renal blood pressure, and stimulate aldosterone secretion from the adrenal glands, thus increasing sodium reabsorption. The juxtaglomerular apparatus consists of four components: (1) an afferent arteriole whose smooth muscle is modified to form myoepithelial cells, which are the juxtaglomerular cells that secrete renin, (2) an efferent arteriole, (3) the macula densa, and (4) and the extraglomerular mesangium.

   Vitamin D is converted in the kidneys to its most active form [1,25-dihydroxycholecalciferol (calcitriol)], which facilitates calcium absorption by the intestine (see Chapter 6, "Endocrine System").

Thus, renal damage can result in reduction of one or more of these five basic functions.

Necropsy Examination of the Kidneys

Examination of the kidneys should include assessment of their position and length relative to those of vertebrae (approximately 2.5 to 3 vertebrae in length) and the abdominal viscera and of their color, contour, topographic features, turgidity, thickness, and degree of adherence of the capsule. The capsule should always be completely stripped from the kidney so that the surface can be examined to evaluate the distribution of cortical lesions. This process is particularly important for localizing small lesions. Kidneys should be incised longitudinally and the cut surfaces examined. Lesions visible on the capsular surface should be evaluated on cut surface to assess whether they are superficial or extend deeply into the underlying parenchyma. On cut surface, the thickness of the cortex relative to normal and relative to the medulla should be assessed, as well as bulging of the parenchyma to assess renal swelling. Color and moistness of the cortex and medulla and the distinctness and intensity of cortical and medullary striations should also be examined on cut surface. Diminution or effacement (i.e., loss of form or features) of the striations is often a key observation in the gross recognition of degenerative and inflammatory lesions in the kidneys. The renal papillae (medullary crest) should be examined, particularly for evidence of erosion or necrosis. Dilatation, inflammation, calculosis, and other lesions of the renal pelvis, ureters, bladder, and urethra should be noted.

Renal Failure

Renal functional capacity can be impaired such that kidneys fail to carry out their normal metabolic and endocrine functions. It is important to remember that the glomerulus, tubules, collecting duct, and capillary blood supply are closely interrelated in each nephron both anatomically and functionally. Alterations in tubular function or structure influence glomerular function and structure and vice versa. For example, necrosis or atrophy of renal tubules results in loss of function of the affected nephrons and secondary atrophy of the glomerulus. In addition, because most of the capillary blood supply to tubules is through postglomerular capillaries, a reduction in glomerular blood flow consequently reduces the blood supply to the tubules.

Renal function can be reduced by prerenal factors such as reduced renal blood flow, circulatory collapse, obstruction of vascular supply to the kidneys, shock, or severe hypovolemia. Renal function also can be impaired by renal disease or by postrenal causes such as obstruction of urine outflow through the lower urinary tract. Impairment of renal function results in the retention of those constituents of plasma that are normally removed by the kidneys. Assays for plasma or serum concentrations of urea, creatinine, and ammonia, the nitrogenous waste products of protein catabolism, are routinely used as indices of diminished renal function. The intravascular increase of these nitrogenous waste products is referred to as **azotemia.** Renal failure can result in intravascular accumulation of other metabolic wastes such as guanidines, phenolic acids, and large molecular weight alcohols (example: myoinositol); reduced blood pH (metabolic acidosis); alterations in plasma ion concentrations, particularly potassium, calcium, and phosphate; and hypertension. The result of renal failure is a toxicosis called **uremia.** Uremia can, therefore, be defined as a syndrome associated with multisystemic clinical signs and lesions due to renal failure.

Animals that die of renal failure usually do so because of the cardiotoxicity of increased serum potassium, metabolic acidosis, and pulmonary edema. Nonrenal lesions of uremia recognizable clinically and at necropsy are useful indicators of renal disease (Table 5-1). The severity of nonrenal lesions of uremia is dependent on the length of time that the animal has survived in the uremic state. Therefore, in acute renal failure, nonrenal lesions are few, whereas in chronic renal failure many lesions can be present. Many of the lesions can be attributed either to endothelial degeneration and necrosis, resulting in thrombosis and infarction, or to the excretion of large concentra-

Table 5-1 Nonrenal Lesions of Uremia

Lesion	Mechanism
Pulmonary edema	Increased vascular permeability
Fibrinous pericarditis	Increased vascular permeability
Ulcerative and hemorrhagic gastritis	Ammonia secretion and vascular necrosis
Ulcerative and necrotic stomatitis	Ammonia secretion in saliva and vascular necrosis
Atrial and aortic thrombosis	Endothelial and subendothelial damage
Hypoplastic anemia	Increased erythrocyte fragility and lack of erythropoietin production
Soft-tissue mineralization (stomach, lungs, pleura, kidneys)	Altered calcium-phosphorus metabolism
Fibrous osteodystrophy	Altered calcium-phosphorus metabolism
Parathyroid hyperplasia	Altered calcium-phosphorus metabolism

tions of ammonia in the saliva and gastric juice. Lesions of uremia include ulcerative and necrotic stomatitis characterized by a brown, foul-smelling, mucoid material adherent to the eroded and ulcerated lingual and oral mucosae (Fig. 5-2). Ulcers are most commonly present on the underside of the tongue. Ulcerative and hemorrhagic lesions often occur in the stomach of dogs and cats and the colon of horses and cattle (Fig. 5-3). Large areas of the gastric or colonic mucosa are often edematous and dark red because of hemorrhage. The gastrointestinal contents can be bloody and smell of ammonia. Microscopically, coagulative necrosis, hemorrhage, and a neutrophilic infiltrate occur in the mucosa. Degeneration, necrosis, and mineralization of the arteriolar intima and media are often present in the gastric mucosa and submucosa (Fig. 5-4).

Increased vascular permeability in uremic patients occasionally results in a fibrinous pericarditis, characterized by fine granular fibrin deposits on the epicardium (visceral pericardium), and diffuse pulmonary edema. In the latter, alveoli contain fibrin-rich fluid and often a mild infiltrate of macrophages and neutrophils. This lesion is called **uremic pneumonitis.**

In the uremic animal, focal subendothelial degeneration can occur in the left atrial endocardium, and less frequently the endothelial surface of the proximal aorta and pulmonary trunk. These arterial lesions, called **mucoarteritis,** appear grossly as finely granular roughened plaques. Mucoarteritis in conjunction with loss of the anticoagulant antithrombin III by glomerular leakage is conducive to the formation of large mural thrombi at these sites. Chronic renal failure often results in reduced production of erythropoietin causing nonregenerative anemia. Uremia-associated increased erythrocytic fragility

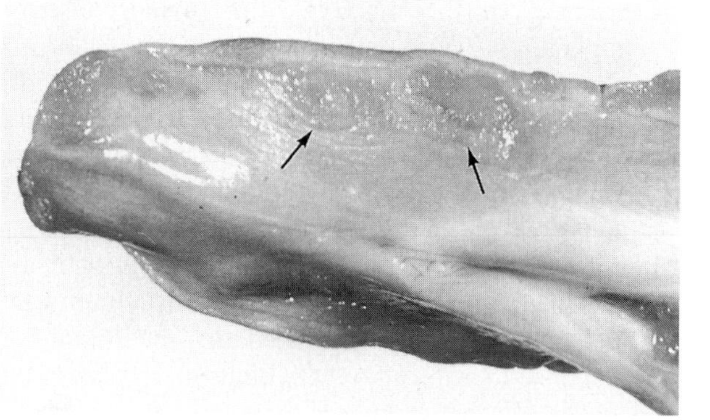

Figure 5-2 Tongue; dog. Ulcerative glossitis. Uremia-induced ulcers *(arrows)* are on the ventral surface of the tongue.

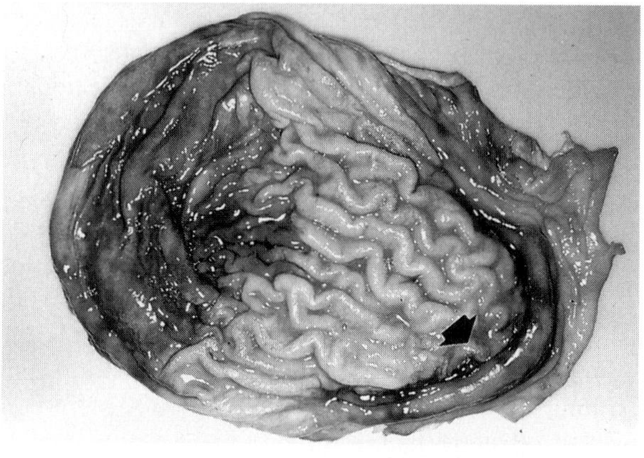

Figure 5-3 Stomach; dog. Uremic gastritis. Because of uremia, the stomach wall is hemorrhagic and contains bloody mucus. Note the edematous mucosal thickening *(arrowhead).*

also contributes to the anemia. Most animals in renal failure have hyperphosphatemia and normocalcemia or hypocalcemia. Alterations in calcium-phosphorus metabolism in the uremic animal are a hallmark of chronic renal failure and result from a complex set of events. When the glomerular filtration rate is chronically reduced to less than 25% of normal, phosphorus is no longer adequately secreted by the kidneys and hyperphosphatemia results.

Because of the Mass Law interactions between serum calcium and phosphorus, ionized calcium concentration in serum is reduced as a result of precipitation of calcium and phosphorus. Reduced ionized serum calcium stimulates parathyroid hormone secretion, causing calcium release from the readily mobilizable calcium stores in the bone and osteoclastic bone resorption. These changes in calcium-phosphorus metabolism are made more severe by the reduced ability of the diseased kidneys to hydroxylate 25-hydroxycholecalciferol to the more active 1,25-dihydroxycholecalciferol **(calcitriol)** resulting in decreased intestinal absorption of calcium. Calcitriol production is further inhibited by hyperphosphatemia. In addition,

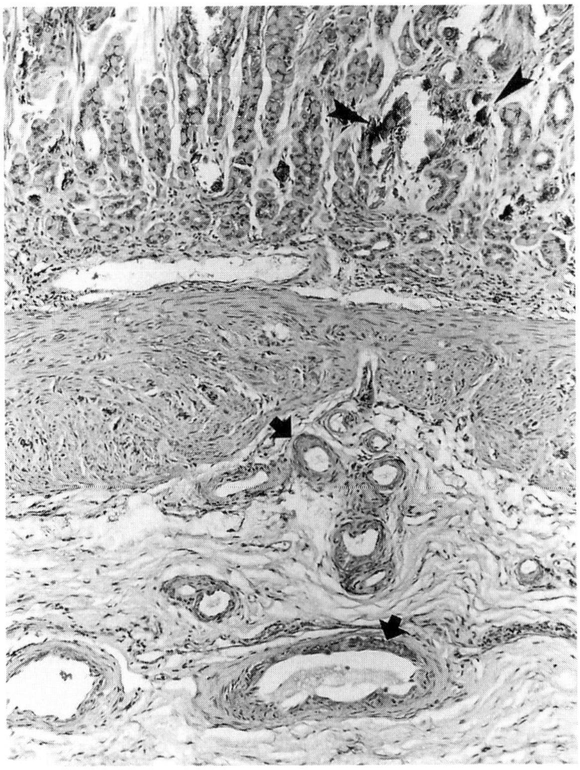

Figure 5-4 Stomach. Uremic gastritis. Submucosal vessels are thickened, hyalinized, and mineralized *(arrows)*. The mucosa has multifocal mineralization of gastric glands *(arrowheads)*. Hematoxylin-eosin (H & E) stain.

calcitriol normally suppresses parathyroid hormone secretion; therefore, reduced calcitriol production further increases parathyroid hormone secretion. With time, these events lead to parathyroid chief cell hyperplasia **(renal secondary hyperparathyroidism),** fibrous osteodystrophy (renal osteodystrophy), and soft tissue calcification. Hyperparathyroidism is further thought to perpetuate and enhance renal disease by stimulating **nephrocalcinosis,** the process by which renal tubular epithelium is damaged by an increase in intracellular calcium. Calcium is precipitated in mitochondria and in tubular basement membranes.

Soft tissue calcification associated with uremia occurs in numerous sites and represents both dystrophic and metastatic calcification. The gastric wall can be gritty when cut because of calcification of the inner and middle layers of the mucosa, as well as the submucosal arterioles. Necrotic arterioles throughout the body are particularly susceptible to calcification during uremia. A characteristic lesion, particularly in dogs, is calcification of the subpleural connective tissue of the cranial intercostal spaces (Fig. 5-5). These lesions are white-gray granular pleural thickenings with a horizontal "ladderlike" arrangement. The intercostal muscles are only superficially calcified. Patchy

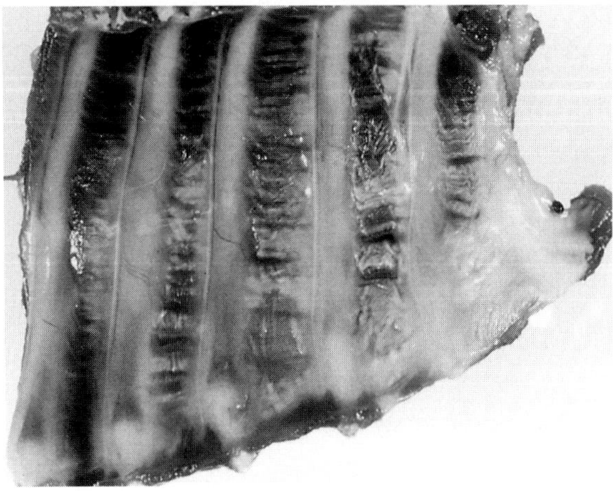

Figure 5-5 Thoracic cavity, parietal pleura; dog. Intercostal mineralization transversely oriented streaks of mineralization are present in the subpleural intercostal connective tissue as a result of chronic uremia.

or diffuse pulmonary calcification results in failure of the lungs to collapse, areas of paleness, and mild to moderate firmness and crunchiness, and can occur occasionally in conjunction with the lesions of uremic pneumonitis. Microscopically, the alveolar septa are calcified and can focally rupture, causing small emphysematous bullae. Although usually not visible at necropsy, calcification occurs in the kidneys. The kidneys can be gritty when cut because of calcification of tubular basement membranes, Bowman's capsules, and necrotic tubular epithelium, especially in the medulla and inner cortex.

Developmental Abnormalities

Renal Aplasia, Hypoplasia, and Dysplasia

Renal aplasia (agenesis) is failure of development of one or both kidneys such that there is no recognizable renal tissue. In these cases, the ureter can be present or absent. If present, the cranial extremity of the ureter begins as a blind pouch. Because life can be sustained when more than one fourth of renal function is maintained, unilateral aplasia is compatible with life provided that the other kidney is normal. Unilateral aplasia can go unnoticed during life and is recognized only at necropsy. Bilateral aplasia, obviously incompatible with life, occurs sporadically. A familial tendency has been observed in Doberman pinscher and beagle dogs.

Renal hypoplasia designates incomplete development of the kidneys such that fewer nephrons, lobules, and calyces are present at birth. Hypoplasia can be unilateral or bilateral; it is rare and is difficult to diagnose either at necropsy or microscopically. Two rigid criteria have been suggested as being required before a diagnosis of renal hypoplasia can be established in human beings: "In the absence of acquired disease, reduction in size of one kidney by more than 50 percent or in total renal mass by more than one-third," and more importantly, "a markedly reduced number of reniculi [renal lobules] and calyces." The latter criterion is likely to be useful only in the evaluation of the kidneys of cattle or pigs, which have renal multipyramidal structure analogous to those in human beings. These anatomic structures (unipyramidal) are fused in most other animal species. In cattle and pigs, the number of renal papillae in the hypoplastic kidney can be compared with those in a normal kidney.

Occasionally, some bovine kidneys are found to have reduced numbers of external lobes, but these kidneys are not hypoplastic and are microscopically and functionally normal; the reduction in external lobes merely represents fusion of lobes. Renal hypoplasia has been documented as an inherited disease of purebred or crossbred Large White pigs in New Zealand and described in foals of various breeds. Hypoplastic kidneys from pigs and foals have a marked reduction in the number of glomeruli. In foals for example, 5 to 12 glomeruli are present per low-power field in affected kidneys compared to 30 to 35 glomeruli per low-power field for normal kidneys from adults. The shrunken, pitted kidneys in young animals, particularly dogs, are often diagnosed as hypoplastic. However, in most of these cases the small kidneys are due to renal fibrosis resulting from renal disease developing at an early age, to progressive juvenile nephropathy, or to dysplasia.

Renal dysplasia is an abnormality of altered structural organization resulting from abnormal differentiation with presence of structures not representative of normal nephrogenesis. Microscopically, five primary features of dysplasia are described: asynchronous differentiation of nephrons, persistence of primitive mesenchyme such that the interstitial connective tissue has a myxomatous appearance, the persistence of metanephric ducts, atypical (adenomatoid) tubular epithelium, and the presence of cartilaginous or osseous tissues. Interstitial fibrosis, renal cysts, and a few enlarged hypercellular glomeruli (compensatory hypertrophy) are seen secondarily to the primary dysplastic changes. Renal dysplasia occurs infrequently and, like renal hypoplasia, must be differentiated from renal fibrosis and progressive juvenile nephropathy. Dysplastic changes can be unilateral or bilateral and can involve much of an affected kidney or occur only as focal lesions. Dysplastic kidneys can be small, misshapen, or both. The number of nephrons, lobules, and calyces are normal. Bilateral renal dysplasia characterized by persistent mesenchyme and atypical tubular development has been described in foals. Cystic renal dysplasia has been described in sheep and is inherited as an autosomal dominant trait.

Progressive juvenile nephropathy (familial renal disease) of Lhaso apso, shih tzu, golden retriever dogs, and perhaps other breeds, could be examples of renal dysplasia. Asynchronous differentiation is often seen and, to a lesser extent, several other lesions of dysplasia. However, until these hereditary lesions of dogs are better characterized, it is probably best to retain the diagnosis of progressive juvenile nephropathy (see Chronic Renal Diseases).

Ectopic and Fused Kidneys

Ectopic kidneys are misplaced from their normal sublumbar location by abnormal migration during fetal development. Ectopic kidneys occur most frequently in pigs and dogs and usually involve only one kidney. Ectopic locations often include the pelvic cavity or inguinal region. Although ectopic kidneys are usually structurally and functionally normal, malposition of the ureter predisposes them to obstruction and secondary hydronephrosis.

Fused (horseshoe) kidneys result from the fusion of the cranial or caudal poles of the kidneys during nephrogenesis. This fusion results in the appearance of one large kidney with two ureters. The histologic structure and function of fused kidneys are usually normal.

Renal Cysts

Congenital renal cysts can occur in cases of renal dysplasia or can occur as a primary entity. Kidneys can have single or multiple cysts. Some cysts cause no alteration in renal function, and are, therefore, considered incidental findings. Such incidental renal cysts are common in pigs and calves and must be differentiated from hydronephrosis.

Cysts can arise anywhere along the nephron and be located in either cortex or medulla. Cysts range from those barely visible to those several centimeters in diameter. Cysts are usually spherical, thin walled, lined by flattened epithelium, and are filled with clear watery fluid. The sources of fluid are glomerular filtrate, transepithelial secretions, or both. When viewed from the renal surface, the cyst wall is pale gray, smooth, and translucent.

Polycystic kidneys have many cysts that involve numerous nephrons such that the kidney can have a "Swiss cheese" appearance when incised (Fig. 5-6). As cysts enlarge, they compress the adjacent parenchyma. When kidneys are polycystic, renal function can be impaired. Congenital polycystic kidneys occur sporadically in many species, but can be inherited as an autosomal dominant lesion in pigs and lambs and can be inherited along with cystic biliary disease in cairn and West Highland white terriers. The lesion is inherited as an autosomal dominant trait in families of Persian cats. A polycystic renal disease with cysts arising from glomeruli has been described in collie puppies.

The pathogenesis of renal cysts is not entirely understood. Once it was proposed that congenital cysts resulted from the failure of nephrons and collecting ducts to unite; however, this theory has not been substantiated. Cysts are likely derived from normal or noncystic segments of the nephron, including Bowman's (urinifer-

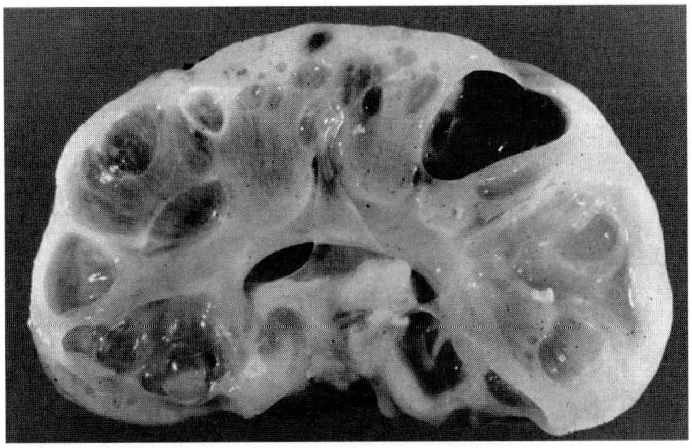

Figure 5-6 Kidney; cat. Polycystic disease. Numerous variably sized cysts are present in the cortex and medulla.

ous) space, renal tubules, and collecting ducts. Although genetic mechanisms can be involved in the pathogenesis of renal cysts, experiments with toxic chemicals indicate that genetic predisposition is not a requirement. Four mechanisms of renal cyst formation are considered plausible. These mechanisms are not mutually exclusive, but several mechanisms often work in concert to form renal cysts. First, obstruction of nephrons can cause increased luminal pressure and secondary dilatation. Second, modifications in extracellular matrix and cell-matrix interactions result in weakened tubular basement membranes allowing saccular dilation of tubules. Third, focal tubular epithelial hyperplasia with production of new basement membranes, increased tubular secretion, and increased intratubular pressure causes development of enlarged, dilated tubules. Fourth, dedifferentiation of tubular epithelial cells results in loss of polarity of cells with abnormal cell arrangements in tubules, reduced tubular fluid absorption, increased intratubular pressure, and dilation of tubules.

Acquired renal cysts can occur as a result of renal interstitial fibrosis (see Chronic Renal Diseases) or other renal diseases that cause intratubular obstruction. These cysts are usually small (1 to 2 mm) and occur primarily in the cortex. In all cases with renal cysts the cysts must be differentiated from hydronephrosis (dilated renal pelvises), especially in pigs and cows with multilobular kidneys.

Inherited Abnormalities in Renal Tubular Function

Inherited abnormalities of tubular metabolism, in transport, or in reabsorption of glucose, amino acids, ions, and proteins have been described in dogs. These diseases are not associated with consistent morphologic changes in the kidneys. The excretion of large quantities of cystine in the urine **(cystinuria)** is a sex-linked inherited disease seen occasionally in purebred or mongrel male dogs. It is of importance because it predisposes affected dogs to calculus formation and obstruction of the lower urinary tract. Primary renal **glucosuria,** an inherited disorder in Norwegian elkhounds and of sporadic occurrence in other dog breeds, occurs when the capacity of tubular epithelial cells to reabsorb glucose is significantly reduced. Glucosuria predisposes dogs to bacterial infections of the lower urinary tract and urinary bladder emphysema, which are splitting of glucose molecules by bacteria, release of CO_2, and absorption of gas into bladder lymphatics. A hereditary generalized defect in tubular reabsorption similar to the **Fanconi syndrome** in human beings has been described in basenji dogs. The underlying tubular defect appears to be abnormal membrane fluidity of the proximal tubular epithelial cell brush borders due to altered lipid content in the cell membrane. Aminoaciduria, glucosuria, proteinuria, increased phosphaturia, and multiple endocrine abnormalities characterize this disease. Histopathologic changes in the kidneys are initially minimal consisting of irregularly sized tubular epithelial cells in the convoluted tubules and loops of Henle. With time, dogs with Fanconi's syndrome develop progressive renal insufficiency and associated renal fibrosis.

Circulatory Disturbances

Renal Blood Supply

The kidney has a rich blood supply. Knowledge of the normal renal blood supply is important in understanding pathogenesis and distribution of various renal lesions. Arterial blood is from the renal arteries. Upon entry at the hilus of the kidney, each renal artery branches into several interlobar arteries that course parallel to the renal pyramids until they turn perpendicular at the corticomedullary junction forming the arcuate arteries. The arcuate arteries send branches, the interlobular arteries, into the renal cortex. A few minor branches of the arcuate arteries also provide some of the blood supply to the medulla. Finally, short vessels, the afferent arterioles, arise from interlobular arteries and sequentially give rise to the glomerular capillary tufts, efferent arterioles, and the peritubular capillary plexus.

Hyperemia and Congestion

As in other organs, **renal hyperemia** and **renal congestion** can be physiologic, active, passive, or hypostatic. Hyperemic kidneys are darker red than normal, can be perceptibly swollen, and ooze blood from the cut surface. At necropsy, unilateral renal hypostatic congestion is present in animals that died in lateral recumbency because of the force of gravity pulling unclotted blood downward.

Hemorrhage

Renal cortical hemorrhages occur in association with many septicemic diseases and result from vasculitis, vascular necrosis, thromboemboli, or disseminated intravascular coagulation. Petechial hemorrhages are com-

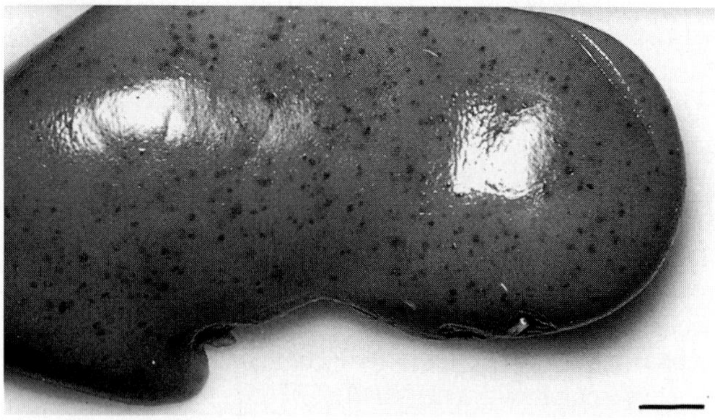

Figure 5-7 Kidney; pig. Renal hemorrhages. Cortical petechial hemorrhages are randomly scattered throughout the kidney. This kidney is from a pig with a septicemic illness (in this case, hog cholera [swine fever]). Bar = 5 mm.

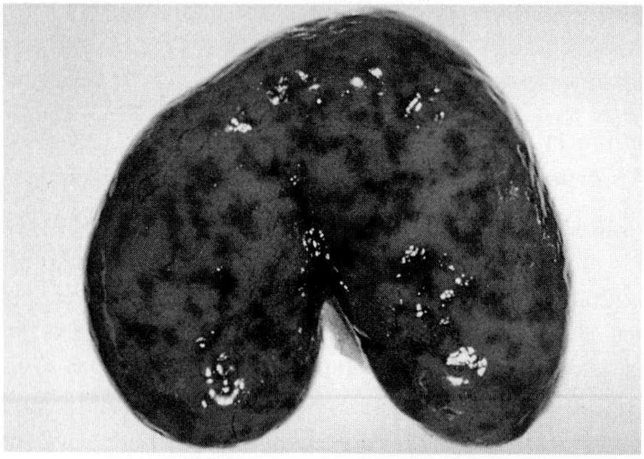

Figure 5-8 Kidney; dog. Renal hemorrhages. Characteristic cortical petechial and ecchymotic hemorrhages from a puppy with herpesvirus canis septicemia.

monly seen on the surface and throughout the cortex of kidneys from pigs that die of septicemia caused by diseases such as hog cholera (swine fever), African swine fever, erysipelas, streptococcal infections, salmonellosis, and other embolic bacterial diseases (Fig. 5-7). Renal cortical ecchymotic hemorrhages associated with multifocal tubular and vascular necrosis are salient and diagnostically important lesions of herpesvirus septicemia of neonatal puppies (Fig. 5-8). Puppies that survive herpesvirus septicemias and reach young adulthood (1 to 3 years of age) can develop clinical signs of chronic renal disease. This renal lesion must be differentiated microscopically from diseases classified as renal dysplasia or progressive juvenile nephropathy because of potential genetic or inheritable aspects of the latter two diseases.

Large intrarenal or subcapsular hemorrhages can result from direct trauma, renal biopsy, bleeding disorders such as hemophilia, and disseminated intravascular coagulation.

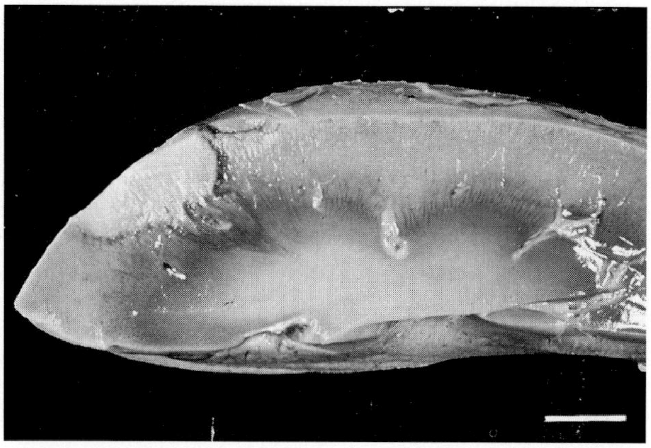

Figure 5-9 Kidney; horse. Acute infarct. The renal cortex contains a pale, wedge-shaped renal infarct. Bar = 1 cm.

Infarction

Renal infarcts are areas of coagulative necrosis that result from the local ischemia of vascular occlusion and usually are due to thromboembolism, mural thrombosis, or aseptic emboli. Grossly, renal infarcts appear red or pale white depending on several factors including the interval after vascular occlusion and whether arteries or veins are occluded (Fig. 5-9). Occlusion of arteries results in infarcts that are initially hemorrhagic and slightly swollen and turn pale yellow-gray within 2 to 3 days because of lysis of erythrocytes and loss of hemoglobin (Fig. 5-10). Pale infarcts have a central area of coagulative necrosis and are usually surrounded by a zone of congestion and hemorrhage along with a pale margin because of a surrounding zone of leukocytes (Fig. 5-11).

Infarcts are often wedge shaped with the base against the cortical surface and the apex pointing toward the medulla conforming to the distribution of the obstructed vessel(s). That appearance, however, might not be apparent when infarcts are extremely large or confluent. Infarcts can involve the cortex only or the cortex and medulla depending on the size of the occluded vessel and the site of obstruction. For example, thrombosis of an arcuate artery, which supplies both cortex and medulla, would result in an infarct involving the cortex and extending partway into the medulla. Thrombosis of a cortical interlobular artery, which supplies mainly the cortex, would result in an infarct of the cortex only. Although less common, infarcts due to venous occlusion are seen occasionally, and they retain their hemorrhagic appearance longer than infarcts resulting from arterial occlusion because of the continued arterial blood flow to the area.

Microscopically, in acute renal infarction, nephrons and interstitium in the central zone of the infarct become necrotic. At the periphery of the infarct, only the proximal tubules, because of their high metabolic rate, are necrotic;

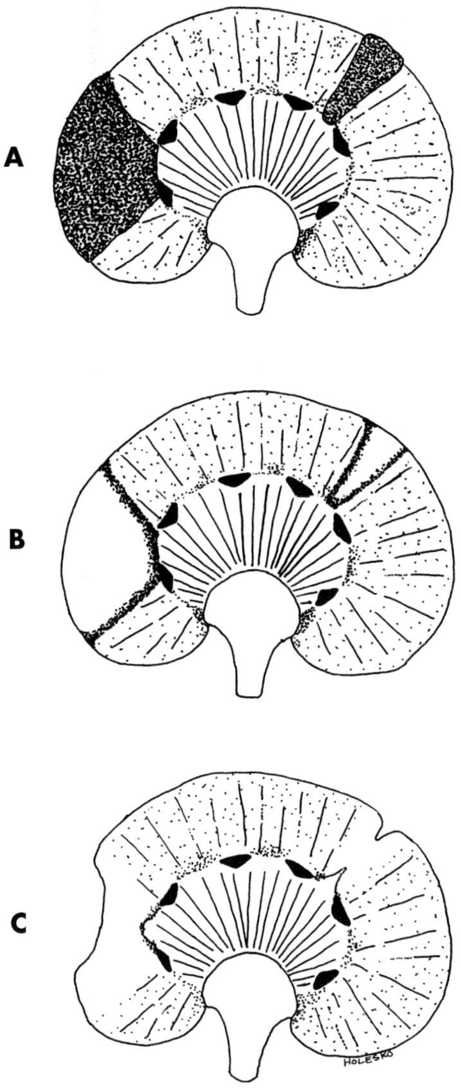

Figure 5-10 Kidney. Renal infarcts. The normal progression of renal infarcts is outlined. **A, B,** Acute renal infarcts. Initially, renal infarcts are swollen and hemorrhagic. In 2 to 3 days, infarcts become pale, surrounded by a zone of hyperemia and hemorrhage. **C,** Chronic infarcts are pale, shrunken, and fibrotic, resulting in distortion of the renal contour.

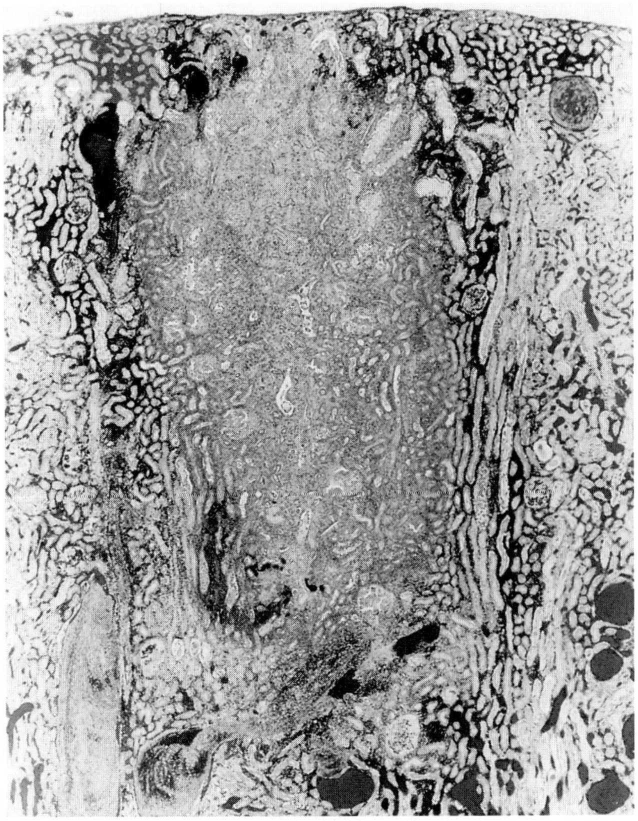

Figure 5-11 Kidney, cortex. Acute infarct. The renal cortex contains an acute infarct with a central zone of coagulation necrosis surrounded by a zone of hyperemia and hemorrhage. H & E stain.

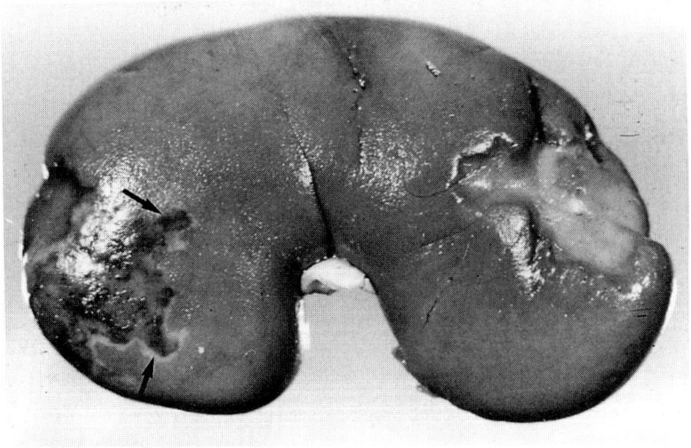

Figure 5-12 Kidney; dog. Multiple renal infarcts. The depressed foci represent healing (scarred) stages of infarction. An acute infarct is at the lower left *(arrows). Courtesy Dr. L. Roth.*

the glomeruli tend to be spared. Along the margin of the necrotic zone, the infiltrate is initially limited and consists of neutrophils with a few macrophages and lymphocytes. Capillaries adjacent to the necrotic area are markedly engorged with blood. Healing of the infarcted area occurs by lysis and phagocytosis of the necrotic tissue and replacement by fibrous connective tissue, leaving a discrete fibrotic scar (Fig. 5-12). Scars range from linear to broad depending on the size of the acute infarct. Various causes of renal scarring and differentiation of scarred lesions are discussed later (see Chronic Renal Diseases).

Endocardial thrombosis (vegetative valvular endocarditis, mural endocarditis) frequently results in thromboembolism of renal vessels because of the great amount of cardiac output (20% to 25%) that goes to the kidneys. Therefore, renal infarcts resulting from thromboemboli are commonly present in cats with left atrial thrombosis associated with cardiomyopathy or in any animal species with endocarditis involving the left heart. In rare cases, emboli can be large enough to occlude the renal artery, causing infarction of the entire kidney, or emboli can occlude the interlobar arteries causing infarction of large segments of cortex and medulla. More commonly, emboli obstruct many smaller vessels (e.g., interlobular arteries) causing multiple small infarcts in the kidneys. In general, renal infarction can occur because of thrombosis resulting from endothelial damage associated with a generalized vascular disease such as polyarteritis nodosa or arteriosclerosis or with cardiovascular collapse and shock. Renal infarcts in horses are rarely due to emboli arising from thrombosed cranial mesenteric arteries associated with migrating larvae of *Strongylus vulgaris*. In such cases, large mural thrombi in the cranial mesenteric artery protrude into the lumen of the aorta, and fragments, when loosened, cause thromboembolism of the kidneys. Thrombosis of pulmonary, coronary, splenic, or renal arteries and resultant infarction are common in dogs with renal amyloidosis primarily because of loss through the urine of plasma anticoagulants such as antithrombin III. Endotoxin-mediated arterial or capillary thrombosis is a common cause of infarction in association with gram-negative sepsis or endotoxic shock.

Septic emboli, particularly those from bacterial valvular endocarditis, can cause renal infarcts as well. Specific examples include *Actinomyces pyogenes* infection in cattle, *Erysipelothrix rhusiopathiae* in pigs, and *Staphylococcus aureus* in small animals. Septic infarcts are initially hemorrhagic, but because of the presence of pyogenic bacteria, the necrotic tissue undergoes liquefactive necrosis and the infarcts can eventually develop into abscesses.

Renal Cortical Necrosis

Renal cortical necrosis results when **disseminated intravascular coagulation (DIC)** causes widespread thrombosis in the glomerular capillaries, the interlobular arteries, and afferent arterioles. This lesion is not to be confused with ischemic acute tubular necrosis discussed in this chapter (see Tubular Necrosis). Partial or complete renal cortical necrosis is usually a bilateral lesion that occurs in all animal species, especially in association with gram-negative septicemias or endotoxemias, and is related to endotoxin-induced endothelial damage, activation of the clotting mechanism, and widespread capillary thrombosis. The lesion can be induced experimentally in animals by two endotoxin injections 24 hours apart and is a manifestation of the generalized **Shwartzman reaction.**

The resulting microthrombosis of vessels throughout the renal cortex results in widespread ischemia and small and large areas of hypoxia-induced coagulation necrosis and hemorrhage. The renal cortex can be diffusely pale with a zone of hyperemia separating the necrotic cortex from the viable medulla, or more often the cortex is a mosaic of large, irregular hemorrhagic areas, resembling hemorrhagic infarcts interspersed with large yellow-gray areas resembling pale infarcts. The necrotic tissue can involve the full width of the cortex or only the outer portion (Fig. 5-13). Thrombi are demonstrable in interlobular and afferent arterioles and glomerular capillaries (Fig. 5-14).

Papillary (Medullary Crest) Necrosis

Necrosis of the renal papillae, or their counterpart the medullary crest, is a response of the inner medulla to ischemia. Papillary necrosis can be a primary lesion or be

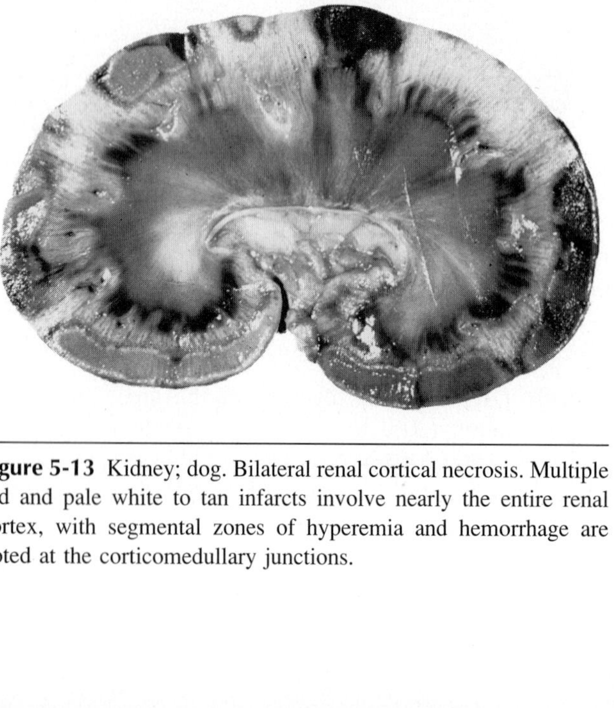

Figure 5-13 Kidney; dog. Bilateral renal cortical necrosis. Multiple red and pale white to tan infarcts involve nearly the entire renal cortex, with segmental zones of hyperemia and hemorrhage are noted at the corticomedullary junctions.

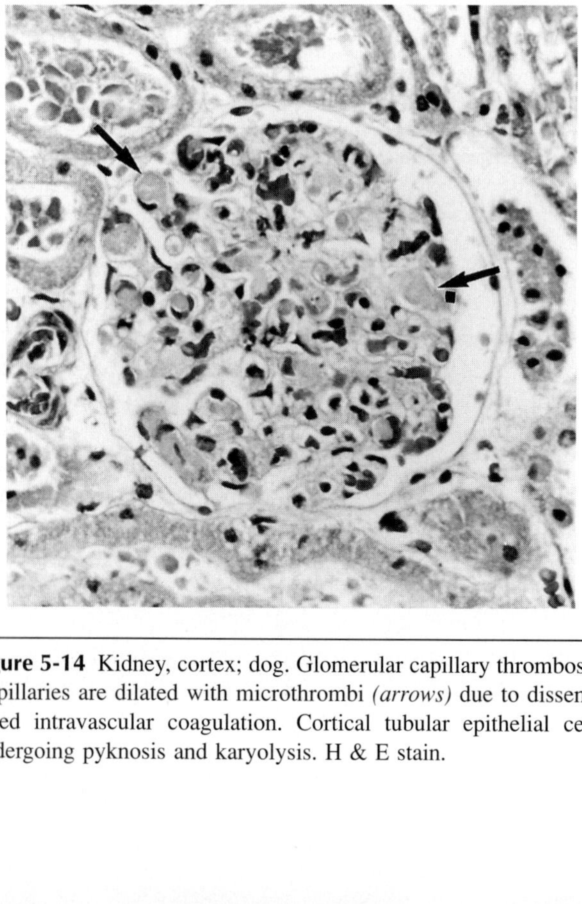

Figure 5-14 Kidney, cortex; dog. Glomerular capillary thrombosis. Capillaries are dilated with microthrombi *(arrows)* due to disseminated intravascular coagulation. Cortical tubular epithelial cells undergoing pyknosis and karyolysis. H & E stain.

secondary to other renal lesions. The inner medulla including the papillae normally is the zone least well perfused with blood of any zones of the kidneys. This outcome is because the inner medulla has little direct perfusion; instead, most of the medullary blood supply is from the cortical blood through the vasa rectae. Because of this limited blood flow, any lesion or disease process that further reduces medullary blood flow can cause ischemic necrosis (infarction) of the papillae.

Papillary necrosis occurs as a primary disease in animals treated with nonsteroidal antiinflammatory-analgesic drugs and is analogous to **analgesic nephropathy** in human beings. The primary disease occurs quite frequently in horses treated for prolonged periods with phenylbutazone or flunixin meglumine. It is of potential importance in dogs and cats because of accidental ingestion of or treatment with ibuprofen, aspirin, or acetaminophen at excessive dosages (see Causes of Acute Tubular Necrosis). Drugs associated with papillary necrosis are sometimes referred to as "papillotoxins." The medullary interstitial cells are the primary targets of papillotoxins. These cells have a key role in synthesis of prostaglandins, antihypertensive factors, and the glycosaminoglycan matrix of the medullary interstitium. Interstitial cell damage decreases prostaglandin synthesis, which reduces normal blood flow and causes ischemia, and modifies the interstitial matrix; the net effect is degenerative changes in tubular epithelial cells in the inner medulla. In addition to its inhibition of prostaglandin biosynthesis, acetaminophen also causes direct oxidative damage to medullary tubular epithelium after covalent binding to the cells, further enhancing necrosis of the renal papillae.

Papillary necrosis also is due to scarring of the outer medulla, medullary amyloidosis, pyelitis, renal pelvic calculi, or with the increased intrapelvic pressure that occurs with obstruction of the lower urinary tract. In addition, papillary necrosis frequently occurs in conjunction with glomerular amyloidosis and in such cases is probably due to decreased postglomerular capillary perfusion and thrombosis, resulting in ischemia of the inner medulla.

Papillary necrosis is usually an incidental finding at necropsy and rarely leads to progressive renal damage and failure. Typically, acute lesions are irregular, discolored areas of necrotic inner medulla sharply delineated from the surviving medullary tissue (Fig. 5-15). The affected tissue, which is undergoing coagulation necrosis, is yellow-gray, green, or pink. With time the necrotic tissue sloughs, resulting in a detached, friable, and discolored tissue fragment in the pelvis. The remaining inner medulla is usually roughened and attenuated as a result of fibrosis (Fig. 5-16). Overlying cortex can be somewhat shrunken because of atrophy of some of the nephrons secondary to the chronic medullary changes. Small pieces of sloughed necrotic medullary tissue pass inconsequentially into the ureter. However, large pieces of sloughed tissue can obstruct the ureter, causing hydronephrosis, or form a nidus for precipitation of minerals, resulting in the formation of pelvic or ureteral calculi.

Tubular Necrosis

Acute tubular degeneration and necrosis, often referred to as **nephrosis,** is the result of ischemic or toxic damage to the renal tubular epithelial cells. Tubular epithelial cells

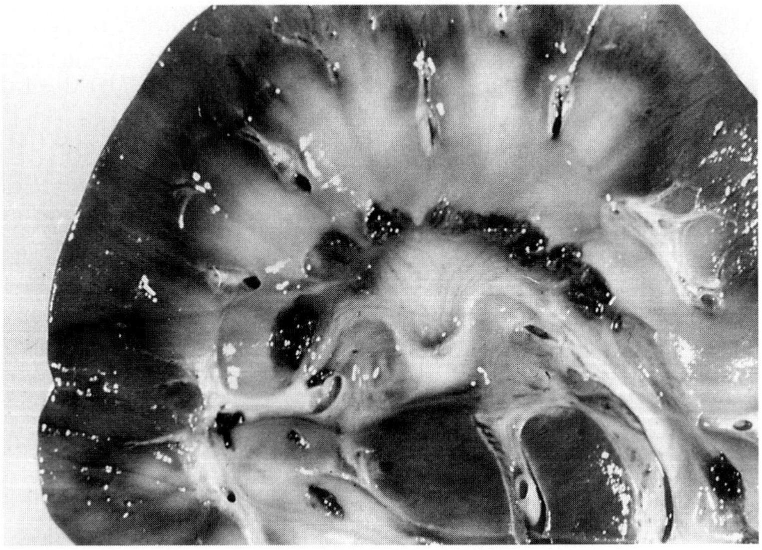

Figure 5-15 Kidney; horse. Papillary (medullary crest) necrosis. Acute coagulation necrosis of the inner medulla is a result of chronic administration of a nonsteroidal anti-inflammatory drug. *Courtesy Dr. L. Roth.*

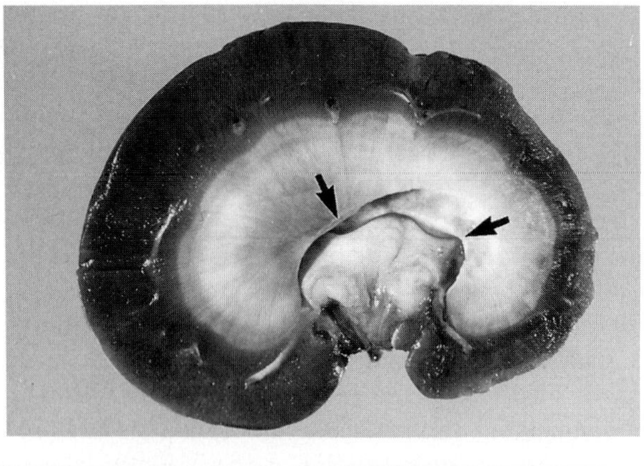

Figure 5-16 Kidney; dog. Chronic papillary (medullary crest) necrosis. The medullary crest is irregularly attenuated *(arrows)*, and there is scarring and contraction of the overlying cortex and medulla.

respond to prolonged ischemia or to nephrotoxins by undergoing degeneration, followed by necrosis and desquamation of the cells into the tubular lumen. The proximal convoluted tubular epithelium is most susceptible to ischemia or toxic injury because of its high metabolic rate. Animals with severe tubular necrosis often have signs of uremia. Characteristically associated with uremia of tubular necrosis origin is a decrease in urine production **(oliguria)** or absence of urine production **(anuria).** Acute tubular necrosis induces oliguria by one or several mechanisms. These mechanisms include the leakage of urine from damaged tubules across disrupted basement membranes into the renal interstitium or intratubular obstruction resulting from desquamated necrotic epithelium. In addition, because of activation of the renin-angiotensin system due to tubular epithelial degeneration and necrosis, particularly affecting outer cortical nephrons, intrarenal vasoconstriction occurs, resulting in decreased glomerular blood flow and filtration and in reduced formation of urine.

At necropsy, the recognition of acute tubular necrosis is often difficult. Nevertheless, initially the kidneys are swollen, the capsular surface is smooth, pale mahogany to beige, and has a slightly translucent appearance. The cut surface of the renal cortex bulges and is usually pale mahogany to beige and excessively moist; striations are muted or accentuated by radially oriented opaque, white streaks. The medulla is pale mahogany to beige or congested. The microscopic appearance of kidneys with acute tubular necrosis can be variable, depending on the severity of the injury, the duration of exposure to the damaging agent, and the length of time between the injury and death. Initially, proximal tubular epithelium is swollen, the microvilli are absent, and the cytoplasm is vacuolated or is granular and intensely eosinophilic, features indicative of coagulation necrosis. In such tubules, the nuclear changes are pyknosis, karyorrhexis, or karyolysis. Necrotic tubular epithelium is subsequently desquamated into tubular lumens resulting in dilated, markedly hypocellular tubules that contain necrotic cellular debris and hyalinized or granular casts (Figs. 5-17 and 5-18).

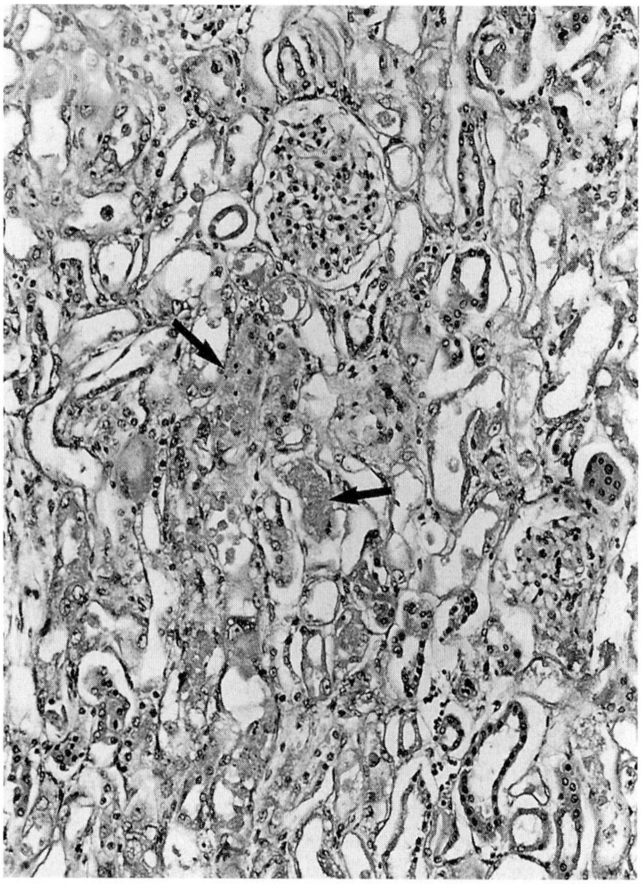

Figure 5-17 Kidney. Acute tubular necrosis. The lesion is characterized by coagulation necrosis of tubular epithelial cells *(arrows)*, dilated hypocellular tubules, and intratubular nuclear and proteinaceous debris. H & E stain.

If the insult to the renal tubules is not lethal to the animal and is removed and the tubular basement membranes remain intact, tubular epithelial regeneration occurs from the surviving epithelium with restitution of renal function. Recent evidence indicates that epidermal growth factor secreted by distal convoluted tubules mediates the tubular repair process. The sequences of events in tubular regeneration have been well documented in an experimental model system of tubular necrosis caused by the nephrotoxin mercuric chloride. In that system, morphologic evidence of regeneration of proximal convoluted tubules is seen within 3 days after a toxic dose. At this time, basement membranes are partially covered with low cuboidal to flattened and elongated epithelial cells that are more basophilic than normal because of the increased concentrations of cytoplasmic ribosomes and

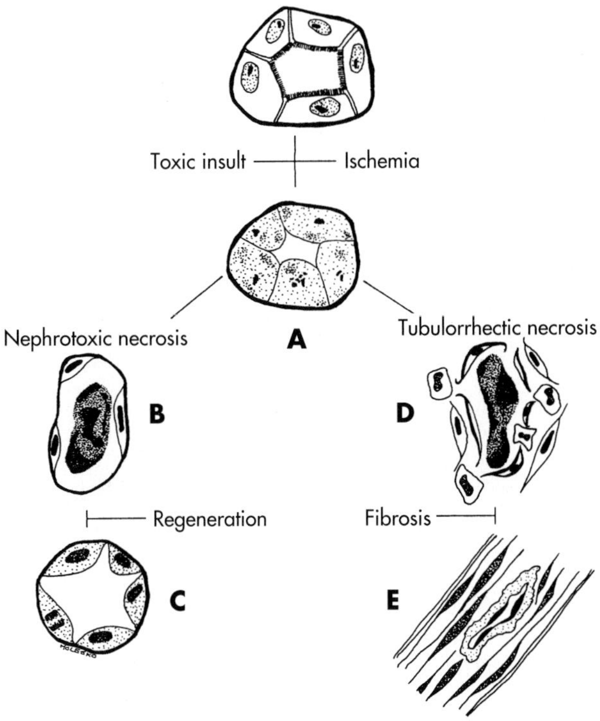

Figure 5-18 Kidney, proximal tubules. Acute tubular necrosis. Acute tubular necrosis results from a nephrotoxin or ischemia. **A,** Both insults cause acute necrosis characterized by cellular swelling, pyknosis, karyorrhexis, and karyolysis. **B,** Subsequent to nephrotoxic necrosis, there is sloughing of necrotic epithelium into the tubular lumina and the basement membranes remain intact allowing, **C,** regeneration to occur. **D,** Ischemia may result in tubulorrhectic necrosis. Necrotic epithelium sloughs into the tubular lumen, the basement membrane is disrupted, macrophages infiltrate, and fibroblasts proliferate. **E,** Fibrosis with tubular atrophy results.

rough endoplasmic reticulum producing protein for repair. Nuclei are hyperchromatic and mitotic figures are present. Regenerating tubules do not function normally, because they lack a brush border and tubular membrane functions. Normal-appearing tubular epithelium subsequently reappears between 7 and 14 days after toxin exposure. Normal renal structure without residual evidence of tubular damage is restored between 21 and 56 days after exposure to the nephrotoxin. Similar time frames for tubular regeneration have been described through sequential renal biopsies from human patients naturally exposed to inorganic mercury and in experimental model systems with other nephrotoxins.

The alternative to regeneration is loss of tubules subjected to nephrotoxins or ischemia. This result is seen if the toxin is not removed, the basement membrane does not remain intact, or adequate tubular epithelium does not survive the toxic dose to allow for complete repair. In those cases, tubules are replaced by fibrous connective tissue. Tubules that remain in an affected site are nonfunctional, can be dilated and lined by flattened epithelium, or be markedly atrophic, appearing shrunken with a collapsed lumen lined by flattened epithelium.

Causes of Acute Tubular Necrosis

As stated earlier, two general mechanisms are responsible for most cases of acute tubular necrosis: ischemia and nephrotoxicity. Markedly reduced renal perfusion from any cause can result in **tubular necrosis.** Severe hypotension is associated with shock and results in preglomerular vasoconstriction and reduced glomerular filtration. The resulting renal ischemia can produce sublethal tubular cell injury and dysfunction or cause cell death by necrosis or apoptosis. Complete ischemia that lasts in excess of 2 hours usually results in tubular necrosis, especially of the proximal convoluted tubules. Cell death is manifested by decreased adenosine triphosphate (ATP) production, increased membrane permeability, calcium ion influx, phospholipase activation, and generation of oxygen radicals. Because mitochondrial respiration is disrupted, further cell membrane damage occurs. Initially, tubular necrosis is randomly distributed in nephrons, but the proximal convoluted tubules are most severely affected. Prolonged ischemia can produce necrosis of epithelium of the proximal and distal convoluted tubules, the loops of Henle, and collecting ducts throughout the cortex, and to a lesser extent, the medulla. Glomeruli often remain morphologically normal even when ischemia is prolonged. A characteristic lesion of ischemic tubular necrosis is disruption of the tubular basement membranes, referred to as **tubulorrhectic necrosis** (Fig. 5-18). Tubular repair in such kidneys is imperfect because regenerating epithelial cells do not have their normal scaffolding. Tubular atrophy and interstitial fibrosis are the results of failed regeneration. Gross and microscopic lesions resemble those previously described (see Tubular Necrosis).

A set of events leading to ischemic tubular necrosis frequently occurs in hypoperfused kidneys complicated by hemoglobinuria or myoglobinuria. **Hemoglobinuria** accompanies episodes of severe **intravascular hemolysis** and **hemoglobinemia** as observed in chronic **copper toxicity** in sheep, **leptospirosis** or **babesiosis** in cattle, **red maple toxicity** in horses, and babesiosis or **autoimmune hemolytic anemia** in dogs. **Myoglobinuria** accompanies acute **rhabdomyolysis** as occurs in **azoturia ("Monday morning disease")** of horses, **capture myopathy** of exotic or wild animals, or severe trauma. In these diseases, serum concentrations of hemoglobin or myoglobin are increased, and these products pass into the glomerular filtrate producing greatly increased concentrations in renal

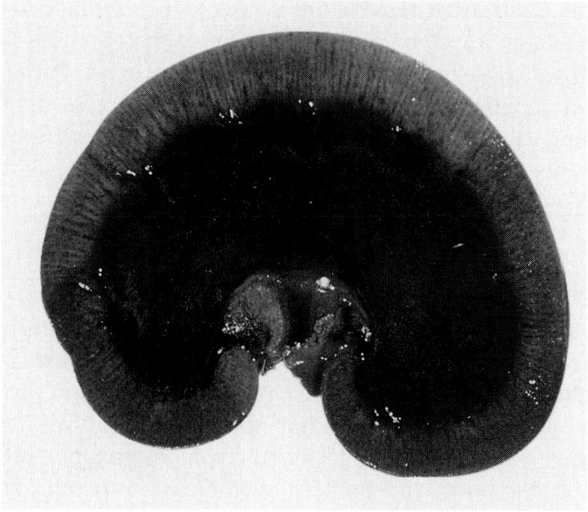

Figure 5-19 Kidney; dog. Hemoglobinuric nephrosis. Diffuse hemoglobin staining of the medulla is due to a severe intravascular hemolytic crisis.

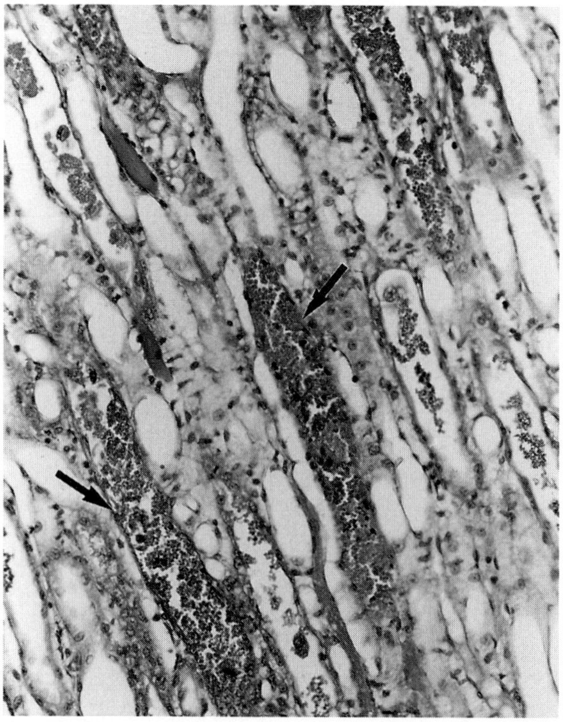

Figure 5-20 Kidney; cow. Myoglobinuric nephrosis. Heme casts *(arrows)* are present in dilated medullary tubules as a result of acute severe rhabdomyolysis. H & E stain.

tubules and causing **hemoglobinuric nephrosis** or **myoglobinuric nephrosis.** Hemoglobin and myoglobin are not nephrotoxic in themselves, and intravenous infusions of these compounds into healthy animals produce no recognizable lesions. However, large concentrations of hemoglobin or myoglobin in the glomerular filtrate can increase the tubular necrosis that occurs as a result of renal ischemia. In the diseases described above (e.g., chronic copper toxicity, rhabdomyolysis), affected animals often have renal ischemia due to shock or severe anemia. Hemoglobinuria and myoglobinuria can have an additive deleterious affect on tubular epithelium undergoing ischemic necrosis.

At necropsy the renal cortices of animals with severe hemoglobinuria or myoglobinuria are diffusely stained red-brown to blue-black and often have intratubular heme casts. These heme casts appear as a red-black stippling of the external surface and continue into the cortex as radially oriented, dark red streaks. The medulla is dark red or has red streaks (Fig. 5-19). Classically, kidneys from sheep with chronic copper toxicity are diffusely and strikingly blue-black and described as "gunmetal blue." Microscopically, tubular epithelial degeneration and necrosis are severe and tubular lumens are filled by abundant orange-red granular refractile material, the characteristic appearance of a heme compound (Fig. 5-20).

In addition to hemoglobin-associated and myoglobin-associated renal changes, increased serum concentrations of bilirubin can be associated with cellular swelling, degeneration, and brown-green pigmentation of the proximal tubular epithelial cells. The term **cholemic nephrosis** has been applied to this lesion; however, its significance is doubtful. Acute tubular necrosis, when seen in association with severe bilirubinemia, the so-called **hepatorenal syndrome,** probably is not due to bile acid or bilirubin retention per se, but to ischemia from prerenal causes such as constriction of renal vessels related to shock or catecholamine release.

Nephrotoxic tubular necrosis is caused by several classes of naturally occurring or synthetic compounds (Box 5-1). Gross and microscopic lesions resemble those described in the section Tubular Necrosis. Nephrotoxins can directly damage renal epithelial cells, particularly the proximal convoluted tubules, and can indirectly stimulate vasoconstriction and ischemia. However, nephrotoxins usually do not damage the tubular basement membranes. In nephrotoxin-associated ischemia, one of the first events in renal tubular cell damage is altered ion transport at the luminal surface. This process results in decreased sodium absorption and increased sodium ions in the distal tubules with stimulation of the renin-angiotensin mechanism causing vasoconstriction and reduced blood flow that result in ischemia and tubular cell damage.

Certain heavy metals, including inorganic mercury, inorganic arsenic, lead, cadmium, and thallium, are nephrotoxins. Common sources of heavy metals include herbicides (arsenic), old paint, batteries, and automobile components (lead), impure petroleum distillates, and other environmental contaminants. Acute tubular necrosis is the result of damage to membranes of proximal convoluted tubular epithelial cells or to mitochondrial damage produced by these toxins. Damage is often related to the

BOX 5-1 COMMON NEPHROTOXINS OF DOMESTIC ANIMALS

Heavy Metals
Mercury
Lead
Arsenic
Cadmium
Bismuth

Antibacterial and Antifungal Agents
Aminoglycosides
- Gentamicin
- Neomycin
- Kanamycin
- Streptomycin
- Tobramycin

Tetracyclines
Amphotericin B

Growth-Promoting Agents
Monensin

Nonsteroidal Antiinflammatory Drugs
Aspirin
Phenylbutazone
Carprofen
Flunixin meglumine
Ibuprofen
Naproxen

Mycotoxins
Ochratoxin A
Citrinin

Plants
Pigweed *(Amaranthus retroflexus)*
Oaks (*Quercus* sp.)
Isotropis sp.
Yellow wood tree *(Terminalia oblongata)*

Oxalates
Ethylene glycol (antifreeze)
Halogeton *(Halogeton glomeratus)*
Greasewood *(Sarcobatus vermiculatus)*
Rhubarb *(Rheum rhaponticum)*
Sorrel, dock (*Rumex* sp.)

Vitamin D
Vitamin D supplements
Calciferol-containing rodenticides
Cestrum diurnum
Solanum sp.
Trisetum sp.

Antineoplastic Compounds
Cisplatin

interaction of these metals with protein sulfhydryl groups. In mercury toxicosis, mercuric ions enter the proximal tubular cells from the luminal side as the ions are present in the glomerular filtrate and from the peritubular sides where the mercuric ions diffuse from the capillary blood, traverse the interstitium and tubular basement membrane, and access the tubular epithelium. Mercuric ions become concentrated in the rough endoplasmic reticulum and cause early tubular changes that include loss of brush borders and dispersion of ribosomes. These changes are followed by mitochondrial swelling and cellular death. Recently, cadmium has been reported to cause cell death in proximal convoluted tubules by apoptosis. The specific metal involved in toxic tubular injury usually cannot be identified by the renal lesions. The exception is lead toxicity, in which the epithelial cells of affected tubules sometimes have acid-fast intranuclear inclusions composed of lead-protein complexes (Fig. 5-21). Acute nephrosis has been reported in sheep after exposure to natural gas condensate, a complex mixture of hydrocarbon compounds. The mechanism of nephrotoxicity was not identified but was not due to heavy metal contaminants.

Certain pharmaceutical agents are nephrotoxic and cause acute tubular necrosis when administered at excessive doses or too frequently. Cisplatin, a platinum-containing cancer chemotherapeutic agent, causes tubular necrosis by direct tubular damage and by reducing renal blood flow via vasoconstriction mediated by the renin-angiotensin mechanism. Aminoglycoside antimicrobials such as gentamicin, neomycin, kanamycin, tobramycin, amikacin, and streptomycin are nephrotoxic by means of one of the mechanisms described below. Relative renal toxicity varies among the different aminoglycoside drugs and correlates with the concentration of the compound in the renal cortex. Neomycin, which is highly nephrotoxic, concentrates to the greatest extent in the renal cortex; streptomycin, the least nephrotoxic, does not concentrate appreciably in the renal cortex. Although gentamicin is intermediate in its nephrotoxic potential between neomycin and streptomycin, tubular toxicity occurs with some frequency because gentamicin is a commonly used drug in veterinary medicine.

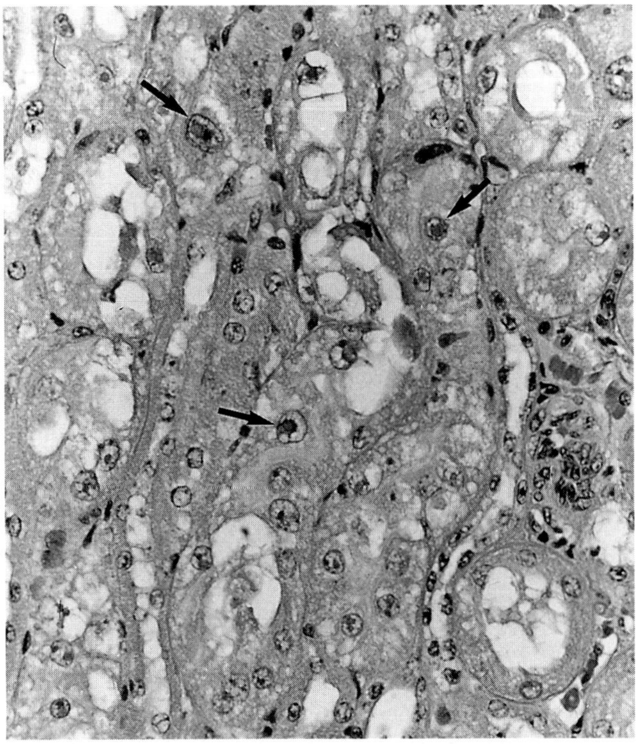

Figure 5-21 Kidney, cortex; rat. Lead nephrosis. Acid-fast intranuclear inclusion bodies *(arrows)* are present in convoluted tubular epithelium as a result of lead intoxication. Acid-fast stain.

The susceptibility of animal species to the nephrotoxic effects of these drugs is variable and is related to differences in susceptibility of renal tubules and to the rate of excretion or inactivation of the drug among animal species. Aminoglycosides become concentrated in lysosomes, and their toxic affects occur after release of large concentrations of the drugs from these organelles. Aminoglycoside toxicosis alters tubular cell membrane transport by the inhibition of sodium-potassium-ATPase, causing an intracellular influx of hydrogen and sodium ions and water. The drugs also inhibit phospholipase activity so that phospholipids accumulate intracellularly, alter mitochondrial function, and inhibit protein synthesis. These biochemical changes are responsible for acute swelling of proximal tubular epithelial cells, mitochondrial swelling, rupture of lysosomes, dilation of endoplasmic reticulum, shedding of the brush border, and cellular death.

Oxytetracycline is occasionally nephrotoxic in cattle and dogs. The mechanism of tubular damage has not been determined, but it is known that large concentrations of tetracycline antibiotics can inhibit mammalian protein synthesis. Renal failure occurs in oxytetracycline toxicosis and is likely the result of tubular obstruction caused by desquamated necrotic tubular epithelium. Amphotericin B, an antifungal polyene antibiotic, is nephrotoxic by the direct disruption of cellular membranes; this membrane damage interferes with normal cholesterol-lipid interactions and causes potassium ion loss, intracellular hydrogen ion accumulation, acute cellular swelling, and necrosis. These renal changes are not confined to cases of overdosage of the drug but can occur in animals given the recommended therapeutic dosage. Sulfonamide-induced tubular necrosis, a common entity in years past, occurs infrequently today because the presently used sulfonamides have greater solubility than those used in the past. Sulfonamides produce tubular epithelial cell necrosis most readily in dehydrated animals. Crystals form in tubules and necrosis is due to direct toxicity to the renal tubular epithelium and to mechanical damage. Fine granular yellow crystalline deposits can be seen grossly in the medullary tubules of affected animals, but the crystalline deposits are dissolved during fixation in aqueous fixatives, such as 10% buffered formalin, and during the processing of tissue for histologic sections. Monensin is an ionophore antibiotic used as a feed additive to control coccidiosis and stimulate weight gains in poultry and cattle. Horses are particularly susceptible to toxicosis with monensin. Although necrosis of striated muscle is the major lesion of the toxicosis (see Chapters 4 and 9, "Cardiovascular System" and "Muscle," respectively), renal tubular degeneration or necrosis can also be due to altered ionic transport in renal tubular epithelial cells and, possibly, to diminished transport of membrane proteins from the cytosol to the cell membrane.

In addition to their association with papillary necrosis, nonsteroidal antiinflammatory drugs (NSAIDs), such as phenylbutazone, aspirin, carprofen, flunixin meglumine, ibuprofen, and naproxen, have been associated with acute renal failure in small animals, especially dogs. As was proposed for papillary necrosis, the mechanism of acute renal failure is related to the NSAIDs' decreasing synthesis of renal prostaglandins. Because prostaglandins are responsible for maintaining normal renal blood flow, NSAID administration results in afferent arteriolar constriction that decreases renal perfusion, resulting in acute tubular degeneration and necrosis and acute renal failure. The overall incidence of NSAID-induced renal failure in small animals is low and is seen most commonly in animals that ingest excessive amounts of the drug or have a concomitant disorder such as dehydration, congestive heart failure, or chronic renal disease.

Among the naturally occurring nephrotoxins are ochratoxins and citrinins, mycotoxins produced by *Aspergillus* sp. and *Penicillium* sp. Ochratoxin A is nephrotoxic for monogastric animals, particularly pigs, and has been associated with tubular degeneration and necrosis. In addition, long-term ingestion results in diffuse renal fibrosis.

Acute tubular necrosis can result from the ingestion of nephrotoxic plants. Several species of pigweed, particularly *Amaranthus retroflexus,* can be responsible for acute tubular necrosis and perirenal edema in pigs and cattle. The toxic principle has not been identified. Ruminants develop tubular necrosis after ingestion of leaves, buds, or acorns from oak trees and shrubs *(Quercus* sp.). The toxic substances are metabolites of tannins; however, the mechanism of tubular damage is unknown. Acutely affected cattle often have swollen, pale kidneys that occasionally have cortical petechial hemorrhages (Fig. 5-22). Perirenal edema is a common lesion, and the body

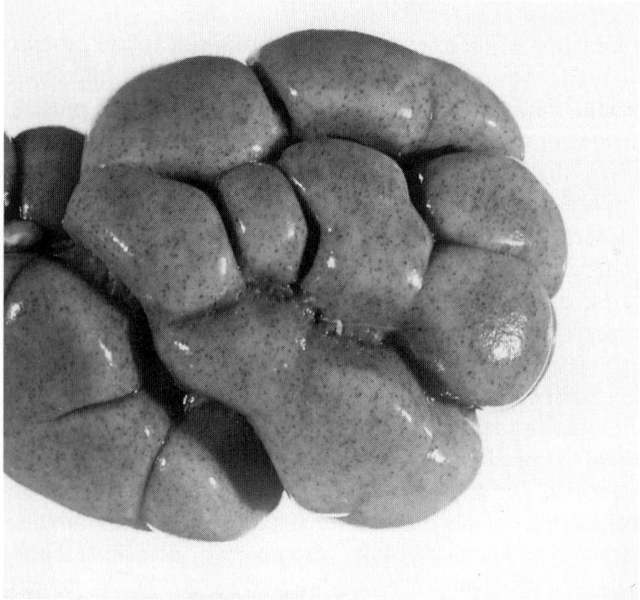

Figure 5-22 Kidney; calf. Oak nephrosis. Acute tubular necrosis is associated with oak toxicity. The kidney is pale, swollen, and moist and has pinpoint hemorrhages throughout the cortex.

cavities contain excessive amounts of a clear fluid. The kidneys in chronic cases are fibrotic, and thus pale, are reduced in size with thinned pale cortices, and have a finely pitted or dimpled surface.

Ingestion of antifreeze is a common cause of acute tubular necrosis in dogs and cats. Ethylene glycol, the major constituent of antifreeze, is readily absorbed from the gastrointestinal tract, and a small percentage is oxidized by hepatic alcohol dehydrogenase to toxic metabolites: glycolaldehyde, glycolic acid, glyoxylate, and oxalate. Ethylene glycol and its toxic metabolic products are filtered by the glomeruli. Acute tubular necrosis is caused by the direct interaction of these toxic metabolites, especially glycolic acid, with tubular epithelium. Of particular significance is that calcium oxalate precipitates as large numbers of pale yellow crystals in renal tubular lumens, tubular epithelial cells, and the interstitium. These crystals cause intrarenal obstruction and degeneration and necrosis of tubular epithelium. Using polarized light, the microscopic identification of large numbers of these birefringent crystals in renal tubules is virtually pathognomonic for ethylene glycol toxicity in dogs and cats. Crystal morphology is apparent with this technique, and crystals appear round to pyramidal and are arranged in rosettes or sheaves.

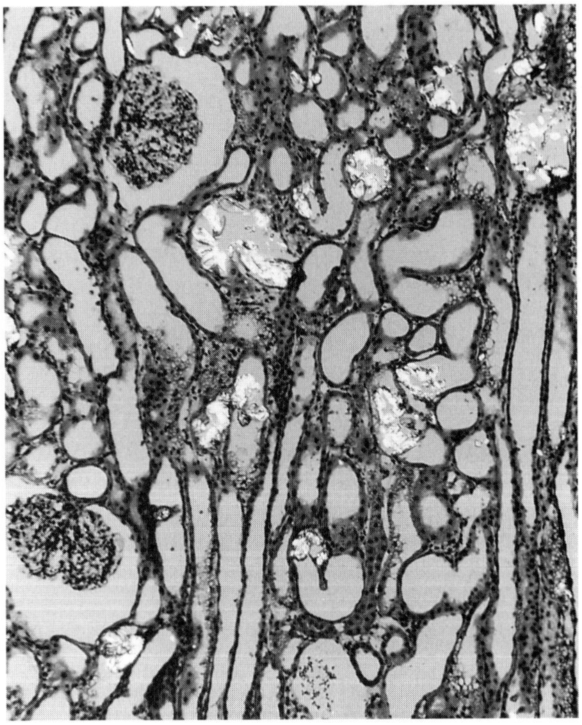

Figure 5-23 Kidney, cortex; sheep. Oxalate nephrosis. Tubular dilatation and tubular necrosis are severe. Numerous tubules contain birefringent calcium oxalate crystals (photographed with polarized light). H & E stain.

Oxalate-induced tubular necrosis also occurs in sheep and cattle after ingestion of toxic quantities of oxalates that accumulate in plants of various genera such as *Halogeton, Sarcobatus, Rheum*, and *Rumex* (Fig. 5-23). After absorption of plant-derived oxalates from the intestine, calcium oxalates form and precipitate in vessel walls and in renal tubules, where they cause obstruction and epithelial cell necrosis. Illness in oxalate poisoning occurs not only because of renal disease, but also because of neuromuscular dysfunction, the result of the hypocalcemia produced by chelation of serum calcium by oxalates. Recently, an oxalate-induced nephrosis was described in Tibetan spaniels with an inherited **hyperoxaluria.**

Nephrosis occurs in dogs and cats given multiple excessive doses of vitamin D (vitamin D intoxication [**vitamin D nephropathy**]) or by accidental ingestion of calciferol-containing rodenticides. In livestock, chronic ingestion of plants such as *Cestrum diurnum* in the southern United States or *Solanum* sp. or *Trisetum* sp. in other countries, each of which contains a chemical with vitamin D–like biologic activity, can also cause nephrosis. Ingestion of excessive amounts of vitamin D can induce hypercalcemia. The subsequent tubular necrosis is the consequence of renal ischemia resulting from vasoconstriction and tubular epithelial cell absorption of calcium, causing mitochondrial calcification, mitochondrial dysfunction, and cellular death. Tubular and glomerular basement membranes are also calcified. Development of lesions depends on the length of time between exposure to rodenticides and death or the duration of continued exposure to vitamin D. In acute cases the kidneys have a smooth capsular surface. Microscopically, tubular epithelium is necrotic and atrophic with a few calcific deposits in tubules scattered randomly throughout the cortex. In more chronic cases, the surface of the kidney is finely granular as a result of fibrosis. White, chalky calcific deposits can be seen within the cortex. Interstitial fibrosis, tubular dilatation and atrophy, glomerular atrophy, and extensive calcification are seen microscopically.

Incidental Lesions of Renal Tubules

Pigment can be present in the renal tubules. In dogs, microscopic granules of hemosiderin frequently are incidental findings in the cytoplasm of proximal convoluted tubules' epithelial cells in kidneys that are otherwise normal. The origin of this pigment is most likely from degradation of hemoglobin resorbed from the glomerular filtrate by proximal tubular epithelium. However, a history or concurrent lesions of a prior hemolytic crisis are often lacking. Fine golden granules of lipofuscin ("wear and tear pigment") can accumulate in renal proximal and distal convoluted tubules of old cattle as well as in striated muscle, resulting in **lipofuscinosis.** Grossly, the renal cortex can have streaks of brown discoloration, but renal function is not affected. **Cloisonné kidneys,** which occur

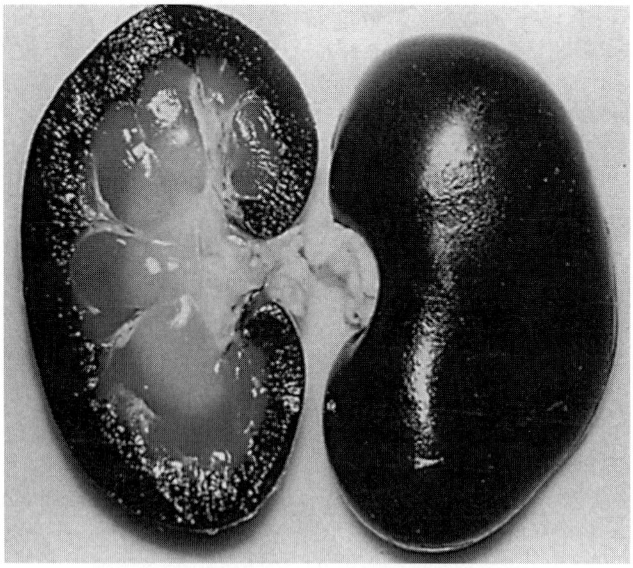

Figure 5-24 Kidney; goat. Cloisonné kidney. The cortex is diffusely black pigmented; the medulla is unaffected.

in goats, have diffuse, intense, black or brown discoloration of the cortex (Fig. 5-24). The medulla is spared. The lesion is the result of tubular membrane thickening due to deposits of ferritin and hemosiderin. Although this lesion is striking, renal function is normal. Other incidental tubular changes include vacuolation of renal tubular epithelium, in the neuronal lysosomal storage diseases such as feline sphingomyelinosis and ovine GM_1 gangliosidosis. In dogs, intranuclear eosinophilic crystalline inclusions occur in renal tubular epithelium. These can be round or rectangular and often greatly distort the nuclei.

Klossiella equi is a sporozoan parasite of the horse. Various stages of schizony can be found microscopically in proximal convoluted tubular epithelium and, to a lesser extent, in glomerular endothelium (Fig. 5-25). Stages of sporogony are present in the epithelial cells of the loop of Henle. Tubules with different coccidial stages occur multifocally and, usually, have no gross lesions and have normal renal function. Occasionally, however, *K. equi* has been associated with multifocal lesions of mild tubular necrosis and with interstitial infiltrates of lymphocytes and plasma cells.

Glomerular Diseases

Glomeruli are complex capillary tufts whose main function is to form a filtrate of plasma that, in its passage through a multifunctional tubular system, is excreted into the lower urinary tract as urine. The glomerular capillary endothelial cells are supported on a basement membrane and are held in their tufted arrangement by the mesangium, a glycoprotein matrix that is formed and maintained by mesangial cells (Fig. 5-26). Mesangial cells are pluripotential mesenchymal cells that are contractile and phagocytic, can synthesize collagen, and are capable of secreting

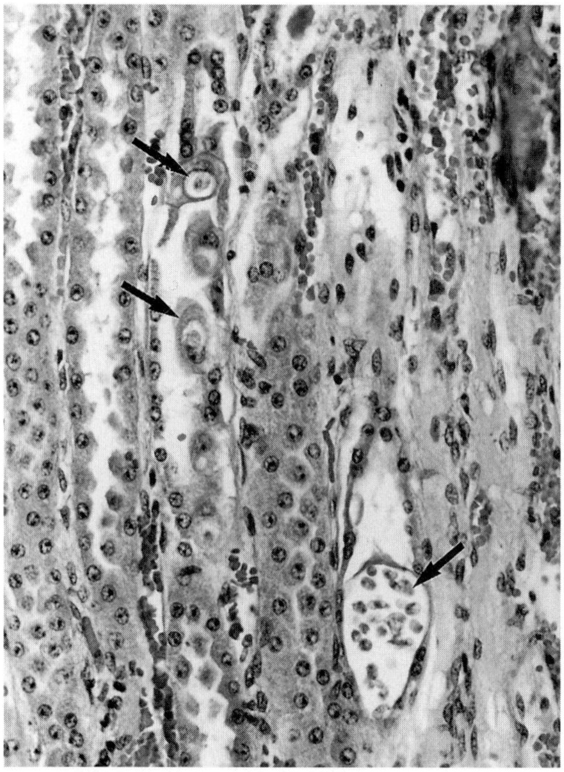

Figure 5-25 Kidney, medulla; horse. *Klossiella equi* infection. Tubular epithelium containing various developmental stages of *K. equi (arrows)*. H & E stain.

inflammatory mediators. Glomerular capillaries are lined by a fenestrated endothelium. The glomerular basement membrane has a thick, dense central layer, the lamina densa, which is covered by thinner, more electron-lucent inner and outer layers, the lamina rara interna and lamina rara externa. The membrane has a network of type IV collagen, which forms a tetrameric porous infrastructure. Numerous glycoproteins, such as acidic proteoglycans and laminin, interact with the collagen fibers to form the complete structure of the membrane. Visceral epithelial cells (podocytes), aligned on the external basement membrane, are responsible for synthesis of basement membrane components and have special cytoplasmic processes (foot processes) that are embedded in the lamina rara externa. Foot processes from adjacent visceral epithelium interdigitate to form filtration slits between them. The endothelium, basement membrane, and filtration slits constitute the glomerular filtration barrier that selectively filters molecules based on size (<70,000 daltons), electrical charge (the more cationic, the more permeable), and capillary pressure. In summary, both size-dependent and charge-dependent filtration is possible because of the porous structure of capillary walls, which is a function of endothelial fenestrations, the collagenous basement membrane superstructure, basement membrane anionic glycoproteins, and filtration slits of the visceral epithelium.

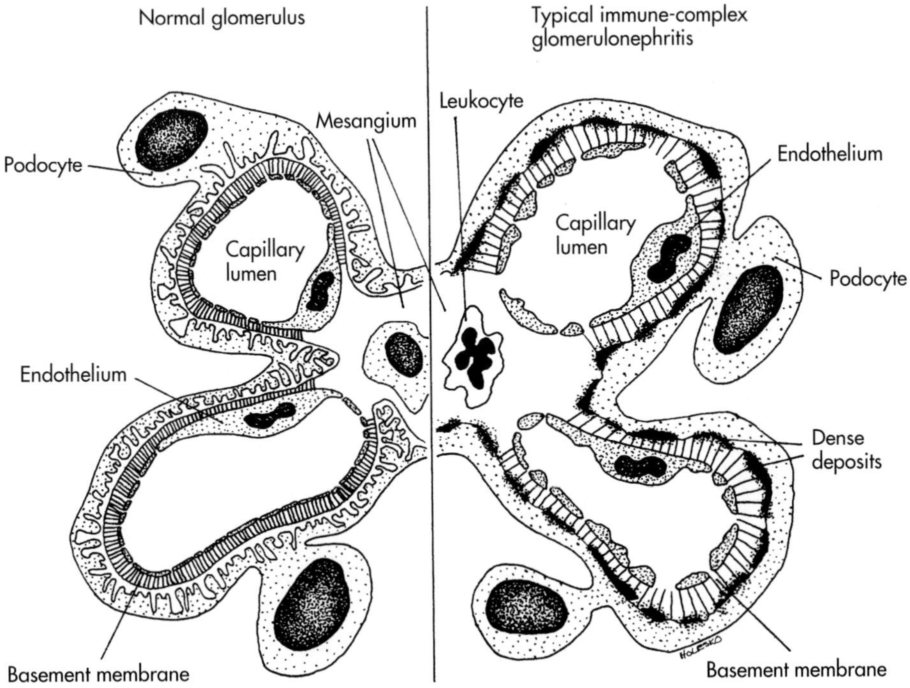

Figure 5-26 Kidney, glomerulus. Normal glomerulus and immune-complex glomerulonephritis. *Left,* normal glomerulus; *right,* a glomerulus with immune-complex glomerulonephritis. Typically, immune-complex glomerulonephritis is characterized by fusion of visceral epithelial (podocyte) foot processes thickening of the capillary basement membranes, leukocyte infiltrates, hypertrophy of endothelium, and dense granular deposits of immune complexes associated with the basement membrane.

Damage to the glomerular filtration barrier can result in renal disease and a variety of clinical signs. A major expression of glomerular disease is the leakage of various low molecular weight (small molecule size) proteins into the glomerular filtrate and subsequently into urine. Renal diseases that result in **proteinuria** are called **protein-losing nephropathies.** A large quantity of plasma protein, particularly albumin, is filtered through the damaged glomerular filtration barrier and overloads the protein reabsorption capabilities of the proximal convoluted tubules to such an extent that protein-rich glomerular filtrate accumulates in the tubular lumina and subsequently appears in the urine. In such diseases, the proximal tubular cells often have microscopic eosinophilic intracytoplasmic bodies referred to as hyaline droplets, which represent accumulations of intracytoplasmic protein absorbed from the filtrate (Fig. 5-27). Microscopically, tubular lumina are often dilated and filled with proteinaceous material. Prolonged, severe renal protein loss results in hypoproteinemia, reduced plasma colloid osmotic (oncotic) pressure, and loss of antithrombin III. Protein-losing nephropathy is one of several causes in animals of severe hypoproteinemia. Prolonged, severe protein-losing nephropathy, the **nephrotic syndrome,** is further characterized by generalized edema, ascites, and pleural effusion.

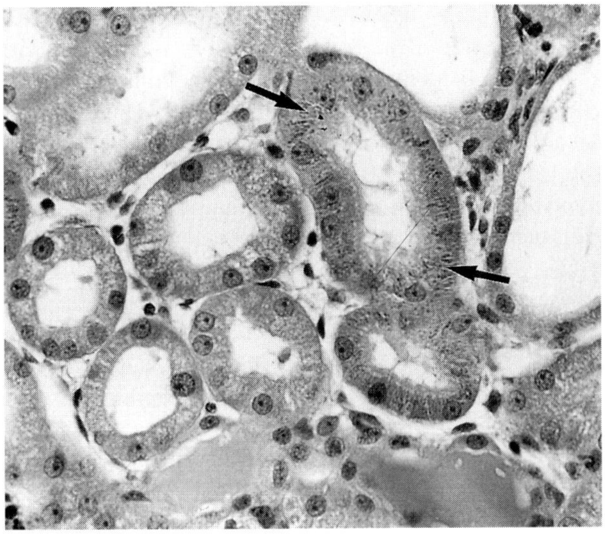

Figure 5-27 Kidney, cortex; dog. Intratubular protein. Because of glomerulonephritis and increased protein in the glomerular filtrate, intracytoplasmic hyalin droplets are present in proximal tubular epithelium *(arrows).* Other tubules contain intraluminal proteinaceous material. H & E stain.

Viral Glomerulitis

Glomerular lesions occur in acute systemic viral diseases such as acute infectious canine hepatitis, septicemic cytomegalovirus infection (inclusion body rhinitis) in neonatal pigs, equine arteritis virus infection, hog cholera, and Newcastle disease in birds. The lesions are mild, usually transient, and result from viral replication in capillary endothelium. Proteinuria is transient. Viral-

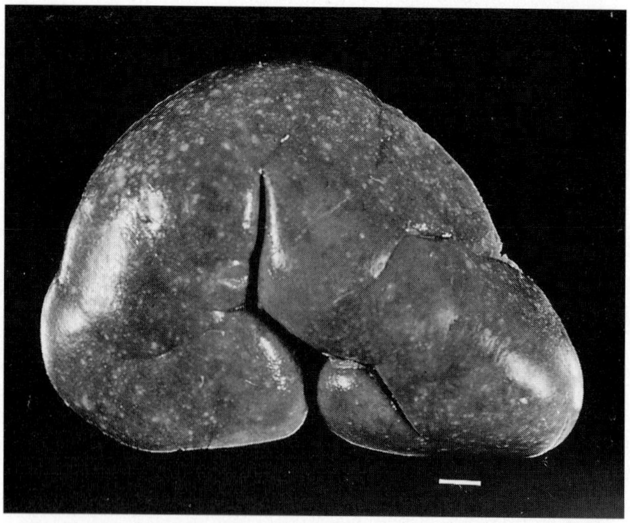

Figure 5-28 Kidney; horse. Embolic nephritis (suppurative glomerulitis). Multiple, small abscesses are randomly scattered throughout the cortex as a result of *Actinobacillus equuli* septicemia. Bar = 1 cm.

induced intranuclear inclusions are present in glomerular capillary endothelium during viremia with infectious canine hepatitis and cytomegalovirus infections. These latter inclusions are usually large, basophilic to magenta, and either fill the nucleus or are separated from the nuclear membrane by a clear halo. In the other diseases, viral antigens can be demonstrated in endothelium, epithelium, or mesangial cells by immunofluorescence or immunohistochemistry. In cases of viral glomerulitis, endothelial hypertrophy, a thickened and edematous mesangium, hemorrhages, and necrosis of endothelium are lesions found at microscopic evaluation. However, some lesions are best demonstrated in electron micrographs. In addition to these lesions, infectious canine hepatitis virus can cause a transient immune-complex glomerulonephritis (see Immune-Mediated Glomerulonephritis) and transient tubulointerstitial nephritis (see Interstitial Nephritis).

Embolic Nephritis (Suppurative Glomerulitis)

Acute **embolic nephritis,** which can also be called **suppurative glomerulitis,** is the result of a bacteremia, in which bacteria randomly lodge in glomeruli and to a lesser extent in interstitial capillaries and cause the formation of multiple foci of inflammation throughout the renal cortex (Fig. 5-28). Microscopically, glomerular capillaries have numerous bacterial colonies. Necrosis and extensive infiltration with neutrophils often obliterate the glomeruli. Glomerular or interstitial hemorrhage can occur as well. As with many other inflammatory diseases, if the affected animals survive, the neutrophilic infiltrates will progressively have increasing numbers of lymphocytes, plasma cells, and macrophages.

A specific example of embolic nephritis is **actinobacillosis** of foals caused by *Actinobacillus equuli.* Foals with actinobacillosis usually die within a few days after birth and have small abscesses in many visceral organs, especially the renal cortex, and a fibrinopurulent polysynovitis.

Embolic nephritis also occurs in other animal species as a result of bacteremia with any of several bacterial species. In pigs, *Erysipelothrix* sp., *Streptococcus* sp., and *Corynebacterium* sp. are frequently isolated from this lesion.

Immune-mediated Glomerulonephritis

Glomerulonephritis results most often from immune-mediated mechanisms, most notably involving antibodies to glomerular basement membranes or the deposition of soluble immune complexes within the glomeruli. Diagnosis of an immune-mediated glomerulonephritis is confirmed by demonstrating immunoglobulin (Ig) and complement components, usually C3, in the glomeruli by immunofluorescent or immunohistochemical techniques.

Antibodies to basement membrane bind to glomerular basement membranes **(antibasement membrane disease)** and damage the glomerulus through fixation of complement and resulting leukocyte infiltration. This mechanism of glomerulonephritis has been well documented in human beings and nonhuman primates but only rarely in other species. To confirm the diagnosis of antibasement membrane disease, Ig and C3 must be demonstrated within glomeruli, and antibodies must be eluted from the kidneys and found to bind to normal glomerular basement membranes of the appropriate species.

Immune-complex glomerulonephritis occurs in association with persistent infections or other diseases that characteristically have a prolonged antigenemia that enhances the formation of soluble immune complexes. In domestic animals, immune-complex glomerulonephritis occurs most commonly in dogs and cats. In a recent study, 77% of dogs with protein-losing glomerular disease had glomerulonephritis, which was presumed to be of immune complex origin. Immune-complex glomerulonephritis is associated with specific viral infections such as feline leukemia virus or feline infectious peritonitis virus, bacterial infections such as pyometra or pyoderma, chronic parasitism such as dirofilariasis, autoimmune diseases such as canine systemic lupus erythematosus, or neoplasia (Box 5-2). However, as in the well-documented disease **feline progressive membranous glomerulonephritis** the specific cause of immune complex glomerulonephritis might never be identifiable. In addition to the role of persistent infections, a familial tendency for development of immune-complex glomerulonephritis was described in a group of related Bernese mountain dogs.

Immune-complex glomerulonephritis is initiated by the formation of soluble immune complexes (antigen-antibody complexes) in the presence of antigen-antibody equivalency or slight antigen excess in the plasma. These

BOX 5-2 DISEASES IN WHICH IMMUNE-COMPLEX GLOMERULONEPHRITIS CAN OCCUR

Dogs	Infectious canine hepatitis
	Chronic hepatitis
	Chronic bacterial diseases
	  Endometritis (pyometra)
	  Pyoderma
	  Prostatitis
	Dirofilariasis
	Borreliosis (Lyme disease)
	Systemic lupus erythematosis
	Polyarteritis
	Autoimmune hemolytic anemia
	Immune-mediated polyarthritis
	Neoplasia
	Hereditary C3 deficiency

Cats	Feline leukemia virus infection Feline infectious peritonitis Feline immunodeficiency virus Progressive polyarteritis Neoplasia Progressive membranous glomerulonephritis
Horses	Equine infectious anemia *Streptococcus* sp.
Cattle	Bovine viral diarrhea Trypanosomiasis
Pigs	Hog cholera African swine fever
Sheep	Hereditary hypocomplementemia in Finnish Landrace lambs

complexes are selectively deposited in the glomerular capillaries where they stimulate complement fixation with formation of C3a, C5a, and C567, which are chemotactic for neutrophils. During early stages, infiltrating neutrophils damage the basement membrane through release of proteinases, arachidonic acid metabolites (such as thromboxane), and oxidants, particularly oxygen-derived free radicals and hydrogen peroxide; in later stages, monocytes infiltrate into the glomeruli and are responsible for continuing damage to the glomeruli by the release of biologically active molecules.

Many specific factors determine the extent of deposition of soluble immune complexes in the glomerular capillary walls. These include persistence of appropriate quantities of immune complexes in the circulation, glomerular permeability, the size and molecular charge of the soluble complexes, and the strength of the bond between the antigen and antibody (avidity). Small or intermediate complexes are the most damaging, since large complexes are removed from circulation through phagocytosis by cells of the mononuclear-phagocyte system in the liver and spleen. An increase in local glomerular vascular permeability is necessary for immune complexes to leave the microcirculation and deposit in the glomerulus. This process is usually facilitated via vasoactive amine release from platelets, basophils, or mast cells. Mast cells or basophils release vasoactive amines by the interaction of the immune complexes with antigen-specific IgE on the surface of these cells, by stimulation of the mast cells or basophils by cationic proteins released from neutrophils, or by the anaphylatoxin activity of C3a and C5a. Platelet activation factor (PAF) is released from immune complex–stimulated mast cells, basophils, or macrophages and causes platelets to release vasoactive amines. Localization of the complexes within the various levels of the basement membrane or in subepithelial locations depends on their molecular charge and avidity. Once small soluble immune complexes are deposited within the capillary wall, they can then become greatly enlarged as a result of interactions of immune complexes with free antibodies, free antigens, complement components, or other immune complexes.

After immune complex deposition, glomerular injury can also occur in the absence of leukocyte infiltration from the aggregation of platelets and activation of Hageman factor with the formation of fibrin thrombi that produce glomerular ischemia. Furthermore, sublytic glomerular epithelial cell and extracellular matrix damage can result directly from the terminal membrane attack complex of the activated complement cascade (C5 to C9), which can cause epithelial detachment and proteinuria.

Finally, if exposure of the glomerulus to immune complexes is short lived, as in a transient infection such as infectious canine hepatitis, immune complexes will be phagocytosed by macrophages or mesangial cells and removed, and the glomerular lesions and clinical signs will resolve. Conversely, continual exposure of glomeruli to soluble immune complexes, such as with persistent viral infections (e.g., feline leukemia virus infection and chronic heartworm disease), can produce progressive glomerular injury with severe lesions and clinical manifestation of glomerular disease.

Ultrastructurally, immune complexes either in the glomerular basement membrane or in a subepithelial location appear as electron-dense bodies (Figs. 5-26 and 5-29). Complexes that are poorly soluble, fairly large, or with high avidity, rather than localizing in capillaries, often enter the mesangium where they can be phagocytosed by macrophages and appear ultrastructurally as dense granular deposits within the mesangial stroma or within macrophages. Other ultrastructural changes commonly seen are loss or effacement of visceral epithelial cell foot processes, cytoplasmic vacuolation, retraction and detachment of visceral epithelium, and infiltrates of neutrophils and monocytes.

A tentative diagnosis of immune-complex glomerulonephritis can be made by demonstration of Ig and C3 in glomerular tufts. In dogs, IgG or IgM are the most common isotypes demonstrated in glomerulonephritis;

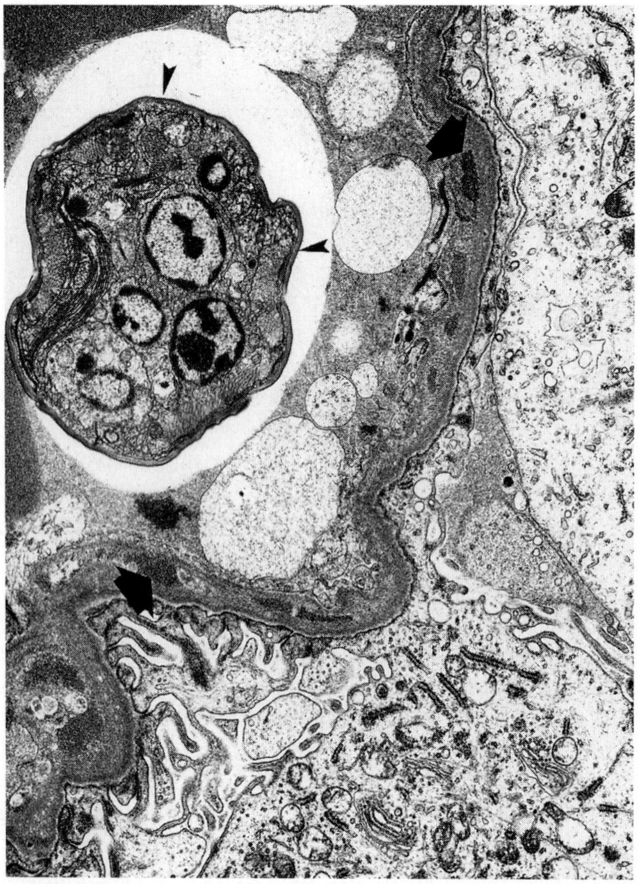

Figure 5-29 Kidney, glomerulus; dog. Immune-complex glomerulonephritis. Electron photomicrograph of a glomerulus with immune-complex deposits due to dirofilariasis. A heartworm microfilaria is present in the capillary lumen *(arrowheads)*. The basement membrane is irregularly thickened and contains granular, electron-dense deposits *(arrows)*. The podocytic foot processes are fused. *Courtesy Dr. N. Cheville.*

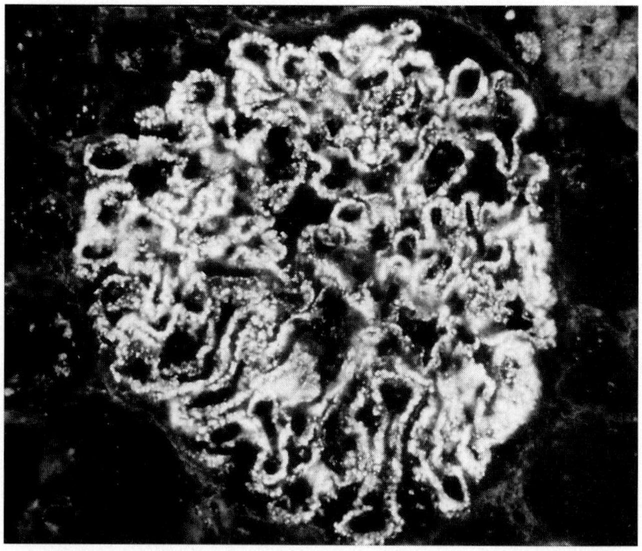

Figure 5-30 Kidney, glomerulus; dog. Immune-complex glomerulonephritis. Intraglomerular immunoglobulin deposits demonstrated by immunofluorescence. Note the granular ("lumpy-bumpy") pattern of fluorescence. *Courtesy Dr. R. Lewis.*

however, combinations of IgG, IgM, and IgA also occur in the glomeruli of some dogs. In one study, IgA was the only Ig found in three dogs with immune-complex glomerulonephritis. Both Ig and C3 are usually seen in a granular ("lumpy-bumpy") pattern using immunofluorescent or immunohistochemical techniques (Fig. 5-30); however, occasionally the deposits have a linear distribution conforming to the basement membranes. The diagnosis of immune-complex glomerulonephritis can be confirmed only by ruling out antibasement membrane disease after demonstrating that the antibodies eluted from glomeruli do not bind to normal glomeruli. Once a diagnosis of immune-complex glomerulonephritis is confirmed, the ideal situation would be to identify the causative antigen present in immune complexes. This process is accomplished by eluting antibodies from diseased glomeruli and attempting to identify their specificity for suspected antigens. For example, antibodies eluted from the glomeruli of dogs with glomerulonephritis associated with severe heartworm disease bind to several *Dirofilaria immitis* antigens including the body wall of adult worms, parasitic uterine fluid, and microfilaria. In most cases of immune-complex glomerulonephritis, the specific causative antigen usually escapes determination. This outcome is the usual case in sheep, in which subclinical lesions of immune-complex glomerulonephritis are common.

Gross lesions of acute immune-complex glomerulonephritis are usually subtle. The kidneys are often slightly swollen, have a smooth capsular surface, are normal color or pale, and have glomeruli that are visible as pinpoint red dots on the cut surface of the cortex. The normal glomeruli of horses are usually visible, so this feature of pinpoint red dots for glomeruli cannot be used for diagnosis in that species. If lesions do not resolve but become subacute to chronic, the renal cortex is somewhat shrunken and the capsular surface has a generalized fine granularity. On cut surface, the cortex can be thinned and granular, and glomeruli can appear as pale pinpoint gray dots. With time, more severe scarring can develop throughout the cortex (see Renal Fibrosis).

Microscopically, immune-complex glomerulonephritis has several histopathologic forms. Although various classifications of glomerulonephritis have been published, the following simple classification is well understood among veterinary pathologists. Lesions in glomeruli may be described as **proliferative, membranous,** or **membranoproliferative.** Glomerular lesion can be distributed **diffusely,** when most of the glomeruli are involved; **focally,** when only a certain proportion of glomeruli are involved;

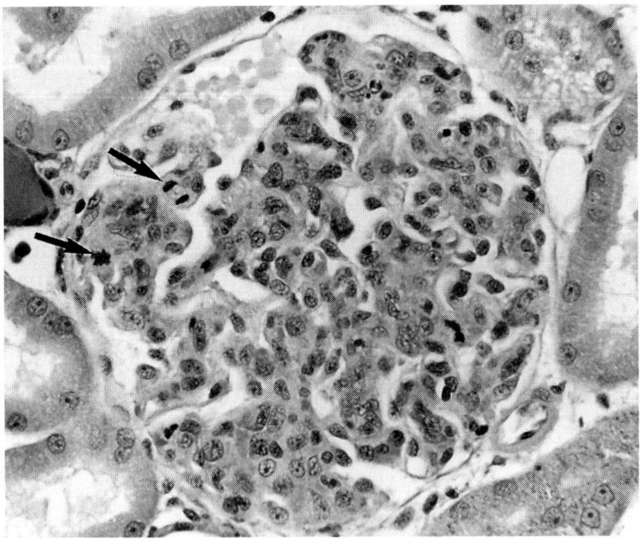

Figure 5-31 Kidney, glomerulus; dog. Proliferative glomerulonephritis. The lesion is characterized by hypercellularity of a glomerulus. There are mitotically active epithelial cells *(arrows)*. H & E stain.

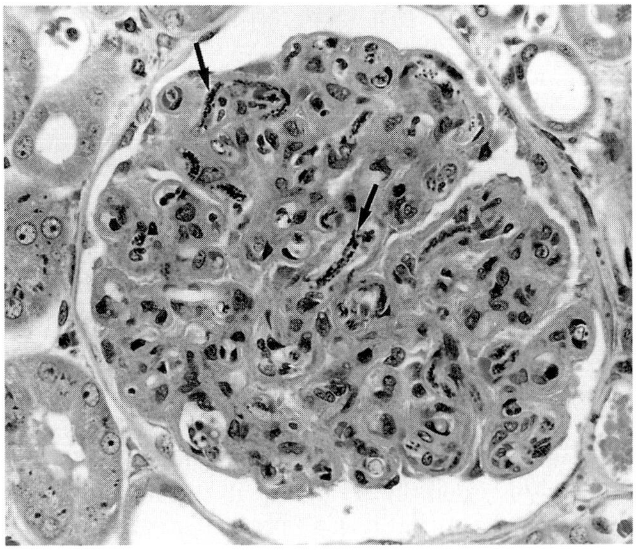

Figure 5-32 Kidney, glomerulus; dog. Membranous glomerulonephritis. The lesion is associated with dirofilariasis and is characterized by generalized hyalin thickening of glomerular capillary basement membranes. Note also microfilaria within vessel lumina *(arrows)*. H & E stain.

globally, when an entire glomerular tuft is involved; and **segmentally,** when only a portion of glomerular tuft is affected. Most of the lesions in immune-complex glomerulonephritis are diffuse, but within an individual affected glomerulus the lesions can be either global or segmental.

- **Proliferative glomerulonephritis** is a form of immune-complex glomerular disease characterized by increased cellularity of the glomerular tufts caused by proliferation of glomerular endothelial, epithelial, and mesangial cells and an influx of neutrophils and other leukocytes involving both the capillary loops and the mesangium (Fig. 5-31).
- **Membranous glomerulonephritis** is characterized by diffuse glomerular capillary basement membrane thickening as the predominant change (Fig. 5-32). This variation is the most common form of immune-complex glomerulonephritis in cats.
- **Membranoproliferative glomerulonephritis** (mesangiocapillary, mesangioproliferative) is characterized by both hypercellularity and capillary basement membrane thickening in affected glomeruli. This variant appears to be the most common morphologic form of immune-complex glomerulonephritis in the dog.

Several other changes in the glomerulus and Bowman's capsule usually accompany the lesions discussed above. These changes include adhesions between the epithelial cells of the glomerular tuft and Bowman's capsule (synechiae), hypertrophy and hyperplasia of the parietal epithelium lining Bowman's capsule, deposition of fibrinogen and fibrinous thrombi in glomerular capillaries, and tubular dilatation with homogeneous proteinaceous fluid. An increase in mesangial matrix is often present along with these described changes. If the damage is mild and the cause is removed, glomeruli can heal without obvious or with minimal residual lesions. However, if the lesion is severe and prolonged, subacute to chronic glomerular changes develop. Bowman's capsule can become thickened and hyalinized. In severe cases, proliferation of parietal epithelium, an influx of monocytes, and deposition of fibrin can occur within Bowman's capsule, resulting in the formation of a semicircular, hypercellular, intraglomerular lesion known as a **glomerular crescent** (Fig. 5-33). The glomerular crescent can also undergo fibrosis, and if Bowman's capsule ruptures, glomerular fibrosis can become continuous with interstitial fibrosis. Interstitial and periglomerular fibrosis and foci of interstitial lymphocytes and plasma cells accompany chronic glomerulonephritis (see Renal Fibrosis).

Glomerulosclerosis

In chronic glomerulonephritis, severely affected glomeruli shrink and become hyalinized because of an increase in fibrous connective tissue and mesangial matrix and a loss of glomerular capillaries (Fig. 5-34). These glomeruli are hypocellular and essentially nonfunctional. This process is referred to as **glomerulosclerosis.** Glomerulosclerosis can be diffuse, involving all glomeruli, or multifocal. In addition, glomerulosclerosis can involve a whole glomerular tuft (global) or only portions of the tuft (segmental) thus appearing as a nodular or segmental hyalinized thickening in affected glomeruli. Because tubules receive their blood supply from the vasa recta, derived from glomerular capillaries and afferent arteriole, glomerulosclerosis reduces the blood flow through the vasa recta thus decreasing oxygen tension in the tubules. The resulting hypoxia is responsible for tubular epithelial cell death via apoptosis that results in tubular atrophy. In addition, chronic proteinuria often accompanies glomerulosclerosis and has been reported to stimulate tubular epithelial cell loss through apoptosis. Numerous factors are associated with and accelerate glomerulosclerosis. These factors include unrestricted protein in the diet, increased glomerular capillary pressure in functional glomeruli in chronically diseased kidneys, and cytokines and platelet-derived growth factors. These factors alter cellular components of the functional glomerular tufts, causing hyperfiltration and damage to endothelium, mesangial cell activation and increased mesangial matrix production, and visceral epithelial cell loss, which allows synechiae (i.e., adhesions between visceral and parietal epithelial cell layers in the glomerulus) to occur.

Glomerulosclerosis is not only the end stage of glomerulonephritis, but can develop in any chronic disease in which severe damage to nephrons or loss of nephron function occurs. Mild multifocal glomerulosclerosis of unknown cause is often an incidental finding in aged animals. Glomerulosclerosis has been documented occasionally in animals with hypertension and diabetes mellitus. In these cases, global or nodular eosinophilic glycoprotein material (hyaline) is deposited in the glomerular mesangium.

Amyloidosis

Amyloid, an insoluble fibrillar protein with a β-pleated sheet conformation, is produced after incomplete proteolysis of several soluble amyloidogenic proteins. The cell responsible for degradation of amyloidogenic proteins is thought to be the macrophage. Amyloid deposits in patients with plasma cell myelomas or other B lymphocyte dyscrasias (called **AL amyloidosis**) are composed of fragments of the light chains of immunoglobulins. In domestic animals, spontaneously occurring amyloidosis is usually an example of what is called **reactive amyloidosis (AA amyloidosis).** This form of the disease is often associated with chronic inflammatory diseases; the amyloid deposits are composed of fragments of a serum acute-phase reactant protein called serum amyloid–associated (SAA) protein. Amyloid fibrils from either source are deposited in tissues along with a glycoprotein called amyloid P-component.

Glomeruli are the most common renal site for deposition of amyloid in most domestic animal species, although the medullary interstitium is a common site for deposition in cats. Renal amyloidosis commonly occurs in association with other diseases, particularly chronic inflammatory or neoplastic diseases. However, idiopathic renal amyloidosis, that is, amyloidosis in which an associated disease process is not recognized, is also described in dogs and cats. The underlying pathogenic mechanisms of idiopathic

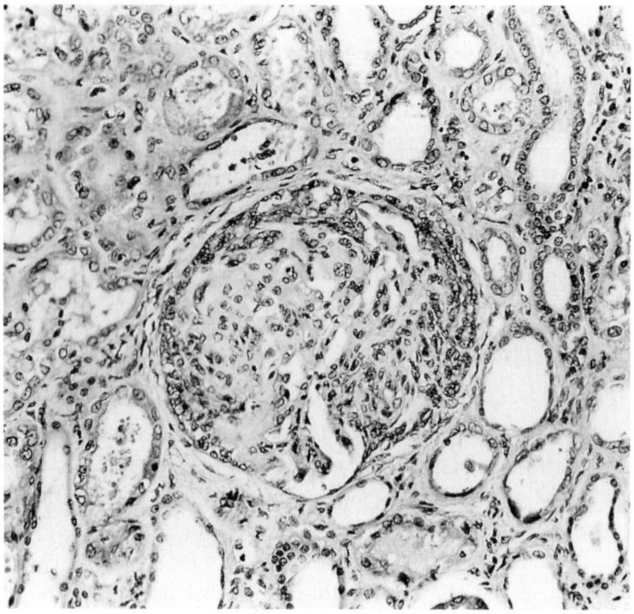

Figure 5-33 Kidney, glomerulus; chimpanzee. Chronic glomerulonephritis. A semicircular hypercellular glomerular crescent is present to the right of the glomerular tuft within *Bowman's capsule.* H & E stain.

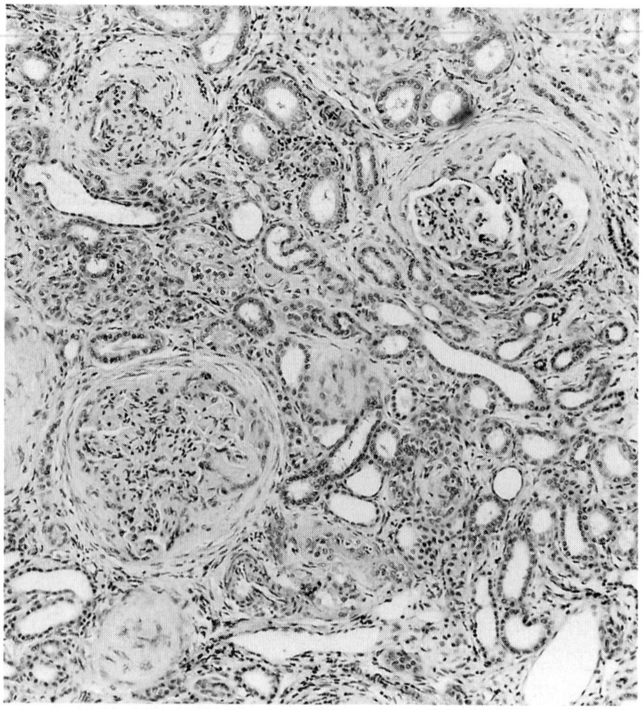

Figure 5-34 Kidney, glomerulus; dog. Glomerulosclerosis. Chronic glomerulonephritis is characterized by various stages of shrinkage, hyalinization, and fibrosis of the glomerular tufts and periglomerular and interstitial fibrosis. H & E stain.

renal amyloidosis are not known. Moreover, proteinuria could be a factor. In a recent study, 23% of dogs that presented with proteinuria had renal amyloidosis. A hereditary predisposition for the development of reactive amyloidosis (AA) has been found in Abyssinian cats and Chinese shar-pei dogs. A familial tendency is suspected as well in Siamese cats, English foxhounds, and beagle dogs. In cattle, renal amyloidosis is nearly always due to chronic systemic infectious disease. Glomerular amyloidosis is a protein-losing nephropathy resulting in marked proteinuria and uremia. It can, like immune-complex glomerulonephritis, result in the nephrotic syndrome. Medullary amyloidosis is usually asymptomatic unless it results in papillary necrosis (see Circulatory Disturbances).

Kidneys affected with glomerular amyloidosis are often enlarged, pale tan to yellow, and have a smooth to finely granular capsular surface. Amyloid-laden glomeruli can be visible as fine tan dots on the capsular and cut surfaces. The cortex can have a finely granular appearance. Treatment of kidneys with an iodine solution, such as Lugol's iodine, in many cases can result in brown staining of glomeruli that become purple when exposed to dilute sulfuric acid (Fig. 5-35). This technique provides a rapid presumptive diagnosis of renal amyloidosis that can be used by veterinarians in clinical practice. Long-standing glomerular amyloidosis results in diminished renal blood flow from the glomeruli to the vasa recta. Such reduced renal vascular perfusion can lead to renal tubular atrophy, degeneration, and diffuse fibrosis. Medullary amyloidosis is usually not grossly recognizable.

Microscopically, glomerular amyloid is deposited in the mesangium and subendothelial locations. Amyloid is relatively acellular and can accumulate segmentally within glomerular tufts; thus, a portion of the normal glomerular architecture is replaced by eosinophilic, homogeneous to slightly fibrillar material (Fig. 5-36). When amyloidosis involves the entire glomerular tuft, the glomerulus is enlarged, capillary lumina become obliterated, and the tuft can appear as a large hypocellular, eosinophilic hyaline sphere. Amyloid can be present in renal tubular basement membranes, and these membranes are hyalinized and thickened. Renal tubules with glomerular amyloidosis are usually markedly dilated and contain proteinaceous material. Amyloid is confirmed microscopically by staining with Congo red stain. When viewed with polarized light, amyloid has green birefringence. Loss of Congo red staining after treatment of a section of affected kidney with potassium permanganate suggests the amyloid is AA-amyloid, i.e., of acute-phase reactant protein origin.

Miscellaneous Glomerular Lesions

Glomerular lipidosis, characterized by small aggregates of lipid-laden foamy macrophages in glomerular tufts, is an occasional incidental finding in dogs. A similar, but more extensive glomerular lipidosis has been described in cats with inherited hyperlipoproteinemia, which is a generalized disease characterized by hyperchylomicronemia, atherosclerosis, and xanthogranulomas in numerous parenchymatous organs, including the kidneys (see Granulomatous Nephritis). Microscopically, glomeruli contain foamy macrophages, characteristic of glomerular lipidosis,

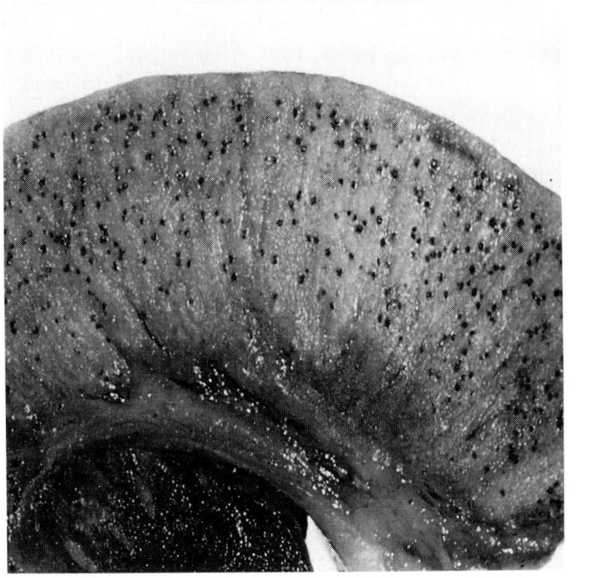

Figure 5-35 Kidney; dog. Amyloidosis. The cut surface of a kidney is stained with Lugol's iodine and treated with sulfuric acid to demonstrate amyloid-infiltrated glomeruli.

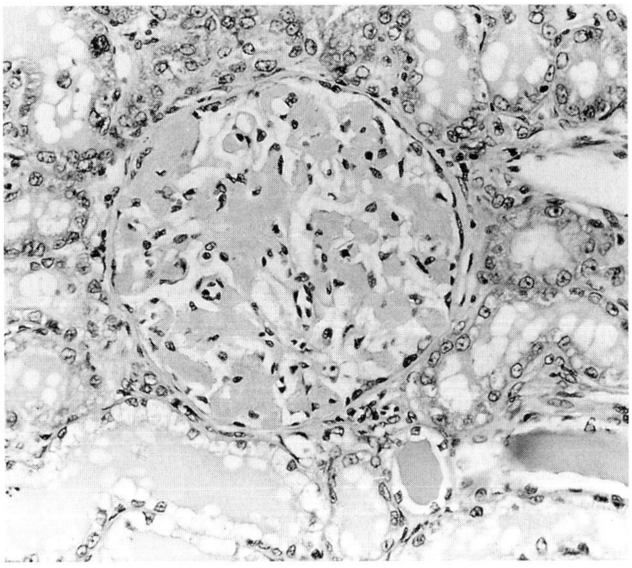

Figure 5-36 Kidney, glomerulus; dog. Amyloidosis. Amyloid is seen as pale eosinophilic homogeneous, hyalinized deposits within the glomerular tuft. Note also the dense proteinaceous material in tubular lumina. H & E stain.

as well as increased mesangium and thickened Bowman's capsule.

An idiopathic **renal glomerular vasculopathy** and **cutaneous vasculopathy** occurs in greyhounds. Affected greyhounds have multifocal erythematous and ulcerated skin lesions and distal limb edema. Variable systemic signs of uremia often accompany the cutaneous lesions. Thrombocytopenia is frequently seen. At necropsy, kidneys from affected dogs are swollen and congested with small cortical petechiae. Microscopically, numerous glomeruli have segmental or global fibrinous thrombi, hemorrhage, and necrosis (Fig. 5-37). At the glomerular vascular pole the walls of afferent arterioles have fibrin deposition and foci of necrosis. The cause of this disease is unknown, but renal lesions are similar to those seen in disseminated intravascular coagulation, thrombotic thrombocytopenic purpura, and hemolytic-anemia syndrome in human beings.

In **canine hyperadrenocorticism** or as a result of excessive exogenous glucocorticoid therapy, proteinuria often develops. Glomerular lesions consist of mild mesangial hypercellularity, synechiae, thickened basement membranes, and effacement of epithelial foot processes. Lesions are devoid of Ig. The cause of this lesion is unknown; however, hypertension has been postulated, because of its occurrence with increased plasma glucocorticoid concentrations.

Tubulointerstitial Disease

Interstitial Nephritis

Aggregates of inflammatory cells can be present in the renal interstitium in various systemic infectious diseases of domestic animals. In many of these diseases, the inflammatory cell infiltrates are visible only microscopically, are not associated with renal failure, and are generally inconsequential (examples are canine erhlichiosis and equine infectious anemia). In other diseases, the renal interstitium is the site of moderate to severe interstitial inflammatory cell infiltrates that are grossly visible and associated with renal failure. When the interstitial inflammation appears to be the primary lesion and there is no evidence of embolic nephritis or pyelonephritis, this lesion has traditionally been called **interstitial nephritis.** More recently, the term **tubulointerstitial nephritis** has been used to acknowledge that inflammatory and degenerative changes in tubules are often present and can actually be involved in the development of the primary lesion. Interstitial nephritis can be acute, subacute, or chronic, and is traditionally associated with a lymphoplasmacytic infiltrate; however, other types of leukocytes can also be present. Chronic interstitial nephritis is associated with renal interstitial fibrosis (see Renal Fibrosis). In addition to interstitial nephritis, leukocytes are also found in the interstitium in pyelonephritis and embolic nephritis. Because of differences in pathogenesis, lesion distribution, and microscopic appearance between those conditions and interstitial nephritis, pyelonephritis and embolic nephritis are considered separate entities (see Embolic Nephritis and Pyelonephritis).

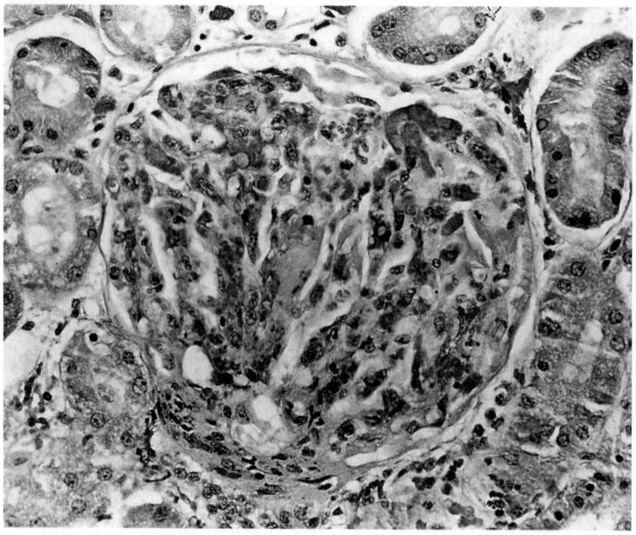

Figure 5-37 Kidney, glomerulus; dog. Glomerular vasculopathy. Necrotic glomerular cells and extensive glomerular capillary thrombosis are present, which is typical of the idiopathic glomerular and cutaneous vasculopathy syndrome in greyhound dogs. H & E stain.

Interstitial nephritis is the result of bacterial and viral septicemias, whereby these infectious agents first infect the kidney tubules and then incite an inflammatory response in the interstitium (Box 5-3). The actual pathogenesis of these lesions is often unknown. The best understood causes of interstitial nephritis in domestic animals are serovars of *Leptospira interrogans.* Serovars *canicola* and *icterohemorrhagiae* are the most common cause of canine **leptospirosis,** whereas serovar *pomona* is the most common cause of the lesion in pigs and occasionally in cattle. Other serovars such as *grippotyphosa* and *bratislava* have also been associated with renal leptospirosis in several animal species. The pathogenesis of leptospirosis is discussed as an example of an acute bacterial interstitial nephritis. Following exposure to the organism, leptospiremia occurs and organisms localize in

BOX 5-3 CAUSES OF INTERSTITIAL NEPHRITIS

Dogs	*Leptospira interrogans* serovars *canicola, icterohemorrhagiae,* and others Infectious canine hepatitis virus, recovery phase
Cattle	*Escherichia coli* septicemia, "white spotted kidney" Malignant catarrhal fever *Theilaria parva*
Horses	Equine viral arteritis
Pigs	*Leptospira interrogans* serovar *pomona* Porcine reproductive and respiratory syndrome
Sheep	Sheeppox

the renal interstitial capillaries, migrate through vascular endothelium, persist in the interstitial spaces, and migrate via the lateral intercellular junctions of tubular epithelial cells to reach renal tubular lumina. Within tubules, leptospires are associated with epithelial microvilli and occur within phagosomes of the epithelium of the proximal and distal convoluted tubules. These tubular epithelial cells undergo degeneration and necrosis as a result of either direct toxic effects of the leptospires or the accompanying interstitial inflammatory reaction. Alhough neutrophils can be present in tubular lumina, the predominant lesion is in the interstitium, which becomes infiltrated with monocytes, macrophages, lymphocytes, and plasma cells. In affected dogs, interstitial plasma cells secrete *Leptospira*-specific antibodies. However, the role of those antibodies in pathogenesis or resolution of the lesion is not known. *Escherichia coli* septicemia in calves can result in interstitial nephritis (so-called **white spotted kidneys**). The pathogenesis is unknown but most likely is similar to that of leptospirosis.

Another well-documented mechanism for the production of interstitial nephritis is the immune response developed to virus of **infectious canine hepatitis** in dogs. During the viremic phase of the disease, virus initially localizes in the glomeruli (viral glomerulitis), producing a transient immune-complex glomerulonephritis. As the dog recovers from the acute phase of the disease and with onset of the systemic immune response, virus disappears from the glomeruli only to reappear in tubular epithelial cells in various portions of the nephron. Virus can persist in tubular epithelium for weeks and months and causes tubular epithelial necrosis as a result of viral-induced cytolysis. This process is followed by a lymphocytic and plasmacytic interstitial nephritis. Basophilic intranuclear inclusions typical of infectious canine hepatitis virus are present in infected renal tubular epithelial cells.

Deposition of immune complexes in or interactions between antibasement membrane antibodies and tubular basement membranes can initiate immune-mediated tubulointerstitial disease in human beings and laboratory animals. Depositions of Ig and complement have rarely been identified in renal tubular basement membranes in domestic animals. At present, the role of immune-mediated mechanisms is questionable as a cause of interstitial nephritis in domestic animals.

Infection with **equine arteritis virus** or **porcine reproductive** and **respiratory syndrome virus** often results in multifocal lymphohistiocytic interstitial nephritis with interstitial edema. Lesions can involve any area in the cortex, but are especially intense at the corticomedullary junction and in the medulla. A severe vasculitis is characterized by fibrinoid necrosis and lymphohistiocytic infiltrates that involve the adventitial and medial layers of cortical and medullary interstitial arteries and veins. Virus can be found in endothelium and in interstitial and vascular macrophages.

Gross lesions of interstitial nephritis can be classified as acute, subacute, or chronic; chronic interstitial nephritis is discussed later (see Renal Fibrosis). The distribution of lesions can be diffuse as in canine leptospirosis (Fig. 5-38) or multifocal as in "white spotted kidneys" of calves due to *Escherichia coli* septicemia (Fig. 5-39), infectious canine hepatitis, malignant catarrhal fever (Fig. 5-40), or porcine leptospirosis. In diffuse interstitial nephritis, kidneys can be swollen and pale tan with a random gray mottling of the capsular surface. The cut surface bulges; gray infiltrates of varying sizes and intensities obscure the normal radially striated cortical architecture. These renal lesions usually are manifested as coalescing gray foci that are particularly intense in the inner cortex. Focal lesions

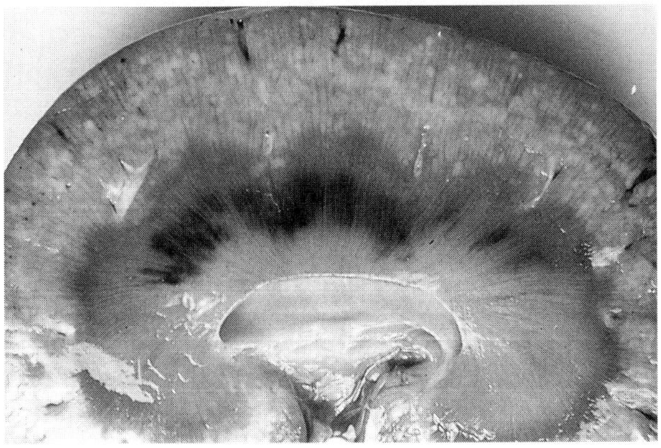

Figure 5-38 Kidney; dog. Interstitial nephritis. Pale foci of inflammatory cellular infiltrate are in the cortex, concentrated near the corticomedullary junction. These lesions are typical for subacute leptospirosis. Note there is a zone of medullary hemorrhage.

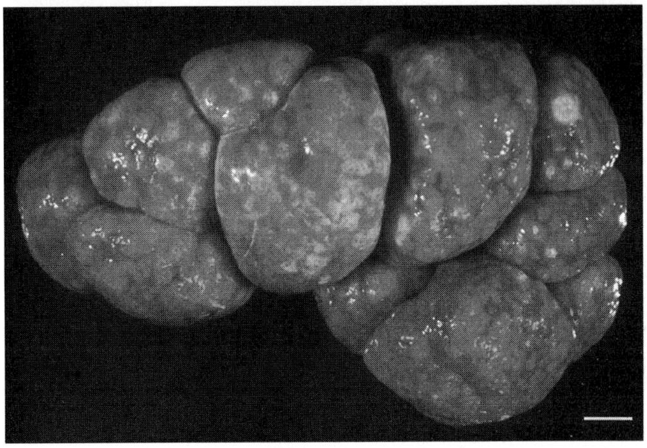

Figure 5-39 Kidney; calf. Multifocal interstitial nephritis (white-spotted kidney). Multiple pale foci of inflammation (2-5 mm in diameter) are randomly scattered throughout the kidney. The capsular surface is irregular due to the cortical inflammation. On cut surface, these foci extend well into the cortex. Bar = 1 cm.

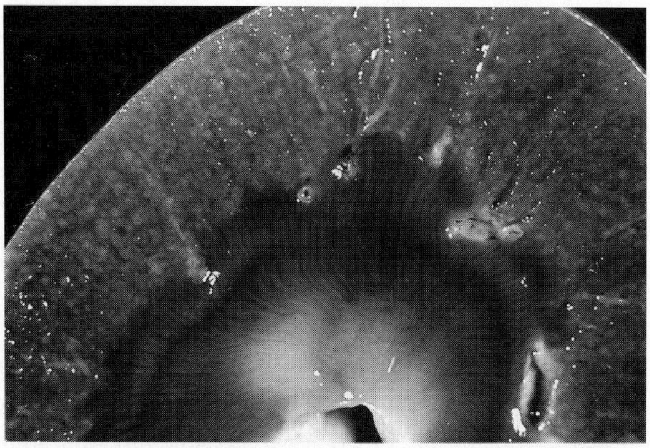

Figure 5-40 Kidney; gaur. Interstitial nephritis. The cortex has multiple, pale, discrete interstitial inflammatory cell infiltrates due to malignant catarrhal fever virus infection. Note that the cortical striations are effaced.

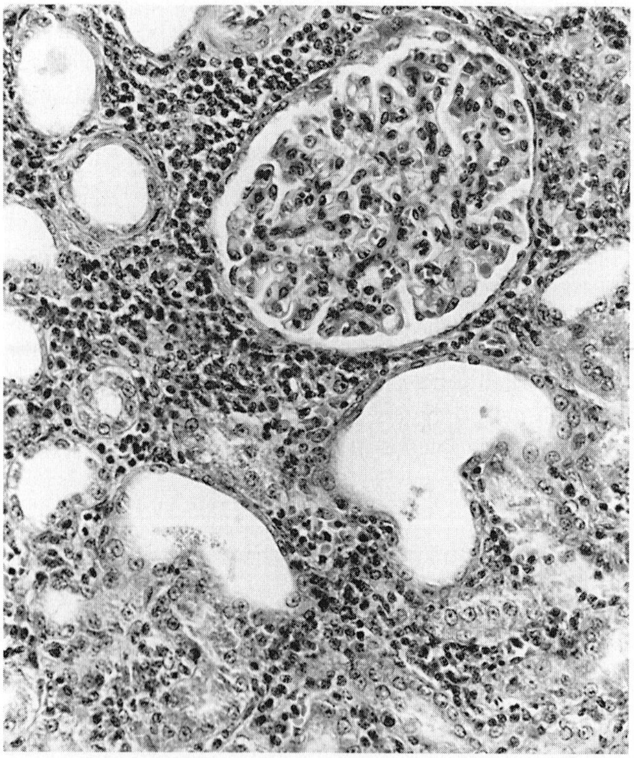

Figure 5-41 Kidney, cortex; dog. Interstitial nephritis. There are extensive lymphoplasmacytic infiltrates in the cortical interstitium due to leptospirosis. Note the normal glomerulus. H & E stain.

of interstitial nephritis are less severe and composed of more discrete gray areas in the cortex and sometimes outer medulla.

Microscopically, aggregates of lymphocytes, plasma cells, and monocytes and a few neutrophils are randomly scattered or intensely localized throughout the edematous interstitium (Figs. 5-41 to 5-42). Tubular epithelial cells

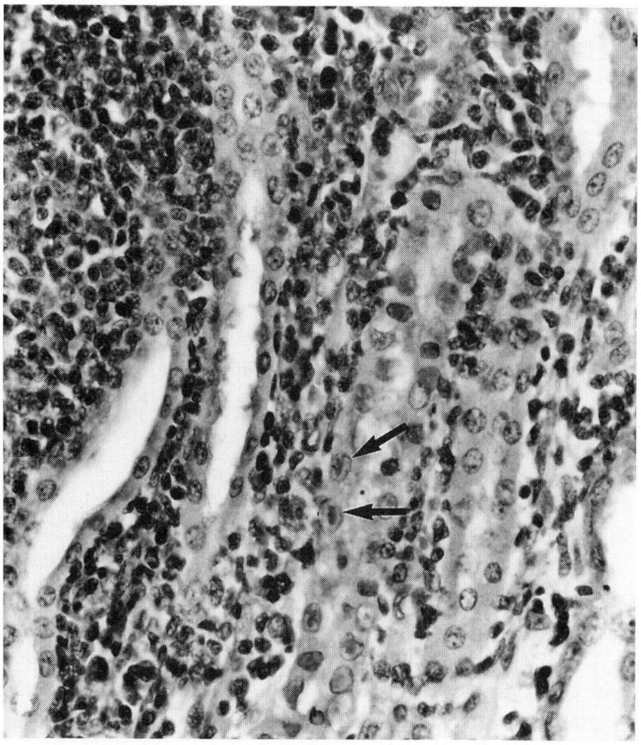

Figure 5-42 Kidney; medulla; dog. Interstitial nephritis. Lesion is typical for the convalescent phase of infectious canine hepatitis. There is an intense lymphoplasmacytic interstitial infiltrate. Renal tubular epithelial cells contain intranuclear inclusion bodies *(arrows)*. H & E stain.

within severely inflamed areas can be degenerate, necrotic, or both.

Granulomatous Nephritis

Granulomatous nephritis is a tubulointerstitial disease that often accompanies chronic systemic diseases that are characterized by multiple granulomas in various organs. In domestic animals, granulomatous nephritis has been associated with a variety of infectious agents including viruses, bacteria, fungi, and parasites. Common to each, however, is the formation of grossly visible granulomas randomly scattered throughout the kidneys, but especially in the cortex.

Cats with **feline infectious peritonitis,** particularly the noneffusive (dry) form, often have multifocal pyogranulomatous nephritis, characterized grossly by multiple, large, irregular, pale gray cortical foci that are firm and granular on cut surface (Fig. 5-43). These lesions are somewhat circumscribed and bulge from the capsular surface. They may be misinterpreted as neoplastic infiltrates such as those associated with renal lymphosarcoma. Microscopically, extensive accumulations of macrophages are interspersed with lymphocytes, plasma cells, and neutrophils (pyogranulomas). The pathogenesis of this lesion is thought to be related to a cell-mediated hypersensitivity (type IV) reaction to feline infectious peritonitis virus. The

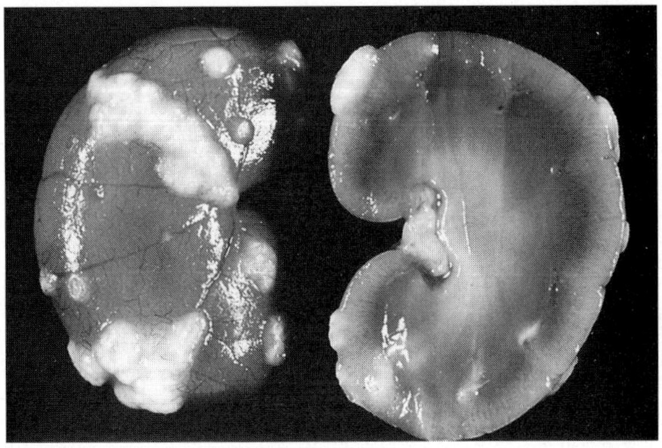

Figure 5-43 Kidney; cat. Granulomatous nephritis. Lesions are typical for the noneffusive dry form of feline infectious peritonitis. There are multifocal, coalescing granulomas that extend into the cortical parenchyma. *Courtesy Dr. D.Y. Cho.*

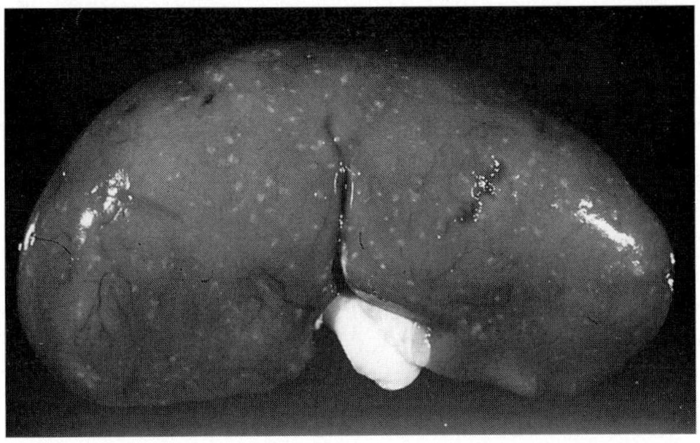

Figure 5-44 Kidney; dog. Granulomatous nephritis. Widespread multifocal, small, discrete granulomatous foci in the renal cortex are due to extensive ascarid larval migration.

immune response causes a granulomatous necrotizing vasculitis and development of pyogranulomas.

Lymphoplasmacytic to granulomatous nephritis occurs in puppies with systemic *Encephalitozoon cuniculi* infection. Microscopically, multifocal interstitial aggregates of lymphocytes, plasma cells, and macrophages are present in the cortex and medulla. Cats with inherited hyperlipoproteinemia have xanthogranulomas in various organs including the kidneys. These lesions are characterized by foamy, lipid-laden macrophages, lymphocytes, plasma cells, and fibrosis interspersed with cleftlike spaces typical of cholesterol deposits (cholesterol clefts). We have observed similar renal xanthogranulomas in dogs with hypothyroidism and severe atherosclerosis.

Granulomatous nephritis is also caused by a variety of granuloma-inducing infectious agents including fungi such as *Aspergillus* sp., Phycomycetes, or *Histoplasma capsulatum;* algae such as *Prototheca* sp.; and higher bacteria such as *Mycobacterium* sp. *Mycobacterium tuberculosis*

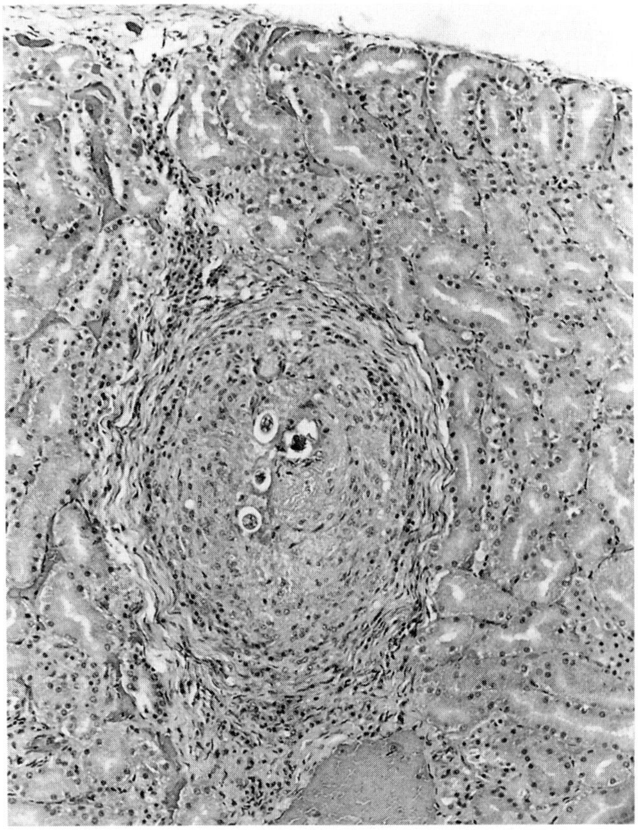

Figure 5-45 Kidney; cortex; dog. Granulomatous nephritis. A mature granuloma contains ascarid larvae. The center contains epithelioid cells and is surrounded by concentrically arranged fibrous connective tissue and inflammatory cells. H & E stain.

can cause granulomatous nephritis, particularly in cattle. Small, gray-white, granulomatous foci (2 to 5 mm) can be scattered randomly throughout the kidneys of animals with generalized miliary tuberculosis. A coarse nodular form of renal tuberculosis also occurs. Kidneys are permeated with large granulomas that can be up to 10 cm in diameter. These foci are white to tan, dry, granular, and can have calcified, caseous centers. Microscopically, lesions are characterized by central foci of necrosis surrounded by epithelioid macrophages and giant cells that contain acid-fast bacteria.

Migratory *Toxocara canis* larvae can induce small, gray to white granulomas (2 to 3 mm) randomly scattered throughout the subcapsular renal cortex of dogs (Fig. 5-44). Such lesions probably are due to cell-mediated immune responses to the migrating larvae and are composed of aggregates of macrophages, lymphocytes, and eosinophils surrounded by fibroblasts within concentrically arranged fibrous connective tissue (Fig. 5-45). In recently acquired lesions, nematode larvae can often be seen in the center of these lesions. Following death, the larvae become fragmented and the debris is phagocytized and eliminated. Lesions heal by fibrosis, leaving a few finely pitted (contracted) foci on the capsular surface.

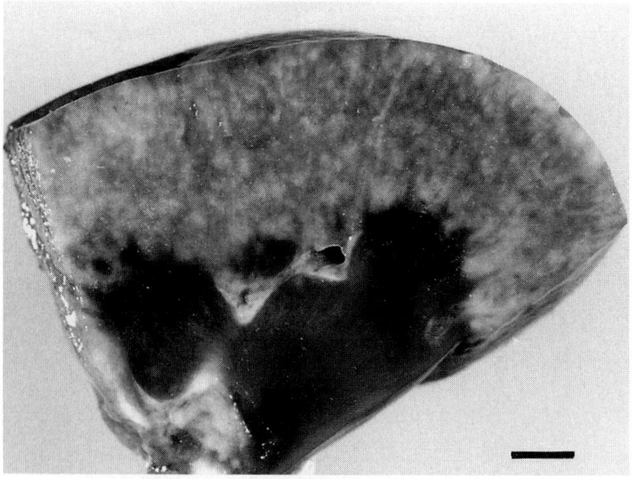

Figure 5-46 Kidney; cow. Granulomatous nephritis. Cortical striations are obliterated by coalescing granulomatous foci associated with hairy vetch toxicosis. Bar = 1 cm.

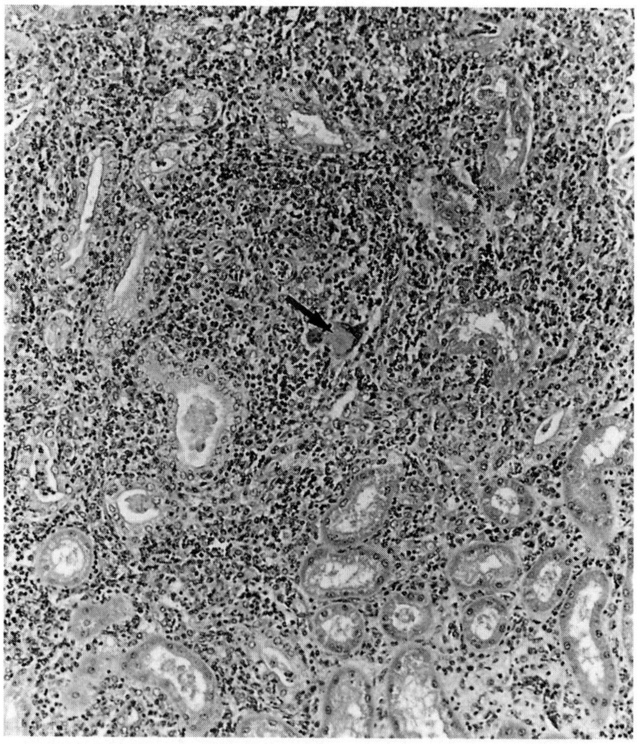

Figure 5-47 Kidney; cortex; cow. Granulomatous nephritis. Lesions associated with hairy vetch toxicosis are characterized by a mixed inflammatory cell infiltrate with renal tubular atrophy and replacement. Note the multinucleated giant cell *(arrow)*. H & E stain.

In cattle, granulomatous nephritis is part of the multisystemic granulomatous disease associated with hairy vetch *(Vicia villosa)* toxicosis. Lesions are characterized by multifocal and coalescing infiltrates of monocytes, lymphocytes, plasma cells, eosinophils, and multinucleated giant cells primarily within the renal cortex (Figs. 5-46 and 5-47).

Pyelonephritis

While **pyelitis** refers to inflammation of the renal pelvis, **pyelonephritis** is inflammation of both the renal pelvis and renal parenchyma and is an excellent example of suppurative tubulointerstitial disease. Each disease usually originates as an extension of a bacterial infection affecting the lower urinary tract (see Lower Urinary Tract) that ascends the ureters to the kidneys and establishes an infection in the pelvis and inner medulla. Rarely, pyelonephritis can result from descending bacterial infections, wherein bacterial infection of the kidneys occurred via the hematogenous route, i.e., embolic nephritis. Ascending infection, however, is by far the most common cause of pyelonephritis. Although cattle do not anatomically have a true renal pelvis, tradition holds that inflammation of the proximal ureter and renal pelvis in cattle is likewise called pyelonephritis.

The pathogenesis of ascending pyelonephritis depends on the abnormal reflux of bacteria-contaminated urine from the lower tract to the renal pelvis and collecting ducts **(vesicoureteral reflux).** Normally, little vesicoureteral reflux occurs during micturition. Vesicoureteral reflux occurs more readily when pressure is increased within the urinary bladder as with urethral obstruction. In addition to physical causes that enhance vesicoureteral reflux, bacterial infection of the lower urinary tract can enhance vesicoureteral reflux by several other mechanisms. When the bladder wall is inflamed (cystitis), the normal competency of the vesicoureteral valve can be compromised, allowing greater freedom for urine to reflux. Cystitis and urethritis, associated with narrowing of the urethra or obstruction by urinary calculi or bladder neoplasms, can increase intracystic pressure and enhanced reflux. Endotoxin liberated from gram-negative bacteria infecting the ureter and bladder can inhibit normal ureteral peristalsis, increasing reflux.

Bacteria that colonize the pelvis can readily infect the inner medulla. The medulla is highly susceptible to bacterial infection because of its poor blood supply (see Papillary Necrosis), its great interstitial osmolality that inhibits neutrophil function, and its large ammonia concentration that inhibits complement activation. Thus, bacteria can randomly infect and ascend collecting ducts, cause tubular epithelial necrosis and hemorrhage, and incite an inflammatory response. Bacterial infection can progressively ascend within tubules and the interstitium until the inflammatory lesions (tubulointerstitial inflammation) extend from pelvis to capsule.

Because most occurrences of pyelonephritis are ascending infections and because females are more susceptible to

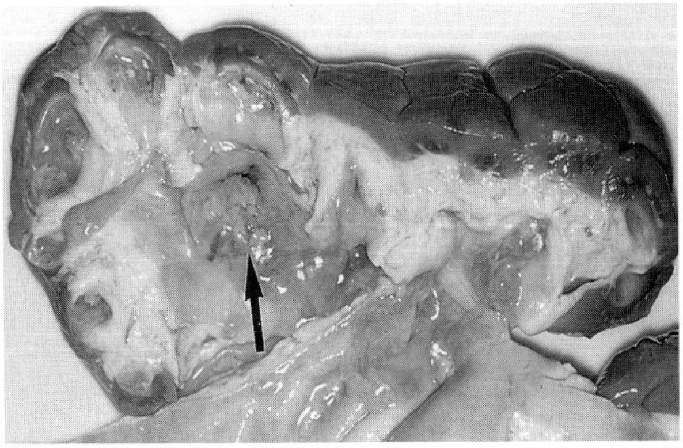

Figure 5-48 Kidney; cow. Pyelonephritis. There are ureteral and pelvic dilatation, pelvic exudate *(arrow)*, and cortical and medullary atrophy.

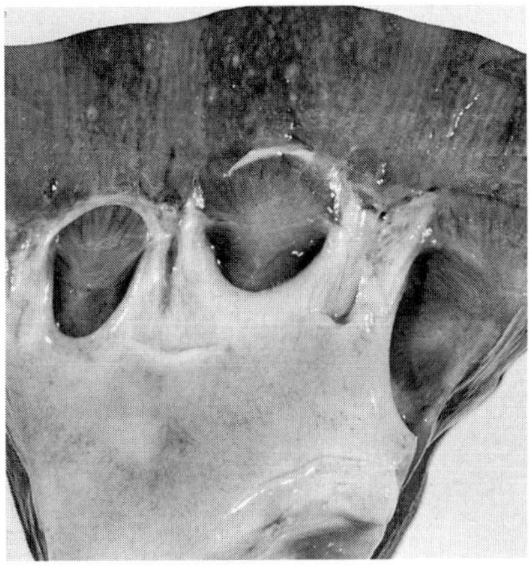

Figure 5-49 Kidney; sow. Pyelonephritis. The pelvic mucosa is hyperemic, the calyces are dilated, the papillae are attenuated, and there are radiating zone of hyperemia and purulent foci in the cortex.

lower urinary tract infections, pyelonephritis occurs more frequently in females than males. *E. coli,* especially uropathogenic strains that produce virulence factors such as α-hemolysin, adhesions, and P fimbria, is one of the most common causes of lower urinary tract disease and pyelonephritis. *Proteus* sp., *Klebsiella* sp., *Staphylococcus* sp., *Streptococcus* sp., and *Pseudomonas aeruginosa* are also common causes of lower urinary tract infection and pyelonephritis in all species. *Corynebacterium renale* and *Eubacterium (Corynebacterium) suis* are specifically pathogenic for the lower urinary tract of cattle and pigs, respectively, and are common causes of pyelonephritis.

A gross diagnosis of pyelonephritis is accomplished by recognizing the existence of acute or chronic pyelitis and the associated inflammation of the renal parenchyma. Pyelonephritis can be unilateral, but it is often bilateral. The pelvic and ureteral mucous membranes can be acutely inflamed, thickened, reddened, roughened or granular, and coated with a thin exudate. The pelvis and ureters can be markedly dilated and have purulent exudate in lumina (Fig. 5-48). The medullary crest (papilla) is often ulcerated and necrotic. Renal involvement is marked by irregular, radially oriented, red or gray streaks involving the medulla, extending toward and often reaching the renal surface (Fig. 5-49). The distribution of lesions in the kidneys is somewhat unique because often patches of inflammation distributed over the renal capsular and cut surfaces are separated from each other by areas of normal renal parenchyma (Fig. 5-50). Inflammation is often most severe at the renal poles. The renal lesions of chronic pyelonephritis, in which an active bacterial infection exists, include most of the elements of acute inflammation described above, as well as extensive necrosis with destruction of the medulla and fibrosis with scarring in a patchy distribution of the outer medulla and cortex. Occasionally, inflammation extends through the surface of the kidneys to produce extensive subcapsular inflammation and localized peritonitis.

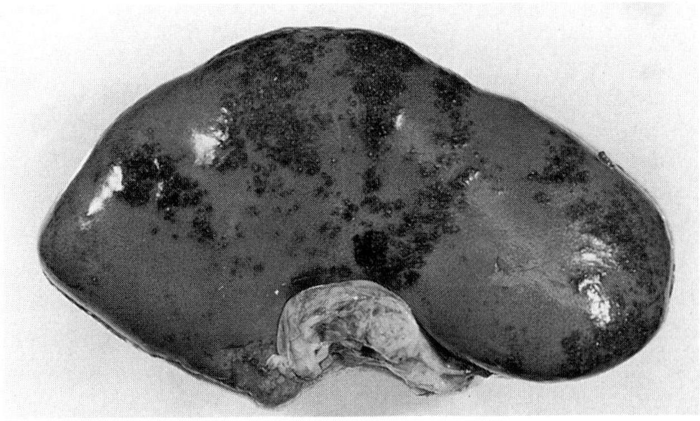

Figure 5-50 Kidney; sow. Pyelonephritis. There are irregularly distributed patches of hyperemia and purulent foci in the subcapsular cortex. The irregular and patchy distribution is a frequent feature of ascending pyelonephritis.

Microscopically, the most severe lesions of pyelonephritis are usually in the inner medulla. The transitional epithelium is usually focally or diffusely necrotic and desquamated. Necrotic debris, fibrin, neutrophils, and bacterial colonies can be adherent to the denuded surface. Medullary tubules are markedly dilated, and their lumina contain neutrophils and bacterial colonies (Fig. 5-51). Focally, the tubular epithelium is necrotic. An intense neutrophilic infiltrate, present in the renal interstitium, can be accompanied by marked interstitial hemorrhages and edema. If obstruction of vasa recta has occurred, coagulative necrosis of the inner medulla (papillary necrosis) can be severe. Similar tubular and interstitial lesions, although less severe, extend radially into the cortical tubules and interstitium. When the lesions become subacute, the severity of the neutrophilic infiltrates

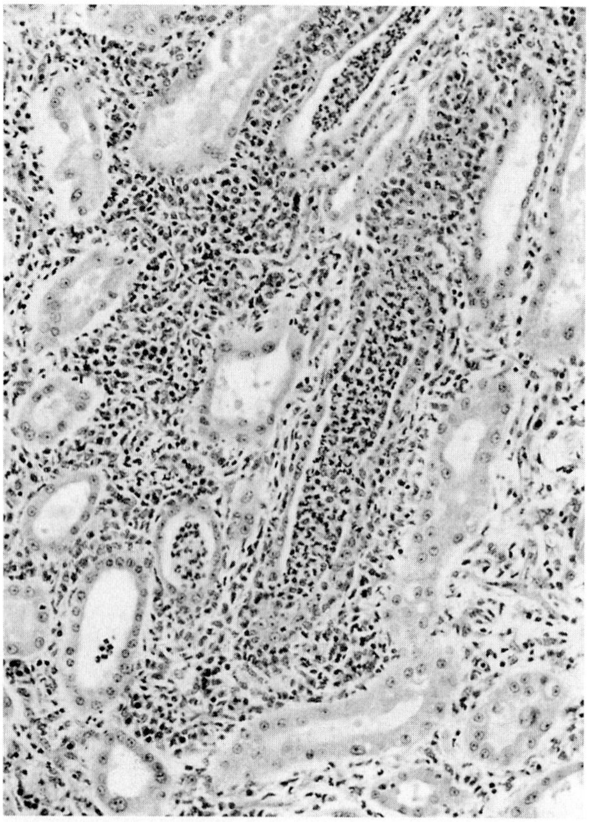

Figure 5-51 Kidney; cow. Pyelonephritis. There is both intratubular and interstitial inflammation. Tubules contain dense neutrophil aggregates. H & E stain.

diminishes and lymphocytes, plasma cells, and monocytes infiltrate the interstitium. Chronic lesions have severe fibrosis (see Renal Fibrosis). If active bacterial infection persists, an intense infiltrate of all inflammatory cell types interspersed with tubular necrosis and fibrosis can be seen.

Hydronephrosis

Hydronephrosis refers to dilatation of the renal pelvis due to obstruction of urine outflow and is associated with increased pelvic pressure, dilatation of the pelvis, and progressive renal parenchymal atrophy. Hydronephrosis occurs in all domestic animals. Obstruction leading to hydronephrosis can occasionally be caused by congenital malformation of the ureter, vesicoureteral junction, or urethra, but the more common causes of hydronephrosis are ureteral or urethral blockage due to urinary tract calculi (see Lower Urinary Tract), chronic inflammation, or neoplasia of the ureter or bladder. Congenitally malpositioned kidneys can result in a kinking of the ureter and obstruction causing hydronephrosis. Hydronephrosis can be unilateral or bilateral. When hydronephrosis is unilateral, cystic enlargement of the kidney can become extensive before the lesion is recognized. If the obstructive process causes partial or intermittent blockage, bilateral

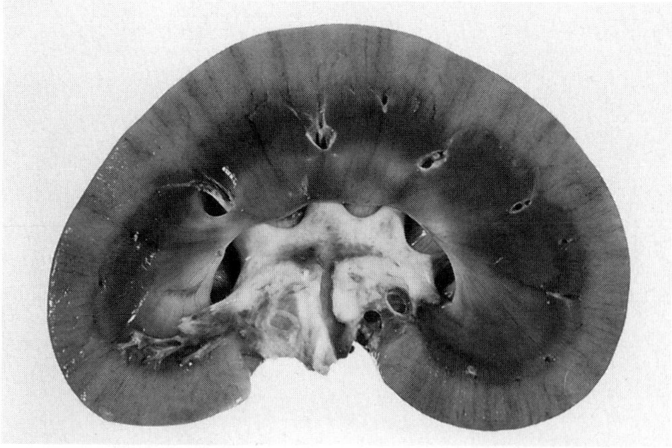

Figure 5-52 Kidney; sheep. Hydronephrosis. Both the pelvis and calyces are dilated, typical of early hydronephrosis.

hydronephrosis can become marked because of continual urine production and pooling of urine in the expanding pelvis. When obstruction is complete, hydronephrosis is limited in development (see below). When the increase in pelvic pressure is substantial and sustained, intratubular pressure is increased and glomerular filtration is markedly reduced; however, even with complete obstruction, glomerular filtrate does not stop completely because of continual reabsorption of the filtrate into the interstitium and lymphatic vessels. When the obstructive lesion is bilateral and complete, death due to uremia occurs before cystic enlargement becomes extensive.

The increased intratubular pressure following ureteral obstruction results in renal tubular dilatation. Glomeruli remain functional, but much of the glomerular filtrate diffuses into the interstitium where it is initially removed via lymphatic vessels and veins. As intrapelvic pressure increases, the interstitial vessels collapse and renal blood flow is reduced, resulting in hypoxia, tubular atrophy due to apoptosis, and, if the pressure increase is continued, interstitial fibrosis. The glomeruli have a relatively normal morphologic appearance for a prolonged period, but eventually become atrophic and sclerotic.

Early changes of hydronephrosis include dilatation of the pelvis and calyces and blunting of the renal crest and papillae (Fig. 5-52). When pelvic dilation is progressive, the kidney silhouette is enlarged and rounder than normal, and the cortex and medulla are progressively thinned (Fig. 5-53). Interstitial vascular obstruction results in cortical ischemia, sometimes infarction, and necrosis. In its most advanced form, the hydronephrotic kidney is a thin-walled (2 to 3 mm thick), fluid-filled sac. The continued pelvic dilation causes loss of tubules by degeneration and atrophy, followed by condensation of interstitial connective tissue and fibrosis of the renal parenchyma. This sac is lined by flattened transitional epithelium, which is spared during lesion development.

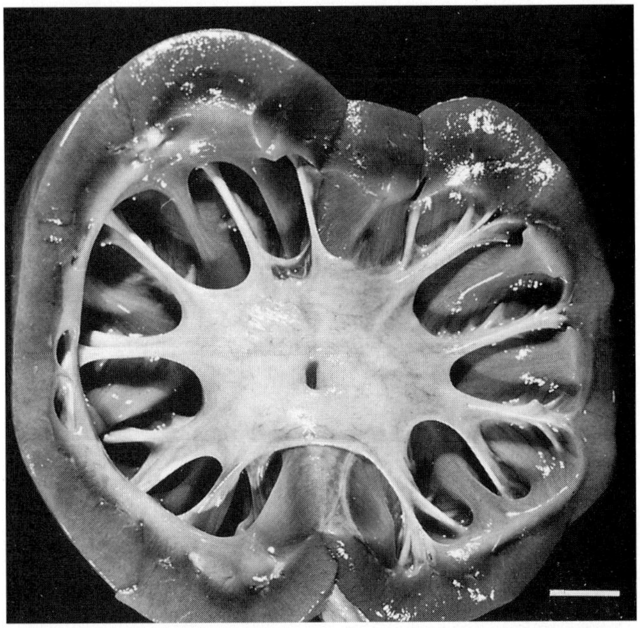

Figure 5-53 Kidney; dog. Hydronephrosis. Advanced hydronephrosis is characterized by marked pelvic and calyceal dilatation and medullary atrophy. The ureter is dilated also. Bar = 1 cm.

Occasionally, a severely hydronephrotic kidney becomes contaminated by bacteria and the thin-walled sac becomes filled with pus instead of urine. This lesion, referred to as **pyonephrosis,** is likely the result of blood-borne bacteria lodging in a hydronephrotic kidney.

Chronic Renal Diseases

Renal Fibrosis (Scarring)

Renal fibrosis can occur as a primary event, but more frequently is a chronic manifestation of the healing phase of a preexisting renal lesion. Renal fibrosis follows many renal lesions including primary inflammation of glomeruli, tubules, or interstitial tissue and degeneration or necrosis of renal tubules. The severity of renal fibrosis usually parallels the intensity of the primary renal disease. The mechanisms by which fibrosis is induced are related to destruction and loss of nephron components by the inflammatory process and the initiation of the healing process. Noninflammatory mechanisms can also incite renal fibrosis. Recent experimental studies have demonstrated that after severe nephrotoxin-induced tubular epithelial cell injury, the remaining cells undergo accelerated apoptosis resulting in tubular atrophy. Interstitial fibroblast proliferation and fibrosis follow the acute process. Sustained proteinuria can also increase tubular epithelial cell apoptosis, leading to tubular atrophy and interstitial fibrosis.

Renal fibrosis and chronic renal disease are the most frequently recognized renal pathologic processes in mature or aging domestic animals, particularly dogs and cats. When renal fibrosis and loss of nephrons are severe, these lesions can be manifested clinically as chronic renal failure and uremia. One of the most common expressions of this chronic disease is the inability of an animal to concentrate urine resulting in frequent urination **(polyuria)** of a dilute urine **(isosthenuria).** Polyuria is accompanied by dehydration and excessive water drinking **(polydipsia).** Hypoplastic anemia occurs as a result of the kidneys' failure to synthesize and secrete erythropoietin. Fibrous osteodystrophy can develop because of abnormal calcium-phosphorus metabolism and renal secondary hyperparathyroidism.

In areas of renal fibrosis, the loss of renal parenchyma includes tubules, glomeruli, and vessels and their replacement by fibrous connective tissue. Therefore, fibrotic kidneys are pale tan to white, shrunken, and firm; excessive adhesions of the capsule to the underlying cortex cause difficulty in removing the capsule from the kidneys. Without careful attention to the pattern of fibrosis, such kidneys can be indiscriminately termed as **chronic interstitial nephritis, end-stage kidney,** or **nephrosclerosis.** However, fibrosis generally follows a pattern characteristic of the antecedent lesion. Fibrosis can be diffuse and finely stippled with pinpoint dimpling and granularity on the capsular surface. In contrast, fibrosis can be coarser as deep and irregularly shaped depressions of the capsular surface in either a diffuse, multifocal, or patchy distribution. In addition to these changes of the capsular surface, the cut surface of the cortex is thinned beneath the capsular surface depressions. In addition, these fibrotic areas are pale tan when compared with more normal parenchyma.

Diffuse fibrosis can be initiated by circulatory disturbances because the blood flow through glomerular capillaries is reduced in chronic glomerulonephritides and amyloidosis. Because most of these primary glomerular lesions involve glomeruli that are diffusely scattered throughout the renal cortex, the distribution of fibrosis secondary to glomerular disease is diffuse and primarily cortical. The capsular surface is stippled or finely granular. Because all components of the nephron are interdependent, glomerular fibrosis and loss of function ultimately results in secondary atrophy of cortical and medullary tubules and fibrosis of the adjoining interstitium.

Diffuse fibrosis with a finely granular pattern can also occur subsequent to widespread necrosis of renal tubular epithelium (acute tubular necrosis) (Fig. 5-54). An example is oak poisoning of cattle, in which severe tubular necrosis also includes the renal tubular basement membrane, resulting in leakage of tubular contents. The loss of the continuity of the basement membrane prevents tubular epithelial cell regeneration. This outcome can be followed by interstitial fibrosis.

Different coarser patterns of renal fibrosis occur when the primary lesion is less evenly distributed in the kidneys. Fibrosis secondary to the tubulointerstitial inflammation of

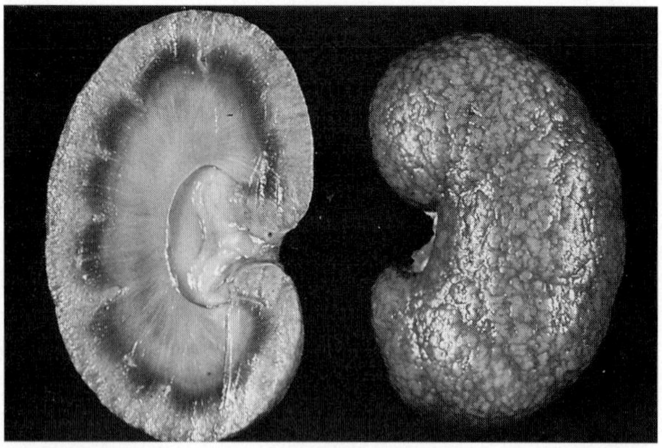

Figure 5-54 Kidney; dog. Fibrosis. Diffuse interstitial fibrosis is present as a finely stippled pattern characterized by fine pitting on the surface and a thin, granular cortex on cut surface. *Courtesy Dr. D.Y. Cho.*

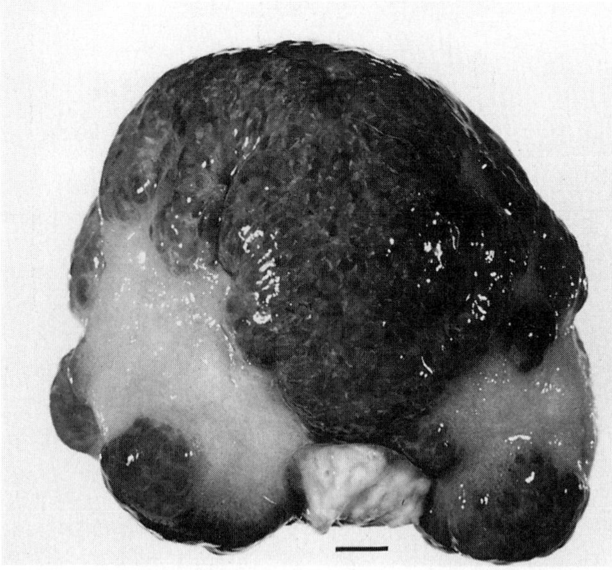

Figure 5-55 Kidney; dog. Fibrosis. There are large patches of advanced cortical scarring at the poles and a finely stippled pattern of fibrosis in the remaining kidney. This pattern suggests previous pyelonephritis. Bar = 1 cm.

pyelonephritis follows the pattern of the acute disease and results in irregularly distributed, patchy scarring that is often deeply depressed on the renal capsular surface and forms linear areas extending through both the cortex and medulla to the pelvis (Fig. 5-55). Like the distribution of the acute lesion, scarring in pyelonephritis can be severe at the poles of the kidneys. The scarring that follows embolic or thrombotic vascular obstruction and infarction is related to the size of the ischemic area caused by vascular compromise (Fig. 5-56).

Ischemia resulting from obstruction of relatively large arterioles causes large areas of coagulative necrosis. Healing results in large, deeply depressed scars that involve primarily the cortex, but can extend into the medulla. Obstruction of smaller arterioles results in small areas of coagulative necrosis that heal as small-diameter pits in the renal surface with an accompanying pale white, linear scar on the cut surface. A coarser pattern of diffuse renal fibrosis occurs in chronic interstitial nephritis and certain progressive juvenile nephropathies of dogs. Both cortex and medulla can be fibrotic, cortical striations are severely distorted or effaced, and the formation of multiple cortical cysts is common.

Microscopically, renal fibrosis is characterized by an increase in interstitial connective tissue and atrophy and disappearance of adjacent renal tubules. Remaining tubules are usually atrophic and have a reduced luminal diameter or can be ectatic, a thickened hyalinized basement membrane, and are lined by flattened epithelium. Even in fibrotic lesions that did not arise from an infectious disease or inflammatory mechanism, foci of

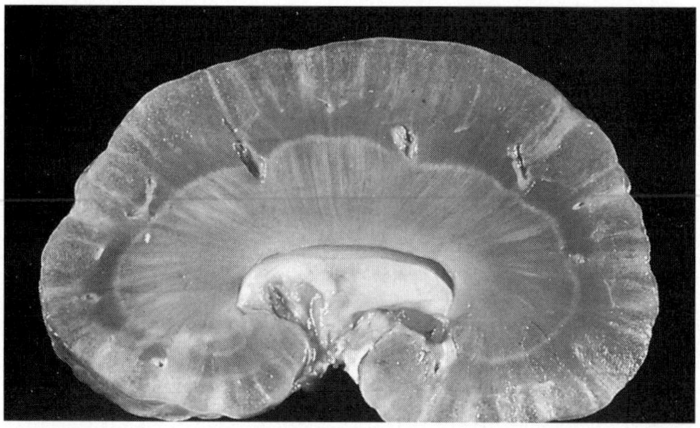

Figure 5-56 Kidney; dog. Fibrosis. There are multiple radial-oriented scars randomly involving the renal cortex, a pattern that suggests previous vascular obstruction.

lymphocytes and plasma cells can be seen randomly scattered throughout the interstitium. The common finding of infiltrating lymphocytes and plasma cells in cases of renal fibrosis has given rise to the often used term, chronic interstitial nephritis (Fig. 5-57). Multiple acquired cysts can be present throughout the cortex and medulla and are lined by flattened epithelial cells. These cysts can be due to either dilated Bowman's capsules and associated atrophic glomerular tufts or to dilated, sequestered, or blocked tubular segments that have become isolated by connective tissue (Fig. 5-58). Glomerulosclerosis is common, particularly in areas of severe interstitial fibrosis. Calcification of vessels, tubular basement membranes, Bowman's

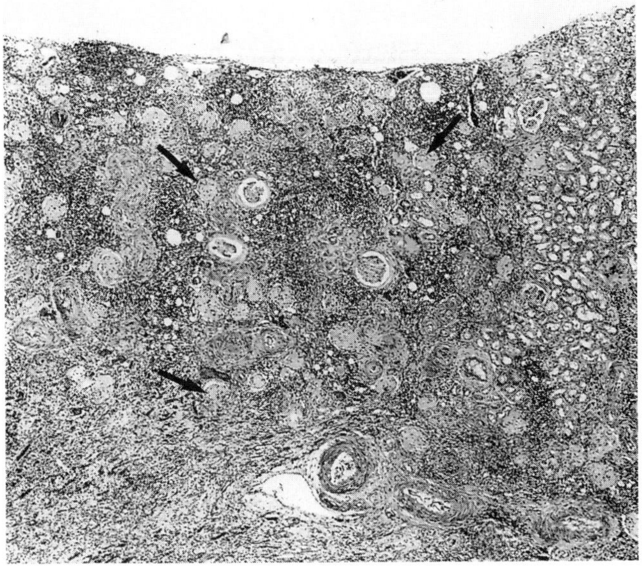

Figure 5-57 Kidney; cortex; dog. Fibrosis. Chronic interstitial nephritis. The lesion is characterized by interstitial fibrosis, tubular atrophy, and interstitial inflammatory cell infiltration. Note the depressed capsular surface due to scarring and the shrunken sclerotic glomeruli *(arrows)*. H & E stain.

capsules, and degenerate tubular epithelium is common in fibrotic kidneys due to alterations in calcium-phosphorus metabolism associated with chronic renal failure.

Progressive Juvenile Nephropathy

The development of severe bilateral renal fibrosis has been described in young dogs of several breeds and referred to as progressive juvenile nephropathy or familial (hereditary) renal disease (Box 5-4). In many dogs a familial tendency is demonstrated, but the mode of inheritance has been determined with certainty in only a few dog breeds. In Samoyeds the lesion is sex-linked; in bull terriers it is autosomal dominant; and in the shih tzu the disease appears to have a simple autosomal recessive inheritance. Although variations exist in microscopic and gross lesions, as well as in the pathogenesis of progressive nephropathy among the different breeds, a typical case is a dog 4 months to 2 years of age that presents with polyuria, polydipsia, and uremia. The clinical presentation and gross lesions are identical to those of chronic renal disease and renal fibrosis in mature or aging dogs.

In the Doberman pinscher, the primary lesion is a glomerulopathy that appears microscopically as a membranoproliferative glomerulonephritis. Later in the clinical course of the disease, the lesions are extensive periglomerular fibrosis, tubular atrophy, and cystic dilatation of Bowman's (uriniferous) space and tubules. In affected Samoyeds and English cocker spaniels, multilamellar splitting of the glomerular basement membrane is due to abnormalities in basement membrane collagen. These

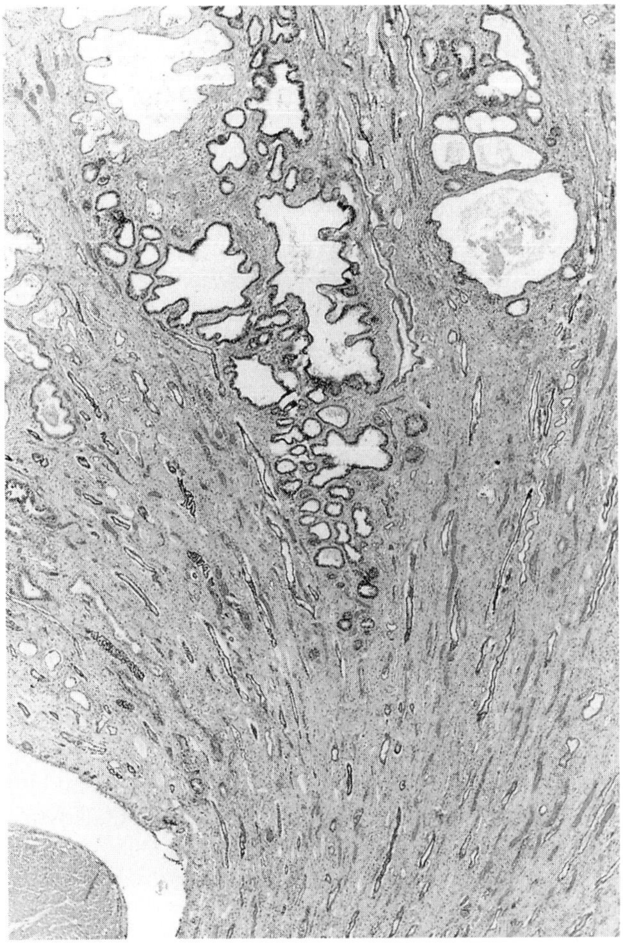

Figure 5-58 Kidney; dog. Multiple acquired cysts. Note the renal interstitial fibrosis with dilated tubules and acquired renal cysts. H & E stain.

BOX 5-4 BREEDS OF DOGS WITH PROGRESSIVE JUVENILE NEPHROPATHY

American cocker spaniels	Standard poodles
English cocker spaniels	Alaskan malmutes
Norwegian elkhounds	Miniature schnauzers
Samoyeds	German shepherds
Doberman pinschers	Keeshounds
Lhaso apsos	Chow chows
Shih tzus	Weimeraners
Soft-coated Wheaten terriers	Golden retrievers
Bull terriers	

lesions progress to severe glomerulosclerosis. In Norwegian elkhounds a tubular disorder of unknown cause has been described and is characterized by progressively tubular atrophy, periglomerular and interstitial fibrosis, and glomerulosclerosis without any indication of a primary glomerular disease. Renal disease has been described in Lhaso apsos, shih tzus, Wheaten terriers, standard poodles, and golden retrievers as a condition resembling renal dysplasia has been reported. Small, shrunken, fetal-like glomeruli composed of small cells with dense nuclei, minimal mesangial tissue, and non-patent capillaries can be seen interspersed with normal, sclerotic, or compensatorily hypertrophied glomeruli. Other lesions include marked interstitial fibrosis and tubular dilatation. Most of the kidneys have minimal inflammatory cell infiltrates. Thus, progressive juvenile nephropathy is a syndrome, the morphologic manifestations of which can be the results of any of several chronic pathologic processes.

Gross renal lesions of progressive juvenile nephropathy are variable among affected breeds and among affected dogs within a breed. Generally, kidneys are markedly shrunken, pale tan to white, and firm. The renal surface can be diffusely pitted and have a fine granular pattern, particularly in those dogs in which glomerular disease is the primary event. In these cases of juvenile nephropathy that are of tubular origin or dysplastic, the renal surface can have patchy, deeply depressed areas of cortical scarring. On the cut surface, the cortex is thin and has linear scars. The medulla is usually diffusely fibrotic. Small (1 to 2 mm), variably sized cysts are seen often in the cortex and the medulla.

Recently, a progressive juvenile nephropathy, similar to that seen in dogs, was described in six young Japanese black cattle. The cattle had a common male ancestor, suggesting a familial basis.

Neoplasia

The prevalence of primary renal neoplasms in domestic animals is less than 1% of the total neoplasms reported. They are usually unilateral and can be of epithelial, mesenchymal, or embryonal origin.

Epithelial Tumors

Renal adenomas are rare. They are incidental findings at necropsy and usually appear as a small, white to yellow, solitary, well-circumscribed mass in the cortex. Microscopically, adenomas are composed of solid sheets, tubules, or papillary proliferations of cuboidal epithelial cells that are uniform in size and have granular eosinophilic cytoplasm and small, round to oval nuclei. Mitotic figures, necrosis, and fibrosis are rare.

Renal carcinomas are the most common primary renal neoplasms and occur most frequently in older dogs. The neoplasms are usually large (up to 20 cm in diameter), spherical to oval, and firm. They often are pale yellow, contain dark areas of hemorrhage and necrosis, and foci of cystic degeneration. The masses usually occupy and obliterate one pole of the kidney and grow by expansion, compressing the adjacent normal renal tissue (Fig. 5-59). Metastasis to the lungs occurs frequently. In German shepherd dogs, a variant of the typical renal carcinoma has been seen in conjunction with nodular dermatofibrosis. The lesions are hereditary and consist of multifocal, bilateral, renal cystadenocarcinomas. As in adenomas, neoplastic cells form solid sheets, tubules, or papillary growth patterns, but the cells in carcinomas are more atypical and anaplastic. Cells vary in shape from cuboidal, columnar, to polyhedral, vary in size, and have clear or granular eosinophilic cytoplasm. Nuclei range from small, round, granular, and uniform to large, oval, vesicular, and pleomorphic. Mitotic figures are numerous. These neoplasms have a moderate fibrovascular stroma.

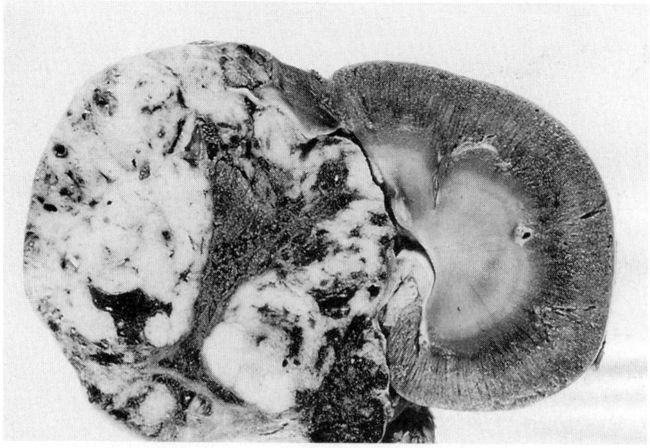

Figure 5-59 Kidney; dog. Renal carcinoma. The neoplasm has infiltrated and replaced one half of the kidney. *Lucke VM, Kelly DF, Vet Pathol 13: 265-276, 1976.*

Transitional cell papillomas and **transitional cell carcinomas** arise in the renal pelvis and lower urinary tract and, when large, can obstruct urinary outflow. Such carcinomas can invade into the kidney. The morphologic features of transitional cell neoplasms will be discussed later with the urinary bladder (see The Lower Urinary Tract).

Mesenchymal and Metastatic Tumors

Occasionally, **fibromas, fibrosarcomas,** or **hemangiosarcomas** originate in the kidneys. Carcinomas and sarcomas **(metastatic tumors)** arising in other organs can metastasize to the kidneys and are characteristically composed of randomly scattered multiple nodules, usually involving both kidneys (Fig. 5-60). Renal lymphosarcoma occurs with some frequency in cattle and cats, particularly as part of generalized or multicentric lymphosarcoma. They appear as single or multiple homogeneous gray-white nodules or as diffuse lymphomatous infiltrates that cause uniform enlargement and pale discoloration of the kidney. Renal lymphosarcoma must be differentiated from the renal granulomas of feline infectious peritonitis by histopathologic examination.

Tumors of Embryonal Origin

Nephroblastomas (embryonal nephroma, Wilms' tumor) are common renal neoplasms of pigs and chickens in which they are usually recognized at slaughter. They occur

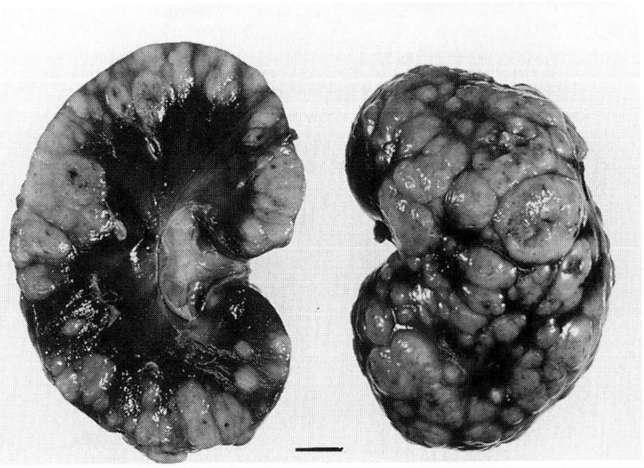

Figure 5-60 Kidney; dog. Metastatic mast cell tumors. Multiple pale, neoplastic nodules are randomly scattered throughout the kidneys. Bar = 1 cm.

in cattle and dogs as well, but less frequently. These neoplasms are of embryonal origin, arise from metanephric blastema, and, thus, occur in young animals. It is speculated that neoplasms result from malignant transformation during normal nephrogenesis or from neoplastic transformation of nests of embryonic tissue that persist in the postnatal kidneys. At necropsy, nephroblastomas can be solitary or multiple masses that often reach a great size and in which recognizable renal tissue can be difficult to detect. They usually are soft to rubbery and gray with foci of hemorrhage. On cut surface they are often lobulated. Because nephroblastomas arise from primitive pluripotential tissue, histologic features vary, but are morphologically similar to the developmental stages of embryonic kidneys. Characteristically, primitive, loose myxomatous mesenchymal tissue predominates. Interspersed in this tissue are primitive tubules lined by elongated, deeply staining cells and structures that resemble primitive glomeruli. Nests of cells resembling the metanephric blastema can be present. Nephroblastomas also have such mesenchymal components as cartilage, bone, skeletal muscle, and adipose tissue.

Parasites

Nematodes

The **giant kidney worm** of dogs *(Dioctophyma renale)* is seen infrequently in dogs in temperate and cold countries worldwide. It is endemic in Canada and in northern regions of the United States. Because of a prolonged and complex life cycle, this nematode is seen only in dogs 2 years old or older. The adult nematode, which can be 100 cm long, resides in the renal pelvis, where it causes severe hemorrhagic or purulent pyelitis and ureteral obstruction. The renal parenchyma can be destroyed, resulting in a kidney that forms a cyst containing the nematode and purulent exudate.

In North America, the **kidney worm** *(Stephanurus dentatus)* of pigs is found most often in adult pigs in southern regions of the United States. The parasite is also a problem in other countries with warm climates. Adult worms normally encyst in perirenal fat; however, some cysts with the nematode can be found in the kidneys. Peripelvic cysts often communicate with the renal pelvis or ureter, and fibrosis and chronic granulation tissue can enclose the parasite.

Capillaria plica and *Capillaria feliscati* have been identified infrequently in dogs and cats worldwide. Typically these nematodes are attached to the renal pelvis, ureter, or bladder of animals of various ages. Microscopic inflammatory cell infiltrates and focal hemorrhages are associated with sites of attachment.

LOWER URINARY TRACT

The lower urinary tract consists of the ureters, urinary bladder, and urethra. The renal pelvis, ureters, and urinary bladder are lined by transitional epithelium, whereas the urethra is lined by transitional epithelium cranially and stratified squamous epithelium immediately cranial to or at the urethral orifice. As in other mucous membranes, the lamina propria has small lymphoid follicles which, following inflammation or antigenic stimulation, can be large enough to be seen grossly as discrete, circular, white foci (1 to 2 mm) in the mucosa. The vesicoureteral valve, created by the oblique passage of the ureter through the wall of the urinary bladder, is an important structure as it normally prevents reflux of urine from the bladder into the ureter and renal pelvis. At death, the urinary bladder can contract to such a degree that the normal bladder wall appears thick at necropsy. The normal mucosa of the lower urinary tract should be smooth and glistening. Urine should be clear except in horses, where, because of the normal presence of mucus or fine crystals, it is cloudy.

Developmental Anomalies

Aplasia and Ectopic Ureters

Ureteral aplasia (agenesis) is rare but can occur alone or in animals with renal aplasia. **Ectopic ureters** are found most frequently in dogs; certain breeds, especially the Siberian husky, are at greater risk. The involved ureter empties into the urethra, vagina, neck of the bladder, vas deferens, prostate, or other secondary sex glands. Ectopic ureters are more subject to obstruction or infection, thus they predispose animals to pyelitis and pyelonephritis. Occasionally, anomalies of the lower urinary tract mucosa are such that transitional epithelium is focally replaced by skin or alimentary tract mucosa.

Patent Urachus

The most common malformation of the urinary bladder is **patent urachus (pervious urachus).** This lesion develops when the fetal urachus fails to close and, therefore, forms a direct channel between the bladder's apex and the umbilicus. Foals are affected most often and have dribbling of urine at the umbilicus. Affected animals have increased susceptibility to bacterial infections of the urinary bladder. Failure of the urachal remnant and the umbilical arteries and vein to involute is frequently observed in cases of "neonatal" omphalitis and can result in a patent urachus. Patent urachus has also occurred because of congenital urethral obstruction. Increased bladder pressure due to the obstruction forces urine out into the urachus.

Occasionally, during urachal closure, the mucosa closes, but closure of the bladder musculature is incomplete. When this occurs, a **bladder diverticulum** (outpouching) of the apex of the bladder can develop. Urine stasis can occur in the diverticulum, predisposing the animal to cystitis or urinary calculi.

Hydroureter and Hydrourethra

Hydroureter and hydrourethra refer to dilatation of the ureter and urethra, respectively, and are due to obstruction of urine outflow by blockage of the ureter(s) or urethra by calculi, chronic inflammation, or neoplasia. Hydroureter can be unilateral or bilateral. Depending on the location of the obstruction, hydronephrosis, hydroureter, and hydrourethra can occur concurrently (see Hydronephrosis).

Urolithiasis

Urinary calculi (uroliths) are concretions formed in the urinary tract and are usually composed of salts of inorganic or organic acids or other materials such as cystine or xanthine. Struvite (magnesium ammonium phosphate hexahydrate), oxalate, apatite, carbonate, silica, urate, cystine, xanthine, or benzocoumarin ("clover stone") calculi have been seen in domestic animals. Calculi can form in the renal pelvis, ureter, or in any portion of the lower urinary tract. Calculi vary in size and shape. Large renal pelvic calculi classically have a "staghorn" appearance because they take the shape of the renal calyces in animal species that have true calyces (Fig. 5-61). These calculi predispose affected animals to pyelitis and pyelonephritis. Urinary bladder calculi can be single or multiple, variable in size (2 mm to 10 cm), and sometimes are composed of a fine, sandlike material that causes cloudy urine. Calculi can have smooth or rough surfaces; they are solid, soft, or friable. Calculi vary in color depending on their composition; however, color is variable among calculi even of the same composition. The calculi can be white to gray (e.g., struvite and oxalate), yellow (e.g., urate, cystine, benzocoumarin, and xanthine), or brown (e.g., silica, urate, and xanthine) depending on their composition. Urolithiasis can cause urinary obstruction or traumatic injury to the urinary bladder mucosa. Lesions of the urinary bladder are manifested as difficult or painful urination **(stranguria; dysuria),** with or without hematuria.

Both males and females are subject to urolithiasis, but calculi cause urinary obstruction more commonly in males because of the narrow urethral diameter and longer urethra of males. When obstruction or dysuria occurs in females, calculi are usually large and located in the renal pelvis or urinary bladder (Fig. 5-62). In males, dysuria can result from large calculi, but urinary tract obstruction with

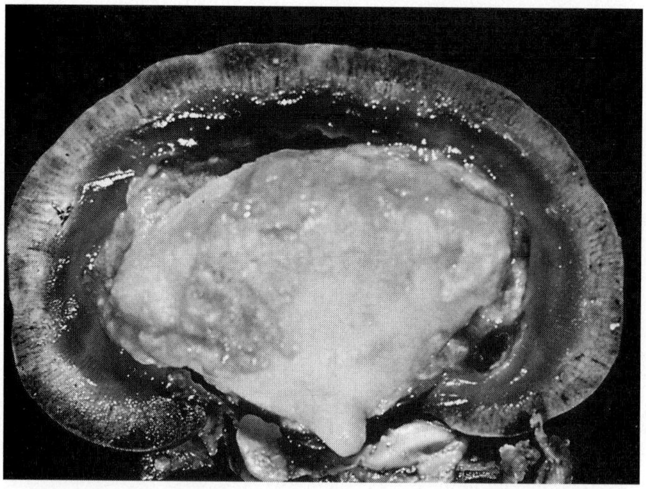

Figure 5-61 Kidney; dog. Urolithiasis. A calculus is filling and distending the renal pelvis and causing extensive erosion and attenuation of the medulla. The apex of the calculus conforms to the ureteral opening.

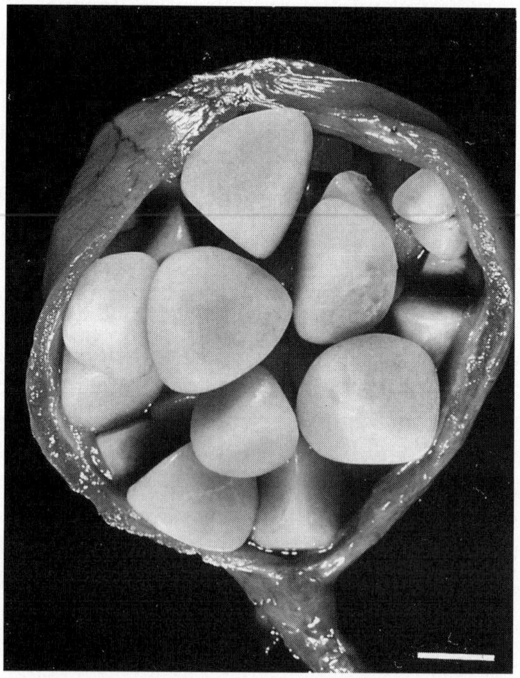

Figure 5-62 Urinary bladder; dog. Urolithiasis. Multiple smooth calculi are present in the urinary bladder. The bladder wall is diffusely thickened (scale in centimeters). Bar = 1 cm.

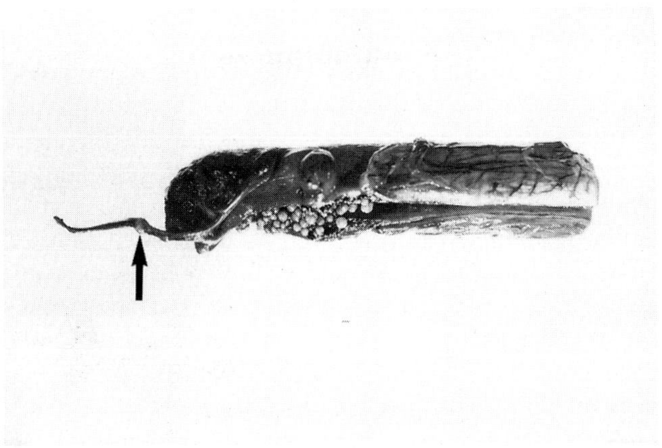

Figure 5-63 Penis; lamb. Urolithiasis. Multiple calculi are in the penile urethra and in the urethral process *(arrow).*

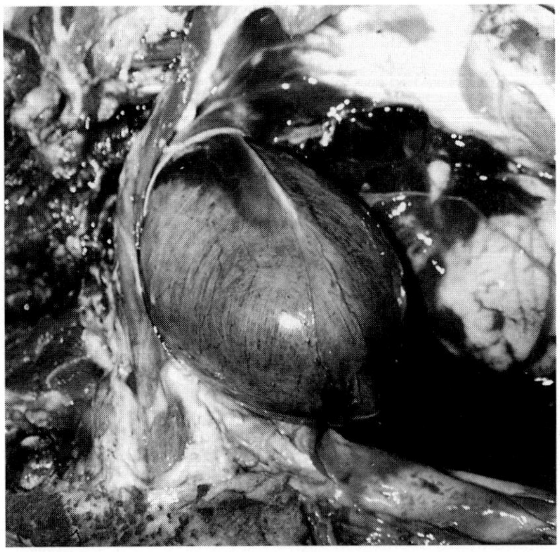

Figure 5-64 Urinary bladder; lamb. Urolithiasis. The bladder is overdistended and turgid as the result of urethral obstruction. Note hemorrhages at the neck and apex of the bladder.

uremia most commonly occurs because of obstruction of the urethra with small calculi. The most common sites of lodgment of urethral calculi vary with the animal species. In male cattle, calculi lodge in the urethra at the ischial arch and at the proximal end of the sigmoid flexure; in rams and wethers, the urethral process (vermiform appendage) is the most common site (Fig. 5-63); and in dogs, calculi lodge proximal to the base of the os penis. In cats, fine struvite crystals (sand) in a rubberlike protein matrix can fill the entire urethra and such calculi are typical for the disease called **feline urologic syndrome.** Urethral calculi are not commonly seen in horses and pigs.

Calculi form as a result of precipitation of salts in urine, usually in association with an organic (protein) matrix. A number of factors can predispose the lower urinary tract to calculus formation. Urine pH is important to the development of calculi in that some salts precipitate more readily at acid pH (oxalates) and others more readily at alkaline pH (struvite and carbonate). Bacterial infections predispose to urolithiasis (particularly struvite calculi in dogs). In one recent study, bacteria were cultured from the lower urinary tract of >60% of dogs with urolithiasis. Bacterial colonies, exfoliated epithelium, or leukocytes can serve as the nidus for the precipitation of mineral constituents. A cell-associated herpesvirus is one of several factors that predispose cats to struvite urolithiasis.

Nutritional and dietary factors have been associated with the formation of urinary calculi. In sheep, diets containing milo or sorghum products, which have large concentrations of phosphate, predispose to struvite urolithiasis. Consumption of dry commercial food rich in magnesium is another predisposing factor for feline urologic syndrome. Ingestion of oxalate-accumulating plants predisposes to oxalate urolithiasis. Vitamin A deficiency can predispose to urolithiasis by inducing squamous metaplasia of transitional epithelium, resulting in desquamated squames that can serve as a nidus for calculi formation. Dehydration, as occurs when water intake is limited, can initiate or increase calculus formation by having the mineral constituents in a supersaturated state in concentrated urine. Supersaturation can be unstable and predispose to spontaneous precipitation. Ingestion of estrogens, such as present in subterranean clover, as well as implantation or injection of estrogens can predispose sheep to so-called clover stones (benzocoumarin) or carbonate calculi.

Hereditary defects that result in urinary excretion of xanthine **(xanthinuria)** or cystine **(cystinuria)** can cause urinary calculi of the appropriate compound (see Inherited Abnormalities in Renal Tubular Function). Urate calculi form most commonly in Dalmatian dogs because of their large urinary excretion of uric acid.

At necropsy, animals that have died of urinary obstruction have greatly distended, turgid or ruptured bladders and dilated ureters and renal pelvises. The bladder wall is thin and often has streaks of or diffuse hemorrhage (Fig. 5-64). When urine is released from the bladder either because of rupture or incision at surgery or necropsy, the wall of the bladder is flaccid, the mucosa is often ulcerated, and the urine contains blood clots. Mucosal ulceration, localized lamina proprial hemorrhage, and mucosal necrosis are usually present in the ureter, bladder, or urethra adjacent to an obstructive calculus. If the bladder ruptures antemortem, blood clots and fibrin are at the site of rupture and in some cases an acute, localized chemical (urine-induced) peritonitis.

Microscopically, inflammation and hemorrhage are present in the lower urinary tract. Lesions are most severe in cases where obstruction has been complete. The mucosa is usually ulcerated, and areas of transitional epithelial cell hyperplasia are interspersed with goblet cells. The lamina propria is usually infiltrated with inflammatory cells. Neutrophils are located at foci of ulceration, and lymphocytes and plasma cells infiltrate perivascularly or uniformly throughout the lamina propria. Hemorrhage is transmural but is most evident in the mucosa and can cause separation of the smooth muscle bundles. Degeneration and necrosis of smooth muscle occurs in severe cases.

Inflammatory Diseases

Acute Cystitis

Inflammation of the urinary bladder **(cystitis)** is common in domestic animals. Because inflammation of the ureter **(ureteritis)** or urethra **(urethritis)** in the absence of cystitis are rare, this discussion concentrates on cystitis. Cystitis can result from several chemical causes. Active metabolites of cyclophosphamide, a drug used to treat neoplastic and immune-mediated diseases of dogs and cats, can cause a sterile hemorrhagic cystitis. Cantharidin toxicosis in horses results from ingestion of blister beetles (*Epicauta* sp.) in alfalfa hay, and hemorrhagic and necrotic cystitis develops as cantharidin is excreted through the urinary tract. Chronic ingestion of bracken fern *(Pteridium aquilinum)* by cattle can result in the syndrome **enzootic hematuria,** which can be manifested as acute urinary bladder hemorrhage, chronic cystitis, or urinary bladder neoplasia. In cats a cell-associated herpesvirus has been found in some cases of mild cystitis. However, for all animal species, bacterial infection of the mucosa is the most common cause of cystitis. Bacterial cystitis is more common in females because their relatively short urethra provides a shorter barrier to ascending infections than the longer and narrow diameter of the male urethra. The bacterial species most commonly associated with cystitis are uropathogenic *Escherichia coli* (α-hemolysin–producing strains) in all animal species; *Corynebacterium renale* in cattle; *Eubacterium (Corynebacterium) suis* in pigs; and *Klebsiella* sp. in horses. In addition, *Proteus* sp., *Streptococcus* sp., and *Staphylococcus* sp. have been isolated from cases of cystitis in several animal species.

Except for the distal urethra, the lower urinary tract is normally free of bacteria. Sterility of the urinary bladder is maintained through normal repeated voiding of urine and because of the antibacterial properties of urine. These antibacterial properties are attributable to the acidic urine of carnivores, secretory IgA, and secreted mucin that inhibit bacterial adhesion, to the large concentration of urea and organic acids, and to high urine osmolality. Cystitis occurs when bacteria are able to overcome normal defense mechanisms and attach to or invade (colonize) the urinary bladder mucosa. Several factors can enhance colonization and predispose animals to cystitis. Colonization is more likely for strains of bacteria that express molecules on their surfaces that enhance adhesion, e.g., the P and type 1 fimbriae of certain strains of *E. coli*. Retention of urine as a result of obstruction or neurogenic causes related to spinal cord diseases often leads to cystitis.

Trauma to the urinary bladder mucosa due to calculi, faulty catheterization, and parturition causes erosion and hemorrhage and predisposes to bacterial invasion of the lamina propria. Hydrolysis of urea by urease-producing bacteria, such as *C. renale* and *E. suis,* releases excessive ammonia that can damage the mucosa. Bacterial growth can be enhanced when glucosuria is present, such as in diabetes mellitus. Urinary bladder emphysema can occur in conjunction with glucosuria-associated cystitis due to fermentation of glucose by certain bacterial species. The gas is absorbed into lymph vessels in the lamina propria, tunica muscularis, and subserosa and small gas bubbles are present throughout the bladder wall. Compromise of the host immune system as found with infection by the immunodeficiency virus can increase susceptibility to bacterial cystitis. Other bacterial virulence factors, such as the *E. coli* hemolysin, enhance pathogenicity and help bacteria overcome antibacterial factors of the urinary bladder and urine.

Once bacteria gain access to the lamina propria, they cause vascular damage and inflammation. Acute cystitis is often described as hemorrhagic, fibrinopurulent, necrotizing, or ulcerative. However, in each case, components of several of these processes are present. The urinary bladder wall often is thickened by edema and an inflammatory cell infiltrate, and diffusely or focally hemorrhagic. Hemorrhage is most common when obstruction is concurrently present or after direct trauma due to catheterization. Urine in such cases is described as cloudy, flocculent, foul-smelling, ammoniacal, and red-tinged. The mucosa can have nonreflectant foci of erosion or ulceration, patches or sheets of adherent exudate and necrotic debris, or adherent blood clots (Fig. 5-65). Microscopically, acute cystitis is characterized by epithelial denudation with bacterial colonies present on the surface. The lamina propria is intensely edematous and has a diffuse neutrophilic infiltrate. Superficial hyperemia and hemorrhage are usually present. A mild perivascular leukocytic infiltrate can occur in the tunica muscularis.

Chronic Cystitis

Chronic cystitis occurs in one of several forms. Often, the lesions are a diffusely thickened, hyperplastic mucosa with goblet cell hyperplasia and a chronic lymphoplasmacytic infiltrate and fibrosis in the lamina propria. Hypertrophy of the tunica muscularis can be observed. This response is particularly common when cystitis is associated with chronic urolithiasis.

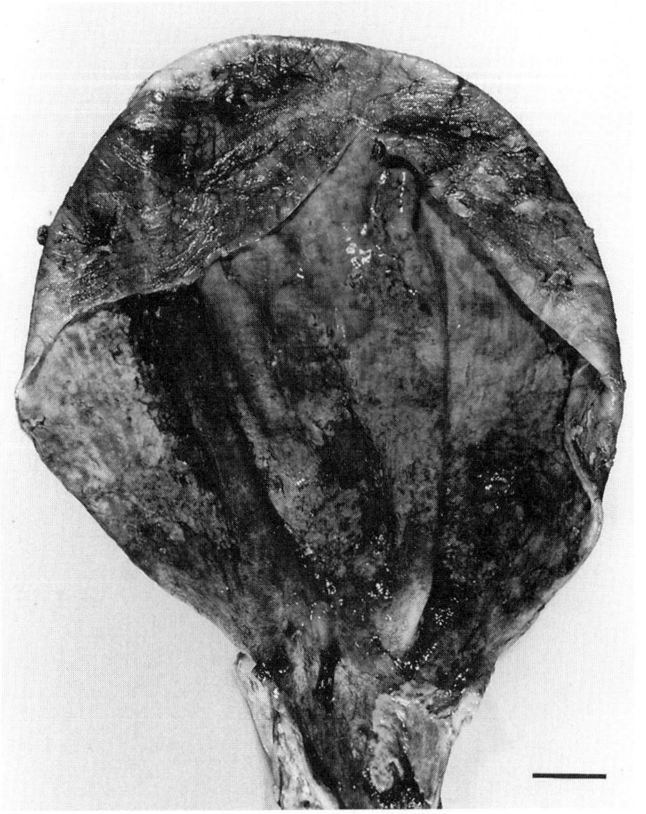

Figure 5-65 Urinary bladder; calf. Acute cystitis. Patchy areas of ulceration are interspersed with inflamed mucosa. Bar = 3 cm.

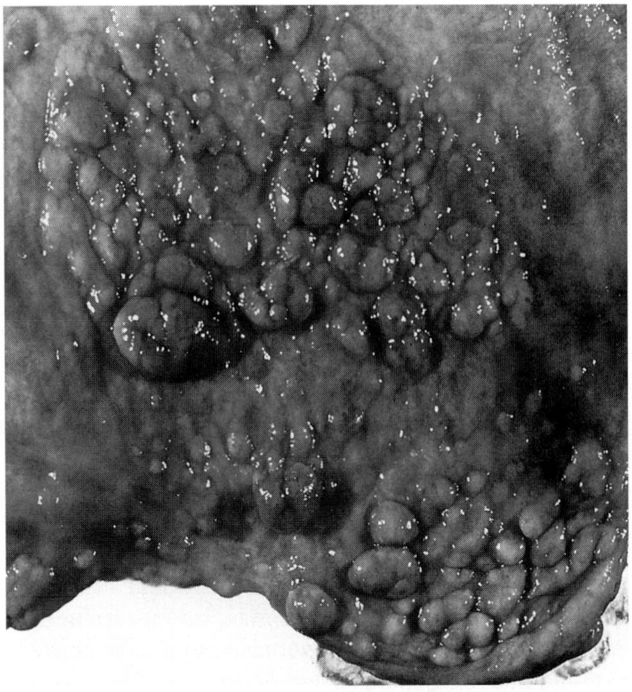

Figure 5-66 Urinary bladder; dog. Chronic cystitis. Multiple polypoid proliferations are seen from the mucosal surface.

Several specific anatomic forms of chronic cystitis can occur. Chronic **polypoid cystitis** is a form found especially in dogs. The mucosa has single or multiple, nodular mucosal masses (Fig. 5-66) composed of fibrous connective tissue and infiltrated with neutrophils and mononuclear leukocytes. The masses are broad based or pedunculated, ulcerated, or covered by hyperplastic epithelium with goblet cell metaplasia. Chronic cystitis also takes the form of disseminated nodular, submucosal lymphoid proliferations (2 to 4 mm in diameter) such that the mucosa has a cobblestone appearance **(follicular cystitis)** (Fig. 5-67). These white-gray lymphoid foci are often surrounded by a zone of hyperemia.

Mycotic Cystitis

Mycotic cystitis is occasionally seen when opportunistic fungi, such as *Candida albicans* or *Aspergillus* sp., colonize the urinary bladder mucosa. Such fungal infections usually occur secondary to chronic bacterial cystitis, especially when animals are immunosuppressed or subjected to prolonged antibiotic therapy. The urinary bladder is usually ulcerated with proliferation of underlying lamina propria; a generalized thickening of the urinary bladder wall is due to extensive inflammation consisting of neutrophils, lymphocytes, plasma cells, macrophages, edema, and fibrosis.

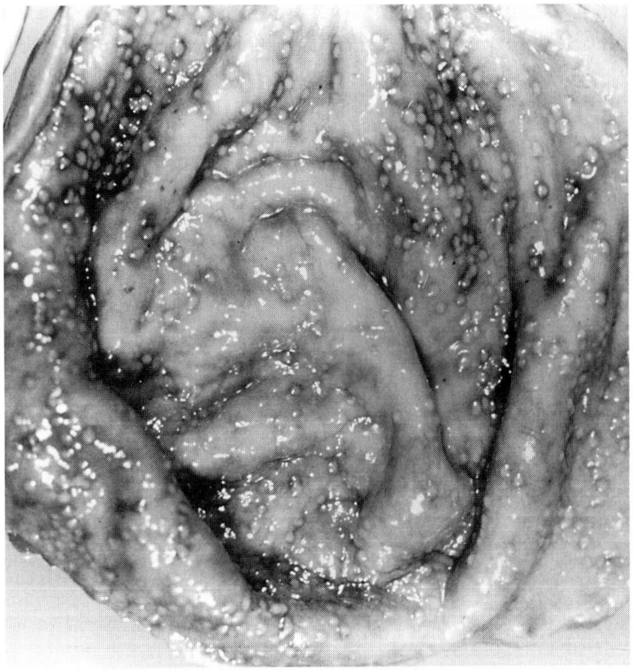

Figure 5-67 Urinary bladder; dog. Chronic cystitis. The lesion is characterized by multiple follicular lymphoid proliferations. *Courtesy Dr. L. Roth.*

Neoplasia

Neoplasms of the lower urinary tract occur predominantly in the urinary bladder. They are observed most frequently in dogs, occasionally in cats, and rarely in other species. Lower urinary tract neoplasms occupy space and often cause mucosal ulceration, resulting in clinical signs of dysuria, hematuria, or obstruction. Urinary bladder neoplasms can invade or block the ureters, causing obstruction of ureteral urine flow, increased ureteral pressure, and hydronephrosis. Urinary bladder neoplasms comprise less than 1% of total canine neoplasms. Most occur in old dogs without a sex predisposition. Many chemicals including intermediate components of aniline dyes, aromatic hydrocarbons, and tryptophan metabolites have been found experimentally or epidemiologically to induce urinary bladder neoplasms. Bracken fern *(Pteridium aquilinum)* contains quercetin, a carcinogen; cattle grazing bracken fern have developed several different neoplasms of the urinary bladder (see Enzootic Hematuria below).

Epithelial Tumors

Epithelial neoplasms are most common and are classified as **transitional cell papillomas, transitional cell carcinomas, squamous cell carcinomas, adenocarcinomas,** and **undifferentiated carcinomas.** Papillomas have a papilliferous or pedunculated appearance. Microscopically, they have a papillary growth pattern consisting of multiple papilliferous fibrous stalks covered by well-differentiated transitional epithelium. Carcinomas are focal, raised nodules or diffuse thickenings of the urinary bladder wall. Transitional cell carcinomas are composed of pleomorphic to anaplastic transitional epithelium. They are observed most commonly in the trigone area of the bladder. Neoplastic transitional cells cover the mucosal surface as irregular layers, readily invade the lamina propria in the form of solid nests and acini (Fig. 5-68), and are found within lymphatic vessels of the submucosal and muscle layers. Squamous cell carcinomas, adenocarcinomas, and unclassified carcinomas most likely arise from transitional epithelium. In the bitch, carcinomas are multicentric in origin, develop not only in the urinary bladder, but also in the urothelium of the ureters, urethra, renal pelvis, and often extend to the vagina and vestibule. Metastasis of urinary bladder carcinomas is most often first to regional lymph nodes at the aortic bifurcation including the deep inguinal, medial iliac, and sacral lymph nodes. Other potential sites of metastasis include lungs and kidneys with metastasis to other parenchymatous organs occurring later.

Mesenchymal Tumors

Mesenchymal tumors including **fibromas, fibrosarcomas, leiomyomas, leiomyosarcomas, rhabdomyosarcomas, lymphosarcomas, hemangiomas,** and **hemangiosarcomas** occur in the lower tract. Leiomyomas are the most common neoplasms and are solitary or multiple, circumscribed, firm, pale white to tan masses in the urinary bladder wall. Leiomyomas have the macroscopic consistency and microscopic appearance of normal smooth muscle. Fibromas arise from lamina proprial connective tissue and project into the bladder lumen as solitary nodules. Primary fibrosarcomas, leiomyosarcomas, hemangiomas, and hemangiosarcomas are rare. Lymphosarcoma occasionally infiltrates the wall, not only of the bladder, but also of the ureters and renal pelves in cattle with malignant lymphoma. Rhabdomyosarcomas are rare but occur in bladders of young dogs (younger than 18 months old) suggesting an embryonal origin. These masses are described as **botryoid** (grapelike) because they are large, fungating masses (4 to 18 cm in diameter) that protrude into the bladder lumen. They infiltrate the urinary bladder wall and can metastasize. Microscopically, the neoplasms are composed of sheets of fusiform cells interspersed with pleomorphic cells. Microscopic demonstration of longitudinal and cross-striations typical of skeletal muscle or immunohistochemical demonstration of

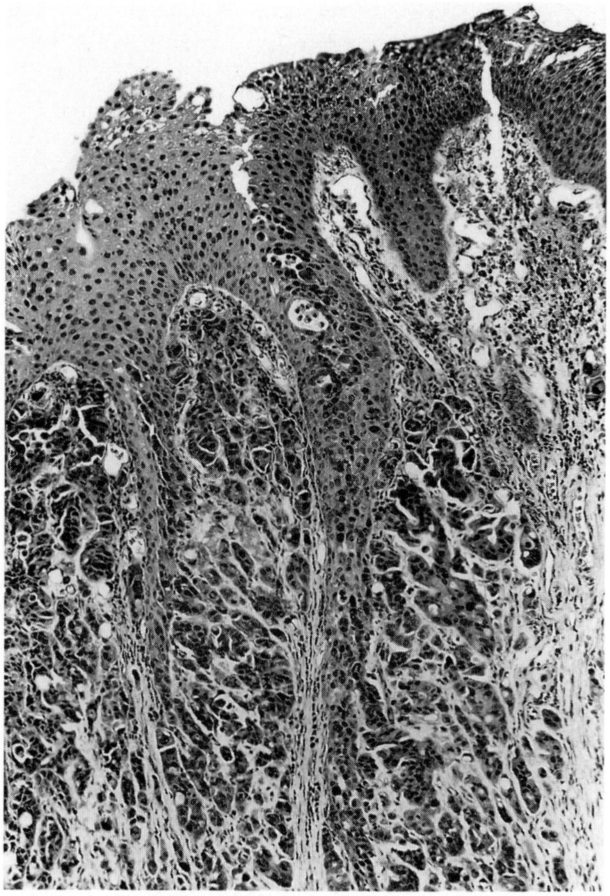

Figure 5-68 Urinary bladder; dog. Transitional cell carcinoma. There is neoplastic transformation of superficial epithelium and infiltration of the lamina propria with neoplastic cells. H & E stain.

the intermediate filament desmin are useful to confirm the diagnosis of rhabdomyosarcoma.

Enzootic Hematuria

Enzootic hematuria is a disease of cattle caused by chronic ingestion of bracken fern *(Pteridium aquilinum)*. The urinary bladder lesion is initially one of hemorrhagic cystitis resulting in marked persistent hematuria, hence the name enzootic hematuria. The mucosa is hemorrhagic with marked capillary congestion and ectasia. With time, epithelial (papillomas or carcinomas), mesenchymal (fibromas, hemangiomas, and their malignant counterparts), or mixed epithelial-mesenchymal neoplasms develop in association with the primary lesions of chronic cystitis. These neoplasms usually ulcerate the mucosa and bleed freely into the lumen.

Suggested Readings

Bach PK Thanh NTY. Renal papillary necrosis—40 years on. Toxicol Pathol 1998; 26:73-91.

Center SA, Smith CA, Wilkinson E, Erb HB, Lewis RM. Clinicopathologic, renal immunofluorescent, and light microscopic features of glomerulonephritis in the dog: 41 cases (1975-1985). J Am Vet Med Assoc 1987; 190:81-90.

Cook AK, Cowgill LD. Clinical and pathological features of protein-losing glomerular disease in the dog: A review of 137 cases (1985-1992). J Am Anim Hosp Assoc 1996; 32:313-322.

Cotran RS, Kumar V, Collins T. Robbins Pathologic Basis of Disease. 6th ed. Philadelphia: WB Saunders, 1999:930-1010.

DiBartola SP, Rutgers HC, Zack PK Tarr MJ. Clinicopathologic findings associated with chronic renal disease in cats: 74 cases (1973-1984). J Am Vet Med Assoc 1987; 190:1196-1202.

DiBartola SP, Tarr MJ, Parker AT, Powers JD, Pultz JA. Clinicopathologic findings in dogs with renal amyloidosis: 59 cases (1976-1986). J Am Vet Med Assoc 1989; 195:358-364.

Divers TJ, Crowell, WA, Duncan JR, Whitlock RH. Acute renal disorders in cattle: A retrospective study of 22 cases. J Am Vet Med Assoc 1982; 181:694-699.

Divers TJ. Diseases of the renal system. In: BP Smith, ed. Large Animal Internal Medicine. 2nd ed. St. Louis: CV Mosby, 1996:953-1000.

Elliott J, Barber PJ. Feline chronic renal failure: Clinical findings in 80 cases diagnosed between 1992 and 1995. J Small Anim Pract 1998; 39:78-85.

Forrester SD, Troy GC. Renal effects of nonsteroidal antiinflammatory drugs. Compendium 1999; 21:910-919.

Grauer GF. Glomerulonephritis. Semin Vet Med Surg 1992; 7:87-197.

Howard JL, Smith RA. Current Veterinary Therapy. Food Animal Practice. 4th ed. Philadelphia: WB Saunders, 1999:619-632.

Ling GH. Lower Urinary Tract Disease of Dogs and Cats. St. Louis, Mosby, 1995.

Ling GV, Ruby AL, Johnson DL, Thurmond M, Franti CE. Renal calculi in dogs and cats: Prevalence, mineral type, breed, age, and gender interrelationships (1981-1993). J Vet Intern Med 1998; 12:11-21.

Maxie GM. The Urinary System. In: Jubb KVF, Kennedy PC, Palmer N, eds. Pathology of Domestic Animals. Vol. 2, 4th ed. San Diego: Academic Press, 1993:447-538.

Mingeot-Leclercq MP, Tulkens PM. Aminoglycosides: Nephrotoxicity. Antimicrob Agents Chemother 1999; 43:1003-1012.

Nagode LA, Chew DJ. Nephrocalcinosis caused by hyperparathyroidism in progression of renal failure: Treatment with calcitriol. Semin Vet Med Surg 1992; 7:202-220.

Picut CA, Lewis RM. Comparative pathology of canine hereditary nephropathies: An interpretive review. Vet Res Commun 1987; 11:561-581.

Rebhun WC, Dill SG, Perdrizet JA, Hatfield CE. Pyelonephritis in cows: 15 cases (1982-1986). J Am Vet Med Assoc 1989; 194:953-955.

Rosol TJ, Capen CC. Pathophysiology of calcium, phosphorus, and magnesium metabolism in animals. Vet Clin North Am Small Anim Pract 1996; 26:1155-1184.

CHAPTER 6

Endocrine System

CHARLES C. CAPEN

INTRODUCTION

Endocrine glands are collections of specialized cells that synthesize, store, and release their secretions directly into the bloodstream. They are sensing and signaling devices located in the extracellular fluid compartment that are capable of responding to changes in the internal and external environments to coordinate a multiplicity of activities that maintain homeostasis.

Endocrine cells that produce polypeptide hormones have a well-developed, rough endoplasmic reticulum that assembles the hormone and a prominent perinuclear Golgi apparatus that packages a hormone into granules for intracellular storage and transport. Secretory granules are unique to polypeptide hormone– and catecholamine-secreting endocrine cells and provide a mechanism for intracellular storage of substantial amounts of preformed active hormone. When the cell receives a signal to secrete hormone, secretory granules are moved to the periphery of the endocrine cell, most likely by the contraction of microfilaments.

Steroid hormone–secreting cells are characterized by large cytoplasmic lipid bodies that contain cholesterol and other precursor molecules. The lipid bodies are in close proximity to an extensive smooth endoplasmic reticulum and large mitochondria. The latter have hydroxylase and dehydrogenase enzyme systems that attach various side chains to the basic steroid nucleus. Steroid-producing cells lack secretory granules and do not store significant amounts of preformed hormone. They depend on continued biosynthesis to maintain the normal secretory rate of a particular hormone.

The histopathologic differentiation among nodular hyperplasia, adenoma, and carcinoma often is more difficult in endocrine glands than in most other organs of the body. However, criteria used to differentiate these proliferative lesions should be established and applied in a uniform manner in the evaluation of proliferative lesions in endocrine glands. For many endocrine glands (especially thyroid C cells, secretory cells of the adrenal medulla, thyroid follicular cells, parathyroid chief cells, endocrine cells of the pancreas, and specific trophic hormone–secreting cells of the adenohypophysis) there appears to be a continuous spectrum of proliferative lesions derived from a specific population of secretory cells between focal ("nodular") hyperplasia and adenomas.

It appears to be a common feature of endocrine glands, especially in laboratory rodents, that prolonged stimulation of a population of secretory cells predisposes to the subsequent development of an increased incidence of neoplasms. Long-continued stimulation can lead to the development of clones of cells within the hyperplastic endocrine glands that grow more rapidly than the remainder and are more susceptible to genetic alterations that can result in neoplastic transformation when exposed to the right combination of promoting agents.

Excessive focal growth of endocrine cells is the consequence of aberrant secretion of either or both of growth- or function-stimulating hormone(s) and has been referred to as "nonneoplastic endocrine hyperplasia." Lesions of this type in endocrine organs are considered to be largely reversible on cessation of the inciting stimulus. Nodules arising in hyperplastic endocrine glands can be polyclonal as well as of clonal origin. Hyperfunction and cellular hypertrophy associated with nonneoplastic endocrine hyperplasia are completely reversible when the overstimulation ceases; however, chronic and severe hyperplasia of endocrine tissues sometimes is not fully reversible.

PATHOGENIC MECHANISMS OF ENDOCRINE DISEASES

Many diseases of the endocrine glands are characterized by dramatic functional disturbances and characteristic clinicopathologic alterations affecting one or several body systems. The affected animal can be presented because of changes that primarily involve the skin (hair loss caused by hypothyroidism), nervous system (seizures caused by hyperinsulinism), urinary system (polyuria caused by diabetes mellitus, diabetes insipidus, and hyperadrenocorticism), or skeletal system (fractures induced by hyperparathyroidism).

Primary Hypofunction of an Endocrine Gland

Hormone secretion is subnormal because of extensive destruction of secretory cells by a disease process, the failure of an endocrine gland to develop properly, or the result of a specific biochemical defect in the synthetic pathway of a hormone. In animals, immune-mediated injury causes hypofunction of several endocrine glands including the parathyroid glands, adrenal cortex, thyroid gland, pancreatic islets, and hypothalamus. Thyroiditis caused by this mechanism is characterized by marked infiltration of lymphocytes and plasmacytes and deposition of electron-dense immune complexes along the follicular basement membranes with subsequent progressive destruction of secretory parenchyma.

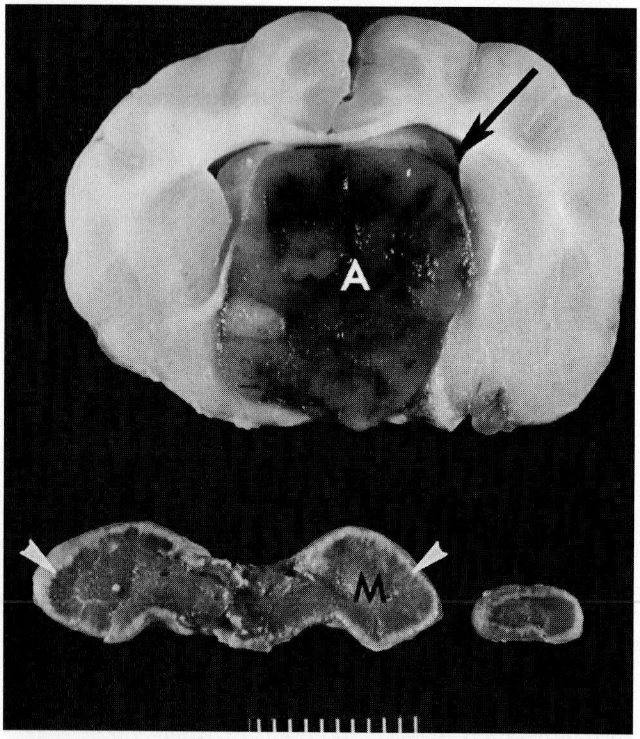

Figure 6-1 Brain; adrenal glands; pituitary gland; dog. Secondary hypofunction of an endocrine gland. A large nonfunctional chromophobe adenoma *(A)* has completely incorporated and destroyed the adenohypophysis and hypothalamus, thereby interrupting the secretion of thyrotropin, adrenocorticotropin, and other pituitary trophic hormones, and extended into the thalamus *(arrow)*. This resulted in severe trophic atrophy of the adrenal cortex *(white arrowheads)*, especially the ACTH-dependent zonae fasciculata and reticularis, and a relatively more prominent medulla *(M)*. Bar = 1 cm.

Failure of development also results in primary hypofunction of an endocrine gland. The classic example of this mechanism in animals is the failure of oropharyngeal ectoderm to differentiate completely into trophic hormone-secreting cells of the adenohypophysis in dogs, resulting in pituitary dwarfism.

Secondary Hypofunction of an Endocrine Gland

In this mechanism a destructive lesion in one organ, such as the pituitary gland, interferes with the secretion of a trophic hormone. This results in hypofunction of the target endocrine gland. Large, endocrinologically inactive pituitary neoplasms in adult dogs, cats, and other animals can interfere with the secretion of the multiple pituitary trophic hormones and result in clinically detectable hypofunction of the adrenal cortex (Fig. 6-1), follicular cells of the thyroid gland, and gonads.

Primary Hyperfunction of an Endocrine Gland

This is one of the most important pathologic mechanisms of endocrine disease in animals. The cells of a lesion, often a neoplasm derived from endocrine cells, synthesize and secrete a hormone autonomously at a rate in excess of the body's ability to use and to degrade, thereby resulting in a syndrome of hormone excess. Examples are summarized in Table 6-1. These include hyperfunction of parathyroid chief cells, thyroid C (parafollicular) cells, beta cells of the pancreatic islets, secretory cells of the adrenal medulla, and follicular cells of the thyroid gland.

Secondary Hyperfunction of an Endocrine Gland

In this mechanism of endocrine disease, a lesion in one organ (e.g., adenohypophysis) secretes an excess of a trophic hormone that leads to long-term stimulation and hypersecretion of a hormone by a target organ. The classic example in animals is the adrenocorticotropic hormone (ACTH)–secreting neoplasm derived from pituitary corticotrophs in dogs (Fig. 6-2). The functional disturbances and lesions primarily are the result of increased blood cortisol concentrations resulting from the ACTH-stimulated hypertrophy and hyperplasia of the zonae fasciculata and reticularis of the adrenal cortex. In some aging dogs with marked adrenal cortical enlargement and functional disturbances of cortisol excess, no gross or

Table 6-1 Primary Hyperfunction of an Endocrine Gland

Neoplasia	Hormone	Lesion/Sign
Thyroid follicular cell adenoma	T_4/T_3	↑ Basal metabolic rate
Parathyroid gland chief cell adenoma	Parathyroid hormone	Fibrous osteodystrophy
Pancreatic β cell adenoma/carcinoma	Insulin	Hypoglycemia
Pheochromocytoma (adrenal medulla)	Norepinephrine	Hypertension
Acidophil adenoma (pituitary gland)	Growth hormone	Acromegaly
C cell adenoma/carcinoma (thyroid gland)	Calcitonin	Osteosclerosis
Adrenal cortical adenoma/carcinoma	Estrogen	Feminization

histopathologic evidence of a neoplasm is present in the pituitary gland. These animals can have a change in negative feedback control due to an age-related increase in monoamine oxidase-β in the hypothalamus and increased metabolism of dopamine. This results in reduced inhibition of ACTH production by the pars intermedia of the pituitary gland, leading to severe corticotroph hyperplasia, increased ACTH concentration in the blood, and long-term stimulation of the adrenal cortex resulting in the syndrome of cortisol excess.

Hypersecretion of Hormones or Hormone-like Factors by Nonendocrine Neoplasms

Certain neoplasms of nonendocrine tissues in both animals and human beings either secrete new humoral substances or hormones that share chemical or biologic characteristics or both with the "native" hormones secreted by an endocrine gland. Most of the recently discovered humoral substances secreted by nonendocrine neoplasms are peptides rather than steroids, iodothyronines, or catecholamines. The nonpeptide hormones require more complex biosynthetic pathways and are infrequently produced by cancer cells. Humoral hypercalcemia of malignancy ("pseudohyperparathyroidism") is a clinical syndrome produced primarily by the autonomous hypersecretion of parathyroid hormone–related peptide (PTH-rP) by cancer cells. PTH-rP interacts with the parathyroid hormone receptor in target cells (e.g., bone and kidneys) and results

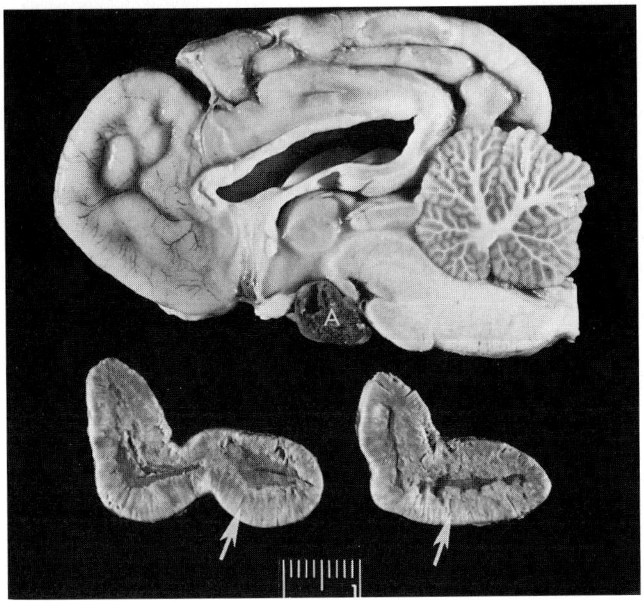

Figure 6-2 Brain; pituitary gland and adrenal glands; dog. Secondary hyperfunction of an endocrine organ. Corticotroph (ACTH-secreting) chromophobe adenoma *(A)* in the pituitary gland and bilateral enlargement of the adrenal glands. The chronic secretion of ACTH has resulted in hypertrophy and hyperplasia of secretory cells of the zonae fasciculata and reticularis in the adrenal cortex *(white arrows)* and an excessive secretion of cortisol. Bar = 1 cm.

in persistent, often life-threatening, hypercalcemia. A well-characterized example of this disease mechanism in animals is the adenocarcinoma of the apocrine glands of the anal sac in dogs. These neoplasms produce PTH-rP that mimic the action of PTH and results in an accelerated mobilization of calcium from bone by osteoclasts leading to the development of persistent hypercalcemia. Serum PTH concentrations are lower in dogs with apocrine carcinomas than in controls and PTH concentrations are undetectable in neoplastic tissue.

Endocrine Dysfunction Due to Failure of Target Cell Response

This mechanism of endocrine disease has been appreciated now that there is a more complete understanding of how hormones interact with target cells to convey their biologic message. A failure of target cells to respond to a hormone can be due either to a lack of adenylate cyclase in the cell membrane or to an alteration in hormone receptors on the cell surface. Hormone is secreted in normal or increased amounts by the cells of the endocrine gland. For example, insulin resistance associated with obesity in both animals and human beings can result from a decrease or down-regulation of receptors on the surface of target cells. The down-regulation of receptors develops in response to a chronic increase in insulin stimulated by the hyperglycemia resulting from excessive food intake. Secretory cells in the corresponding endocrine gland (i.e., pancreatic islets) undergo compensatory hypertrophy and hyperplasia in an attempt to secrete additional hormone.

An interesting form of hypoparathyroidism has been reported in human patients in whom the inability of target cells to respond is due to a defect in the cyclic adenosine monophosphate (cAMP)-mediated signal transduction that results from inactivating mutations of specific nucleotide regulatory protein in the cell membrane. Human patients with pseudohypoparathyroidism develop hypocalcemia and hyperphosphatemia in spite of hyperplastic parathyroid glands and increased blood concentration of PTH.

Endocrine Hyperactivity Due to Diseases of Other Organs

The best characterized example is the hyperparathyroidism that develops as a result of chronic renal failure or nutritional imbalance. In the renal form, retention of phosphorus occurs early, resulting in a reciprocal decline in serum calcium and parathyroid stimulation. Subsequently, the progressive destruction of cells of the proximal convoluted tubules interferes with the metabolic activation of vitamin D by 1α-hydroxylase in the kidneys leading to decreased intestinal calcium absorption and continued parathyroid stimulation. This rate-limiting step in the metabolic activation of vitamin D is controlled by multiple factors including parathyroid hormone, serum phosphorus, and several other hormones. The intestinal absorption of calcium is impaired and results in the development of progressive hypocalcemia; the hypocalcemia leads to long-term parathyroid gland stimulation and, subsequently, to the development of generalized demineralization of the skeleton. Nutritional hyperparathyroidism develops in animals fed abnormal diets that are either too low in calcium, too high in phosphorus, or deficient in cholecalciferol (e.g., in new world nonhuman primates).

Hyperfunction of an endocrine organ also can result from hormonal imbalances induced by xenobiotic chemicals. For example, in rodents during chronic toxicity testing, hyperactivity of the pituitary gland can occur that results in increased incidence of neoplasms in the gonads or mammary glands. An excess production of luteinizing hormone (LH), usually due to disruption of negative feedback control by estrogen or testosterone, increases the incidence of tubulostromal adenomas and granulosa cell neoplasms in the ovaries of mice and Leydig (interstitial) adenomas of the testes in rats.

Failure of Fetal Endocrine Function

Subnormal function of the fetal endocrine system, seen especially in ruminants, can disrupt normal fetal development and result in prolonged gestation. In Guernsey and Jersey cattle a genetically determined failure of development (aplasia) of the adenohypophysis has been described, although the neurohypophysis develops normally. This aplasia results in a lack of fetal pituitary trophic hormone secretion during the last trimester and hypoplasia of target endocrine organs, namely the adrenal cortex, gonads, and follicular cells of the thyroid gland. Fetal development is normal up to approximately 7 months of gestation, but fetal growth subsequently ceases irrespective of how long the viable fetus is retained in the uterus.

Prolongation of the gestation period occurs in ewes that ingest the plant *Veratrum californicum* early in gestation. Toxins in the plant cause extensive malformations of the central nervous system (CNS) and hypothalamus in lambs. Although the adenohypophysis is present, it is unable to secrete normal amounts of trophic hormones (ACTH) because it lacks the necessary fine control derived from the releasing hormones of the hypothalamus. Target endocrine organs in the fetus are hypoplastic and the adrenal cortex does not differentiate completely into the three distinctive zones that secrete corticosteroid hormones.

V. californicum plant contains potent steroidal alkaloids that inhibit neural tube development when ingested by the ewe between the 9th and 14th days of gestation. Cyclopia and extensive CNS malformations are found in lambs. Arrhinencephalia and lack of development of nasal bones accompany the formation of a proboscis-like structure. The lambs retained in the uterus continue to grow beyond the normal gestation period.

The concepts that have emerged from the study of these two valuable experiments of nature are (1) fetal hormones are necessary for final growth and development of the fetus in certain animals, and (2) normal parturition at term in these species requires an intact fetal hypothalamic-adenohypophyseal-adrenocortical axis working in concert with trophoblasts of the placenta.

Although the presence or absence of functional adenohypophyseal tissue determines whether the fetus continues to grow in utero, the pathogenesis of prolongation of the gestational interval is similar in these two examples. The subnormal development of the fetal adrenal cortex in the calves and lambs results in an inadequate secretion of cortisol and a failure to induce 17α-hydroxylase in the placenta that converts precursor molecules, such as progesterone, to estrogen. Thus the dam's circulating progesterone is maintained near mid-gestational concentrations and the marked increase in estrogens that normally occurs at term and results in parturition is missing. The estrogen surge when it occurs stimulates a synthesis of prostaglandins in the uterus, which results in the smooth muscle contractions and biochemical changes in collagen along the birth canal that normally permit delivery of the fetus.

Endocrine Dysfunction Resulting from Abnormal Degradation of Hormone

Decreased Degradation

The rate of secretion of a hormone by an endocrine gland can be normal with this mechanism, but because of the decreased rate of degradation, blood concentrations are persistently increased, thereby simulating a syndrome of hypersecretion. The classic example of this mechanism is the syndrome of feminization due to hyperestrogenism and from decreased hepatic degradation of estrogens in patients with cirrhosis. Chronic renal disease in dogs occasionally is associated with hypercalcemia, due in part to a decrease in the ability of the diseased kidneys to degrade PTH (along with a decrease in urinary excretion of calcium).

Increased Degradation

In laboratory rodents the long-term administration of various xenobiotics (i.e., phenobarbital and others) results in the induction of hepatic enzymes (e.g., thyroxine [T_4] uridine diphosphate glucuronyl transferase) that increase the rate of degradation of thyroxine. This chronic disruption of the thyroid-pituitary gland axis results in an increased TSH secretion. In rodents, especially male rats, the development of thyroid follicular cell neoplasms often is increased in chronic toxicity and oncogenicity studies with certain new drugs and chemicals.

Iatrogenic Syndromes of Hormone Excess

The administration of an exogenous hormone can influence the activity of target cells either directly or indirectly and results in important functional disturbances. It is well recognized that the chronic administration of potent preparations of adrenal cortical steroids at inappropriately

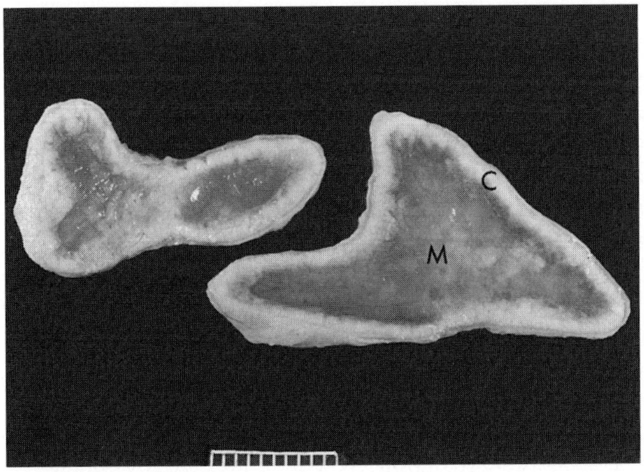

Figure 6-3 Adrenal glands; dog. Iatrogenic syndrome of hormone excess. Hyperadrenocorticism, caused by long-term administration of exogenous corticosteroids, has resulted in marked trophic atrophy of the ACTH-dependent zona fasciculata and zona reticularis of the adrenal cortex *(C)*. The adrenal medulla *(M)* occupies a relatively greater percentage of the atrophic adrenal gland than of a normal adrenal. Bar = 1 cm.

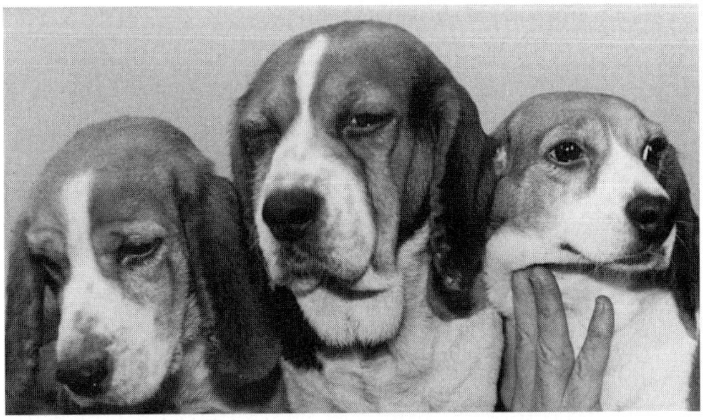

Figure 6-4 Iatrogenic acromegaly; beagle, *center* (compared with unaffected littermates, *left* and *right*). Note the coarseness of the facial features and the marked thickening and folding of the skin of the face. These characteristic changes are the result of the protein anabolic effects of somatotropin (produced by hyperplastic ductular epithelial cells) that has been stimulated by the exogenous administration of medroxyprogesterone acetate. *Courtesy of Dr. P. Concannon.*

large daily doses (for the symptomatic treatment of various diseases) can produce most of the functional disturbances associated with an endogenous hypersecretion of cortisol. Increased concentrations of exogenous cortisol result in marked atrophy of the adrenal cortex, particularly the ACTH-dependent zona fasciculata and zona reticularis (Fig. 6-3). Similarly, the administration of excessively large doses of insulin can result in hypoglycemia, and an excess of T_4 or triiodothyronine (T_3) can result in hyperthyroidism, especially in certain species (e.g., cats) that have limited capacity to conjugate T_4 with glucuronic acid and, thus, enhance biliary excretion.

The administration of progestogens to dogs indirectly results in a syndrome of growth hormone excess. For example, the injection of medroxyprogesterone acetate for the prevention of estrus in dogs stimulates the expression of the growth hormone gene in the mammary glands and results in elevated circulating growth hormone concentrations producing many of the clinical manifestations of acromegaly. The excessive skin folds (Fig. 6-4), expansion of interdigital spaces, and abdominal enlargement in dogs with iatrogenic acromegaly are related to the protein anabolic effects of growth hormone.

PITUITARY GLAND (HYPOPHYSIS)

The **adenohypophysis** consists of three portions: the pars distalis, pars tuberalis, and pars intermedia (Fig. 6-5). In many animal species, the adenohypophysis completely surrounds the pars nervosa of the neurohypophyseal system. The pars distalis is the largest and is composed of the populations of different endocrine cells that secrete the

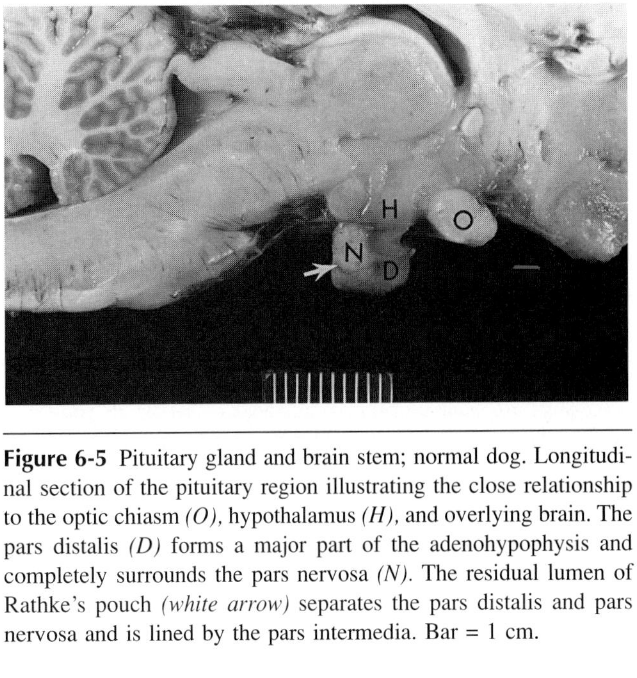

Figure 6-5 Pituitary gland and brain stem; normal dog. Longitudinal section of the pituitary region illustrating the close relationship to the optic chiasm *(O)*, hypothalamus *(H)*, and overlying brain. The pars distalis *(D)* forms a major part of the adenohypophysis and completely surrounds the pars nervosa *(N)*. The residual lumen of Rathke's pouch *(white arrow)* separates the pars distalis and pars nervosa and is lined by the pars intermedia. Bar = 1 cm.

pituitary trophic hormones. The secretory cells are surrounded by abundant capillaries (Fig. 6-6).

The pars tuberalis consists of dorsal projections of cells along the infundibular stalk. It functions primarily as a scaffold for the capillary network of the hypophyseal portal system in its course from the median eminence to the pars distalis. The pars intermedia is located between the pars distalis and pars nervosa; it lines the residual lumen of Rathke's pouch and has two populations of cells

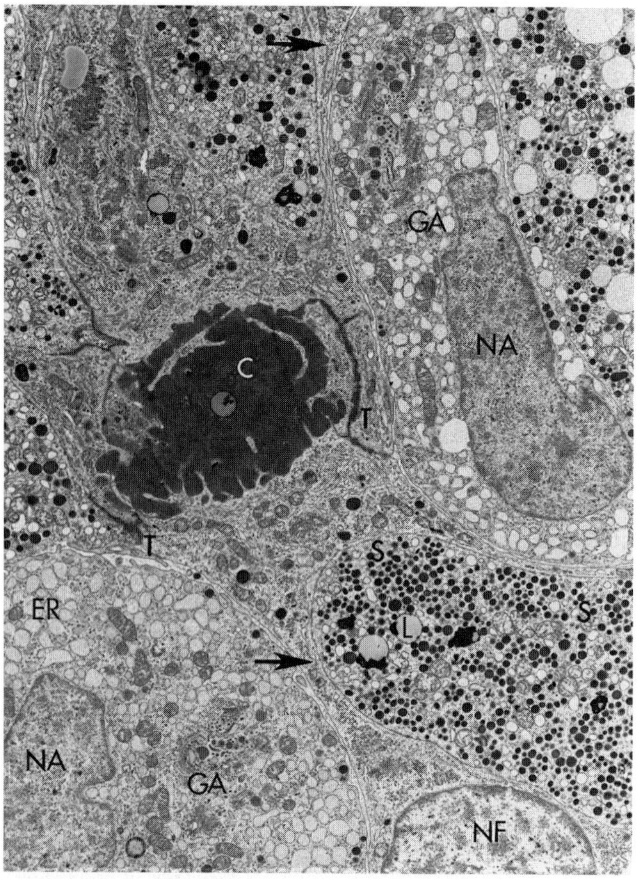

Figure 6-6 Pituitary gland, pars distalis; normal dog. Follicular cells *(NF)* in the pars distalis form a framework and extend cytoplasmic processes *(arrows)* around extracellular accumulations of colloid *(C)*. Adjacent follicular cells are joined by prominent terminal bars *(T)*. Acidophils in the storage phase of the secretory cycle contain numerous large, uniformly electron-dense secretory granules *(S)*, scattered lipofuscin *(L)* bodies, but a small amount of endoplasmic reticulum *(ER)*, and a small Golgi apparatus. Hypertrophied acidophils *(NA)* have few mature secretory granules but many distended profiles of endoplasmic reticulum and large Golgi apparatuses *(GA)* associated with prosecretory granules in the process of formation. TEM ×7500.

in certain species. In the dog, one of these cell types (B cell) synthesizes and secretes ACTH.

A specific population of endocrine cells is present in the pars distalis (and in the pars intermedia of dogs for ACTH) that synthesizes, processes, and secretes each of the pituitary trophic hormones. Secretory cells in the adenohypophysis are classified as acidophils, basophils, and chromophobes based on the reactions of their secretory granules with pH-dependent histochemical stains. Based on contemporary specific immunocytochemical staining, acidophils can be further subclassified functionally into somatotrophs that secrete growth hormone (GH; somatotrophin) and luteotrophs that secrete luteotropic hormone (LTH; prolactin). Their granules contain simple protein hormones. Basophils include both gonadotrophs that secrete LH and follicle-stimulating hormone (FSH) and thyrotrophs that secrete thyrotropic hormone (thyroid-stimulating hormone [TSH]). Chromophobes are pituitary cells that by light microscopy do not have stainable cytoplasmic secretory granules. They include the pituitary cells involved with the synthesis of ACTH and melanocyte-stimulating hormone (MSH) in some species, nonsecretory follicular (stellate) cells (Fig. 6-6), degranulated chromophils (acidophils and basophils) in the actively synthesizing phase of the secretory cycle, and undifferentiated stem cells of the adenohypophysis.

Each type of endocrine cell in the adenohypophysis is under the control of a specific releasing hormone or factor from the hypothalamus. These releasing hormones are small peptides synthesized and secreted by neurons of the hypothalamus. They are transported by axonal processes to the median eminence where they are released into capillaries and are conveyed by the hypophyseal portal system to specific endocrine cells in the adenohypophysis. Each hormone stimulates the rapid release of secretory granules containing a specific preformed trophic hormone.

The **neurohypophysis** is subdivided into three anatomic parts. The pars nervosa (posterior lobe) represents the distal component of the neurohypophyseal system. The infundibular stalk joins the pars nervosa to the overlying hypothalamus and is composed of axonal processes from neurosecretory neurons. It is composed of numerous capillaries, supported by modified glial cells (pituicytes), which are termination sites for the nonmyelinated axonal processes of neurosecretory neurons in the hypothalamus. The neurohypophyseal hormones (i.e., oxytocin and antidiuretic hormone) are synthesized in the cell body of hypothalamic neurons, packaged into secretory granules, transported by long axonal processes, and released into the bloodstream in the pars nervosa.

Neurosecretory neurons in the hypothalamus secrete hormone in response to neural input from higher centers resulting in hormonal secretion. Antidiuretic hormone (ADH or vasopressin) and oxytocin are nonapeptides synthesized by neurons situated either in the supraoptic or paraventricular nuclei of the hypothalamus. ADH and its corresponding neurophysin appear to be synthesized as part of a common larger biosynthetic precursor molecule, termed **propressophysin.** The hormones are packaged with a corresponding binding protein (i.e., neurophysin) into membrane-limited neurosecretory granules and transported to the pars nervosa for release into the circulation.

Developmental Disturbances of Adenohypophysis

Pituitary Cyst

Pituitary dwarfism in dogs usually is associated with a failure of the oropharyngeal ectoderm of Rathke's pouch to differentiate into trophic hormone-secreting cells of the pars distalis. This results in a progressively enlarging,

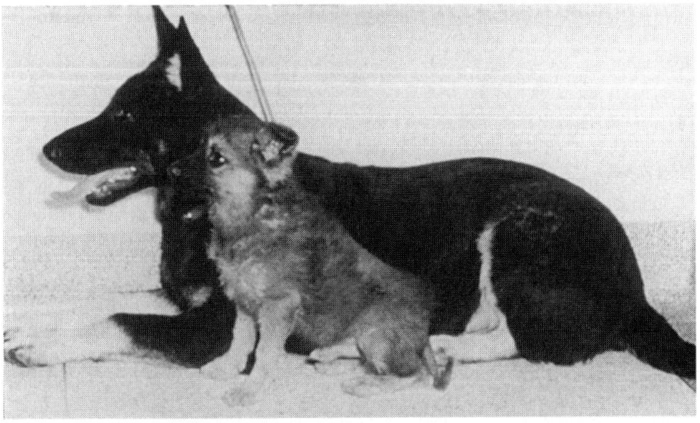

Figure 6-7 Panhypopituitarism ("pituitary dwarfism"); 5-month-old German shepherd and littermate. The unaffected littermate weighed 27.3 kg while the dwarf puppy weighed only 4 kg. The pituitary dwarf has retained the puppy haircoat.

multiloculated cyst in the sella turcica and an absence of the adenohypophysis.

Juvenile panhypopituitarism occurs most frequently in German shepherd dogs, but it has been reported in spitz, toy pinscher, and Carelian bear dogs. The dwarf pups appear normal from birth to about 2 months of age. Subsequently, the slower growth, retention of puppy hair coat, and lack of primary guard hairs gradually become evident (Fig. 6-7). A bilaterally symmetric alopecia develops gradually and often progresses to complete alopecia except for the head and tufts of hair on the legs. There is progressive hyperpigmentation of the skin until the skin is uniformly brown-black over most of the body. Adult German shepherd dogs with panhypopituitarism vary in size from as small as 2 kg to nearly half normal size, apparently depending on whether the failure of formation of the adenohypophysis is nearly or only partially complete.

The mode of inheritance is a simple autosomal recessive. The activity of somatomedin (a nonspecies-specific, cartilage growth-promoting peptide whose production in the liver and plasma activity are controlled by somatotropin) is low in dwarf dogs. Intermediate somatomedin activity is present in the phenotypically normal ancestors suspected to be heterozygous carriers. Assays for somatomedin provide a useful indirect measurement of circulating growth hormone activity in dogs with suspected pituitary dwarfism if canine growth hormone assays are not available.

NEOPLASMS OF ADENOHYPOPHYSIS

Adenomas of Pars Intermedia

Adenoma derived from cells of the pars intermedia is the most common type of pituitary gland neoplasm in horses, the second most common type in dogs, and rare in other species. Adenomas develop in older horses, more frequently in females. Nonbrachycephalic breeds of dogs have adenomas of the pars intermedia more often than brachycephalic breeds.

Two cell populations have been identified in the pars intermedia of normal dogs by immunocytochemistry. The predominant cell type (A cell) stains strongly for α-MSH as in the pars intermedia of other species. A second cell type (B cell) in the canine pars intermedia stains intensely for ACTH but not for α-MSH. This second cell population accounts for the high bioactive ACTH concentration found in the pars intermedia of dogs and most likely gives rise to corticotroph adenomas of the pars intermedia in dogs with the syndrome of cortisol excess.

In dogs, adenomas of the pars intermedia result in only a moderate enlargement of the pituitary gland. The pars distalis is readily identifiable and sharply demarcated from the anterior margin of the neoplasm, usually by an incomplete layer of condensed stroma. The neoplasm can extend across the residual hypophyseal lumen and result in compression atrophy, but it usually does not invade the pars distalis. The posterior lobe is incorporated within the neoplasm, but the infundibular stalk is intact.

Adenomas of the pars intermedia in dogs either are functionally inactive and associated with varying degrees of hypopituitarism and diabetes insipidus or endocrinologically active and secrete excessive ACTH, leading to bilateral adrenal cortical hyperplasia and a syndrome of cortisol excess. Endocrinologically active (ACTH-secreting) adenomas of the pars intermedia in dogs have prominent groups of corticotrophs that have abundant eosinophilic cytoplasm and more widely scattered follicles.

In horses, adenomas of the pars intermedia often are large neoplasms that extend out of the sella turcica and severely compress the overlying hypothalamus. The adenomas are yellow to white, multinodular, and enclose the pars nervosa. When the neoplasm is incised, the pars distalis usually can be identified as a compressed subcapsular rim of tissue on the anterior margin. A sharp line of demarcation remains between the neoplasm and the compressed pars distalis.

The neoplastic cells arranged in cords and nests along the capillaries and connective tissue septa are large, cylindrical, spindle-shaped, or polyhedral with an oval hyperchromatic nucleus. The pattern is often reminiscent of that of the prominent pars intermedia of normal horses. More cuboidal neoplastic cells occasionally form follicular structures that have dense eosinophilic colloid (Fig. 6-8). The clinical syndrome associated with neoplasms of the pars intermedia in horses is characterized by polyuria, polydipsia, ravenous appetite, muscle weakness, somnolence, intermittent hyperpyrexia, and generalized hyperhidrosis. The affected horses often develop a striking hypertrichosis ("hirsutism") because of failure to seasonally shed hair. The hair over most of the trunk and extremities is long (up to 10 to 12 cm), abnormally thick, wavy, and often matted (Fig. 6-9).

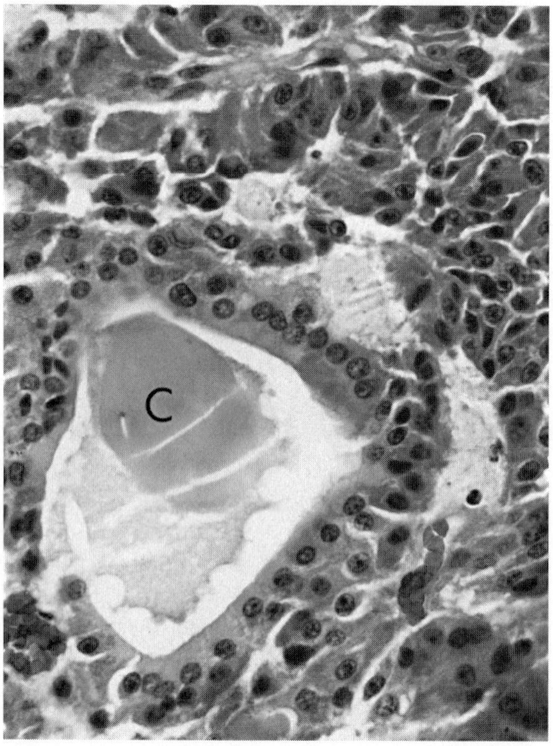

Figure 6-8 Pituitary glands, pars intermedia; horse. Adenoma. The follicle is lined by cuboidal cells and contains colloid *(C)*. H & E stain.

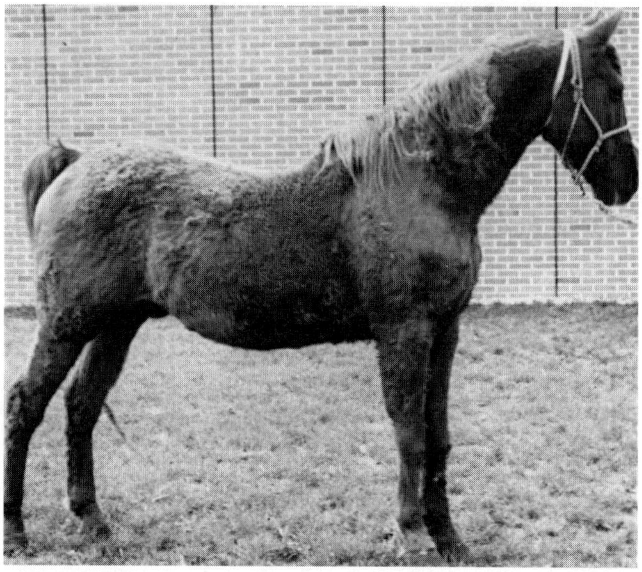

Figure 6-9 Horse. The hirsutism is the result of a failure of shedding due to an adenoma of the pars intermedia.

Horses with larger neoplasms sometimes have hyperglycemia (insulin-resistant) and glycosuria, probably the result of a down-regulation of insulin receptors on target cells induced by the chronic excessive intake of feed and hyperinsulinemia. The disturbances in carbohydrate metabolism, ravenous appetite, hypertrichosis, and hyperhidrosis are considered to be primarily a reflection of deranged hypothalamic function caused by compression of the overlying hypothalamus by the large pituitary neoplasms. The hypothalamus is the primary center for homeostatic regulation of body temperature, appetite, and cyclic shedding of hair.

In addition to their space-occupying effects, some adenomas of the pars intermedia are endocrinologically active. Plasma cortisol and immunoreactive adrenocorticotropin (iACTH, molecular weight 4,500) concentrations can be modestly elevated in horses with pars intermedia adenomas. The cortisol concentrations often lack the normal diurnal rhythm and are not suppressed by either large or small doses of dexamethasone.

The modest increases of plasma immunoreactive ACTH (4,500 daltons) appear to be due to the different processing of pro-opiomelanocortin (POMC) in neoplasms derived from cells of the pars intermedia. This could explain the normal or slightly increased blood cortisol concentrations and normal or mildly hyperplastic adrenal cortices observed in some horses with adenomas of the pars intermedia. The concentrations of ACTH in the neoplasm have been reported to be six times that of the normal pars intermedia and only approached the concentrations found in the pars distalis of normal horses. The plasma and neoplasm concentrations of pars intermedia–derived peptides (CLIP [corticotrophin-like intermediate lobe peptide], α-MSH, β-MSH, and β-endorphin [β-END]) are disproportionately increased (40 times or more) compared with those of ACTH, apparently as the result of selective posttranslational processing of POMC in a manner similar to that of the normal pars intermedia.

Adenomas of the pars intermedia have immunocytochemical staining similar to that of the nonneoplastic equine pars intermedia. The findings include a strong, diffuse cytoplasmic reaction for POMC, a moderate strong reaction for α-MSH and β-END, a weak reaction for ACTH, and negative immunostaining for prolactin, glial fibrillary acidic protein, and neuron-specific enolase. Two antisera directed against different parts of the *N*-terminal fragment of human (h) POMC differed in their immunoreactivity. Anti-h^{1-48} *N*-POMC had stronger immunostaining of the neoplastic cells than did antisera h^{1-76} *N*-POMC.

These immunocytochemical findings support the biochemical studies that suggest horses with pituitary adenomas derived from the cells of the pars intermedia develop a unique clinical syndrome that is the result of hypothalamic and neurohypophyseal derangement and of an autonomous production of excess amounts of POMC-derived peptides. Although many of the functional disturbances in horses with pituitary adenomas (e.g., diabetes insipidus, polyphagia, hyperpyrexia, hyperhidrosis, and hirsutism) appear to be the result of hypothalamic or neurohypophyseal dysfunction, other behavioral signs (e.g., docility and diminished responsiveness to painful stimuli) could be related to increased plasma and cerebrospinal fluid (CSF) concentrations of β-END. The clinical syndrome in horses with pituitary neoplasms is distinctly different than that of Cushing's disease in dogs, cats, and human patients.

ACTH-secreting (Corticotroph) Adenoma

Functional (endocrinologically active) neoplasms arising in the pituitary gland most likely are derived from corticotroph (ACTH-secreting) cells in either the pars distalis or the pars intermedia of dogs. These neoplasms cause a clinical syndrome of cortisol excess (Cushing's disease). These neoplasms are encountered most frequently in dogs, particularly in adult to aged boxers, Boston terriers, and dachshunds.

The pituitary gland is consistently enlarged (Fig. 6-2); however, neither the occurrence nor the severity of functional disturbances appear to be directly related to the size of the neoplasm. Because the diaphragma sella is incomplete in the dog, the line of least resistance favors dorsal expansion of the gradually enlarging pituitary gland mass. This results in invagination into the infundibular cavity, dilation of the infundibular recess and the third ventricle with eventual compression or replacement of the hypothalamus, and possible extension of the neoplasm into the thalamus (Fig. 6-1).

Bilateral enlargement of the adrenal glands occurs in dogs with functional corticotroph adenomas (Fig. 6-2). This enlargement is due to cortical hyperplasia, primarily of the zona fasciculata and zona reticularis. Nodules of yellow-orange cortical tissue often are found outside the capsule as well as extending down into and compressing the adrenal medulla.

Pituitary corticotroph adenomas are composed of well-differentiated, large or small, chromophobic cells supported by fine connective tissue septa. The cytoplasm of the neoplastic cells usually is devoid of secretory granules, but stains immunocytochemically for ACTH and MSH. Hormone-containing secretory granules can be demonstrated by electron microscopy in functional corticotroph adenomas of dogs.

Endocrinologically Inactive Chromophobe Adenoma

Nonfunctional pituitary neoplasms occur in dogs, cats, laboratory rodents, and parakeets but are uncommon in other species. Although chromophobe adenomas seem endocrinologically inactive, they can cause significant functional disturbances and clinical signs by virtue of

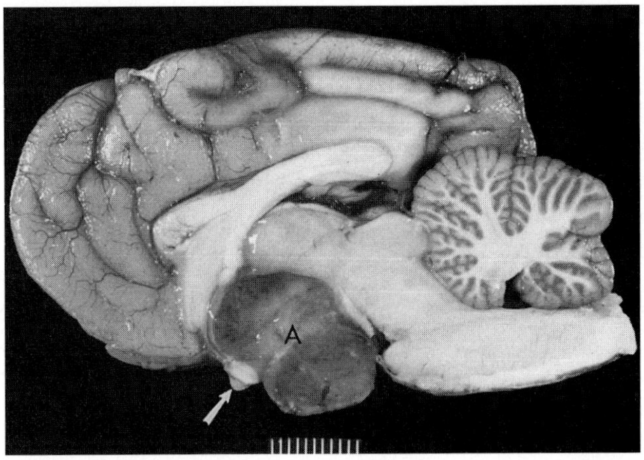

Figure 6-10 Pituitary gland; dog. Adenoma. A large pituitary adenoma *(A)* extends dorsally and compresses the overlying brain. The optic chiasm *(white arrow)* also is severely compressed. The adenohypophysis, neurohypophysis, and hypothalamus have been destroyed by the neoplasm. Bar = 1 cm.

compression atrophy of adjacent portions of the pituitary gland and dorsal extension into the overlying brain (Fig. 6-10). The clinical disturbances result either from the lack of secretion of pituitary trophic hormones and diminished target organ function (e.g., adrenal cortex; see Fig. 6-1) or dysfunction of the CNS. Affected animals often have decreased spontaneous activity, have incoordination and other disturbances of balance, are weak, and sometimes collapse after exercise. Chronically affected animals are blind and have dilated and fixed pupils due to compression and disruption of the optic nerves by dorsal extension of the pituitary neoplasms (Fig. 6-10). Endocrinologically inactive pituitary adenomas often become large before they cause clinical signs or kill the animal (see Figs. 6-1 and 6-10).

Clinical signs associated with nonfunctional pituitary adenomas and hypopituitarism are not specific and could be confused with other disorders of the CNS, such as brain neoplasms and encephalitis, or with chronic renal disease. There is no effect on body stature associated with compression of the pars distalis and interference with growth hormone secretion, because these neoplasms usually arise in adult animals that have already completed their growth. However, atrophy of the skin and loss of muscle mass could be related, in part, to a lack of the protein anabolic effects of growth hormone. Interference with the secretion of pituitary trophic hormones often leads to a reduced basal metabolic rate due to decreased TSH secretion and to hypoglycemia because of trophic atrophy of the adrenal cortex (see Fig. 6-1).

Craniopharyngioma

Craniopharyngioma is a benign neoplasm that is derived from epithelial remnants of the oropharyngeal ectoderm of the craniopharyngeal duct (Rathke's pouch). It often occurs in animals younger than those with other types of pituitary neoplasms and is present in either a suprasellar or infrasellar location. Craniopharyngioma is one cause of panhypopituitarism and dwarfism in young dogs, since it causes subnormal secretion of somatotrophin and other trophic hormones at an early age, before closure of the growth plates.

It has been proposed recently that some pleomorphic neoplasms in the suprasellar region of younger dogs be classified as germ cell tumors rather than craniopharyngiomas. The diagnosis of germ cell tumors was based on three criteria: (1) midline suprasellar location, (2) presence within the tumor of several distinct cell types (one population resembling a seminoma or dysgerminoma and others suggesting teratomatous differentiation into secretory glandular and squamous elements), and (3) positive staining for alpha-fetoprotein.

Craniopharyngiomas and suprasellar germ cell tumors often are large and grow along the ventral aspect of the brain, where they can surround several cranial nerves. In addition, they extend dorsally into the hypothalamus and thalamus (Fig. 6-11). The resulting clinical signs often are due to a combination of the following:

1. A lack of secretion of pituitary trophic hormones resulting in trophic atrophy and subnormal function of the adrenal cortex and thyroid gland, atrophy of the gonads, and failure to attain somatic maturation due to a lack of secretion of growth hormone
2. Disturbances in water metabolism (polyuria, polydipsia, low urine specific gravity, and osmolality) from an interference in the synthesis and release of antidiuretic hormone (ADH) by the large neoplasm
3. Deficits in cranial nerve function
4. CNS dysfunction due to extension into the overlying brain.

Microscopically, craniopharyngiomas have alternating solid and cystic areas. The solid areas are composed of nests of epithelial cells (cuboidal, columnar, or squamous) with focal areas of mineralization. The cystic spaces are lined by either columnar or squamous cells and contain keratin debris and colloid.

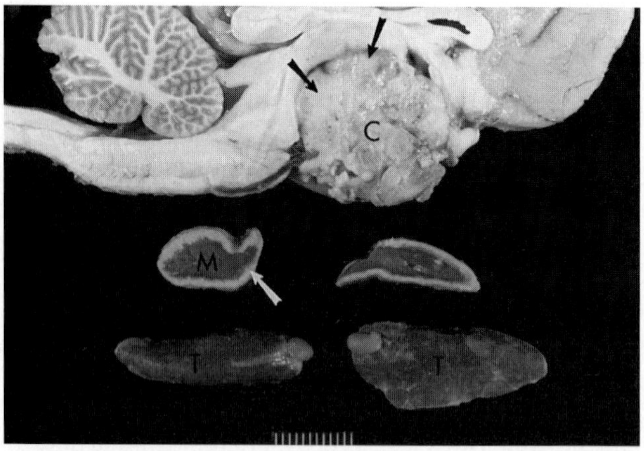

Figure 6-11 Pituitary area, adrenal glands, thyroid glands; dog. Craniopharyngioma. The neoplasm has extended dorsally through the hypothalamus and compresses the thalamus *(black arrows)*. The neoplasm has also destroyed the adenohypophysis and neurohypophysis, resulting in severe trophic atrophy of the adrenal cortex *(white arrow)*. The adrenal glands consist predominantly of medulla *(M)* surrounded by a thin rim of cortex (capsule plus zona glomerulosa). Although the thyroid follicular cells are atrophic, the overall gland *(T)* size is within normal limits because of colloid involution of the follicles. Bar = 1 cm.

Pituitary Gland Carcinoma

Pituitary gland carcinomas are uncommon neoplasms compared with adenomas but have been seen in older dogs and cows. They usually are endocrinologically inactive, but can cause significant functional disturbances by destruction of the pars distalis and neurohypophyseal system, leading to panhypopituitarism and diabetes insipidus. Carcinomas are large and invade extensively into the overlying brain, along the ventral aspect of the cranial cavity, and into the sphenoid bone of the sella turcica where they cause osteolysis. Metastases occur infrequently to regional lymph nodes or to distant sites such as the spleen or liver. Carcinomas are highly cellular and often have large areas of hemorrhage and necrosis. Giant cells, nuclear pleomorphism, and mitotic figures are encountered more frequently than in adenomas.

DISORDERS OF NEUROHYPOPHYSIS

Diabetes Insipidus

Diabetes insipidus results when inadequate ADH is produced or target cells in the kidneys lack the biochemical pathways necessary to respond to the secretion of normal or increased circulating concentrations of ADH. The hypophyseal form of diabetes insipidus results from compression and destruction of the pars nervosa, infundibular stalk, or supraoptic nucleus in the hypothalamus. The disruption of ADH synthesis or secretion in hypophyseal diabetes insipidus results from a large pituitary neoplasm, a dorsally expanding cyst, or inflammatory granuloma, and by traumatic injury to the skull with hemorrhage and glial proliferation in the neurohypophyseal tissues. Compression or disruption of the posterior lobe, infundibular stalk, and hypothalamus by neoplastic cells interrupts the transport of ADH in nonmyelinated axons from its site of production, primarily in the supraoptic nucleus of the hypothalamus, to the site of release in the capillary plexus of the pars nervosa.

Animals with diabetes insipidus excrete large volumes of hypotonic urine, which in turn obliges them to drink equally large amounts of water to prevent dehydration and hyperosmolality of body fluids. Urine osmolality is decreased below normal plasma osmolality (approximately 300 mOsm/kg) in both hypophyseal and nephrogenic forms of diabetes insipidus. In response to water deprivation, urine osmolality remains below that of the plasma in both forms of diabetes insipidus in contrast to increased osmolality observed in normal animals. Urine osmolality is increased above that of plasma in response to exogenous ADH in the hypophyseal form, but this increase does not occur in nephrogenic diabetes insipidus, a useful feature in differential diagnosis.

ADRENAL CORTEX

Structure and Function

The adrenal glands of mammals consist of two distinct parts that differ not only in morphology and function but also in embryologic origin. Because of their close structural relationships, the outer cortex and inner medulla of the adrenal glands usually have been considered parts of one organ. The adrenal cortex develops from cells of the coelomic epithelium that are of mesodermal origin. The chromaffin tissue and sympathetic ganglion cells of the adrenal medulla are derived from ectoderm of the neural crest.

The adrenal cortex of normal dogs is firm, yellow, and of nearly uniform thickness. The soft, brown medulla is surrounded by the cortex. In normal dogs the cortical/medulla ratio is approximately 2:1. The adrenal glands are richly vascularized, and a sinusoidal network about the cell columns of the adrenal cortex empties into the venous tree at the periphery of the medulla.

The adrenal cortex microscopically and functionally is subdivided into three layers or zones, although the demarcation between zones often is not distinct. The zona glomerulosa (multiformis) (outer zone) is composed of columns of cells adjacent to the capsule that have a sigmoid or arclike arrangement. It represents about 10% to 15% of the cortex and is responsible for the secretion of mineralocorticoid hormones. The secretory cells of the zona fasciculata (middle zone) are arranged in long anastomosing cords separated by numerous small capillaries. This zone comprises about 65% to 70% of the cortex, is composed of cells that contain abundant cytoplasmic lipid, and is responsible for the secretion of the glucocorticoid hormones. The zona reticularis (inner zone) accounts for the remaining 15% of the cortex. The secretory cells, arranged in small groups surrounded by capillaries, are responsible for the secretion of sex steroids.

Mineralocorticoids are adrenal steroids that principally affect ion transport by epithelial cells and cause excretion of potassium and conservation of sodium. The most potent and important naturally occurring mineralocorticoid is aldosterone. The enzymatically controlled electrolyte "pumps" in epithelial cells of the renal tubule and sweat glands respond to mineralocorticoids by conserving sodium and chloride and by excreting potassium. In the distal convoluted tubule of the mammalian nephron, a cation-exchange mechanism is responsible for the resorption of sodium from the glomerular filtrate and secretion of potassium into the lumen. These reactions are accelerated by mineralocorticoids but still proceed, although at a much slower rate, in their absence (Fig. 6-12). A lack of secretion of mineralocorticoids (such as in the Addison's-like disease of dogs) can result in a lethal retention of potassium and loss of sodium (Fig. 6-12).

Cortisol and lesser amounts of corticosterone are the most important naturally occurring glucocorticoid hormones secreted by the adrenal glands in many animal species. In general, the actions of glucocorticoids on carbohydrate, protein, and lipid metabolism result in a sparing of glucose and a tendency to hyperglycemia and increased glucose production. In addition, glucocorticoids decrease lipogenesis and increase lipolysis in adipose tissue, which results in release of glycerol and free fatty acids.

Glucocorticoids also function to suppress both inflammatory and immunologic responses and, thereby, reduce the associated necrosis and fibroplasia. However, under

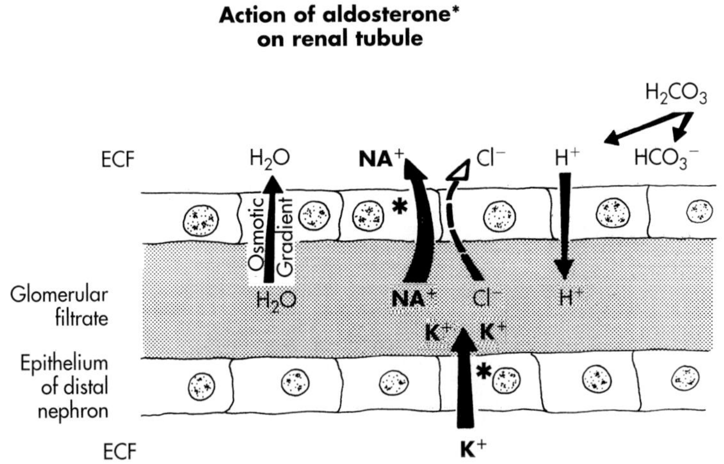

Figure 6-12 Aldosterone secreted by the zona glomerulosa of the adrenal cortex acts on the distal portions of the nephron to increase tubular excretion of potassium and increase resorption of sodium (and secondarily chloride). The resulting osmotic gradient facilitates movement of water from the glomerular filtrate into the extracellular fluid.

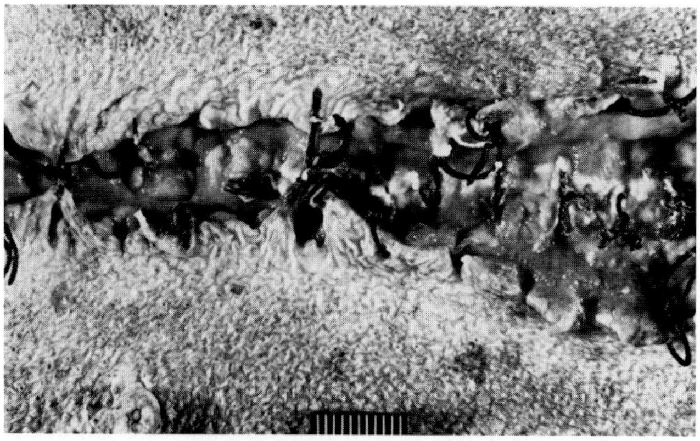

Figure 6-13 Skin; dog. Dehiscence of surgical wound. Wounds heal slowly in dogs with cortisol excess because of an inhibition of fibroblastic proliferation. Bar = 1 cm.

the influence of increased concentrations of glucocorticoids, an animal has reduced resistance to bacterial, viral, and fungal diseases. Glucocorticoids can impair the immunologic response at any stage from the initial interaction and processing of antigens by cells of the macrophage-monocyte system through the induction and proliferation of immunocompetent lymphocytes and subsequent antibody production. Inhibition by glucocorticoids of a number of functions of lymphoid cells forms part of the basis for suppression of the immunologic response.

Glucocorticoids exert a profound negative effect on wound healing. Dogs with hypercortisolism can have wound dehiscence (Fig. 6-13). The basic mechanism is inhibition of fibroblast proliferation and collagen synthesis, leading to a decrease in scar tissue formation.

Sex hormones (e.g., progesterone, estrogens, and androgens) are synthesized in small amounts by secretory cells of the zona reticularis of the adrenal cortex. An excessive secretion of adrenal sex steroids associated with a neoplasm arising in the zona reticularis can occur infrequently, resulting in clinical manifestations of virilism, precocious sexual development, or feminization (effects dependent on which steroid is secreted in excess, the sex of the patient, and the age at onset).

Developmental Disturbances

Hypoplasia of the adrenal cortex is seen secondary to maldevelopment of the hypophysis associated with anencephaly, in some cases of cyclopia, and in hypophyseal aplasia. The adrenal cortices are small but the adrenal medulla is normal.

Degenerative and Inflammatory Lesions

Calcification of the Adrenal Glands

Extensive deposits of calcium salts occur frequently in the adrenal glands of adult cats. The cause is unknown. The calcium deposits, although often bilateral and extensive, usually are not associated with clinical signs. A few dogs with extensive calcification and degeneration of the adrenal glands die suddenly after relatively minor stress. Extensively calcified adrenal glands are coarsely nodular, firm, and mottled, and have multiple, yellow-white, gritty foci throughout the cortex. Some have large areas of necrosis with calcium deposits adjacent to areas of nodular regenerative hyperplasia. These hypertrophic cortical cells have abundant lipid in their expanded cytoplasmic area and appear to be able to maintain near-normal blood cortisol concentrations.

Amyloid

Amyloid deposition in the adrenal glands occurs in all species and usually involves only the cortex. The affected adrenal cortices often are widened and the amyloid deposits are grossly visible as translucent areas. Amyloid deposition begins around the sinusoids in the inner portions of the zona fasciculata and often is largely confined to this zone. Signs of adrenal cortical insufficiency usually are not observed.

Adrenalitis

Bacterial and parasitic agents frequently localize in the adrenal glands and produce varying degrees of inflammation and necrosis. Focal inflammations usually are suppurative, arising in the course of bacterial septicemias. The adrenal capsule provides an effective barrier against direct invasion by inflammatory reactions in adjacent tissue. Granulomatous adrenalitis due to *Histoplasma capsulatum, Coccidioides immitis,* or *Cryptococcus neoformans* occasionally occurs in dogs and cats. Multiple granulomas with central areas of necrosis and calcification can destroy nearly the entire adrenal cortex. *Toxoplasma gondii* produces necrosis with an infiltration of histiocytes in the adrenal cortex of many species of animals. Experimental evidence suggests that the large local concentration of antiinflammatory steroids in the adrenal cortex (e.g., cortisol and corticosterone) suppresses local cell-mediated immunity and permits the progressive growth of certain fungi (e.g., *H. capsulatum, C. immitis*), protozoa (e.g., *Babesia darlingi, B. jellisoni,* or *Toxoplasma gondii*), and bacteria (e.g., *Mycobacterium tuberculosis*).

Hyperplasia and Neoplasia of Adrenal Cortex

Accessory Adrenal Tissue

Accessory cortical nodules are common in the adrenal glands of adult to aged animals and are found in the capsule, cortex, and medulla. Many of these nodules arise either as evaginations of the cortex into the capsule and surrounding periadrenal fat or invaginations of the cortex into the medulla.

Hyperplasia

Nodular hyperplasia is common in the adrenal glands as well-defined spherical nodules in the cortex or attached to the capsule (Fig. 6-14). Hyperplastic nodules are usually

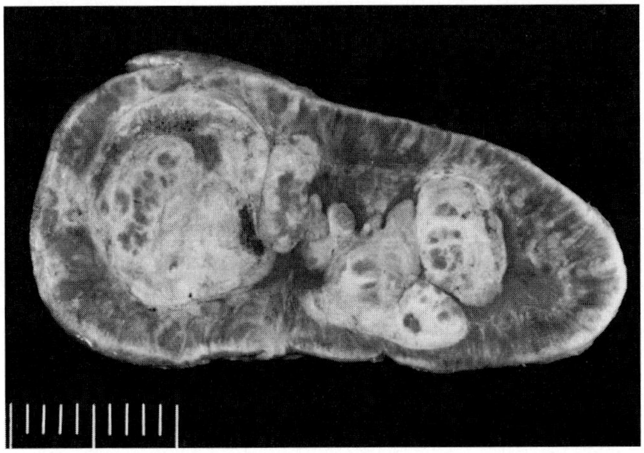

Figure 6-14 Adrenal gland; dog. Nodular adrenal cortical hyperplasia. Multiple discrete nodules of cortical hyperplasia extend into the medulla. Bar = 1 cm.

multiple, bilateral, and yellow and involve any of the three zones of the cortex. Histologically, the nodules near the capsule resemble zona multiformis (glomerulosa) and sometimes have areas that resemble zona fasciculata. The lipid content in these hyperplastic nodules is retained in circumstances that reduce the amount of lipid in the normal adrenal cortex. Hyperplastic cortical nodules are most common in older horses, dogs, and cats. Nodular hyperplasia of the zona reticularis has been seen in animals with functional disturbances suggestive of androgen excess (e.g., greater muscle mass, well-developed crest, hypertrophy of clitoris, and involution of mammary gland).

Diffuse cortical hyperplasia results in a uniform, usually bilateral, enlargement of the adrenal cortices. Marked hypertrophy and hyperplasia of cells of the zona fasciculata and zona reticularis occur in response to an autonomous hypersecretion of ACTH by a corticotroph adenoma of the pituitary gland (Fig. 6-2). The cytoplasm of the hyperplastic cells of the zona fasciculata is vacuolated because of the lipid content. Cells of the outer zona multiformis (glomerulosa) can be compressed by the expansion of the inner two zones. Nodular hyperplasia can be present in a diffusely hyperplastic cortex.

Cortical Adenomas

Adenomas of the adrenal cortex occur most frequently in older dogs and only sporadically in horses, cattle, and sheep. Castrated male goats have a greater incidence of cortical adenomas than intact males. Although usually incidental findings at necropsy, the neoplasms occasionally are endocrinologically active. Cortical adenomas are well demarcated, usually a single nodule in one adrenal gland. Larger cortical adenomas are yellow to red, distort the contour of the gland, compress the adjacent cortical parenchyma, and are partially or completely encapsulated. Cortical adenomas often develop in an adrenal gland with multiple nodules of hyperplasia and adenomas are difficult to differentiate grossly from hyperplastic nodules. However, nodular hyperplasia consists of multiple small foci, usually in both adrenal glands with no encapsulation, and, often, associated with extracapsular nodules of hyperplastic cortical tissue. Cortical adenomas are composed of well-differentiated cells that resemble secretory cells of the normal zona fasciculata or zona reticularis. The abundant cytoplasm of neoplastic cells is lightly eosinophilic, often vacuolated, and filled with lipid droplets. Adenomas are partially or completely surrounded by a fibrous connective tissue capsule of varying thickness and a rim of compressed cortical parenchyma with collapsed stroma.

Cortical Carcinomas

Adrenal cortical carcinomas occur less frequently than adenomas and have been reported most often in cattle and older dogs but occur infrequently in other species. Carcinomas develop in adult to older dogs with no apparent breed or sex prevalence. Adrenal carcinomas are larger than adenomas and are more likely to be bilateral. In dogs, they are composed of a variegated, yellow-red, friable tissue and can invade extensively into surrounding tissues and into the wall of the caudal vena cava resulting in thrombus formation. Carcinomas attain considerable size in cattle (up to 10 cm or more in diameter) and have multiple areas of calcification or ossification.

Carcinomas are composed of more highly pleomorphic secretory cells than adenomas and are subdivided by a fine fibrovascular stroma. The affected adrenal gland usually is obliterated completely by the carcinoma. The pattern of growth of neoplastic cells varies between neoplasms and within the same carcinoma and includes trabecular, lobular, and focal. Neoplastic cells usually are large and polyhedral and have prominent nucleoli and densely eosinophilic or vacuolated cytoplasm.

Carcinomas and adenomas of the adrenal cortex in dogs occasionally are functional and secrete excessive amounts of cortisol. The clinical syndrome produced by excessive secretion by adrenal cortical carcinomas can be complicated by signs produced by compression of adjacent organs where the neoplasm is large, by invasion into the aorta or caudal vena cava that can lead to intraabdominal hemorrhage, and by metastases to distant sites (e.g., liver, kidneys, mesenteric lymph nodes, and lungs). Functional cortical adenomas and carcinomas are responsible for the severe atrophy of the adrenal cortex of the contralateral adrenal gland because of negative feedback inhibition of the pituitary ACTH secretion by the increased blood cortisol concentrations. The atrophic cortex consists primarily of the adrenal capsule and zona glomerulosa (multiformis) (Fig. 6-15). Atrophy is also present in the remnants of the adrenal cortex compressed by functional adenomas. The adrenal medulla appears more prominent because of the lack of cortical tissue (Fig. 6-15).

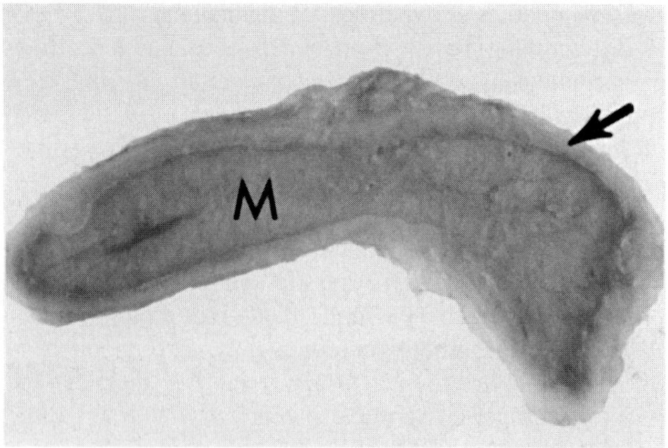

Figure 6-15 Adrenal gland; dog. Cortical atrophy. The adrenal cortex is markedly thinned *(arrow)* as a result of severe trophic atrophy and consists of the zona glomerulosa and a thickened fibrous capsule. The adrenal medulla *(M)* is relatively more prominent because of the trophic atrophy of the cortex.

Adrenal Gland Neoplasms in Ferrets

Adrenal gland neoplasms are being recognized with greater frequency in ferrets as more are being kept as pets and living longer. The adrenal gland enlargements are either bilateral (approximately 45%) as a result of diffuse (most frequent) or nodular hyperplasia or unilateral (approximately 55%) as a result of adrenal cortical carcinoma or cortical adenoma. Clinical signs in ferrets with adrenal cortical neoplasms include vulvar enlargement, bilaterally symmetric alopecia especially on the ventral abdomen and medial aspects of the rear legs, polyuria, polydipsia, and the presence of a palpable mass at the cranial pole of the kidneys (left side greater frequency than right). Adrenal gland neoplasms develop in adult ferrets (mean age 5 years) with females more frequently affected than males (sex ratio ≥2:1). The history frequently includes the information that the ferrets underwent gonadectomy at an early age (5 or 6 weeks). Other functional disturbances including anemia, thrombocytopenia, pyometra, and endometrial hyperplasia are consistent with an overproduction of estrogenic steroids by the adrenal gland neoplasms. Some of the functional disturbances resemble those seen in intact females with persistent or prolonged estrus; ferrets are seasonally polyestrous and are induced ovulators. About one third of ferrets with adrenal cortical neoplasms also have neoplasms derived from the insulin-producing beta cells of the pancreatic islets. These neoplasms can produce increased concentrations of serum insulin resulting in hypoglycemia that can lead to seizures, episodic lethargy, ptyalism, ataxia, and hind leg weakness.

The most consistent endocrinologic change in ferrets with adrenal gland neoplasms is increased plasma concentrations of estradiol-17β. It is presumed that the estradiol-17β is produced directly by the neoplastic cells, but an alternative possibility would be that the adrenal gland neoplasms secrete androgenic steroids that are aromatized in the skin and possibly elsewhere to estrogenic steroids. No increase in circulating estradiol-17β concentrations is found in response to exogenous ACTH, but plasma concentrations decrease after adrenalectomy. Plasma cortisol and corticosterone concentrations in ferrets with adrenal gland neoplasms either are in the normal range or below and are not increased greatly in response to exogenous ACTH. Plasma cortisol is not decreased after unilateral adrenalectomy, and the contralateral adrenal cortex is not atrophic as would be expected if the adrenal gland neoplasm was secreting excess cortisol. The clinical signs in ferrets with adrenal cortical neoplasms can be effectively reversed by adrenalectomy (especially of the left side if there is no macroscopic enlargement) but not by chemotherapy with mitotane (*o,p'*-DDD). Complete regrowth of hair usually occurs by 2 to 3 months after adrenalectomy.

Hypercortisolism (Cushing's Disease or Syndrome)

The clinical manifestations and lesions associated with the syndrome of hyperadrenocorticism primarily result from chronic overproduction of cortisol by hyperactive cells of adrenal cortices. Affected dogs develop a spectrum of functional disturbances and lesions from the combined glyconeogenetic, lipolytic, protein catabolic, and antiinflammatory effects of the glucocorticoid hormones on many organs. The disease is insidious and slowly progressive. Cortisol excess is one of the most common endocrinopathies in adult and aged dogs, occurs infrequently in cats, but rarely in other domestic animals.

The increase in circulating cortisol concentrations in dogs with hyperadrenocorticism can result from one of several different pathogenic mechanisms. The most common cause is a functional corticotroph (ACTH-secreting) adenoma of the pituitary gland that causes bilateral adrenal cortical hypertrophy and hyperplasia (see Fig. 6-2). The cortex of each adrenal gland is widened considerably as a result of diffuse and nodular hyperplasia, primarily in the zona fasciculata. Functional adrenal gland neoplasms are an infrequent (10% to 15% of cases) cause of the Cushing's syndrome of cortisol excess in the dog. Many of the clinical signs and lesions of the naturally occurring hyperadrenocorticism can be induced by the long-term, daily administration of large doses of corticosteroids, as in the treatment of other diseases. To accurately separate the different pathogenetic mechanisms responsible for cortisol excess, plasma cortisol concentrations must be evaluated with the animal in the basal state and after dexamethasone (large or small dose) suppression and ACTH stimulation.

Functional Disturbances and Lesions of Cortisol Excess

The appetite and intake of food often are increased as a direct result of either the hypercortisolism or damage due

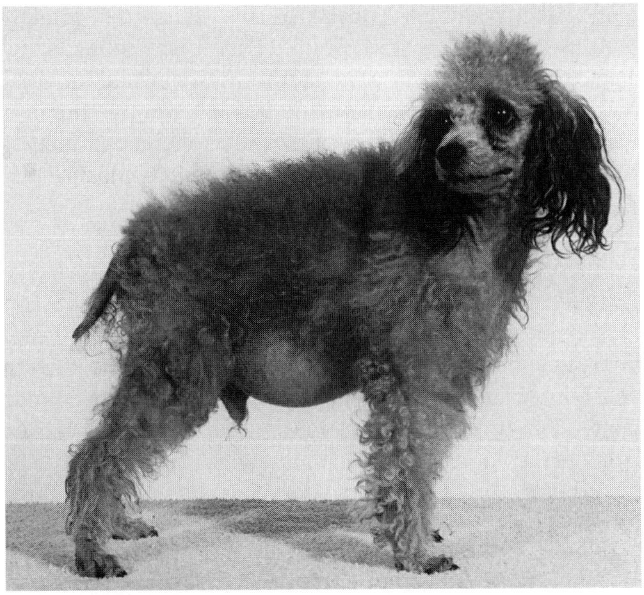

Figure 6-16 Cushing's-like disease of hypercortisolism in a poodle due to idiopathic adrenal cortical hyperplasia. Muscle asthenia is evident by the pendulous abdomen. Alopecia is present on the abdomen, ventral cervical region, and tail.

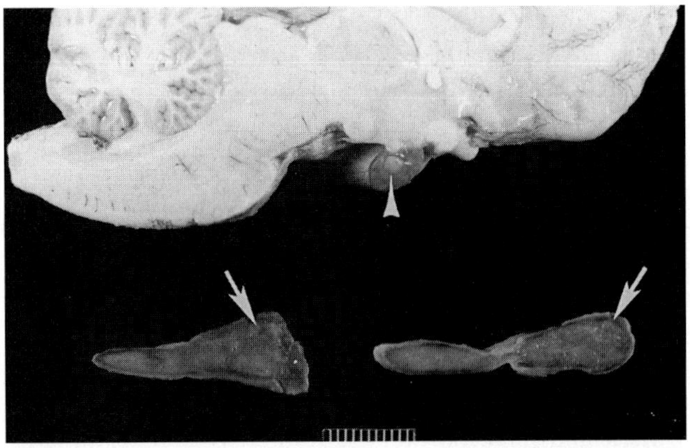

Figure 6-17 Brain stem and pituitary gland; adrenal glands; dog. Cortical atrophy. Bilateral atrophy of all three cortical layers *(white arrows)* is characteristic of hypoadrenocorticism. The pituitary gland *(white arrowhead)* was grossly normal with microscopic evidence of corticotroph hyperplasia. Bar = 1 cm.

to compression of hypothalamic appetite centers by a large dorsally expanding pituitary gland neoplasm. The muscles of the extremities and abdomen are weakened and atrophied, resulting in gradual abdominal enlargement (Fig. 6-16), lordosis, muscle trembling, and a straight-legged, skeletal-braced posture assumed to support the body's weight. Hepatomegaly caused by increased deposits of fat and glycogen can contribute to the development of the distended, often pendulous, abdomen. The muscular asthenia and wasting are the result of increased catabolism of structural proteins combined with diminished protein synthesis under the influence of long-term cortisol excess. Cutaneous lesions occur frequently in dogs with hyperadrenocorticism. The initial changes in the skin often are observed over points of wear (e.g., neck, flanks, behind the ears) and over bony prominences. These initial cutaneous changes spread in a bilaterally symmetric pattern to involve a significant percentage of the body surface. Cutaneous lesions caused by excessive cortisol include atrophy of the epidermis and pilosebaceous apparatus, combined with loss of collagen and elastin in the dermis and subcutis. Cutaneous calcification ("calcinosis cutis") is a characteristic lesion in dogs with hypercortisolism (up to 30%). Numerous calcium crystals are deposited along collagen and elastin fibers in the dermis and can protrude through the atrophic and thinned epidermis. These calcium deposits occur in dogs with normal blood calcium and phosphorus concentrations. This manifestation of hypercortisolism most likely is related to the glyconeogenetic and protein catabolic action of cortisol, resulting in the rearrangement of the molecular structure of such proteins as collagen and elastin, and the formation of an organic matrix that attracts and binds calcium. Severe calcification also occurs in other tissues such as the lungs, active skeletal muscles, and the wall of the stomach.

Hypoadrenocorticism (Addison's Disease)

Chronic adrenocortical insufficiency was the first recognized endocrine disease. Dogs with hypoadrenocorticism have bilateral adrenocortical atrophy involving all layers of the adrenal cortex. Production of all three classes of corticosteroids (mineralocorticoids, glucocorticoids, and adrenal sex steroids) is deficient. The adrenal cortex is reduced to one tenth or less of its normal thickness and consists primarily of the adrenal capsule (Fig. 6-17). Thus, the adrenal medulla becomes relatively more prominent and, along with the capsule, makes up the bulk of the remaining adrenal gland.

The precise pathogenesis of idiopathic adrenal cortical atrophy is unknown, but the lesion is most likely immune mediated. Early in the disease multiple foci of lymphocytes and plasma cells are interspersed between the adrenal sinusoids and parenchymal cells. The entire three zones of the cortex are nearly absent in dogs that die from untreated hypoadrenocorticism. The capsule is thickened by collapse of the adrenal cortex and fibroblastic proliferation. Pituitary gland lesions have not been observed in dogs with idiopathic adrenal cortical atrophy in which all three zones of the adrenal cortex are atrophic, including the zona multiformis (glomerulosa) that is not under ACTH control. By comparison, atrophy of the adrenal cortex due to a destructive pituitary gland lesion that decreases ACTH secretion is characterized by severe atrophy only of the inner two cortical zones. The zona multiformis remains intact (see Fig. 6-1), and these animals do not have electrolyte abnormalities since the secretion of aldosterone remains within normal limits.

Chronic adrenal gland insufficiency is recognized as a distinct and common endocrinopathy of dogs. Idiopathic adrenal cortical insufficiency occurs more frequently in young adult dogs and most likely has an immune-mediated pathogenesis. The synthesis and secretion of mineralocorticoids are reduced, resulting in marked alterations of serum potassium, sodium, and chloride concentrations. Less potassium is excreted by the kidneys (hypokaluria), resulting in a severe hyperkalemia (Fig. 6-12). Less sodium and chloride are reabsorbed from renal tubules, leading to varying degrees of hypernatremia and hyperchloruria and a corresponding decline in blood concentrations of these ions. The severe hyperkalemia frequently produces marked cardiovascular disturbances. The pronounced bradycardia that develops in some dogs (heart rate of 50 or fewer beats per minute) does not change with exercise, but does predispose to weakness and circulatory collapse after minimal exertion.

A decreased production of glucocorticoids results in several characteristic functional disturbances of hypoadrenocorticism. A failure of gluconeogenesis and increased sensitivity to insulin contributes to the development of moderate hypoglycemia. Hyperpigmentation of the skin occurs in some dogs with long-standing adrenocortical insufficiency and is a common finding in Addison's disease of human beings. This lesion results from a lack of negative feedback on the pituitary gland and the increased release of ACTH (and possibly MSH). The plasma cortisol concentrations in dogs with hypoadrenocorticism are low and range from 0.1 to 1.5 μg/dl. Because of the severe atrophy of the adrenal cortex, little or no increase in blood cortisol concentration results after the administration of ACTH.

ADRENAL MEDULLA

The adrenal medulla is derived from neuroectoderm of the neural crest and produces catecholamine hormones. The main biosynthetic pathway for catecholamines in mammals starts with tyrosine that is converted first to 1-dihydroxyphenylalanine (dopa) by tyrosine hydroxylase. Dopa is then decarboxylated to 3,4-dihydroxyphenylethylamine (dopamine) by 3,4-amino acid decarboxylase and the dopamine, which subsequently undergoes beta-hydroxylation (by dopamine beta-oxidase) to norepinephrine. In mammals the medulla is completely surrounded by the adrenal cortex, and venous blood from the cortex bathes the medullary cells. This blood has the greatest concentration of corticosteroids of any fluid in the body. This close anatomic association between the adrenal cortex and medulla in mammals is not fortuitous because the *N*-methylating enzyme (phenylethanolamine-*N*-methyl transferase) that converts norepinephrine to epinephrine is corticosteroid hormone dependent.

Proliferative Lesions

Adrenal Medullary Hyperplasia

Diffuse or nodular adrenal medullary hyperplasia appears to precede the development of pheochromocytoma in bulls and human beings with C cell neoplasms of the thyroid gland. The proliferated chromaffin cells are nonencapsulated but compress the surrounding adrenal cortex. The hyperplastic cells are round to oval and have a lightly basophilic cytoplasm. Some bulls with prominent diffuse medullary hyperplasia often have a few small nodules of proliferated medullary cells (Fig. 6-18). Medullary hyperplasia is diagnosed on the basis of these criteria: an increased adrenal weight, a decrease in corticomedullary

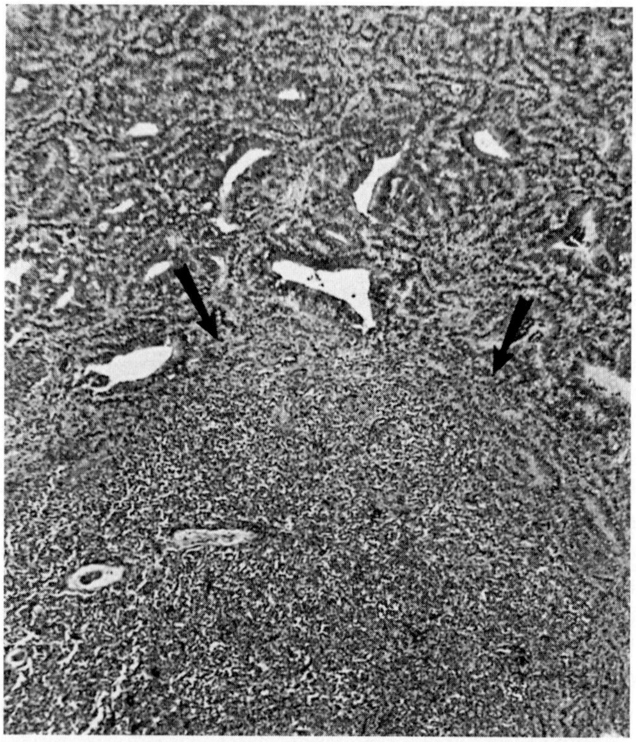

Figure 6-18 Adrenal medulla; bull. Bilateral diffuse hyperplasia of adrenal medulla in a bull with a concomitant C cell carcinoma of the thyroid gland. The expanded adrenal medulla *(bottom)* compress the surrounding adrenal cortex *(arrows)*. H & E stain. *Yarrington JT, Capen CC. Ultrastructural and biochemical evaluation of adrenal medullary hyperplasia and pheochromocytoma in aged bulls. Vet Pathol 1981; 18:316-325.*

tyrosine —(tyrosine hydroxylase)→ 1-dihydroxyphenylalanine (dopa) —(3,4-amino acid decarboxylase)→ 3,4-dihydroxyphenyl-ethylamine (dopamine) —(dopamine beta-oxidase)→ norepineph ratio due to an increase in the size and number of medullary cells, and numerous mitotic figures in the adrenal medulla.

Neoplasms

Neuroblastomas and Ganglioneuromas

Neuroblastomas usually occur in young animals, arise from primitive neuroectodermal cells, and form a large intraabdominal mass. Ganglioneuromas usually are small neoplasms that have well-differentiated multipolar ganglion cells and neurofibrils. Neuroblastomas are composed of small neoplastic cells that have a hyperchromatic nucleus and a scant amount of cytoplasm and thus resemble lymphocytes. They tend to aggregate about vessels to form pseudorosettes. Neurofibrils or unmyelinated nerve fibers can be demonstrated in neuroblastomas.

Ganglioneuromas are benign neoplasms composed of multipolar ganglion cells and neurofibrils and have a prominent fibrous connective tissue stroma. The surrounding adrenal cortex is often severely compressed. Occasionally, neoplastic cells in adrenal medullary neoplasms differentiate into two cell lines, resulting in pheochromocytoma and ganglioneuroma in the same adrenal gland.

Pheochromocytoma

Pheochromocytomas are the most common neoplasms in the adrenal medulla of animals, occurring most often in cattle and dogs and infrequently in other species. Pheochromocytomas in bulls and human beings sometimes develop concurrently with calcitonin-secreting C cell neoplasms of the thyroid gland. Malignant pheochromocytomas invade through the capsule of an adrenal gland and into adjacent structures (e.g., caudal vena cava) or metastasize to distant sites (e.g., liver, regional lymph nodes, or lungs).

Pheochromocytomas are neoplasms of catecholamine-secreting ("chromaffin") cells. They usually are located in the adrenal medulla of animals (rarely can be located at extraadrenal sites in the abdomen) and are unilateral or bilateral. Pheochromocytomas often are large (10 cm or more in diameter) and replace most of the affected adrenal gland. Smaller neoplasms are completely surrounded by a thin, compressed rim of adrenal cortex. Large pheochromocytomas are multilobular and are variegated and light brown to yellow-red, as a result of areas of hemorrhage and necrosis.

Neoplastic cells in pheochromocytomas vary from small, round to polyhedral cells to large pleomorphic cells with multiple hyperchromatic nuclei. The cytoplasm is lightly eosinophilic, finely granular, and often indistinct. Pheochromocytomas are composed of either epinephrine- or norepinephrine-secreting cells or both cell types.

Functional pheochromocytomas have been reported infrequently in animals. Tachycardia, edema, and cardiac hypertrophy observed in several dogs and horses with pheochromocytomas were attributed to excessive catecholamine secretion. Arteriolar sclerosis and widespread medial hyperplasia of arterioles has been reported in dogs with pheochromocytomas and clinical signs suggestive of paroxysmal hypertension. Hypertension was detected in 43% of dogs with pheochromocytomas; all hypertensive dogs had concurrent diseases that could have contributed to the increase in blood pressure. Infrequently, hyperadrenocorticism occurs concurrently in dogs with pheochromocytoma and could contribute to the development of hypertension, particularly during digital manipulation of the affected adrenal gland during surgery.

Norepinephrine is the principal catecholamine extracted from pheochromocytomas in dogs. This is similar to the finding in normal pups, in which norepinephrine is the predominant catecholamine; in adult dogs, epinephrine predominates in adrenal medullary tissues. The catecholamine content of pheochromocytomas in bulls with concurrent C cell neoplasms of the thyroid gland was greater than in the normal adrenal medulla. Urinary excretion of vanillylmandelic acid and free unconjugated catecholamines are increased in bulls with pheochromocytomas.

THYROID GLAND

Thyroid Follicular Cells

The thyroid gland in most animal species occurs as two lobes on the lateral surfaces of the trachea. In pigs, the main lobe of the thyroid gland is on the midline in the ventral cervical region with dorsolateral projections from each side. In dogs, the right lobe of the thyroid gland is situated slightly cranial to the left lobe and almost touches the caudal aspect of the larynx.

The thyroid gland is the largest of the endocrine organs that function exclusively as an endocrine gland. The basic histologic structure of the thyroid gland is unique among endocrine glands and consists of follicles of varying size (20 to 250 μm) that contain colloid produced by the follicular cells. The follicular cells are cuboidal to columnar, and are orientated so that their secretory pole is directed toward the lumen of the follicle. An extensive network of interfollicular and intrafollicular capillaries provides the follicular cells with an abundant blood supply. Follicular cells have extensive profiles of rough endoplasmic reticulum for synthesis and a large Golgi apparatus for packaging of substantial amounts of protein that are then transported into the follicular lumen. The luminal side of follicular cells in contact with the colloid is modified by the formation of numerous microvilli (Fig. 6-19).

The synthesis of thyroid hormones is unique among those of the endocrine glands because the final assembly of hormone occurs extracellularly within the follicular lumen. Follicular cells trap essential raw materials, such as iodide from the blood by a sodium-iodide symporter in the basolateral plasma membrane, transport them rapidly against a concentration gradient to the lumen, where the

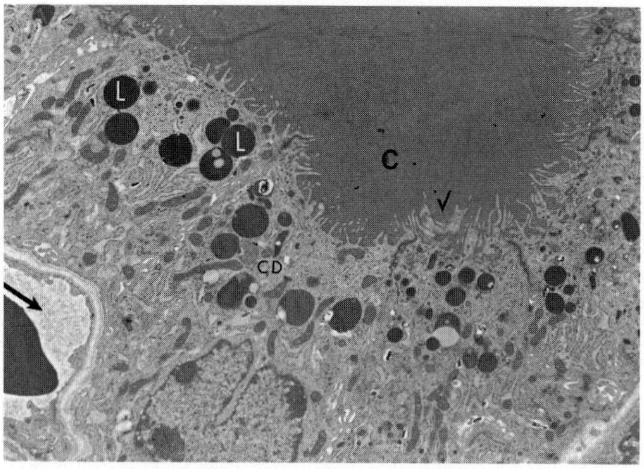

Figure 6-19 Thyroid gland; normal dog. Thyroid follicular cells with long microvilli *(V)* that extend into the colloid *(C)* in follicular lumen. Numerous lysosomes *(L)* and colloid droplets *(CD)* are present in the apical portion of the follicular cells. An interfollicular capillary *(arrow)* is present at the base of the follicle. TEM.

iodine is oxidized by thyroperoxidase in the microvilli to reactive iodine (I_2) (Fig. 6-20). The assembly of thyroid hormones within the follicular lumen is made possible by a unique protein (thyroglobulin). Thyroglobulin is a high-molecular-weight (600,000 to 750,000 daltons) glycoprotein synthesized in successive subunits on the ribosomes of the endoplasmic reticulum in follicular cells. The constituent amino acids (tyrosine and others) and carbohydrates (i.e., mannose, fructose, galactose) are derived from the circulation. Recently synthesized thyroglobulin (17S) leaves the Golgi apparatus and is packaged into apical vesicles that are extruded into the follicular lumen (Fig. 6-20). The amino acid tyrosine, an essential component of thyroid hormones, is incorporated within the molecular structure of thyroglobulin. Iodine is bound to tyrosyl residues in thyroglobulin at the apical surface of follicular cells to form, successively, monoiodotyrosine (MIT) and diiodotyrosine (DIT). The resulting MIT and DIT combine to form the two biologically active iodothyronines (thyroxine [T_4], triiodothyronine [T_3]) secreted by the thyroid gland.

The secretion of thyroid hormones into the bloodstream from colloid is initiated by elongation of microvilli and formation of pseudopodia on the luminal surface follicular cells. These elongated cytoplasmic projections are increased in response to pituitary thyrotropin (TSH), extend into the follicular lumen, and indiscriminately phagocytose adjacent colloid. Colloid droplets within follicular cells fuse with numerous lysosomes. T_3 and T_4 are released from the thyroglobulin molecule, diffuse from the follicular cell, and enter into adjacent capillaries. Negative feedback control of thyroid hormone secretion is accomplished by the coordinated response by the adenohypophysis and certain hypothalamic nuclei to circulating concentrations of T_4 and T_3.

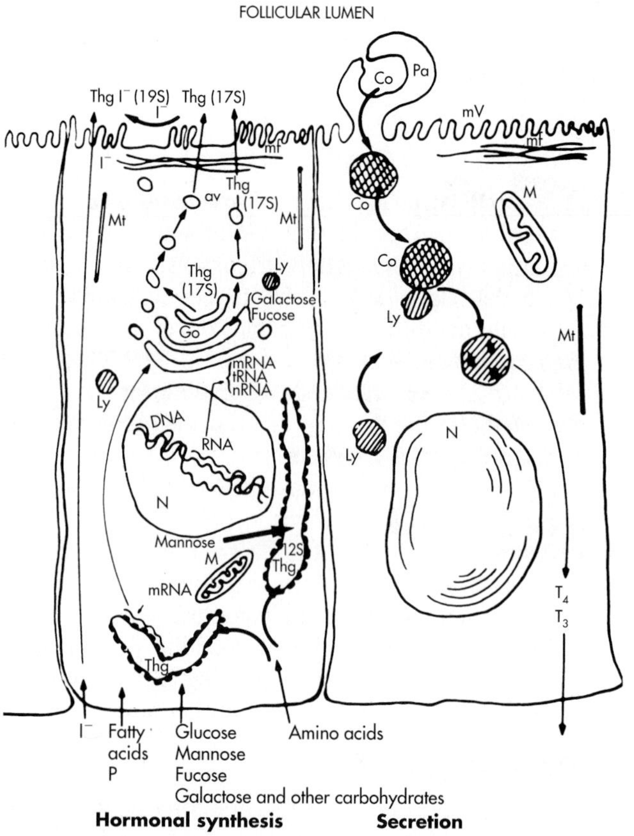

Figure 6-20 Thyroid follicular cells illustrating two-way traffic of materials from capillaries into the follicular lumen. Raw materials, such as iodine, are concentrated by follicular cells and rapidly transported into the lumen (*left side* of drawing). Amino acids (tyrosine and others) and sugars are assembled by follicular cells into thyroglobulin, packaged into apical vesicles *(av)* and released into the lumen. The iodination of tyrosyl residues with the thyroglobulin molecule to form thyroid hormones occurs within the follicular lumen. Elongation of microvilli and endocytosis of colloid by follicular cells occur in response to TSH stimulation (*right side* of drawing). The intracellular colloid droplets *(Co)* fuse with lysosomal bodies *(Ly)*, active thyroid hormone is enzymatically cleaved from thyroglobulin, and free T_4 and T_3 are released into the circulation. *Bastenie PA, Ermans AM, Bonnyns M, et al. Lymphocytic thyroiditis as an autoimmune disease. In: Good RA, Day SB, Yunis JJ, eds. Molecular pathology. Springfield, IL: Charles C Thomas, 1975.*

Thyrotropin (TTH or TSH) is conveyed to thyroid follicular cells where it binds to the basilar aspect of the cell, activates adenyl cyclase, and increases the rate of all biochemical reactions concerned with the biosynthesis and secretion of thyroidal hormones. If the secretion of TSH is sustained (hours or days), thyroid follicular cells become more columnar and follicular lumina become smaller as a result of increased uptake of colloid by endocytosis (Fig. 6-21). Numerous periodic acid–Schiff (PAS)-positive colloid droplets are present in the luminal aspect of the hypertrophied follicular cells. The converse (of what has

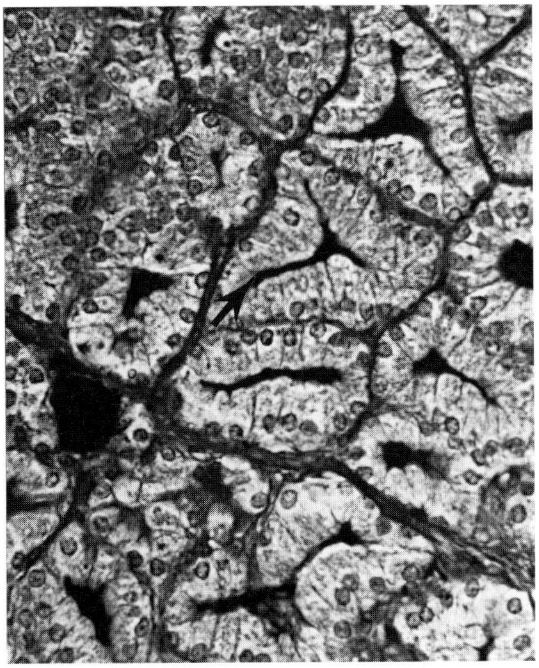

Figure 6-21 Thyroid gland; dog. Hyperplasia. Follicular cells 8 hours after TSH stimulation are columnar, and many follicles are nearly depleted of colloid and are partially collapsed *(arrow)*. H & E stain.

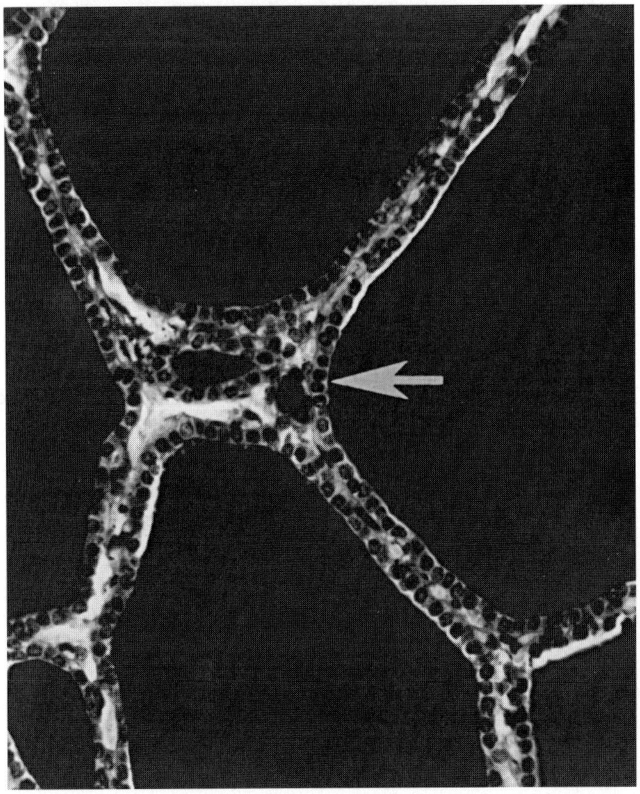

Figure 6-22 Thyroid gland; dog. Atrophy. Thyroid follicular cells after long-term administration of exogenous thyroxine *(arrow)* are cuboidal. Thyroid follicles are distended with dense colloid. H & E stain.

been just described) occurs in the thyroid gland in response to an increase in circulating thyroid hormone (T_4 and T_3) and a corresponding decrease in circulating pituitary TSH. Thyroid follicles become enlarged and distended with colloid as a result of decreased TSH-mediated endocytosis of colloid. Follicular cells lining the involuted follicles are low cuboidal, and few endocytotic vacuoles are at the interface between the colloid and follicular cells (Fig. 6-22).

T_4 and T_3, once released into the circulation, act on many different target cells in the body. The overall functions of T_4 and T_3 are similar, although much of the biologic activity appears to be the result of monodeiodination of T_4 (a prohormone) of the thyroid hormones to 3,5,3′-triiodothyronine (T_3) before interacting with high-affinity nuclear receptors in target cells. In certain diseases (protein starvation, the neonatal period, hepatic and renal disease, febrile illness, etc.), T_4 is preferentially monodeiodinated to 3,3′,5′-triiodothyronine ("reverse T_3"). Because "reverse T_3" produced by target cells is biologically inactive, monodeiodination to form "reverse T_3" provides a mechanism to attenuate the overall metabolic effects of thyroid hormones. The subcellular mechanism of action of thyroid hormones resembles that of steroids in that free hormone enters target cells and binds initially to cytosol-binding proteins and, subsequently, to high-affinity nuclear receptors. Binding of thyroid hormone to receptors on the inner mitochondrial membrane is responsible for the early activation of energy metabolism and increased oxidative phosphorylation.

Developmental Disturbances

Accessory Thyroid Tissue

The thyroid gland originates embryologically as a thickened plate of epithelium in the ventral aspect of the pharynx. Because of the complex embryogenesis of the thyroid, this leads to the frequent occurrence of accessory thyroid tissue. This accessory thyroid tissue is most frequently located in the mediastinum, but can be located anywhere from the base of the tongue to the diaphragm. About 50% of adult dogs have nodules of accessory thyroid tissue embedded in the fat around the base of the heart and origin of the aorta. The follicular structure and function are the same as those of the main thyroid lobes. Attempts to induce hypothyroidism in the dog by surgical thyroidectomy are not successful because the accessory thyroids readily respond to the prompt increase in endogenous TSH secretion and can undergo sufficient hyperplasia to sustain adequate hormone production. This accessory thyroid tissue has undergone neoplastic transformation.

Thyroglossal Duct Cysts

Thyroglossal duct cysts develop most frequently in dogs and pigs and occasionally in other animals. They form as a result of persistence of portions of the midline embryologic primordia of the thyroid gland, which migrates caudally from the ventral aspect of the primitive pharynx to form the postnatal thyroid lobes. These cysts are present in the ventral aspect of the cervical region in dogs as fluctuant masses. They rupture and form a tract to the exterior. Their lining epithelium consists of multiple layers of follicular cells in which are occasionally found colloid-containing follicles. These cells sometimes undergo neoplastic transformation and give rise to papillary carcinomas.

Degenerative and Inflammatory Lesions

Idiopathic Follicular Atrophy ("Collapse")

In follicular atrophy, the loss of follicular epithelium and disruption of follicles is progressive and the gland is replaced by adipose connective tissue with only a minimal inflammatory response. The gland usually is smaller and lighter in color than normal. The early lesion in dogs with mild clinical signs of hypothyroidism appears to be confined to one part of the thyroid gland. This affected part has small follicles lined by tall columnar follicular cells and with little colloid. A more advanced form of follicular atrophy is present in dogs with clinical hypothyroidism and low blood concentrations of thyroidal hormones. These thyroid glands are markedly reduced in size and are composed predominantly of adipose connective tissue with only a few clusters of small follicles containing vacuolated colloid.

Lymphocytic (Immune-mediated) Thyroiditis

Lymphocytic thyroiditis in dogs, obese strains of chickens, nonhuman primates, and Buffalo rats closely resembles Hashimoto's disease in human beings. Although the exact pathogenetic mechanism in the dog is not completely established, evidence suggests a polygenic pattern of inheritance similar to that observed in human beings. The immunologic basis of the development of chronic lymphocytic thyroiditis in both human beings and dogs appears to be through production of autoantibodies usually directed against thyroglobulin or a microsomal antigen (thyroperoxidase) and infrequently against the TSH receptor protein, nuclear antigen, and a second colloid antigen from thyroid follicular cells. Thyroglobulin autoantibodies have been found in 48% of pet dogs with hypothyroidism. Laboratory beagle dogs with naturally occurring lymphocytic thyroiditis also have circulating thyroidal autoantibodies, but the focal thyroiditis usually is not associated with clinical signs of hypothyroidism.

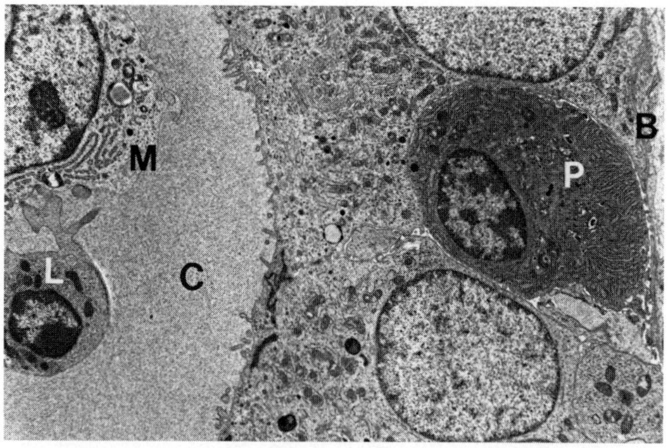

Figure 6-23 Lymphocytic thyroiditis in a dog with severe hypothyroidism. A lymphocyte *(L)* and macrophage *(M)* are present in the colloid *(C)* of a thyroid follicle. A plasma cell *(P)* within the follicular basement membrane *(B)* is infiltrating between thyroid follicular cells. TEM. *Gosselin SJ, Capen CC, Martin SL, Krakowka S. Autoimmune lymphocytic thyroiditis in dogs. Vet Immunol Immunopathol 1982; 3:185-201.*

Microscopic alterations consist of multifocal to diffuse infiltrates of lymphocytes, plasma cells, and macrophages and, sometimes, lymphoid nodules. Thyroid follicles are small and lined by columnar epithelial cells; lymphocytes, macrophages, and degenerate follicular cells are often present in vacuolated colloid (Fig. 6-23). Thyroid C cells are present as small nests or nodules between follicles and often are more prominent than those in normal dogs. Some remaining follicular cells appear to be transformed into large oxyphilic cells with densely eosinophilic granular cytoplasm.

Goiter

Hyperplasia of Thyroid Follicular Cells ("Goiter")

Goiter is a clinical term used to describe a nonneoplastic and noninflammatory enlargement of the thyroid gland. It develops in all domestic mammals, birds, and other submammalian vertebrates as a result of hyperplasia of follicular cells. Certain forms of thyroid hyperplasia, especially nodular, are difficult to differentiate from adenomas. The major pathogenic mechanisms for the development of thyroid hyperplasia include iodine-deficient diets, goitrogenic compounds that interfere with thyroxinogenesis, excess dietary iodide, and genetically determined defects in the enzymes or thyroglobulin that are essential for the biosynthesis of thyroidal hormones. All these result in inadequate thyroxine synthesis and decreased blood concentrations of T_4 and T_3. This decreased concentration of thyroid hormone is detected by the hypothalamus, which in turn stimulates the pituitary gland to increase the secretion of TSH, which results in hypertrophy and hyperplasia of follicular cells.

Diffuse Hyperplastic and Colloid Goiter

Dietary iodine deficiency that resulted in diffuse hyperplastic goiter was common in many areas of the world before the widespread addition of iodized salt to animal diets. Iodine-deficient goiter still occurs worldwide in domestic animals, but cases are sporadic and few animals are affected. Marginally iodine-deficient diets that contain goitrogenic compounds can cause severe thyroid follicular cell hyperplasia and goiter. Goitrogenic substances include thiouracil, sulfonamides, anions of the Hofmeister series, and a number of plants of the family *Brassicacceae.* Offspring of females fed iodine-deficient diets are likely to develop severe thyroidal follicular cell hyperplasia and have clinical signs of hypothyroidism. Both lateral lobes of the thyroid gland are uniformly enlarged in young animals as a result of diffuse hypertrophy and hyperplasia of follicular cells (Fig. 6-21). The enlargements, when extensive, result in palpable or visible swellings in the cranial cervical area. The affected lobes are firm and dark red because an extensive interfollicular capillary network develops under the influence of long-term TSH stimulation.

Colloid goiter represents the involutionary phase of diffuse hyperplastic goiter in young adult and adult animals. The markedly hyperplastic follicular cells continue to produce colloid, but endocytosis of colloid from the lumen is decreased. This is a consequence of the diminished pituitary TSH concentrations produced in response to the return of blood T_4 and T_3 concentrations to normal. Both thyroid lobes are diffusely enlarged but are more translucent and lighter in color than in hyperplastic goiter. These differences in macroscopic appearances are the result of less vascularity in colloid goiter and development of macrofollicles distended with colloid.

Colloid goiter develops either after sufficient amounts of iodide have been added to the diet or after the requirements for thyroid hormones have diminished in an older animal. Blood T_4 and T_3 concentrations return to normal, and the secretion of TSH by the pituitary gland is correspondingly decreased. Follicles are progressively distended (Fig. 6-22) with densely eosinophilic colloid due to diminished TSH-induced endocytosis. The follicular cells lining the macrofollicles are flattened and atrophic. The interface between the colloid and luminal surface of the follicular cells is smooth and the cells lack the characteristic endocytotic vacuoles of actively secreting thyroid follicular cells. Some involuted follicles in colloid goiter have remnants of the papillary projections of follicular cells extending into their lumens.

The changes in diffuse hyperplastic and colloid goiters are consistent throughout the diffusely enlarged thyroid lobes. Follicles are irregular in size and shape in hyperplastic goiter because they contain varying amounts of colloid that is lightly eosinophilic and vacuolated. Some follicles collapse because of the lack of colloid. Their lining epithelial cells are columnar and have a deeply eosinophilic cytoplasm and small hyperchromatic nuclei that often are situated in the basilar portion of the cell. The follicles are lined by single or multiple layers of hyperplastic follicular cells that, in some follicles, form papillary projections into the lumen (Fig. 6-24). Similar proliferative changes are present in ectopic thyroid tissue in the neck and mediastinum.

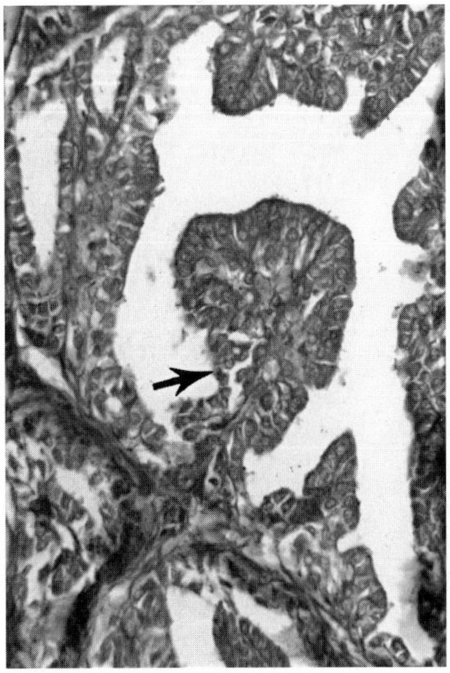

Figure 6-24 Thyroid gland, dog. Hyperplastic goiter. Papillary projection *(arrow)* extends into follicular lumen. The partial collapse of follicles is the result of increased endocytosis of colloid. H & E stain.

Although seemingly paradoxic, an excess of iodide in the diet also can result in thyroid hyperplasia in animals and human beings. Foals of mares fed dry seaweed containing excessive iodide develop thyroid hyperplasia and clinically evident goiter. The thyroid glands of the young are exposed to greater blood iodide concentrations than in the dam because iodide is concentrated first by the placenta and then by the mammary gland. Increased blood iodide interferes with one or more steps of thyroidal hormone synthesis and secretion, leading to lowered blood T_4 and T_3 concentrations with a compensatory increase in pituitary TSH secretion. Excess iodine appears to particularly block the release of T_3 and T_4 by interfering with proteolysis of colloid by lysosomal enzymes in thyroid follicular cells.

Multifocal Nodular Hyperplasia

Multifocal nodular hyperplasia in thyroid glands of old horses, cats, and dogs appears as multiple, white to tan

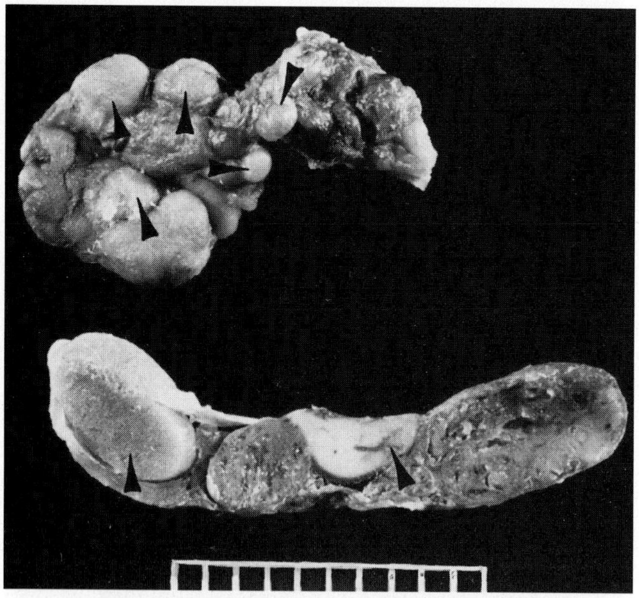

Figure 6-25 Thyroid glands; cat. Hyperplasia, hyperthyroidism. Multinodular follicular cell hyperplasia *(arrowheads)* involves both thyroid lobes. Bar = 1 cm.

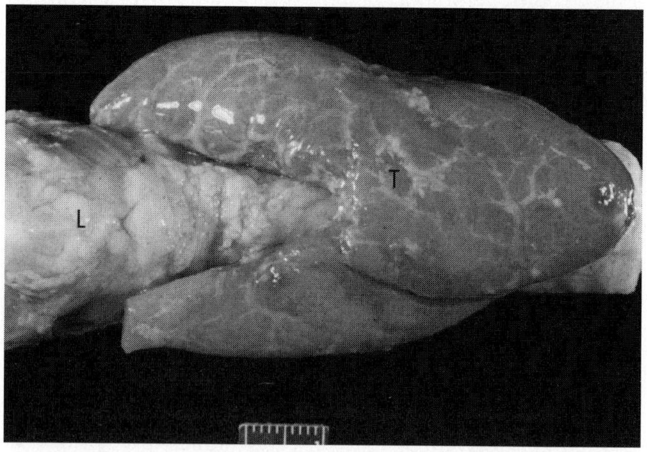

Figure 6-26 Thyroid gland; lamb. Congenital dyshormonogenetic goiter. The symmetrically enlarged thyroid *(T)* lobes are fused on the midline beneath the larynx *(L)* and trachea. Bar = 1 cm.

nodules of variable size (Fig. 6-25) giving affected lobes a moderately enlarged and irregular contour. Multifocal nodular goiter in most animals (except cats) is endocrinologically inactive and is an incidental lesion at necropsy. However, functional thyroid adenomas often develop in a thyroid gland of aged cats with hyperthyroidism and multinodular hyperplasia of follicular cells. In contrast to thyroid adenomas, the areas of nodular hyperplasia are not encapsulated and cause minimal to no compression of adjacent parenchyma. Thus, nodular goiter consists of multiple foci of hyperplastic follicular cells that are sharply demarcated but not encapsulated from the adjacent thyroid tissue.

The microscopic appearance of nodular hyperplasia often is variable. Some hyperplastic follicular cells form small follicles with little or no colloid. Other nodules are composed of larger, irregularly shaped follicles lined by one or more layers of columnar cells that form papillary projections into the lumen. Some of the follicles have undergone colloid involution and are filled with densely eosinophilic colloid. These changes appear to be the result of alternating periods of hyperplasia and colloid involution in the thyroid glands of aged animals.

Congenital Dyshormonogenetic Goiter

Congenital dyshormonogenetic goiter in sheep (Corriedale, Dorset Horn, Merino, and Romney breeds), Afrikander cattle, and Saanen dwarf goats is inherited as an autosomal recessive trait. The subnormal growth rate, absence of normal wool development or a rough, sparse hair coat, subcutaneous myxedematous swellings, weakness, and sluggish behavior suggest that the affected young are clinically hypothyroid. Most lambs with congenital goiter either die shortly after birth or are markedly sensitive to the effects of adverse environmental conditions, particularly cold.

Thyroid lobes are symmetrically enlarged at birth because of an intense diffuse hyperplasia of follicular cells (Fig. 6-26). Thyroid follicles are lined by tall columnar cells, but often are collapsed because of lack of colloid resulting from the marked endocytotic activity. The tall columnar follicular cells lining thyroid follicles have dilated profiles of rough endoplasmic reticulum and large mitochondria, dense (lysosomal) granules associated with the Golgi apparatus, but few thyroglobulin-containing apical vesicles are present near the luminal plasma membrane. Numerous long microvilli extend into the follicular lumen.

Although thyroidal uptake and turnover of ^{131}I are greatly increased compared with euthyroid controls, circulating T_4 and T_3 concentrations are consistently low. The lack of a defect in the iodide transport mechanism and organification or dehalogenation, plus an absence of normal 19S thyroglobulin in goitrous thyroids and only minute amounts of thyroglobulin-related antigens (0.01% of normal) suggest an impairment in thyroglobulin biosynthesis. A closely related or similar defect occurs in congenital goiter of sheep, cattle, and goats.

Neoplasms of the Thyroid Gland

Follicular Cell Adenoma

Adenomas usually are white to tan, small, solid nodules that are well demarcated from the adjacent thyroid parenchyma. The affected thyroid lobe is only moderately enlarged and distorted; usually only a single adenoma is present in a thyroid lobe. A distinct, white, fibrous connective tissue capsule of variable thickness separates the adenoma from the compressed parenchyma. Some thyroid adenomas are composed of thin-walled cysts filled with a yellow to red fluid. Their external surfaces are smooth and covered by an extensive network of blood vessels. Small masses of neoplastic tissue remain in the wall and form rugose projections into the cyst. Adenomas are classified into follicular and papillary types; the follicular type is more common in the thyroid gland of animals.

Follicular Cell Carcinoma

In dogs, thyroid carcinomas occur more often than adenomas, but in cats adenomas are more common. Boxer dogs develop thyroidal carcinomas more frequently than any other breed, but beagle and golden retriever dogs have a significant risk for the development of thyroid carcinoma. Approximately 60% of thyroid carcinomas in dogs are detectable clinically by palpation as a firm mass in the neck and by evidence of respiratory distress due to compression of the trachea. Carcinomas become fixed in position by extensive local invasion of adjacent structures, whereas adenomas (which do not invade) are freely movable under the skin. Neoplasms of thyroid origin also occur in accessory thyroidal tissue that is located anywhere from the base of the tongue to the cranial mediastinum.

Thyroid carcinomas often grow rapidly and invade adjacent structures, such as the trachea, esophagus, and larynx. The earliest and most frequent site of metastasis is to the lungs because thyroid carcinomas early in the course of development invade branches of the thyroid vein. The retropharyngeal and caudal cervical lymph nodes are infrequent sites of metastases.

Hyperthyroidism

Proliferative lesions that secrete excess thyroidal hormones (e.g., adenomas and multinodular hyperplasia) are common in the thyroid glands of adult and aged cats. Follicular cell adenomas, which often develop in a thyroid gland with multinodular hyperplasia, are encountered more commonly than thyroid carcinomas. In aged cats, a syndrome of hyperthyroidism associated with multinodular hyperplasia, adenomas, or carcinomas derived from follicular cells of the thyroid gland is being recognized more frequently. Follicles in the rim of thyroid tissue around a functional adenoma are markedly enlarged and distended with an accumulation of colloid ("colloid involution"). The follicular cells are low cuboidal and atrophic with little evidence of endocytotic activity in response to the increased circulating concentrations of thyroid hormones. In cats with solitary adenomas, the opposite thyroid lobe should be carefully examined for evidence of nodular hyperplasia or "microadenomas." These small foci of multinodular hyperplasia of follicular cells can be the cause of recurrence of hyperthyroidism several months to a year or more after surgical removal of a functional adenoma.

Hyperthyroidism in cats also occurs in association with bilateral multinodular ("adenomatous") hyperplasia ("goiter"). These multiple areas of thyroidal cell hyperplasia usually cause only slight enlargement of the affected lobe(s) (see Fig. 6-25). In contrast to adenomas, the areas of nodular hyperplasia are not encapsulated and the adjacent thyroid tissue is not compressed. Microscopically, hyperplastic nodules are composed of irregularly shaped, colloid-filled follicles lined by cuboidal follicular cells. These multiple nodules of follicular cell hyperplasia are considered a preneoplastic lesion as they can coalesce and form a thyroid follicular cell adenoma.

Since the late 1970s there has been a dramatic increase in the incidence of neoplasms and other focal proliferative lesions of the thyroid glands of cats that have resulted in hyperthyroidism. Hyperthyroidism is one of the two most common endocrine diseases in adult to aged cats (diabetes mellitus being the other). Before 1980, clinical hyperthyroidism was diagnosed infrequently in cats. The reason for the apparent increased incidence is uncertain but appears to be related, in part, to (1) a larger population of old cats receiving veterinary medical care, (2) improved assays for thyroid hormones, (3) detailed characterization of the clinical syndrome, and (4) increased awareness by veterinary clinicians of its common occurrence in adult to aged cats. In addition, there does appear to be a "real" increase in the incidence of feline hyperthyroidism over the past 30 years. Potential risk factors that have been reported include a predominantly indoor environment, regular treatment with flea powders, exposures to herbicides and fertilizers, a diet primarily of canned food, and non-Siamese breeds (10 times greater occurrence). It has been suggested that wide variations (excessive to inadequate) in dietary iodine intake over prolonged periods could play a role in the pathogenesis of thyroid disorders in cats.

The disease in cats is mechanistically different from Graves' disease in human patients in that hyperthyroid cats do not have increased circulating concentrations of thyroid-stimulating immunoglobulins comparable to long-acting thyroid stimulator (LATS) (an autoantibody that binds to the TSH receptor and activates follicular cells in human beings). Purified immunoglobulin G (IgG) prepared from hyperthyroid cats significantly increased ^{3}H-thymidine incorporation into DNA and stimulated thyroid follicular cell proliferation 15-fold but did not stimulate intracellular cAMP production. The ^{3}H-thymidine incorporation could be inhibited completely by a specific TSH receptor blocking antibody. These data suggest that increased titers of thyroid growth-stimulating immunoglobulins are present in cats with hyperthyroidism and most likely act by the TSH receptor. This important thyroid disease in cats most closely resembles toxic nodular goiter in human patients. Hyperplastic and neoplastic thyroid tissue from cats is transplantable into athymic (nude) mice and continues to overproduce T_4 and T_3 in a subcutaneous location.

Cats with hyperthyroidism usually have markedly increased serum T_4 and T_3 concentrations. The serum T_4 concentration in cats with hyperthyroidism range from 3.4 to 30 μg/dl (normal range 1.5 to 5 μg/dl), and serum T_3 concentrations range from 179 to 470 ng/dl (normal 60 to 200 ng/dl). Moderately increased serum enzyme activities, including serum alanine aminotransferase (ALT, SGPT), serum aspartate aminotransferase (AST, SGOT) and especially alkaline phosphatase, occur in hyperthyroid cats.

Hyperthyroid cats often have disturbances of calcium homeostasis and diffuse chief cell hyperplasia in the parathyroid glands. Blood ionized (not total) calcium and plasma creatinine concentrations are significantly decreased and plasma phosphate and intact parathyroid hormone concentrations are increased compared with reference ranges. Hyperparathyroidism occurred in 77% of hyperthyroid cats with parathyroid hormone concentrations elevated up to 19 times the upper limit of the reference range. Hyperphosphatemia was present in approximately 40% of hyperthyroid cats. The mechanisms for the development of hyperphosphatemia in feline hyperthyroidism are uncertain but could be related, in part, to polyphagia with increased intestinal phosphorus absorption, increased catabolism of muscle proteins, and release of phosphorus due to the gluconeogenic effects of the increased thyroid hormone concentrations, and increased bone resorption with release of phosphorus into the blood. The hyperparathyroidism and chief cell hyperplasia appear to be related to the reciprocal decline in circulating amounts of ionized calcium in response to the hyperphosphatemia. An increased blood phosphate also could decrease the renal 1α-hydroxylase activity and decrease the production of the active form of vitamin D, thereby reducing intestinal calcium absorption. However, circulating concentrations of 1,25-$(OH)_2$-dihydroxycholecalciferol were not decreased in a limited number of hyperthyroid cats evaluated.

Thyroid neoplasms in the dog can secrete sufficient thyroidal hormones to produce mild clinical signs of hyperthyroidism, including weight loss, polyphagia, weakness and fatigue, intolerance to heat, and nervousness. In general, the likelihood of developing clinical hyperthyroidism associated with thyroid neoplasms in animals depends on (1) the capability of neoplastic cells to synthesize T_4 and T_3 (e.g., well-differentiated thyroid neoplasms that form follicles and produce colloid are more likely to synthesize thyroid hormones than poorly differentiated solid neoplasms) and (2) the extent of increase of circulating concentrations of T_4 and T_3, which depends on a balance between the rate of secretion of thyroid hormones by the neoplasm and the rate of degradation of thyroid hormones. Dogs have a much more efficient enterohepatic excretory mechanism for thyroid hormones than cats that is difficult to overload; therefore, clinical hyperthyroidism in dogs with functional thyroid (follicular cell) neoplasms is infrequent. Cats are very sensitive to phenol and phenol derivatives and have a poor ability to conjugate phenolic compounds (such as T_4) with glucuronic acid and excrete the T_4 glucuronide into the bile. The capacity of conjugation of T_3 with sulfate is limited and easily overloaded.

Hypothyroidism

Hypothyroidism is a well-recognized and clinically important disease in dogs but is encountered only occasionally in other animals. Although the disease occurs in many adult purebred and mixed breed dogs, certain breeds (golden retriever, Doberman pinscher, dachshund, Shetland sheep dog, Irish setter, miniature schnauzer, cocker spaniel, and Airedale) are more commonly affected. Hypothyroidism in dogs usually is the result of primary lesions in the thyroid gland, particularly lymphocytic thyroiditis and idiopathic follicular collapse. Less common causes of hypothyroidism include bilateral nonfunctional thyroidal cell neoplasms and severe iodine-deficient goiter. Hypothyroidism due to long-standing pituitary gland or hypothalamic lesions that prevent the release of either TSH or thyrotropin-releasing hormone (TRH) is encountered infrequently in the dog. In these cases the thyroid gland is moderately reduced in size and composed of colloid-distended follicles lined by flattened follicular cells.

Many functional disturbances associated with hypothyroidism are due to a reduction in basal metabolic rate. A gain in body weight without an associated change in appetite occurs in some hypothyroid dogs. Thinning of the hair coat is often accompanied by a bilaterally symmetric alopecia. Areas affected initially by hair loss are those receiving frictional wear such as the tail and cervical area.

Hyperkeratosis is a consistent finding in hypothyroidism and results in an increased scaliness of the skin. When severe, it occurs as circular scaling patches resembling seborrhea. Microscopically, hyperkeratosis (Fig. 6-27) involves the external root sheath, resulting in follicular keratosis. Hyperpigmentation, especially in such localized areas of alopecia as the dorsal aspect of the nose and distal portion of the tail, occurs in many dogs with hypothyroidism. Myxedema occurs and is the result of accumulation of mucins (neutral and acid mucopolysaccharides combined with protein) in the dermis and subcutis. These substances bind considerable amounts of water, which results in marked thickening of the skin. Microscopically, mucins appear as granular or fibrillar material in H & E–stained sections.

Abnormalities in reproduction include lack of libido, reduction in sperm count, abnormal or absent estrus cycles, and reduced conception rates. The spermatogenic epithelium in the testes is often markedly atrophic in chronic hypothyroidism.

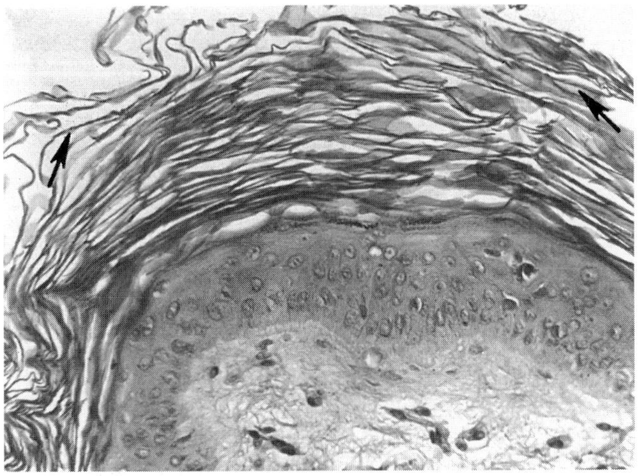

Figure 6-27 Skin; dog. Hypothyroidism. Hyperkeratosis *(arrows)* resulting in the thickening of the epidermis of the skin. H & E stain.

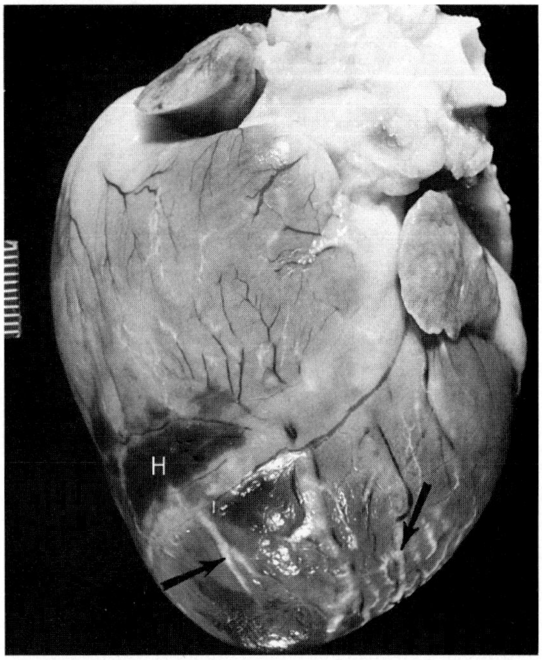

Figure 6-28 Heart; dog. Hypothyroidism with marked hyperlipidemia associated with severe primary hypothyroidism. Hypothyroidism. Note coronary atherosclerosis *(arrows)* with areas of ischemic necrosis and hemorrhage of myocardium *(H)*. Bar = 1 cm.

Hypothyroidism in dogs is accompanied by decreased circulating thyroidal hormone concentrations and decreased ^{131}I uptake by the thyroid gland. In dogs with hypothyroidism, the T_4 concentration is usually below 0.8 μg/dl (normal 1.5 to 3.4 μg/dl) and that of T_3 is below 50 ng/dl (normal 48 to 150 ng/dl). In the euthyroid dog the T_4 concentrations will at least double 8 hours after intravenous or intramuscular injection of TSH. In dogs with hypothyroidism, the T_4 concentrations do not change significantly after injection of TSH.

The serum cholesterol concentration often is increased greatly (300 to 900 mg/dl) in many hypothyroid dogs (normal serum cholesterol 40 to 80 mg/dl). The marked hypercholesterolemia in long-standing and severe hypothyroidism results in a variety of secondary lesions, including atherosclerosis, hepatomegaly, and glomerular and corneal lipidosis. Atherosclerosis of coronary (Fig. 6-28) and cerebral vessels develops in dogs that have severe hypothyroidism and long-standing hyperlipidemia.

Thyroid C (Parafollicular) Cells

Calcitonin is secreted by a second endocrine cell population, C (parafollicular) cells, in the mammalian thyroid gland. These cells are situated either in the follicular wall within the basement membrane between follicular cells (Fig. 6-29) or as small groups of cells adjacent to interfollicular capillaries between follicles. C cells do not border the follicular colloid directly, and their secretory pole is oriented toward the interfollicular capillaries. The distinctive feature of C cells is the presence of numerous small, membrane-limited secretory granules in their cytoplasm (Fig. 6-29). Immunocytochemical techniques have localized the calcitonin activity of C cells to these secretory granules.

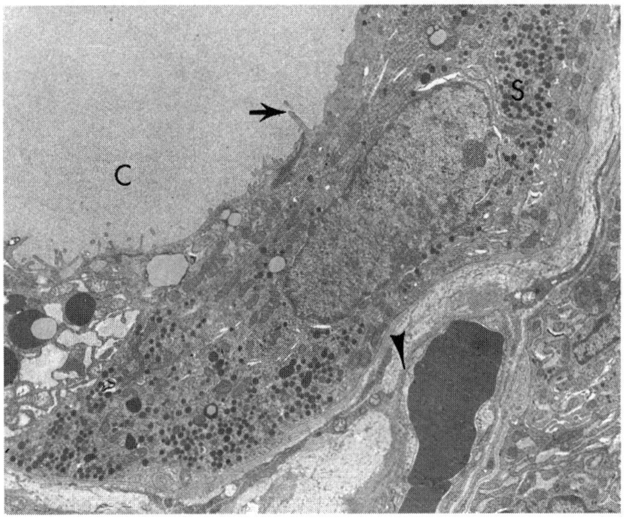

Figure 6-29 Thyroid gland; normal dog. Thyroid C (parafollicular) cell with numerous secretory granules *(S)* and moderate development of Golgi apparatus and rough endoplasmic reticulum. Microvilli from follicular cells *(arrow)* extend into the colloid of the follicular lumen *(C)*. The secretory polarity of the C cell is directed toward an interfollicular capillary *(arrowhead)* with fenestrae. TEM.

Calcitonin is a polypeptide hormone, and the calcium ion concentration in plasma and extracellular fluids is the principal physiologic stimulus for the secretion of calcitonin by C cells. The rate of secretion of calcitonin is

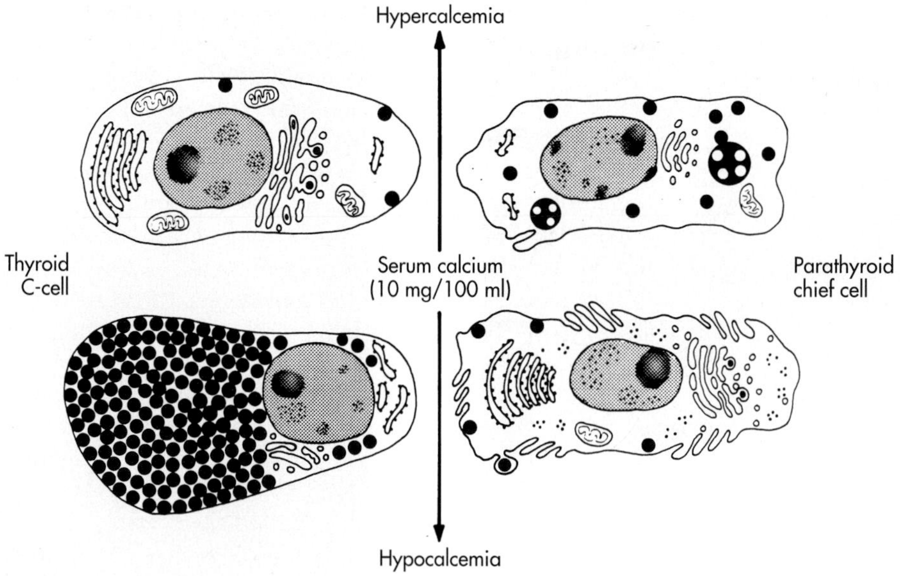

Figure 6-30 Response of thyroid C cells and parathyroid chief cells to hypercalcemia and hypocalcemia. C cells accumulate secretory granules in response to hypocalcemia, whereas chief cells are nearly degranulated but have an increased development of synthetic and secretory organelles. In response to hypercalcemia, C cells are degranulated, and parathyroid chief cells are predominantly in the inactive stage of the secretory cycle.

increased greatly in response to increased blood calcium concentrations.

C cells store substantial amounts of calcitonin in their cytoplasm, and in response to hypercalcemia the hormone is discharged rapidly from C cells into interfollicular capillaries (Fig. 6-30). Hyperplasia of C cells occurs in response to long-term hypercalcemia. When the blood calcium concentration is reduced, the stimulus for calcitonin secretion is diminished, and numerous secretory granules accumulate in the cytoplasm of C cells (Fig. 6-30). Calcitonin exerts its function by interacting with target cells located primarily in bone and kidneys. The actions of parathyroid hormone and calcitonin are antagonistic on bone resorption but synergistic in decreasing the renal tubular reabsorption of phosphorus.

Thyroid C (Ultimobranchial) Cell Neoplasms

Neoplasms derived from C cells of the thyroid gland are most frequently encountered in adult to aged bulls (but not in cows fed similar diets), certain strains of laboratory rats, occasionally in horses and dogs, but infrequently in other species. A high percentage of aged bulls fed calcium-rich diets develop C cell neoplasms (30%) or hyperplasia of C cells and ultimobranchial derivatives (15% to 20%). The incidence of C cell neoplasms increases with advancing age in bulls and has been associated with the development of increased vertebral bone density. The syndrome of C cells neoplasms in bulls shares many similarities with that of medullary thyroid carcinoma in human beings. Multiple endocrine neoplasms, especially bilateral pheochromocytomas and occasionally pituitary adenomas, have also been present in bulls and human beings with C cell neoplasms. A diffuse or nodular hyperplasia in the adrenal medulla precedes the development of pheochromocytoma.

Adenomas. C cell adenomas occur as discrete, single or multiple, gray to tan nodules in one or both thyroid lobes. Adenomas are smaller (approximately 1 to 3 cm in diameter) than carcinomas and are separated from the adjacent compressed thyroid gland parenchyma by a thin, fibrous connective tissue capsule. Larger C cell adenomas replace most of the thyroid lobe, but a rim of dark, brown-red thyroid gland often is present on one side (Fig. 6-31). Microscopically, a thyroid C cell adenoma is a discrete, expansive mass of cells larger than a colloid-distended follicle. The adenoma is well circumscribed or partially encapsulated, and adjacent follicles are compressed to varying degrees. The neoplastic C cells are well differentiated and have abundant to clear, palely eosinophilic cytoplasm.

Carcinomas. Thyroid C cell carcinomas result in extensive multinodular enlargements of one or both thyroid lobes and can replace the entire thyroid gland. Thyroid C cell neoplasms in bulls, other animal species, and human beings are firm, and, in some areas, the stroma consists of dense bands of fibrous connective tissue. Multiple metastases occur to the cranial cervical lymph nodes. These are usually large (Fig. 6-32) and have areas of necrosis and hemorrhage. Pulmonary metastases appear as

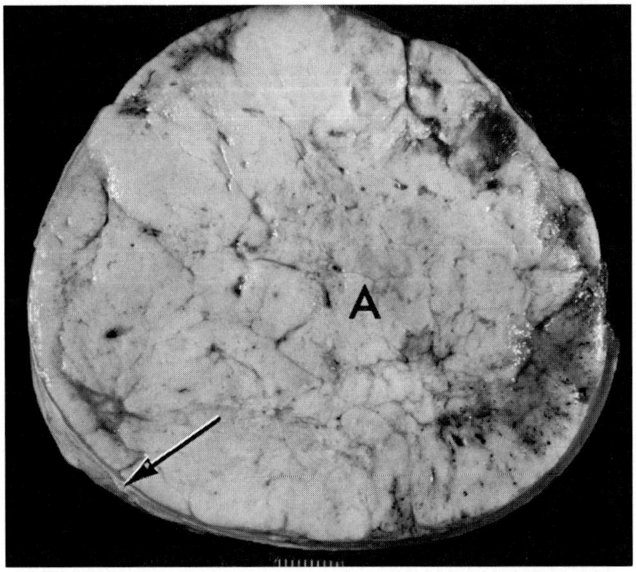

Figure 6-31 Thyroid gland; horse. Adenoma. The adenoma *(A)* is confined by the thyroid capsule and a rim of compressed thyroid gland *(arrow)* at the periphery of the mass. Bar = 1 cm.

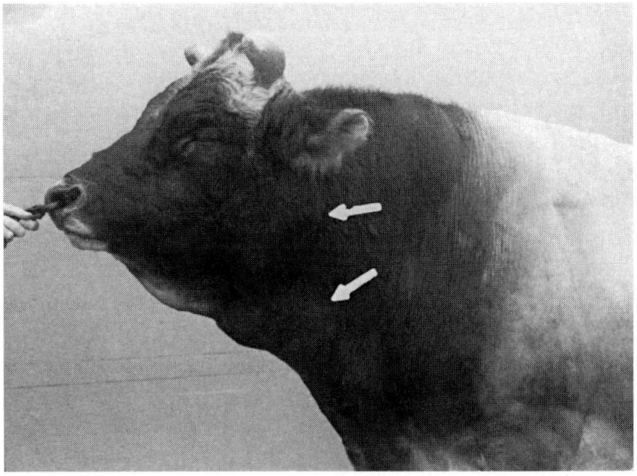

Figure 6-32 Jersey bull. C cell carcinoma with multiple metastases to anterior cervical lymph nodes. Note the swellings in the neck *(arrows)* as a result of the metastases.

discrete tan nodules and occur infrequently. C cell carcinomas are composed of neoplastic cells that are more pleomorphic than cells of C cell adenomas. The carcinomatous cells are poorly differentiated, polyhedral to spindle shaped, and have palely eosinophilic, finely granular, indistinct cytoplasm. Both adenomas and carcinomas have deposits of amyloid.

The etiology of C cell neoplasms is unknown, but the chronic stimulation of C cells by large concentrations of calcium absorbed from the digestive tract can be responsible for their high incidence. A significant decline in the incidence of C cell neoplasms occurs when the excessive calcium intake of bulls is reduced. Cows fed similar rations rarely develop proliferative lesions of C cells because of the greater physiologic requirements of pregnancy and lactation for calcium.

Ultimobranchial neoplasms in the thyroid glands of bulls often have a more complex histologic structure than the typical C cell (medullary) carcinoma in human beings, dogs, horses, and many strains of laboratory rats. The neoplasm is composed of differentiated C cells arranged as focal accumulations of neoplastic cells that have an abundant palely eosinophilic cytoplasm either within the wall of the thyroid and ultimobranchial follicles or present as larger solid nodules. Ultimobranchial thyroid neoplasms often are accompanied by a multifocal hyperplasia of C cells in other parts of the thyroid lobes and hilus. The neoplastic C cells often are embedded in an increased amount of hyalinized stroma with deposits of amyloid in some neoplasms. Portions of this thyroid neoplasm in bulls that are derived from less differentiated ultimobranchial remnants consist of follicle-like structures, cysts, and tubules composed of immature small basophilic cells. These neoplasms in bulls and other species closely resemble undifferentiated or stem cells of the normal ultimobranchial body that can differentiate into both C cells and follicular cells. Thyroid follicles and cribriform structures with colloid-like material formed by cells resembling differentiated follicular cells often are present in the neoplasms in close association with these more primitive ultimobranchial-derived structures. The heterogeneous histologic structure of ultimobranchial neoplasms in bulls resembles a variant of thyroid carcinoma in human beings. This neoplasm, designated as an intermediate type of differentiated carcinoma, has structural and immunocytochemical characteristics of both C cells (medullary) and follicular carcinomas.

The source of the localized amyloid deposits in the thyroid C cell neoplasms is uncertain, but the amyloid appears to be produced by the neoplastic cells, and amyloid deposits are not present in other organs. Amyloid deposition is consistently associated with medullary thyroid carcinoma in human beings, and amyloid has been reported also in certain other endocrine neoplasms. Amyloid in C cell neoplasms is present between neoplastic cells, around vessels, and in the interstitium. Amyloid has been observed in bulls, horses, dogs, and laboratory rats, but in varying amounts (minimal to substantial) from case to case. Chemical differences exist between amyloid fibrils of immunoglobulin origin and those produced by endocrine neoplasms.

PARATHYROID GLANDS

Parathyroid glands in most animal species consist of two pairs of glands situated in the cranial cervical region. The dog and cat have both the external and internal parathyroid glands located near the thyroid gland. Other animal

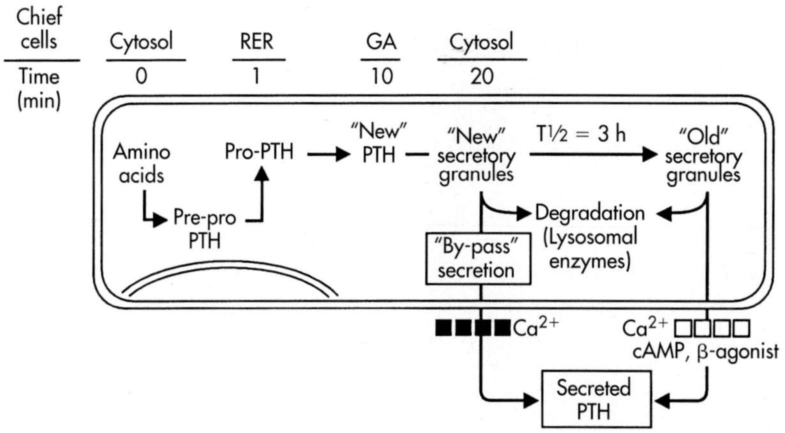

Figure 6-33 Bypass secretion of parathyroid hormone in response to increased demand signaled by decreased blood calcium ion concentration. Recently synthesized and processed active PTH can be released directly and not enter the storage pool of mature ("old") secretory granules in the cytoplasm of chief cells. PTH from the storage pool can be mobilized by cAMP and β-agonists (such as epinephrine, norepinephrine, and isoproterenol), as well as by lowered blood calcium ion, whereas secretion from the pool of recently synthesized PTH can be stimulated only by a decreased calcium ion concentration. *RER,* rough endoplasmic reticulum; *GA,* Golgi apparatus.

species, such as the pig and laboratory rat, have only a single pair of parathyroid glands cranial to the thyroid gland, embedded either in the thymus in young animals or in adipose connective tissue in adult animals. In cattle and sheep, the larger external parathyroid gland is located a considerable distance cranial to the thyroid gland in the loose connective tissue along the common carotid artery. The smaller internal parathyroid glands are situated on the dorsal and medial surface of the thyroid gland. In horses, the larger ("lower") parathyroid gland is located a considerable distance from the thyroid gland in the caudal cervical region near the bifurcation of the bicarotid trunk at the level of the first rib, while the smaller ("upper") parathyroid gland is situated near the thyroid gland.

The parathyroid glands consist of a single type of secretory cell that produces one hormone. The parathyroid glands of animals and human beings are composed predominantly of chief cells in different stages of secretory activity or in transition to oxyphilic cells in certain species. Oxyphilic cells increase in number with advancing age and often form nodules in the parathyroid glands of aged animals. They are larger than chief cells, and their abundant cytoplasm is filled with numerous large, often bizarre-shaped mitochondria.

Biologically active PTH secreted by chief cells is a straight-chain polypeptide consisting of 84 amino acid residues with a molecular weight of approximately 9,500. Secretory cells in the parathyroid glands of most animals store relatively small amounts of preformed hormone but are capable of responding to minor fluctuations in calcium ion concentration by rapidly altering the rate of hormonal secretion and, more slowly, by altering the rate of hormonal synthesis (Fig. 6-33). In contrast to most endocrine organs, which are under complex control, the parathyroid glands have a unique feedback control system based primarily on the concentration of calcium (and, to a lesser extent, of magnesium) ion in blood. Calcium ion concentration controls not only the rate of biosynthesis and secretion of parathyroid hormone but also other metabolic and intracellular degradative processes within chief cells. Increased calcium ion concentration in extracellular fluids rapidly inhibits the uptake of amino acids by chief cells, synthesis of proPTH and conversion to PTH, and secretion of stored PTH (Fig. 6-33).

Parathyroid hormone is the principal hormone involved in the minute-to-minute, fine regulation of blood calcium concentration (total and ionic calcium) in mammals. It does this by directly influencing the function of target cells located primarily in bone and kidneys and indirectly acting in the intestine to maintain plasma calcium concentration sufficient to ensure the optimal functioning of a wide variety of body cells. The overall action of PTH on bone is to mobilize calcium into extracellular fluids (Fig. 6-34). The response of bone to PTH is the result of increasing the activity of osteoclasts and osteocytes existing in bone.

PTH has a rapid (within 5 to 10 minutes) and direct effect on renal tubular function, leading to decreased reabsorption of phosphate and consequently the development of phosphaturia. The site of action where PTH blocks tubular reabsorption of phosphate has been determined to be the proximal tubule. The ability of PTH to enhance the

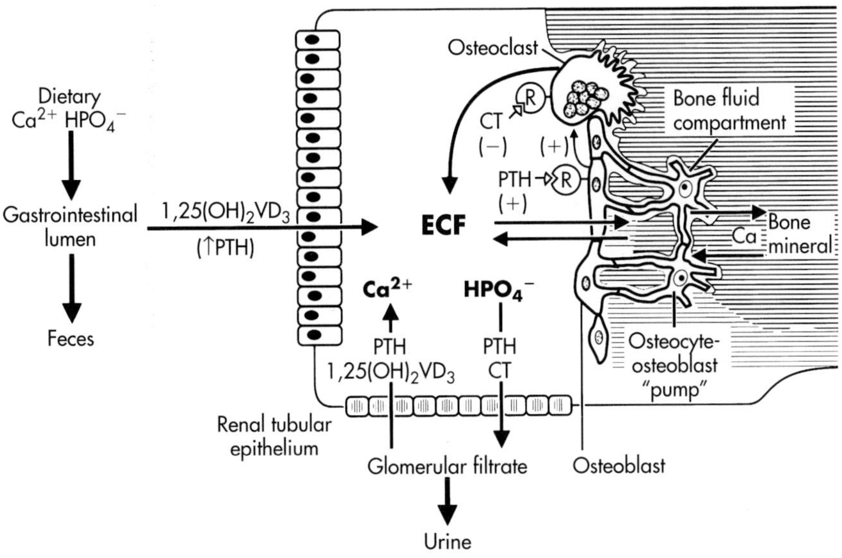

Figure 6-34 Interrelation of parathyroid hormone *(PTH)*, calcitonin *(CT)*, and 1,25-dihydroxycholecalciferol (1,25-$[OH]_2D_3$) in hormonal regulation of calcium and phosphorus in extracellular fluids.

renal absorption of calcium also is of considerable importance in the maintenance of calcium homeostasis. This effect of PTH upon tubular reabsorption of calcium appears to be due to a direct action on the distal convoluted tubule. Calcitonin and parathyroid hormone, acting in concert, provide a dual negative feedback control mechanism to maintain within narrow limits the concentration of calcium in extracellular fluids.

The third major hormone involved in the regulation of calcium metabolism and skeletal remodeling is cholecalciferol or vitamin D_3 (Fig. 6-34). Cholecalciferol is ingested in small amounts in the diet and can be synthesized in the epidermis from precursor molecules (e.g., 7-dehydrocholesterol) through a provitamin D_3 intermediate form. The active metabolites of vitamin D increase the absorption of calcium and phosphorus from the intestine and, thereby, maintain adequate concentrations of these electrolytes in the extracellular fluids as required for the appropriate mineralization of bone matrix. From a functional point of view, vitamin D brings about the retention of sufficient mineral ions to ensure mineralization of bone matrix, whereas PTH maintains the proper ratio of calcium to phosphorus in extracellular fluids. The major target tissue for 1,25-$(OH)_2D_3$ is the mucosa of the small intestine, where the vitamin increases the active transcellular transport of calcium (proximal small intestine) and phosphorus (distal small intestine).

Developmental Disturbances

Parathyroid Cysts

Small cysts within the parenchyma of the parathyroid glands or in the immediate vicinity of the glands occur frequently in dogs but only occasionally in other animal species (Fig. 6-35). Parathyroid gland cysts are usually

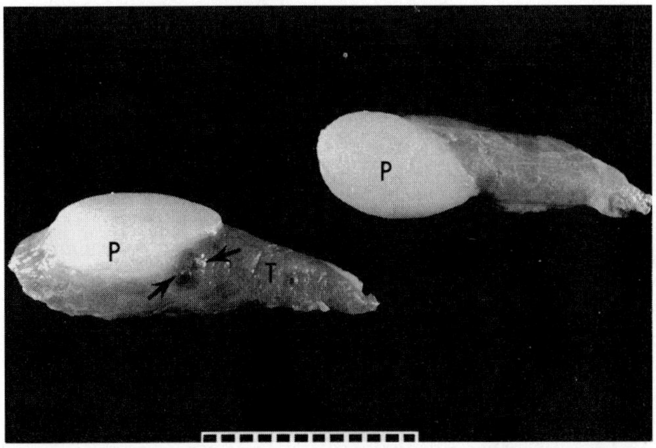

Figure 6-35 Parathyroid gland; dog. Parathyroid cyst. The parathyroid cyst *(arrows)* was formed from the persistent and distended embryonic duct that connects parathyroid-thymic primordia in the III and IV pharyngeal pouches (Kürsteiner's cyst). *T*, thyroid gland. Hyperplastic parathyroids *(P)* from a dog with chronic renal failure. Bar = 1 cm.

multiloculated, lined by a cuboidal to columnar (often ciliated) epithelium, and are filled with a densely eosinophilic proteinic material. Parathyroid gland cysts (Kürsteiner's cysts) appear to develop from persistent and dilated remnants of the duct that connects the parathyroid and thymic primordia during embryonic development. Parathyroid gland cysts are distinct from midline cysts derived from remnants of the thyroglossal duct. The latter are lined by multilayered thyroidogenic epithelium that often has colloid-containing follicles. The cysts are usually located near the midline, from the base of the tongue to the mediastinum.

Degenerative Lesions of Parathyroid Chief Cells
Multinucleated Syncytial Cells

A unique multinucleated syncytial giant cell can develop in parathyroid glands of dogs and rats. These cells are often more numerous near the periphery of the parathyroid glands. However, considerable numbers can be present in the more central portions of some glands. The number of syncytial cells varies considerably between parathyroid glands in the same animal and can equal one half of the parenchyma of the gland. These cells appear to form by the fusion of the cytoplasm of adjacent chief cells. The cytoplasm is densely eosinophilic and homogeneous and the plasma membrane is often indistinct. The oval nuclei are smaller and more hyperchromatic than the adjacent chief cells. The etiology and functional significance of syncytial chief cells is uncertain, but they usually are incidental findings.

Inflammatory Lesions and Hypoparathyroidism
Lymphocytic Parathyroiditis and Hypoparathyroidism

In hypoparathyroidism, either the parathyroid glands secrete subnormal amounts of PTH or the hormone secreted is unable to interact with target cells. Hypoparathyroidism has been recognized in dogs, particularly in smaller breeds such as schnauzers and terriers, but infrequently in other animal species. Idiopathic hypoparathyroidism in adult dogs usually is caused by a diffuse lymphocytic parathyroiditis and is characterized by extensive degeneration of chief cells and replacement fibrosis. Mild lesions include infiltrates of lymphocytes and plasma cells and nodular hyperplasia of chief cells. Later, the parathyroid gland is completely replaced by lymphocytes, fibroblasts, and neocapillaries with only a few viable chief cells (Fig. 6-36).

Lymphocytic parathyroiditis develops by an immune-mediated mechanism, since a similar destruction of parathyroid gland parenchyma and lymphocytic infiltration has been produced in dogs by the injection of emulsions of parathyroid gland in adjuvant. Other infrequent causes of hypoparathyroidism include invasion and destruction of parathyroid glands by primary or metastatic neoplasms and trophic atrophy of parathyroid glands resulting from long-term hypercalcemia. Also, the parathyroid glands are sometimes damaged or inadvertently removed during surgery involving the thyroid glands.

The functional disturbances and clinical manifestations of hypoparathyroidism primarily are the result of increased neuromuscular excitability and tetany. Because of the lack of PTH, bone resorption is decreased and blood calcium concentrations diminish progressively to 4 to 6 mg/dl (Fig. 6-37). Affected animals are restless, nervous, ataxic, weak, and have intermittent tremors of separate muscle groups. Tremors can progress to generalized tetany and convulsive seizures. Concurrently, blood phosphorus concentrations are increased because of increased renal tubular reabsorption.

Hyperplasia of Chief Cells
Hyperparathyroidism Secondary to Nutritional Imbalances

Nutritional hyperparathyroidism occurs commonly in cats, dogs, certain nonhuman primates, horses, domestic and captive birds, and reptiles. The increased secretion of parathyroid hormone is a compensatory mechanism induced

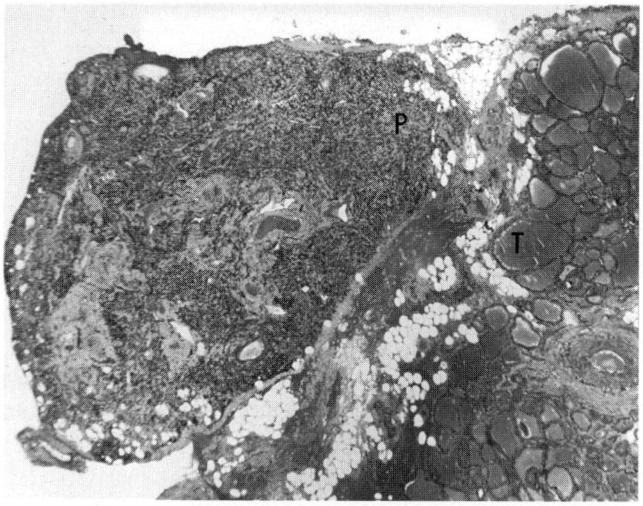

Figure 6-36 Parathyroid gland, dog. Diffuse lymphocytic parathyroiditis *(P)*. The external parathyroid gland has been completely replaced by lymphocytes, plasma cells, fibroblasts, and neocapillaries. *T*, thyroid gland. H & E stain.

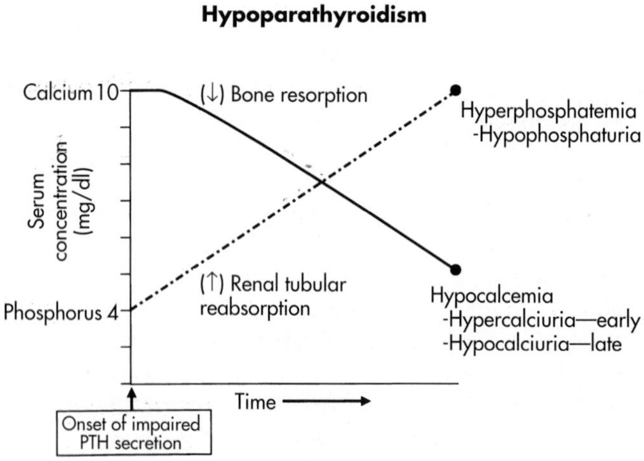

Figure 6-37 Alterations in serum and phosphorus in response to an inadequate secretion of parathyroid hormone. A progressive increase in serum phosphorus and a marked decline in the concentrations of serum calcium has resulted in increased neuromuscular excitability and tetany.

by nutritional imbalances. Such imbalances occur in diets low in calcium or diets with an excess of phosphorus and normal or low content of calcium, and in New World primates housed indoors and fed diets with inadequate amounts of vitamin D_3. The significant result is hypocalcemia, which stimulates the parathyroid glands. Blood phosphorus concentration, when elevated, contributes indirectly to parathyroid stimulation by decreasing blood calcium.

In response to the diet-induced hypocalcemia, chief cells undergo hypertrophy and hyperplasia with increased amounts of lightly eosinophilic or vacuolated cytoplasm. The organelles involved with protein synthesis (endoplasmic reticulum) and packaging of secretory products (Golgi apparatus) are well developed. Many chronically stimulated chief cells with well-developed secretory organelles accumulate glycogen after 5 to 14 weeks.

The most frequent nutritional imbalance causing hyperparathyroidism in horses is the ingestion of excessive amounts of phosphorus. Hyperphosphatemia stimulates the parathyroid gland indirectly by the lowering of blood calcium. Horses that develop the disease usually have been fed grain diets with below-average-quality roughage. Evidence of excessive phosphorus intake might be difficult to determine as the excess phosphorus could have been supplied as a bran supplement to the grain ration. The diet is usually palatable and nutritious except for the excessive phosphorus and marginal or deficient calcium content. A diet deficient in calcium fails to supply the daily calcium requirement, and hypocalcemia develops even though a greater proportion of calcium ingested is absorbed. Changes in concentrations of calcium and phosphorus in urine are more consistent and useful in the clinical diagnosis of nutritional secondary hyperparthyroidism in horses than changes in blood concentrations of these minerals. The increased secretion of PTH acts on normal kidneys to markedly increase urinary phosphorus excretion but to decrease calcium loss in the urine.

Hyperparathyroidism Due to Renal Disease

Hyperparathyroidism as a complication of chronic renal failure is characterized by excessive production of parathyroid hormone in response to chronic hypocalcemia. When the renal disease is extensive enough to reduce the glomerular filtration rate, phosphorus is retained and hyperphosphatemia develops. The increased blood phosphorus concentration contributes to parathyroid stimulation by decreasing blood calcium. Chronic renal disease impairs the production of 1,25-$(OH)_2D_3$ by the kidneys and, thereby, diminishes intestinal calcium transport and increases mobilization of calcium from the skeleton. All parathyroid glands undergo marked chief cell hyperplasia, and the bones subsequently develop varying degrees of generalized fibrous osteodystrophy.

Acute Parathyroid Stimulation: Hypocalcemia Associated with Parturition

Parturient paresis in dairy cattle is a complex metabolic disease characterized by the development of severe hypocalcemia and hypophosphatemia near the time of parturition and the initiation of lactation. The serum calcium concentration decreases to less than 50% of normal in spite of an increased secretion of PTH by the cow's parathyroid glands. Bone resorption remains minimal and few osteoclasts are present on bone surfaces. Biochemical and ultrastructural studies in cows indicate that the parathyroid glands are capable of responding to the acute hypocalcemia by increased development of cellular organelles for hormonal synthesis and by the increased secretion of parathyroid hormone.

The composition of the diet fed to dairy cows is a significant factor in the pathogenesis of parturient hypocalcemia. Diets with excessive celcium have been incriminated as significantly increasing the incidence of the disease. Conversely, diets low in calcium or diets supplemented with therapeutic doses of vitamin D reduce the incidence of parturient hypocalcemia. Calcium homeostasis in pregnant cows fed an excessive calcium diet appears to be maintained principally by intestinal calcium absorption (Fig. 6-38). This greater reliance on intestinal absorption rather than on PTH-stimulated bone resorption probably is a significant factor in the more frequent development of profound hypocalcemia near parturition in cows fed excessive calcium prepartal diets.

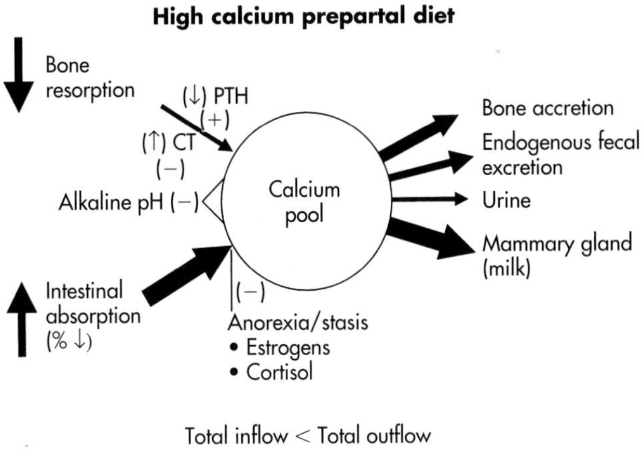

Figure 6-38 Calcium homeostasis in cows fed a high-calcium prepartal diet. The calcium homeostasis is primarily dependent on intestinal calcium absorption. The rate of bone resorption is low, and parathyroid glands are inactive. Anorexia and gastrointestinal stasis that often occur near parturition interrupts the major inflow into the extracellular fluid calcium pool. Outflow of calcium with the onset of lactation exceeds the rate of inflow into the calcium pool, and the cows develop a progressive hypocalcemia and paresis.

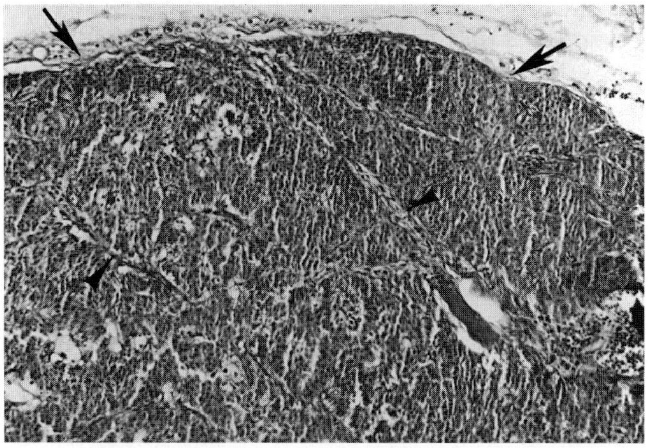

Figure 6-39 Parathyroid gland; dog. Adenoma. Closely packed chief cells are formed into small groups by fine fibrous septa containing capillaries *(arrowheads)*. A thin capsule of fibrous connective tissue *(arrows)* surrounds the neoplasm. H & E stain.

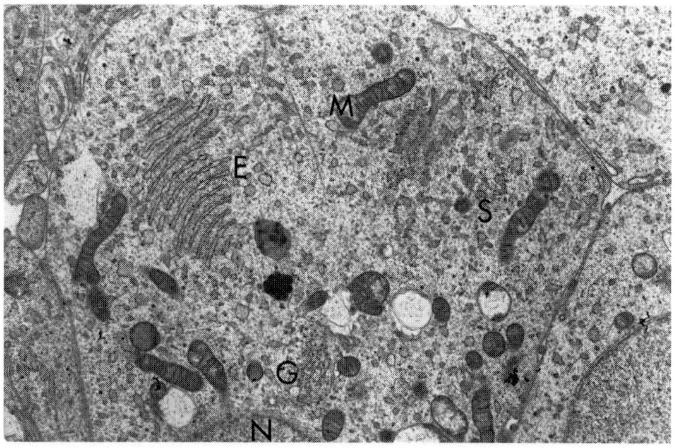

Figure 6-40 Parathyroid gland; dog. Adenoma. Active chief cells have large lamellar arrays of rough endoplasmic reticulum *(E)*, prominent Golgi apparatus *(G)*, and large mitochondria *(M)* but few secretory granules *(S)*. *N*, nucleus of chief cell. TEM. ×7100.

An increased prepartal secretion of calcitonin in cows that develop parturient hypocalcemia ("milk fever"), especially those fed excessive calcium diets, could be a factor that contributes to the inability of increased PTH concentrations to mobilize calcium rapidly from skeletal reserves and maintain blood calcium concentrations during the critical period near parturition. The thyroidal content of calcitonin is reduced, many C cells are degranulated, and plasma concentrations of calcitonin often are increased in cows before the development of profound hypocalcemia.

Functional Neoplasms of Chief Cells: Primary Hyperparathyroidism

Adenomas and carcinomas of parathyroid glands often secrete excessive amounts of parathyroid hormone, resulting in a syndrome of primary hyperparathyroidism. A prolonged increased secretion of PTH accelerates osteolytic and osteoclastic bone resorption. Mineral is removed from the skeleton at an accelerated rate, and bone is replaced by immature fibrous connective tissue. The lesions of fibrous osteodystrophy are generalized throughout the skeleton, but are accentuated in certain areas (e.g., maxilla, mandible, and subperiosteal areas of long bones).

Adenomas of parathyroid glands are encountered in older animals, particularly dogs and infrequently in certain strains of rats, but parathyroid carcinomas are uncommon. Chief cell adenomas usually cause considerable enlargement of a single parathyroid gland that is grossly light brown to red and located either in the cervical region by the thyroid gland or, infrequently, within the thoracic cavity near the base of the heart. Parathyroid adenomas are encapsulated and sharply demarcated from the adjacent thyroid gland.

Parathyroid gland adenomas are composed of closely packed small groups of chief cells enclosed by delicate vascular connective tissue septa that have many capillaries (Fig. 6-39). The chief cells are round to polyhedral and have palely eosinophilic cytoplasm. The expanded cytoplasm of neoplastic chief cells has few electron-dense secretory granules but prominent arrays of endoplasmic reticulum and Golgi complexes (Fig. 6-40).

The functional disturbances observed with endocrinologically active chief cell neoplasms are primarily the result of hypercalcemia and weakening of bones by excessive PTH-stimulated resorption of calcium. Cortical bone is thinned as a result of increased resorption by osteoclasts stimulated by the autonomous secretion of parathyroid hormone (Fig. 6-41). Lameness is due to fractures of long bones that occur after relatively minor physical trauma. Compression fractures occur in vertebral bodies, resulting in pressure on the spinal cord and nerves that leads to motor or sensory dysfunction or both. Facial hyperostosis due to extensive osteoblastic proliferation and deposition of poorly mineralized osteoid and loosening or loss of teeth from alveolar sockets has been observed in dogs with primary hyperparathyroidism. Hypercalcemia results in anorexia, vomiting, constipation, depression, polyuria, polydipsia, and generalized muscular weakness due to decreased neuromuscular excitability.

The most practical laboratory test to aid in the diagnosis of primary hyperparathyroidism is quantitation of total blood calcium and phosphorus and circulating concentrations of parathyroid hormone (*N*-terminal or immunoradiometric [IRMA] assay). Dogs with primary hyperparathyroidism have greatly increased blood calcium concentrations (12 to 20 mg/dl or above). The blood phosphorus is low (4 mg/dl or less) or in the low-normal range because of inhibition of renal tubular reabsorption of phosphorus by the autonomous secretion of PTH. The urinary excretion of calcium and phosphorus is increased

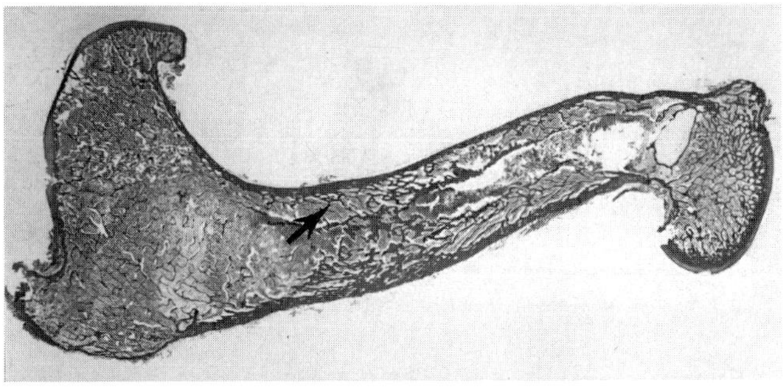

Figure 6-41 Humerus; dog. Primary hyperparathyroidism. Severe thinning of cortical bone and large resorptive cavities *(arrow)* results from localized resorption of bone by osteoclasts.

and can predispose to the development of nephrocalcinosis and urolithiasis.

Humoral Hypercalcemia of Malignancy: Pseudohyperparathyroidism

Hypercalcemia is a common disorder in animals with many causes. The most common form is cancer-associated hypercalcemia. Three mechanisms by which the serum calcium is increased by neoplasms are (1) humoral hypercalcemia of malignancy (HHM), (2) hypercalcemia induced by metastases of solid neoplasms to bone, and (3) hematologic malignancies. Hypercalcemia results from an imbalance of calcium released from bones, calcium excreted by the kidneys, or calcium absorbed from the intestinal tract.

The clinical signs of hypercalcemia are similar regardless of underlying cause and depend on the rapidity of onset of increased concentrations of serum ionized calcium. Animals with serum calcium values in excess of 16 mg/dl (4 mmol/L) generally have the most severe clinical signs. Exceptions to this rule occur, and some animals with severe hypercalcemia have only mild clinical signs. Horses and rabbits have normal total serum calcium concentrations greater than those found in other domestic animals, which should be considered before hypercalcemia is diagnosed in these species. Metabolic acidosis enhances the severity of clinical signs since it results in an increase in the ionized fraction of serum calcium. Increased serum ionized calcium induces clinical signs relating to the gastrointestinal, neuromuscular, cardiovascular, and renal systems.

A syndrome of HHM in aged, primarily female dogs with adenocarcinomas derived from apocrine glands of the anal sac has been characterized. The dogs have persistent hypercalcemia (mean 16.2 mg/dl) and often mild hypophosphatemia, both of which return to normal following surgical excision of the neoplasm. The hypercalcemia persists after removal of the parathyroid glands, suggesting that the humoral factor produced by neoplastic cells does not stimulate an increased secretion of PTH. Increased circulating concentrations of parathyroid hormone–related protein (PTH-rP) have been observed in hypercalcemic dogs with anal sac apocrine gland adenocarcinomas. The neoplasms are malignant and most have metastasized to iliac and sublumbar lymph nodes by the time of initial presentation. Clinical signs include generalized muscular weakness, anorexia, vomiting, bradycardia, depression, polyuria, and polydipsia. These signs are primarily the result of severe hypercalcemia.

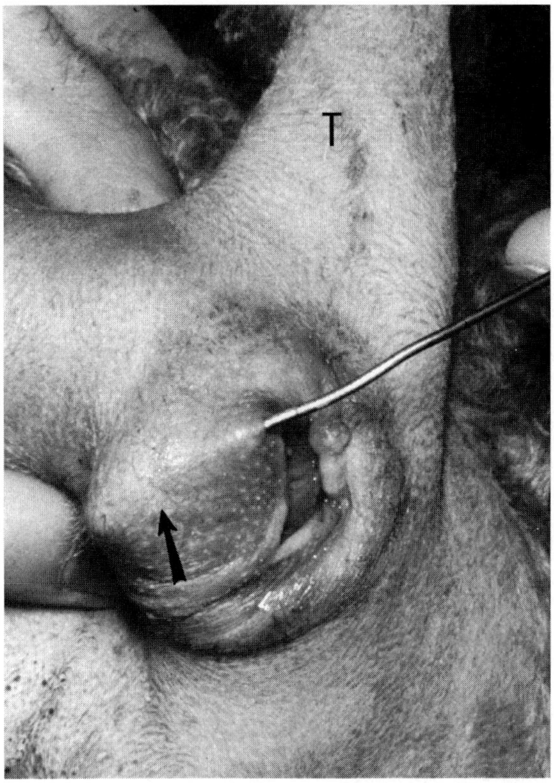

Figure 6-42 Perirectal region; dog. Adenocarcinoma. Small adenocarcinoma *(arrow)* derived from apocrine glands of the anal sac enlarges the region and protrudes as a nodular lesion. *T*, tail.

Apocrine gland adenocarcinoma develops as a firm mass, usually unilateral, ventrolateral to the anus, close to the anal sac but not attached to the overlying skin (Fig. 6-42). The neoplasm arises in the wall of the anal sac and projects as a variably size mass into its lumen (Fig. 6-43).

This unique adenocarcinoma forms glandular acini and papillary projections of apical cytoplasm that extend into the lumen (Fig. 6-44). It is histologically distinct from the more common perianal (circumanal) gland tumor. The majority of neoplasms are histologically bimorphic and contain glandular and solid areas. The solid pattern

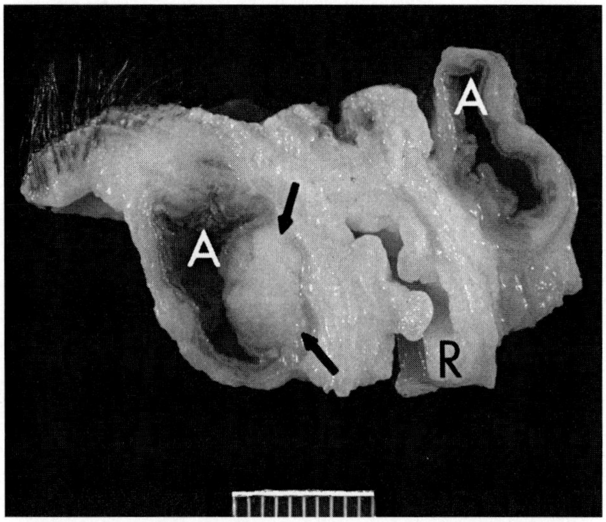

Figure 6-43 Perineum (transverse section); dog. Adenocarcinoma. A neoplasm derived from apocrine glands of the anal sac is present as a 1-cm diameter nodule *(arrows)* arising in the wall of the left anal sac and protruding into its lumen. Anal sacs *(A)* are present on both sides of the rectum *(R)*. Bar = 1 cm. *Meuten DJ, Cooper BJ, Capen CC, et al. Hypercalcemia associated with an adenocarcinoma derived from the aprocrine glands of the anal sac. Vet Pathol 1981; 18:454-471.*

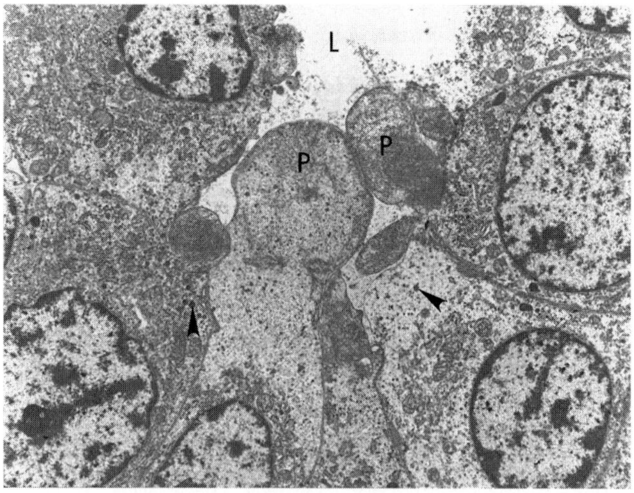

Figure 6-44 Anal sac; dog. Adenocarcinoma. Projections *(P)* of apical cytoplasm extend into the lumen *(L)* of acinus. Small membrane-limited secretory granules *(arrowheads)* are present in the cytoplasm. TEM. *Meuten DJ, Capen CC, Kociba GJ, Chew DJ. Ultrastructural evaluation of an adenocarcinoma derived from apocrine glands of the anal sac associated with hypercalcemia in dogs. Am J Pathol 1982; 107:167-175.*

is characterized by sheets, microlobules, and packets separated by a thin fibrovascular stroma. Pseudorosettes are common in solid areas adjacent to small blood vessels.

The parathyroid glands are small, difficult to locate, or undetectable grossly. The parathyroid glands respond to the persistent cancer-associated hypercalcemia by trophic atrophy. Atrophic parathyroid glands in dogs with HHM are characterized by narrow cords of inactive chief cells with an abundant fibrous connective tissue stroma and widened perivascular spaces. Thyroid C cells in respose to the persistent elevation in blood calcium undergo either diffuse or nodular hyperplasia.

Renal calcification has been detected microscopically in approximately 90% of dogs with HHM and anal sac apocrine gland adenocarcinomas, particularly when the calcium × phosphorus product is 50 or greater. Tubular calcification is most pronounced near the corticomedullary junction but is present also in cortical and inner medullary tubules, Bowman's capsule, and glomerular tufts. Calcification also occurs in the fundic gastric mucosa and endocardium.

Excessive secretion of biologically active PTH-rP plays a central role in the pathogenesis of hypercalcemia in most forms of HHM; however, cytokines such as interleukin-1 (IL-1), tumor necrosis factor-α, or transforming growth factors-α and -β or 1,25-dihydroxyvitamin D can have synergistic or cooperative actions with PTH-rP. Before PTH-rP was identified, it was well understood that nonparathyroid neoplasms associated with humoral hypercalcemia of malignancy induced a syndrome that mimicked primary hyperparathyroidism due to secretion of a PTH-like factor that was antigenically unrelated to PTH. Purification of the PTH-like activity from the adenocarcinoma derived from apocrine glands of the anal sac in dogs and multiple human neoplasms associated with HHM resulted in the discovery of PTH-rP. PTH-rP also can be demonstrated in a number of normal tissues by immunohistochemical and biochemical analysis, where it appears to function primarily as a paracrine factor.

Hypercalcemia Associated with Lymphosarcoma

Lymphosarcoma is the most common neoplasm associated with hypercalcemia in dogs and cats. Estimates of the prevalence of hypercalcemia in dogs with lymphosarcoma vary from 20% to 40%. Peripheral lymph node enlargement is present in some cases; cranial mediastinal or visceral nodes usually are involved. The hypercalcemia results from the production by neoplastic cells of humoral substances or from physical disruption of trabecular bone by lymphosarcoma in bone marrow, or from both mechanisms. Serum immunoreactive PTH concentrations have been subnormal, and plasma prostaglandin E_2 concentrations did not differ from those of controls.

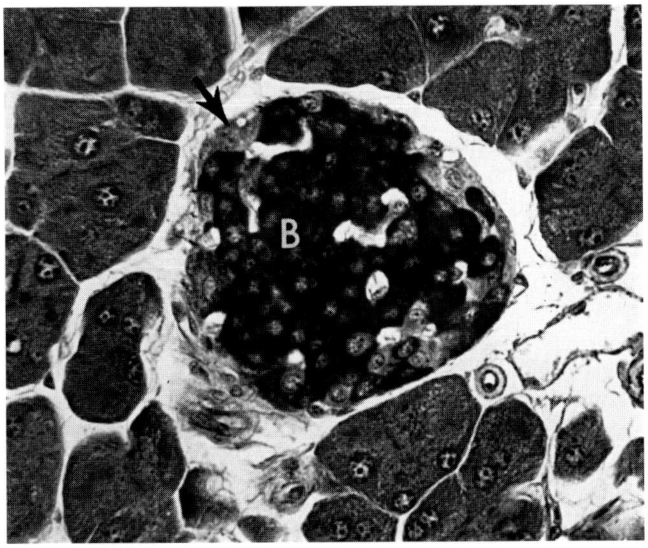

Figure 6-45 Pancreatic islet; dog. Normal. Gomori's aldehyde fuchsin stains the centrally located beta cells *(B)* surrounded by a thin rim of poorly staining alpha and delta cells *(arrow)* at the periphery. The islets are surrounded by the exocrine pancreas.

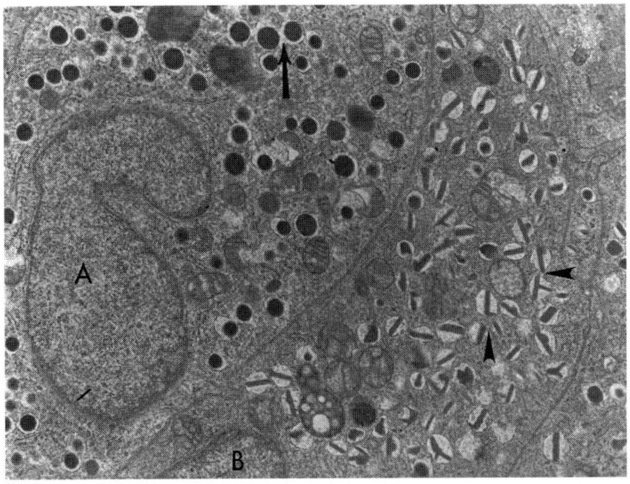

Figure 6-46 Pancreatic islet; normal dog. Differences in secretion granules between beta *(B)* and alpha *(A)* cells; the internal cores of secretion granules in beta cells *(arrowheads)* are bar- or Y-shaped with a prominent space between the limiting membrane and internal core. Secretion granules of the glucagon-secreting alpha cell have an electron-dense, circular, internal core with a narrow submembranous space *(arrow)*. TEM.

Most dogs with lymphoma and HHM have significantly increased circulating PTH-rP concentrations, but concentrations are lower (2 to 15 pmol) than in dogs with carcinomas and HHM, but there is no correlation with serum calcium concentration. This indicates that PTH-rP is an important marker in dogs with HHM and lymphoma, but is not the sole humoral factor responsible for the stimulation of osteoclasts and development of hypercalcemia. It is likely that cytokines such as IL-1 or tumor necrosis factor function synergistically with PTH-rP to induce HHM in dogs with lymphoma. Some dogs and human patients with lymphoma and hypercalcemia have increased serum 1,25-dihydroxyvitamin D concentrations that could be responsible for or contribute to the induction of hypercalcemia. Parathyroid hormone (*N*-terminal) concentrations in dogs with lymphoma and hypercalcemia usually are in the normal range; however, a few dogs have concentrations increased slightly out of the normal range.

Neoplasms Metastatic to Bone

Solid neoplasms that metastasize widely to bone and grow locally can produce hypercalcemia by inducing local bone resorption. This is not common in animals, but is an important cause of cancer-associated hypercalcemia in human beings, particularly patients with breast and lung carcinomas.

The pathogenesis of enhanced bone resorption is not well understood, but the two primary mechanisms include (1) secretion of cytokines or factors that stimulate local bone resorption, and (2) indirect stimulation of bone resorption by tumor-induced cytokine secretion from local immune or bone cells. Cytokines or factors that are secreted by neoplastic cells and stimulate local bone resorption include PTH-rP, transforming growth factor-α and -β, and prostaglandins (especially prostaglandin E_2).

PANCREATIC ISLETS

The endocrine function of the pancreas is performed by small groups of cells ("islets of Langerhans") that are completely surrounded by acinar (exocrine) cells that produce digestive enzymes (Fig. 6-45). During embryonic development of the pancreas, a close relationship exists between the endocrine and exocrine portions. Evidence suggests that islet, acinar, and ductal cells arise from a common multipotential precursor cell. In early embryonic development the endocrine cells are integrated within the exocrine matrix of the pancreatic bud. They subsequently accumulate in nonvascularized clusters and later become separated from the exocrine tissue and independently vascularized.

The pancreatic islets of normal animals contain multiple types of cells. Beta cells, the predominant secretory cell, function in the biosynthesis of insulin but co-secrete islet amyloid polypeptide. F cells or PP cells in the islets secrete pancreatic polypeptide. The glucagon-secreting alpha cells are less numerous. The different cell types of the endocrine pancreas can be differentiated by immunohistochemical techniques (Fig. 6-45) and by electron microscopy (Fig. 6-46). Alpha, beta, and delta cells have well-developed rough endoplasmic reticulum and Golgi apparatus that participate in the biosynthesis of polypeptide hormones, and numerous secretory ("storage") granules are present in the cytoplasm. Each type of endocrine cell in the pancreatic islets has secretory granules with distinct characteristics that can be used to identify the cell types (Fig. 6-46); however, immunocytologic identification of the specific islet hormone is a more accurate method of identifying the different cell types in the pancreatic islets.

The major physiologic stimulus for the release of insulin from beta cells is glucose. An appropriate concentration of calcium ion in extracellular fluids is required for induction of insulin release from beta cells.

Insulin is a powerful hormone that has broad biologic influences and affects either directly or indirectly the structure and function of every organ in the body. Tissues especially responsive to insulin include skeletal and cardiac muscle, adipose tissue, fibroblasts, hepatocytes, leukocytes, mammary glands, cartilage, bone, skin, aorta, pituitary gland, and peripheral nerves. The principal function of insulin is to stimulate anabolic reactions involving carbohydrates, fats, proteins, and nucleic acids. It catalyzes the formation of macromolecules used in cell structure, energy stores, and regulation of many cell functions. Hepatocytes, adipose cells, and muscle are three principal target sites for insulin. In general, insulin increases the transfer of glucose and certain other monosaccharides, some amino acids and fatty acids, and potassium and magnesium ions across the plasma membrane of target cells. It also enhances glucose oxidation and glycogenesis and stimulates lipogenesis and the formation of ATP, DNA, and RNA. Insulin also decreases the rate of lipolysis, proteolysis, ketogenesis, and gluconeogenesis.

Glucagon is a hormone that stimulates energy release from target cells and is secreted in response to a reduction in blood glucose concentration. It mobilizes stores of energy-yielding nutrients by increasing glycogenolysis, gluconeogenesis, and lipolysis, thereby increasing the blood concentration of glucose. At physiologic concentrations, glucagon increases both hepatic glycogenolysis and gluconeogenesis. Insulin and glucagon act in concert to maintain the concentration of glucose in extracellular fluids within relatively narrow limits. A "glucose sensor" in the pancreatic islets controls the relative mixture of these two biologic antagonists. Glucagon controls glucose influx into the extracellular space from the hepatocytes, and insulin controls glucose efflux from the extracellular space into such insulin-sensitive tissues as adipose cells, muscle, and hepatocytes.

Hypofunction: Diabetes Mellitus

Diabetes mellitus is a metabolic disorder that results from diminished availability of insulin for normal function of many cells of the body. In some cases, increased concentrations of glucagon contribute to development of the persistent hyperglycemia. Insulin unavailability could be due to degenerative changes in beta cells of the pancreatic islets, reduced effectiveness of the hormone due to the formation of anti-insulin antibodies or inactive complexes, damage to beta cells from immune-mediated islet cytotoxicity, or inappropriate secretion of hormones by neoplasms in other endocrine organs.

Diabetes mellitus is a common endocrinopathy in dogs with a reported incidence of 1:200. Most cases of spontaneous diabetes occur in mature dogs and in females approximately twice as often as males. An increased incidence of diabetes mellitus has been observed in certain small breeds of dogs, such as miniature poodles, Dachshund, and terriers, but nearly all breeds of dogs can be affected.

In the pathogenesis of diabetes mellitus, several factors are responsible for the decreased available insulin. The destruction of islets secondary to severe pancreatitis or the selective degeneration of islet cells are the most common causes in animals. In dogs, the pancreatic islets are often destroyed because of inflammation of the exocrine pancreas. Chronic relapsing pancreatitis with progressive loss of both exocrine and endocrine cells and replacement by fibrous connective tissue is a frequent cause of diabetes mellitus. In these dogs, the pancreas becomes firm, multinodular, and after a recent relapse has scattered areas of hemorrhage and necrosis (Fig. 6-47). Later in the course of the disease, all that remains of the pancreas is a thin fibrous band or nodule near the duodenum and stomach (Fig. 6-48). In other cases, beta cells are reduced in

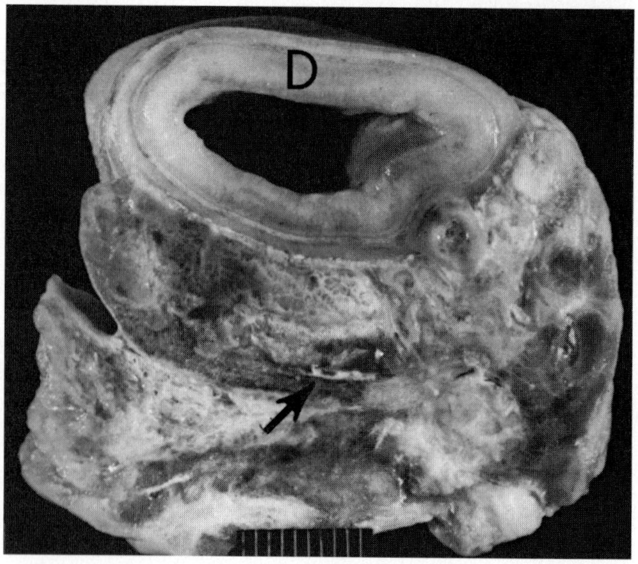

Figure 6-47 Pancreas; dog. Chronic relapsing pancreatitis. The pancreas is multinodular and firm with areas of hemorrhage *(arrow)* and necrosis. *D*, duodenum. Bar = 1 cm.

number and remaining cells have vacuolated cytoplasm. When disease is chronic, the islets are difficult to find. Immune-mediated isletitis characterized by a progressive lymphoplasmacytic infiltration and selective destruction of endocrine cells of the islets is another cause of diabetes mellitus in human beings (type 1), rodent models, and occasionally in dogs.

Development of diabetes mellitus in young dogs is the result of idiopathic atrophy of the pancreas, acute pancreatitis with necrosis and hemorrhage, and aplasia of pancreatic islets. The pancreas with idiopathic atrophy is reduced to a third or less of its size. Hypoplasia of pancreatic islets has caused diabetes mellitus in young dogs (2 to 3 months of age). The islets are absent, but the pancreatic acini and ducts are present and functional.

Cats with diabetes mellitus usually have specific degenerative lesions localized selectively in the islets of Langerhans, whereas the remainder of the pancreas appears normal. The selective deposition of amyloid in islets, resulting in degenerative changes in alpha and beta cells, is the most common pancreatic lesion in cats with diabetes. Scattered amyloid deposits in pancreatic islets that increase progressively with age occur in the pancreatic islets of many cats without clinically apparent diabetes mellitus. Islet amyloid polypeptide (IAPP) (37 amino acids) and insulin are both secreted by B cells.

The IAPP in cats (also human beings and racoons) has a unique amino acid sequence (amino acids 25 to 28: alanine, isoleucine, leucine, and serine) that predispose to polymerization and accumulation in pancreatic islets. As the insoluble amyloid fibers progressively accumulate in the islets, it disrupts B cells and surrounds islet capillaries, leading to subsequent degeneration of islet cells.

Another lesion in the pancreatic islets of cats with diabetes mellitus is hydropic (vacuolar) degeneration of the beta and alpha cells (Fig. 6-49). The cytoplasm of beta cells is distended by massive accumulation of glycogen particles (Fig. 6-50). Vacuolar degeneration with glycogen accumulation in cats appears to develop in beta cells in response to long-term overstimulation ("exhaustion") because of peripheral insulin resistance.

The onset of diabetes is insidious, and the clinical course is often chronic. The signs in dogs most often associated with diabetes mellitus include polydipsia, polyuria, increased feed consumption, loss of weight, bilateral cataracts, and weakness. The disturbances in water metabolism primarily have an osmotic basis. In dogs

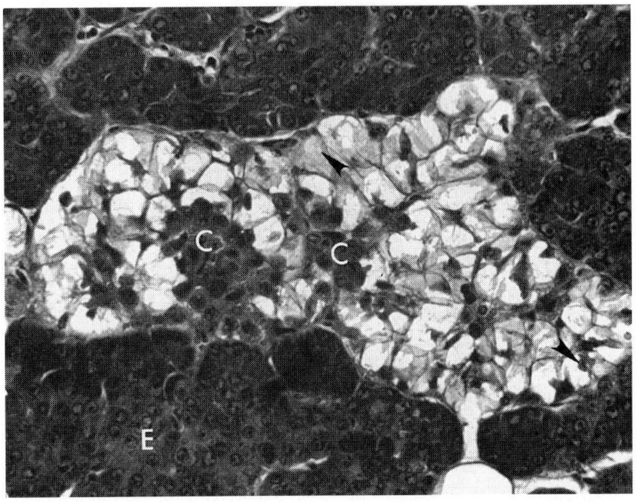

Figure 6-49 Pancreas; islet, cat. Hydropic ("vacuolar") degeneration. Discrete vacuoles *(arrowheads)* are present in the cytoplasm of beta cells. A few viable secretory cells remain adjacent to several capillaries *(C)*. *E,* exocrine pancreas. H & E stain.

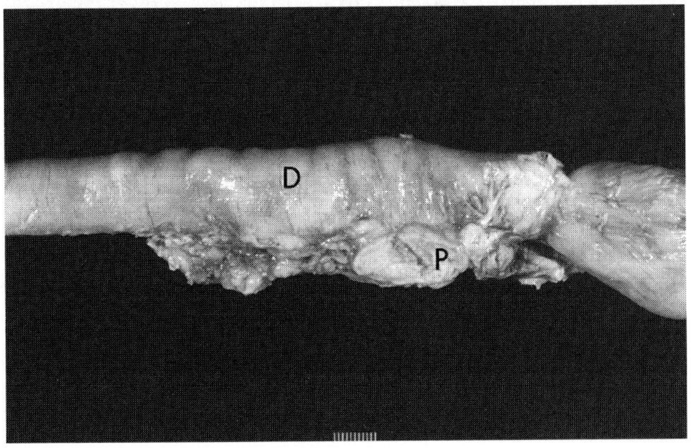

Figure 6-48 Pancreas; dog. Chronic pancreatitis. The parenchyma of the pancreas *(P)* is almost completely replaced by fibrous connective tissue in "end-stage" pancreatitis. *D,* duodenum. Bar = 1 cm.

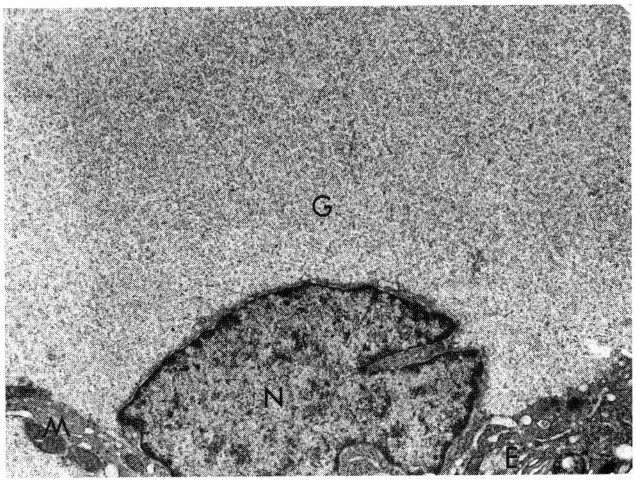

Figure 6-50 Pancreas, islet; cat. Glycogen accumulation in beta cell. The nucleus *(N)* and secretory organelles are displaced to the periphery of the beta cell by the accumulation of glycogen *(G)* particles. *M,* mitochondria, *E,* endoplasmic reticulum. ×4000.

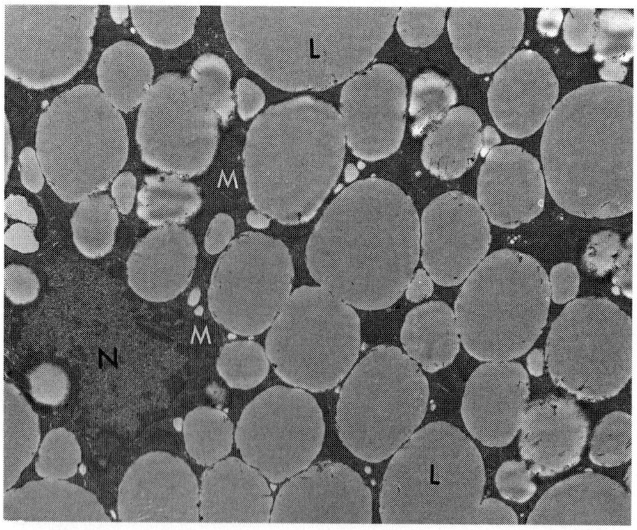

Figure 6-51 Liver; dog. Fatty degeneration. The cytoplasm contains multiple large lipid droplets *(L)* that have displaced the nucleus *(N)* peripherally and compressed cytoplasmic organelles such as mitochondria *(M)*. TEM. ×6600.

with persistent hyperglycemia and glycosuria, the renal tubular epithelium is unable to concentrate the urine effectively against the osmotic attraction of glucose in the glomerular filtrate.

Diabetic animals have diminished resistance to bacterial and fungal infections and often develop chronic or recurrent infections such as suppurative cystitis, prostatitis, bronchopneumonia, and dermatitis. This increased susceptibility to infection in patients with poorly controlled diabetes can be related in part to impaired chemotactic, phagocytic, and microbicidal functions and decreased adherence of polymorphonuclear leukocytes. The impaired microbicidal function of leukocytes can have a metabolic basis resulting from the diminished cellular energy production from glucose. These defects in leukocyte function are at least partially corrected by appropriate treatment. Radiographic evidence of emphysematous cystitis is strongly suggestive of diabetes mellitus. Infections of the urinary bladder with glucose-fermenting organisms, such as *Proteus* sp., *Aerobacter aerogenes,* and *Escherichia coli,* result in gas formation in the wall and lumen. Emphysema also develops in the gallbladder wall in some diabetic dogs.

Hepatomegaly occurs as a result of fatty degeneration and cirrhosis. Lipids accumulate in the liver as the result of increased fat mobilization and hepatocytes, injured by ketonemia, have decreased utilization of fats. Individual hepatocytes are greatly enlarged by multiple droplets of neutral lipid (Fig. 6-51). If the accumulation of lipid is extensive and long-standing, cirrhosis develops. The liver remains enlarged, and its surface becomes coarsely nodular because of extensive remodeling of hepatic parenchyma (Fig. 6-52). Individual hepatocytes degenerate and are replaced by regenerative and hyperplastic nodules and interlobular fibrosis. Icterus and bilirubinuria often accompany severe cirrhosis.

Cataracts often develop in dogs with poorly controlled diabetes mellitus. They are stellate ("asteroid") in shape (Fig. 6-53) and initially appear along the suture lines of lenticular fibers. Cataract formation in the diabetic patient is related to the unique sorbitol pathway by which glucose is metabolized in the lens. Glucose is first converted to sorbitol by the enzyme aldose reductase and, subsequently, to fructose by sorbitol dehydrogenase. These sugar alcohols accumulate within the lens and result in an intracellular accumulation of solute and hypertonicity. The initial structural change in the lens consists of swelling and hydropic degeneration of lenticular fibers. Swelling of lenticular fibers continues in long-standing cases of diabetes mellitus until the majority of lenticular fibers are affected. Later, macromolecular aggregation or precipitation of normally translucent lenticular proteins develops accompanied by disruption of lenticular fibers and formation of interfibrillar clefts. This results in the diffuse, often bilateral, opacity of the lens observed in animals with chronic diabetes mellitus.

Other extrapancreatic lesions of diabetes mellitus, such as chronic renal disease, blindness, and gangrene, are the result of microangiopathy characterized by thickening of the capillary basement membrane. Dogs with long-standing, poorly controlled, spontaneous diabetes mellitus develop nodular or diffuse glomerulosclerosis characterized by PAS-positive fibrillar deposits of glycoprotein that sometimes form spherical nodules in the glomerular capillary tufts. Other renal lesions include accumulation of glycogen within cells of Henle's loop (intracytoplasmic) and distal convoluted tubule (intranuclear) (Fig. 6-54).

Complete expression of the complex metabolic disturbances in diabetes mellitus appears to be the result of a bihormonal abnormality. Although a relative or absolute deficiency of insulin action in response to a rising extracellular glucose concentration has been long recognized as the sine qua non of diabetes mellitus, the importance of an absolute or relative increase of glucagon secretion in some forms of the disease in certain species has been appreciated only recently. Hyperglucagonemia in diabetic patients can be the result of increased secretion of pancreatic glucagon, enteroglucagon, or both. An increased blood glucagon concentration contributes to the severe endogenous hyperglycemia by mobilizing hepatic stores of glucose and to the development of ketoacidosis by increasing the oxidation of fatty acids by hepatocytes. The major glucoregulatory consequence of insulin deficiency is reduction of movement of glucose into insulin-sensitive tissues (e.g., liver, fat, and muscle) with a corresponding increase in hepatic glucose production, resulting in marked endogenous hyperglycemia.

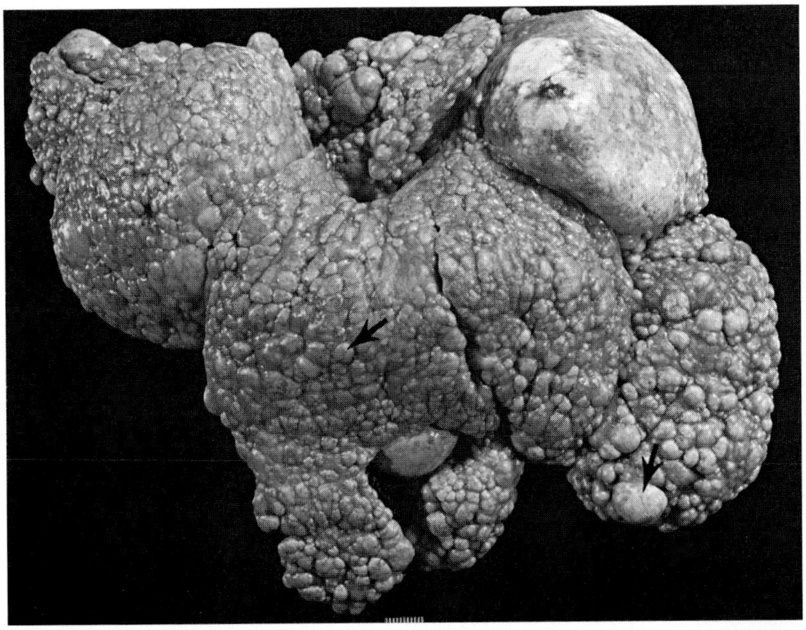

Figure 6-52 Liver; dog. Cirrhosis. All lobes of the liver are considerably enlarged, firm, and have a coarsely nodular surface. The nodules *(arrows)* represent areas of regenerative hyperplasia of hepatocytes. Bar = 1 cm.

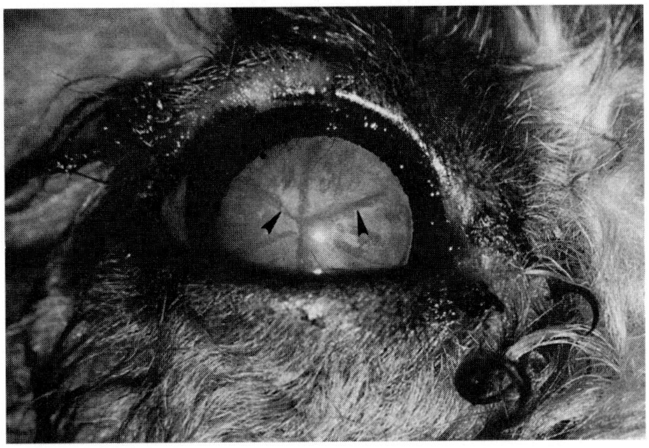

Figure 6-53 Eyeball, lens; dog. Diabetes mellitus. Early stellate lesion *(arrowheads)* along the sutures of the lens.

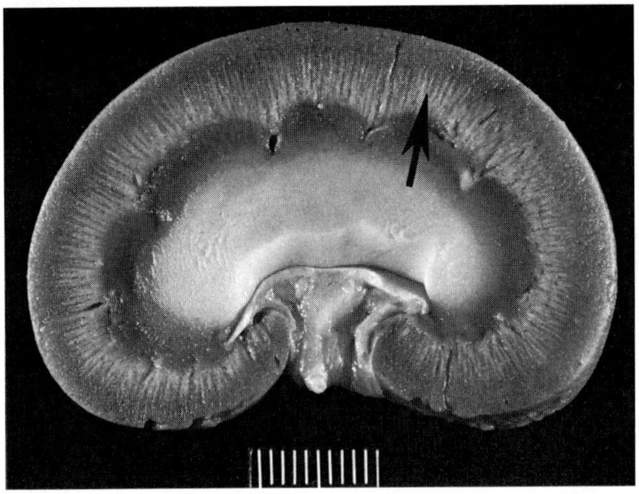

Figure 6-54 Kidney, dog. Glycogen "nephrosis," diabetes mellitus. The radially arranged light areas in the inner cortex of the kidney *(arrow)* represent prominent tubules with an abnormal accumulation of glycogen. Bar = 1 cm.

Hyperfunction of Pancreatic Islets

Beta Cell (Insulin-Secreting) Neoplasms

The neoplasms most frequently arising in pancreatic islets are adenomas and carcinomas derived from beta cells. These neoplasms often are endocrinologically active and produce dramatic functional disturbances. Other pancreatic neoplasms appear to be derived from multipotential ductal epithelial cells that differentiate into one of the several other cell types of the pancreatic islets. Beta cell neoplasms are seen most frequently in dogs 5 to 12 years of age (mean 9 years). These neoplasms also occur in older cattle and have been associated with periodic convulsions.

Adenoma of the beta cells of the pancreatic islets ("insulinomas") is usually a single yellow to dark red, spherical, small (1 to 3 cm) nodule. The neoplasms are of similar consistency to or slightly firmer than that of the surrounding pancreas. Adenomas occur as single or less often multiple nodules in one or multiple lobes of the pancreas. A thin layer of fibrous connective tissue separates the adenoma from the adjacent parenchyma (Fig. 6-55).

Carcinomas of the pancreatic islets are more common in dogs than adenomas and are more common in the duodenal (right) lobe of the pancreas. Carcinomas of the pancreatic islets can be differentiated from adenomas by their larger size, multilobular appearance, extensive invasion of adjacent parenchyma and lymph vessels, and

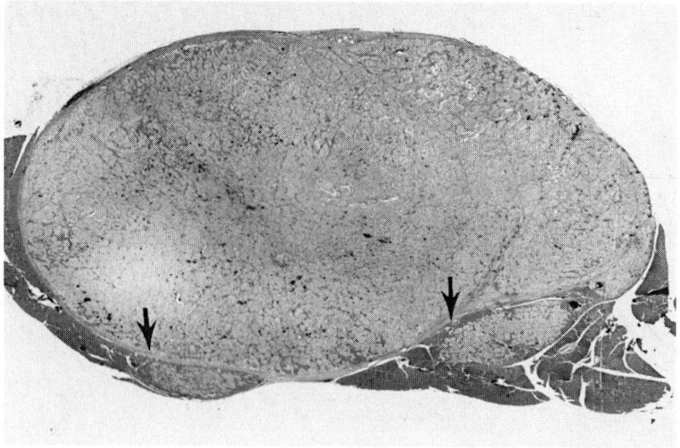

Figure 6-55 Pancreas, islet; dog. Beta cell adenoma. The thin fibrous capsule around the adenoma is incomplete at several points *(arrows)* where there is intermingling of islet and acinar epithelial cells.

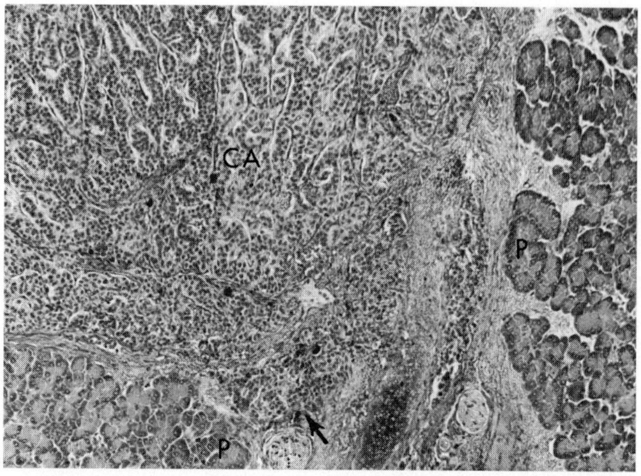

Figure 6-56 Pancreas, islet; dog. Beta cell carcinoma. Neuroendocrine packeting of neoplastic cells *(CA)* and invasion of carcinoma through the fibrous capsule *(arrows)* into adjacent exocrine pancreas. *P,* exocrine pancreas. H & E stain.

metastases in extrapancreatic sites such as regional lymph nodes (e.g., duodenal, mesenteric, hepatic, and splenic), liver, mesentery, and omentum.

Islet cell adenomas are sharply delineated and surrounded by a thin capsule of fibrous connective tissue (Fig. 6-55). Small nests of acinar epithelial cells are sometimes present throughout the neoplasm, but are more common at the periphery. Numerous connective tissue septa containing small capillaries radiate from the capsule into the neoplasm and subdivide the neoplasm into small lobules or packets. The neoplastic cells are well differentiated, varying from round to polyhedral, have a palely eosinophilic and finely granular cytoplasm, and indistinct cellular membranes.

Islet cell carcinomas are consistently larger than adenomas, are multilobular, and invade into and through the fibrous capsule of the pancreas (Fig. 6-56). The dense bands of fibrous tissue that course through the neoplasm give rise to fine connective tissue septa containing capillaries that subdivide the neoplasm into small cords or lobules. The well-differentiated neoplastic cells in islet cell carcinomas are closely packed but are less uniform in size and shape than cells of adenomas. They are round to polyhedral and have a granular eosinophilic cytoplasm. Mitotic figures are not numerous. Microscopic evidence of distinct local tissue invasion is the principal criteria for the diagnosis of islet cell carcinoma.

Cells composing functional islet cell neoplasms in dogs usually have ultrastructural, histochemical, and immunocytochemical characteristics of beta cells. The neoplastic beta cells are electron dense because of the numerous cytoplasmic organelles.

The clinical alterations observed with functional beta cell neoplasms are the result of excessive insulin secretion and the development of severe hypoglycemia. The clinical signs are not specific for the hyperinsulinism produced by beta cell neoplasms. Initial signs include weakness, fatigue after vigorous exercise, generalized muscular twitching and weakness, ataxia, mental confusion, and changes of temperament. The dogs are easily agitated and have intermittent periods of excitability and restlessness. Periodic convulsive seizures of the tonic-clonic type occur later in the disease and increase progressively in frequency and intensity.

The predominance of clinical signs relating to the CNS demonstrates the primary dependence of the brain on the metabolism of glucose for energy. The failure to recognize that dogs with functional islet cell neoplasms can present with clinical signs suggesting primary disease of the nervous system has frequently led to the misdiagnoses of idiopathic epilepsy, brain neoplasm, or other organic neurologic disease. Repeated episodes of prolonged and severe hypoglycemia result in neuronal necrosis and permanent neurologic disability with terminal coma and eventually death.

Non–Beta (Gastrin-Secreting) Islet Cell Neoplasms

Gastrin-secreting, non–beta islet cell neoplasms of the pancreas have been reported in human beings, dogs, and cats. The hypersecretion of gastrin in human beings results in the well-documented Zollinger-Ellison syndrome consisting of hypersecretion of gastric acid and recurrent peptic ulceration in the gastrointestinal tract. The non–beta islet cell neoplasms derived from ectopic APUD (**a**mine **p**recursor **u**ptake **d**ecarboxylase) cells in the pancreas produce an excess of gastrin, which normally is secreted by cells of the antral and duodenal mucosa. The incidence of gastrin-secreting pancreatic neoplasms in dogs and cats is uncertain, but it appears to be uncommon compared with insulin-secreting beta cell neoplasms. In the comparatively few cases studied in the dog and cat, the clinical signs have included anorexia, vomiting of blood-tinged material, intermittent diarrhea, progressive weight loss, and dehydration. The prominent functional disturbances are the result of the multiple ulcerations of the gastrointestinal mucosa due to the gastric acid hypersecretion stimulated by gastrin.

Animals with Zollinger-Ellison-like syndrome have had single or multiple variably sized neoplasms in the pancreas. The neoplasms are firm, have increased amounts of fibrous connective tissue, and partial encapsulation, but the neoplasm usually extends into the surrounding pancreas.

The basic histologic pattern of pancreatic islet cell neoplasms in animals is similar irrespective of whether they are secreting insulin or gastrin. Three histologic patterns of non–beta cell islet neoplasms are recognized in dogs: the ribbon or trabecular pattern, solid nests of cells with a delicate highly vascularized stroma, and an acinar pattern with arrangement of cuboidal neoplastic cells around a central lumen. The stroma is prominent and hyalinized in some gastrin-secreting neoplasms.

Gastrin-secreting islet cell neoplasms in dogs invade locally into the adjacent pancreas and often metastasize to regional lymph nodes and to the liver. These dogs have either single or multiple ulcerations in the gastric or duodenal mucosa, or both, and with blood in the lumen.

Other non–beta islet cell neoplasms reported in animals are the glucagon-secreting alpha cell neoplasms. Glucagonomas have been reported rarely in dogs and are associated with superficial necrolytic dermatitis.

CHEMORECEPTOR ORGANS

Chemoreceptor tissue is present at several sites in the body including the carotid body, aortic bodies, nodose ganglion of the vagus nerve, ciliary ganglion in the orbit, pancreas, bodies on the internal jugular vein below the middle ear, and glomus jugular along the recurrent branch of the glossopharyngeal nerve. The chemoreceptor organs are sensitive barometers of changes in the blood carbon dioxide content, pH, and oxygen tension, thereby aiding in the regulation of respiration and circulation. Carotid and aortic bodies can initiate an increase in the depth, minute volume, and rate of respiration via parasympathetic nerves and an increased heart rate and elevated arterial blood pressure via the sympathetic nervous system. The bodies are composed of parenchymal (chemoreceptor) cells and stellate (sustentacular) cells. Nerve endings with synaptic vesicles as well as nerve fibers occur in close association with the chemoreceptor cells.

Although chemoreceptor tissue appears to be widely distributed in the body, neoplasms develop principally in the aortic and carotid bodies of animals. Aortic body chemodectomas are encountered more frequently in animals than those of the carotid body, but the reverse is true for human beings. These neoplasms develop primarily in dogs and infrequently in cats and cattle. Brachycephalic breeds of dogs such as the boxer and Boston terrier are highly predisposed to develop neoplasms of the aortic and carotid bodies.

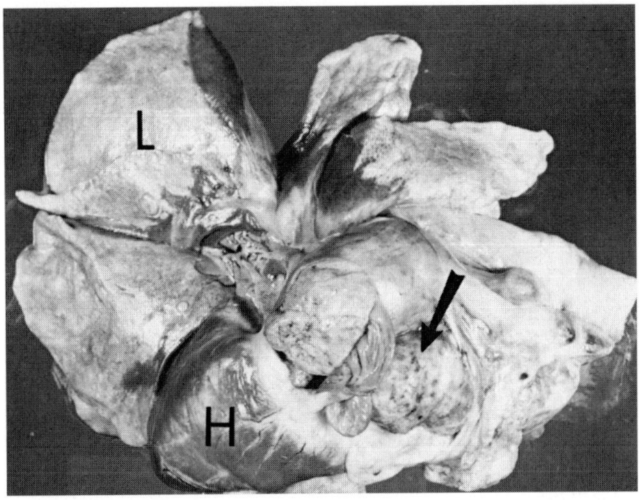

Figure 6-57 Aortic body; dog. Carcinoma. Multiple nodules *(arrow)* are at the base of the heart, *(H)*. *L,* diaphragmatic lobe of lung.

Neoplasms

Neoplasms of Aortic Body

Aortic body neoplasms appear most frequently as a single mass or as multiple nodules near the base of the heart. They vary considerably in size (from 0.5 to 12.5 cm) with carcinomas, in general, being larger than adenomas. Solitary small adenomas either are attached to the adventitia of the pulmonary artery and ascending aorta or are embedded in the adipose connective tissue between these major vessels. They have a smooth external surface and on cross section are white and mottled with red to brown areas. Larger adenomas can indent the atria or displace the trachea, are multilobular, and partially surround the major vessels at the base of the heart. Aortic body carcinomas are less frequent than adenomas in dogs. Carcinomas infiltrate the wall of the pulmonary artery and form papillary projections into the lumen or invade through the wall into the lumen of the atria (Fig. 6-57). Although neoplastic cells often invade blood vessels, metastases to the lungs and liver occur infrequently in dogs with aortic body carcinomas.

Neoplasms of the aortic bodies in animals are not functional (i.e., they do not secrete excess hormone into the circulation), but as a space-occupying lesion they can produce a variety of functional disturbances. Larger aortic body adenomas and carcinomas put pressure on the atria, vena cava, or both and cause manifestations of cardiac decompensation. More aortic body neoplasms than carotid body neoplasms are benign. Aortic body carcinomas invade locally into the atria, pericardium, and adjacent vessels.

Neoplasms of Carotid Body

Carotid body neoplasms arise near the bifurcation of the common carotid artery in the cranial cervical area. They are usually unilateral, only rarely bilateral, and are slow growing. Adenomas vary from approximately 1 to 4 cm in diameter, are well encapsulated, and have a smooth external surface. The bifurcation of the carotid artery is incorporated in the mass, and neoplastic cells are firmly adherent to the tunica adventitia. Adenomas are firm, white with scattered areas of hemorrhage, and are extremely vascular.

Carotid body carcinomas are larger, more coarsely multinodular than adenomas, invade the capsule, and penetrate into the walls of adjacent blood and lymph vessels. The external jugular vein and some cranial nerves can be incorporated into the neoplasm. Metastases of carotid body carcinomas occur in approximately 30% of cases and have been found in the lungs, tracheobronchial and mediastinal lymph nodes, liver, pancreas, and kidneys. Multicentric neoplastic transformation of chemoreceptor tissue (aortic and carotid bodies) occurs frequently in brachycephalic breeds of dogs.

The microscopic features of chemoreceptor neoplasms ("chemodectomas") are essentially similar whether they are derived from either the carotid or aortic body. The neoplasm is subdivided into lobules by prominent branching trabeculae of connective tissue that originate from the fibrous capsule and are further subdivided into smaller nests by fine septa of collagenous and reticulin fibers and small capillaries. Neoplastic cells are commonly aligned along and around small capillaries and are discrete, round to polyhedral, closely packed, and have palely eosinophilic, finely granular, and often vacuolated cytoplasm.

Although the etiology of carotid and aortic body neoplasms is unknown, a genetic predisposition aggravated by chronic hypoxia could account for the greater risk of development in certain brachycephalic breeds such as the boxer and Boston terrier. Carotid bodies of several mammalian species, including dogs, have developed hyperplastic foci when the animals are subjected to the chronic hypoxia of high altitude. Human beings living at high altitudes have 10 times the frequency of chemodectomas as those residing at sea level.

Heart-Base Neoplasms Derived from Ectopic Thyroid Gland Tissue

Adenomas and carcinomas derived from ectopic thyroid gland account for approximately 5% to 10% of "heart-base" neoplasms in dogs. They often compress or invade structures in the cranial mediastinum near the base of the heart (Fig. 6-58). Areas of ectopic thyroid gland neoplasms have a compact cellular (solid) pattern that is difficult to distinguish histologically from aortic body neoplasms. Cells of ectopic thyroid gland neoplasms generally are smaller than those of aortic body neoplasms and have more hyperchromatic nuclei and an eosinophilic cytoplasm. Thyroidal neoplasms of follicular cells are not consistently subdivided into small packets by fine strands of connective tissue. Giant cells are infrequent in ectopic thyroid gland neoplasms, and the stroma is not prominent. Usually, primitive follicular structures or colloid-containing follicles can be demonstrated in ectopic thyroid gland neoplasms but not in aortic body neoplasms.

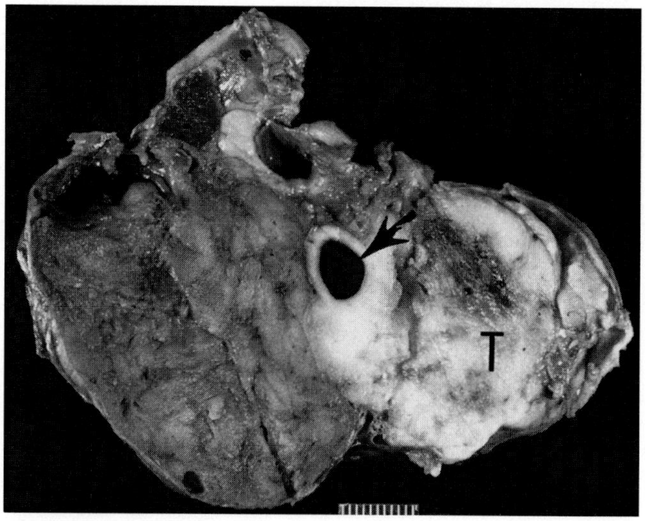

Figure 6-58 Ectopic thyroid tissue; dog. Carcinoma. Neoplastic tissue *(T)* surrounds the trachea *(arrow)* and other structures in the cranial mediastinum. Bar = 1 cm.

References

General considerations

Aurbach GD. Inherited disorders of hormone resistance. In: Desnick RJ, et al., eds. Animal Models of Inherited Metabolic Diseases. New York: Alan R. Liss, 1982.

Binns W, James LF, Shupe JL, Evertte G. A congenital cyclopian-type malformation in lambs induced by maternal ingestion of a range plant, *Veratrum californicum*. Am J Vet Res 1963; 24:1164-1175.

Capen CC. Mechanistic data and risk assessment of selected toxic end points of the thyroid gland. Toxicol Pathol 1997; 25:39-48.

Capen CC. Toxic responses of the endocrine system. In: Klaassen CD, ed. Casarett and Doull's Toxicology: The Basic Science of Poisons. 5th edition. New York: McGraw Hill, 1995:617-640.

Capen CC, Rosol TJ. Pathobiology of parathyroid hormone and parathyroid hormone–related protein: Introduction and evolving concepts. In: LiVolsi VA, DeLellis RA, eds. Pathology of the Thyroid and Parathyroid Gland: An Update. Philadelphia: Williams & Wilkins, 1993:1-33.

Chan L, O'Malley BW. Mechanism of action of the sex steroid hormones. N Engl J Med 1976; 294:1322-1328.

Clegg ED, Cook JC, Chapin RE, Foster PMD, Daston GP. Leydig cell hyperplasia and adenoma formation: Mechanisms and relevance to humans. Reprod Toxicol 1997; 11:107-121.

Cox RI. The endocrinologic changes of gestation and parturition in the sheep. In: Brandly CA, et al., eds. Advances in Veterinary Science and Comparative Medicine. Vol. 19. New York: Academic Press, 1975.

Curran PG, DeGroot LJ. The effect of hepatic enzyme-inducing drugs on thyroid hormones and the thyroid gland. Endocr Rev 1991; 12:135-150.

Gosselin SJ, Capen CC, Krakowka S, Martin SL. Lymphocytic thyroiditis in dogs: Induction with local graft-versus-host reaction. Am J Vet Res 1981; 42:1856-1864.

Gosselin SJ, Capen CC, Martin SL. Histopathologic and ultrastructural evaluation of thyroid lesions associated with hypothyroidism in dogs. Vet Pathol 1981; 18:299-309.

Gosselin SJ, Capen CC, Martin SL, Krakowka S. Autoimmune lymphocytic thyroiditis in dogs. Vet Immunol Immunopathol 1982; 3:185-201.

Holzworth J, Theran P, Carpenter JF, Harpster NK, Todoroff RJ. Hyperthyroidism in the cat: Ten cases. J Am Vet Med Assoc 1980; 176:345-353.

Hotz KJ, Wilson AGE, Thake DC, Roloff MV, Capen CC, Kronenberg JM, Brewster DW. Mechanism of thiazopyr-induced effects on thyroid hormone homeostasis in male Sprague-Dawley rats. Toxicol Appl Pharmacol 1997; 142:133-142.

Kennedy PC, Kendrick JW, Stormont C. Adenohypophyseal aplasia, an inherited defect associated with abnormal gestation in Guernsey cattle. Cornell Vet 1957; 47:160-178.

Leav I, Schiller AL, Rijnberg A, Legg MA, de Kinderen PJ. Adenomas and carcinomas of the canine and feline thyroid. Am J Pathol 1976; 83:61-122.

McClain RM, Posch RC, Bosakowski T, Armstrong JM. Studies on the mode of action for thyroid gland tumor promotion in rats by phenobarbital. Toxicol Appl Pharmacol 1988; 94:254-265.

McClain RM, Levin AA, Posch R, Downing JC. The effects of phenobarbital on the metabolism and excretion of thyroxine in rats. Toxicol Appl Pharmacol 1989; 99:216-228.

Meuten DJ, Capen CC, Kociba GJ, Chew DJ. Ultrastructural evaluation of an adenocarcinoma derived from apocrine glands of the anal sac associated with hypercalcemia in dogs. Am J Pathol 1982; 107:167-175.

Pammenter M, Albrecht C, Kiebenberg vdW, van Jaarsveld P. Afrikander cattle congenital goiter: Characteristics of its morphology and iodoprotein pattern. Endocrinology 1978; 102:954-965.

Studer H, Derwahl M. Mechanisms of nonneoplastic endocrine hyperplasia—A changing concept: A review focused on the thyroid gland. Endocrine Rev 1995;16:411-425.

van Herle AJ, Vassart G, Dunmont JE. Control of thyroglobulin synthesis and secretion. N Engl J Med 1979; 301:239-249.

van Voorthuizen WF, Dinsort C, Flavell RA, de Vijlder JJM, Vassart G. Abnormal cellular localization of thyroglobulin mRNA associated with hereditary congenital goiter and thyroglobulin deficiency. Proc Natl Acad Sci USA 1978; 75:74-78.

Vogelgesand G, Harmeyer J, vonGrabe C. Measurements of intestinal calcium uptake in pigs with vitamin D-dependent rickets. In: Nuclear Techniques in Animal Production and Health. Vienna: Proc Joint JAEA/FAO, 1976.

Pituitary gland

Boujon CE, Bestetti GE, Meier HP, Straub R, Junker U, Rossi GL. Equine pituitary adenoma: A functional and morphological study. J Comp Pathol 1993; 109:163-178.

Capen CC, Martin SL, Koestner A. Neoplasms in the adenohypophysis of dogs: A clinical and pathologic study. Path Vet 1967; 4:301-325.

Capen CC. Tumors of the endocrine glands. In: Moulton JE, ed. Tumors in Domestic Animals. 3rd ed. Los Angeles: University of California Press, 1990.

Capen CC, Koestner A. Functional chromophobe adenomas of the canine adenohypophysis. An ultrastructural evaluation of a neoplasm of pituitary corticotrophs. Vet Pathol 1967; 4:326-347.

Capen CC, Martin SL. Animal model: Hyperadrenocorticism (Cushing's-like syndrome and disease in dogs). Am J Pathol 1975; 81:459-462.

Halmi NS, Peterson ME, Colurso GJ, Liotta AS, Kreiger DT. Pituitary intermediate lobe in dogs: Two cell types and high bioactive adrenocorticotrophin content. Science 1981; 211:72-74.

Hare WR. Primary suprasellar germ cell tumor in a dog. J Am Vet Med Assoc 1993; 203: 1432-1433.

Heinrichs M, Baumgärtner W, Capen CC. Immunocytochemical demonstration of proopiomelanocortin-derived peptides in pituitary adenomas of the pars intermedia in horses. Vet Pathol 1990; 27:419-425.

Loeb WF, Capen CC, Johnson LE. Adenomas of the pars intermedia associated with hyperglycemia and glycosuria in two horses. Cornell Vet 1966; 56:623-639.

Millington WR, Dybdal NO, Dawson R, Jr., Manzini C, Mueller GP. Equine Cushing's disease: differential regulation of β-endorphin processing in tumors of the intermediate pituitary. Endocrinology 1988; 123:1598-1604.

Muller GH. Pituitary dwarfism: Cutaneous manifestions of an endocrine disorder. Vet Clin North Am 1979; 9:41-48.

Orth DN, Holscher MA, Wilson MG, Nicholson W E, Plue RE, Mount CD. Equine Cushing's disease: Plasma immunoreactive proopiolipomelanocortin peptide and cortisol levels basally and in response to diagnostic tests. Endocrinology 1982; 110:1430-1442.

Valentine BA, Summers BA, de Lahunta A, White CL, III, Kuhajda FF. Suprasellar germ cell tumors in the dog: A report of five cases and review of the literature. Acta Neuropathol 1988; 76:94-100.

Wilson MG, Nicholson WE, Holscher MA, Sherrell BJ, Mount CD, Orth DN. Proopiolipomelanocortin peptides in normal pituitary, pituitary tumor, and plasma of normal and Cushing's horses. Endocrinology 1982; 110:941-954.

Adrenal cortex

Anderson MP, Capen CC. Diseases of the Endocrine System. In: Benirschke K, et al., eds. Pathology of Laboratory Animals. Vol. 1. New York: Springer-Verlag, 1978:423-508.

Hullinger RL. Adrenal cortex of the dog (Canis familiaris). Histomorphological changes during growth, maturity, and aging. Zbl Vet Med C Anat Histol Embryol 1978; 7:1-27.

Lawrence HJ, Gould WJ, Flanders JA, Rowland PH, Yeager AE. Unilateral adrenalectomy as a treatment for adrenocortical tumors in ferrets: Five cases (1990-1992). J Am Vet Med Assoc 1993; 203:267-270.

Mulnix JA. Hypoadrenocorticism in the dog. J Am Anim Hosp Assoc 1971; 7:220-241.

Peterson ME, Gilbertson SR, Drucker WD. Plasma cortisol response to exogenous ACTH in 22 dogs with hyperadrenocorticism caused by adrenocortical neoplasia. J Am Vet Med Assoc 1982; 180:542-544.

Rosenthal KL, Peterson ME, Quesenberry KE, Hillyer EV, Beeber NL, Moroff SD, Lothrop CD, Jr. Hyperadrenocorticism associated with adrenocortical tumor or nodular hyperplasia of the adrenal gland in ferrets: 50 Cases (1987-1991). J Am Vet Med Assoc 1993; 203:271-275.

Schaer M, Chen CL. A clinical survey of 48 dogs with adrenocortical hypofunction. J Am Anim Hosp Assoc 1983; 19:443-452.

Weiss CA, Scott MV. Clinical aspects and surgical treatment of hyperadrenocorticism in the domestic ferret: 94 cases (1994-1996). J Am Anim Hosp Assoc 1997; 33:487-493.

Williams B, Heffess C. Proliferative lesions of the ferret adrenal cortex. Vet Pathol 1994; 31:5.

Adrenal medulla

Barthez PY, Marks SL, Woo J, Feldman EC, Matteucci M. Pheochromocytoma in dogs: 61 cases (1984-1995). J Vet Intern Med 1997; 11:272-278.

Howard EB, Nielsen SW. Pheochromocytomas associated with hypertensive lesions in dogs. J Am Vet Med Assoc 1965; 147:245-252.

Sponenberg DP, McEntee K. Pheochromocytomas and ultimobranchial (C cell) neoplasms in the bull: Evidence of autosomal dominant inheritance in the Guernsey breed. Vet Pathol 1983; 20:396-400.

von Dehn BJ, Nelson RW, Feldman EC, Griffey SM. Pheochromocytoma and hyperadrenocorticism in dogs: Six cases (1982-1992). J Am Vet Med Assoc 1995; 207:322.

Yarrington JT, Capen CC. Ultrastructural and biochemical evaluation of adrenal medullary hyperplasia and pheochromocytoma in aged bulls. Vet Pathol 1981; 18:316-325.

Thyroid follicular cells

Barber PJ, Elliott J. Study of calcium homeostasis in feline hyperthyroidism. J Small Anim Pract 1996; 37:575-582.

Bastenie PA, Ermans AM, Bonnyns M, Neve P, Delespesse G. Lymphocytic thyroiditis as an autoimmune disease. In: Good RA, et al., eds. Molecular Pathology. Springfield, Ill.: Charles C. Thomas, 1975.

Brown RS, Keating P, Livingston PG, Bullock L. Thyroid growth immunoglobulins in feline hyperthyroidism. Thyroid 1992; 2:125.

Gerber H, Peter H, Ferguson DC, Peterson ME. Etiopathology of feline toxic nodular goiter. Vet Clin North Am Small Anim Pract 1994; 24:541-565.

Gosselin SJ, Capen CC, Martin SL. Histopathologic and ultrastructural evaluation of thyroid lesions associated with hypothyroidism in dogs. Vet Path 1981; 18:299-309.

Gosselin SJ, Martin SL, Capen CC, Targowski SP. Biochemical and immunological investigations of hypothyroidism in dogs. Can J Comp Med 1980; 44:158-168.

Gosselin SJ, Capen CC, Martin SL, Krakowka S. Autoimmune lymphocytic thyroiditis in dogs. Vet Immunol Immunopathol 1982; 3:185-201.

Holzworth J, Theran P, Carpenter JL, Harpster NK, Rodoroff RJ. Hyperthyroidism in the cat: Ten cases. J Am Vet Med Assoc 1980; 176:345-353.

Jernigan AD. Idiosyncrasies of feline drug metabolism. In: Proceedings of the 12th Annual Kal Kan Symposium for Treatment of Small Animal Diseases. Kal Kan Foods, Inc, Vernon, CA, 1989.

Johnson LA, Ford HC, Tarttelin MF, et al. Iodine content of commercially prepared cat foods. N Z Vet J 1992; 40:18-20.

Leav I, Schiller AI, Rijnberk A, Legg MA, der Kinderen PJ. Adenomas and carcinomas of the canine and feline thyroid. Am J Pathol 1976; 83:61-94.

Martin SL, Capen CC. Hypothyroidism and the skin. In: Muller GH, ed. Veterinary Clinics of North America: Symposium on Skin and Internal Disease. Vol. 9. Philadelphia: Saunders, 1979:29-40.

Peter HJ, Gerber H, Studer H, Smeds S. Pathogenesis of heterogeneity in human multinodular goiter: A study on growth and function of thyroid tissue transplanted onto nude mice. J Clin Invest 1985; 76:1992-2002.

Peterson ME, Kintzer PP, Cavanagh PG, Fox PR, Ferguson DC, Johnson GF, Becker DV. Feline hyperthyroidism: Pretreatment clinical and laboratory evaluation of 131 cases. J Am Vet Med Assoc 1983; 183:103-110.

Peterson ME, Livingston P, Brown RS. Lack of circulating thyroid stimulating immunoglobulins in cats with hyperthyroidism. Vet Immunol Immunopathol 1987; 16:277-282.

Peterson ME. Diagnosis and treatment of feline hyperthyroidism. In: van Marthens E, ed. Proceedings of the 6th Kal Kan Symposium for Treatment of Small Animal Disease. Kal Kan Foods, Inc, Vernon, CA, 1983:63-66.

Rojko JL, Hoover EA, Martin SL. Histopathologic interpretation of cutaneous biopsies from dogs with various dermatologic disorders. Vet Pathol 1978; 579-589.

Scarlett JM. Epidemiology of thyroid diseases of dogs and cats. Vet Clin North Am Small Anim Pract 1994; 24:477-486.

Thyroid C cells

Black HE, Capen CC, Young DM. Ultimobranchial thyroid neoplasms in bulls. A syndrome resembling medullary thyroid carcinoma in man. Cancer 1973; 32:865-878.

Bordi C, Anversa P, Vitali-Mazza L. Ultrastructural study of a calcitonin-secreting tumor: Cytology of the tumor cells and origin of amyloid. Virchows Arch 1972; 357:145-161.

Capen CC. Metabolic bone and disease calcium regulating hormones. In: Newton CD, Nunamaker DM, eds. Textbook of Small Animal Orthopaedics. Philadelphia: Lippincott, 1985:673-722.

Ljungberg O, Bondeson L, Bondeson A-G. Differentiated thyroid carcinoma, intermediate type: A new tumor entity with features of follicular and parafollicular cell carcinoma. Hum Pathol 1984; 15:218-228.

Ljungberg O, Ericsson U-B, Bondeson L, Thorell J. A compound follicular-parafollicular cell carcinoma of the thyroid: A new tumor entity? Cancer 1983; 52:1053-1061.

Manning PC Jr, Molnar GD, Black BM, Priestly JT, Woolner LB. Pheochromocytoma, hyperparathyroidism and thyroid carcinoma occurring coincidentally. N Engl J Med 1963; 268:68-72.

McDermott FT, Hart JAL. Medullary carcinoma of the thyroid with hypocalcaemia: Clinical and ultrastructural observations. Br J Surg 1970; 57:657-661.

Pearse AGE, Ewen SWB, Polak JM. The genesis of apud amyloid in endocrine polypeptide tumours: Histochemical distinction from immunamyloid. Virchows Arch B 1972; 10:93-107.

Zarrin K. Naturally occurring parafollicular cell carcinoma of the thyroids in dogs. A histological and ultrastructural study. Vet Pathol 1977; 14:556-566.

Parathyroid gland

Black HE, Capen CC, Yarrington JT, Rowland GN. Effect of a high calcium prepartal diet on calcium homeostatic mechanisms in thyroid glands, bone, and intestine of cows. Lab Invest 1973; 29:437-448.

Capen CC. Functional and fine structural relationships of parathyroid glands. Adv Vet Sci Comp Med 1975; 19:249-286.

Capen CC, Young DM. The ultrastructure of the parathyroid glands and thyroid parafollicular cells of cows with parturient paresis and hypocalcemia. Lab Invest 1967; 17:717-737.

Capen CC, Rosol TJ. Pathobiology of parathyroid hormone and parathyroid hormone-related protein: Introduction and evolving concepts. In: LiVolsi VA, DeLellis RA, eds. Pathology of the Thyroid and Parathyroid Gland: An Update. Philadelphia: Williams & Wilkins, 1993:1-33.

Capen CC, Cole CR, Hibbs JW. Influences of vitamin D on calcium metabolism and the parathyroid glands of cattle. Fed Proc 1968; 27:142-152.

Garrett IR. Bone destruction in cancer. Semin Oncol 1993; 20:4-9.

Gröne A, Werkmeister JR, Steinmeyer CL, Capen CC, Rosol TJ. Parathyroid hormone-related protein in normal and neoplastic canine tissues: Immunohistochemical localization and biochemical extraction. Vet Pathol 1994; 31:308-315.

Gröne A, Weckmann MT, Steinmeyer CL, Capen CC, Rosol TJ. Altered parathyroid hormone-related protein secretion and MRNA expression in squamous cell carcinoma cells *in vitro*. Eur J Endocrinol 1996; 135:498-505.

Heath H, Weller RE, Mundy GR. Canine lymphosarcoma: A model for study of the hypercalcemia of cancer. Calcif Tissue Int 1980; 30:127-133.

Hunt RD, Garcia FG, Hegsted DM. A comparison of vitamin D_2 and D_3 in New World primates. I. Production and regression of osteodystrophia fibrosa. Lab Anim Care 1967; 16:222-234.

Krook L, Barrett RB. Simian bone disease—a secondary hyperparathyroidism. Cornell Vet 1962; 52:459-492.

Merryman JI, Capen CC, McCauley LK, Werkmeister JR, Suter MM, Rosol TJ. Regulation of parathyroid hormone-related protein production by a squamous carcinoma cell line *in vitro*. Lab Invest 1993; 69:347-354.

Merryman JI, DeWille J, Werkmeister JR, Capen CC, Rosol TJ. Effects of transforming growth factor-beta on PTRrP production and RNA expression by a squamous carcinoma cell line *in vitro*. Endocrinology 1994; 134:2424-2430.

Meuten DJ, Capen CC, Kociba GJ, Cooper BJ. Hypercalcemia of malignancy: Hypercalcemia associated with an adenocarcinoma of the apocrine glands of the anal sac. Am J Pathol 1982; 108:366-370.

Meuten DJ, Capen CC, Thompson KG, Serge GV. Syncytial cells in canine parathyroid glands. Vet Pathol 1984; 21:463-468.

Meuten DJ, Kociba GJ, Capen CC, Chew DJ, Segre GV, Levin L, Tashjian AJ Jr, Voelkel EF, Nagode LA. Hypercalcemia in dogs with lymphosarcoma: Biochemical, ultrastructural and histomorphometric investigations. Lab Invest 1983; 49:553-562.

Meuten DJ, Segre GV, Capen CC, Kociba GJ, Voelkel EF, Levine L, Tashjian AH Jr, Chew DJ, Nagode LA. Hypercalcemia in dogs with adenocarcinoma derived from aprocine glands of anal sac: Biochemical and histomorphometric investigations. Lab Invest 1983; 48: 428-435.

Moseley JM, Gillespie MT. Parathyroid hormone-related protein. Crit Rev Clin Lab Sci 1995; 32:299-343.

Powell GJ, Southby J, Danks JA, Stillwell RG, Hayman JA, Henderson MA, Bennett RC, Martin TJ. Localization of parathyroid hormone-related protein in breast cancer metastases: Increased incidence in bone compared to other sites. Cancer Res 1991; 51-3059-3061.

Rosol TJ, Capen CC. Biology of disease: Mechanisms of cancer-induced hypercalcemia. Lab Invest 1992; 67:680-702.

Rosol TJ, Chew DJ, Nagode LA, Capen CC. Pathophysiology of calcium metabolism. Vet Clin Pathol 1995; 24:49-63.

Rosol TJ, Nagode LA, Couto CG, Hammer AS, Chew DJ, Peterson JL, Ayl RD, Steinmeyer CL, Capen CC. Parathyroid hormone (PTH)-related protein, PTH, and 1,25-dihydroxyvitamin D in dogs with cancer-associated hypercalcemia. Endocrinology 1992; 131:1157-1164.

Seymour JF, Gagel RF. Calcitriol: The major humoral mediator of hypercalcemia in Hodgkin's and non-Hodgkin's lymphomas. Blood 1993; 82:1383-1394.

Strewler GJ, Nissenson RA. Nonparathyroid Hypercalcemia. Adv Intern Med 1987; 32:235-258.

Weir EC, Burtis WJ, Morris CA, Brady TG, Insogna KL. Isolation of 16,000-dalton parathyroid hormone-like proteins from two animal tumors causing humoral hypercalcemia of malignancy. Endocrinology 1988; 123:2744-2751.

Pancreatic islets

Capen CC, Martin SL. Hyperinsulinism in dogs with neoplasia of the pancreatic islets: A clinical, pathologic, and ultrastructural study. Pathol Vet 1969; 6:309-341.

Ehrhart N, Withrow SJ, Ehrhart EJ, Wimsatt JH. Pancreatic beta cell tumor in ferrets: 20 cases (1986-1994). J Am Vet Med Assoc 1996; 209:1737-1740.

Happe' RP, van der Gaag I, Lamers CBHW, van Toorenburg J, Renfeld JF, Larsson LI. Zollinger-Ellison syndrome in three dogs. Vet Pathol 1980; 17:177-186.

Jergens AE, Shaw D P. Hyperinsulinism and hypoglycemia associated with pancreatic islet cell tumor in a ferret. J Am Vet Med Assoc 1989; 194:269-271.

Johnson KH, O'Brien TD, Betsholtz C, Westermark P. Biology of disease: Islet amyloid polypeptide: Mechanisms of amyloidogenesis in the pancreatic islets and potential roles in diabetes mellitus. Lab Invest 1992; 66:522-535.

Johnson KH, O'Brien TD, Betsholtz C, Westermark P. Islet amyloid, islet-amyloid polypeptide, and diabetes mellitus. N Engl J Med 1989; 321:513-518.

Johnson KH, Osborne CA, Barnes DM. Intracellular substance with some amyloid staining affinities in pancreatic acinar cells of a cat with amyloidosis. Pathol Vet 1970; 7:153-162.

Luttgen PJ, Storts RW, Rogers KS, Morton LD. Insulinoma in a ferret. J Am Vet Med Assoc 1986; 189:920-921.

Marini RP, Ryden EV, Rosenblad WD, Murphy JC, Fox JG. Functional islet cell tumor in six ferrets. J Am Vet Med Assoc 1993; 202:430-433.

Meier H. Diabetes mellitus in animals. Diabetes 1960; 9:485-489.

O'Brien TD, Butler PC, Westermark P, Johnson KH. Islet amyloid polypeptide: A review of its biology and potential roles in the pathogenesis of diabetes mellitus. Vet Pathol 1993; 30:317-332.

Chemoreceptor organs

Bloom F. Structure and histogenesis of tumors of the aortic bodies in dogs with a consideration of the morphology of the aortic and carotid bodies. Arch Pathol 1943; 36:1-12.

Cheville NF. Ultrastructure of canine carotid body and aortic body tumors: Comparison with tissues of thyroid and parathyroid origin. Vet Pathol 1972; 9:166-189.

Edwards C, Heath D, Harris P, Castillo Y, Kruger H, Arias-Stella J. The carotid body in animals at high altitude. J Pathol 1971; 104:231-238.

Johnson KH. Aortic body tumors in the dog. J Am Vet Med Assoc 1968; 152:154-160.

CHAPTER 7

The Hemopoietic System

Gene P. Searcy

STRUCTURE AND FUNCTION

The hemopoietic system includes all the cells that arise from stem cells in the bone marrow and organs such as the thymus, lymph nodes, and spleen, where cells are sequestered for conditioning, proliferation, and function. The bone marrow, spleen, and lymph nodes share certain basic anatomic features. For example, specialized fibroblast-like reticular cells extend long filamentous processes that provide a scaffolding arrangement to support populations of cells. In addition to physical support, these cells also provide a microenvironment that attracts the appropriate circulating cells and enables them to multiply or differentiate into cells of a particular lineage. Within the reticular networks of these organs are thin-walled sinuses that control movement of cells and large molecules. These sinuses are located between arterioles and venules in the bone marrow and spleen, but contain lymph within lymph nodes. Macrophages, derived from monocytes, are found in most of these reticular cell networks where they perform a wide variety of functions. They, collectively, are part of the monocyte-macrophage or **mononuclear phagocyte system.**

Hemopoiesis within the bone marrow remains active throughout life and constantly produces new cells in the blood. It is particularly efficient in entrapping circulating stem cells and nurturing them. Expression of cell membrane glycoproteins, in response to growth factors, facilitates the binding of hemopoietic cells to reticular cells and to intercellular adhesive proteins such as fibronectin and fibrinogen. The up- and down-regulation of these adhesive mechanisms is the basis for homing of stem cells to the bone marrow and eventual release of their progeny into the blood. In the 1950s, it was shown that bone marrow–derived cells injected into irradiated mice formed splenic colonies. These colonies contained varying numbers of erythrocytic, granulocytic, megakaryocytic, and undifferentiated cells. It was eventually proven that each of these colonies arose from a single stem cell capable of renewal and differentiation. Similar findings were confirmed in other animals and in human beings. By use of chromosomal markers, it was shown that lymphoid stem cells arose from a more pluripotent stem cell that was also the origin of hemopoietic cells (myeloid stem cells) (Fig. 7-1). Techniques that facilitate growth of hemopoietic cells in liquid culture have enabled investigators to study humoral mediators that control differentiation and maturation of blood cells. A compartment of stem cells committed to erythropoiesis was recognized and further subdivided into burst-forming units–erythroid (BFU-E) and colony-forming units–erythroid (CFU-E). The former is under control of interleukin 3 (IL-3) and erythropoietin, whereas CFU-E proliferation occurs in response to erythropoietin. In a similar manner, the stem cells that give rise to granulocytes and monocytes are known as colony-forming units–granulocyte-monocyte (CFU-GM) (Fig. 7-1). These are under the control of several mediators called colony-stimulating factors (CSF). Megakaryocyte-committed colonies (CFU-Meg) arise from stem cells also under control of specific mediators including thrombopoietin produced by the liver and kidneys. It can now be appreciated that hematologic findings after bone marrow injury vary depending on the stage of differentiation of the affected stem cells. For example, the diversity of bone marrow and blood disorders in feline leukemia virus (FeLV)–infected cats results from variation in the viral disturbance of hemopoietic cells.

Significant insight into diseases of the hemopoietic system may be gained by simply submitting blood for hematologic examination. Indeed, a complete hemogram is frequently of greater value than the necropsy in understanding disease mechanisms of the hemopoietic system. Learning to evaluate blood smears is a valuable addition to the information gained from the physical examination of an animal. Lymph node and bone marrow aspirates are also frequently indicated when studying disorders of the hemopoietic system.

RESPONSES OF THE HEMOPOIETIC SYSTEM

Like other organs, the bone marrow, lymph nodes, and spleen may undergo atrophy, hyperplasia, hypertrophy, and neoplasia. **Atrophy** of the bone marrow hemopoietic cell population follows certain types of injury and results in failure of erythropoiesis (causing anemia), granulopoiesis (causing neutropenia), and thrombopoiesis (causing thrombocytopenia). Occasionally, injury to stem cells results in complete failure of hemopoiesis with resultant **pancytopenia.** Splenic atrophy is uncommon, but does occur in older

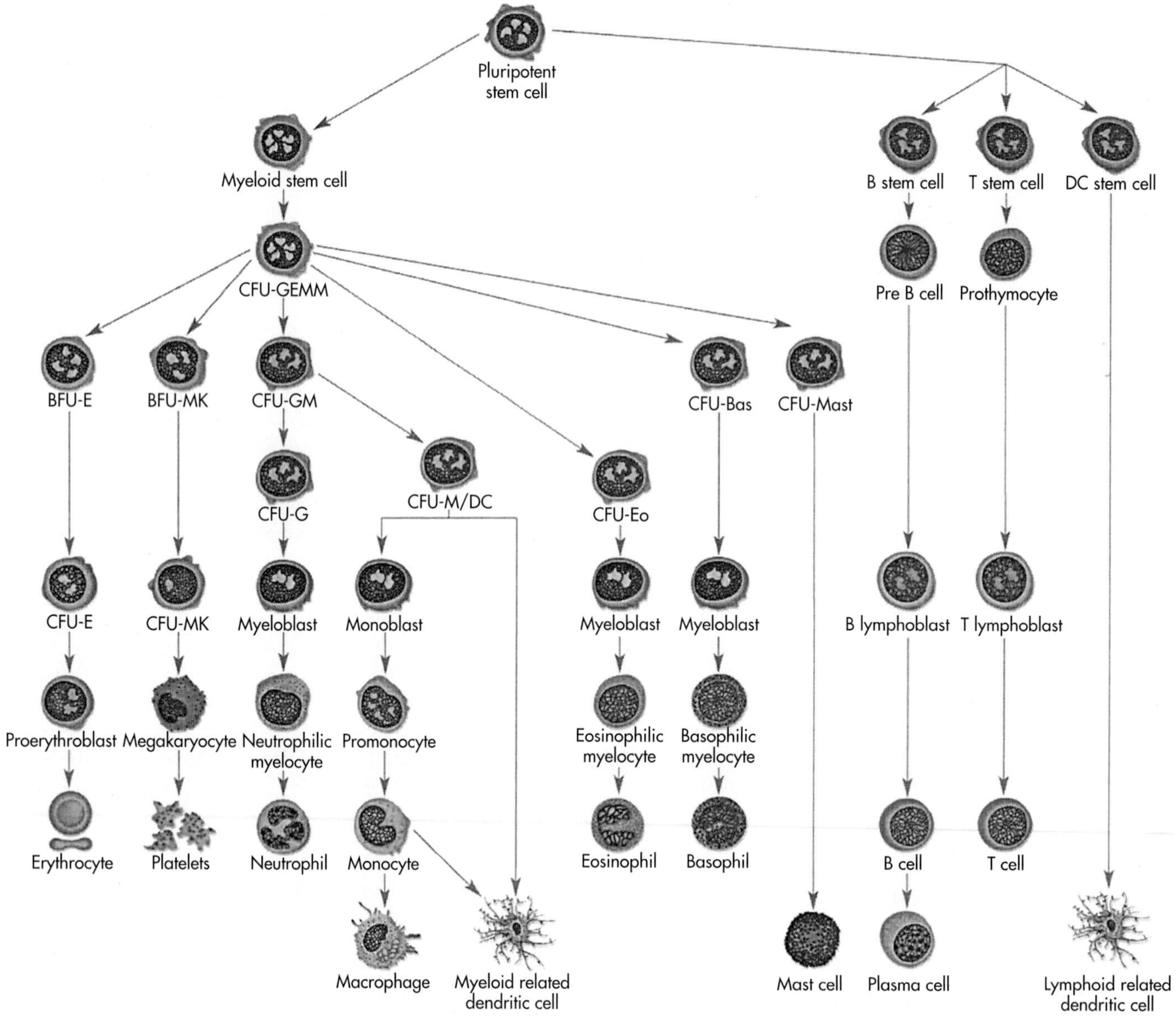

Figure 7-1 Hematopoietic cascade. *CFU-GEMM,* colony-forming unit–granulocyte, erythroid, macrophage, megakaryocyte; *BFU-E,* burst-forming unit–erythroid; *CFU-E,* colony-forming unit–erythroid; *CFU-Meg,* colony-forming unit–megakaryocyte; *CFU-GM,* colony-forming unit–granulocyte-macrophage; *CFU-G,* colony-forming unit–granulocyte; *CFU-M,* colony-forming unit–monocyte; *CFU-Eo,* colony-forming unit–eosinophil; *CFU-Bas,* colony-forming unit–basophil; *GM-CSF,* granulocyte-macrophage colony-stimulating factor; *M-CSF,* macrophage colony-stimulating factor; *G-CSF,* granulocyte colony-stimulating factor; *SCF,* stem cell factor; *EPO,* erythropoietin; *TPO,* thrombopoietin; *IL,* interleukin. *From Chart of Hemopoiesis, Immunex Corporation, Seattle, Washington.*

animals, and is usually of little consequence. Certain viruses and toxins as well as malnutrition can cause thymic and lymph node atrophy, which impairs immune functions.

Hypertrophy of bone marrow is most unlikely in animals because hemopoietic tissue is enclosed by bone. (In children with congenital hemolytic anemias, some flat bones may become enlarged as a result of years of erythroid hyperplasia). **Hyperplasia** of the splenic lymphocyte or macrophage populations also results in splenic hypertrophy; when this occurs, the spleen is firm and fleshy when incised. Lymph node enlargement secondary to cellular proliferation or hyperplasia occurs in response to inflammation and antigenic stimulation. Hypertrophy of superficial lymph nodes is usually confined to the node receiving lymph from that area of injury or inflammation. Generalized lymph node hyperplasia and hypertrophy is uncommon and occurs with systemic infections of some duration.

Hyperplasia of bone marrow hemopoietic tissue occurs following prolonged hemorrhage or hemolysis and bacterial infections. The hemopoietic tissue expands and replaces adipocytes; yellow marrow becomes red, extending from the ends of long bones along the endosteum. Extramedullary hemopoiesis in organs such as the liver and spleen frequently accompanies hyperplasia of the bone marrow.

The hemopoietic system in some species, such as the cat, has a significant incidence of **neoplasia.** Although not universally practiced, the foundational terminology for neoplastic diseases as taught in general pathology can be applied to the hemopoietic system and is used in this chapter. Sarcomas of bone marrow can be derived from erythrocytic, granulocytic, megakaryocytic, lymphocytic, and plasma cell populations. Sarcomas of bone marrow are unique in pathology because they may release neoplastic cells into the blood. It follows that identification of the sarcoma can be made by identifying the leukemic cells in blood smears. Frequently, however, bone marrow aspiration is required to identify the sarcoma; veterinarians should be capable of obtaining these samples. Lymphosarcomas arise in any organ but, as would be expected, frequently cause lymph node enlargement. Superficial lymph node aspirates for cytology, and biopsies for histology, usually allow differentiation of lymphosarcoma from lymphadenitis or hyperplasia.

ERYTHROCYTE DISORDERS

Erythrocytosis

Erythrocytosis is an increase in erythrocyte number, hemoglobin concentration, and packed cell volume; it may be classified as relative or absolute.

Relative Erythrocytosis

Relative erythrocytosis is the result of dehydration or hemoconcentration in which extracellular fluid imbalance leads to contraction of the plasma compartment. Although the hematocrit, hemoglobin concentration, and erythrocyte number are increased, the total erythrocyte mass is normal. Plasma proteins are affected by shifts in fluid volume in the same manner as erythrocytes. Estimation of the hematocrit or packed cell volume and plasma protein provide some assessment of the degree of dehydration.

Absolute Erythrocytosis

Absolute erythrocytosis is an actual increase in erythrocyte number. It can be further classified as primary or secondary erythrocytosis. Primary erythrocytosis is the result of proliferation of marrow erythroid precursors that are no longer influenced by erythropoietin; this form of erythrocytosis may represent the escape of a clone of such cells from normal control mechanisms. Although the disease is uncommon, it has been described in young to middle aged dogs and in cats. Hematocrits in dogs have ranged from 0.65 to 0.85 L/L (65% to 85%).

Secondary erythrocytosis results from excessive production of erythropoietin. Appropriate production of erythropoietin occurs in response to hypoxemia. It probably occurs to a mild degree in older dogs with cardiac or pulmonary disease. Occasionally, it can result where there is congenital anomalous transposition of major vessels, and a significant percentage of the erythrocytes bypass the pulmonary circulation. Erythrocytosis due to inappropriate production of erythropoietin in the absence of hypoxia occurs as a part of a paraneoplastic syndrome. Although rare, this syndrome has been reported in dogs with renal and extrarenal neoplasms.

The clinical signs of absolute erythrocytosis include markedly cyanotic oral mucous membranes and depression. The increased viscosity of the blood causes impaired blood flow, cyanosis, and a tendency for thrombosis. Necropsy findings include marked generalized congestion, thrombosis of major vessels, and hyperplastic bone marrow.

Anemia

Mechanisms of Anemia

Anemia is the reduction of erythrocyte numbers in an animal for that particular age, species, breed, and geographic location. Erythrocyte numbers decrease in neonatal animals following ingestion of colostrum; this decrease continues during the period of rapid body growth. The age at which erythrocyte numbers begin to increase, as well as the age at which adult levels are reached, varies among species. In dogs, adult values are usually reached between 4 and 6 months of age; in horses, this occurs at approximately 1 year of age. In most species, erythrocytes are larger at birth and mean corpuscular volumes (MCVs) decline as fetal erythrocytes are replaced within 8 to 10 weeks. It is important that these factors be considered when assessing hemograms in young animals. Factors such as malnutrition and parasitism delay the age at which adult erythrocyte numbers are reached. Breed influences erythrocyte numbers in horses and dogs. Draught horses have lower erythrocyte numbers than those of racing breeds. Some breeds of dogs such as greyhounds and whippets have higher erythrocyte numbers than most other breeds. Animals residing at higher altitudes have higher erythrocyte counts. While assessing hemograms from animals, these factors must be taken into consideration and assessment made as to what erythrocyte values might have been before the current illness.

Anemia is a significant indicator of underlying disease and should be investigated in a routine, logical manner. The initial decision is whether the anemia is regenerative or nonregenerative based on the presence or absence of indicators of compensatory erythropoiesis. Regenerative anemias result from hemorrhage or hemolysis, which is followed by stimulation of the bone marrow with release of immature erythrocytes. A blood film contains large immature erythrocytes that vary in size (anisocytosis). The

Table 7-1 Nomenclature of Erythrocyte Shapes and Associated Diseases

Term	Description	Disease Association
Discocyte	Normal bioconcave disk Degree of central pallor varies with species	None
Macrocyte	Large erythrocyte	Release of immature cells in response to blood loss Congenital in some poodle dogs
Polychromasia	Diffuse blue erythrocytes on Wright-Giemsa stains	Release of immature cells in response to blood loss
Reticulocyte	Erythrocyte containing precipitated strands of RNA with supravital stains	Release of immature cells in response to blood loss
Nuclear remnant	Small, single, black-staining, round inclusion in various locations within erythrocyte	Response to blood loss; splenic malfunction
Basophilic stippling	Punctate precipitate in cytoplasm	Response to blood loss in ruminants; lead poisoning
Microcyte	Small erythrocyte	Iron deficiency
Hypochromia	Erythrocyte with thin rim of pale peripheral hemoglobin and large amount of central pallor	Iron deficiency
Echinocyte (I-III)	Spiculate erythrocyte with short, equally spaced projections over entire surface	Usually an in vitro artefact Uremia Electrolyte depletion in horses
Spherocyte	Small, dense erythrocyte lacking central pallor	Immune-mediated hemolysis; senescent erythrocytes; accompany poikilocytosis
Heinz bodies	Round, pale structures on the internal surface of the membrane, stain prominently with new methylene blue. They may project from the surface and when numerous may be free in the plasma	Oxidative injury and precipitation of globin and membrane skeletal proteins. Common in cats because of several amino acids containing sulfhydryl groups in their globin chains
Poikilocyte	Nonspecific term for abnormally shaped erythrocyte	See more specific terms
Acanthocyte	Erythrocyte with projections of variable length at variable intervals around the cell	Splenic disease; hemangiosarcomas
Schizocytes	Small, irregular erythrocyte fragment that may have two or three pointed extremities	Intravascular coagulation; vasculitis
Eccenterocyte	Hemoglobin displaced to one side of cell	Hemolytic anemias induced by chemicals
Keratocyte	Half-moon shape with spicules	Intravascular coagulation
Dacrocyte	Teardrop cell	Myelofibrosis

immature erythrocytes stain blue (polychromasia), and polychromasia is a most useful indicator of compensatory erythropoiesis. Additional morphologic indicators of rapid erythropoiesis include metarubricytes and rubricytes, and in ruminants, basophilic stippling (Table 7-1). Incubation of blood with supravital stains (such as new methylene blue) causes aggregation of mitochondria, ribosomes, and remnants of the Golgi bodies in immature erythrocytes into the blue strands characteristic of reticulocytes. Absolute reticulocyte counts (obtained by multiplying the percentage of reticulocytes by the erythrocyte count) greater than 80×10^6/L in dogs and 60×10^6/L in cats are consistent with a regenerative response. In dogs, a reticulocyte production index (RPI), similar to that used in human beings, may be calculated to compensate for the relative increase in the percentage of reticulocytes in an anemic animal and the prolonged maturation time of the more immature reticulocytes.

$$\text{RPI} = \%\ \text{Reticulocytes} \times \frac{\text{Observed Hct}}{\text{Normal Hct}} \times \frac{1}{\text{Blood maturation time (days)}}$$

The maturation time of reticulocytes in the blood is estimated as 1 day at a hematocrit of 45 L/L (45%), 1.5 days at 35 L/L (35%), 2 days at 25 L/L (25%), and 2.5 days at 15 L/L (15%). An RPI greater than 2 is consistent with a regenerative response. Unfortunately, the formula is not standardized for other species.

Special precautions are necessary when counting reticulocytes in cats because of the appearance of punctate reticulocytes, as well as aggregate reticulocytes. As the name implies, punctate erythrocytes contain noncoalescing blue dots. The aggregate forms are representative of immature erythrocytes, whereas the punctate forms are descendants of the aggregate type. The latter may persist for several days and indicate earlier responsive erythropoiesis. Reticulocytes appear in the blood within 2 to 3 days after hemorrhage or hemolysis. On initial examination, animals with hemolytic anemias usually have evidence of compensatory erythropoiesis; this may not be true if animals are presented because of hemorrhage. Evaluation of anemia in horses is complicated because the horse does not release reticulocytes from the bone marrow. Intense erythrogenesis in horses may increase the MCV and red cell distribution width (RDW); however, examination of bone marrow aspirates may also be necessary to assess erythropoietic rate.

Regenerative Anemias

After establishing that an anemia is regenerative (i.e., the result of erythrocyte loss), it is necessary to differentiate anemia due to hemorrhage from that due to hemolysis. Such differentiation is often difficult; a good history and thorough examination of the animal are required to detect occult hemorrhage, e.g., bleeding into body cavities and large muscle masses. Significant bleeding at the free gingival margin of thrombocytopenic dogs may go undetected because the blood is lost by constant swallowing. Commercial tablets for detection of hemoglobin in feces are extremely sensitive and will detect the hemoglobin present in meat ingested by carnivores. It may be necessary to place animals in which gastrointestinal bleeding is suspected on cereal diets before testing their feces for occult blood. Routine urinalysis will detect bleeding into the urinary tract; samples obtained during urination are preferred because samples obtained by cystocentesis from dogs and cats frequently contain erythrocytes.

When hemorrhage has occurred within the previous 36 to 48 hours, hypoproteinemia occurs concurrently with the anemia; as fluid enters the vascular compartment to maintain blood pressure, the dilution that results in anemia also causes hypoproteinemia. In species with a storage spleen, such as the horse, splenic contraction initially compensates for erythrocyte loss, but dilution of plasma proteins begins within minutes.

Detection of hemolysis may also be difficult. Icteric mucous membranes and bilirubin and hemoglobin in plasma and urine indicate hemolysis. Because dogs are able to conjugate and excrete large amounts of bilirubin rapidly, they only have products of hemolysis in the blood after a hemolytic crisis. Bilirubinuria is a more constant finding. Blood smears may have erythrocyte alterations suggestive of hemolysis such as spherocytes in the canine immune-mediated hemolytic anemias. The reticulocyte response after hemolysis due to erythrophagocytosis is usually greater than that after hemorrhage because of the efficient salvage of iron from hemoglobin and the release of cytokines from activated macrophages.

Hemorrhagic Anemias

An important consequence of chronic hemorrhage is the exhaustion of iron stores, which results in impaired erythropoiesis. This can occur in parasitic diseases such as bovine pediculosis, severe flea infestations of puppies and kittens, and hookworms in puppies. Chronic immune-mediated thrombocytopenia in dogs and gastrointestinal neoplasms in older animals may also cause iron deficiency owing to chronic extracorporeal hemorrhage. Bleeding intestinal carcinomas and lymphosarcomas in dogs deserve special emphasis; these neoplasms should be considered immediately when the hemogram has features suggestive of iron deficiency.

Hemolytic Anemias

Most hemolytic anemias in animals are acquired after injury to erythrocytes by infectious agents, antibodies, or strong oxidizing agents. Inherited hemolytic anemias, however, result from an intracellular defect confined to a single protein and are less common. The severity of the inherited hemolytic anemias varies depending on the abnormal protein and the location of the abnormality within the molecule. These anemias in animals can result from abnormalities in heme synthesis, membrane skeletal proteins, and glycolytic enzymes.

Intracellular Defects. In animals, inherited mutations in enzymes involved in heme synthesis occur and result in accumulations of precursor porphyrin molecules. **Congenital erythropoietic porphyria,** transmitted as an autosomal recessive trait, occurs in Holstein and shorthorn cattle and is characterized by red-brown discoloration of teeth, bones, and urine due to accumulation of porphyrins. Because of the circulation of the photodynamic porphyrins in blood, these animals have lesions of photosensitization of the nonpigmented skin and hemolytic anemia. All affected tissues, including erythrocytes, exhibit fluorescence with ultraviolet light. The premature destruction of developing and mature erythrocytes is caused by the accumulation of excess porphyrins. Bovine **erythropoietic protoporphyria** is an inherited disorder of heme synthetase, a terminal enzyme of the heme synthetic pathway, resulting in the accumulation of protoporphyrins in tissues and erythrocytes. It is inherited as an autosomal recessive trait and is confined to Limousin or Limousin-cross cattle. Photosensitivity is the only clinical manifestation of the disease; there is no discoloration of teeth and bone or anemia. A congenital porphyria described in Siamese and domestic short-haired cats resembles congenital erythropoietic porphyria in cattle. These cats have brown teeth, photosensitization, and hemolytic anemia.

Inherited disorders of the erythrocyte membrane skeleton are rare in animals, in contrast to human beings, where they are more numerous and precisely defined. The erythrocyte membrane consists of an outer lipid bilayer and an inner skeleton consisting of long fibrillar proteins that form a mesh on the cytoplasmic side of the lipid bilayer. The two are linked by integral membrane proteins that extend vertically across the lipid membrane and attach to skeletal proteins below. Band 3 is the most important integral protein linking the lipid membrane to the protein skeleton. A disorder similar to hereditary spherocytosis in human beings occurs in Japanese black cattle as a result of the absence of band 3. The affected cattle have spontaneous shedding of microspheres from the erythrocyte membrane, moderate hemolytic anemia, and retarded growth.

Inherited glycolytic enzyme abnormalities in erythrocytes occur in animals. **Pyruvate kinase deficiency** in basenji, beagle, West Highland, white terrier, cairn terrier, and American Eskimo dogs and Abyssinian cats results in severe hemolytic anemia with marked reticulocytosis. This distal block in the Embden-Meyerhof pathway results in inadequate synthesis of adenosine triphosphate (ATP) and shortened erythrocyte life span. Many of these animals develop myelofibrosis and osteosclerosis. Affected dogs die at 3 to 5 years of age because of impaired erythropoiesis and liver disease resulting from hemochromatosis. A single nucleotide deletion has been detected in the gene for one of the pyruvate kinase enzymes in basenji dogs, and a genetic test using polymerase chain reaction (PCR) amplification of genomic DNA has been developed for this breed of dog. **Phosphofructokinase (PFK) deficiency** has been described in English springer spaniel and American cocker spaniel dogs. Affected dogs have mild to moderate hemolytic anemia with elevated numbers of reticulocytes. Hemolytic crises occur and are characterized by lethargy, fever, and pallor of mucous membranes. PFK-deficient erythrocytes are sensitive to changes in pH and are rendered more susceptible to hemolysis during periods of exercise, when panting results in alkalemia. There are three genes that code for PFK enzymes; they are designated M in muscle and erythrocytes, L in liver, and P in platelets. A point mutation in the gene coding for the M enzyme results in an unstable, truncated molecule. Based on this finding, normal, carrier, and affected dogs can be differentiated using PCR amplification of the affected gene.

Most hemolytic anemias in animals are caused by partial or complete phagocytosis of erythrocytes by macrophages of the mononuclear phagocyte system. By tradition, this mechanism has been termed extravascular hemolysis, in contrast to intravascular hemolysis in which erythrocyte lysis occurs within the blood vessels. The concept of partial phagocytosis is important. Here, the erythrocyte loses a portion of its membrane and has a decreased surface area relative to its volume. This change in shape from disk-to-sphere results in decreased deformability of the cells. Erythrocytes must be extremely pliable to traverse the splenic red pulp and sinusoidal walls (Fig. 7-2); spherocytes, therefore, tend to be retained in the spleen in close association with macrophages with risk of further injury and eventual destruction.

Erythrocyte-macrophage interaction with spherocyte formation is important for the destruction of aged erythrocytes. This interaction is significantly mediated by antibody fixation to erythrocyte membrane proteins, which become exposed as the cells age. Following erythrophagocytosis, the enzymes within phagolysosomes dissolve the erythrocytes and hemoglobin is degraded, releasing bilirubin and iron from the porphyrin part of the molecule. The bilirubin is transported in the plasma combined with albumin to the liver. The iron is bound to plasma transferrin and transported to the marrow, where it is taken up by receptors on red cell precursors.

In intravascular erythrocyte lysis, hemoglobin released into the plasma is immediately bound to haptoglobin, its

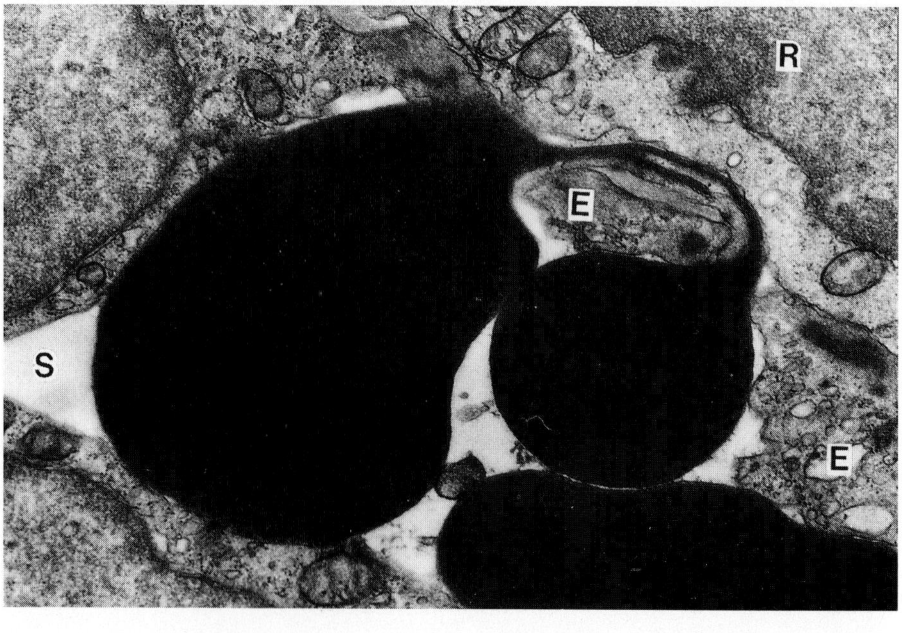

Figure 7-2 Electron micrograph. Spleen; rabbit. The deformability of an erythrocyte is shown as it passes through two apertures of basement membrane. Two globular portions of the erythrocyte are in a sinus *(S)*. An attenuated connecting portion lies deep in the basement membrane. *E*, endothelial cells; *R*, reticular cell. *From Burke JS, Simon GT. Am J Pathol 1970; 58:127-155.*

principal transport protein. The hemoglobin-haptoglobin complex is then removed by hepatocytes and the hemoglobin is degraded. Hemoglobinuria, an important indicator of intravascular hemolysis, is only visible when the haptoglobin binding capacity is exceeded.

Infectious Causes. Infectious agents that cause hemolytic anemia include viruses, bacteria, rickettsiae, and protozoa. Mechanisms of erythrocyte destruction by some of these agents involve antibody fixation to the erythrocyte membrane, with subsequent phagocytosis by macrophages.

Equine infectious anemia. Equine infectious anemia is a disease of horses, mules, and donkeys caused by an arthropod-borne retrovirus. Horses may die of anemia during the initial viremia or may recover to undergo subsequent episodes of viremia and anemia. The virus replicates in macrophages and possibly other cells, which eventually release large amounts of virus into the extracellular fluid. Each subsequent hemolytic crisis is caused by a new antigenic variant of the virus. Hemolysis is assumed to be immune mediated, as C3 complement is present on erythrocytes, presumably following adsorption of virus, antibody fixation, and complement activation, which leads to erythrophagocytosis. Later in the course of the disease, compensatory erythropoiesis is inhibited, presumably by the mechanisms responsible for the anemia of chronic inflammation.

During the viremic phase, horses with equine infectious anemia are markedly depressed and have fever, icterus, dependent pitting edema, and pallor of mucous membranes. Petechiae are frequently present on the ventral surface of the tongue and conjunctivae. Hemograms taken during periods of anemia reveal severely reduced erythrocyte numbers and hematocrits as low as 0.10 L/L (10%). There is usually bilirubinemia. The only indication of compensatory erythropoiesis may be an increased MCV and RDW. The accompanying leukopenia is caused by neutropenia and a marginal lymphopenia. Monocytes occasionally contain erythrocytes; larger numbers of such cells can be seen in smears of buffy coat. Thrombocytopenia is evident within 1 or 2 days of viral inoculation, but the mechanism is unclear. At this stage, the bone marrow has marked erythroid hyperplasia but megakaryocytes do not appear increased, suggesting that the thrombocytopenia may, in part, be due to impaired thrombopoiesis. As the disease progresses, the erythropoietic rate declines and there is accumulation of hemosiderin-laden macrophages and plasma cells in the bone marrow and spleen. Confirmation of a diagnosis of equine infectious anemia is by means of an agar-gel immunodiffusion test, in which a precipitin line develops in the presence of serum antibody to tissue culture–derived antigen.

Animals dying during hemolytic crises have icterus, anemia, and widespread hemorrhages. In more chronic cases, emaciated animals have serous atrophy of fat. The spleen and liver are enlarged, dark and turgid, and they and other organs have superficial subcapsular hemorrhages (Fig. 7-3). Petechiae are evident beneath the renal capsule and throughout the cortex and medulla. The bone marrow is dark red as a result of replacement of fat by hemopoietic tissue; the extent of replacement is an indication of the duration of the anemia. The severity of microscopic lesions is dependent on the chronicity of the disease and are most significant in the spleen, liver, and bone marrow. As would be anticipated, microscopic findings of the spleen are predominantly influenced by the number and activity of macrophages, which is a reflection of the duration of the disease and the frequency of hemolytic episodes. Hemosiderin-laden macrophages persist for months to years; therefore, large numbers are consistent with chronicity. Kupffer cell hyperplasia with hemosiderin stores and periportal infiltrates of lymphocytes are the most

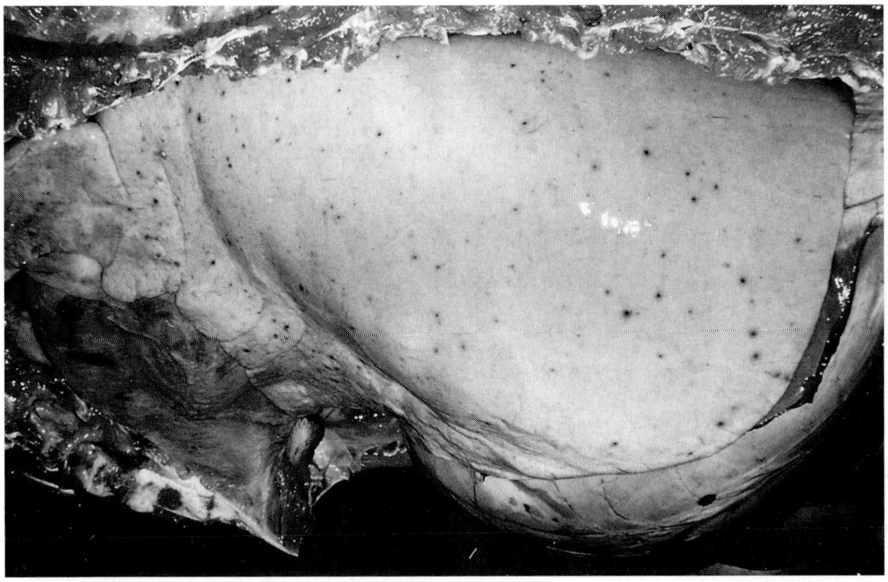

Figure 7-3 Lung; horse. Equine infectious anemia. Focal hemorrhages are visible beneath the visceral pleura.

significant changes in the liver. Bone marrow histologic findings vary depending on the duration of the disease. In most animals, the marrow is cellular because of the replacement of fat by intense, orderly erythropoiesis. Granulocytes are relatively less numerous and plasma cells are increased. As in the spleen, hemosiderin-laden macrophages are present in large numbers in chronic cases.

Leptospirosis. Leptospirosis is a disease of domestic animals, rodents, and human beings caused by serovars of *Leptospira interrogans.* The organisms are ubiquitous, occurring throughout the world wherever the environmental conditions are favorable. Leptospires may survive for months under ideal conditions of moist soil and stagnant water. Leptospires are best visualized by dark-field microscopy of fluids, in which they appear as delicate motile spirilla.

Leptospires are not highly host specific; thus, several serovars may cause disease in several different species. In species serving as maintenance hosts (carriers), the organisms persist in the kidneys or genital tract as a reservoir for contamination of the environment by urine and discharges following abortion. There then may be infection of other animals of the maintenance host species or incidental hosts that are less susceptible to that particular serovar. There is considerable overlap in clinical signs, laboratory results, and necropsy findings in the disease caused by different serovars in different animals.

Infection occurs percutaneously and via mucosal surfaces and is followed by leptospiremia; organisms then localize in the kidney, liver, and pregnant uterus. During the bacteremic phase, animals may become icteric as a result of a combination of hemolysis and liver injury. In calves, the icterus is mainly due to intravascular hemolysis; hemoglobinuria may be transient or persist for several days depending on the rate and extent of hemolysis. In cows, there is agalactia and blood-tinged milk. Abortion may occur in the acute phase or during convalescence. The fetus that dies before abortion is frequently decomposed. In dairy cows, a subacute form of the disease causes fever and decreased milk production. The udder is flabby and the milk resembles colostrum. In swine, the most significant form of leptospirosis is abortion and birth of weak piglets; the dead piglets are heavily infected with leptospires. Venereal infection of sows with some serovars causes infertility. Leptospirosis in swine and cattle causes a chronic interstitial nephritis that is most commonly observed at slaughter. A variety of serovars in horses cause liver and kidney disease in foals, abortion in mares, and chronic uveitis.

Dogs are the maintenance host for the *Leptospira canicola* serovar; however, vaccination has significantly reduced the incidence of disease. The *Leptospira icterohemorrhagia serovar,* acquired from the environment contaminated by rats, causes acute hepatic injury, which results in hyperbilirubinemia and elevated concentrations of liver enzymes in serum. This septicemic phase of disease can be very severe and cause rapid death in pups. Following septicemia, all serovars in dogs localize in the kidney. Leptospires in the kidney cause a focal to diffuse interstitial nephritis, initially characterized by hyperemia, edema, and endothelial cell swelling, and later by interstitial accumulation of lymphocytes and plasma cells. Although renal injury may be severe, death from renal failure is uncommon; animals that survive may excrete organisms in the urine for years.

In the laboratory diagnosis of leptospirosis, precautions must be taken to protect human beings from infection and to optimize the methods for isolation of such a fragile organism. The long-standing practice of demonstrating organisms by dark-field microscopy of fluids and tissue emulsions is now regarded as less sensitive compared with newer procedures such as immunofluorescence of urine or homogenates of fetal lung, kidney, or placenta.

The most prominent findings in ruminants that die of acute leptospirosis are the results of intravascular hemolysis. These include anemia, icterus, pulmonary edema, and a pale, friable, bile-stained liver. The kidneys are swollen and dark from hemoglobin staining; later in the course of the disease, there are pale foci caused by interstitial cell infiltrates. Widespread ecchymotic hemorrhages may be present.

Dogs dying of the acute disease have widespread hemorrhages and focal hepatic necrosis. The kidneys are most consistently affected and in the acute disease are swollen, with subcapsular and cortical ecchymotic hemorrhages. Microscopic lesions at this stage include tubular epithelial degeneration and necrosis and interstitial edema. This is followed by infiltration of lymphocytes and plasma cells. With time, the kidneys become shrunken and have varying degrees of cortical fibrosis.

Babesioses. Babesioses are tick-borne diseases caused by protozoa of the genus *Babesia.* They occur in all domestic animals, including recently domesticated species such as North American elk *(Cervus elaphus)* and wildlife ruminants, principally in warmer climates that are suitable for the tick vectors. These protozoa can cause an acute syndrome characterized by hemolytic anemia and injury to multiple organs, a chronic syndrome associated with anemia and weight loss, and a carrier state. Calves less than 3 months of age are resistant to *Babesia* infections; in dogs, the acute disease occurs in pups. The speciation of *Babesia* is difficult because of incomplete knowledge of many of the isolates; however, *B. bigemina, B. bovis, B. divergens,* and *B. major* occur in cattle; *B. caballi,* and *B. equi* occur in horses; *B. canis* and *B. gibsoni* occur in dogs; and *B. foliata, B. motasi,* and *B. ovis* occur in sheep.

Babesia produce acute disease by two principal mechanisms: hemolysis and circulatory disturbances. Babesia invade erythrocytes and cause intravascular and macrophage-mediated hemolysis. The precise mechanisms of intravascular hemolysis are unclear but are assumed to be directly attributable to the protozoa, because correlation exists between the severity of the parasitemia and the

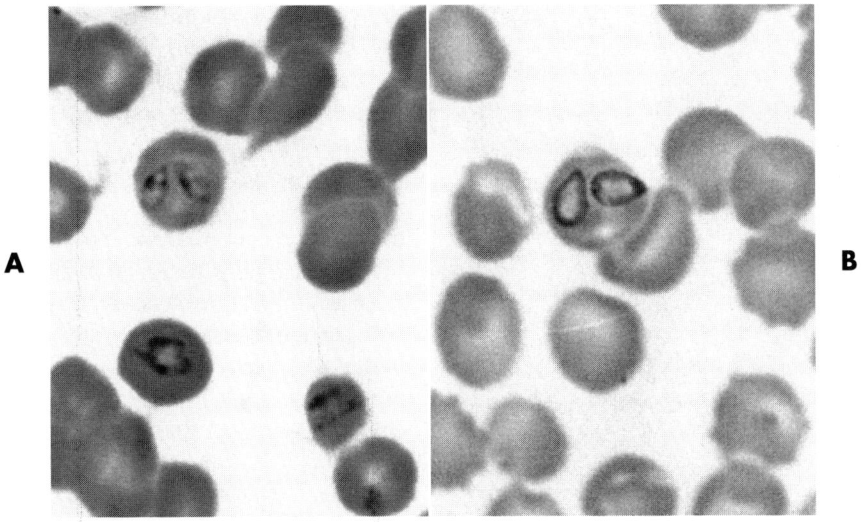

Figure 7-4 Babesiosis. **A,** Blood smear; horse. **B,** Blood smear; dog. Wright-Giemsa stain. *Courtesy of M. D. Campbell.*

severity of anemia, hemoglobinemia, and hemoglobinuria. Phagocytosis of parasitized erythrocytes may be enhanced by antibody in the later stages of disease, as some *Babesia*-infected animals have positive direct antiglobulin tests and lowered complement levels.

B. bovis and *B. canis,* in addition to causing hemolysis, initiate events resulting in circulatory shock. The organisms activate plasma vasodilatory agents, such as kallikrein and bradykinin, resulting in sludging of blood in the microvasculature. Tissue hypoxia and widespread inflammation damage multiple organs because of the unchecked host responses mediated by cytokines, nitric acid, free oxygen radicals, eicosanoids, and platelet-activating factor.

The wide variety of clinical signs of babesiosis is due to variations in pathogenicity of the organisms and susceptibility of the animals. The organisms usually appear in erythrocytes within 8 to 16 days following vector-transmitted infection; this appearance is accompanied by fever. Animals become listless, dehydrated, and weak with hemoglobinuria and icterus. Subcutaneous edema of the lower abdomen and thorax is detected in horses. *B. bovis* infections in cattle and *B. canis* infections in dogs result in nervous signs such as mania, recumbency with paddling of limbs, and coma, most likely the result of circulatory disturbances caused by occlusion of cerebral capillaries and resultant ischemia. If animals recover from the acute form of babesiosis, they have variable, unpredictable relapses. Others experience chronic disease characterized by unthriftiness and weight loss.

Laboratory findings in animals with acute babesiosis are those of anemia with intense erythropoiesis and protozoa visible in erythrocytes. Infected erythrocytes are large and most numerous in the feather edge of blood films. In vivo, infected erythrocytes accumulate in capillaries; therefore, blood films prepared from capillary blood, as from an ear or tail incision, are useful for finding round to pyriform organisms (Fig. 7-4). The percentage of parasitized erythrocytes detected is significantly increased after Percoll gradient separation of the larger cells. In the later stages of disease, leukocyte counts increase because of lymphocytosis. During the period of severe anemia, serum concentrations of liver enzymes, such as alanine and aspartate aminotransferases (ALT and AST), and bilirubin are elevated. Serologic tests are available to assist in diagnosing babesiosis; these are most useful in animals with chronic disease when organisms are difficult to find. The indirect fluorescent antibody test is widely used and highly specific but is not very sensitive. Agglutination tests, including hemagglutination, capillary, slide, and card tests, are sensitive methods of detecting antibodies.

At necropsy, animals dying of the acute disease have marked splenomegaly, jaundice, hemoglobinuria, swollen hemoglobin-stained kidneys, and subepicardial and subendocardial hemorrhages. The gallbladder is usually distended with thick bile. A striking feature of *B. bovis* infections is congestion of gray matter throughout the brain, which is readily visible compared with the white matter. Parasitized erythrocytes are best visualized on impression smears of kidney, brain, and skeletal muscle. Microscopic findings in the liver and kidney are typical of a hemolytic crisis and include degeneration and loss of periacinar hepatocytes and cholestasis, and hemoglobinuric nephrosis with degeneration of tubular epithelium. Erythroid hyperplasia is present in the bone marrow. In animals that survive the acute disease, there is hemosiderin accumulation in the liver, kidney, spleen, and bone marrow.

Anaplasmosis. Anaplasmosis is a disease of cattle and sheep caused by organisms of the genus *Anaplasma,* order Rickettsiales. In cattle, *A. marginale* causes severe hemolytic anemia, whereas *A. centrale* is less pathogenic. Bo-

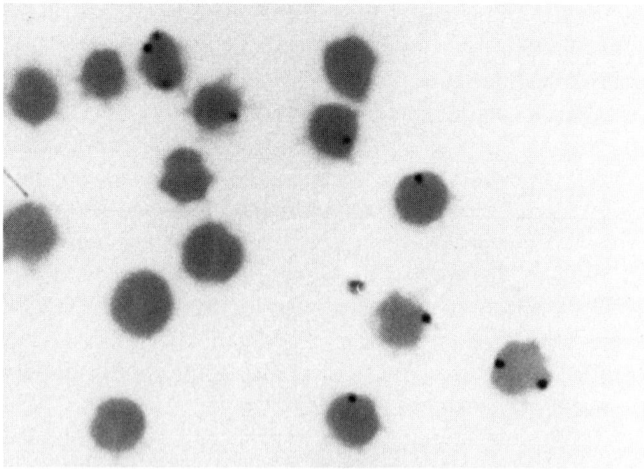

Figure 7-5 Blood smear; cow. Anaplasmosis. Discrete, round organisms are visible at the periphery of erythrocytes. Wright-Giemsa stain. *Courtesy of M.D. Campbell.*

vine anaplasmosis is economically significant in Australia, the United States, South America, and Russia; *A. ovis* (of sheep and goats) causes significant disease in the Mediterranean region. The organisms are transmitted by ticks and mechanically by biting flies and hypodermic needles.

Mechanisms of disease induced by *Anaplasma* organisms involve penetration of the erythrocyte, in which the membrane of the red cell invaginates and engulfs the organisms within a vesicle. The parasite then divides by binary or multiple fission into new infective units. Later, pores form in the erythrocyte membrane through which organisms escape to infect other cells. It is suspected that the organism can proceed through these stages and exert its effects on the red cell by release of hydrolytic enzymes. The presence of *Anaplasma* proteins on the erythrocyte results in the formation of antibodies that subsequently affix to the erythrocyte and interact with macrophage receptors. The observation that noninfected erythrocytes are also destroyed would suggest that antibodies are produced that interact with normal erythrocyte membrane proteins.

Young animals are susceptible to infection but do not develop disease. The immunity that develops following infection is tolerant of a carrier state that results in a reservoir of domestic and wild ruminants that can infect other animals. Splenectomy of carrier animals results in marked parasitemia and acute hemolysis.

The incubation period of anaplasmosis is 1 to 3 months, followed by hemolytic anemia. Affected animals have pale, icteric mucosae, are depressed and weak, and have reduced exercise tolerance. In contrast to babesiosis, there is no hemoglobinuria. Some animals that recover remain debilitated.

Laboratory findings are anemia of varying severity with hematocrits as low as 0.10 to 0.15 L/L (10% to 15%). When the disease is severe, as many as 50% to 60% of the erythrocytes contain organisms (Fig. 7-5). There may be one or more dark blue to black organisms, of 0.3 to 1 μm in diameter, per erythrocyte. They must be differentiated from nuclear remnants, which are usually not as numerous, vary more in size, and occur as single inclusions. The anemia is usually regenerative with elevated MCV, abundant polychromasia, basophilic stippling, and reticulocytosis. There may be moderate neutrophilia. During brisk hemolysis, there is hyperbilirubinemia. Recovery from acute anaplasmosis results in persistent infection in which animals serve as reservoirs for transmission within herds. Assays to identify carrier animals use PCR technology and enzyme-linked immunosorbent assays (ELISA) to detect the PCR products.

Animals dying of acute anaplasmosis have blood of low viscosity, pale to icteric tissues, an enlarged turgid spleen, and an icteric liver with a distended gallbladder.

Eperythrozoonoses. Eperythrozoonoses are diseases caused by erythrocytic parasites within the order Rickettsiales, family Bartonellaceae. A carrier state exists in sheep, cattle, swine, and llamas in which there can be occasional occurrences of hemolytic anemia. Transmission of the organisms from animal to animal has not been as extensively studied as that of babesiosis and anaplasmosis, but the greatest incidence of disease in sheep and swine accompanies heavy ectoparasite infestations. The mechanism of disease appears similar to those of other red cell parasites, wherein immune-mediated hemolysis within macrophages follows attachment of the organisms to erythrocytes.

The disease in sheep and swine has a seasonal incidence corresponding to the peak occurrence of biting insects. However, it can also occur at other times of the year, as a recrudescence in a carrier animal secondary to another disease. In both sheep and swine, sudden death of one or two animals is followed by anemia in other animals within the herd. *Eperythrozoon wenyoni* in cattle is less pathogenic than *Eperythrozoon ovis* and *Eperythrozoon suis;* infection appears to be widespread, but it rarely causes disease.

It is imperative that blood samples and smears be taken from anemic sheep or swine before euthanasia, because detection of the organism in blood smears after death is difficult. In acute disease, the anemia may be severe and significantly regenerative, and many organisms are found on erythrocytes as well as free between erythrocytes. In less severe infections, the anemia may be mild, and it is necessary to search to find the few parasitized cells. Regardless of the degree of parasitemia, infected erythrocytes usually harbor several organisms, frequently within one portion of the cell (Figs. 7-6 and 7-7). The organisms closely resemble *Hemobartonella felis;* they tend to be ring forms with pale centers except on the edge of the cell, where they appear bacillary. Identification of the organisms requires a good-quality blood smear without stain precipitate and the use of an oil immersion, 100x lens. An ELISA assay has been developed to detect antibodies to *E. suis.*

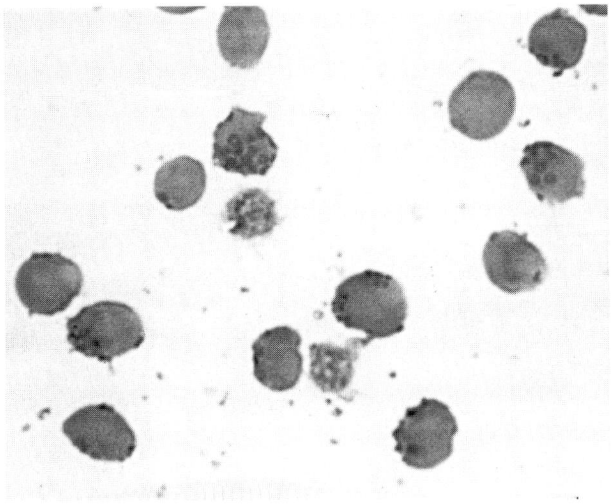

Figure 7-6 Blood smear; pig. Eperythrozoonosis. Note that organisms are adhered to the erythrocytes and in the plasma. Wright-Giemsa stain.

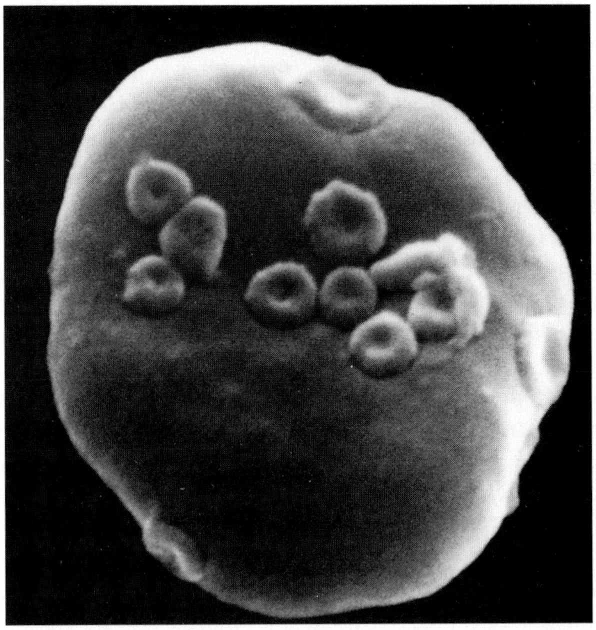

Figure 7-7 Scanning electron micrograph. Blood; calf. *Eperythrozoon* organisms adhered to an erythrocyte.

In animals dying of eperythrozoonosis, the findings are typical of macrophage-mediated hemolysis with obvious anemia, icterus, splenomegaly, and distended gallbladder. Microscopic lesions in the spleen include congestion, erythrophagia, macrophage hyperplasia, and hemopoiesis. Plasma cell numbers are increased in the spleen. Bone marrow has varying degrees of erythroid hyperplasia; the severity reflects the duration of hemolysis.

Trypanosomiasis. Trypanosomiasis is caused by flagellated protozoa that occur in the blood and occasionally in tissues of animals and human beings. They have widespread geographic distribution but cause significant disease in warmer climatic areas, such as Africa and South America. The principal pathogens of animals are *Trypanosoma congolense, Trypanosoma vivax,* and *Trypanosoma brucei,* whereas trypanosomes such as *Trypanosoma melophagium* in sheep and *Trypanosoma theileri* in cattle are widespread and nonpathogenic. Trypanosomes normally survive and are nonpathogenic in wildlife reservoir hosts. They are transmitted to other animals by arthropod vectors, such as the tsetse fly, in which the organism survives in the salivary glands for the life of the fly. Other biting insects transmit trypanosomes mechanically.

The mechanisms by which trypanosomes cause disease are complex and incompletely studied. The considerable variation in the severity of the disease is due to factors such as strain of organism and immunocompetence of the host. Some trypanosomial species induce rapidly fatal disease, others cause chronic debilitating disease, and some allow complete recovery with significant immunity. Because some African native cattle have considerable resistance to trypanosomes, clearer insight into these parasite-host interactions would be of considerable significance in learning to control infections in more susceptible cattle. Trypanosomes escape from the host's immune response following development of new cell membrane proteins, which results in waves of parasitemia and chronic disease.

Cattle with acute trypanosomiasis have significant anemia that initially is regenerative, with macrocytosis, reticulocytosis, and bone marrow erythroid hyperplasia. With time, the anemia becomes less regenerative. Platelet numbers are between 100 and 200×10^9/L. There is a significant leukopenia caused by neutropenia and lymphopenia. Plasma protein concentrations are reduced because of hypoalbuminemia. The extent of parasitemia is readily apparent with *T. vivax* and *T. theileri* infections because the organisms are present in large numbers in the blood (Fig. 7-8). This is in contrast to *T. congolense,* which localizes within the vasculature of the brain and skeletal muscle. Cattle with *T. congolense* infections develop chronic debilitating disease; they have scruffy haircoats, appear "potbellied," and have fever, intermittent diarrhea, and exercise intolerance. Mortality is greater with *T. vivax* infections, usually from intercurrent acute infectious diseases such as salmonellosis.

Necropsy findings in cattle with trypanosome infections include cachexia, generalized edema with increased fluid in body cavities, and generalized lymph node enlargement. Bronchopneumonia, a flabby heart, and serous atrophy of pericardial fat may be present. Liver and kidneys are symmetrically enlarged. The lymph nodes are enlarged up to four times normal size because of lymphoid hyperplasia, and most of the fatty bone marrow is replaced by red hemopoietic tissue. The spleen is enlarged because of lymphoid hyperplasia and is firm when incised.

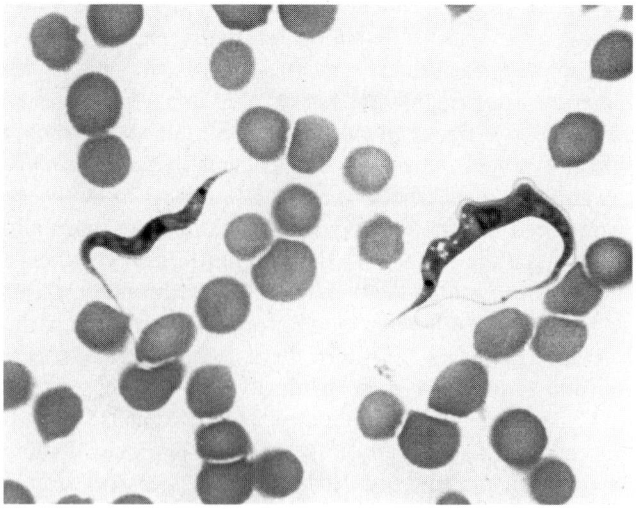

Figure 7-8 Blood smear; calf. *Trypanosoma theileri.* Wright-Giemsa stain.

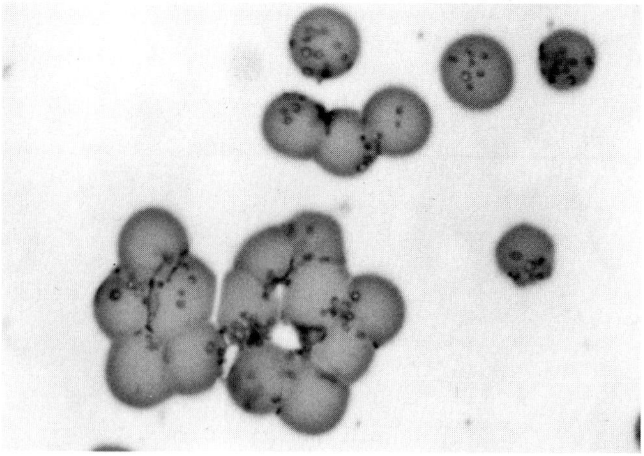

Figure 7-9 Blood smear; cat. Hemobartonellosis. Wright-Giemsa stain.

T. cruzi infection (Chagas' disease) occurs in dogs in the southern United States. Reservoir hosts include raccoons, opossums, armadillos, and skunks, and transmission to dogs is by hemipteran insects. Clinical signs include tachycardia, pale mucous membranes, ascites, and lymph node enlargement. Laboratory evaluation involves finding trypanosomes in the peripheral blood, buffy coat smears, and lymph node aspirates or biopsies. Postmortem findings include those of cardiac failure, i.e., pulmonary edema, ascites, and chronic passive congestion of the liver. Cardiac lesions, most pronounced in the right heart, include multiple yellow to white myocardial foci (myocardial necrosis and myocarditis) and, in chronic cases, myocardial flaccidity and dilatation.

Hemobartonellosis. Hemobartonellosis is caused by organisms (family Bartonellaceae, order Rickettsiales)that resemble *Eperythrozoon* species in most respects. They are widespread geographically and occur in rats, cattle, goats, and dogs but are of most significance in the cat as the cause of feline infectious anemia. Transmission is probably due to bloodsucking arthropods. *Haemobartonella* organisms should always be searched for in dogs following splenectomy, but, even if they are present, they may not significantly shorten the lifespan of the erythrocytes.

Hemobartonellosis in the cat may cause an acute hemolytic, regenerative anemia with marked parasitemia. *Haemobartonella felis*–erythrocyte membrane interactions are assumed to provoke immune-mediated erythrophagocytosis in the spleen, liver, and bone marrow. Cats with the acute form of the disease are weak and depressed and have pale, icteric, mucous membranes. Hematologic findings in these cats are a regenerative anemia with hematocrits as low as 0.10 L/L (10%). Detection of *H. felis* in erythrocytes requires a correctly stained blood film of good quality and an experienced examiner. Differentiation of the organism from artifact may be difficult, especially when the organisms are rod forms on the edge of the erythrocyte. Finding ring forms away from the cell periphery is very helpful in distinguishing organisms from artifacts (Fig. 7-9). When *H. felis* is present on erythrocytes of chronically ill cats with nonregenerative anemias, other underlying disease mechanisms, especially feline leukemia and immunodeficiency virus infections, should be investigated.

Cats dying of hemolytic anemia due to *H. felis* have pale mucous membranes with or without icterus. There is usually splenomegaly, and bone marrow fat is partially replaced by red hemopoietic tissue as a result of erythroid hyperplasia.

Cytauxzoonosis. Cytauxzoonosis, caused by *Cytauxzoon felis,* a protozoal organism in the order Piroplasmida, family Theileriidae, is an acute, fatal disease of domestic cats in the southern United States. The mechanism of natural transmission is unknown, although arthropods are most likely vectors. Experimental transmission has been achieved by injection of blood or tissue homogenates from infected cats into normal cats. The domestic cat is probably an unusual or "dead end" host for this organism, and the bobcat (*Lynx rufus*) may be the reservoir host.

C. felis undergoes schizogony within macrophages that enlarge and accumulate within the walls of veins, eventually causing occlusion of the vessels. Merozoites are released and enter erythrocytes. Cats become acutely ill with fever, pallor, and icterus and usually die within 2 to 3 days. Hematologic findings include moderate to marked hemolytic anemia and neutropenia. The organisms within

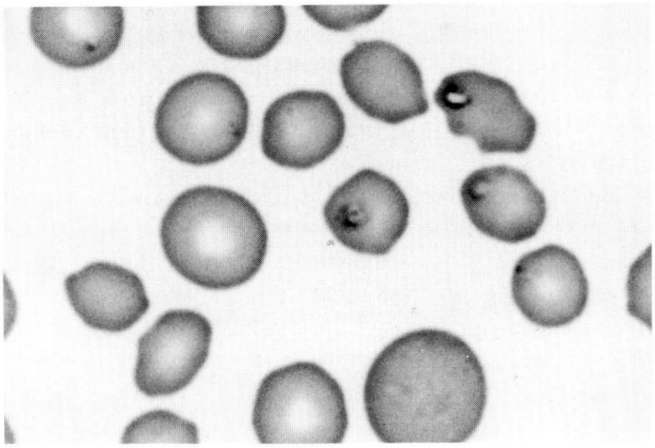

Figure 7-10 Blood smear; cat. Cytauxzoonosis. The protozoa are bipolar, oval or "signet ring" forms, 1.0 to 1.5 μm in diameter. Wright-Giemsa stain. *Courtesy of D.A. Schmidt.*

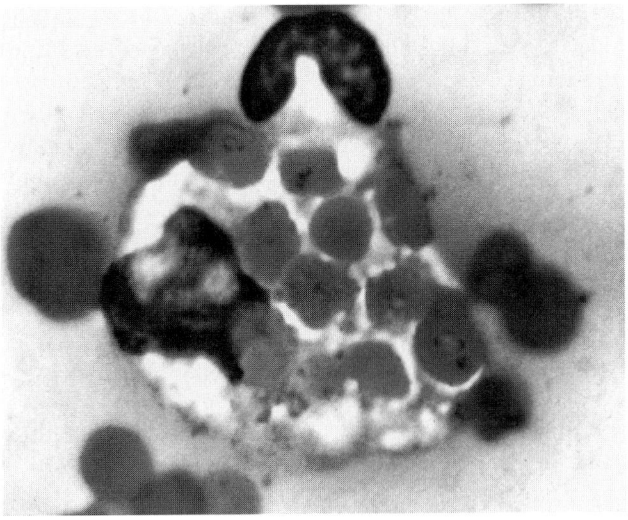

Figure 7-11 Bone marrow aspirate; cat. Cytauxzoonosis. A macrophage has phagocytosed erythrocytes containing *Cytauxzoon felis* organisms. *Courtesy of J.W. Harvey.*

erythrocytes are "signet ring" shaped or bipolar oval forms 1 to 1.5 μ in diameter (Fig. 7-10). In Wright-Giemsa–stained smears, the protozoal cytoplasm stains light blue, whereas the nucleus is darkened or purple. Erythrophagocytosis is a prominent finding in bone marrow aspirates and impression smears of the spleen (Fig. 7-11); these preparations are also useful for demonstration of schizonts of developing *C. felis* organisms in macrophages.

Induced by Chemicals. Hemolytic anemias can be induced by chemicals that inhibit erythrocyte metabolism or that cause denaturation and precipitation of hemoglobin and proteins in the membrane skeleton of the erythrocyte. The erythrocyte, as an anucleate cell, survives by constantly generating ATP from glucose metabolism through the Embden-Meyerhof pathway. This energy is needed to maintain erythrocyte cation content, iron of hemoglobin in the divalent form, sulfhydryl groups of hemoglobin and enzymes in the reduced form, and membrane integrity. The erythrocyte membrane consists of a lipid bilayer in which certain proteins are attached to an underlying cytoskeleton. The latter provides the membrane with both its strength and its flexibility, allowing it to withstand shearing and deforming stress in capillaries and while traversing the walls of sinusoids. Any disruption of the membrane cytoskeleton may lead to hemolysis.

An important aspect of erythrocyte metabolism, in relation to injury by oxidative toxins, is the capacity to maintain a reducing environment by efficient antioxidant mechanisms. These mechanisms involve the enzymes methemoglobin reductase and glutathione peroxidase, as well as reduced pyridine nucleotides nicotinamide-adenine dinucleotide (NADH) and NADH phosphate (NADPH). Oxidant injury to erythrocytes in animals usually occurs because of overloading of the reducing capacity of the erythrocyte subsequent to ingestion of the offending substance. Methemoglobin formation appears to be a prerequisite in the evolution and precipitation of denatured hemoglobin to form Heinz bodies. It is suspected that the precipitated, denatured hemoglobin results in further oxidation of membrane proteins and inhibition of several erythrocyte enzymes. The end result is erythrocyte injury leading to cation leak, loss of deformability, and fixation of immunoglobulin to altered membrane proteins. Both macrophage-mediated erythrocyte destruction and intravascular lysis follow.

Onions contain an agent capable of causing oxidative hemolytic anemia. Indeed, some of the earliest veterinary records of disease and death in North American horses and cattle were associated with the ingestion of wild onions. Poisoning occasionally occurs in cattle when onions are incorporated into the ration, and in dogs that ingest onions in cooked food or chew raw onions. Clinical findings include acute hemolytic anemia with pallor, icterus, and weakness. Hemoglobinuria has occurred in cattle that have ingested large quantities of onions.

Cats are prone to erythrocyte oxidative injury because their globin chains contain more sulfhydryl-containing amino acids than those of other mammals. For this reason, Heinz bodies are frequently present in feline erythrocytes. Until recently, **propylene glycol,** was a common additive to commercial pet foods and induced Heinz body formation in cat erythrocytes. Drugs such as aspirin and related products contain strong oxidants that can cause hemolytic anemia in cats.

Oxidative injury to erythrocytes has occurred in horses following the ingestion of leaves and bark of **red maple trees** (*Acer rubrum*). Experiments in which marine birds ingested crude oil have produced significant hemoglobin oxidative injury with Heinz body formation and hemolysis. These phenomena are most likely significant in birds involved with oil spills. Heinz body hemolytic anemias may occur in dogs as a result of **zinc toxicity,** following ingestion of zinc nuts, bolts, and pennies.

Hematologic findings in animals with oxidative erythrocyte disorders include varying degrees of anemia and compensatory erythropoiesis. The important diagnostic feature of these anemias is the presence of Heinz bodies in erythrocytes. In Wright's-Giemsa–stained blood films, these are discrete protrusions from the cell membrane or tiny pale spherules under the cell membrane (Fig. 7-12). These inclusions are more readily visible on new methylene blue–stained smears. Eccentrocytes—erythrocytes with hemoglobin concentrated in one portion of the cell—occur subsequent to erythrocyte oxidative injury in dogs (Fig. 7-12). Animals dying of Heinz body hemolytic anemia have generalized pallor and icterus. There is usually pulmonary edema with frothy fluid in the trachea. The spleen is enlarged and turgid. The liver is usually enlarged and icteric, and the gallbladder is distended with bile.

Copper poisoning and hemolysis occur when copper is present in the plasma at concentrations exceeding the binding capacity of its transport proteins, albumin and ceruloplasmin. This occurs in sheep, cattle, and swine following release of copper from the liver. At lower concentrations, copper inhibits erythrocyte enzymes of the Embden-Meyerhof pathway, which results in ATP depletion and erythrocyte lysis. At higher concentrations, copper inhibits enzymes within the hexose-monophosphate shunt, leading to impaired glutathione metabolism, and as a consequence, Heinz body formation. Anemia in all species most likely results from a combination of these mechanisms, which lead to hemolysis followed by hemoglobinemia and hemoglobinuria.

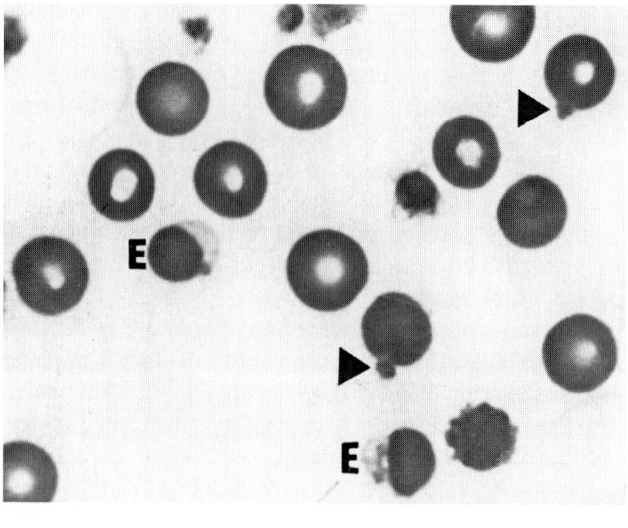

Figure 7-12 Blood smear; dog. Eccentrocytes *(E)* and erythrocytes containing Heinz bodies *(arrowheads)* in a dog with hemolytic anemia from the ingestion of onions. Wright-Giemsa stain.

Hemograms from animals with copper toxicity reveal severe anemia. The hemoglobin concentration may be elevated in relation to the hematocrit and erythrocyte count owing to the measurement of plasma hemoglobin. Inspection of blood films can confirm severe anemia and may reveal Heinz bodies; however, sheep may die from copper toxicity before compensatory erythropoiesis becomes evident.

Hypophosphatemic hemolytic anemia occurs as postparturient hemoglobinuria in the dairy cow 3 to 8 weeks after parturition. It also occurs in beef cattle and nonpostpartum cattle consuming phosphorus-deficient diets. One or two animals with hemolytic anemia may indicate an underlying nutritional disorder in a herd. Cattle dying in hemolytic crises have generalized pallor, icterus, watery blood, pulmonary edema, and fluid in serous cavities. The liver is enlarged, turgid, and pale; the gallbladder is distended with bile; and the spleen is enlarged and congested.

Erythrocytes require inorganic phosphorus for incorporation into phosphorylated intermediate molecules within the Embden-Meyerhof pathway and for synthesis of ATP. Inorganic phosphorus also exerts control over the reaction rate of a key enzyme in the pathway (phosphofructokinase). In phosphate depletion, the erythrocytic glycolytic rate is slowed, and ATP synthesis declines. The structure and function of erythrocytes are no doubt compromised, and when plasma phosphorus concentrations reach a critical level, hemolysis occurs. Intravascular hemolysis, indicated by hemoglobinuria is a common finding, but phagocytosis of abnormal erythrocytes (extravascular hemolysis) probably also occurs.

Laboratory findings include hemoglobinemia and hemoglobinuria. The anemia may be severe with hematocrits as low as 0.10 L/L (10%). In acutely ill animals, there are few immature erythrocytes present on blood smears, but in cattle with hemolysis of several days' duration, moderate to marked reticulocyte responses are seen. Serum phosphorus concentrations in hemoglobinemic animals may be normal, perhaps because phosphates from the hydrolysis of intracellular phosphates released by lysed erythrocytes are measured in the assay. In these cases, it is advisable to do serum phosphorus analyses on other animals in the herd. In the author's experience with a herd of beef cattle with hemolytic anemia in one cow, the serum phosphorus concentration was 1.40 mmol/L (4.34 mg/dl) in the affected cow. However, in 18 other animals in the herd, the mean phosphorus concentration was 0.97

mmol/L (3 mg/dl) with a range of 0.38 to 1.65 mmol/L (1.18 to 5.1 mg/dl) compared with normal reference values of 1.08 to 2.76 mmol/L (3.34 to 8.54 mg/dl).

Immunologically Mediated

Neonatal alloimmune hemolytic anemia. Neonatal alloimmune hemolytic anemia (neonatal isoerythrolysis) occurs in foals that acquire antierythrocyte antibody in colostrum from mares that have been sensitized to erythrocyte antigens released from the fetus, which inherited them from the sire. Foal erythrocytes enter the maternal circulation at sites of focal placental hemorrhage, or the mare may have been sensitized to foal red cells during a previous parturition. The incidence of the disease is approximately 1% in thoroughbred horses and about 2% in standardbred horses. Some blood groups are more antigenic than others; blood groups Aa in the A system and Qa in the Q system are very immunogenic in mares which are Aa–, Qa–, or both. Severely affected foals become lethargic and weak as early as 8 to 10 hours after birth or at anytime over the succeeding 4 to 5 days. They have pale, icteric mucous membranes and if hemolysis is severe, hemoglobinuria. Hematocrits from affected foals may be as low as 12 to 15 L/L (12% to 15%). Within a few days, erythroid hyperplasia is evident in the bone marrow. Serum bilirubin concentrations are usually increased. Foals that die during a hemolytic crisis are markedly icteric and have splenomegaly.

Kittens of blood group A born to queens of blood group B are at risk for neonatal hemolysis. Cats with blood group B have naturally occurring antibodies to the A antigen. Fortunately, blood group B is rare in most cats; however, neonatal hemolysis has occurred in Persian and related breeds and should be considered as a possible cause of the fading kitten syndrome and neonatal death.

Idiopathic immune-mediated hemolytic anemia. Idiopathic immune-mediated hemolytic anemia is the most common type of hemolytic anemia in dogs but also occurs in other species. The etiology of most cases of canine immune-mediated hemolytic anemia is unknown. It is possible that the offending antibody develops because infectious agents (such as viruses) or foreign substances (such as drugs) alter erythrocyte membrane proteins. Circulating immune complexes of these antigens may be adsorbed to erythrocyte membranes. In a controlled study, it was found there was a higher incidence of this disease in dogs recently vaccinated against canine distemper, adenovirus type 2, leptospirosis, parainfluenza, and parvovirus.

The decreased survival of antibody-coated erythrocytes is mostly due to the fact that macrophages, principally in the spleen, but also in the liver (Kupffer cells) and bone marrow, have receptors for the Fc region of IgG. Partial phagocytosis, due to removal of portions of the erythrocyte membrane with the highest concentration of antibody, results in transformation of erythrocytes from biconcave disks to spheres; spherocytosis is the hallmark of this disease. Spherocytes are readily recognized in smears of canine blood as small erythrocytes lacking central pallor. It would seem logical to expect a direct correlation between the numbers of spherocytes and the rate of hemolysis.

When the disease is acute, however, and spherocytes predominate, the macrophage population, especially in the spleen, may be inadequate pending the arrival of monocytes and their maturation to activated macrophages. Spherocytic erythrocytes are at risk for phagocytosis because they are no longer pliable or deformable and are retained in the spleen, in close proximity to macrophages. As these cells accumulate in the spleen, lactic acid from erythrocyte glycolysis causes a drop in the pH of the red pulp, and the function of erythrocyte glycolytic enzymes is impaired.

The IgG class of antibody is the most significant cause of canine immunohemolytic anemia. As demonstrated in human beings, it is most likely that there is a direct correlation between the quantity of IgG bound to erythrocytes and hemolysis. The antibody may also fix complement-enhancing phagocytosis. Occasionally, dogs in a hemolytic crisis have hemoglobinemia and hemoglobinuria consistent with complement-mediated injury to the erythrocyte membrane followed by leakage of hemoglobin into the plasma. IgM antibodies are particularly efficient at binding complement and may also be present on erythrocytes of these animals.

Frequently dogs with immune-mediated hemolytic anemia are acutely ill and recumbent, but the disease may occur in a subclinical form. Acutely ill dogs have pale mucosae with or without icterus, and some may vomit and have a fever. A drop of blood should be placed on a slide to look for agglutination (Fig. 7-13). Should it occur, hemoglobinuria is a grave sign. These animals should be

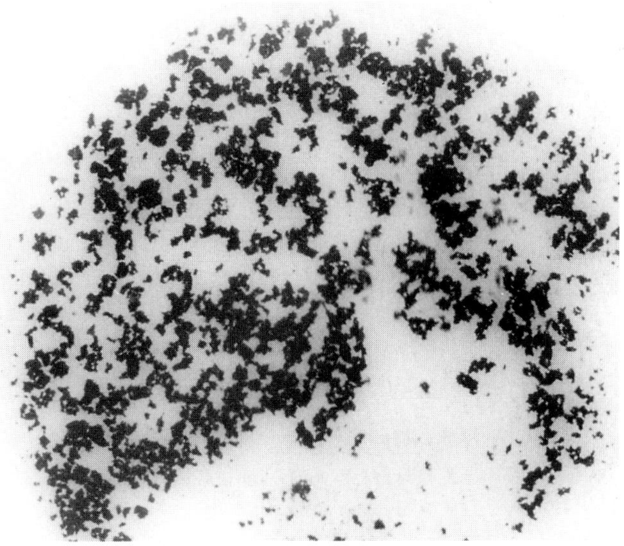

Figure 7-13 Blood; dog. Immune-mediated hemolytic anemia. Erythrocyte agglutination in a drop of blood.

recognized as emergency cases requiring rapid diagnosis and treatment.

Laboratory examination is essential for an accurate diagnosis of this disease. The degree of anemia is variable but may be severe with hematocrits of 0.05 to 0.15 L/L (5% to 15%). Thus, practicing veterinarians must do the studies necessary for diagnosis as there is no time to send blood to a laboratory. In most dogs, the anemia is regenerative at the time of presentation; however, in very acute cases, there will be spherocytosis without polychromasia in blood smears. Occasionally dogs with immune-mediated hemolytic anemia remain reticulocytopenic or compensatory erythropoiesis is delayed. In these dogs, bone marrow should be examined. Usually there is phagocytosis of erythrocytes, and metarubricytes and rubricytes are present (Fig. 7-14), indicating that inadequate compensatory erythropoiesis is due to phagocytosis of erythrocyte precursors.

Obviously, the prognosis is guarded in these reticulocytopenic dogs. The blood in the tube and the stained blood film must be critically examined for agglutination of erythrocytes. Agglutinated erythrocytes are most easily detected in the thicker areas of the blood smear where they occur as irregular clumps, which must not be confused with the linear formations of erythrocytes in rouleaux. The presence of polychromatophilic erythrocytes in the clumps indicates agglutination because these cells do not participate in rouleaux. One of the most striking features of the erythrocytes, visible at low magnification, is marked anisocytosis. This extreme variation in erythrocyte diameter is due to the presence of macrocytic, immature erythrocytes lus small spherocytes (Fig. 7-15).

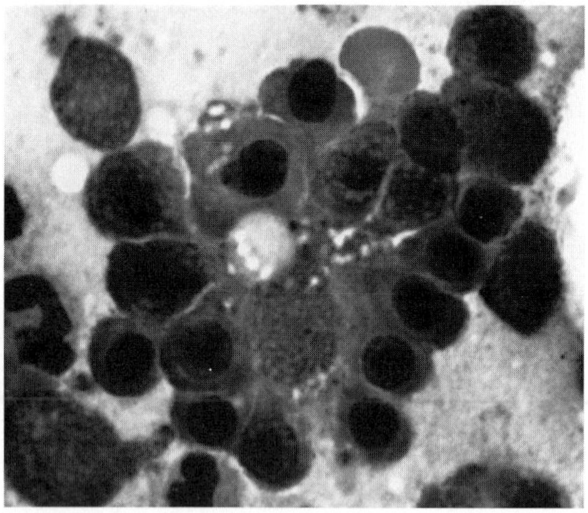

Figure 7-14 Bone marrow aspirate; dog. A reticulocytopenic dog with immune-mediated hemolytic anemia. Note the macrophage with adherent metarubricytes. Wright-Giemsa stain.

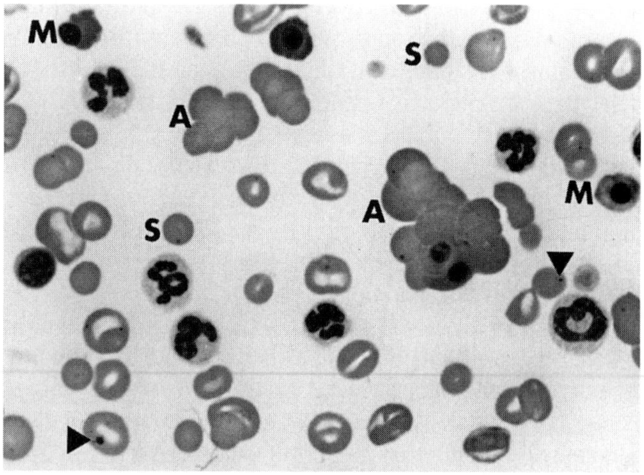

Figure 7-15 Blood smear; dog. Immune-mediated hemolytic anemia. Agglutination of erythrocytes *(A)*, spherocytes *(S)*, metarubricytes *(M)*, nuclear remnants *(arrowheads)*. Wright-Giemsa stain.

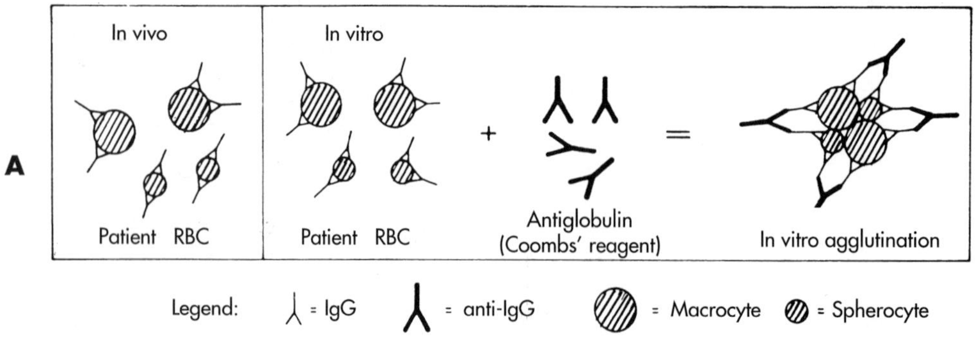

Figure 7-16 Direct antiglobulin test (DAT). **A,** Red blood cells *(RBC)* of patient are coated with antibody in vivo. **B,** In vitro detection of antibody is accomplished by adding heterologous antiglobulin reagent, resulting in cross-linking of RBCs and microscopic or macroscopic agglutination. *From Lewis RM, Picut CA.* Hematologic disorders. *In: Veterinary Clinical Immunology: From Classroom to Clinics. Philadelphia: Lea & Febiger, 1989:9.*

Polychromasia is usually pronounced, and metarubricytes and rubricytes may be present. Platelets may be reduced because of concurrent immune-mediated thrombocytopenia. If platelets are not involved, their numbers will be increased and some may be enlarged. Neutrophilia is also common and appears to accompany the reticulocyte response. Occasionally dogs have leukocyte counts in excess of 50×10^9/L (50,000/mm^3) because of neutrophilia and monocytosis. The monocytosis is a reflection of traffic from the bone marrow to the spleen where monocytes become macrophages capable of erythrophagocytosis.

The direct antiglobulin test (DAT; Coombs' test) is a hemagglutination assay for antibody or complement bound to erythrocytes (Fig. 7-16). Washed saline suspensions of erythrocytes are incubated at 37° and 4° C with antisera containing goat- or rabbit-derived antibody for canine IgG, IgM, and complement C3. The assay should be conducted in microtiter trays, using serial doubling dilutions of the antisera. This will overcome the prozone effect in which false-negative results occur because excess antibodies prevent the cross-linking necessary for agglutination. The reported titer should be the last dilution causing agglutination of the patients' erythrocytes; this gives a rough estimate of the quantity of antibodies coating the erythrocytes.

Although this test is justified as part of the laboratory investigation of this disease, the results must be interpreted carefully in the context of other laboratory and clinical findings. Dogs treated previously with glucocorticoid drugs frequently have a negative test result. Test results may also be negative when antibody molecules are of low avidity and are lost during erythrocyte washings or when the numbers of antibody molecules are too low to be detected. A negative DAT result in the presence of hematologic and clinical findings consistent with immune-mediated hemolytic anemia should not preclude the diagnosis. Flow cytometry may replace the DAT in the future because it detects lower numbers of antibody molecules on erythrocytes.

In the early stages of the disease, bone marrow aspirates have erythroid hyperplasia and varying amounts of erythrophagocytosis (Fig. 7-17). Megakaryocyte numbers are usually increased. When the disease is of longer duration, or following relapses, there may be an increase in hemosiderin-laden macrophages and plasma cells. In dogs with severe hemolysis, there will be hyperbilirubinemia and elevated serum ALT activity due to hypoxic hepatocyte injury.

Postmortem findings in dogs with immune-mediated hemolytic anemia include pale tissues, mild to moderate icterus, pulmonary edema, and frothy tracheal fluid. The heart may be rounded and dilated if the anemia was of some duration; the liver is usually enlarged and pale, and the gallbladder is distended. The spleen is enlarged and is usually firm and meaty when incised. In more acute cases, the enlarged spleen may be turgid. Lymph nodes are enlarged and hyperplastic in the acute disease but are small in dogs treated with glucocorticoid drugs. Thrombosis of pulmonary vessels is present in some dogs. In dogs with thrombocytopenia, hemorrhages are present on the serosal surfaces and on capsular surfaces of visceral organs. The bone marrow has varying amounts of red marrow extending from the ends and endosteal surfaces of long bones, reflecting the duration of compensatory erythropoiesis.

Histologically, macrophages in the liver, spleen, and bone marrow contain hemosiderin. There is a direct relationship between the numbers of hemosiderin-containing macrophages and the duration of the disease. The red pulp of the spleen is occupied by erythroid precursor cells in various stages of differentiation, megakaryocytes, macrophages, and plasma cells. There is periacinar vacuolation and necrosis of hepatocytes due to anemia. Bile plugs are in canaliculi. Fibrin thrombi may be present within capillaries of several organs.

DATs have been performed on cats with a variety of diseases. The incidence of positive test results has been much greater than the incidence of hemolytic anemia. Most of these cats have nonregenerative anemia due to chronic diseases such as feline leukemia or immunodeficiency virus infections. Blood films from these cats have erythrocytic agglutination. The combination of erythrocyte agglutination and positive DATs in cats with chronic diseases may be due to adherence of antigen-antibody complexes to erythrocytes.

Occasionally, hemolytic anemias are encountered in horses that have negative tests for equine infectious anemia by the agar-gel immunodiffusion test. An immune-mediated pathogenesis should be suspected; some are idiopathic, some have antipenicillin antibodies on erythrocytes, and some animals have occult lymphosarcoma.

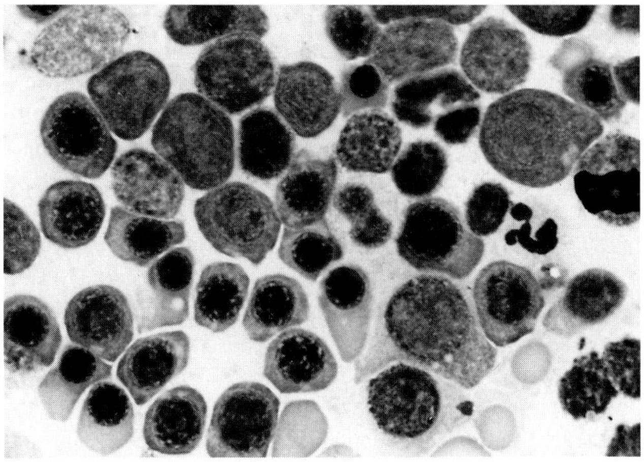

Figure 7-17 Bone marrow aspirate; dog. Immune-mediated hemolytic anemia has resulted in erythroid hyperplasia. Wright-Giemsa stain.

Studies of autoimmune hemolytic anemia in human beings with lymphocytic leukemia have provided evidence that the offending antibodies are products of the B lymphocyte neoplastic clones.

Nonregenerative Anemias

Anemias due to impaired erythropoiesis are the most common anemias in animals and human beings. For this reason, the hemogram is essential as an integral part of a thorough clinical examination because nonregenerative anemia is an indicator of occult disease. Dogs with liver disease, for example, are frequently anemic; additional laboratory tests are required to define the underlying disorder. Bone marrow examination is indicated in animals with significant nonregenerative anemia when an underlying disease is not apparent.

Anemia of Chronic Disease. The anemia of chronic disease (ACD) is an anemia that accompanies chronic inflammatory or neoplastic disorders. The anemia is primarily due to impaired erythropoiesis, which results in low reticulocyte production. The mechanisms by which chronic inflammation and neoplasia impair erythropoiesis are obscure and undoubtedly complex. However, studies of cytokines produced in inflammatory disorders, such as rheumatoid arthritis in human beings, have helped to define the mechanisms by which erythropoiesis is inhibited in ACD. Serum concentrations of interleukin 1 (IL-1), a polypeptide with a wide variety of activities in inflammation and immunity, are elevated in ACD. IL-1 inhibits erythropoiesis indirectly by stimulating T lymphocytes to produce interferon-γ, which has been shown to directly inhibit erythroid precursor cells in culture.

Tumor necrosis factor, another cytokine with a significant role in inflammation and the immune response, causes a nonregenerative anemia when administered to animals and inhibition of the growth of erythrocyte precursor cells in culture. It is possible that other cytokines that help to regulate inflammatory and immune responses also impair erythropoiesis. Although erythropoietin concentrations are elevated in ACD, they are decreased in comparison with the concentrations measured in equally anemic individuals without ACD. There is experimental evidence of inhibition of erythropoietin production by IL-1 and tumor necrosis factor, thus amplifying their contribution to the development of ACD. The anemia of ACD is often accompanied by low serum iron in the presence of adequate stores of iron in the monocyte-macrophage system. It is now suspected that the delayed release of iron from macrophages follows the cytokine-mediated inhibition of erythropoiesis. Animals in renal failure are frequently anemic principally because of inadequate production of erythropoietin by the kidney. The mechanisms of anemia in chronic liver disease are as yet unknown.

Animals with ACD usually have a mild to moderate anemia with quantitative erythrocyte parameters reduced by 10% to 30% (occasionally lower in dogs with renal failure). Despite the decreased availability of iron, the erythrocyte indices are usually normal. Alterations in shape of erythrocytes occur in cats and dogs with chronic liver disease and include elongated erythrocytes with short irregular projections and acanthocytes (Fig. 7-18). In chronic inflammatory disorders, concentrations of plasma proteins are frequently increased and the albumin/globulin ratio is decreased because of increased gamma globulin. Bone marrow aspirates usually have normal granulocyte/erythrocyte ratios. Granulocytic hyperplasia may be present in animals with chronic suppurative inflammation somewhere in the body.

Hemosiderin deposits, visible microscopically as gold, nugget-like clumps in unstained marrow aspirates, may be increased. If these are not visible, iron stores should be assessed using Prussian blue–stained marrow smears as this reaction stains ferritin as well as hemosiderin.

Nutritional Deficiency Anemias. Nutritional deficiency anemias are uncommon in domestic animals. Because piglets have low iron stores at birth and a rapid rate of growth, they become iron deficient **(iron deficiency anemia),** anemic, and severely debilitated if they do not receive a supplement of iron soon after birth. Parenteral administration of iron is now common in swine, and iron deficiency anemias occur only sporadically, for example, when administration of iron to a litter of piglets has been overlooked. Iron-deficient piglets have retarded growth, dyspnea, and lethargy at around 3 weeks of age. The skin and mucosae are pale, and edema of the head and forelimbs may be present. Hematologic findings include erythrocyte numbers as low as 3 or 4×10^9/L (3 or $4 \times 10^6/mm^3$), hemoglobin concentrations of 20 to 40 g/L (2 to 4 g/dl), and hematocrits as low as 0.08 L/L (8%). MCV may be reduced to approximately 40 fL, mean corpuscular hemoglobin (MCH) to 20 pg, and mean corpuscular

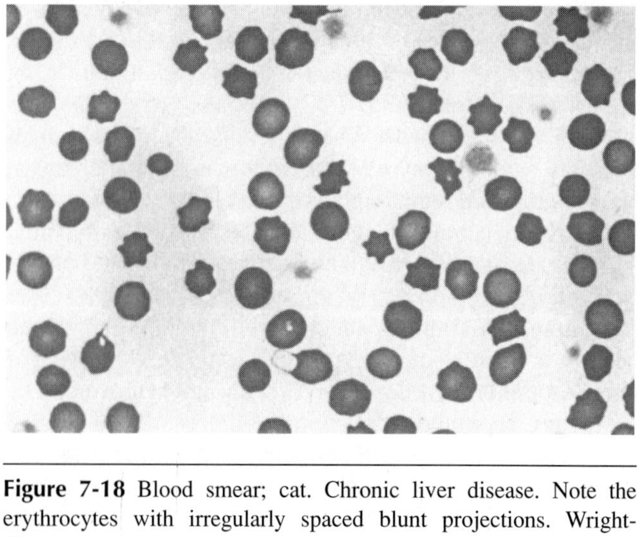

Figure 7-18 Blood smear; cat. Chronic liver disease. Note the erythrocytes with irregularly spaced blunt projections. Wright-Giemsa stain.

hemoglobin concentration (MCHC) to 280 g/L. Blood films from these animals may have microcytic, hypochromic erythrocytes and poikilocytes. There is often marked thrombocytosis. Serum iron concentrations are decreased and may be as low as 5 μmol/L (28 μg/dl). Bone marrow aspirates have an accumulation of rubricytes and metarubricytes because of inadequate transport of iron for hemoglobin synthesis.

Nutritional iron deficiencies are rare in other species; a more common occurrence is iron deficiency secondary to chronic hemorrhage. Chronic hemorrhage may be caused by blood-sucking parasites such as hookworms *(Ancylostoma caninum)* and fleas *(Echidnophaga gallinacea)* in dogs and *Haemonchosis* in cattle and sheep. Bleeding from mucosal surfaces, principally in dogs, can exhaust iron stores. Laboratory findings of hypochromic, microcytic anemia suggest occult bleeding from lesions such as intestinal neoplasms or the result of chronic immune-mediated thrombocytopenia.

Aplastic Pancytopenia. Aplastic pancytopenias are a group of disorders characterized by pancytopenia and hypocellular bone marrow. They occur in cats with leukemia virus infections and sporadically as an idiopathic disorder in dogs. Pure erythrocytic aplasia is the term used to describe failure of erythropoiesis while granulopoiesis and thrombopoiesis are normal. Dogs with pure erythrocytic aplasia initially may develop trilineage aplasia. These disorders result from injury to pluripotential stem cells. Laboratory studies of human patients have provided increasing evidence for immune-mediated stem cell injury. Patient T lymphocytes in culture overproduced both interferon-γ and tumor necrosis factor, cytokines that inhibit in vitro hemopoietic colony formation. When secreted into the marrow microenvironment, they inhibit stem cell proliferation by effects on the mitotic cycle and by apoptosis. The events that initiate immune-mediated stem cell injury are less clear. Recent viral infections and exposure to drugs have been linked to the occurrence of aplastic pancytopenia in human beings. Chemical injury to stem cells by agents such as benzene and related compounds is documented in human beings and experimental animals.

Dogs are particularly prone to estrogen toxicity. This may occur as endogenous hyperestrogenism, as in animals with Sertoli cell tumors, or as a result of estrogen therapy. These dogs initially have neutrophilia and thrombocytosis, followed by thrombocytopenia and anemia. Dogs may recover any time if estrogen concentrations in the body return to normal; the disease, however, may become irreversible in some dogs, and then they become pancytopenic.

Owners bring dogs with pancytopenia to veterinarians for a variety of reasons including hemorrhage, infection, or lethargy and depression. Aspiration of bone marrow may be unsuccessful in obtaining particles of hemopoietic tissue, but smears should be made from any tissue within the needle as it may contain traces of bone marrow. If bone marrow tissue is obtained, it frequently consists of stromal cells with low numbers of hemopoietic cells (Fig. 7-19), fibrous tissue, and numerous hemosiderin-laden macrophages. Core bone marrow biopsies should be obtained from these dogs, fixed in 10% buffered neutral formalin, embedded in paraffin, and sections stained with hematoxylin and eosin (H & E) to evaluate cellularity. These biopsies are hypocellular and have variable amounts of fibrous tissue (Fig. 7-20).

Ehrlichiosis. Ehrlichiosis is a tick-transmitted rickettsial disease affecting several species of animals and human beings. In dogs, disease is caused by *Ehrlichia canis, Ehrlichia chaffeensis, Ehrlichia risticii, Ehrlichia ewingii, Ehrlichia equi,* and *Ehrlichia phagocytophilia,* and in horses by *Ehrlichia equi* and *Ehrlichia risticii. E. risticii*

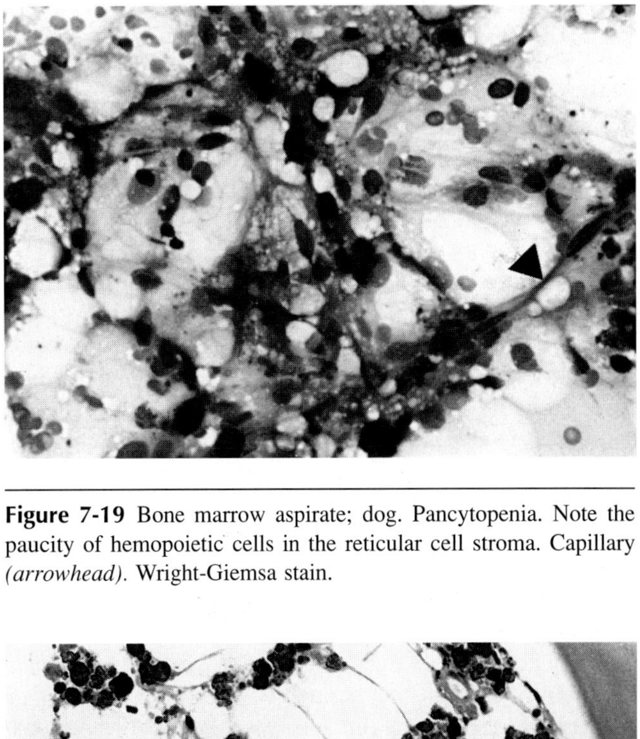

Figure 7-19 Bone marrow aspirate; dog. Pancytopenia. Note the paucity of hemopoietic cells in the reticular cell stroma. Capillary *(arrowhead).* Wright-Giemsa stain.

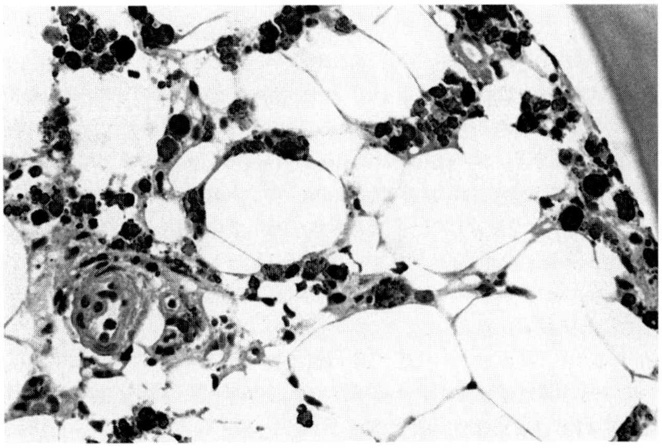

Figure 7-20 Bone marrow core biopsy; dog. Pancytopenia. There is little evidence of hemopoiesis; most of the cells are hemosiderin-laden macrophages and adipocytes. Hematoxylin-eosin (H & E) stain.

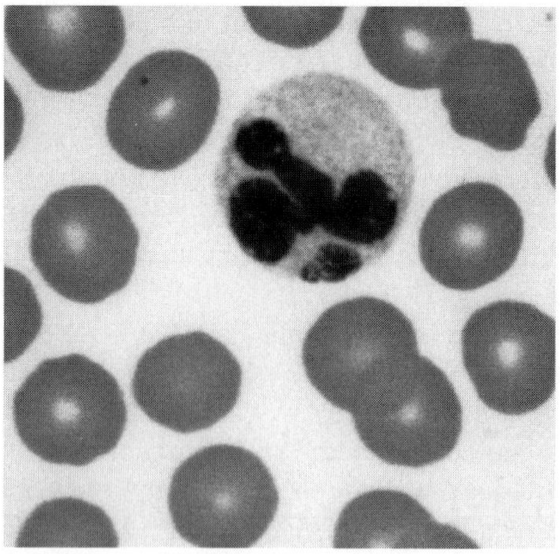

Figure 7-21 Blood smear; dog. Ehrlichiosis. An *Ehrlichia* morula within a neutrophil. Wright-Giemsa stain. *Courtesy of P. S. MacWilliams.*

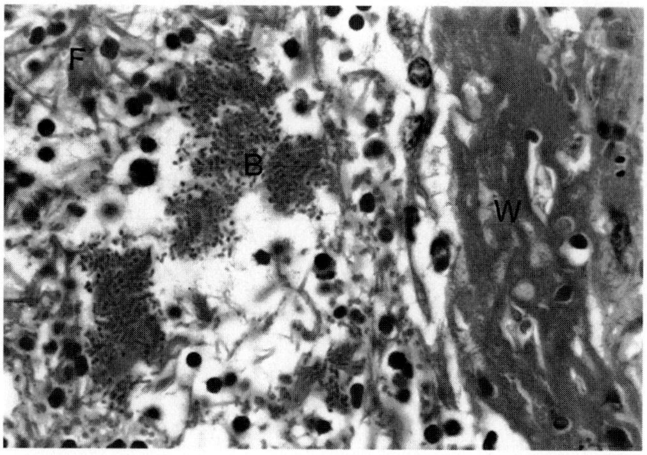

Figure 7-22 Lung; cow. Septic embolus in a neutropenic animal with bracken fern toxicity. *W,* damaged vessel wall; *B,* bacteria; and *F,* fibrin filaments. H & E stain.

causes fever, diarrhea, and leukopenia in horses and is discussed with the gastrointestinal system (Potomac horse fever). *Ehrlichia platys* causes canine cyclic thrombocytopenia and is discussed with those disorders. Most studies of natural and experimental disease have involved *E. canis,* a parasite of monocytes, macrophages, and lymphocytes.The arthropod vector of *E. canis* is the brown dog tick, *Rhipicephalus sanguineous.* Following an incubation period of 8 to 20 days, *E. canis* induces acute disease in which organisms infect monocytes and then spread throughout the mononuclear phagocyte system. This is followed by endothelial invasion, which results in vasculitis. The disease then enters a subclinical phase, from which dogs may either recover or go on to develop pancytopenic bone marrow failure. In transmission studies using blood from *E. canis*–infected dogs, some dogs developed and then spontaneously overcame subclinical infections.

Clinical findings during the acute phase of canine ehrlichiosis are nonspecific and include fever, ocular and nasal discharges, anorexia, and lymph node enlargement. The subclinical phase lasts from 40 to 120 days and is characterized by signs of multisystemic disease including the musculoskeletal, ocular, and nervous systems. Ehrlichiosis in German shepherd dogs causes a severe hemorrhagic disorder. This unique susceptibility has been attributed to depressed cell-mediated immunity to *E. canis* in this breed.

Laboratory findings in the acute phase of canine ehrlichisosis include consistent thrombocytopenia with large platelets and nonregenerative anemia. *Babesia canis* infection may be present concurrently and can result in regenerative anemia. Morulae of *Ehrlichia* species may be visible in the acute phase of the disease in neutrophils, lymphocytes, and monocytes (Fig. 7-21). Examination of buffy coat smears is helpful for finding the organism. In some dogs, lymphocytosis develops as the disease progresses. Pancytopenia develops in the chronic phases of the disease, and bone marrow examination reveals depletion of erythrocytic, granulocytic, and megakaryocytic cells (but persistence of plasma cells). Other significant laboratory findings include hypergammaglobulinemia and hypoalbuminemia. Serum concentrations of liver enzymes may be elevated in the acute phase of the disease.

Serologic diagnosis of ehrlichiosis is based on the indirect fluorescent antibody test. Antigenic cross-reactivity occurs between some *Ehrlichia* species; Western immunoblotting and PCR are specific.

Necropsy findings vary with the stage of the disease. In the acute disease there are widespread petechiae and ecchymoses, with splenomegaly and lymphadenomegaly. Chronically infected dogs are emaciated. The bone marrow is hyperplastic and red in the acute disease but becomes hypoplastic and pale in the chronic disease. Histologic findings include generalized perivascular plasma cell infiltration, which is most pronounced in the chronic disease. Multifocal, nonsuppurative meningoencephalitis, interstitial pneumonia, and glomerulonephritis are present in most dogs. *Ehrlichia* organisms are difficult to detect histologically; examination of Wright-Giemsa–stained impression smears of lung, liver, lymph nodes, and spleen is a more effective method for detecting the morulae of *Ehrlichia* in macrophages.

E. equi infection produces a disease in horses similar to the canine disease, but mortality is low. Equine ehrlichiosis is characterized by fever, anorexia, depression, edema of the legs, and ataxia. Laboratory findings include a mild anemia, leukopenia, and thrombocytopenia. Morulae of the organisms may be visible in the cytoplasm of neutrophils and eosinophils. Necropsy findings include petechiae and ecchymoses and icterus of the subcutaneous tissues and fascia.

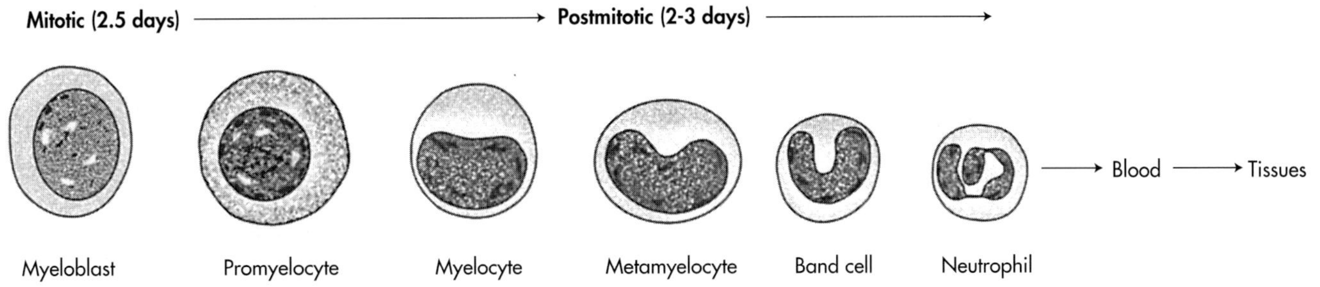

Figure 7-23 Development of the neutrophil. *Modified from Bainton DF, Ullyot JL, Farquhar MG.* The development of neutrophilic polymorphonuclear leukocytes in human bone marrow. *J Exp Med 1971; 134:907.*

Stress leukogram
· neutrophilia
· monocytosis
· lymphopenia
· eosinopenia

Bracken fern poisoning. Bracken fern poisoning is a pancytopenic disease of cattle and horses that follows several weeks of ingestion of the green plant or hay containing the fern. In both species, it causes hemopoietic stem cell injury; in horses, however, the thiaminase in the plant causes nervous system dysfunction before significant changes in the hemopoietic system. In cattle, hemorrhage is the main sign of disease. There is low morbidity and high mortality. Laboratory findings include leukopenia and thrombocytopenia. The severity of the anemia reflects the duration of toxic inhibition of stem cells, and the amount of hemorrhage is the consequence of thrombocytopenia. Postmortem findings are dominated by numerous hemorrhages in all tissues. Because animals are leukopenic, bacterial emboli frequently occur, and these cause renal infarcts (Fig. 7-22). Bone marrow is obviously nonreactive (appearing pink and watery) and is hypocellular.

Myeloproliferative Disorders. Myeloproliferative disorders are bone marrow diseases in which disturbance of one hemopoietic cell type interferes with differentiation of that cell line as well as other hemopoietic cells arising from the same stem cell. An erythrocytic sarcoma, for example, invariably results in anemia and may cause leukopenia and thrombocytopenia. In the same manner, granulocytic and plasma cell sarcomas also interfere with erythropoiesis. The myeloproliferative disorders are discussed in more detail later in this chapter.

LEUKOCYTE DISORDERS

Leukocyte Counts

The total and differential leukocyte counts should be an integral part of clinical evaluations. Correlation of these data with clinical findings can confirm or exclude diseases characterized by significant inflammation, necrosis, or both. Knowledge of neutrophil kinetics in health and disease allows assessment of the duration and severity of inflammatory processes. Animals that are ill and under stress, or receiving glucocorticoid drugs, have characteristic changes in the leukocyte profile; these include neutrophilia, eosinopenia, and lymphopenia. In the dog, there is also a monocytosis. Reversal of these changes implies recovery from the stressful state and a favorable prognosis. Examination of blood monocytes provides insight into the activity of the mononuclear phagocyte system; these cells play a vital role in chronic inflammation and hemolytic anemias.

Neutrophils

Because of their significance in defense against infections, evaluation of numbers and age of neutrophils is particularly valuable in disease assessment. To interpret changes in these parameters, one must be cognizant of species variations in neutrophil kinetics in health and disease. Neutrophils or neutrophilic granulocytes are produced in the bone marrow, and it is useful conceptually to consider granulopoiesis as occurring in compartments or pools—the mitotic and postmitotic maturation and storage pools (Fig. 7-23). In the circulating compartment, neutrophils may marginate along vascular endothelium or be free in the blood. In the dog, horse, and calf the two pools are of equal size; in cats, the marginated pool is larger than the circulating pool. The size of the circulating pool (i.e., total neutrophil numbers) is a reflection of the rates at which cells enter the blood from the bone marrow and leave the blood to enter the tissues. Blood therefore serves as a vehicle to transport neutrophils, with a transit time of approximately 10 hours. Following migration into tissues, neutrophils do not reenter capillaries. There is continual removal of neutrophils from the blood as they migrate across mucus membranes, particularly the alimentary tract and into other tissues.

Table 7-2 Leukocyte Responses in Benign Diseases

Species	Normal Neutrophil/ Lymphocyte Ratio	Maximum Expected Leukocytosis × 10^9/L
Dog	2.4	120
Cat	1.5	75
Foal	1.4	70
Horse	1.2	60
Pig	0.7	35
Goat	0.6	30
Sheep	0.5	25
Calf	1.0	50
Cow	0.5	25

From Valli VEO. The hemopoietic system. In: Jubb KVF, Kennedy PC, Palmer N, eds. Pathology of Domestic Animals. Vol. 3, 4th ed. San Diego, Calif.: Academic Press, 1993:113.

Table 7-3 A Species Comparison of Granulocyte Kinetics in Mastitis

Hemogram	Cow	Bitch
WBC × 10^9/L	3.18	23.90
Neutrophil × 10^9/L	0.50	18.50
Band neutrophils × 10^9/L	0.78	4.80
Metamyelocytes × 10^9/L	0.35	0.00
Lymphocytes × 10^9/L	1.50	0.60

WBC, white blood cells.

The ability of animals to respond to increased tissue demand for neutrophils varies according to the species and can be predicted from the numbers of circulating neutrophils or the neutrophil/lymphocyte ratio (Table 7-2). Animals with greater numbers of circulating neutrophils in health are able to produce and deliver the most neutrophils to tissues. Animals respond to a greater tissue demand for neutrophils by releasing mature cells from the bone marrow postmitotic maturation and storage pool, followed, if necessary, by the premature release of immature cells to the circulating pool. At the same time, humoral mediators including granulocyte macrophage–colony stimulating factor (GM-CSF) and IL-3 stimulate differentiation of pluripotent stem cells into the committed neutrophil mitotic pool (Fig. 7-1). Therefore, the degree of neutrophilia or neutropenia, as well as the numbers of band and metamyelocyte neutrophils in a given species, provides insight into the duration and severity of an inflammatory process. Reference to Table 7-2 allows one to predict that the greatest neutrophilia, without release of band neutrophils in response to inflammation, would occur in the dog; whereas a lesser neutrophilia, with increased need for band neutrophils, would occur in the cow.

In very severe inflammations, sequestration of the entire circulating neutrophil pool and most of the marrow postmitotic maturation and storage pool into the site of inflammation may occur, and circulating band and metamyelocyte neutrophil numbers approximate or exceed mature neutrophils. This is a more common occurrence in the cow and horse than in the dog and cat. From another perspective, these changes occur with less severe inflammatory processes in the cow and horse than in the cat and dog. In Table 7-3, leukocyte profiles of a cow and a bitch, each with severe mastitis of short duration, illustrate that depletion of the marrow neutrophil storage pool is greatest in the cow.

The rate of restoration of the marrow neutrophil postmitotic maturation and storage pool and the blood neutrophil pool is determined by the severity of the inflammatory process and the rate and degree to which it is contained. If the infection is rapidly contained, neutrophil numbers return to normal and band neutrophils disappear. However, if the infection is not contained, stem cells are committed to continue production of neutrophils. Bone marrow hypertrophy occurs until more neutrophils are released than are required, resulting in neutrophilia. These inflammatory processes can then be considered as moderately severe and of long duration.

One could predict that greater neutrophilia would occur in carnivores than in herbivores, with severe to moderately severe inflammatory processes of long duration. A dog with severe inflammation of some duration may have a leukocyte count of 80 to 100×10^9/L (80 to $100 \times 10^3/mm^3$) with neutrophilia, minimal numbers of band neutrophils, and monocytosis. Neutrophil production in such an animal has reached a new steady state, in which neutrophil production per kilogram of body weight per hour is several times greater than normal. In cattle, a total leukocyte count greater than 30×10^9/L ($30 \times 10^3/mm^3$) because of neutrophilia is unusual. Calves and foals less than 3 to 5 months of age can mount a greater neutrophilia than adults.

A good illustration of neutrophil kinetics in disease is that of a bitch with endometritis, in which the initial leukocyte profile is compared with one 24 to 48 hours following hysterectomy (Table 7-4). Rapid neutrophil sequestration into the uterus leads to partial depletion of the marrow postmitotic maturation and storage pool; this is evident from the total leukocyte count and mature and band neutrophil numbers. The leukocyte profile following hysterectomy indicates output from the expanded neutrophil mitotic and postmitotic pools. The total leukocyte count is rapidly elevated because the tissue site of sequestration (the uterus) has been removed. The neutrophilia gradually subsides over a 2- to 3-week period. Neutrophilia with varying degrees of left shift (band neutrophil increase) occurs with bacterial and fungal infections, immune-mediated inflammation such as polyarthritis, tissue necrosis, and severe hemolysis.

Neutropenia result from depletion of the circulating and marrow postmitotic maturation and storage pools in

Table 7-4 Comparison of Leukocyte Profiles from a Bitch with Endometritis Before and 24 Hours After Hysterectomy

Hemogram	Before Hysterectomy	After Hysterectomy
WBC × 10^9/L	42.78	72.35
Neutrophils × 10^9/L	28.63	56.73
Band Neutrophils × 10^9/L	9.54	10.32
Lymphocytes × 10^9/L	0.96	1.20
Monocytes × 10^9/L	3.65	4.10

WBC, white blood cells.

animals with overwhelming infections. Although admittedly rare, immune-mediated neutropenias occur and should be considered in chronically neutropenic animals. Bone marrow aspirates may confirm phagocytosis of neutrophils by macrophages. Bone marrow disorders may result in neutropenia. In parvoviral infections of cats and dogs, neutropenia is due to sequestration of neutrophils into the gut subsequent to epithelial necrosis and impaired neutrophil production resulting from stem cell injury. Neutropenia also results from all the forms of stem cell injury. Neutropenia is a frequent manifestation of feline leukemia virus infections. In contrast to parvoviral neutropenia, feline leukemia viral neutropenia is of longer duration and can be cyclic. The feline immunodeficiency virus is also a significant cause of neutropenia. Aspirates and core biopsies of bone marrow should be examined in persistently neutropenic animals.

Neutrophil dysfunction has been documented in human beings with diabetes mellitus and uremia. As in human beings, impaired movement and phagocytic defects of neutrophils probably occur in animals with these disorders. Congenital leukocyte function disorders have been described in human beings, Irish setter dogs, and Holstein cattle. These are characterized by recurrent bacterial and fungal infections and persistent neutrophilia in the young. The neutrophils have a defect in the integrin CD11/CD18 that is responsible for adhesion of neutrophils to surfaces and also serves a receptor for complement C3b. Neutrophils with this defective integrin are unable to migrate across capillary walls into tissues. Recurrent bacterial and fungal infections have also been described in Doberman pinscher dogs in which neutrophils had normal phagocytic function but impaired bactericidal ability.

Eosinophils

Eosinophilopoiesis in the bone marrow resembles that of neutrophils; however, infiltration of tissues by eosinophils is somewhat independent of other leukocytes. Three cytokines, IL-3, IL-5, and GM-CSF are particularly important in regulating the production of eosinophils (Fig. 7-1). There is now good evidence that eosinophils are attracted to tissues as part of a T lymphocyte–mediated immune response to certain antigens, most notably allergens and those of helminths. T helper lymphocytes are involved in the production of IL-5, which stimulates the release of eosinophils from the marrow and up-regulates eosinophil membrane adhesion molecules, resulting in increased adhesion to endothelial cells at the site of inflammation. Once eosinophils arrive at a site of inflammation, they may undergo apoptosis and be rapidly phagocytosed by macrophages, but if they are stimulated by IL-3, IL-5, and GM-CSF, they survive for prolonged periods and also become responsive to other activating agents.

Eosinophils are predominately tissue cells, especially in those tissues with an epithelium exposed to the external environment, such as in the respiratory and gastrointestinal tracts. Consequently, it is possible to have marked bone marrow eosinophilopoiesis and tissue eosinophilia without significantly increased numbers of circulating eosinophils; their blood transit time is short.

Eosinophil granules have constituents similar to other granulocytes; however, their specific effector molecules are the most important. Major basic protein, the most abundant cationic eosinophil protein, is toxic to helminths, tumor cells, and host cells. Eosinophil peroxidase is toxic to helminths, protozoa, bacteria, tumor cells, and host cells, whereas eosinophilic cationic protein has bactericidal and helminthotoxic activities.

It is now apparent that eosinophils defend against large, nonphagocytosable organisms such as parasites. It would appear that eosinophil numbers in the blood vary depending on geographic locale; this may reflect variations in parasite burdens. Initial binding of eosinophils to helminths can be mediated by antiparasite IgG, IgE antibodies, or by C3b that have been deposited on the surfaces of parasites.

Another function of eosinophils on body surfaces is the modulation of inflammatory reactions involving mast cells, basophils, and IgE antibodies. Products of activated mast cells serve as chemoattractant molecules for eosinophils in the initial events following exposure to antigen, but their importance in promoting eosinophilia is uncertain. At sites of hypersensitivity inflammation, eosinophils neutralize histamine and are capable of inhibiting mast cell degranulation.

A number of syndromes occur in animals with marked tissue eosinophilia with or without concurrent blood eosinophilia. These include pulmonary eosinophilia and eosinophilic enteritis in dogs and cats, eosinophilic granulomatous inflammation of the alimentary tract and skin in horses, and a variety of neoplastic diseases. Although these may be responses to allergens, the mechanisms responsible for recruitment of eosinophils in many of these disorders are unclear.

Eosinopenia is a common occurrence in animals, usually in response to stress or the administration of glucocorticoid drugs, most likely due to inhibition of T lymphocyte subsets that modulate eosinophil movement and functions.

Basophils and Mast Cells

Similar to eosinophils, basophils and mast cells are specialized effector cells of the immune system. They share the membrane glycoprotein CD45 with other cells in the bone marrow, an indication that mast cells are derived from hemopoietic stem cells. Mast cells leave the bone marrow as undifferentiated cells to assume their unique structure and function after homing to tissue sites such as beneath epithelial surfaces. The mast cell–committed progenitor cell appears to be a nongranulated, mononuclear cell sharing certain properties with monocytic cells.

There is no clear understanding of basophil and mast cell functions in some inflammatory states. It is likely, however, that they have critical roles in the expression of host resistance to certain parasites and that this role may vary according to factors such as species of parasite, host, and site of inflammation. There is extensive evidence that basophils and mast cells and their mediators are primary effectors of allergic inflammation. Basophils and mast cells have IgE binding sites, and following formation of IgE-antigen complexes, activation of the cells results in secretion of their histamine, neutral proteases, and cytokines that are responsible for most of the early events that characterize allergic reactions of the respiratory tract, intestine, and skin. The growing evidence that IgE binding initiates synthesis and secretion of several cytokines by human basophils and mast cells supports the hypothesis that these cells play both proinflammatory and immunomodulatory roles in allergic disorders.

Basophilia is rare in animals but is occasionally seen concurrently with eosinophilia. This is to be expected because basophils and eosinophils share many immunophenotypic properties. Occasionally basophils and mast cells are seen with eosinophils in transtracheal washes of dogs and horses with intermittent or chronic bronchitis, presumably hypersensitivity disorders. The same is true in transtracheal washes from dogs containing *Oslerus osleri* larvae.

Monocytes and Macrophages

Monocytes are produced in bone marrow and then are transported in the blood to tissues and body cavities, where they rapidly differentiate into macrophages. In the bone marrow, monoblasts, promonocytes, and monocytes can be identified based on monoclonal antibodies recognizing cell surface glycoproteins (immunophenotyping), and by the staining of their lysosomal enzymes. Monocytes remain in the bone marrow approximately 24 hours before entering the peripheral blood. In humans beings, blood monocytes are distributed into circulating (approximately 40%) and marginated (approximately 60%) pools. In the normal steady state, the proportion of monocytes migrating to various organs corresponds approximately to the size of the organ.

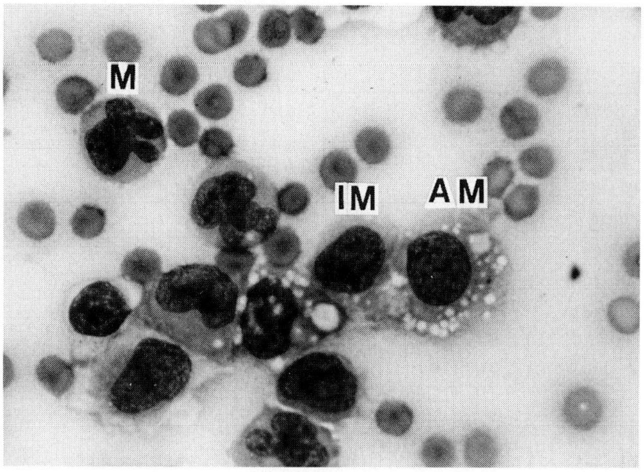

Figure 7-24 Aspirate from a subcutaneous hematoma in a dog. Note the transition from monocytes *(M)* to immature macrophages *(IM)* and activated macrophages *(AM)*. Wright-Giemsa stain.

Macrophages are derived from monocytes that undergo biochemical and immunophenotypic changes peculiar to the diverse purposes of the liver, spleen, bone marrow, lymph nodes, lungs, central nervous system, and other tissues containing components of the mononuclear phagocyte system. This diversity includes the highly phagocytic activity of Kupffer cells in the liver, in contrast to macrophages with purely secretory activity in support of the immune response or hemopoiesis. The morphologic transitions from monocytes to resting and activated macrophages may be evident in fine-needle aspirates of hematomas (Fig. 7-24). Tissue macrophage populations are constantly being renewed; the turnover time for Kupffer cells is approximately 5 to 6 days. The rate of monocyte migration to inflammatory sites has been shown to increase to compensate for increased requirement and turnover of macrophages.

Macrophages play a vital role in the immune response. They display foreign antigens on their surface in a form that can be recognized by antigen-specific T lymphocytes. T lymphocytes in turn can secrete cytokines that activate macrophages, which are then more efficient at phagocytosis and cytocidal functions. Macrophages and lymphocytes, therefore, are mutually interactive.

Bone marrow macrophages not only secrete growth factors vital to hemopoiesis, but no doubt exert local control over stem cells within the hemopoietic microenvironment. Macrophages are the central cells in erythroblastic islands, where by means of the cytoadhesive protein fibronectin, they nurture erythroid precursor cells. The erythroid cells migrate along macrophage membrane extensions until they reach a marrow sinusoid. The island macrophage also ingests nuclei extruded by metarubricytes as they enter sinusoids.

Monocytosis in hematograms of animals is indicative of an increased demand for macrophages in the tissues. This is especially evident in hemolytic anemias; blood smears from cats with severe *Hemobartonella felis* infections or dogs with immune-mediated hemolytic anemia frequently have numerous monocytes en route to the spleen. Monocytosis (2 to 8×10^9/L) (2 to 8×10^3/mm^3) may be present in established suppurative inflammatory states, such as pyometra in dogs and traumatic pericarditis in cattle. Monocytosis (1 to 3×10^9/L) (1 to 3×10^3/mm^3) occurs in dogs following administration of glucocorticoid drugs.

MYELOPROLIFERATIVE DISORDERS

The myeloproliferative disorders refer to neoplastic transformation of one or more of the descendants of the myeloid stem cell (Fig. 7-1). Myeloproliferative disorders may result in release of abnormal cells into the peripheral blood (leukemia), or they may cause pancytopenia because of the interference with hemopoiesis. Frequently there is a combination of abnormal hemopoiesis and leukemia. Neoplasia of one myeloid cell line will cause impaired differentiation within that population and may interfere with the differentiation and maturation of the other cell lines. Most discussions of myeloproliferative disorders exclude lymphoid neoplasms, although those that arise in bone marrow would be myeloproliferative disorders; lymphosarcomas and lymphocytic leukemias are considered in the discussion of lymph nodes. The abnormal B lymphocyte precursors of plasma cell sarcomas have unique properties that enable them to colonize the hemopoietic microenvironment and will be considered with the myeloproliferative disorders.

Knowledge of the mechanisms responsible for neoplastic transformation of hemopoietic pluripotential or unipotential cells has, in part, emerged from studies of the human myeloproliferative disorders. Leukemias arise when normal bone marrow cells acquire somatic mutations that confer a selective growth advantage on the mutated cells. The study of chromosomal abnormalities including translocations, inversions, deletions or duplications, and gain or loss of entire chromosomes in the leukemic cells, has identified regions of chromosomes that are susceptible to these abnormalities. The genes that occupy these regions are being cloned and studied to determine the mechanisms responsible for pathogenesis of the leukemia. Leukemic cell proliferation may be driven by cytokines such as IL-1 and tumor necrosis factor. The tumor cells may produce their own growth factors or induce production of growth factors by neighboring cells. The leukemias have been classified as acute or chronic based on clinical course and degree of differentiation of the neoplastic cells. The acute myeloid leukemias, because of poorly differentiated cells in the blood and bone marrow, are difficult to classify and to differentiate from lymphocytic leukemias. To this end, the French-American-British (FAB) classification of the human leukemias, based on light and electron microscopy, cytochemistry, and immunophenotyping of the cells, has been applied to the animal leukemias.

In human beings, the stimulus for accurate identification of these cells has been to develop treatment protocols that are most efficacious for the particular type of leukemia. The clinical relevance of applying the FAB classification to the leukemias in animals is unknown, in part because of the rarity of acute myeloid tumors in animals in comparison with human beings. An additional problem is the difficulty in achieving conformity among pathologists with respect to identification of blast cells and identification of cell lineages in the bone marrow. Counting 1000 nucleated cells in bone marrow may be necessary in some animals.

Occasionally many of the cells are insufficiently differentiated and do not contain the enzymes used for cytochemical classification, or they are genetically altered and fail to express certain enzymes or membrane glycoproteins; these are classified as undifferentiated sarcomas. Myeloid leukemias occur in most domestic animals but at a much lower incidence than the lymphoid leukemias. Although the terms myeloid and myelogenous refer to all hemopoietic cells exclusive of lymphocytes (Fig. 7-1), when discussing the leukemias, their use is restricted to neutrophil precursors.

Acute Leukemias

Acute Myelogenous Leukemia

Acute myelogenous leukemia (M1 and M2) is identified by stains that react with cytoplasmic enzymes. In the FAB classification, they are subclassified into acute myeloblastic leukemias without maturation (M1) and with maturation (M2). The latter have a greater number of cells with a few cytoplasmic granules typical of immature promyelocytes. Affected dogs and cats are usually in good condition with recent onset of anorexia, depression, or weight loss; some may have evidence of bleeding such as epistaxis. Hematologic findings may include nonregenerative anemia, thrombocytopenia, and neutropenia. Frequently there are variable numbers of cells in the blood that are difficult to differentiate from lymphoblasts. There may be morphologic features that indicate a lineage, but special stains are necessary (Table 7-5) for accurate identification.

Bone marrow aspirates are dominated by one population of cells that is usually less differentiated than those in the blood. As expected, the cells are mostly blast cells, which have staining characteristics consistent with granulocyte precursor cells; by careful study, they may be subclassified as M1 or M2. Numerous cells are in mitosis.

Table 7-5 Cytochemistry for Acute Myeloid Leukemias

Reaction	Normal Cells Manifesting Reaction	Diagnostic Utility
Myeloperoxidase	Neutrophil series Eosinophils (cyanide resistant) Basophils ± Monocytes ±	Myeloblastic leukemia without maturation—1 Myeloblastic leukemia with maturation—2
Sudan black B	Neutrophil series Monocytes ±	M1, M2
Chloracetate esterase	Neutrophil series Monocytes ±	M1, M2
Nonspecific esterase (α-napthyl acetate substrate or α-napthyl butyrate)	Monocytes (inhibited by sodium fluoride)	Monocyte leukemias Monocytic leukemia, differentiated—M5 Monocytic leukemia, poorly differentiated—M5 (acute monoblastic) Myelomonocytic leukemia—??
Periodic acid–Schiff		Erythroleukemia—M6 Acute lymphatic leukemias

Used with permission of R. D. Brunning, MD, Department of Pathology, University of Minnesota.

At necropsy, tissue pallor and petechiae are seen if the animals are thrombocytopenic. The spleen may be uniformly enlarged. The fat in the medullary cavities of long bones is replaced by yellowish white to red, firm tissue. Histologically, the spleen and bone marrow are filled by large, round cells, which require cytologic examination and cytochemical staining to identify them and differentiate them from lymphoblasts.

Promyelocytic Leukemia

Promyelocytic leukemia (M3) is also a rare neoplasm of dogs and cats. It shares clinical, hematologic, and necropsy findings with the acute myeloblastic leukemias. The cells are granulated and therefore classified as promyelocytes. A complicating feature in the human promyelocytic leukemias, which most likely occurs in animals, is the release of procoagulant proteins that may initiate intravascular coagulation, fibrinolysis, and thrombosis.

Myelomonocytic Leukemia

Myelomonocytic leukemia (M4) is a concurrent leukemia of neutrophil and monocyte precursors. Detailed morphologic study and cytochemical staining of cells in the blood and bone marrow are required to identify at least 20% involvement by both cell lines. These are rare neoplasms of dogs, cats, and horses and have similar clinical and necropsy findings with the other acute myeloid leukemias (Fig. 7-25).

Monocytic Leukemia

Monocytic leukemia (M5) occurs infrequently in dogs, cats, horses, and cattle. Affected animals have recent weight loss, anorexia, and depression. Hematologic findings include nonregenerative anemia with variable concurrence of neutropenia, neutrophilia, and thrombocytopenia. There are usually atypical cells in the blood, and some have nuclear shapes suggestive of that of monocytes (Fig. 7-26); cytochemical staining is necessary to confirm their lineage (Table 7-5). Bone marrow aspirates also have large numbers of these atypical cells as well as blast cells. The other cell lines committed to hemopoiesis are depleted. Necropsy findings are similar to the other leukemias; however, there may be more extensive involvement of other organs including the spleen, liver, lungs, lymph nodes, and kidneys. Nodules may be visible protruding from the surface and throughout the parenchyma of the liver and lung. Microscopically, the masses

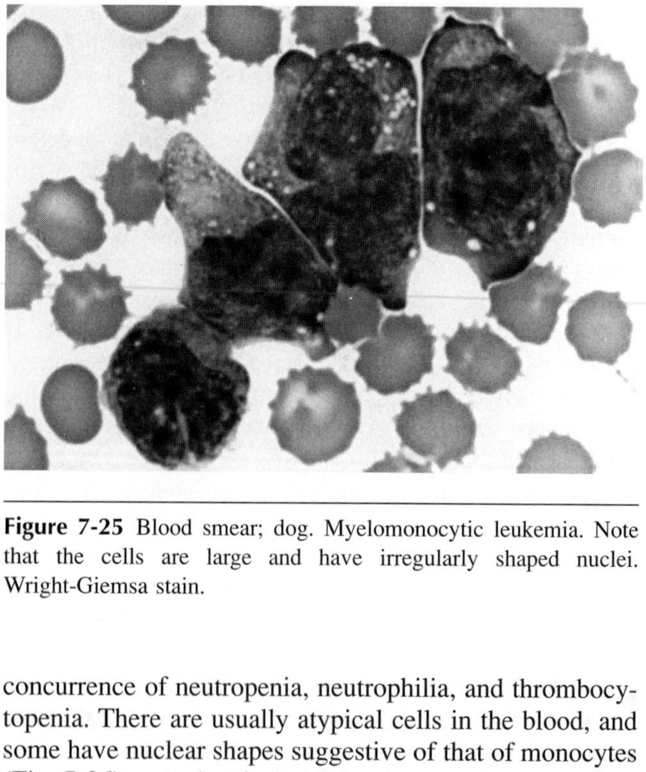

Figure 7-25 Blood smear; dog. Myelomonocytic leukemia. Note that the cells are large and have irregularly shaped nuclei. Wright-Giemsa stain.

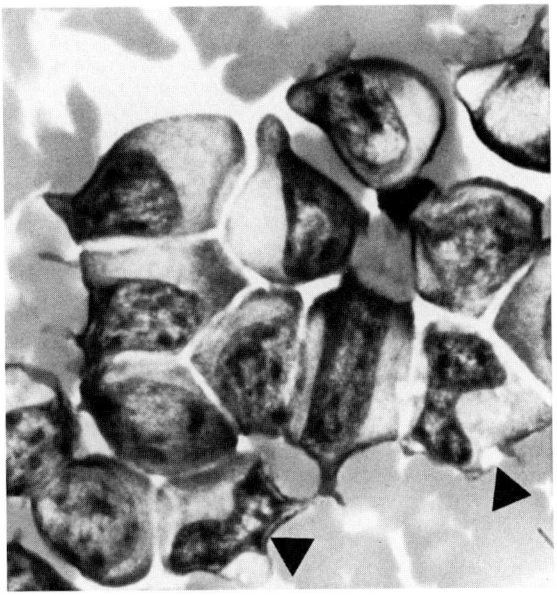

Figure 7-26 Blood smear; horse. Monocytic leukemia. Note the group of large cells with variable nucleus/cytoplasm ratios; two cells resemble monocytes *(arrowheads)*. Wright-Giemsa stain. *Courtesy of C.E. Monteith.*

consist of numerous large, round cells with large nuclei similar to those in the blood and bone marrow.

Malignant Histiocytosis

Malignant histiocytosis is a disease of dogs and cats characterized by neoplastic proliferation of macrophages in many organs including the skin (see Chapter 11). Dogs with malignant histiocytosis may have anorexia, weight loss, lethargy, and anemia. Generalized lymph node enlargement is common. Persistent regenerative hemolytic anemia with or without thrombocytopenia may mimic the immune-mediated cytopenias; however, there is no agglutination and the direct antiglobulin test is negative. Hyperferritinemia has been reported in human beings and a dog with malignant histiocytosis; the neoplastic histiocytes are presumed to synthesize and secrete ferritin.

Lymph node aspirates have a dominant population of large cells, which may have irregular nuclei and vacuolated cytoplasm; erythrophagocytosis may have occurred. Bone marrow aspirates have orderly erythropoiesis and granulopoiesis with lowered granulocyte/erythrocyte ratios similar to those in erythroid hyperplasia in anemic animals. Variable numbers of large cells resembling those in lymph node aspirates are present, and some contain phagocytosed erythrocytes or hemosiderin. The cells stain with α-napthyl acetate esterase, which is characteristic of cells of monocyte-macrophage lineage. At necropsy, there may be widespread hemorrhages in thrombocytopenic dogs. Lymph nodes are enlarged and firm, and there is frequently splenomegaly and hepatomegaly. Numerous

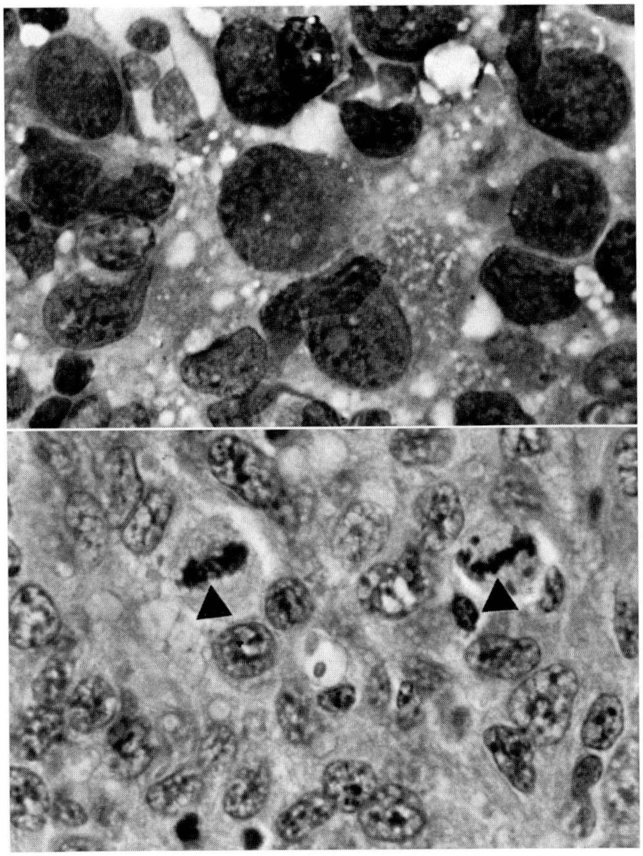

Figure 7-27 **A,** Impression smear of the spleen; dog. Malignant histiocytosis. Wright-Giemsa stain. **B,** Spleen; dog. Malignant histiocytosis. Note the mitotic figures *(arrowheads)*. H & E stain.

round to spindle-shaped cells and abundant erythrophagia are found on microscopic examination of the lymph nodes, liver, and splenic red pulp (Fig. 7-27).

A histiocytic proliferative disease occurring in Burnese mountain dogs is characterized by infiltration of the skin and lymph nodes by histiocytes. The disease can be rapidly progressive in some dogs in which there are nodular masses in the lungs, liver, lymph nodes, and spleen. The masses contain large pleomorphic cells and giant cells. Phagocytosis of erythrocytes and neutrophils is consistent with cells of macrophage lineage. Analysis of pedigrees of affected Bernese mountain dogs has provided strong evidence for inheritance of this disease.

Erythrocytic Sarcoma

Erythrocytic sarcoma (M6) (erythremic myelosis) in cats is characterized by lethargy, pallor, and a variety of hematologic abnormalities including a severe, nonregenerative anemia with hematocrits as low as 0.06 L/L (6%). The MCV is frequently high, but polychromatophilic erythrocytes and reticulocytes are absent or present in low numbers for an anemia of this magnitude. Blood films

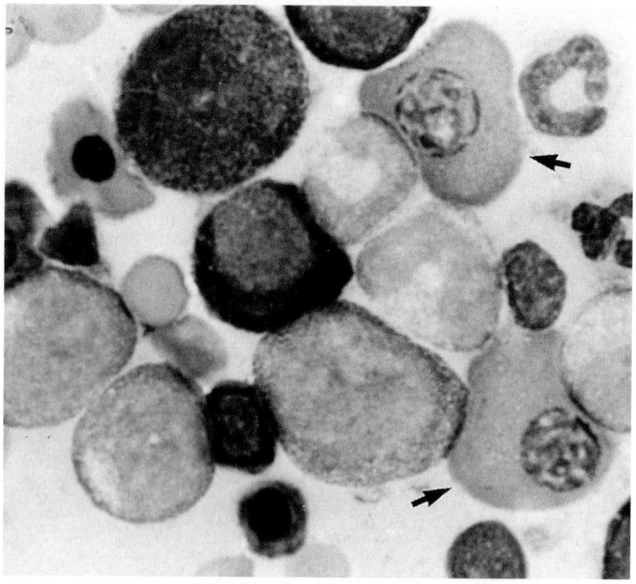

Figure 7-28 Bone marrow; cat. Erythrocytic sarcoma. Asynchronous nuclear-cytoplasmic maturation in erythrocytic precursors. Note the large coarse nuclei in cells with a full complement of hemoglobin *(arrows)*. Wright-Giemsa stain.

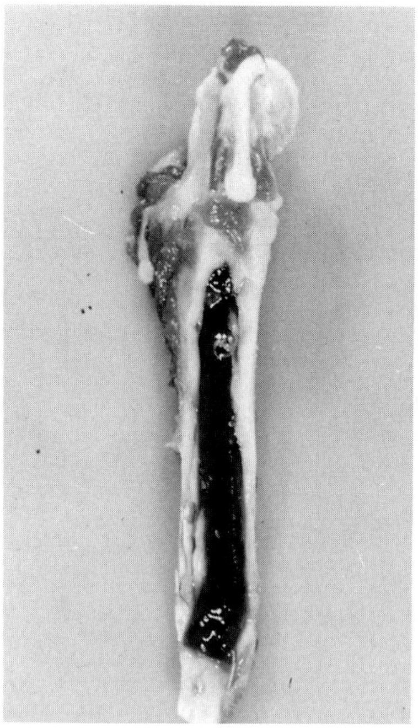

Figure 7-29 Femur; cat. Erythrocytic sarcoma. The bone marrow cavity is completely occupied by firm tissue.

often contain erythrocyte precursors in various stage of differentiation. Metarubricytes without polychromasia may be present in the peripheral blood, indicating an arrest at a late stage of erythrogenesis. Peripheral blood of other cats may contain only an occasional large atypical cell that is difficult to classify. Asynchronous development of the nucleus and cytoplasm of erythrocyte precursors is often evident in blood and marrow smears of cats with erythrocytic sarcomas. This is a poorly understood manifestation of impaired nuclear division and maturation (simulating that seen in cobalamin and folic acid deficiency). It results in asynchronous cell development, evident as an immature nucleus in hemoglobinated (i.e., mature) cytoplasm (Fig. 7-28). This defect in nuclear division results in large erythrocytes that electronic cell counters record as a high MCV. Bone marrow from cats with erythrocytic sarcomas contains a preponderance of erythrocytic precursor cells. Nuclear-cytoplasmic asynchrony is most evident in nucleated erythrocytes containing hemoglobin.

In addition to watery blood at necropsy, there are striking abnormalities in bone marrow cavities. In a sagittally cut femur, the medullary cavity is partially to completely filled by firm, red tissue. When interpreting these changes in bone marrow at necropsy, reference to the hematologic findings of nonregenerative anemia will help to differentiate hyperplasia from neoplasia. Impression smears should be made for cytologic evaluation and samples placed in 10% neutral buffered formalin for histologic evaluation (Fig. 7-29). Splenomegaly and hepatomegaly may also be present, most often in cats with many circulating neoplastic cells.

Megakaryoblastic Leukemia

Megakaryoblastic leukemia (M7) is a rare disease of dogs and cats. There is usually a rapid clinical course with variable degrees of pancytopenia. Bone marrow aspirates are highly cellular with large numbers of blast cells and pleomorphic megakaryocytes in various stages of differentiation. In most reports, animals have low to normal numbers of platelets. This indicates that platelet synthesis by neoplastic megakaryocytes is impaired. Numerous cells are in mitosis. At necropsy, there is tissue pallor, lymph node enlargement, and splenomegaly. Impression smears for cytology and histologic sections of lymph nodes, spleen, and liver have infiltrates of cells similar to those observed in the bone marrow. Immunohistochemical staining for von Willebrand factor and platelet integrin beta 3 (GPIIIa) confirm that a portion of the blast cells are megakaryocytes and that most are pleomorphic megakaryocytes. Some blast cells may not produce these proteins.

Plasma Cell Sarcoma

Plasma cell sarcoma is not common but does occur in dogs and cats. There are two basic disease mechanisms in animals with plasma cell sarcomas; one is caused by neoplastic cell proliferation, the other is the result of protein released from the neoplastic plasma cells. Although plasma cell neoplasms have been described in other tissues, most reside in the bone marrow where they interfere with hemopoiesis and erode endosteal bone by focal osteolysis. Although the lymph nodes and the lamina propria of the gut are the richest sources of normal plasma cells, they are not the sites where plasma cell sarcomas occur. The bone marrow microenvironment possesses distinct mechanisms for capturing genetically abnormal pre–B lymphocytes via stromal adhesive proteins and nurturing their differentiation into a population of plasma cells no longer capable of division or travel. Cytokines produced by the neoplastic plasma cells and others produced by bone marrow stromal cells favor preferential proliferation of the neoplastic clone. IL-6, produced by bone marrow stromal cells, is particularly important in the recruitment of abnormal pre-B lymphocytes and coordination of the cytokines responsible for their maturation. IL-6 also promotes longevity of the tumor cells by delaying apoptosis. IL-6 normally plays a central role in coordinating the cytokines responsible for osteoclastic activity and in this disease promotes localized bone resorption to accommodate the expanding tumor.

Most plasma cell sarcomas secrete protein. Because the neoplastic cells arise from transformation of one cell, the protein molecules are similar and represent partial to complete immunoglobulin molecules of one class. Serum electrophoretograms have a large, narrow-based peak in the **β-γ** region (monoclonal gammopathies), in contrast to the large broad-based globulin peaks in animals with chronic infections (polyclonal gammopathies) (Fig. 7-30). Occasionally dogs with chronic infections such as ehrlichiosis and blastomycosis have monoclonal gammopathies. Hyperviscosity of the plasma is a reflection of the quantity and structural properties of the protein and therefore is more severe if cells are producing IgM molecules rather than IgG or IgA molecules. Plasma viscosity can be simply assessed by comparing the rate at which the patient's plasma and normal plasma at 37° C drain from warmed (37° C) pipettes. In dogs, plasma hyperviscosity causes retinal hemorrhages, glomerular disease, and depression.

Epistaxis and melena have been observed in dogs with plasma cell sarcoma. Bleeding is presumed to be caused by effects of the abnormal protein on platelets and coagulation proteins. When hyperviscosity is severe, bleeding can result from distention and rupture of small vessels coupled with impaired primary and secondary hemostasis.

In dogs, renal disease is caused by the effects of hyperproteinemia on glomeruli and deposition of protein in tubules. The precise effects on the kidney depend on the molecular weight of the proteins involved and, hence, their filterability. Neoplastic plasma cells frequently fail to

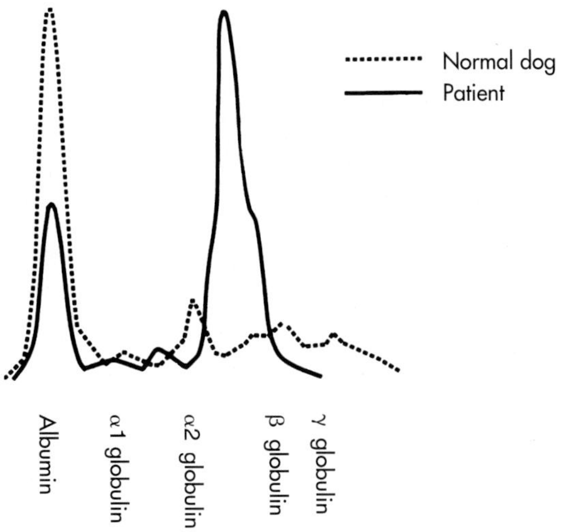

Figure 7-30 Serum electrophoretogram; dog. Plasma cell sarcoma. Note the spikelike pattern of the protein secreted by the neoplastic cells.

assemble normal combinations of light and heavy chain molecules, resulting in release into the circulation of light chains or low-molecular-weight proteins that appear in the urine. Quantitation of the urinary proteins may be achieved by heat precipitation or more sensitive immunoprecipitation assays.

Animals with plasma cell sarcomas have mild to moderate nonregenerative anemia, or pancytopenia if the marrow is severely involved. Extensive erythrocytic rouleaux formation and a diffuse, intercellular, proteinaceous precipitate are evident in blood films when protein content is in excess of 115 g/L (11.5 g/dl). Marrow and splenic aspirates may have increased numbers of plasma cells in varying stages of differentiation. In some cases, differentiation of neoplasia from prolonged antigenic stimulation of the immune system is difficult, and all laboratory and clinical findings must be taken into consideration. If the cells have abnormal morphology (for example, binucleate cells), and there is interference with hemopoiesis, or focal osteolysis, a diagnosis of neoplasia should be made.

At necropsy, plasma cell sarcomas appear as soft, gelatinous, pink to red masses in bone marrow spaces including those of the vertebrae; neoplasms may have eroded bone and extended into the surrounding soft tissue. Microscopically, the tumors are composed of sheets of atypical to well-differentiated plasma cells (Fig. 7-31).

Chronic Leukemias

The chronic leukemias are characterized by a long clinical course with large numbers of circulating cells that are more differentiated than those in the acute leukemias.

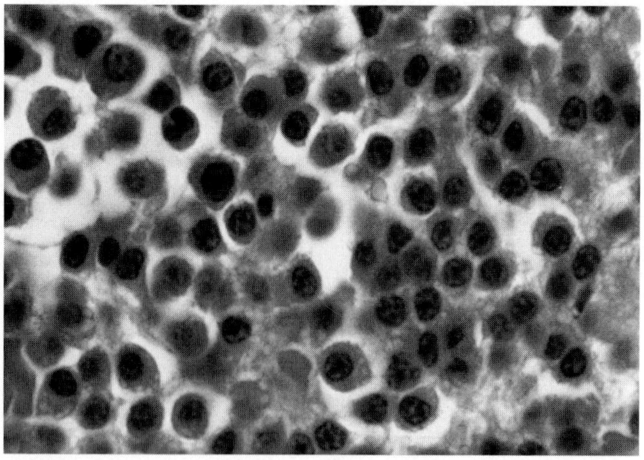

Figure 7-31 Bone marrow; dog. Plasma cell sarcoma. Note that the hemopoietic cells have been completely replaced by plasma cells. H & E stain.

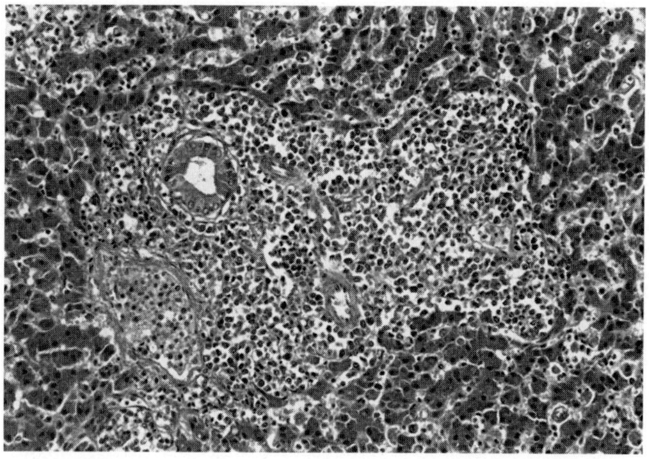

Figure 7-32 Liver; dog. Chronic granulocytic leukemia. Note the accumulation of neoplastic cells in the portal area. H & E stain.

Chronic Granulocytic Leukemia

Chronic granulocytic leukemia is rare in animals, but occurs in cats infected with feline leukemia virus, and dogs and horses. Dogs are debilitated and the spleen may be so enlarged that it is detectable by palpation. There is a nonregenerative anemia, marked leukocytosis, and a variable incidence of thrombocytopenia. Leukocyte counts vary from 50×10^9/L (50×10^3/mm^3) to as high as 200×10^9/L (200×10^3/mm^3). Neutrophilic leukemias are most common; however, eosinophilic leukemias have been reported in cats infected with the feline leukemia virus. Basophilic leukemias are rare. Giant neutrophils and band neutrophils with impaired segmentation may be present. Myelocytes, promyelocytes, and myeloblasts are usually identified by thorough smear examination. Bone marrow aspirates and core biopsies are highly cellular with very high granulocyte/erythrocyte ratios. Megakaryocyte numbers become reduced late in the course of the disease.

At necropsy, these animals are usually emaciated. Dogs have marked splenomegaly and lymph nodes are frequently enlarged. The bone marrow cavities are completely filled with red tissue. Histologically, granulocytes have infiltrated into the spleen, liver, and lymph nodes. The differentiation of neutrophilic leukemia from a chronic inflammatory response (leukemoid reaction) may be difficult. Extravascular accumulations of cells in the liver, kidney, and other organs, a disproportionate number of immature granulocytes in the peripheral blood, and thrombocytopenia support a diagnosis of chronic granulocytic leukemia (Fig. 7-32).

Chronic Megakaryocytic Sarcoma

Chronic megakaryocytic sarcoma is rare but may occur in cats infected with the feline leukemia virus. Platelet counts are high and may exceed 2000×10^9/L (2000×10^3/mm^3) with marked variation in platelet size and numbers of alpha granules. The marked thrombocytosis may cause thrombosis. A macrocytic nonregenerative anemia may be present. In bone marrow aspirates, there are numerous megakaryocytes in all stages of development and nuclear-cytoplasmic asynchrony of erythrocytic precursors. At necropsy, these cats have generalized tissue pallor, splenomegaly, hepatomegaly, and bone marrow cavities occupied by solid red tissue. Microscopically, marked accumulations of megakaryocytes occur in the splenic red pulp, hepatic sinusoids, and lymph nodes (Fig. 7-33).

Mast Cell Leukemia

Mast cell leukemia is a rare disease of dogs, with a somewhat higher incidence in cats. Clinical signs resulting from excess production of histamine include vomition and diarrhea. Splenomegaly occurs in most cats with mast cell leukemia. Variable numbers of mast cells are found in blood smears, and buffy coat preparations should be examined. Gastric and duodenal ulceration are usually seen at necropsy. The spleen is consistently enlarged and firm, and there is often hepatomegaly. Large numbers of mast cells infiltrate the splenic red pulp, and occupy hepatic sinusoids and parenchyma, bone marrow, and kidneys (Fig. 7-34).

Myelodysplastic Syndromes

The myelodysplastic syndromes in human beings are characterized by peripheral blood cytopenias, ineffective hemopoiesis, and hypercellular marrow. A similar syndrome occurs with feline leukemia virus infection. Affected cats are anorectic, inappetent, and febrile. Hematologic findings include nonregenerative anemia and neutropenia. Thrombocytopenia is rare. In chronic feline cases, there may be cyclic neutropenia. Bone marrow

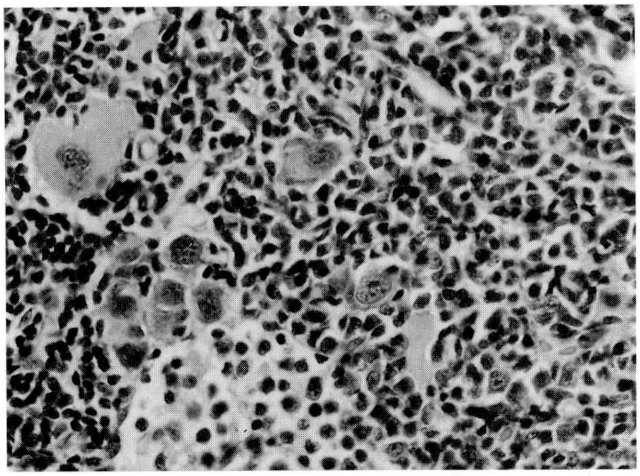

Figure 7-33 Lymph node; cat. Chronic megakaryocytic sarcoma. Note the accumulation of megakaryocytes in various stages of differentiation. H & E stain.

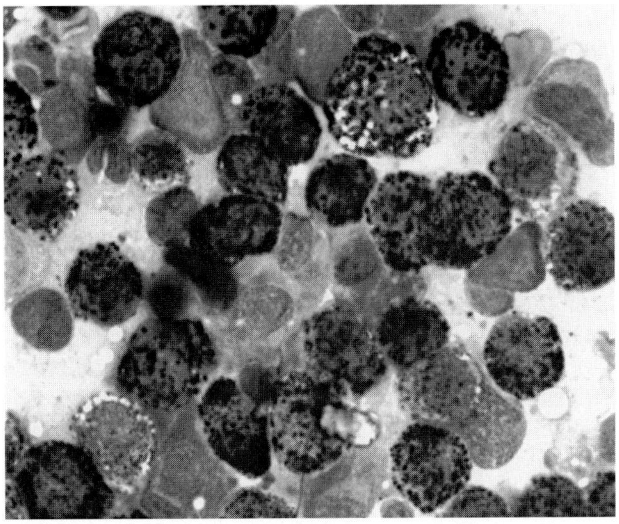

Figure 7-34 Bone marrow aspirate; dog. Mast cell sarcoma. Note the numerous mast cells with many cytoplasmic granules among hemopoietic cells.

aspirates are cellular in spite of depletion of the neutrophilic postmitotic maturation and storage pool; granulopoiesis is usually arrested at the myelocyte stage. In human beings, the myeloproliferative disorders frequently progress to myelogenous leukemia. Although marrow fibrosis has been reported in cats, most are euthanatized before the disease progresses to overt leukemia.

PLATELET DISORDERS

Structure and Function

Platelets are small, anucleate granular cells that adhere to subendothelial collagen in the walls of injured blood vessels in the initial phase of hemostasis. They may vary in size, especially in cats, but are approximately one third to one half the diameter of erythrocytes. Platelet release into the lumina of bone marrow sinusoids occurs by rapid fragmentation of mature megakaryocyte cytoplasm intimately associated with the sinusoidal wall. Some observers believe that an important portion of normal thrombocytopoiesis occurs by orderly fragmentation of megakaryocytes lodged in pulmonary alveolar capillaries. Platelets circulate for approximately 8 days. Equine platelets stain less prominently and may be difficult to see on blood films.

Although anuclear, platelets are metabolically active and have a cytoskeleton containing actin and myosin. They also have numerous granules, which after platelet activation, release their contents into a canalicular system that communicates with the external membrane. Bovine platelets are unique in having a poorly developed canalicular system; they secrete granular constituents directly onto the surface. Following endothelial injury, platelets arrest bleeding by adhering to exposed, subendothelial collagen. Adherence occurs when von Willebrand protein, anchored in the subendothelial matrix, binds to the platelet transmembrane glycoprotein Ib-IX integrin. Integrins are heterodimeric glycoproteins that link the intracellular skeletal proteins to extracellular adhesive proteins. Once adhered, the platelets are immediately activated and secrete granular constituents, causing nearby platelets to aggregate to the adhered platelets. Platelet activation results in expression of the $\alpha_{IIb}\beta_{III}$ integrin, which is then capable of binding large adhesive proteins such as fibrinogen and von Willebrand factor, which form bridges between adjacent platelets. The in vitro assessment of platelet aggregation is possible using specialized photometers (aggregometers). The platelet plug is then stabilized by fibrin. When platelet numbers are sufficiently reduced or platelet function is impaired, erythrocytes seep through capillary walls. Further consideration of the role of platelets in hemostasis is found in the Coagulation Disorders discussion.

Thrombocytosis

Platelet numbers fluctuate in the blood of animals and increase substantially in response to most hemopoietic stimuli. This may reflect the intimate apposition of megakaryocytes to sinusoidal walls in the bone marrow. Normal reference values for platelets in animals vary, ranging from 100 to 600×10^9/L (100 to $600 \times 10^3/mm^3$) in the horse to 200 to 900×10^9/L (200 to $900 \times 10^3/mm^3$) in the dog. Neutrophilia and anemia with reticulocytosis are usually accompanied by thrombocytosis. Thrombocytosis in which platelets exceed 1000×10^9/L ($100 \times 10^3/mm^3$) is rare but occasionally occurs in cats infected with feline leukemia virus, and thrombosis is a possible consequence.

Thrombocytopenia

Thrombocytopenia is an important disorder in animals. When electronic cell counters record low platelet numbers, it is important that this result be confirmed by blood film examination because tiny clots commonly occur in animal blood samples and may result in a spurious diagnosis of thrombocytopenia. Microscopic examination of a stained blood film should routinely include the feather edge, where platelet clumps are visible when tiny clots are present in the blood sample. The simplest method for an approximate estimate of platelet numbers on a blood film is as follows: each platelet identified in a 1000 magnification oil immersion objective field, containing a monolayer of erythrocytes, represents approximately 20×10^9 platelets per liter (20×10^3/mm^3).

Thrombocytopenia, similar to neutropenia or anemia, may be due to premature cellular destruction or impaired production. Platelet life span may be decreased because of consumption of platelets following their adhesion to injured vascular endothelium (e.g., in diseases such as infectious canine hepatitis and hog cholera). Platelet adhesion followed by platelet activation may initiate intravascular coagulation and further platelet consumption. Thrombocytopenia due to phagocytosis of antibody-coated platelets may occur alone, or it may accompany other immune-mediated diseases such as hemolytic anemia and systemic lupus erythematosus. The possible mechanisms resulting in antibody adherence to platelets are similar to those described for immune-mediated hemolytic anemias. An isoimmune thrombocytopenia occurs in neonatal piglets at 1 to 3 days following ingestion of colostrum. The syndrome is characterized by severe hemorrhage and high mortality.

A cyclic thrombocytopenia occurs in dogs as a result of infection of platelets by *Ehrlichia platys,* an organism presumably transmitted by ticks. Following experimental intravenous infection in dogs, there is an incubation period of 8 to 15 days. At that time, many platelets contain morulae of *E. platys,* resulting in a marked thrombocytopenia. Platelet numbers return to normal in 3 to 4 days after disappearance of the organism. Parasitemia and the resultant thrombocytopenia subsequently recur at 1- to 2-week intervals. Immunocytochemical staining can specifically identify *E. platys* in platelets, and *E. platys* antibodies are detected by an indirect serum fluorescent antibody test.

Thrombocytopenia as a result of failure of platelet production can occur in any bone marrow disorder. More detailed information is presented under Aplastic Pancytopenia and Myeloproliferative Disorders. Estrogen toxicity in dogs is frequently detected clinically by hemorrhages that are typical of thrombocytopenia. The same is true of bracken fern poisoning in cattle. The cardinal clinical signs of thrombocytopenia are petechiation, best observed on mucosae and ocular sclerae. The skin of dogs has petechial to diffuse hemorrhages. Mucosal bleeding at the free gingival margin and into the intestine is significant in canine thrombocytopenia and may not be observed by pet owners. Epistaxis is also common in thrombocytopenic animals, and hemorrhage can be severe following surgery or trauma.

Thrombocytopenic dogs with spontaneous bleeding have platelet numbers ranging from undetectable to approximately 50×10^9/L (50×10^3/mm^3). When the thrombocytopenia is the result of platelet destruction, increased numbers of megakaryocytes in various stages of development are present in the bone marrow. Young megakaryocytes are large, mononuclear or binuclear cells with a thin rim of deeply basophilic cytoplasm. In contrast, mature megakaryocytes are larger with multiple nuclei and abundant granular cytoplasm.

Unlike the erythrocyte direct antiglobulin test, tests for antiplatelet antibody have been difficult to develop. Because platelet alpha granules contain immunoglobulin, it is necessary to detect surface-bound immunoglobulin for evidence of immune-mediated platelet destruction. An ELISA assay has been used to detect platelet surface immunoglobulin in dogs with idiopathic thrombocytopenia. Some dogs had immunoglobulin bound to the $\alpha_{IIb}\beta_{III}$ integrin.

Platelet Function Disorders

Platelet function disorders are characterized by spontaneous occurrence of petechiae and mucosal bleeding, and life-threatening hemorrhage following surgery, despite normal platelet counts. These functional defects may be congenital or acquired, and result from impaired platelet secretion, adhesion, or aggregation. The ability of the platelets to adhere to subendothelial collagen in spite of a high shear rate from rapid blood flow in arterioles is mediated by the von Willebrand cytoadhesive protein. Congenital absence or decrease in this protein results in von Willebrand's disease (discussed below).

Platelet secretion, adhesion, aggregation, and prostaglandin metabolism are impaired in uremia, and are responsible for the mucosal hemorrhage that tends to occur in animals with renal failure. In human patients with uremia, mobilization of calcium from storage pools within platelets following platelet activation is reduced and may be the reason for the decreased function of membrane glycoproteins responsible for adhesion and aggregation. Platelet aggregation is impaired following the administration of aspirin and related compounds because of inhibited thromboxane synthesis from arachidonic acid. Bovine platelets synthesize little thromboxane, and platelet function is unaffected by the administration of aspirin. Inherited bleeding disorders with impaired in vitro platelet aggregation occur in human beings and animals. They result from abnormal structure or expression of the $\alpha_{IIb}\beta_{III}$ integrin following platelet activation. The structural abnormalities in the integrin in human patients range from complete absence of one or both molecules to a single point mutation in one molecule, which results in impaired binding of fibrinogen. The bleeding disorder in Great Pyrenees dogs is attributed to markedly reduced numbers of $\alpha_{IIb}\beta_{III}$ glycoproteins on platelets, whereas the impaired platelet aggregation that occurs in Simmental cattle is due to delayed expression of the receptor, which if given enough time, will bind fibrinogen following activation. A disorder of fibrinogen receptor activation may also be present in bleeding basset hound and spitz dogs.

Platelet aggregates are most likely unstable and disintegrate before stabilization of the platelet plug by fibrinogen. Delayed activation of the integrin may occur as the result of a mutation in the short cytoplasmic portion of one of the integrin molecules or a defect in intracellular signaling mechanisms. A bleeding Simmental calf was also found to have truncated von Willebrand protein, which would exacerbate the effects of inadequate platelet aggregation. A platelet aggregation defect responsible for hemorrhage in Japanese black cattle is due to a storage pool deficiency because affected animals lack platelet alpha granules. A similar disorder in bleeding American cocker spaniel dogs is characterized by an inadequate content of adenosine diphosphate (ADP) in platelets; ADP released following platelet activation is an important activating agent for nearby platelets, thus facilitating platelet aggregation.

COAGULATION DISORDERS

Coagulation Cascade

Platelet disorders cause seepage bleeding from mucosal surfaces, the result of inadequate initial plugging at sites of endothelial disruption. In disorders of coagulation the failure of fibrin synthesis within platelet aggregates results in inadequate stabilization of the platelet plug. Prolonged bleeding then occurs after temporary occlusion of the injured vessel wall by the unstable platelet plug.

The familiar cascading sequence of coagulation has undergone significant revision over the past decade. It is now apparent, for example, that platelet and endothelial cell surfaces provide a framework for assembly and interaction of coagulation proteins. Traditionally, the cascade hypothesis of coagulation has been subdivided into intrinsic and extrinsic pathways; these are now known to be highly interdependent. The general principle, that coagulation events are all directed toward the conversion of fibrinogen to fibrin, remains unchanged. Fibrinogen, an acute-phase reactant, is synthesized in hepatocytes, circulates in plasma, and is located in platelet and megakaryocyte alpha granules.

Certain coagulation proteins (prothrombin and factors VII, IX, and X) and proteins C and S (inhibitors of coagulation) are vitamin K dependent factors. To become functional, the vitamin K–dependent proteins must undergo carboxylation of selected glutamic acid residues. This reaction is catalyzed within hepatocytes by the vitamin K–dependent enzyme γ-glutamylcarboxylase. These carboxylated glutamic acid residues avidly bind calcium ions, which in turn maintain the precise shapes of the proteins, necessary for them to bind to phospholipids exposed on activated platelets. Following cleavage of a specific activation domain, vitamin K–dependent proteins become functional serine proteases and then assume a structure that exposes their catalytic domains.

Factors V and VIII are homologous cofactors for the vitamin K–dependent serine proteases. Both molecules are activated (designated Va and VIIIa) by thrombin. Factor VIIIa participates in assembling factor IX and calcium in close proximity to factor X on the platelet surface (Fig. 7-35). This facilitates factor IXa activation of factor X. Factor VIIIa is rendered inactive following further cleavage by thrombin or protein C. Factor V activation and inactivation mechanisms are similar to those of factor VIII. Factor Va serves to assemble factor Xa and calcium on platelets so as to facilitate the factor Xa–catalyzed conversion of prothrombin to thrombin (Fig. 7-35).

It is now evident that cell surfaces play a vital role in coagulation. Platelets have surface receptors for factors V, VIII, IX, and X, which become exposed following platelet activation by thrombin (Fig. 7-35). Platelet activation also causes exposure of phospholipids normally found on the internal aspect of the platelet membrane. A further event following platelet activation is the shedding of membrane particles from platelet surfaces, which most likely also serve as sites for assembly of coagulation proteins.

The traditional view of initiation of coagulation by activation of factor XII in the intrinsic pathway has been modified by recent research. It now appears that essentially all coagulation in vivo is initiated by the extrinsic pathway. A key component of extrinsic pathway activation is tissue factor, a transmembrane polypeptide that acts as a cell surface receptor for factor VII. It is found on cells surrounding blood vessels; it does not occur on endothelial cells or circulate in plasma. Therefore, binding of factor VII by tissue factor occurs whenever there is trauma to tissues. The extrinsic and intrinsic pathways are now known to be highly interdependent because the tissue factor–factor VII complex not only activates factor X but also factor IX (Fig. 7-35). Tissue factor pathway activity is controlled by a lipoprotein-associated coagulation inhibitor (LACI) also known as extrinsic pathway inhibitor (EPI).

Thrombin is the most important component in sustaining coagulation and is the chief activator of factor XI. Thrombin also activates factors V and VIII as well as factor XIII (Fig. 7-35). Factor XIII is responsible for the stabilization of fibrin.

Down-regulation of coagulation is vital to normal hemostasis and, like the initiation of coagulation, initially occurs on cell surfaces. Endothelial cells are most important because they express the transmembrane protein thrombomodulin, a receptor for thrombin. Thrombin

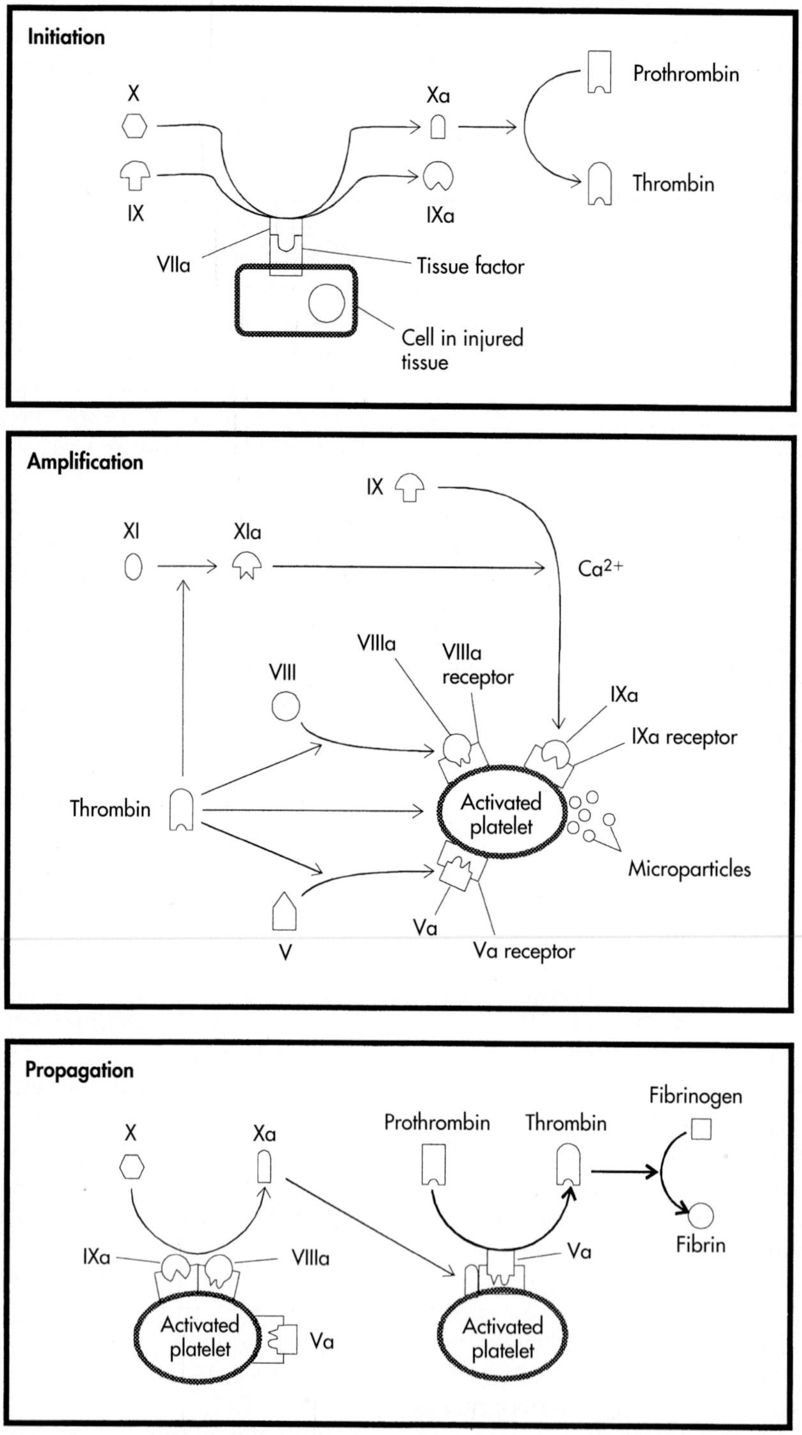

Figure 7-35 Three-stage model of coagulation is suggested by knowledge of the underlying molecular biology. Clotting is initiated *(top)* by tissue factor (TF)–Factor VIIa surface complexes, which activate factor X (and also factor IX). The result is the generation of a small amount of thrombin. In turn, thrombin activates platelets *(middle)* and promotes the activation and assembly of coagulation factors and cofactors on the platelet surface. In this way, the stage is set for augmented generation of factor Xa, thrombin and fibrin *(bottom)*. Not shown are the effects of inhibitors of coagulation: lipoprotein-associated coagulation inhibitor, also known as extrinsic pathway inhibitor *(EPI)*, inhibits the TF-VIIa-Xa complex. Antithrombin III controls thrombin in amplification and propagation phases of clotting. *From Roberts HR, Lozier JN. New perspectives on the coagulation cascade. Hosp Pract 1992; 27:97-112.*

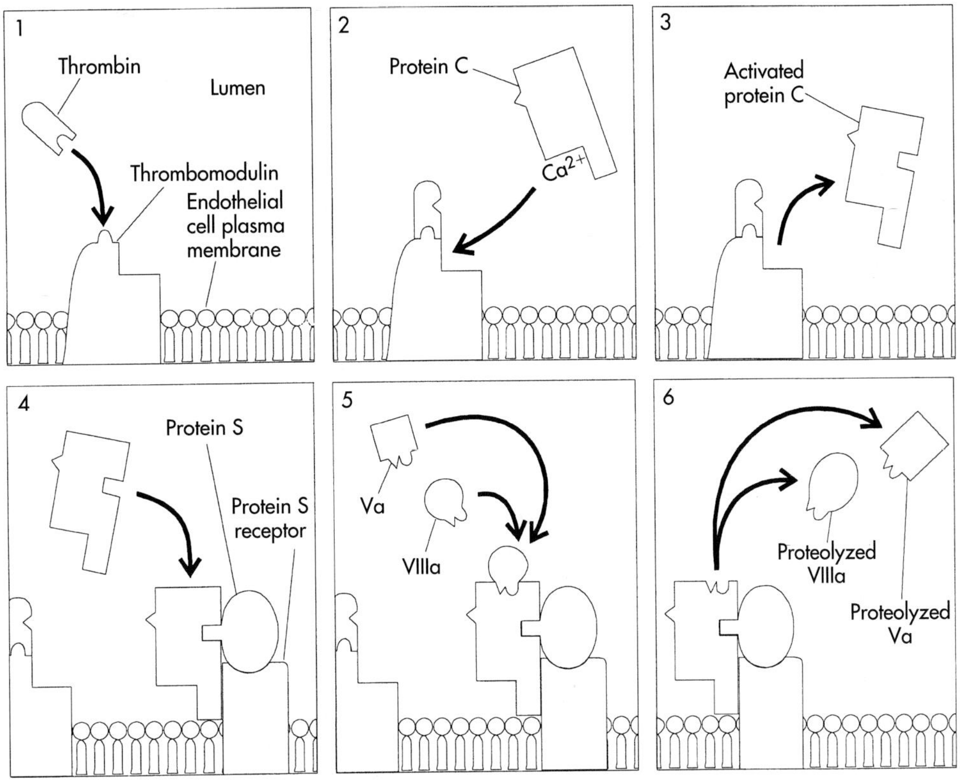

Figure 7-36 Down-regulation of clotting is one of the multiple roles endothelial cells play in hemostasis. Thrombomodulin, an endothelial transmembrane protein, binds thrombin *(1)*. The resulting complex captures protein C through electrostatic attraction between calcium ions on protein C and a negative region on thrombomodulin *(2)*. The bound protein C is proteolytically activated *(3)*; it then binds to nearby protein S on endothelial cells or platelets *(4)*. In the C-S complex, activated protein C is capable of inactivating factors Va and VIIa *(5* and *6)*. *From Roberts HR, Lozier JN. New perspectives on the coagulation cascade. Hosp Pract 1992; 27:97-112.*

bound to thrombomodulin activates protein C. In turn, activated protein C, with protein S as a cofactor, inactivates factors Va and VIIIa (Fig. 7-36). Activated protein C also promotes dissolution of clots. Antithrombin III is an important inhibitor of coagulation factor activities by forming complexes with the activated zymogens in the presence of heparin. The fibrinolytic system is a series of reactions similar to those of coagulation, in which zymogens are activated, resulting in proteolysis of fibrin. Fibrinolysis is achieved by a potent plasma proteolytic enzyme, plasmin. Its precursor plasminogen, an inert zymogen, is synthesized in the liver and then released into the blood. Plasminogen activators convert plasminogen to plasmin. Plasmin digests fibrinogen and fibrin and also degrades von Willebrand factor and factors V and VIII. An intensely proteolytic enzyme such as plasmin must be kept under constant control; this is achieved primarily by α_2-antiplasmin, which forms a stable complex with plasmin.

Coagulation disorders, because of inadequate synthesis or altered function of one or more coagulation proteins, may be congenital or acquired. The congenital, inherited disorders usually appear in young animals, but if the defect is mild, it may not become apparent until severe hemorrhage occurs following injury or surgery. Congenital coagulopathies usually involve a single defect in a single protein; acquired disorders usually affect more than one protein.

Congenital Coagulation Disorders

The congenital coagulation disorders result from molecular lesions in coagulation proteins. In the broadest sense, there may be inadequate synthesis of a normal molecule or synthesis of an abnormal molecule in which an abnormality in a strategic location interferes with function. The latter situation may result from a purine or pyrimidine base change in DNA. Most coagulation factors undergo postribosomal modification, such as cleavage of a portion of the molecule before it becomes functional, and this process also may be abnormal.

Factor XII Deficiency

Factor XII deficiency occurs in cats as an autosomal recessive trait and occasionally has been reported in dogs.

Feline heterozygotes have approximately 50% activity, whereas homozygotes have no measurable factor XII. Homozygotes have prolonged activated partial thromboplastin times (APTTs) but no clinical evidence of bleeding. Attempts to characterize the defect have found no apparent deletion of genomic DNA sequences or transcriptional or splicing abnormalities, suggesting that abnormal factor XII synthesis in cats may be due to premature termination of ribosomal amino acid assembly.

Factor XI Deficiency

Factor XI deficiency occurs in Holstein cattle and in Great Pyrenees, English springer spaniel, and Kerry blue terrier dogs. It is transmitted as an autosomal recessive gene in cattle. Spontaneous hemorrhage is insignificant in affected animals but can be severe following surgery. Homozygous factor XI–deficient animals have prolonged whole blood clotting times, APTTs, and lack of factor XI activity. Heterozygous animals have approximately 50% of normal factor XI activity.

Factor IX Deficiency (Hemophilia B)

Factor IX deficiency occurs in dogs and cats. The inheritance is sex linked, because the gene is present on the X chromosome. Affected males have low factor IX activity, and carrier females have 40% to 60% of normal activity. A wide variety of defects account for hemophilia B in different human families. Some patients have normal levels of factor IX antigen but low levels of factor IX activity (i.e., a poorly functioning protein). This can result from a single amino acid substitution that may distort one of the many changes the molecule must undergo before becoming functional. For example, in one factor IX–deficient patient, a strategic amino acid substitution prevents cleavage of a portion of the molecule, normally removed as part of the molecular rearrangement necessary for function. The abnormal factor IX molecule is not only larger but nonfunctional.

It should now be apparent that factor IX and other factor deficiencies in animals may result from a wide range of molecular lesions that have yet to be clarified. Bleeding in male Labrador retriever pups has recently been attributed to complete deletion of the factor IX gene. Canine hemophilia B closely mimics the human disease and serves as an important model for gene therapy studies. Intramuscular injections of an adeno-associated viral vector expressing canine factor IX into factor IX–deficient dogs has resulted in stable (>1 year), expression of biologically active factor IX in the circulation of the animals.

Hemorrhage in factor IX deficiency is mild in cats and small dogs and more severe in large dogs, presumably because of the greater degrees of trauma in large weight-bearing animals. Laboratory findings in factor IX–deficient animals are normal one-stage prothrombin times (OSPTs), prolonged APTTs, and activated clotting times (ACTs). In mildly affected animals, it may be necessary to dilute the plasma to reveal a prolonged APTT.

Factor VIII Deficiency (Hemophilia A)

Factor VIII deficiency is an important disease in dogs and has been described in most breeds and mongrels. It also occurs in horses, cattle, sheep, and cats, and in all species, it is an X chromosome–linked recessive trait. Bleeding may be severe in large dogs and horses. Hemarthroses, subcutaneous hematomas, and bleeding into the central nervous system and body cavities may occur to varying degrees in factor VIII deficiency. Laboratory evaluation reveals long APTTs and ACTs. Factor VIII activity is low, and von Willebrand factor levels are normal. Carrier female animals have approximately 50% factor VIII activity and normal levels of von Willebrand factor.

von Willebrand's Disease

von Willebrand's disease is an inherited abnormality of von Willebrand glycoprotein synthesis. It is generally acknowledged as the most significant hemostatic disorder in human beings and in many breeds of dogs; it also occurs in cats and horses. It was described in swine in the 1940s, and affected animals have been used extensively in research of von Willebrand's disease.

The von Willebrand protein or factor (vWF) is synthesized as a prepropolypeptide in endothelial cells and megakaryocytes. The human gene encoding the protein is located on chromosome 12. The mature canine subunit of 2813 amino acids is glycosylated and joined to other subunits by disulfide bonds to form multimers with molecular weights as high as 10 to 20×10^6; very large molecules. Immunochemical methods used to study this protein in human beings have also been used in dogs and cats, revealing similar multimeric patterns. The glycoprotein is found in plasma, megakaryocytes, platelets, subendothelium, and endothelial cells. In the plasma, von Willebrand protein forms a complex with factor VIII, which increases the concentration of factor VIII at sites of vascular injury and protects it from proteolytic degradation. Although dogs with low plasma concentrations of vWF have reduced factor VIII activity, this activity is reduced less than in human patients and does not appear to increase the risk of hemorrhage. Platelet von Willebrand glycoprotein is primarily located in alpha granules and is secreted onto the surface following platelet activation.

Mature vWF functions to facilitate adhesion of platelets to exposed vascular subendothelium following injury. This is especially important in small vessels with rapid blood flow (high shear rate). The most important platelet vWF receptor is the glycoprotein Ib–IX (GPIb-IX) complex. As is frequently true, a bleeding disorder due to quantitative and qualitative disorders of GPIb-IX (Bernard-Soulier syndrome) in human beings greatly facilitated our understanding of the function of the von Willebrand glycoprotein. As might be anticipated, the largest vWF molecules have the most GPIb-IX binding sites, and bleeding times are prolonged in human beings and dogs unable to assemble large multimers.

Laboratory assessment of animals suspected of having von Willebrand's disease is achieved by quantitative and multimeric analysis. Plasma vWF concentrations are measured by an ELISA using polyclonal antibodies specific for canine vWF. By convention, the protein measured in this assay is referred to as von Willebrand antigen (vWF:Ag). Assessment of the multimeric structure of the protein is achieved by electrophoresis followed by application of antibodies to vWF.

Intensive study of human beings with von Willebrand's disease has established that there is molecular heterogeneity among families. This suggests that similar heterogeneity occurs among breeds of dogs, and breed differences are now being characterized. Most forms of the disease are one of three types. Type I, the most common in dogs, is characterized by decreased levels of a normal multimeric glycoprotein pattern. In type II, dogs lack the large multimers. Type III dogs have very low or no detectable von Willebrand glycoprotein. The genetic defect responsible for type III von Willebrand's disease in Dutch Kooiker dogs is due to a splice site mutation at the first position of the donor splice site sequence of intron 16. The mutation results in the generation of a stop codon in the propeptide and failure of synthesis of the mature subunit. The genetic defect responsible for type I von Willebrand's disease in Doberman pinscher dogs is due to a G to A mutation at the end of exon 43. This nucleotide change allows approximately 10% to 20% of the normal amount of vWF to be synthesized in homozygous mutant animals. A PCR-based test for this mutation can differentiate homozygous normal, carrier, and affected dogs.

Thus, animals with von Willebrand's disease have a bleeding disorder consistent with impaired platelet adhesion. Epistaxis, oozing of blood from mucous membranes, petechiation, and serious postoperative hemorrhage are the most common findings. Despite being a congenital defect, variation in the expression of von Willebrand's disease may result in bleeding in some mature dogs; dogs with mild forms of von Willebrand's disease may only bleed because of another disorder such as urinary or intestinal tract carcinomas or inflammation of a mucosal surface.

Acquired Coagulation Disorders

Toxicities resulting in hemorrhage most commonly follow ingestion of one of a group of related substances—the coumarins. Coumarins are synthesized by molds in sweet clover and are used in rodenticides. Sweet clover poisoning is most common in cattle but can also occur in sheep and horses. Dogs and cats that accidentally ingest rodenticides develop life-threatening hemorrhages. Development of resistance to the coumarins has initiated development of more potent "second-generation" anticoagulant rodenticides. Repeated ingestion of coumarins is necessary to exhaust vitamin K stores, whereas the second-generation anticoagulants (such as brodifacoum and bromadiolone) cause significant bleeding following a single ingestion.

Coumarins and Related Compounds

Coumarins and related compounds interfere with the vitamin K–dependent coagulation factors II, VII, IX, and X. As described in the review of hemostasis, the calcium and phospholipid binding properties of these proteins follows posttranslational carboxylation of the gamma carbon on glutamic acid. Vitamin K is a cofactor in the carboxylation reaction becoming oxidized as the reaction proceeds. Coumarin compounds interrupt the vitamin K oxidation-reduction cycle, resulting in exhaustion of the vitamin and incomplete carboxylation of coagulation factors.

The clinical signs in vitamin K–deficient animals vary depending on the degree and location of hemorrhage. Spontaneous bleeding causes large hematomas and hemarthroses. Cattle with sweet clover poisoning bleed severely following minor surgery. Calves born to dams ingesting moldy sweet clover may die of internal hemorrhage at birth, although the dam is unaffected. Human infants are also susceptible to vitamin K deficiency causing hemorrhage, presumably a result of inadequate dietary intake of the vitamin (e.g., low levels of Vitamin K in milk) before intestinal colonization with vitamin K–producing bacteria.

Rodenticide toxicity in dogs causes a broad spectrum of clinical signs resulting from hypovolemia from hemorrhage, organ dysfunction, or bleeding into body cavities. Hemorrhage into the brain may produce neurologic dysfunction and occasionally sudden death. Hemarthrosis causes acute lameness. Hematomas occur following venipunctures and trauma.

Vitamin K–deficient animals have long OSPTs. The OSPT may also be used to monitor hemostasis in cattle ingesting sweet clover. The short half-life of factor VII (relative to prothrombin and factors IX and X) results in prolongation of the OSPT prior to APTT prolongation. However, times in both tests are usually prolonged when animals are presented with hemorrhage from vitamin K antagonists. Animals that die following coumarin or rodenticide toxicity reveal massive hemorrhages in body cavities and joints and along fascial planes.

Liver Disease

Liver disease in which there is inadequate synthesis of coagulation factors, can cause severe bleeding. It is apparent that significant depletion of these factors only occurs either late in progressive liver diseases when most of the organ is destroyed, or in cases of acute, overwhelming hepatocyte necrosis. Accurate laboratory assessment of coagulation factor function in animals with liver disease is difficult because this may be complicated by subnormal platelet function and concurrent disseminated intravascular coagulation with fibrinolysis. Severe acute liver disease in dogs may prolong both OSPT and APTT, whereas partially compensated chronic hepatic disease may only cause slight prolongation of the APTT.

Disseminated Intravascular Coagulation

Disseminated intravascular coagulation and fibrinolysis is an important coagulation disorder in veterinary medicine. It is the result of an intriguing array of intermediary mechanisms in neoplastic diseases, overwhelming viral and bacterial infections, severe hemolysis, and other disorders. These disorders induce the unregulated and excessive generation of thrombin, which is the most important factor in the pathogenesis of disseminated intravascular coagulation (DIC). The overexpression of thrombin results in the consumption of coagulation factors that are its substrates, such as fibrinogen, factor V, and factor VIII. Thrombin binds to its receptors on platelets and endothelial cells and is a potent agonist inducing platelet activation and aggregation. Thrombin also induces endothelial cells to release tissue plasminogen activator. Newly formed fibrin stimulates the production of plasmin from plasminogen and results in aggressive fibrinolysis. Therefore the clinical and laboratory manifestations of DIC result from the overexpression of thrombin and plasmin. The overexpression of thrombin with relatively reduced expression of plasmin may result in either large-vessel thrombosis or microvascular fibrin deposition leading to organ dysfunction and ischemic necrosis. Excessive thrombin generation with vigorous secondary fibrinolysis may result in increased consumption of hemostatic factors and bleeding. Both the bleeding and thrombotic manifestations of DIC are well-documented postmortem findings in animals.

THE THYMUS AND LYMPH NODES

Structure and Function

The thymus, a lymphoepithelial organ within the mediastinum of young animals, is essential for the development and function of the immune system. The epithelial portions are derived from branchial pouches, whereas lymphocytes arise in bone marrow and travel to the thymus in the blood. The thymus provides an architecturally organized microenvironment for the development of mature T lymphocytes, which normally constitute 70% to 80% of peripheral blood lymphocytes. Precursor bone marrow–derived lymphocytes or prothymocytes migrate to the thymus, where they undergo differentiation into mature T lymphocytes. The gland consists of subcapsular, cortical, and medullary zones, and prothymocytes in afferent blood migrate from the subcapsular zone to the medulla before leaving through efferent blood vessels and lymphatics.

During intrathymic migration, lymphocytes receive signals to undergo proliferation, receptor gene rearrangement, positive selection for major histocompatibility complex (MHC) restriction, negative selection for deletion of self-reactive and defective cells, and molecular and functional maturation. Many lymphocytes undergo apoptosis during migration, ensuring that only MHC-restricted and self-tolerant T cells leave the thymus. MHC restriction ensures that T cells will only interact with those cells that present antigen associated with MHC molecules on their surfaces.

The thymic stromal epithelial cells, bone marrow–derived macrophages, and reticular cells play a key role in the development and differentiation of T lymphocytes. Thymic epithelial cells secrete a variety of polypeptides, including thymic hormones and cytokines, and form cell-cell contacts mediated by adhesion molecules. The thymus also participates in bidirectional hormonal interactions involving the thymic epithelium and the hypothalmus-pituitary axis. Adenohypophyseal hormones include prolactin, growth hormone, thyroid-stimulating hormone, and adrenocorticotrophic hormone; the latter two influence thymic epithelium through their respective target organs.

MHC molecules are expressed by many of the nonlymphoid cells in the thymus and may be necessary for the selection of the mature T cell repertoire. Within the cortex, thymocytes mature from a triple-negative stage in which they lack cell surface glycoproteins CD3, CD4, and CD8 to double-positive cells expressing CD4 and CD8 along with CD3. During cortical migration, the cell's antigen receptor (T cell receptor) forms as a heterodimer. In the medulla, they become single-positive cells expressing either CD4 (helper) or CD8 (suppressor-cytotoxic) markers (Fig. 7-37). The CD4 and CD8 transmembrane glycoproteins mediate cell-cell adhesion and may initiate signal transduction. As T lymphocyte development occurs, they in turn promote maintenance of thymic stromal integrity; lack of thymocyte transition from a triple-negative to double-positive state inhibits the development of a distinct cortex, and lack of thymocyte transition from double-positive to single-positive inhibits the development of the thymic medulla.

Following release from the thymus into the blood, T cells travel to the splenic periarteriolar lymphatic sheaths and the cortical areas around germinal centers in lymph nodes. The critical balance of production and distribution of T lymphocytes is extremely important in immune homeostasis, so much so that immunodeficiency or autoimmunity may result from inadequate or overzealous activity of a particular subset.

The thymus is large prior to birth and involutes following sexual maturity; the lymphoid and epithelial components are gradually replaced by loose connective tissue and fat. Recent studies of human centenarians have shown that virgin T cells continue to be processed, and thymic remnants or other lymphoid organs continue to produce and select high numbers of T cells.

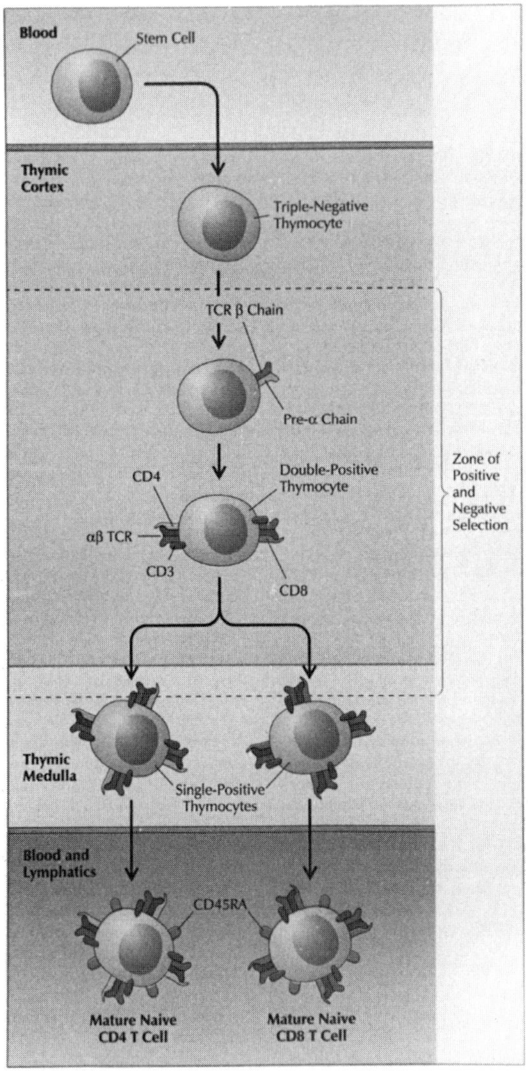

Figure 7-37 Thymopoiesis is the intricate process by which hemopoietic stem cells percolate through thymic epithelium from cortex to medulla, maturing into T lymphocytes. Starting as triple-negative, the cells become double-positive—expressing both CD4 and CD8, along with the signal transducer CD3—and then single-positive, committed to CD4 or CD8. The cell's antigen receptor (the T cell receptor, or TCR) becomes a heterodimer consisting most commonly of α and β chains. Not shown is the proliferation by which a single stem cell expands into thousands of thymocytes, which are then winnowed down to a relative few that are neither strongly autoreactive nor completely unreactive with self-antigens. Mature T cells emerge with a naïve phenotype characterized by expression of a protein termed DC45RA that is thought to mark T cells that have never been activated by antigen in the periphery. *From Haynes BF, Hale LP. Thymic function, aging, and AIDS. Hosp Pract 1999; 34:59-88.*

Thymic Disorders

Developmental Disorders of the Thymus

Included in this discussion are the congenital disorders that result in inadequate T lymphocyte function, as well as those resulting in B lymphocyte and plasma cell dysfunction. Many have been described in human beings and have been invaluable in learning more about mechanisms of immunity and immune regulation. The animal counterparts of immunodeficiency serve as valuable models in comparative immunology research. Combined immunodeficiencies (CIDs) are diseases affecting both B and T lymphocytes.

Combined Immunodeficiency. **Equine CID** is a genetic disorder occurring in Arabian or partly Arabian foals. It is inherited as an autosomal recessive trait, meaning that both the sire and dam are carriers of the defective gene. It has been determined that CID occurs in approximately 2% of Arabian foals and that approximately 25% of Arabian horses carry the gene. There is failure of functional B and T lymphocyte production, so foals are remarkably susceptible to a variety of microbial agents and usually die before 5 months of age. Adenoviruses that are typically resisted by normal foals are major causes of death in foals with CID. The viral infection is frequently complicated by various bacterial or protozoal infections that typically result in pneumonia.

The underlying biochemical basis for failure of B and T lymphocyte differentiation must occur at an early stage of lymphocyte development. In children, this is the result of adenosine deaminase deficiency, which may cause impaired DNA synthesis in lymphocytes. This enzyme is not deficient in affected foals; the exact mechanism of their lymphocyte stem cell failure is unknown.

Affected foals frequently have profuse nasal discharge, unthrifty haircoat, loss of condition, pneumonia, and occasionally diarrhea. Confirmatory diagnosis of CID in such a foal requires evidence of the following: persistent lymphopenia, absence of serum immunoglobulin, or hypoplastic lymphoid tissue. Varying degrees of neutrophilia and left shift and a mild anemia occur and probably result from chronic inflammation. Lymphopenia is marked and persistent and usually less than 0.8 to 1×10^9/L (0.8 to $1 \times 10^3/mm^3$). Serum IgM, which is normally present in newborn foals, is undetectable. Maternally derived IgG declines to very low concentrations by approximately 3 months of age. Necropsy findings are severe bronchopneumonia in combination with a small spleen and lymph nodes. The thymus may be difficult to identify or may consist of a few isolated lobules within the mediastinal fat. The spleen has marked reduction in the white pulp owing to absence of germinal centers and periarteriolar lymphocytic sheaths. Lymph nodes are similarly depleted of lymphocytes. The thymus usually consists of a few islands of lymphocyte-like cells and thymic corpuscles.

X-linked severe combined immunodeficiency has been reported in basset hounds. The affected male pups lack mature, functional T cells. The animals have a normal serum level of IgM but low or undetectable IgG and IgA. The thymus of these dogs is small and often obscured by mediastinal fat. Tonsils, lymph nodes, and Peyer's patches usually cannot be identified at necropsy. Microscopically, the thymic tissue consists of small dysplastic lobules with a variable number of Hassall's corpuscles.

An immunodeficiency syndrome in juvenile llamas is characterized by wasting and susceptibility to chronic diseases that fail to respond to therapy. There is a mild nonregenerative anemia, unless the llamas have concurrent eperythrozoonosis, in which case the anemia may be severe and regenerative. Affected llamas have low serum IgG concentrations and poor response to vaccination with *Clostridium perfringens* C toxoid. There is marked depletion of lymphocytes in the paracortical regions of lymph nodes.

Inflammatory and Degenerative Disorders of the Thymus

Injury to the thymus resulting in variable degrees of immunodeficiency may be caused by infectious agents (usually viruses), toxins, neoplasia, malnutrition, and aging. The feline leukemia virus (FELV) and immunodeficiency virus (FIV), are examples of agents that infect T lymphocytes, resulting in chronic, respiratory, and digestive system infections. Viruses with similar capabilities are those of canine distemper, bovine virus diarrhea, equine rhinopneumonitis (equine herpesvirus-1), and feline parvovirus. Previous reference has been made to the importance of T lymphocyte surface glycoproteins; one of these (CD4) is the receptor for attachment of the human acquired immunodeficiency (AIDS) virus. In FIV-infected cats, there is depletion of CD4 lymphocytes, and this results in reversal of the CD4/CD8 T lymphocyte ratio. In FIV-infected cats, the thymic cortex has a high viral load early after infection and lymphoid follicles become hyperplastic; later there is lymphoid depletion and follicular involution. As would be anticipated, thymic and lymph node atrophy are apparent at necropsy in animals with these viral infections.

Environmental toxins such as polychlorinated biphenyls, lead, and mercury have a suppressive effect on the immune system. Thymic function is impaired in severe dietary protein deficiencies of young animals, leading to reduced immunoglobulin synthesis.

A syndrome termed **idiopathic thymic hemorrhage** has been reported involving the thymus, thymic mediastinum, and thymic remnants in young dogs. Affected dogs die unexpectedly of massive mediastinal hemorrhage and hypovolemic shock. The etiology of this disorder is unknown.

Thymic cysts can be found within the developing and mature thymus and in thymic remnants in the anterior mediastinum. These cysts represent developmental remnants of branchial arch epithelium and are usually of no significance.

Neoplastic Disorders of the Thymus

Since the thymus has both lymphoid and epithelial components, it is possible for either or both to be neoplastically transformed. **Thymic lymphosarcoma** is a T lymphocyte neoplasm of young animals, particularly cats and cattle, with a much lower incidence in dogs. Clinical findings reflect the presence of a large mass in the thoracic cavity. Thoracic aspirates have many medium to large lymphocytes, which frequently have vacuolated cytoplasm, a feature unique to neoplastic lymphocytes in fluid. When present, mitoses are a significant indication of neoplasia.

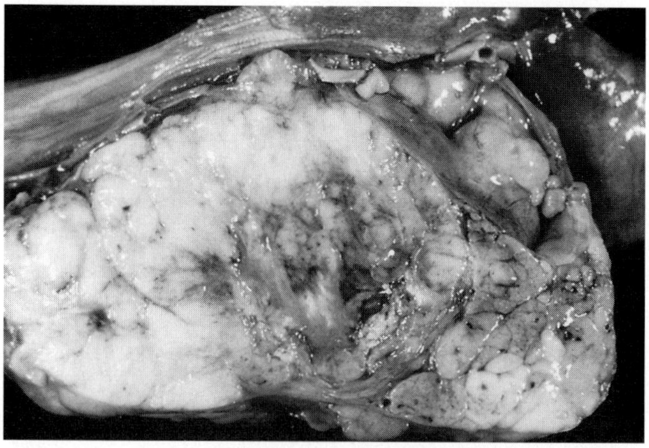

Figure 7-38 Thymus; cat. Lymphosarcoma. The large tumor has been transected and lies immediately cranial and ventral to the lungs.

Bovine thymic lymphosarcoma most often occurs in beef cattle 6 to 24 months of age and is characterized by massive thymic enlargement. The etiology is unknown, and concurrent leukemia is unusual. The thymus is an important site of lymphosarcoma in cats. The tumors are large, white or gray mediastinal masses that displace adjacent structures and result in fluid accumulation (Fig. 7-38). In cats, the thoracic fluid is frequently chylous because of lipid accumulations. Microscopically, these tumors are diffuse lymphosarcomas dominated by large lymphocytes that are homogeneous in size, shape, nuclear morphology, and nuclear/cytoplasmic ratio.

Thymomas are primary neoplasms of thymic epithelial cells and are accompanied by varying proportions of nonneoplastic lymphocytes (thymocytes). They grow slowly and are uncommon but occur in dogs, cats, cattle, and sheep. In dogs, a paraneoplastic syndrome of myasthenia gravis and megaesophagus may accompany thymomas. They are usually encapsulated, nodular, firm masses with soft and cystic areas, located in the cranial mediastinum. They are cytologically heterogeneous with small lymphocytes and round to spindle-shaped epithelial cells singly or in clumps. Variable numbers of mast cells, plasma cells, eosinophils, neutrophils, and macrophages

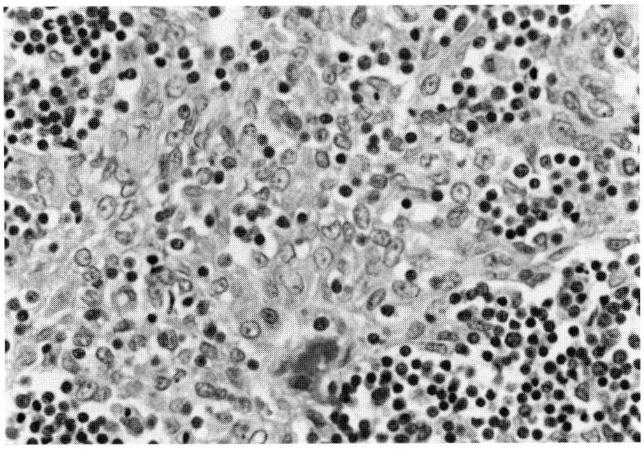

Figure 7-39 Thymoma; dog. Note the neoplastic thymic epithelial cells and numerous small lymphocytes. H & E stain.

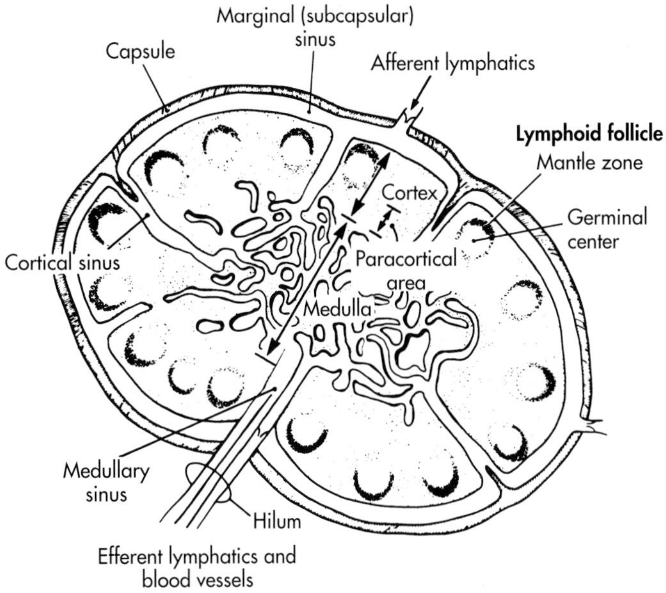

Figure 7-40 Schematic view of the organization of the lymph node. *From Miller KB. Reactive lymphocyte disorders and lymphadenopathy. In: Handin RI, Stossel TP, Lux SE, eds. Blood: Principles and Practice of Hematology. Philadelphia: JB Lippincott, 1995:662.*

may be present. Histologically, connective tissue trabeculae of variable thickness subdivide the mass into lobules composed of solid sheets and cords of round to spindle-shaped epithelial cells. Variable numbers of predominantly small lymphocytes are present accompanied by smaller numbers of medium and large lymphocytes (Fig. 7-39). The cystic structures are lined by epithelial cells, which may be ciliated.

THE LYMPH NODES

Structure and Function

Lymph nodes are ideally suited for surveillance and immune function. Lymph transports antigens from a wide area of tissue to lymph nodes, where they are concentrated among phagocytes and lymphocytes. Patrolling lymphocytes enter lymph nodes by migrating through walls of specialized venules, and they leave in efferent lymph within a few hours if they do not encounter an antigen they recognize. The successful encounter of lymphocytes with antigen is assisted by antigen-presenting cells that display antigens in highly immunogenic forms. Lymph nodes therefore serve to introduce lymph-borne antigen to blood-borne lymphocytes to enhance antigen detection and presentation.

Lymph nodes are traditionally divided into three regions: the superficial cortex, the deep cortex or paracortex, and the medulla (Fig. 7-40). Within the cortex are B cell and T cell domains. The B cell–dependent cortex consists of follicles that may be immunologically inactive (primary follicles) or active (secondary follicles or germinal centers). Germinal centers consist of a central pale zone of large lymphocytes and macrophages within a zone of small lymphocytes. The T cell–dependent paracortex is situated between and deep to the B cell follicles. From a functional viewpoint, there are three spaces within each region: an intralymphatic space, an intravascular space, and an interstitium. The boundaries of these spaces are formed by vascular and lymphatic endothelial cells, which control the movement of cells, antigens, and cytokines.

Afferent lymphatics penetrate the capsule and enter the subcapsular space. The subcapsular space connects with medullary sinuses that eventually converge on the efferent lymphatics. Unless these sinuses are particularly distended with lymph, they and their thin endothelium are usually microscopically imperceptible. A striking feature of the intravascular space is the concentration of lymphocytes within venules characterized by high endothelial cells. At these sites, B and T lymphocytes migrate into the interstitium. This controlled migration of blood cells is mediated by surface glycoproteins, which become expressed on activated lymphocytes and bind to appropriate glycoproteins expressed on endothelial cells. Although the factors and cell types involved in the induction and maintenance of the specialized high endothelial cells, are not well characterized, the important components appear to be cytokines produced locally or supplied by afferent lymph, extracellular matrix proteins surrounding the high endothelial cells, and interdigitating dendritic cells.

The lymphoid cells within lymph nodes are classified on a morphologic basis as small lymphocytes, large lymphocytes, and plasma cells. The use of monoclonal antibodies for cell surface protein recognition has allowed subclassification of lymphocytes within these groups. The T cell marker CD3 is conserved across species lines and is an intracytoplasmic portion of a T cell transmembrane receptor that mediates signal transduction. A similar marker system, CD79a, exists on B lymphocytes. These markers can be identified in formalin-fixed paraffin wax–embedded specimens by means of fluorescent immunocytochemistry.

The accessory or nonlymphoid cells in lymph nodes act in harmony with B and T lymphocytes throughout the immune response. There are several groups of accessory cells in lymph nodes that are recognizable mainly by morphology and location. The perception of where they come from relative to their function is most interesting and of central significance to immunology. The macrophages that are closely associated with sinus endothelial cells are differentiated, bone marrow–derived monocytes with morphologic and cytochemical characteristics of macrophages. Interdigitating cells within the paracortical nodules have numerous fingerlike cytoplasmic projections that intertwine with those of their neighbors. They also appear to be of bone marrow origin, but if they are monocyte derived, they undergo differentiation to assume characteristics distinct from classic macrophages.

Follicular dendritic cells are probably non-marrow-derived stromal cells found in follicles following antigenic stimulation. They too have numerous branching projections. These accessory cells collaborate in the complex process of digesting and presenting antigenic particles. Nonlymphoid dendritic cells originate in the bone marrow and migrate to various tissues where they undergo differentiation and assume characteristics unique to that environment. Ultimately, they may trap antigen and carry it to the nearest lymph node. There is good evidence that the Langerhans' cells of the skin follow such a route and ultimately become interdigitating cells in the nearest lymph node.

Lymph nodes may undergo atrophy or hypertrophy or may become the site of focal or diffuse inflammation (lymphadenitis). They may become enlarged because of lymphoid neoplasia or metastatic tumor cell proliferation. It is essential that enlarged lymph nodes be examined microscopically. For superficial nodes, this is easily accomplished by aspiration using 22- to 25-gauge needles, with expulsion of the cell suspension onto glass slides. The fragility of lymphocytes necessitates gentle spreading techniques to prevent distortion and disintegration of the cells. Aspirates may be stained with Wright-Giemsa or new methylene blue stains. The ease of lymph node aspiration and staining provides veterinary clinicians the opportunity to become proficient in lymph node cytology. Aspirates provide excellent cellular detail, but, for the study of architectural derangements, removal of the node for histologic evaluation is necessary. The surgeon must handle lymph nodes carefully to minimize artifacts. A portion of one end of the node should be removed and used to prepare impression smears. The remainder of the node should be placed in fixative fluid, with the capsule intact, for 1 hour. This period of fixation prevents bulging of the node through the capsule, which occurs when lymph nodes are cut without prior fixation. The lymph node should then be sliced transversely into parallel sections to ensure penetration of the fixative fluid.

Establishing a prioritized list of differential diagnoses for lymph node disorders can best be approached systematically by determining the size of the lymph node(s) and if they are enlarged, whether the enlargement is uniform or nodular. If a lymph node(s) is enlarged, it is called **lymphadenomegaly;** if a node(s) is small or absent it is called **lymph node hypoplasia, lymph node aplasia,** or **lymph node atrophy** depending on the cause. Lymphadenomegaly may be localized involving a single node or generalized involving many nodes. These categories are summarized in Table 7-6.

Table 7-6 Diseases or Conditions Causing Enlarged or Small Lymph Nodes

	Mechanism of Alteration	
Lymph Node Size	Removal of Cells/Foreign Material	Proliferation of Cells
Localized enlargement	Local/regional infections Regional neoplastic metastases	Primary neoplastic disease Metastatic neoplastic diseases Antigenic stimulation Lymphoid/macrophage hyperplasia
Generalized enlargement	Bacteremia/septicemia Hemotropic parasitic diseases Immune-mediated diseases Chronic infectious diseases	Chronic antigenic stimulation Metastatic neoplastic disease Hemotropic parasitic diseases Lymphoid/macrophage hyperplasia Immune-mediated diseases Chronic infectious diseases

Lymphocyte and Lymph Node Disorders

Developmental Disorders of Lymph Nodes

The congenital immunodeficiency syndromes include developmental disorders of lymph nodes and are discussed with Developmental Disorders of the Thymus.

Degenerative Disorders of Lymph Nodes

Atrophy of lymph nodes and bronchial and gut-associated lymphoid tissues may result from viral infections, toxins, and malnutrition. Examples of these are discussed with degenerative disorders of the thymus. Degenerative processes associated with aging also result in impaired function and decreased numbers of lymphocytes, resulting in deficient immunologic responses.

Hyperplasia of Lymph Nodes

The arrival of large numbers of antigens in a lymph node results in increased blood supply, increased numbers of macrophages, and recruitment of many lymphocytes. Superficial lymph nodes become palpably enlarged. Lymphocytes transform to large cells, which undergo cell division. Depending on the nature of the antigen, the transformed cells will mature into T lymphocytes or plasma cells. In comparison to normal lymph nodes, aspirates of hyperplastic nodes have greater variation in lymphocyte morphology because of increased numbers of large lymphocytes among the predominate population of small lymphocytes. There are also increased numbers of macrohages, which may be antigen-presenting cells, and a few neutrophils. Mitotic figures are not common. The nuclear chromatin pattern of lymphocytes is variable in hyperplastic lymph nodes. Plasma cells are usually evident and are valuable indicators of recent stimulation of the node by antigens that stimulate antibody synthesis (Fig. 7-41). In contrast to hyperplastic nodes, aspirates of lymphosarcomatous nodes may have many disintegrated cells. The aspirates are frequently a sheet of densely packed, uniformly sized lymphocytes that may require additional staining. Intact cells are usually large with uniformly large nuclei and a thin rim of cytoplasm. The nucleochromatin pattern is uniform throughout, and mitotic figures are frequently increased. There is greater variation in nucleolar shape and size in nuclei of neoplastic lymphocytes.

The histologic findings in hyperplastic lymph nodes reflect the duration of stimulation. The venules with high endothelium are prominent, reflecting increased lymphocyte adhesion and migration shortly after the arrival of antigen. Germinal centers with numerous debris-laden macrophages become prominent in secondary follicles (Fig. 7-42). The T cell population is increased; as a result, the paracortex is expanded. Within a few days, increased numbers of plasma cells may be detected in medullary cords. Chronically stimulated nodes have increased numbers of follicles with irregular contours. Differentiation of benign hyperplasia from neoplasia may be difficult, but nodal architecture, especially the subcapsular sinus, is retained in hyperplastic nodes. The subcapsular sinus is regularly infiltrated in lymphosarcoma.

Inflammatory Disorders of Lymph Nodes

Many of the gross and microscopic findings in lymphadenitis include those of hyperplasia because of antigenic stimulation. In addition, the numbers of neutrophils, monocytes, and macrophages are increased. Lymph node aspirates and biopsy specimens should be thoroughly examined for the presence of organisms. In some bacterial and mycotic infections, the node is mostly occupied by neutrophils, and excision of the capsule exposes an abscess.

Caseous Lymphadenitis. Caseous lymphadenitis is a specific lymphadenitis of sheep and goats caused by *Corynebac-*

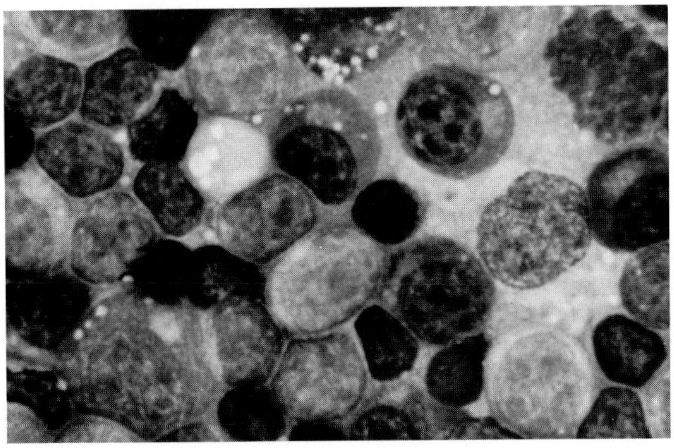

Figure 7-41 Lymph node aspirate; dog. Hyperplasia. Note the increased numbers of large lymphocytes and plasma cells. Wright-Giemsa stain.

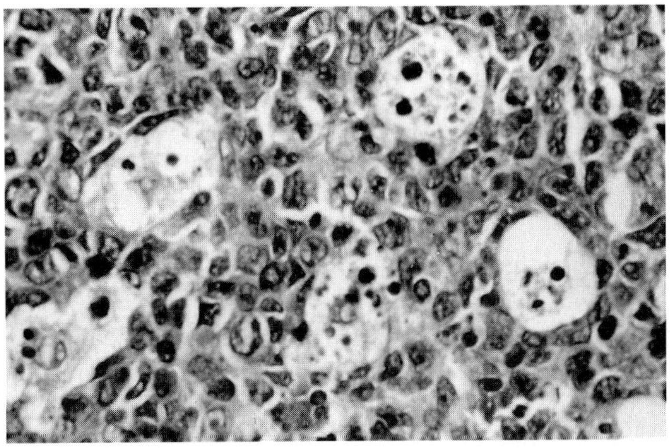

Figure 7-42 Lymph node; Hyperplasia. Note the debris-laden macrophages in the germinal center of a lymphoid follicle, indicating apoptosis of lymphocytes. H & E stain.

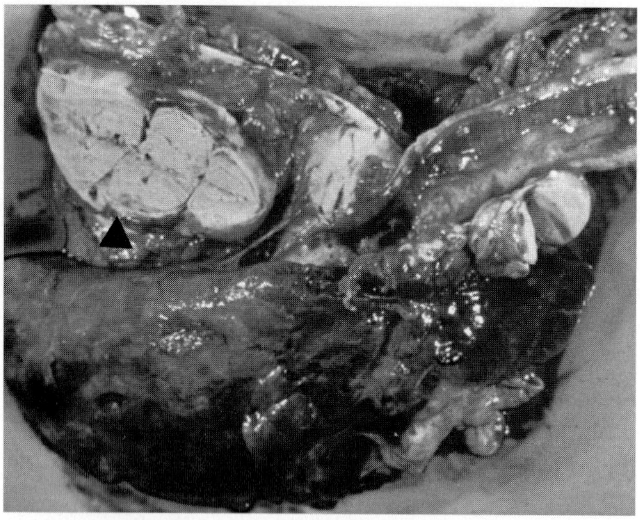

Figure 7-43 Lung; sheep. Caseous lymphadenitis. Note that the incised caudal mediastinal lymph nodes are completely filled with caseous material *(arrowhead). Courtesy of D.M. Middleton.*

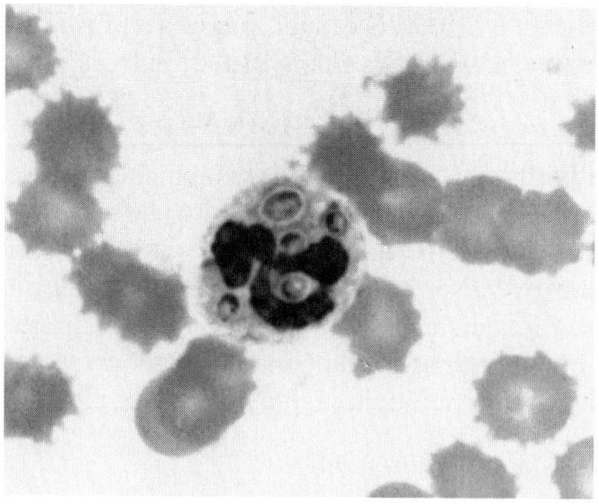

Figure 7-44 Blood smear; dog. Histoplasmosis. Note the *Histoplasma capsulatum* organisms in the neutrophil. Wright-Giemsa stain. *Courtesy of M.D. Campbell.*

terium pseudotuberculosis, which is also the cause of ulcerative lymphangitis in cattle and horses and pectoral abscesses in horses. It is suspected that the organism lives within the intestine and enters the skin through wounds contaminated with soil containing fecal material or purulent discharges. In sheep, abscesses occur in superficial lymph nodes, and these may rupture and discharge thick, green pus. Most sheep do not become ill; debilitation occurs only in a small percentage of sheep in which infection involves internal lymph nodes and other organs.

The encapsulated abscesses of ovine cutaneous lymphadenitis are characteristically green and caseous, with concentric rings resembling those of an onion (Fig. 7-43). Similar abscesses may be found in the lungs, especially in older sheep. The abscesses in goats are usually more numerous and frequently involve lymph nodes of the head and neck.

Histoplasmosis. Histoplasmosis is a diffuse disease of the monocyte-macrophage system caused by *Histoplasma capsulatum.* A dimorphic fungus, it grows as a mold in soil and as a yeast in animal tissues. The fungus is distributed throughout the world, in major river valleys, in temperate and tropical climates; it grows especially well in soil enriched by bird feces. The highest incidence of disease is in dogs; the incidence is lower in cats.

In most animals, the organism is inhaled and results in a mild; self-limiting infection with hypertrophy of tracheobronchial lymph nodes in asymptomatic dogs and cats. Because the fungus is confined to monocytes and macrophages, spread beyond the respiratory tract is assumed to occur by hematogenous and lymphatic dissemination of infected cells. Disseminated histoplasmosis in dogs and cats results in gastrointestinal or liver disease of long duration. There are several reports of ocular involvement in feline disseminated histoplasmosis.

Disseminated histoplasmosis is characterized by neutrophilia and monocytosis in some animals. Nonregenerative anemia is common because of the chronic inflammation. Biochemical changes include increased activity of serum alkaline phosphatase and hyperbilirubinemia. The total serum protein may be low, normal, or elevated, depending on factors such as the extent and duration of the diarrhea and emaciation. Regardless of the total protein concentration, a shift in the albumin/globulin ratio occurs because of hypergammaglobulinemia secondary to the immune response.

Cytology is useful for the diagnosis of histoplasmosis. The least invasive procedures include examination of cells of buffy coat, body fluids, and tracheal wash preparations and aspirates of bone marrow and lymph nodes. The organisms are visible in monocytes, neutrophils, and macrophages (Fig. 7-44).

Dogs dying of this disease are emaciated. The large bowel is thickened with mucosal corrugations caused by infiltration of the submucosa and lamina propria with macrophages, lymphocytes, and plasma cells. Lymph nodes are enlarged and, in contrast to lymphosarcoma, are firm when incised. The spleen and liver are enlarged and firm, and the liver is diffusely gray.

Epizootic Lymphangitis. Epizootic lymphangitis or equine histoplasmosis is a chronic suppurative lymphadenitis of solipeds caused by *Histoplasma farciminosus.* It occurs in

Mediterranean countries, Asia, and Africa. The fungal organisms exist in the soil and enter the body through contaminated wounds. Fungal spores are also inhaled and cause lesions of the upper and lower respiratory tracts. Keratoconjunctivitis may result from transmission of the organism by flies.

The lesions, in most locations, are nodules that eventually discharge a mucopurulent exudate. The organism is evident in smears of the exudate as globose to oval yeasts 2 to 3 μm in diameter. Spontaneous recovery may occur; however, horses are often euthanatized because of debility. At necropsy, suppurative and granulomatous lesions are most numerous in the skin, with occasional dissemination to the lungs, liver, and spleen.

Leishmaniasis. Leishmaniasis, like histoplasmosis, is a disseminated disease of the monocyte macrophage system caused by protozoa in the genus *Leishmania*. It occurs in human beings, dogs, and other animals and is confined to endemic areas including parts of Europe, the Mediterranean countries, the Middle East, Africa, and Central and South America. It may be seen in any part of the world in dogs that have resided in endemic areas. The protozoa proliferate by binary fission in the gut of the sand fly and become flagellated organisms that are introduced to mammals by insect bites; they then assume a nonflagellated form in macrophages.

The cutaneous lesions in dogs are ulcers at the site of insect bites. These ulcers are directly attributable to proliferation of the organism within macrophages, the accumulation of neutrophils, lymphocytes, and plasma cells, and focal disruption of the dermis and epidermis. In the visceral form of the disease, dogs are emaciated and have generalized enlargement of lymph nodes. Lymph node aspirates contain macrophages with organisms. Dogs have a nonregenerative anemia and a polyclonal hypergammaglobulinemia with total serum protein concentrations that may exceed 100 g/L (10 g/dl).

At necropsy, dogs with visceral leishmaniasis are emaciated and have enlarged, liver, spleen, and lymph nodes. The bone marrow is usually hyperplastic. In impression smears of these enlarged organs, macrophages contain numerous round organisms approximately 2 μm in diameter. A vesicular nucleus and a small kinetoplast aid in distinguishing them from *Histoplasma capsulatum* (Fig. 7-45).

Porcine Circovirus Lymphadenitis. Porcine circovirus lymphadenitis is a newly recognized disease of growing pigs. The disease, termed **post weaning multisystemic wasting syndrome** (PWMS), results in poor growth of affected pigs. Virus infection causes generalized enlargement of all lymph nodes and microscopically results in granulomatous inflammation with the formation of giant cells in lymphoid tissues including lymph nodes, spleen,

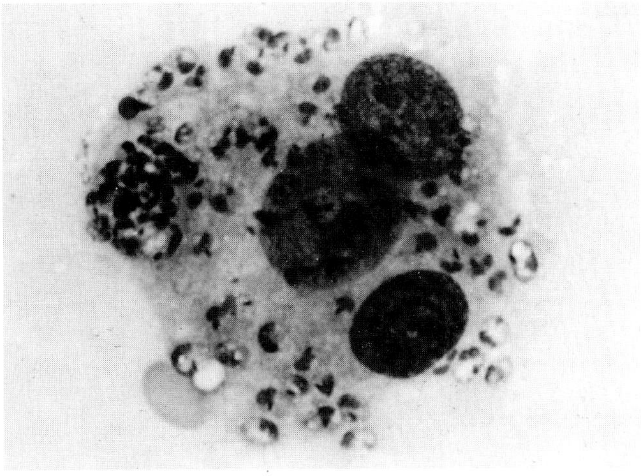

Figure 7-45 Lymph node aspirate; dog. Leishmaniasis. The macrophage contains numerous *Leishmania* organisms. Wright-Giemsa stain.

tonsil, and thymus. Basophilic cytoplasmic inclusions are present within macrophages.

Neoplastic Lymphocyte Disorders

Neoplastic lymphocyte disorders occur as leukemia, characterized by neoplastic cells in the blood and bone marrow, and lymphosarcoma in which there are tumors in soft tissue. In animals with leukemia, the presence of tumor in bone marrow may result in interference with hemopoiesis evident as one or more of anemia, neutropenia, and thrombocytopenia. Animals with lymphosarcoma frequently have a normal hemogram with the exception of a mild, nonregenerative anemia in some animals because of chronic disease. However, animals with lymphosarcoma most likely have some neoplastic lymphocytes in the circulation, and an absolute lymphocytosis occurs in approximately 20% of cases. Therefore, attempts to separate the two disorders may not be justified.

Lymphocytic Leukemia. Although leukemias in human beings are now classified as acute when caused by large lymphocytes (without regard to duration of the disease), in animals, lymphocytic leukemias caused by large, poorly differentiated, lymphocytes have a shorter clinical course than those with chronic leukemias caused by small lymphocytes.

Acute lymphocytic leukemias occur in all species, and the cells may be of B or T cell origin. With the exception of calves, most affected animals have minimal lymph node enlargement. Cats and dogs are presented to veterinarians for nonspecific signs of illness including anorexia and lethargy. Animals with leukemia are ill because of sequestration of cells with rapid metabolic rates in capillary beds, thus denying normal cells access to glucose and other substrates. When the tumor has replaced

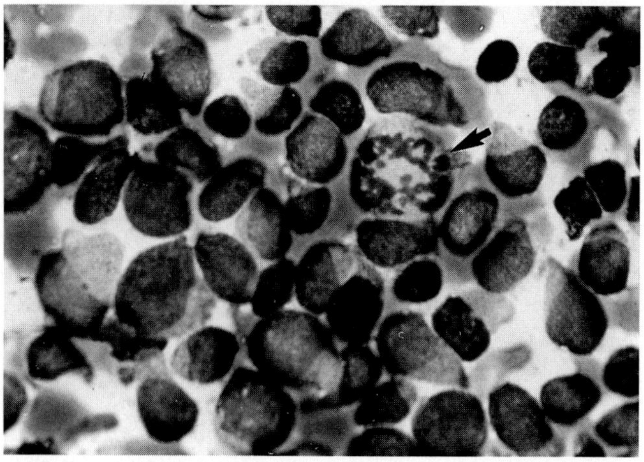

Figure 7-46 Bone-marrow; dog. Lymphosarcoma. There is complete displacement of hemopoietic cells by neoplastic cells. Note the cell in mitosis *(arrow)*. Wright-Giemsa stain.

hemopoietic tissue in the bone marrow, the hemogram findings include anemia, neutropenia, and thrombocytopenia. Blood smears have predominantly large lymphocytes, and although the numbers of leukocytes may be within reference range, they more commonly exceed 50×10^9/L (50×10^3/mm^3). The cells are uniformly large with large nuclei and prominent nucleoli. Disintegrated neoplastic cells are common, most likely because of their fragility. Bone marrow aspirates frequently yield fleshy marrow particles in which lymphocytes, similar to those present in the blood, predominate (Fig. 7-46). They are differentiated from granulocytes by cytochemical staining (Table 7-5).

At necropsy, animals with acute lymphocytic leukemia have varying degrees of pallor. Calves have generalized lymph node enlargement, hepatomegaly, and splenomegaly, in contrast to other species where lymph nodes are mildly or irregularly enlarged and the liver and spleen are mildly enlarged. The spleen is firm and fleshy. In calves, the marrow cavities are frequently fully occupied by tumor in which areas of necrosis may be present. In dogs and cats, the marrow may be partially or completely replaced by yellow-white tissue whose consistency is firmer than that of fat. Histologically, the bone marrow is dominated by a homogeneous population of large cells with large spaces within the nucleochromatin and one or more large nucleoli.

Cytologic evaluation of marrow imprints allows more precise identification of the cells and is helpful in distinguishing neoplastic erythroid precursors from lymphocytes in cats. Thus at necropsy, tissues for both fixation and cytology should be taken. In the liver, sinusoids frequently contain large lymphocytes in larger numbers than expected because of sequestration of the tumor cells at low rates of blood flow; colonies of these cells may be established in portal areas. There is frequently a diffuse population of large lymphocytes in the red pulp of the spleen.

Chronic lymphocytic leukemia is less common in comparison to acute lymphocytic leukemia. It is characterized by a persistent increase in circulating small lymphocytes and vague, nonspecific, clinical findings. It occurs in older cats, dogs, and cattle. Hemograms have a mild nonregenerative anemia. The degree of neutropenia and thrombocytopenia is an indication of the extent of bone marrow occupied by lymphocytes. Lymphocyte counts are variable and range from 10×10^9/L to 100×10^9/L (10×10^3/mm^3 to 100×10^3/mm^3). The cells are small to medium-sized lymphocytes. These cells occasionally produce immunoglobulin, and the laboratory findings are similar to those seen with secretory plasma cell sarcomas in which there is marked hyperproteinemia. Occasionally, in dogs and cats, the cell type consists of lymphocytes with cytoplasmic granules. Bone marrow aspirates are frequently very cellular and dominated by lymphocytes morphologically similar to those in the blood.

At necropsy, animals with chronic lymphocytic leukemia frequently have tissue pallor. There may be mild enlargement of lymph nodes and liver. The spleen may be markedly enlarged and fleshy when incised. White tumor nodules may be present on the liver and kidney. Microscopically, the tumor nodules are densely packed with small lymphocytes with scant cytoplasm. These cells are crowded in portal areas in the liver and form dense foci in the kidneys and other organs. Lymph node lesions are characterized by dense populations of small lymphocytes occupying significant portions of the node. These obliterate the normal architecture in the cortex, resulting in a monotonous expanse of lymphocytes without follicles.

LYMPHOSARCOMA. Lymphosarcoma is a significant disease in domestic animals, with species-dependent variations in etiology, tumor distribution, and clinical and necropsy findings. Animals with lymphosarcoma may or may not be leukemic, i.e., have neoplastic cells in bone marrow and blood.

The National Cancer Institute Working Formulation classification system for human lymphosarcomas has been applied to animal lymphosarcomas. The precepts of the Working Formulation are that lymphosarcomas of small cells with low mitotic rate have a low rate of progression and thus respond poorly to therapy, whereas lymphosarcomas of larger cells with high proliferative rates are potentially curable diseases. The system requires the identification and correlation of tumor cell types and tumor growth patterns. The neoplasms are thus graded as low-grade (indolent clinical course), intermediate-grade, and high-grade (aggressive clinical course) lymphosarcomas.

Staining of lymphosarcoma cells with monoclonal antibodies has facilitated identification of cell lineages. This has prognostic significance; dogs with B cell

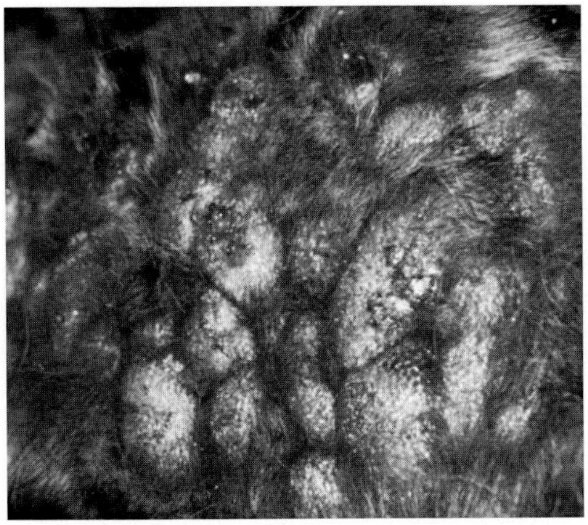

Figure 7-47 Skin; dog. Cutaneous (epitheliotropic) lymphosarcoma. *Courtesy of D. Joffe.*

lymphosarcomas have a better prognosis than those with T cell neoplasms. Immunophenotyping also allows identification of non–B cell, non–T cell lymphosarcomas. Cellular proliferation is being evaluated as a prognostic indicator in a variety of tumors using antibodies specific to cellular proliferating antigens. Proliferating cell nuclear antigen (PCNA), a protein associated with DNA polymerase that is expressed only in the nuclei of cells actively synthesizing DNA, is one of several proliferation markers that may prove useful in the identification of neoplastic lymphocytes. The appearance and location of tumors at necropsy, cytologic and histologic microscopic appearance, and immunophenotyping are all used in the study of lymphosarcoma.

Canine lymphosarcoma. In dogs, lymphosarcoma occurs predominantly in middle-aged animals. It occurs in multicentric, alimentary, cutaneous,and mediastinal forms, with the multicentric form most common. In all forms of the disease, dogs are anorexic and lethargic, eventually becoming cachectic. The **multicentric** form leads to generalized enlargement of lymph nodes, with or without hepatic and splenic enlargement and infiltration of bone marrow. Dogs with mediastinal disease are dyspneic and have reduced exercise tolerance. In the **alimentary form,** vomition, diarrhea, and blood in the stool are observed. Nodules, plaques,and ulcers are present in the skin of dogs with the **cutaneous form** of lymphosarcoma (Fig. 7-47). Occasionally, dogs are presented to veterinarians because of polyuria and polydypsia. These dogs have hypercalcemia, and frequently azotemia, as a result of hypercalcemic nephropathy. Hypercalcemia occurs in 10% to 20% of dogs with lymphosarcoma; most of these are T lymphocyte tumors.

Mild to moderate nonregenerative anemia is observed, and the anemia may be microcytic and hypochromic with mild reticulocytosis, because bleeding tumors of the intestines have depleted the dog's iron stores. Aspirates should be obtained from enlarged lymph nodes, liver, spleen, and the bone marrow, if suspect cells are noted on the blood film. Lymph node aspirates from dogs with lymphosarcoma have a preponderance of large lymphocytes of uniform morphology. These cells are usually fragile, and as a result, the aspirate may contain numerous naked nuclei and free cytoplasmic fragments. The nuclei in intact cells are large with a mantle of scant coarse cytoplasm. Nuclear chromatin is finely stippled, and rectangular and triangular nucleoli are common. Cells in mitosis are more numerous than in hyperplastic nodes. Lymphosarcoma of liver is obvious if numerous large lymphocytes are present. The diagnosis is more difficult in splenic aspirates, which may also have normal lymphocytes, plasma cells, and numerous erythrocytes. Aspirates of bone marrow may be large and fleshy if the bone marrow cavity is occupied by lymphosarcoma. Evaluation of the degree to which hemopoietic cells have been replaced by lymphocytes in these aspirates is done by examination under a 10× objective.

Necropsy findings in canine lymphosarcoma vary with the form of the disease. When lymph nodes are enlarged, they are white-gray and bulge when incised. Similar tissue is frequently present in the spleen and liver. Long bones should be sawn sagittally to check the extent of replacement of fat and hemopoietic tissue by tumor. Histologic differentiation of lymph node hyperplasia from neoplasia may be difficult. In neoplastic areas, there is a significant portion of the node in which normal architecture is completely effaced by cells with large open nuclei and prominent nucleoli. Frequently there are many lymphocytes in mitosis. Infiltration of lymphocytes into the subcapsular sinus and through the capsule into the adjacent fat is consistent with lymphosarcoma.

Cutaneous lymphosarcoma occurs in two forms—epitheliotropic and nonepitheliotropic. Epitheliotropic cutaneous lymphosarcoma is characterized by infiltration of neoplastic T lymphocytes into the epidermis and adnexal epithelium. The lymphocytes have clear cytoplasm with large pale nuclei that are often pleomorphic. The nonepitheliotropic tumors are characterized by B cell or T cell infiltration into the dermis and subcutis. Histologically, the majority of nonepitheliotropic lymphosarcomas consist of large lymphocytes, but immunoblastic and histiocytic types also occur.

Feline lymphosarcoma. Lymphosarcoma is one manifestation of several hemopoietic diseases caused by the feline leukemia virus (FLV). Cats become infected when the virus first colonizes the pharyngeal epithelium and pharyngeal lymphoid tissue. The virus evokes an immune response in most cats, which results in neutralization of the virus at this stage. The virus replicates in the spleen, lymph nodes, and gut-associated lymphoid tissue in cats that are unable to mount an effective immune response and then replicates in bone marrow cells and intestinal crypt epithelial cells. Viremia and excretion of virus into saliva and urine follows infection of neutrophils and platelets and widespread epithelial infection. Persistent viremias are most likely in kittens, in cats in crowded unsanitary conditions, and in immunosuppressed cats.

FLV is a retrovirus that contains a single strand of RNA and the enzyme reverse transcriptase, enclosed in a lipoprotein envelope. Reverse transcriptase enables the virus to make a DNA copy of the viral RNA, which is then incorporated into the host cell's DNA. The viral DNA may be transcribed with host cell DNA or remain dormant and be passed to daughter cells. The virus may replicate at any time, usually following some form of stress.

Persistently viremic cats are immunosuppressed and may develop other infectious diseases, bone marrow disorders, or lymphosarcomas. The lymphosarcomas have been classified as **multicentric, thymic, alimentary,** and **miscellaneous;** the latter includes ocular, renal, and neural forms. Lymphocytes with abnormal morphology may be found in blood or bone marrow from cats with any form of lymphosarcoma.

The clinical expression of lymphosarcoma varies with the form of the disease, i.e., the location of the tumor or tumors. Nonspecific signs include pallor of mucous membranes, lethargy, and wasting. Cats with thymic lymphosarcoma have dyspnea and a noncompressible thorax. Cats with internal lymph node enlargement, hepatomegaly, or intestinal lymphosarcoma may have palpable abdominal masses. Cats with renal lymphosarcoma may be presented in renal failure.

Laboratory findings in feline lymphosarcoma include nonregenerative anemia, regardless of the form of the disease. If the bone marrow is involved, there may be neutropenia, thrombocytopenia, and anemia as the tumor replaces hemopoietic tissue. Frequently dyserythropoiesis due to impaired nuclear maturation is reflected in a high mean corpuscular volume, despite reticulocytopenia, and the release of an occasional rubricyte or metarubicyte with asynchronous maturation of nucleus and cytoplasm (discussed with erythrocytic sarcomas). Occasionally, small numbers of *Haemobartonella felis* organisms are evident on erythrocytes, most likely as a result of the immunosuppressive effects of the virus. Blood films from these animals should be scanned at low magnification to search for abnormal nucleated cells. Agglutination of erythrocytes is also frequently observed while scanning the slide, perhaps as a result of circulating FLV-antibody complexes. Lymphocytes from cats with lymphosarcoma and leukemia are usually larger than normal large lymphocytes. They have large nuclei relative to cytoplasm, and nuclear shapes may be irregular. Aspirates of bone marrow and fine-needle aspirates of palpable masses should be examined in cats suspected of having lymphosarcoma. The bone marrow aspirates may have variable numbers of immature lymphocytes, and in some instances, complete replacement of hemopoietic cells by the tumor. Cats with abdominal masses are frequently emaciated, which facilitates immobilization and fine-needle aspiration of the tumors. If the masses are lymph nodes, the aspirates contain mainly large lymphocytes, some of which are in mitosis.

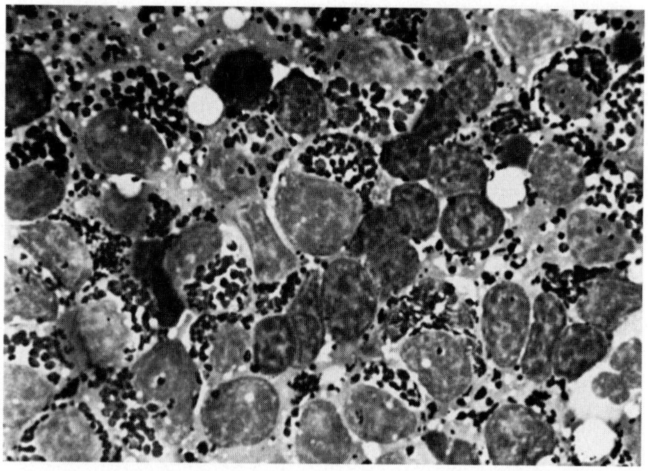

Figure 7-48 Impression smear of lymph node; cat. Granular lymphocyte lymphosarcoma. Note that the predominant cells are lymphocytes with large cytoplasmic granules. Wright-Giemsa stain.

With liver and kidney lymphosarcomas, aspirates contain numerous lymphocytes among hepatocytes and renal tubular epithelial cells, respectively. A form of lymphosarcoma characterized by cells with cytoplasmic granules occurs in the intestine and spleen. The feline leukemia virus has not been isolated from these tumors. Granular lymphocytes are heterogeneous with respect to granule size and number and cytochemical and histochemical reactions. These are tumors of cytotoxic T lymphocytes and natural killer cells (Fig. 7-48).

At necropsy, cats with lymphosarcoma may have diffuse or nodular enlargement of organs such as the liver, kidneys, thymus, and lymph nodes. If enlarged lymph nodes are incised, the surface is soft white and bulges. With thymic lymphosarcomas, a large, gray, soft mass is present in the thoracic cavity (Fig. 7-38). Marrow cavities of long bones are occupied by yellow-white tissue in animals with lymphosarcoma involving the bone marrow. Impression smears should be made of these tissues to augment the histologic examination.

Bovine lymphosarcoma. Enzootic bovine lymphosarcoma is a disease of adult cattle caused by the bovine leukemia virus (BLV), an RNA retrovirus similar to other oncogenic viruses. Its behavior differs from the feline virus because of minimal viral expression in spite of persistence within lymphocytes for the life of the animal. Transmission of the virus is mostly horizontal because of transmission of infected lymphocytes as opposed to transmission of free virus in secretions. Following establishment of infection, circulating antibody appears and is present throughout life. Blood-sucking arthropods or other mechanical means of transferring small numbers of infected lymphocytes are the principal means of spread. The disease has a much higher incidence in dairy cattle in comparison to beef cattle, presumably because dairy cattle husbandry favors viral transmission. Herd surveys have revealed high rates of infection but low incidence of disease.

Clinical expression of enzootic bovine lymphosarcoma has a peak incidence of 6 to 8 years and reflects the location of tumors. Enlargement of one or more superficial lymph nodes is common, and enlarged abdominal and pelvic lymph nodes may be found on rectal palpation. Unilateral or bilateral exophthalmos occurs following involvement of retrobulbar lymphoid tissue. Involvement of the digestive tract may cause persistent diarrhea, and involvement of the right heart may cause congestive heart failure. Nervous system lymphosarcoma is most frequently manifested as posterior paresis or paralysis because of pressure by the extradural mass on the cauda equina or on the lumbar spinal cord or its nerve roots. In addition to the distribution of lesions as described above, most cattle have lesions of lymphosarcoma in the liver and spleen. Involvement of the bone marrow and leukemia may occur in the terminal stages of the disease. Persistent lymphocytosis develops in approximately 30% of infected animals and may last for many years without, or prior to, clinical expression of the disease. Serologic detection of BLV antibody assists in differentiating BLV-induced lymphocytosis from the lymphocytosis induced by chronic bacterial infections.

The etiology of sporadic lymphosarcoma is unknown. The thymic form is characterized by large cranial thoracic masses, respiratory distress, and weight loss in cattle less than 2 years of age. The juvenile form is a disseminated lymphosarcoma and has been reported in fetuses and in calves up to 6 months of age. Lesions are generalized lymph node enlargement, depression, weight loss, and frequently leukemia with markedly elevated numbers of lymphocytes accompanied by anemia and neutropenia. The cutaneous form is rare, occurs in young cattle, and consists of discrete cutaneous plaques or large scabby lesions.

Necropsy findings in all forms of bovine lymphosarcoma reveal characteristic tumors whose location depends on the form of the disease. Enlarged lymph nodes bulge when incised to reveal soft, gray-white tissue that may exude a milky fluid. Large masses, as in thymic lymphosarcoma, may contain areas of necrosis. In addition to tumors in lymph nodes, liver, and spleen, cardiac involvement in enzootic bovine lymphosarcoma is most common in the right atrium, with possible extension to the ventricular myocardium. Abomasal involvement results in a variably thickened wall, with a tendency for mucosal ulceration.

Equine lymphosarcoma. The incidence of lymphosarcoma in horses is lower than that of cattle, dogs, and cats. The distribution of lymphosarcoma in the horse is variable; reports of concurrent leukemia vary from rare to more than 50%. With the exception of the cutaneous disease, most forms result in debility with anemia, hypoproteinemia, and dependent edema. The **multicentric form** is characterized by irregular involvement of peripheral lymph nodes with tumor masses in the mediastinum and abdomen. **Cutaneous** and **subcutaneous lymphosarcoma** in horses, as in other species, are chronic diseases without leukemia or internal organ involvement. The subcutaneous tumors are multiple, well-circumscribed, yellow to white firm nodules in various locations over the body, often involving tendons at joint surfaces.

The **alimentary form** of equine lymphosarcoma is a wasting syndrome, presumably due to involvement of the small intestine, resulting in malabsorption. The large intestine and numerous lymph nodes including thoracic lymph nodes may be involved. The neoplastic lymphocytes from the bowel and enlarged adjacent lymph nodes are frequently plasmacytoid; mitotic figures are rare. **Splenic lymphosarcoma** in the horse is characterized by massive organ enlargement; some cases are leukemic with lymphocyte counts in excess of 100×10^9/L ($100 \times 10^3/mm^3$). In contrast to the alimentary form, most tumors in the other forms are composed of large lymphocytes. Immunophenotyping has identified both B and T lymphocytes in these tumors, with a predominance of neoplastic B lymphocytes. A significant number of diffuse, large B cell lymphosarcomas contain large numbers of T cells and are classified as T cell–rich B cell lymphosarcomas. With the exception of splenic lymphosarcomas, most tumors have some degree of fibrous tissue proliferation. Occasionally, horses with lymphosarcoma have regenerative anemia characterized by an elevated MCV, RDW, and marrow erythroid hyperplasia, in the absence of hemorrhage. Splenic sequestration of erythrocytes could occur in massively enlarged spleens; however, some horses are positive for the direct antiglobulin (Coombs') test consistent with an immune-mediated mechanism of hemolysis.

THE SPLEEN

Structure and Function

The blood supply to the spleen and its sievelike anatomic structure render it an efficient organ for monitoring viability of cells, particularly erythrocytes. Splenic immune functions include trapping of blood-borne antigens with subsequent macrophage T and B lymphocyte responses resulting in the production of antibody and B memory cells.

Spleens have been classified as storage or defense spleens. Although it would be safe to assume that the organ serves both functions, in many species one function often predominates. A spleen that is relatively large, rich in smooth muscle, but poor in lymphoid tissue, such as in the horse, is primarily a storage spleen. In contrast, a smaller spleen that is poor in trabeculae but rich in lymphoid tissue may be regarded as a defense spleen. The rabbit and human spleens are examples of the latter; those of cats, dogs, and cattle have considerable storage capability.

Fundamental to splenic structure and function are the afferent and efferent blood vessels and the white and red pulp. The white pulp consists of lymphocytes and macrophages surrounding central arterioles (periarteriolar lymphoid sheaths). Lymphocytes surrounding arterioles are derived from the thymus (T cells), and those in germinal centers are B cells derived from the bone marrow. In intimate apposition to the germinal center is a corona of B cells surrounded by a mantle zone that merges with the periarteriolar lymphoid sheath. The mantle zone consists of B and T lymphocytes that constantly interchange with those in the blood.

The red pulp is a meshwork of specialized fibroblast-like cells with long, interdigitating filamentous projections called **reticular cells.** Interspersed among the reticular cells are numerous macrophages. The vascular components of the red pulp vary among species, based on the presence or absence of thin-walled venous sinuses. The sinusal spleen of the dog has sinuses, one endothelial cell layer thick, which link terminal arterioles to venules. The endothelial cells contain contractile filaments, which on activation, create gaps between the cell margins to facilitate passage of cells. Their adventitial surface is partially covered by the filamentous projections of reticular cells. The reticular cells, therefore, have a significant effect on the rate of passage of erythrocytes, leukocytes, and platelets through the sinus wall. In the feline and equine nonsinusal spleens, cells are deposited from terminal arterioles into the red pulp, where they traverse the reticular cell–macrophage meshwork before entering terminal venules. The red pulp reticular cells in the canine and equine spleen have an extraordinary large complement of filaments, especially intermediate filaments, and are rich in adrenergic nerve fibers. These contractile cells are ideally suited to shunt blood through the red pulp into the venous circulation or, when appropriate, to facilitate storage of large numbers of erythrocytes and platelets.

A particularly dense population of macrophages (the periarteriolar macrophage sheath) is adjacent to terminal arterioles in the red pulp. This arrangement favors efficient trapping of antigenic material from the plasma, as well as surveillance of passing erythrocytes. The red pulp–reticular cell and macrophage populations retain immature erythrocytes to allow maturation. Erythrocyte inclusions such as nuclear remnants, Heinz bodies, or rickettsial organisms are removed as the cells make their way among the macrophages and through sinusoid walls in sinusal spleens. In dogs, large numbers of nuclear remnants in erythrocytes are a good indication of splenic malfunction. Splenic macrophages have IgG receptors and they remove entire erythrocytes, or portions of erythrocyte membranes, and platelets in immune-mediated hemolytic anemias and thrombocytopenias. In addition to surveillance of cells as they pass through the spleen, it is also responsible for removal of bacteria during bacteremia and septicemia and rickettsial organisms. Resurgence of infections such as anaplasmosis, eperythrozoonosis, and hemobartonellosis may occur following splenectomy.

Splenic Disorders

Atrophy and Enlargement of the Spleen

Atrophy and enlargement of the spleen may be difficult to distinguish from normal variations in organ size. The common causes of splenic atrophy and enlargement among domestic animal species are listed in Table 7-7. **Atrophy** results from mechanisms such as hemosiderosis, old age, wasting diseases, and induration following prolonged splenic congestion. Viral diseases such as bovine virus diarrhea and drugs such as corticosteroids destroy lymphocytes, resulting in splenic atrophy. The atrophic spleen is small and firm, with a shriveled capsule. Accumulation of iron and calcium as siderotic nodules beneath the capsule is a frequent finding in the spleen of old dogs (Fig. 7-49). Hemosiderin is frequently present within splenic macrophages, especially following prolonged congestion. Episodes of hemolysis mediated by splenic erythrophagocytosis and chronic inflammatory states result in increased numbers of hemosiderin-laden macrophages.

Rupture of the spleen occurs frequently in dogs. The spleen may exist in two or more portions with various irregular fibrotic fissures reflecting trauma at some time in the animal's life.

An enlarged, uniform spleen **(splenomegaly)** is a common postmortem finding in animals and occurs following congestion, hyperplasia, or neoplasia. Congested spleens are turgid and ooze dark blood when incised, features which are accentuated if autolysis is rapid as in anthrax. Splenomegaly due to proliferation of cells results in a meaty spleen with little oozing of blood when incised.

Splenomegaly from splenic congestion occurs in animals euthanatized with barbiturates, in acute hemolytic anemias due to retention of erythrocytes in the red pulp, and in septicemias and enterotoxemias. This nonspecific reaction in septicemias may be caused by the organisms as well as products of the inflammatory response. Microscopically, the major change is congestion and expansion of the red pulp, which may then be far larger than the white pulp. In septicemias, neutrophils may be present throughout the red and white pulp.

Torsion of the spleen results in marked congestion and splenomegaly due to occlusion of the splenic vein.

Table 7-7 Causes of Splenic Atrophy or Enlargement (Splenomegaly) in Animals

Atrophy
Cachexia
Old age
Viral diseases
Corticosteroid drugs
Hemosiderosis

Splenomegaly

	Firm spleen (increased cellularity)	*Blood-filled spleen*
Cattle and sheep	Salmonellosis Lymphosarcoma Babesiosis (subacute) Anaplasmosis Trypanosomiasis	Anthrax Congestion Septicemias Toxemias Babesiosis (acute)
Horses	Equine infectious anemia Lymphosarcoma Metastatic melanoma Immune-mediated hemolytic anemia Salmonellosis	Anthrax
Pigs	Salmonellosis Erysipelas Lymphosarcoma Eperythrozoonosis African swine fever	Congestion Torsion Septicemias
Dogs and cats	Lymphosarcoma Immune-mediated hemolytic anemia Histoplasmosis Amyloidosis Leishmaniasis Mast cell sarcoma (cats) Lymphoid hyperplasia* Myelogenous leukemia Malignant histiocytosis Erythrocyte sarcoma (cats)	Barbiturates Torsion (dogs) Hemangiomas* Hemangiosarcomas*

*Nodular
Modified from Valli VEO. The hematopoietic system. In: Jubb KVF, Kennedy PC, Palmer N, eds. Pathology of Domestic Animals. 4th ed. New York: Academic Press, 1993:101.

Ultimately, occlusion of the artery occurs, resulting in ischemia, which is followed by hemolysis and diffusion of hemoglobin through the devitalized splenic capsule. This process results in hemoglobinemia and hemoglobinuria.

Splenomegaly due to cellular proliferation results in a firm spleen. This occurs in chronic hemolytic anemias in which the gradual accumulation of macrophages results in a less congested and more cellular red pulp. Numerous erythroid progenitor cells (extramedullary hemopoiesis) may contribute to the cellularity. Splenitis and septic thrombosis of the splenic vein may be observed in cattle with traumatic reticuloperitonitis. The cut surface of the spleen has irregular white to yellow areas due to abscesses and necrosis (Fig. 7-50). Microscopically, these areas consist of necrosis with neutrophils and foci of mixed bacterial populations.

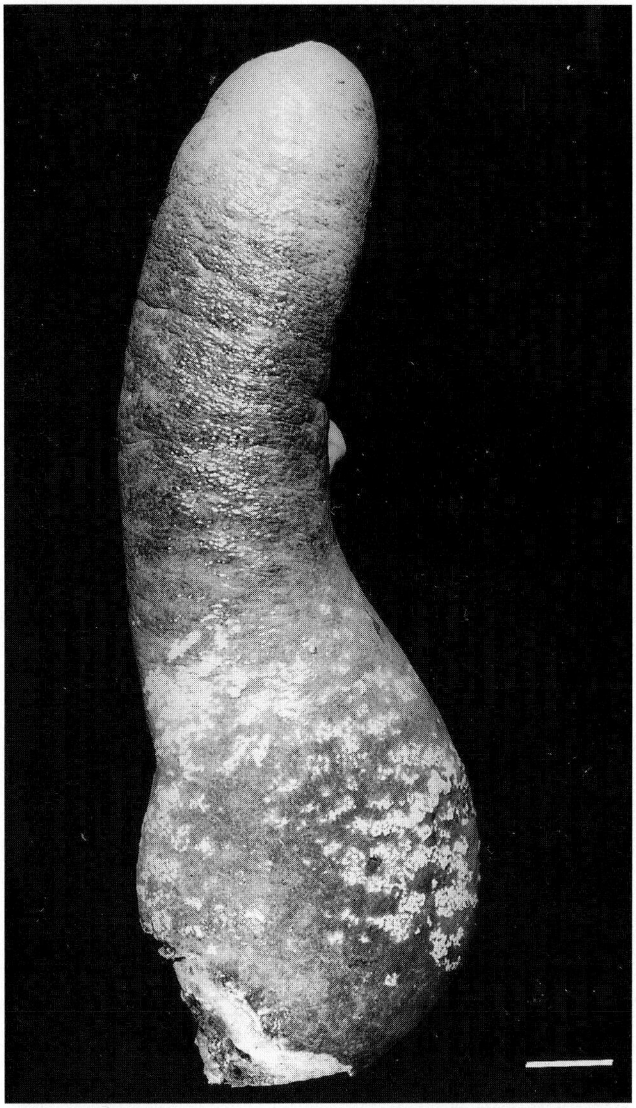

Figure 7-49 Spleen; dog. Subcapsular siderocalcific nodules formed by deposits of iron and calcium. Bar = 2 cm. *Courtesy of G.L. Mason.*

Diffuse infiltration of neoplastic cells into the spleen results in a uniformly firm spleen and occurs in lymphocytic, granulocytic, and mast cell leukemias and in plasma cell sarcomas. Microscopically, the red pulp is completely occupied by tumor cells, and there is usually effacement of lymphoid follicles in the white pulp.

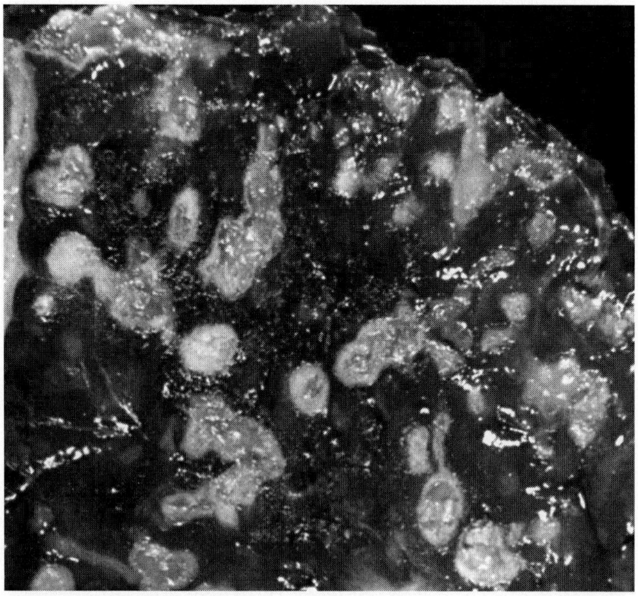

Figure 7-50 Spleen; cow. Abscesses and areas of necrosis in the spleen caused by bacteremia from septic thrombosis of the portal vein. *Courtesy of E.G. Clark.*

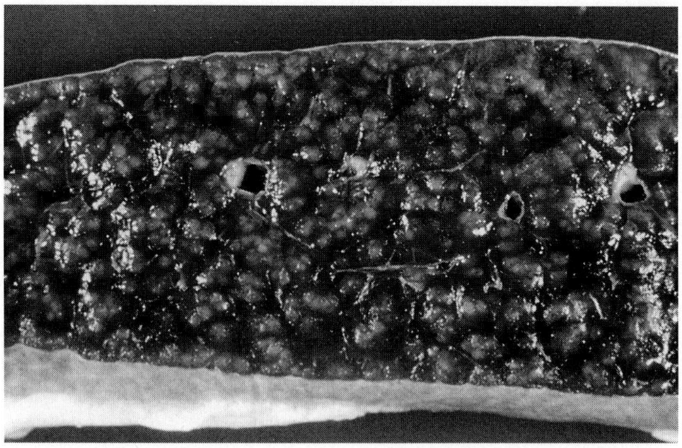

Figure 7-51 Spleen; pig. Leptospirosis. Nodular hyperplasia. *Courtesy of E.G. Clark.*

A spleen enlarged for any reason is prone to thrombosis and infarction. This occurs because blood flow is compromised by congestion or infiltration of the red pulp by cells. In granulocytic leukemias and plasma cell sarcomas, the thrombotic process is enhanced by factors that contribute to intravascular coagulation. In septicemias, blood flow may be compromised by swelling and proliferation of endothelial cells. Infectious and immune-mediated causes of vasculitis and intravascular coagulation and thrombosis may result in splenic infarcts. Thrombosis of splenic vessels can occur in animals with valvular endocarditis and, if septic, abscesses and necrosis are potential sequelae.

Nodular Disorders of the Spleen

The presence of discrete nodules beneath the capsule or that protrude from the cut surface of the spleen is indicative of benign nodular lymphoid hyperplasia (Fig. 7-51). It is most common in the dog but is seen in all species. The nodules may be up to 2 cm in diameter, and they vary from gray to red pink. The largest nodules may have yellow centers because of necrosis.

Splenic hematomas are common in dogs, but the cause is often not obvious at necropsy. Small hematomas must be differentiated from nodular hyperplasia and large ones from hemangiomas and hemangiosarcomas.

Neoplastic Disorders of the Spleen

The endothelial cell neoplasms, hemangiomas, and hemangiosarcomas, occur in the spleen. They occur frequently in older dogs of the large breeds and are prone to rupture and cause significant intraperitoneal hemorrhage. The presence of anemia with reticulocytosis in many of these dogs is indicative of bleeding from these tumors over a period of time.

Splenic involvement in bovine lymphosarcoma is variable, but a significant incidence occurs in both the enzootic and juvenile forms of the disease. A high incidence of splenic involvement occurs in canine, feline, and equine lymphosarcoma. In most cases, the organ is uniformly enlarged, and microscopically the white pulp follicles are displaced and the red pulp is occupied by neoplastic lymphocytes. Discrete masses of lymphosarcoma can occur in the spleen and are white to yellow when incised (Fig. 7-52).

Granulocytic leukemia in the dog usually results in marked splenomegaly caused by infiltration and proliferation of neoplastic granulocytes. Plasma cell sarcomas in dogs, and mast cell and erythrocytic sarcomas in cats, frequently result in splenomegaly. Splenic aspirates are more commonly being attempted in dogs, cats, and horses and are a valuable adjunct to bone marrow aspirates for diagnosis of hemopoietic cell sarcomas. In contrast to aspirates from normal spleens, which reveal many erythrocytes, lymphocytes of varying size, and a few macrophages, aspirates, or imprints from fresh tissue at postmortem examination from neoplastically infiltrated spleens are dominated by a homogeneous population of sarcoma cells.

The splenic parenchyma is not fertile ground for the establishment of metastatic carcinomas, and they are only occasionally found late in the course of disseminated

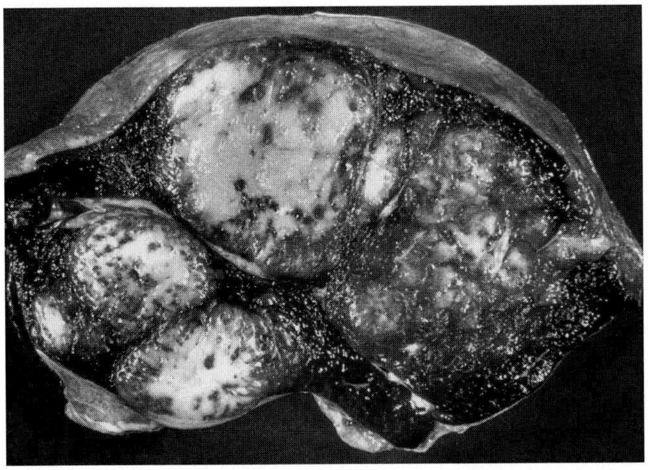

Figure 7-52 Spleen; horse. Lymphosarcoma. *Courtesy of E.G. Clark.*

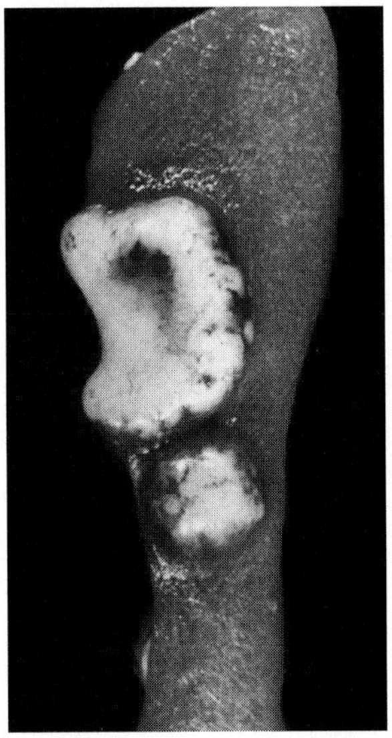

Figure 7-53 Spleen; cat. Metastatic bronchogenic carcinoma. *Courtesy of E.G. Clark.*

neoplastic disease. Although uncommon, implantation of mesotheliomas and carcinomas to the splenic capsule can occur (Fig. 7-53).

Acknowledgments

I wish to thank Ian Shirley and Kathy Kaspell for preparation of photographs. The chapter "The Hematopoietic System," written by V.E.O. Valli in the fourth edition of the book, *Pathology of Domestic Animals,* edited by K.V.F. Jubb, Peter C. Kennedy, and Nigel Palmer, was an important source of information and is hereby acknowledged. I also wish to thank Drs. Marion Jackson and Dorothy Middleton for reading portions of the manuscript, and Dr. V.E.O. Valli for personal communications.

Suggested Readings

Atwater SW, Powers BE, Park RD, et al. Thymoma in dogs: 23 cases (1980-1991). J Am Vet Med Assoc 1994; 205:1007-1013.

Berent LM, Messick JB, Cooper SK. Detection of *Haemobartonella felis* in cats with experimentally induced acute and chronic infections, using a polymerase chain reaction assay. Am J Vet Res 1998; 59:1215-1220.

Boudreaux MK, Crager C, Dillon AR, et al. Identification of an intrinsic platelet function defect in Spitz dogs. J Vet Int Med 1994; 8:93-98.

Boudreaux MK, Kvam K, Dillon AR, et al. Type I Glanzmann's thrombasthenia in a Great Pyrenees dog. Vet Pathol 1996; 33:503-511.

Callan MB, Bennett JS, Phillips DK, et al. Inherited platelet δ-storage pool disease in dogs causing severe bleeding: An animal model for specific ADP deficiency. Thromb Haemost 1995; 74:949-953.

Calverley DC, Liebman HA. Disseminated intravascular coagulation. In: Hoffman R, Benz EJ, Shattil SJ, et al. eds. Hematology. Basic Principles and Practice. 3rd ed. New York: Churchill Livingstone, 2000:1983.

Catalfamo JL, Raymond SL, White JG, et al. Defective platelet-fibrinogen interaction in hereditary canine thrombopathia. Blood 1986; 67:1568-1577.

Colbatzky F, Hermanns W. Acute megakaryoblastic leukemia in one cat and two dogs. Vet Pathol 1993; 30:186-194.

Comazzi S, Paltrinieri S, Manfredi MT, et al. Diagnosis of canine babesiosis by Percoll gradient separation of parastized erythrocytes. J Vet Diagn Invest 1999; 11:102-104.

Dardenne M, Savino W. Control of thymus physiology by peptidic hormones and neuropeptides. Immunology Today 1994; 15:514-523.

Duncan JR, Prasse KW, Mahaffey EA. Veterinary Laboratory Medicine, Clinical Pathology. 3rd ed. Ames, Iowa: Iowa University Press, 1994.

Duval D, Giger U. Vaccine-associated immune-mediated hemolytic anemia in the dog. J Vet Intern Med 1996; 10:290-295.

Estrow Z, Kurzrock R, Talpaz M. Cytokines and their antagonists in myeloid disorders. Semin Hematol 1995; 32:220-231.

Fisher DJ, Naydan D, Werner LL, et al. Immunophenotyping lymphomas in dogs: A comparison of results from fine needle aspirate and needle biopsy samples. Vet Clin Pathol 1995; 24:118-123.

Franceschi C, Monti D, Sansoni P, et al. The immunology of exceptional individuals: The lesson of centenarians. Immunology Today 1995; 16:12-16.

Frojmovic MM, Wong T, Searcy GP. Platelets from bleeding Simmental cattle have a long delay in both ADP-activated expression of GpIIB-IIIA receptors and fibrinogen-dependent platelet aggregation. Thromb Haemost 1996; 76:1047-1052.

Fushuku S, Okamoto K, Deguchi E, et al. Changes of platelet cytoskeleton proteins following platelet aggregation induced by collagen and platelet membrane glycoprotein in Japanese black cattle with δ-storage pool deficiency. J Vet Med Sci 1998; 60:1107-1112.

Gale KR, Dimmock CM, Gartside M, et al. Anaplasma marginale: Detection of carrier cattle by PCR-ELISA. Int J Parasitol 1996; 26:1103-1109.

Giger U, Bucheler J. Transfusion of type-A and type-B blood to cats. J Am Vet Med Assoc 1991; 198:411-418.

Girard JP, Springer TA. High endothelial venules (HEVs): Specialized endothelium for lymphocyte migration. Immunology Today 1995; 16:449-457.

Grindem CB, Page RL, Ammerman BE, et al. Immunophenotypic comparison of blood and lymph node from dogs with lymphoma. Vet Clin Pathol 1998; 27:16-20.

Guglielmino R, Canese MG, Miniscalco B, et al. Comparison of clinical, morphological, immunophenotypical and cytochemical characteristics of LGL leukemia/lymphoma in dog, cat and human. Eur J Histochem 1997; 41(Suppl 2):23-24.

Harvey JW. Canine thrombocytic Ehrlichiosis. In: Greene CE, ed. Infectious Diseases of the Dog and Cat. 2nd ed. Philadelphia: Saunders, 1998:147.

Haynes BF, Hale LP. Thymic function, aging, and AIDS. Hosp Pract 1999; 34:59-88.

Herzog RW, Hagstrom JM, Yang EY, et al. Long-term phenotypic correction of hemophilia B in a large animal model of AAV-mediated gene transfer. Blood 1998; 92(Supp 1):153a. [Abstract].

Hinrichs U, Puhl S, Rutteman GR, et al. Lymphangiosarcomas in cats: A retrospective study of 12 cases. Vet Pathol 1999; 36:164-167.

Hoover JP, Walker DB, Hedges JD. Cytauxzoonosis in cats: Eight cases (1985-1992). J Am Vet Med Assoc 1994; 205:455-460.

Hutchison JM, Garry FB, Belknap EB, et al. Prospective characterization of the clinicopathologic and immunologic features of an immundeficiency syndrome affecting juvenile llamas. Vet Immunol Immunopathol 1995; 49:209-227.

Inaba M, Yawata A, Koshino I, et al. Defective anion transport and marked spherocytosis with membrane instability caused by hereditary total deficiency of red cell band 3 in cattle due to a nonsense mutation. J Clin Invest 1996; 97:1804-1817.

Jain NC, Blue JT, Grindem CB, et al. Proposed criteria for classification of acute myleoid leukemia in dogs and cats. Vet Clin Pathol 1990; 20:63-82.

Jandl JH. Blood: Textbook of Hematology. 2nd ed. Boston: Little, Brown, & Company, 1996.

Janeway CA, Travers P. Immunobiology: The Immune System in Health and Disease. 3rd ed. New York: Garland, 1997.

Kariya K, Konno A, Ishida T. Perforin-like immunoreactivity in four cases of lymphoma of large granular lymphocytes in the cat. Vet Pathol 1997; 34:156-159.

Kaushansky K. Thrombopoietin. N Engl J Med 1998; 339:746-754.

Kelley LC, Mahaffey EA. Equine malignant lymphomas: Morphologic and immunohistochemical classification. Vet Pathol 1998; 35: 241-252.

Knowler C, Giger U, Dodds WJ, et al. Factor XI deficiency in Kerry blue terriers. J Am Vet Med Assoc 1994; 205:1557-1561.

Krantz SB. Pathogenesis and treatment of the anemia of chronic disease. Am J Med Sci 1994; 307:353-359.

Landsverk T, Mcl.Press C. immune system. In: Dellmann HD, Eurell JA, eds. Veterinary Histology. 5th ed. Baltimore: Williams & Wilkins, 1998:128.

Latimer KS, Bounous DI, Collatos C, et al. Extreme eosinophilia with disseminated eosinophilic granulomatous disease in a horse. Vet Clin Pathol 1996; 25:23-26.

Lewis DC, Meyers KM. Studies of platelet-bound and serum platelet-bindable immunoglobulins in dogs with idiopathic thrombocytopenic purpura. Exp Hematol 1996; 24:696-701.

Lewis DC, Meyers KM, Callan MB, et al. Detection of platelet-bound and serum platelet-bindable antibodies for diagnosis of idiopathic thrombocytopenic purpura in dogs. J Am Vet Med Assoc 1995; 206: 47-52.

Lobetti RG. Canine babesiosis. Compend Contin Educ Pract Vet 1998; 20:418-430.

Magnarelli LA, Van Andel AE, Ijdo JW, et al. Serologic testing of horses for granulocytic ehrlichiosis, using indirect flourescent antibody staining and immunoblot analysis. Am J Vet Res 1999; 60:631-635.

Marone G, Casolaro V, Patella V, et al. Molecular and cellular biology of mast cells and basophils. Int Arch Allergy Immunol 1997; 114:207-217.

Milner RJ, Pearson J, Nesbit JW, et al. Immunophenotypic classification of canine malignant lymphoma on formalin-fixed paraffin wax-embedded tissue by means of CD3 and CD79a markers. Onderstepoort J Vet Res 1996; 63:309-313.

Neer TM. Ehrlichiosis. In: Greene CE, ed. Infectious Diseases of the Dog and Cat. 2nd ed. Philadelphia: Saunders, 1998:139.

Newlands CE, Houston DM, Vasconcelos DY. Hperferritinemia associated with malignant histiocytosis in a dog. J Am Vet Med Assoc 1994; 205:849-851.

Raskin RE, Krehbiel JD. Prevalence of leukemic blood and bone marrow in dogs with multicentric lymphoma. J Am Vet Med Assoc 1989; 194:1427-1429.

Rieger M, Schwarz HP, Turecek PL. Identification of the genetic defect in type III von Willebrand factor deficient Dutch Kooiker dogs. Blood 1997; 90(Suppl 1):468a. [Abstract].

Rikihisa Y, Kawhahara M, Wen B, et al. Western immunoblot analysis of *Haembobartonella muris* and comparison of the 16S rRNA gene sequences of *H. muris, H. felis* and *Eperythrozoon suis.* J Clin Microbiol 1997; 35: 823-829.

Rothenberg ME. Eosinophilia. N Engl J Med 1998; 338:1592-1600.

Schaer M, Harvey JW, Calerwood-Mays M, et al. Pyruvate kinase deficiency causing hemolytic anemia with secondary hemochromatosis in a Cairn terrier. J Am Anim Hosp Assoc 1992; 28:233-239.

Smith BF, Stedman H, Rajpurohit Y, et al. Molecular basis of canine muscle type phosphofructokinase deficiency. J Biol Chem 1996; 271:20070-20074.

Sreedhara R, Itagaki I, Hakim RM. Uremic patients have decreased shear-induced aggregation mediated by decreased availablity of glycoprotein IIb-IIIa receptors. Am J Kidney Dis 1996; 27:355-364.

Steele KE, Saunders GK, Coleman GD. T-cell-rich B-cell lymphoma in a cat. Vet Pathol 1997; 34:47-49.

Sthoeger ZM, Sthoeger D, Shtalrid M, et al. Mechanism of autoimmune hemolytic anemia in chronic lymphocytic leukemia. Am J Hematol 1993; 43:259-264.

Valli VEO. The hematopoietic system. In: Jubb KVF, Kennedy PC, Palmer N, eds. Pathology of Domestic Animals. Vol 3, 4th ed. San Diego, Calif.: Academic Press, 1993:101.

Venta PJ, Li J Schall WD, et al. A leaky splice site junction mutation causes recessively inherited type I von Willebrand's disease in the Doberman pinscher. J Vet Intern Med. 2000; 14:10-19.

Walkowiak B, Borkowska E, Koziolkiewicz W, et al. Platelet membrane fluidity and intraplatelet Ca^{2+} mobilization are affected in uraemia. Eur J Haematol 1997; 58:350-356.

Walton RM, Burkhard MJ, Frank AA, et al. Malignant histiocytosis in a domestic cat: Cytomorphologic and immunohistochemical features. Vet Clin Pathol 1997; 26:56-60.

Whitney KM, Lothrop CD. Genetic test for pyruvate kinase deficiency of Basenjis. J Am Vet Med Assoc 1995; 207:918-921.

Zeleznik-Le NJ, Nucifora G, Rowley JD. The molecular biology of myeloproliferative disorders as revealed by chromosomal abnormalities. Semin Hematol 1995; 32:201-219.

Lymph Nodes

Ellis J, Hassard L, Clark E, et al. Isolation of circovirus from lesions of pigs with postweaning multisystemic wasting syndrome. Can Vet J 1998; 39:44-51.

Ellis J, Krakowka S, Lairmore M, et al. Reproduction of lesions of postweaning multisystemic wasting syndrome in gnotobiotic piglets. J Vet Diagn Invest 1999; 11:3-14.

Kiupel M, Stevenson GW, Mittal SK, et al. Circovirus-like viral associated disease in weaned pigs in Indiana. Vet Pathol 1998; 35:303-307.

Morozov I, Sirinarumitr T, Sorden SD, et al. Detection of a novel strain of porcine circovirus in pigs with postweaning multisystemic wasting syndrome. J Clin Microbiol 1998; 36:2535-2541.

Spleen

Day MJ, Lucke VM, Pearson H. A review of pathological diagnoses made from 87 canine splenic biopsies. J Small Anim Pract 1995; 36:426-433.

DiBartola SP, Tarr MJ, Webb DM, Giger U. Familial renal amyloidosis in Chinese Shar Pei dogs. J Am Vet Med Assoc 1990; 197:483-487.

Hardie EM, Vaden SL, Spaulding K, Malarkey DE. Splenic infarction in 16 dogs: A retrospective study. J Vet Intern Med 1995; 9:141-148.

Hendrick MJ, Brooks JJ, Bruce EH. Six cases of malignant fibrous histiocytoma of the canine. Vet Pathol 1992; 29:351-354.

Kapatkin AS, Mullen HS, Matthiesen DT, Patnaik AK. Leiomyosarcoma in dogs: 44 cases (1983-1988). J Am Vet Med Assoc 1992; 201:1077-1079.

McGee ED, Fritz DL, Ezzell JW, et al. Anthrax in a dog. Vet Pathol 1994; 31:471-473.

Neath PJ, Brockman DJ, Saunders HM. Retrospective analysis of 19 cases of isolated torsion of the splenic pedicle in dogs. J Small Anim Pract 1997; 38:387-392.

Risoe C, Hall C, Smiseth OA. Blood volume changes in liver and spleen during cardiogenic shock in dogs. Am J Physiol 1991; 261(6 Pt2): H1763-1768.

Spangler WL, Culbertson MR. Prevalence, type, and importance of splenic diseases in dogs: 1,480 cases (1985-1989). J Am Vet Med Assoc 1992; 200:829-834.

Spangler WL, Culbertson MR, Kass PH. Primary mesenchymal (nonangiomatous/nonlymphomatous) neoplasms occurring in the canine spleen: Anatomic classification, immunohistochemistry, and mitotic activity correlated with patient survival. Vet Pathol 1994; 31:37-47.

Spangler WL, Kass PH. Pathologic and prognostic characteristics of splenomegaly in dogs due to fibrohistiocytic nodules: 98 cases. Vet Pathol 1998; 35:488-498.

Wood CA, Moore AS, Gliatto JM, et al. Prognosis for dogs with stage I or II splenic hemangiosarcoma treated by splenectomy alone: 32 cases (1991-1993). J Am Anim Hosp Assoc 1998; 34:417-421.

Zhao D, Yamaguchi R, Tateyama S, et al. Canine splenic hemangiosarcoma with abdominal dissemination. J Vet Med Sci 1994; 56:753-755.

Bone Marrow

Raskin RE. Myelopoiesis and myeloproliferative disorders. Vet Clin North Am Small Anim Pract 1996; 26:1023-1042.

Thymus

Beeson D, Bond AP, Corlett L, et al. Thymus, thymoma, and specific T cells in myasthenia gravis. Ann N Y Acad Sci 1998; 841:371-387.

Bradley GA, Tye J, Lozano-Alarcon F, et al. Hemopericardium in a dog due to hemorrhage originating in a heart base thymic remnant. J Vet Diagn Invest 1992; 4:211.

Coolman BR, Brewer WG, D'Andrea GH, Lenz SD. Severe idiopathic thymic hemorrhage in two littermate dogs. J Am Vet Med Assoc 1994; 205:1152-1153.

Day MJ. Review of thymic pathology in 30 cats and 36 dogs. J Small Anim Pract 1997; 38:393-403.

Gores BR, Berg J, Carpenter JL, Aronsohn MG. Surgical treatment of thymoma in cats: 12 cases (1987-1992). J Am Vet Med Assoc 1994; 204:1782-1785.

Rusbridge C, White RN, Elwood CM, Wheeler SJ. Treatment of acquired myasthenia gravis associated with thymoma in two dogs. J Small Anim Pract 1996; 37:376-380.

van der Linde-Sipman JS, van Dijk JE. Hematomas in the thymus in dogs. Vet Pathol 1987; 24:59-61.

Vincent A, Willcox N, Hill M, et al. Determinant spreading and immune responses to acetylcholine receptors in myasthenia gravis. Immunol Rev 1998; 164:157-168.

CHAPTER **8**

The Nervous System

RALPH W. STORTS
DONALD L. MONTGOMERY

CENTRAL NERVOUS SYSTEM

Structure and Function

The central nervous system (CNS) consists of a parenchyma containing neurons, neuroglia, blood vessels, ependymal cells, and choroid plexus. The exterior of the CNS is covered by the meninges. Except for the meninges, these components are arranged to form two basic parts of the CNS, the gray and white matter. The gray matter is typified by numerous neuronal cell bodies plus a feltwork of intermingled axons and dendrites, their synaptic junctions, and processes of oligodendroglia, astrocytes, and microglia. This network of processes in the gray matter is referred to as the **neuropil.** The white matter is characterized by prominently myelinated axons that extend from neuronal cell bodies of the gray matter, plus the presence of oligodendroglia, astrocytes, and microglia.

Neuroglia include astrocytes, oligodenroglia, microglia, and ependymal cells. The meninges, which consists of the dura mater, arachnoid membrane/subarachnoid space, and pia mater, form an outer covering of the brain and spinal cord. The neuroglia and meninges are discussed in detail below.

The cellular elements of the CNS vary in their susceptibility to injury. Neurons are the most sensitive. The more resistant glial cells often react to injury by an increase in size, number, or both. Because the response of the neuron to injury is frequently necrosis followed by its disappearance, in chronic diseases the response of the glia to injury may be more obvious microscopically.

Neurons

Neuronal cell bodies vary considerably in size and shape, from very small lymphocyte-like granule cells of the cerebellar cortex to the large neurons of the lateral vestibular nucleus and ventral gray matter of the spinal cord. Their nuclei tend to be vesicular to spherical in shape, are usually centrally located, and often, particularly in large neurons, contain a prominent central nucleolus. Focal arrays of rough endoplasmic reticulum and polysomes termed Nissl substance are characteristic features (Figs. 8-1 and 8-2). Nissl substance is responsible for the production of proteins that are involved in many vital processes including development of cytoskeletal components that are involved in axoplasmic transport (flow of axoplasm along axons) and regeneration of peripheral nerves.

REACTION TO INJURY. The appearance of the neuronal cell body can vary according to the injury that occurs. Characteristic changes of the neuronal cell body are associated with axonal injury (central chromatolysis), ischemia (ischemic cell change), lysosomal enzyme deficiencies (enlargement of the cell body resulting from alteration of lysosomes), aging (accumulation of lipofuscin pigment), and certain neuronal degenerative diseases (excess accumulation of neurofilaments). Additionally, special features accompany certain viral infections (intranuclear or intracytoplasmic inclusion body formation or both [as with intracytoplasmic Negri body formation in rabies]) and prominent cytoplasmic vacuolation (typical of spongiform encephalopathies such as scrapie).

RESPONSE OF NEURONS FOLLOWING INJURY TO THEIR AXONS THAT EXTEND TO THE PERIPHERY. An example of this type of injury involves somatic motor neurons whose cell bodies are located in the brain and spinal cord with axons extending peripherally in peripheral nerves to innervate skeletal muscle. Axons of motor neurons whose cell bodies are located in the brain are in cranial nerves III, IV, V, VI, VII, IX, X, XI, and XII, while axons of spinal motor neurons, with cell bodies in the ventral gray matter of the spinal cord, are located in ventral spinal nerves. After axonal injury (e.g., crush or transection), the change that occurs in the cell body is referred to as **central chromatolysis** or the **axonal reaction.** Central chromatolysis is indicative of enhanced synthesis of transport and structural proteins required for regeneration of the axon and reestablishment of fast and slow axonal transport systems. The extent to which central chromatolysis develops is related to the degree and location of axonal injury. It is more prominent, and can even be followed by neuronal death, the more severe the axonal injury and the closer the axonal injury is to the cell body. The time required for recovery of cell bodies can be several months and in most cases will vary

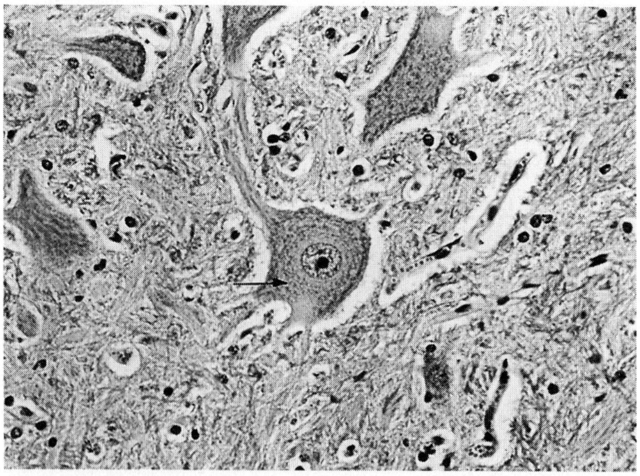

Figure 8-1 Spinal cord, ventral horn; dog. Normal animal. This normal motor neuron *(center)* has a centrally positioned nucleus and contains cytoplasmic Nissl substance *(arrow)*. H & E stain.

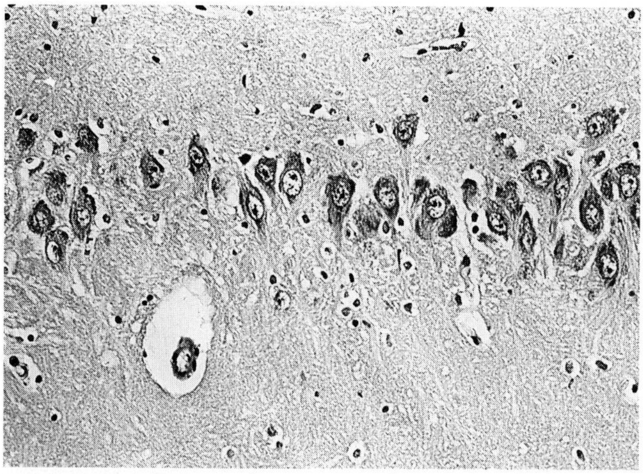

Figure 8-2 Hippocampus, pyramidal neurons; normal dog. The pyramidal neurons are normal, are smaller, and have less prominent Nissl substance than the motor neurons depicted in Fig. 8-1. H & E stain.

from 3 to 6 months, depending on the severity of the axonal injury and the length of axon regenerated.

Microscopically, central chromatolysis is characterized by swelling of the neuronal cell body, dispersion of central Nissl substance, and peripheral displacement of the nucleus (Fig. 8-3, and see Figs. 8-36 and 8-47). Onset is within 24 to 48 hours and reaches its maximum in about 18 days following axonal injury. The change in the axon distal to the point of injury, which is referred to as **Wallerian degeneration,** is first evident within 24 hours of injury. Wallerian degeneration is initially characterized by irregularity of the axonal diameter that is followed after 48 to 72 hours by fragmentation of the axon and myelin along its length. This axonal alteration is followed by disintegration, and usually there is no evidence of the axon remaining by the second week after the injury.

Changes in the myelin sheath surrounding myelinated axons are evident by 28 to 96 hours after injury when axonal disintegration is well advanced. Initially, there are irregularities in the sheath accompanied by folding, lamellar splitting, fracturing, and fragmentation. The fragmented components of the sheath can form droplets (termed ellipsoids), which surround and enclose isolated fragments and debris of the former axon. Both axonal and myelin debris are then removed by macrophages through phagocytosis. Degeneration of myelin is usually completed by the end of the second week, although evidence of myelin debris can be detectable up to 1 to 3 months after axonal injury (i.e., the time required for macrophages to phagocytose and clear the debris).

If the neuronal cell body survives the injury to its axon, regeneration from the proximal stump can occur. The degree of axonal regeneration depends on the status of the endoneurial tube distal to the original point of injury. The normal endoneurial tube and its contents consist (from outside inward) of (1) a connective tissue investment referred to as the endoneurium, (2) the basement membrane that surrounds the Schwann cell plus the Schwann cell cytoplasm, (3) the myelin sheath of myelinated axons, and (4) the axon. Approximately 24 to 72 hours after axonal injury, the endoneurial tube, formed by persisting basement membrane and endoneurium, contains degenerating remnants of the previously existing axon along with Schwann cells. Schwann cells begin to proliferate and eventually form a longitudinal column of cells referred to as the **bands of Büngner.**

If the endoneurial tube remains intact, as can occur following compression injury to a peripheral nerve, neural regeneration through the formation of axonal sprouts can occur. A regenerating sprout from the proximal axonal stump can enter the column of Schwann cells and regenerate uninterrupted along its original pathway to the periphery, reestablishing innervation with an end organ (e.g., skeletal muscle). Such axons can also become remyelinated and regain their physiologic function of impulse transmission. Because of axoplasmic flow, a regenerating neuron lengthens at a rate of approximately 1 to 4 mm per day. Although the time required for axonal regeneration can vary depending on the length of axon to be regenerated, examples of times required for morphologic and functional recovery following crush injury of a peripheral nerve are 250 to 300 and 456 to 486 days, respectively. If, however, the integrity of the endoneurial tube is destroyed, as would occur after complete severance of a peripheral nerve, regeneration might not occur. In such a case, the proximal axonal stump might not reach the distal endoneurial tube because of fibrous connective tissue proliferation (scar formation) at the site of axonal

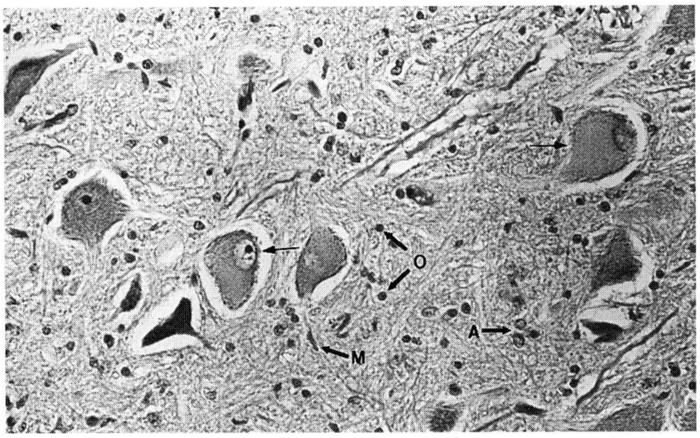

Figure 8-3 Neurons, facial nucleus; dog. Central chromatolysis. Compare with Fig. 8-1. Two cells have eccentric nuclei *(arrows);* neurons in the center and to the right have pale central cytoplasm. The cell body of the neuron to the right is also swollen. Note the normal astrocytic *(A),* oligodendroglial *(O),* and microglial *(M)* nuclei. H & E stain.

severance. Regenerating axons may also enter inappropriate endoneurial tubes resulting in improper impulse transmission (e.g., a sensory neuron axonal sprout entering an endoneurial tube intended for a nerve innervating a muscle).

Response of Neurons Following Injury to Their Axons That Remain Within the CNS. The response of the cell body after injury of axons that remain within the CNS (e.g., upper motor neurons) can vary. Upper motor neurons make up the motor system confined to the CNS that is responsible for initiation of voluntary movement, maintenance of tone for support of the body against gravity, and regulation of posture. Some cell bodies have central chromatolysis; others initially have central chromatolysis followed by atrophy and death (e.g., by apoptosis), and others undergo atrophy. Infrequently, central chromatolysis can result from causes other than specific axonal injury (e.g., with avian encephalomyelitis and dietary niacin deficiency in human beings).

Wallerian degeneration within the CNS is similar to that described for the peripheral nervous system (PNS), except that in the CNS degenerated axons and myelin sheaths can remain for months before complete removal. Affected axons and their myelin sheaths undergo a rather characteristic series of changes as they degenerate. Initially, axons form linear and bulbous swellings at, and some distance from, the site of injury (Figs. 8-4 and 8-5). The axonal enlargements can be seen as early as a few hours at the site of injury and remain prominent, particularly for the first week or so. The surrounding myelin sheath is usually distended to create a space between the sheath and the axonal swelling (Fig. 8-4). Progressively, such affected axons and myelin sheaths fragment along their length (Fig.

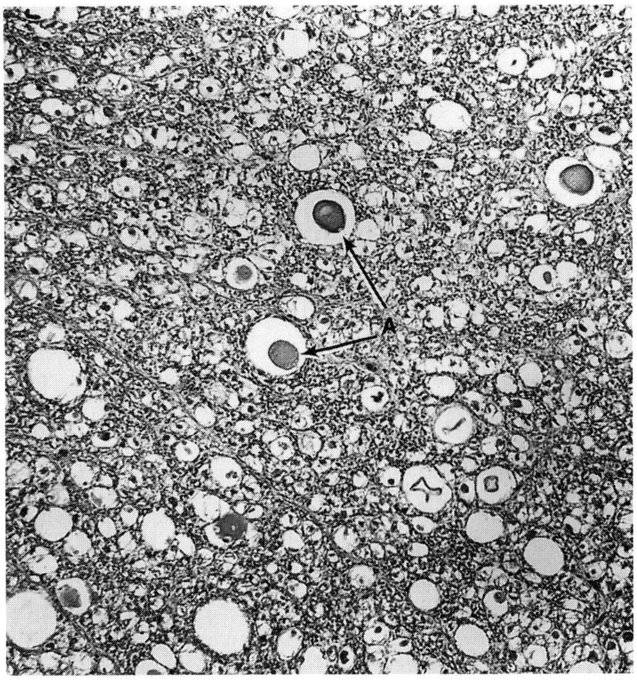

Figure 8-4 Spinal cord, lumbar; cow with posterior paralysis for 2 days secondary to trauma. Wallerian degeneration of axons in the white matter. Several axons *(A)* are markedly swollen and their myelin sheaths are distended. Empty spaces may indicate absence of axons that have longitudinally separated at the plane of section. H & E stain.

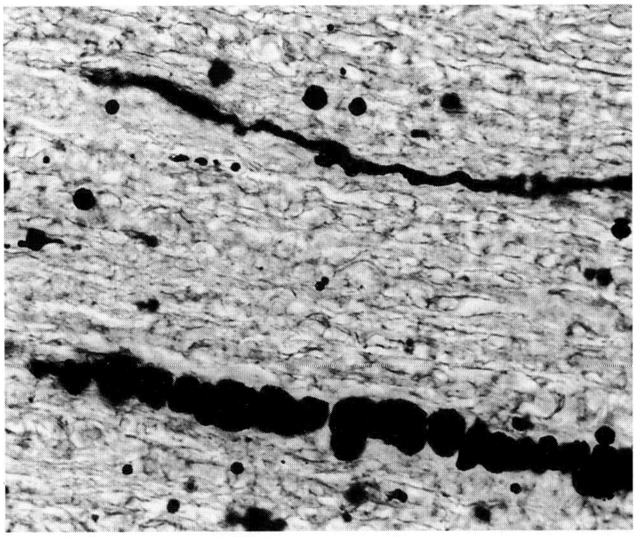

Figure 8-5 Spinal cord, white matter; cow. Wallerian degeneration. Two myelinated axons are degenerated. The top one is minimally enlarged while the lower axon is markedly swollen and undergoing fragmentation. Also, note the focal myelin debris. Marchi method for degenerating myelin. *Courtesy Dr. M. D. McGavin.*

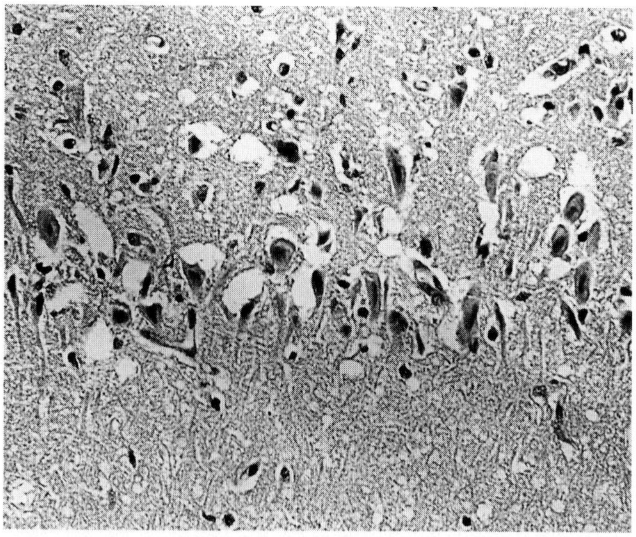

Figure 8-6 Hippocampus, pyramidal neurons; dog. Cerebral ischemia caused by cardiac arrest. Compare with Fig. 8-2. The hippocampal pyramidal neurons have shrunken cell bodies and dark, shrunken nuclei typical of the ischemic cell change. The pericellular space is prominent, in part, because of swelling of astroglial processes. H & E stain.

8-5) forming **ellipsoids** as in the PNS and eventually are removed through degeneration and phagocytosis, leaving an empty space, or one containing myelin debris or macrophages or both. With time and continued degeneration, most of the lesion will consist of enlarged empty spaces. The absence of swollen axons in such dilated spaces, especially in the early stages after CNS trauma, does not necessarily mean that the entire axon has degenerated and been removed, which can require several months. It might instead be the site of separation of an enlarged axon from the adjacent axon at the level of the section being examined.

Ischemic Neuronal Injury. Neurons are dependent on a continuous supply of oxygen to remain viable and if the supply is interrupted for several minutes, the most susceptible neurons will degenerate. Ischemic neuron injury (also referred to as ischemic cell change) occurs following ischemia that can result from obstruction of blood flow to the CNS or reduction in the available oxygen in the blood. This type of neuronal lesion can also result from metabolic disturbances other than ischemia, such as in nutritional deficiencies and toxicities that ultimately interfere with oxygen utilization. In hematoxylin and eosin (H & E) stained sections, the neuronal cell body is shrunken and deeply eosinophilic. The nucleus is reduced in size, often is triangular, and is pyknotic (stains dark blue). The nucleolus might not be detectable. Perineuronal and perivascular spaces are prominent because of swelling of astrocytic processes (Fig. 8-6). In contrast to neurons, some cells such as astrocytes swell following ischemia because of the increased uptake of sodium and chloride ions and water. It is important to remember that such swelling depends upon the cell being viable and still having a semipermeable plasma membrane, even though its function is abnormal. If the degree and duration of the ischemia is sufficiently severe to result in cell death, the plasma membrane becomes fully permeable and the cell does not swell, but becomes shriveled or shrunken and undergoes disintegration, as described for the ischemic cell change of neurons. It should also be emphasized that cells of the CNS are not equally sensitive to ischemia, and the degree of ischemia that causes swelling or death for one cell (e.g., astrocyte) is not the same as that for another cell (e.g., neuron) (see Circulatory Disturbances).

Astrocytes

Astrocytes have traditionally been classified into two types based on morphology. Protoplasmic astrocytes are located primarily in gray matter, whereas fibrous astrocytes occur chiefly in white matter. More recently, astrocytes have been classified as type 1 or type 2 based on cell markers and functions, mainly in cell culture. Similarities exist between type 1 and protoplasmic astrocytes and between type 2 and fibrous astrocytes, but these two classifications are not mutually inclusive. Microscopically, astrocytes have relatively large vesicular nuclei, indistinct or inapparent nucleoli, and no discernible cytoplasm with routine (H & E) staining (Fig. 8-3). With suitable special stains, metallic impregnation, or immunohistochemical staining for glial fibrillary acidic protein (GFAP), the major intermediate filament in astrocytes, cytoplasmic processes are prominent. Processes vary from short, bushlike to long branching processes in protoplasmic and fibrous astrocytes, respectively.

Astrocytes are the most numerous cell type in the CNS. In the CNS, reparative processes after injury such as inflammation and necrosis are facilitated by astrocytes and are analogous to those reparative processes associated with fibroblasts in other organ systems. Astrocytes serve as the main stromal cell population used for repair, but do not synthesize collagen fibers. Instead, repair is facilitated by abundant proliferating astrocytic cell processes containing intermediate filaments composed of GFAP (see following text for more detail). Fibroblasts, however, are an important structural component of the meninges which cover the gyri, are pulled into the sulci by blood vessels, and follow blood vessels into the brain parenchyma before the blood-brain barrier is formed. These fibroblasts can participate in local reparative processes following meningitis and other types of chronic injury that induce fibroplasia and can also give rise to meningeal neoplasms.

Structurally, astrocytic processes provide support for other cellular elements and ensheathe and insulate synapses. A dense meshwork of processes forms the **glia limitans** beneath the pia mater and is also variably prominent in subependymal areas. Processes of astrocytes **(foot processes)** also terminate on blood vessels throughout the CNS. Astrocytes have other diverse functions that can be grouped in three categories: (1) brain development, (2) homeostasis of the microenvironment, and (3) regulation of and participation in immune reactions. During development, cells termed **radial glia** provide a scaffold and guidance for migrating neurons. When development is completed, radial glia mature into astrocytes. Astrocytes secrete growth factors and extracellular matrix molecules that play a role not only in development but also in repair of the CNS. The microenvironment of the CNS must be under strict controls to maintain normal function. Primary roles of astrocytes are regulation of ionic and water balance, antioxidant defense, uptake and metabolism of neurotransmitters, and metabolism or sequestration of toxins that include ammonia, heavy metals, and neurotransmitters such as glutamate that are potential neurotoxins. Finally, interactions between astrocytes, microglia, and neurons orchestrate immune reactions in the brain. In this regard, astrocytes can express major histocompatibility (MHC) class I and II antigens, a variety of cytokines and chemokines, and adhesion molecules that modulate inflammatory events in the CNS.

Reactions to Injury. Common astrocytic reactions in CNS injury are swelling and hypertrophy (astrogliosis). Swelling is an acute response and could be the sole change or may progress with time to hypertrophy. Swollen astrocytes have clear-staining or vacuolated cytoplasm. If injury is severe, astrocytic processes fragment and disappear followed by lysis of the cell body. Hypertrophied astrocytes, often referred to as "reactive," represent a response to a more protracted injury to the CNS. Because of increases in intermediate filaments, mainly GFAP, the cytoplasm becomes apparent along with increased length and branching of the processes with H & E staining. The increase of intermediate filaments and consequently the intensity of GFAP immunohistochemical staining in these cells is so dramatic that some have defined reactive astrocytes on the basis of this change. In protracted degenerative conditions, astrocytes termed **gemistocytes** can be observed. These cells have eccentric nuclei and abundant pink homogeneous cytoplasm with routine H & E staining (Fig. 8-7). Astrocytic proliferation (astrocytosis) can occur in CNS injury but in most instances, proliferative capacity is limited. When it occurs, the most dramatic examples of astrocytosis are associated with attempts to "wall-off" abscesses and neoplasms or to fill in cavitated areas (porencephaly) that result following necrosis of large foci of neural tissue.

Oligodendroglia

Oligodendroglia are located in both the white and gray matter of the CNS and are termed interfascicular oligodendroglia and perineuronal satellite oligodendroglia, respectively. Interfascicular oligodendroglia are prominent in the white matter, where they tend to be aligned in rows

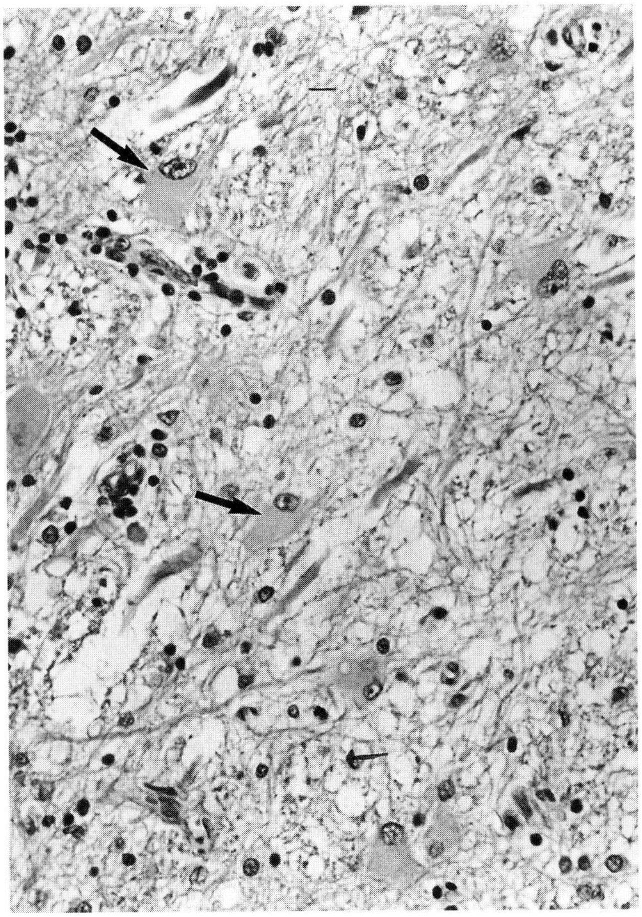

Figure 8-7 Cerebellum, deep cerebellar white matter; cat. Focal chronic lesion secondary to unilateral inner ear infection. Note the prominent gemistocytic astrocytes *(arrows)* with eccentric nuclei, homogeneous cytoplasm, and variably extended processes. Holzer's stain.

parallel to myelinated axons and are responsible for the formation and maintenance of the myelin sheaths. One oligodendroglial cell can radially extend as many as 50 different processes, each of which can myelinate segments (internodes) of many different axons. These cells have been compared to neurons with regard to their total cell size in that their processes occupy much more space than the cell body. Oligodendroglia also influence maturation and maintenance of axons, as well as inhibit regeneration of established myelinated axons. Perineuronal satellite oligodendroglia surround neuronal cell bodies in the gray matter, where they may regulate the perineuronal microenvironment, and are also around blood vessels. When the perineuronal microenvironment is altered or neuron cells bodies are injured, perineuronal satellite oligodendroglia hypertrophy and proliferate in a process referred to as **satellitosis** in an attempt to regulate the environmental perturbation.

The mature, small oligodendrocyte has a spherical, hyperchromatic nucleus similar to that of a lymphocyte. As with astrocytes, the cell body and processes of this cell do not stain with conventional (H & E) staining methods (see Fig. 8-3), and can only be demonstrated following special procedures that include metallic (silver) impregnation.

Reaction to Injury. Reaction to injury includes degeneration and proliferation. Both perineuronal and interfascicular oligodendroglia degenerate; however, only perineuronal oligodendroglia and myelin precursor cells (not interfascicular oligodendroglia) can proliferate. Degeneration of interfascicular oligodendroglia, which can have several causes (including ischemia, infection by certain viruses, toxicities, and certain immunologic processes), can result in selective degeneration of myelin sheaths referred to as primary demyelination. Frequently, however, oligodendroglial injury is not selective, as might occur after diffuse CNS injury resulting from trauma. In such cases, oligodendroglia and other tissue components including axons are damaged, and the myelin degeneration is termed secondary demyelination (Wallerian degeneration). Myelin precursors cells, which mature into interfascicular oligodendroglia, can also proliferate in response to noncytocidal injury and become involved in remyelination following demyelination. The role that perineuronal oligodendroglia (satellite cells) play in normal neuronal function and neuronal injury has not been definitively clarified.

Microglia

The origin of microglia in the CNS has been debated for years. The current consensus is that the cells originate from circulating monocytes that enter and populate the CNS during development and early postnatal life, analogous to the monocyte/macrophage system in other organs. After entry into the CNS, the cells become **amoeboid microglia,** phagocytosing effete cells and cellular debris during remodeling and maturation of the CNS. Amoeboid cells then enter a quiescent stage and transform into **ramified microglia.** Ramified microglia constitute up to 20% of the glial cells and are present throughout the mature CNS, serving as sentinels of brain injury. Ramified microglia, also called resting cells, are most numerous in perineuronal and perivascular areas and in interfascicular locations in white matter. Evidence of pinocytosis in ramified cells suggests some role in maintaining the neural microenvironment. The principal function of microglia, however, is participation in immunoregulation and in degenerative and inflammatory diseases of the CNS. The CNS also contains macrophages, distinct from microglia, mainly in leptomeninges, choroid plexus, and perivascular areas. These macrophages differentiate from blood monocytes involved in normal "leukocytic trafficking" through the CNS and can be involved in immunologic and phagocytic responses to disease processes and infectious organisms.

Ramified microglia have small, hyperchromatic ovoid, rod-, or comma-shaped nuclei and no appreciable cytoplasm with routine H & E staining. With special labeling techniques or metallic impregnation, ramified cells have few delicate branching processes. The small hyperchromatic nuclei and nuclear shape distinguish microglia from astrocytes and oligodendrocytes (see Fig. 8-3).

Table 8-1 Comparison of Ameboid, Ramified, Activated, and Reactive Microglia

	Ameboid	Ramified	Activated	Reactive
Phagocytosis	++	−	+	++
Complement receptors	++	±	+	++
MHC class I	++	−	+	++
MHC class II	±	−	−	++

MHC = major histocompatibility complex.

Reaction to Injury. Microglia are the first cells to react to CNS injury, and the magnitude of the response is graded to correlate with the severity of damage. After injury, ramified microglia progress through a stage of activation, becoming fully immunocompetent reactive cells (Table 8-1). These reactive or **rod cells** readily proliferate, either focally forming **glial nodules** or more diffusely depending on the nature of the injury. As mentioned, in concert with astrocytes and neurons, microglia help coordinate inflammatory events in the CNS. Resident microglia and blood-derived macrophages express major histocompatibility complex (MHC) class I and II antigens, serve as antigen-presenting cells, and possess a broad armament of adhesion molecules, cytokines, and chemokines. Once activated, these cells can also produce nitric oxide, reactive oxygen intermediates, and other chemical mediators of inflammation that can damage the CNS if not under strict control. When tissue necrosis occurs, foamy lipid-laden macrophages, sometimes termed "gitter cells" (see Fig. 8-20) accumulate in the damaged CNS. Macrophages assume this "foamy" appearance because they phagocytize necrotic cellular debris. The origin of these cells is still controversial. Some studies indicate that these are derived from blood-borne monocytes gaining access to the CNS following severe injury, disruption of the blood-brain barrier, and tissue destruction.

Ependyma, Choroid Plexus, Secretion and Absorption of CSF, and Barriers of the CNS

The ependyma is a single-layered, cuboidal to columnar, ciliated epithelium that lines the ventricles and mesencephalic aqueduct of the brain, and central canal of the spinal cord. This layer of cells is therefore situated between the cerebrospinal fluid (CSF) and nervous tissue. Ependymal cells have cilia that project into the CSF and beat in a coordinated manner in the direction of CSF flow. Other structures, referred to as circumventricular organs (CVO), which include the choroid plexus, are covered by highly specialized ependymal cells. The ependymal cells of the choroid plexus are less prominently ciliated and have specialized tight junctions (zonulae occludentes) that are a functional part of the **blood-CSF barrier** discussed in the following text. In contrast to the choroid plexus, junctions between the conventional ependymal cells include gap junctions, and zonulae and fasciae adherentes, that permit movement of materials (e.g., proteins and tracers such as ferritin and horseradish peroxidase) from the CSF into the extracellular space of the brain. This cellular lining, however, is not a static membrane and does have a barrier function in that it regulates several processes that involve interaction between the CSF and brain parenchyma. Proposed functional activities include regulation of fluid homeostasis between the ventricular cavities and the brain parenchyma. This homeostasis has been proposed to include secretion and absorption of CSF, endocytosis, phagocytosis, and metabolism of substances such as iron resulting from the lysis of erythrocytes following hemorrhage. Finally, ependymal cells possess the structural and enzymatic characteristics necessary for scavenging and detoxifying a wide variety of substances in the CSF.

During embryonic development, the medial wall of the lateral ventricle (choroid fissure), the roof of the third ventricle, and the lower part of the roof of the fourth ventricle consist of a single layer of ependymal cells that is adherent on its outer surface to the pia mater. This ependyma-pia union forms the **tela choroidea,** providing an anchor for the **choroid plexus,** which is formed by an invagination of this bilayered membrane into the ventricular spaces.

The important function of the choroid plexus is production of the CSF. It should be noted, however, that fluid from other sources (e.g., secretion by the ependyma, interstitial fluid of the brain, and ultrafiltrate of the blood) has also been reported to contribute to the formation of CSF. Removal of CSF has traditionally been proposed to occur via the arachnoid granulations, which are focal extensions of the subarachnoid space into dural venous sinuses. More recent evidence indicates that other routes of drainage also exist, which vary in different species. These routes include a more direct movement of CSF into the circulation of the brain, as well as drainage of CSF into the lymph vessels that surround the CNS.

The apposing surfaces of the epithelial cells that cover the choroid plexus form tight junctions (zonulae occludentes). This barrier, along with the tight junctions that form between the cells of the arachnoid membrane, make up the blood-CSF barrier. Tight junctions between endothelial cells of cerebral blood vessels form the **blood-brain barrier.** It should be noted that the blood vessels of the choroid plexus and the dura mater are fenestrated, which explains the location of tight junctions between the epithelium of the choroid plexus and cells of the arachnoid membrane. It has also been demonstrated that astrocytes, whose processes intimately surround blood vessels of the brain, are responsible for inducing endothelial cells to form this barrier.

Reaction to Injury. Responses of ependymal cells to injury include atrophy, degeneration, and necrosis. Atrophy usually occurs in response to enlargement of the ventricles as occurs with hydrocephalus. The cilia and microvilli of affected cells are reduced in number, and there is also a reduction in cellular organelles such as endoplasmic reticulum and mitochondria. An additional lesion that accompanies ventricular enlargement is stretching and tearing of the lining ependyma, regardless of whether the hydrocephalus is internal (obstruction within the ventricular system), external (obstruction external to the ventricular system), or secondary to cerebral atrophy (hydrocephalus ex vacuo, or compensating hydrocephalus) (see Anomalies and Malformations). In such instances, the resulting areas of ependymal discontinuity result in the subependymal parenchyma being directly exposed to the CSF. Unfortunately, mammalian ependymal cells are more like neurons than other neuroglia in that they do not regenerate and therefore do not repair the denuded areas. After 1 to 2 weeks, astrogliosis, which varies greatly in degree and uniformity, occurs in the exposed areas. Astrogliosis can extend into the ventricular space or be minimal in extent and confined to the subventricular area.

Inflammation of the ependyma (ependymitis) can also occur, with infection being the most common cause. Organisms most commonly gain entrance to the ependyma via the circulation (hematogenous), by direct contamination (e.g., rupture of a cerebral abscess into the ventricular system), and by retrograde reflux through the lateral apertures of infected CSF from the subarachnoid space in cases of meningitis. In the case of bacterial infection, the suppurative exudate that forms in the CSF can cause obstructive hydrocephalus, although the development of hydrocephalus cannot always be explained on the basis of obstruction. The proposed mechanism involves impairment of ependymal fluid and ion transport, resulting in reduced absorption of CSF (e.g., by brain capillaries as noted above).

Meninges

The meninges, which enclose the CNS, consist of three layers: the dura mater, the arachnoid mater, and the pia mater. The arachnoid and pia mater are frequently referred to together as the leptomeninges. They form a single functional compartment called the subarachnoid space that contains the CSF and blood vessels. The meninges form a protective covering for the CNS and provide a scaffolding that supports nerves and blood vessels that enter and leave the brain and spinal cord. They also provide an external envelope filled with CSF having a specific gravity close to that of the CNS that provides additional protection.

The **dura mater,** once referred to as the pachymeninx (thick meninges), is a strong and dense collagenous membrane. It differs in its relationship to the surrounding bone in the cranium versus the vertebral canal. In the cranium, the dura consists of two layers that are fused with each other. The outer layer serves as the periosteum of the cranial bone, except in the areas of the venous sinuses (surrounded by dura) and falx cerebri, which is the membrane that extends ventrally between the two cerebral hemispheres. At the level of the foramen magnum, the two layers become separated, with the outer layer continuing to function as the periosteum of the vertebral (spinal) canal and the inner layer forming the free dural membrane that surrounds the spinal cord. The inner aspect of dura mater is lined by elongated, flattened mesothelial-like cells. There is no epidural or extradural space in the cranial vault meninges as there is in the spinal cord meninges, except in the neonate.

The **arachnoid mater** is a thin, but multilayered membrane composed of cells that overlap one another. It contains no blood vessels and has an outer smooth surface formed by mesothelial-like cells that abut similar cells in the dura. The arachnoid membrane is also characterized by tight junctions (zonulae occludentes) between its cells, although other junctions (zonulae adherentes, maculae adherentes, and gap junctions) have also been described. The specialized tight junctions of this membrane form, along with the choroid plexus, the blood-CSF barrier of the CNS. The inner surface of the arachnoid membrane is separated from the pia mater by a space (subarachnoid space) that is traversed by many thin trabeculae (arachnoid trabeculae) that anchor the inner arachnoid membrane to the pia mater. CSF occupies the subarachnoid space. Blood vessels run in the subarachnoid space and penetrate through the pia mater (described in the following text) to enter or exit the brain or spinal cord.

The **pia mater** is closely adherent to the surface of the brain and spinal cord and is penetrated by a large number of blood vessels that supply the underlying nervous tissue. The pia mater consists of flat, thin overlapping connective tissue cells (fibroblasts) that are separated from the underlying neural tissue by variable amounts of loose collagen fibers and the glia limitans. The glia limitans, which covers the outer surface of the brain and spinal cord and is situated immediately subjacent to the pia mater, consists of astrocytic foot processes and basement membrane. In many areas the pia (which lacks a basal lamina) is only one cell layer thick and has fenestrations, so that the glia limitans is exposed directly to the subarachnoid space. Pial and arachnoid cells also ensheathe blood vessels, collagen bundles, and nerves that are within, or cross, the subarachnoid space. Macrophages also occur throughout the leptomeninges (i.e., a term used to describe the combined pia and arachnoid layers; also referred to as the pia-arachnoid layer or pia-arachnoid).

Reaction to Injury. Pathologic processes that initially involve the meninges, most commonly the leptomeninges, can secondarily invade the CNS because of the close relationship between the two tissues. Conversely, processes that primarily affect the CNS can secondarily affect the meninges, most commonly the leptomeninges.

Meningitis refers to inflammation of the meninges. In common usage the term generally refers to inflammation of the leptomeninges (the pia mater, subarachnoid space and adjacent arachnoid mater) in contrast to inflammation of the dura mater, which is referred to as pachymeningitis. Leptomeningitis can be acute, subacute, or chronic and, depending on the cause, suppurative, nonsuppurative, or granulomatous (see Inflammation of the Central Nervous System). Infectious agents spread to the meninges by the same routes (e.g., hematogenous, direct extension, leukocytic trafficking) that result in infection of the brain excluding retrograde axonal transport, which occurs with some viral infections (e.g., rabies virus). Inflammation of specific parts of the dura mater of the cranial cavity can occur in the external dura (periosteal dura) following osteomyelitis, formation of extradural abscesses, and skull fracture, and involve the inner dura in association with leptomeningitis.

Other meningeal lesions include a fibroblast-like proliferation of the inner dural mesothelial-like cells, arachnoid cells, and cells of the pia mater in response to irritation. Additional lesions likely related to aging or degeneration include formation of cellular nests on the outer surface (mesothelial-like cells) of the arachnoid membrane, mineralization of the arachnoid membrane in human beings, and mineralization plus ossification of the dura mater of the spinal cord in both human beings and dogs. The lesion in the dog, which tends to affect the ventral cervical and lumbar dura mater, is most commonly encountered in large breeds, although smaller breeds can be affected. The clinical significance of this lesion has been debated but not decided.

Anomalies and Malformations

Anencephaly

Anencephaly literally means an absence of the brain, but in many instances of so-called anencephaly only the rostral part of the brain (cerebral hemispheres) is absent, or very rudimentary, and to varying degrees the brain stem is preserved. Thus, this abnormality is best designated **prosencephalic hypoplasia** (Fig. 8-8). Such anomalies result from an abnormal development of the rostral aspect of the neural tube. Although the cause for these anomalies is largely unknown, anencephaly has been reported to be associated with anomalies in other body systems in calves. Additionally, anencephaly, following initial cranium bifidum (see following text) and exencephaly (protrusion of brain not covered by skin; or meninges), has been reported to occur in rat fetuses after exposure of the

Anencephaly
- rat Fetuses after exposure of pregnant dam to
↳ excess vitamin A
↳ cyclophosphamide

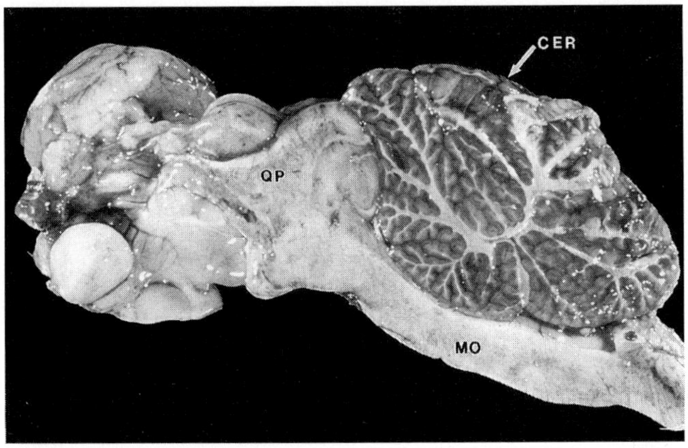

Figure 8-8 Brain, markedly underdeveloped cerebral hemispheres; quadrigeminal plate *(QP)*, cerebellum *(CER)*, and medulla oblongata *(MO)*; calf. Prosencephalic hypoplasia. Only the caudal components of the brain are clearly recognizable.

pregnant dam to excessive concentrations of vitamin A and cyclophosphamide.

Hydrocephalus

Hydrocephalus typically refers to an increased accumulation of CSF within the ventricular system. It can result from obstruction within the ventricular system (noncommunicating form), or when there is communication of CSF with the subarachnoid space where the CSF can be in excess (communicating form).

Obstruction within the ventricular system at, or rostral to, the lateral apertures of the fourth ventricle results in noncommunicating hydrocephalus. An area of particular vulnerability for obstruction is the mesencephalic aqueduct (Fig. 8-9). When congenital, this type of hydrocephalus can be associated with an enlargement (doming) of the cranium if obstruction occurs before the sutures have fused, and the enlarged head can cause dystocia. Hydrocephalus of this type has a predisposition for certain breeds of dogs, being most common in toy breeds and brachycephalic dogs. Acquired noncommunicating hydrocephalus has been associated with obstruction of any of the following: the lateral apertures of the fourth ventricle, the aqueduct, or the interventricular foramen. Causes of obstruction include infection or inflammation (see Lesions Resulting From Viral Infection of the Fetus), neoplasia, and, uncommonly, cholesteatomas in the choroid plexus of the horse (Fig. 8-10). As stated previously, noncommunicating hydrocephalus can occur without the presence of typical obstruction to CSF flow (see Ependyma, Choroid Plexus, Secretion and Absorption of CSF, and Barriers of the CNS).

Communicating hydrocephalus, in which CSF of the ventricular system communicates with the subarachnoid space, is the least common of the two forms. A recent hypothesis proposes that this type of hydrocephalus is caused by a decreased expansion of intracranial arteries

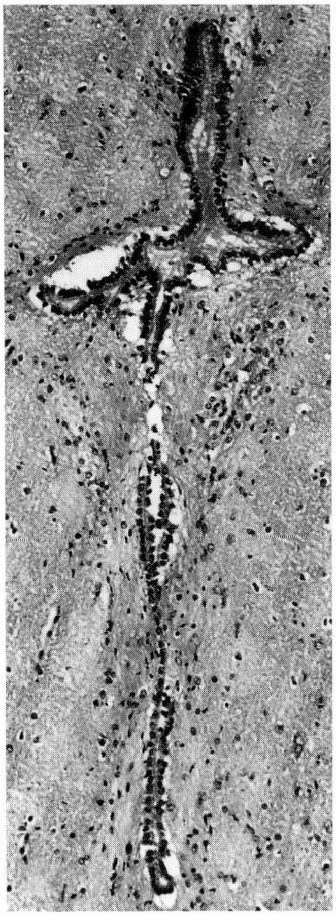

Figure 8-9 Brain, mesencephalon; young cat. Stenotic mesencephalic aqueduct causing hydrocephalus. Undetermined cause. Note the stenosis and discontinuity of the mesencephalic aqueduct. H & E stain.

during systole as a result of reduced compliance involving the arterial walls, or the subarachnoid space, and is referred to as "restricted arterial pulsation hydrocephalus." Because the intracranial arteries cannot fully expand, pressure gradient develops in which there is greater pressure within the brain tissue and the ventricles than outside the brain. Several causes have been advanced, including arteritis, subarachnoid hemorrhage, and meningitis.

In a third type of hydrocephalus, referred to as **hydrocephalus ex vacuo** (or compensating hydrocephalus), the increase in size of the lateral ventricles, with increase in volume of CSF, is secondary to absence or loss of cerebral tissue. This type of hydrocephalus can occur any time there is lack of development or destruction and loss of cerebral tissue surrounding the lateral ventricles. Examples include certain anomalies (hydranencephaly) (see Fig. 8-12) plus some storage diseases (e.g., ceroid-lipofuscinosis), and aging of the CNS, both of which are associated with cerebral atrophy. Interference in flow, or increased pressure, of the CSF would not be expected in this type of hydrocephalus.

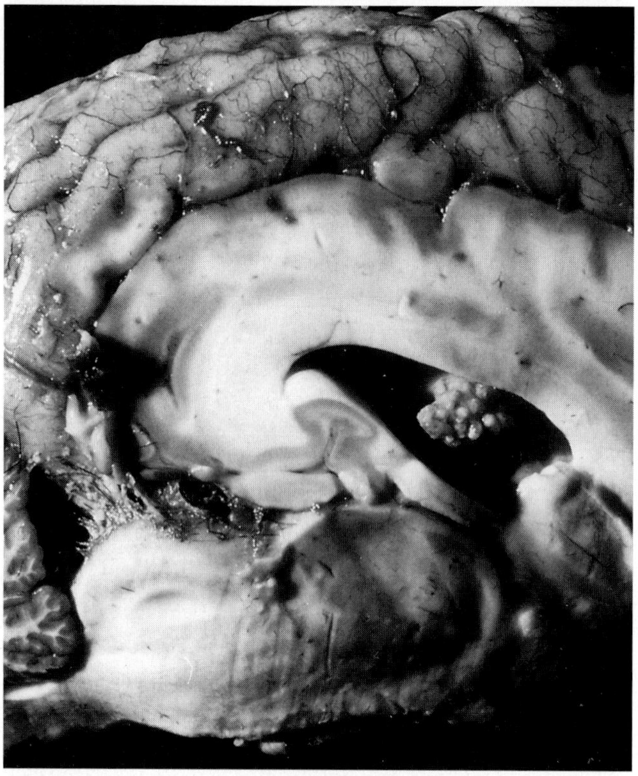

Figure 8-10 Brain, lateral ventricle; horse. Cholesteatoma of choroid plexus. The cholesteatoma consists of firm nodules containing cholesterol crystals and granulomatous inflammation. *Courtesy Dr. M. D. McGavin.*

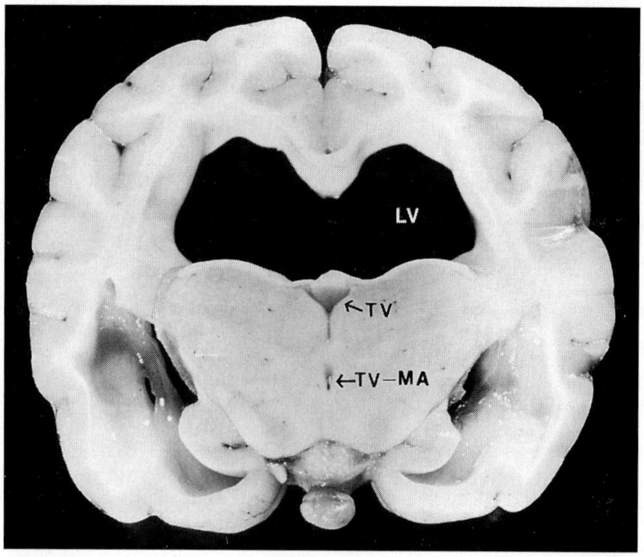

Figure 8-11 Brain, junction between parietal and occipital lobes, level of thalamus; dog. Hydrocephalus. Bilateral dilatation of lateral ventricles dorsally *(LV),* and ventrolaterally. The fornix has separated and lies on the flattened floor of the ventricle. Note that the third ventricle *(TV)* and junctional area between the third ventricle and mesencephalic aqueduct *(TV-MA)* are not enlarged and are possibly even reduced in size, suggesting that the obstruction may be at, or rostral, to this plane of section.

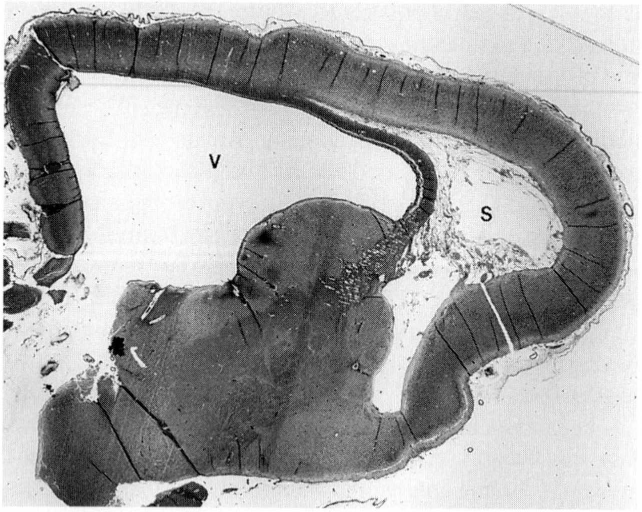

Figure 8-12 Brain (transverse section), junction between parietal and frontal lobes, level of corpus striatum; lamb infected in utero with Cache valley bunyavirus. Hydranencephaly. A prominent space *(S)* has replaced the central part of the cerebral parenchyma. The lateral ventricle *(V)* is enlarged as a result of the reduced resistance (hydrocephalus ex vacuo). H & E stain. *Courtesy Dr. J. F. Edwards.*

Lesions associated with either of the first two forms of hydrocephalus, but particularly the noncommunicating form, include prominent enlargement of the ventricular system proximal to the point of obstruction (Fig. 8-11). White matter adjacent to the dilated lateral ventricles is reduced in thickness, although the gray matter can retain a relatively normal appearance. The ependyma can become atrophied and focally discontinuous (see Ependyma, Choroid Plexus, Secretion and Absorption of CSF, and Barriers of the CNS). Other lesions include atrophy with fenestration of the interventricular septum (septum pellucidum), atrophy of the hippocampus in the floor of the lateral ventricles, flattening of surface gyri, and caudal displacement of the brain, which can cause herniation of the cerebellum through the foramen magnum. The resulting coning of the cerebellum can be accompanied by necrosis of cells in the cerebellar folia due to circulatory obstruction.

Hydranencephaly

Hydranencephaly, unlike hydrocephalus, is characterized by a cavitation in the area normally occupied by the white matter of the cerebral hemispheres and results from lack of proper development of this part of the cerebrum (Fig. 8-12). The cavitation results from destruction of immature progenitor cells whose loss prevents normal development. Hydranencephaly is often quite severe with very little tissue present between the expanded ventricular lining and the outer meninges. Such a lesion grossly appears as a thin-walled sac. Because of the lack of resistance, the

Hydranencephaly
• Calf: • Fetal Akabane (V)
• Fetal BVD (V)
• lamb: • Fetal bluetongue (V)
• Fetal border disease (V)
• Fetal Rift valley fever (V)
• Fetal Wesselbron disease (V)
• in utero copper deficiency

ventricles expand into this space (hydrocephalus ex vacuo), and the ependymal lining remains relatively preserved or may be variably defective. The cranium and meninges are generally unaltered.

Causes include fetal viral infection (e.g., Akabane and bovine virus diarrhea viral infection in calves; and blue tongue, border disease, Rift Valley fever, and Wesselsbron disease viral infections in lambs) and nutritional copper deficiency (affecting the ovine fetus in utero).

Another term, **porencephaly,** refers to a cleft or cyst in the wall of the cerebral hemisphere that typically communicates with the brain surface (e.g., subarachnoid space), but can also communicate with the lateral ventricle of the brain.

Syringomyelia

Syringomyelia is defined as a tubular cavitation (syrinx) in the spinal cord not lined by ependyma, but separate from the central canal. It can extend over several spinal cord segments. The lesion is well known in human beings and has also been described in the dog (weimaraner breed) and calves. The syrinx can communicate with the central canal but should not be confused with hydromyelia, which means dilatation of the central canal. The lesion can extend rostrally and affect the medulla (syringobulbia) and pons (syringopontia) in the human being. The cavity contains fluid and is unlined, except for varying degrees of mural astrocytosis that is usually very mild in the weimaraner dog. Proposed causes include presence of an anomalous vascular pattern that results in a low-grade ischemia, as well as trauma, infection, and neoplasia that cause parenchymal degeneration and cavitation.

Dysraphic Anomalies

Dysraphia. Dysraphia literally means an abnormal seam and usually refers to a defective closure of the neural tube during development. This defect, which can occur at any point along the tube, is exemplified by anencephaly, prosencephalic hypoplasia, cranium bifidum, and spina bifida.

Cranium Bifidum. Cranium bifidum is characterized by a dorsal midline cranial defect through which meningeal and brain tissue can protrude. The protruded material, which forms a sac (-cele), is covered by skin and can be lined by meninges (meningocele) (Fig. 8-13), or meninges accompanied by a part of the brain (meningoencephalocele). Causes of the these malformations include inheritance in pigs and cats and treatment of pregnant cats with griseofulvin.

Spina Bifida. Spina bifida is the spinal counterpart of cranium bifidum. This lesion, which frequently tends to affect the caudal spine, is characterized by a dorsal defect in one to several vertebrae of the dorsal spinal column. The lesion results from a defective closure of the neural tube.

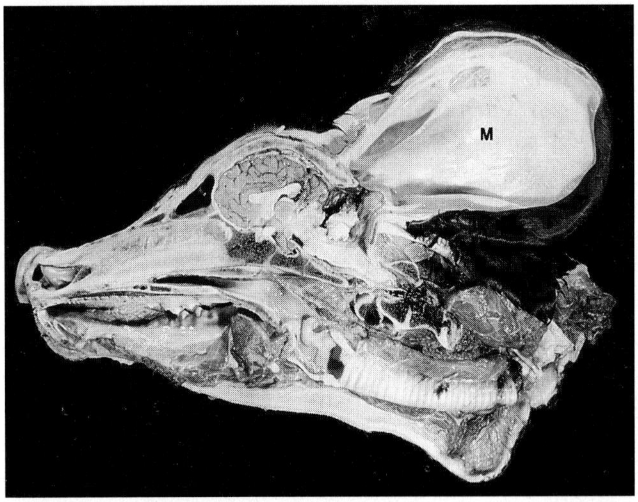

Figure 8-13 Brain, cranium bifidum; calf. Meningocele *(M)*. A defect in the caudal skull has resulted in continuity between the cranial cavity and a large external pouch covered by skin. The pouch is lined by a meningeal membrane continuous with that surrounding the brain.

There can be no herniation of the meninges or spinal cord through the defect (spina bifida occulta), or herniation of either meninges (meningocele) or meninges and spinal cord (meningomyelocele) can occur, forming a sac covered with skin. The lesion has been detected in several species, including horses, calves, sheep, dogs (especially English bulldog), and cats, particularly the Manx breed, in which it is inherited as an autosomal dominant trait. An additional lesion, **myeloschisis,** is similar to spina bifida except in its severe form results from failure of the entire spinal neural tube to close. This lesion is therefore characterized by lack of development of the entire dorsal vertebral column.

Lesions Resulting from Viral Infection of the Fetus

Viruses can affect the fetus directly or indirectly (i.e., only the dam or the placenta is infected, and fetal lesions occur secondarily). Direct infection can induce malformation by affecting organogenesis in the developing embryo, immature cells of the fetus, or differentiated cells of the fetus.

Viral Effect on Organogenesis. Two examples of this type of viral teratology include (1) microencephaly (abnormally small brain) and myeloschisis (see Spina Bifida) caused by influenza viral infection and (2) myeloschisis caused by Newcastle disease viral infection, both in young chicken embryos.

Viral Effect on Immature Cells. Lesions due to parvoviral infection have been detected in the rat, hamster, cat, and ferret (rat virus); cat and ferret (feline infectious enteritis virus [feline panleukopenia virus]) and mouse (minute virus). Grossly, the size of the cerebellum is reduced (cerebellar hypoplasia); the reduction in size varies in severity depending on the age and developmental stage of the brain when the host (e.g., fetus or neonate) is infected. The viruses involved have an affinity for and destroy cells undergoing mitosis (mitocidal virus). The viruses primarily infect cells of the external granular layer of the cerebellum (e.g., in the cat) that are still dividing during the late gestational and early neonatal periods. Necrosis of these cells prevents their normal migration to form the internal granular layer. In addition to the loss of the external granular layer, there is degeneration and loss of Purkinje cells that are postmitotic, but immature (see Fig. 8-45 for similar lesion). Reasons for degeneration of Purkinje cells might include infection by the virus or lack of normal development of the cerebellar cortex. The Purkinje cells can also be malpositioned (e.g., located in the molecular layer) as a result of the viral-induced alteration in development of the cerebellar cortex.

Congenital defects in neonatal calves can result from fetal infection with bovine virus diarrhea virus (a pestivirus). The primary lesion is a cerebellar hypoplasia-atrophy (Fig. 8-14), but other lesions of the CNS also can occur, including porencephaly, hydranencephaly (associated with early inflammation), and dysmyelination (see Disorders of Myelin Formation and Maintenance). The type of lesion depends on the age of the fetus and therefore the stage of CNS development at the time of infection. Early retinal inflammation followed by degeneration can also occur when fetuses are infected in utero. The cerebellar lesion, which follows infection at 150 days of gestation (midtrimester), is considered to involve two

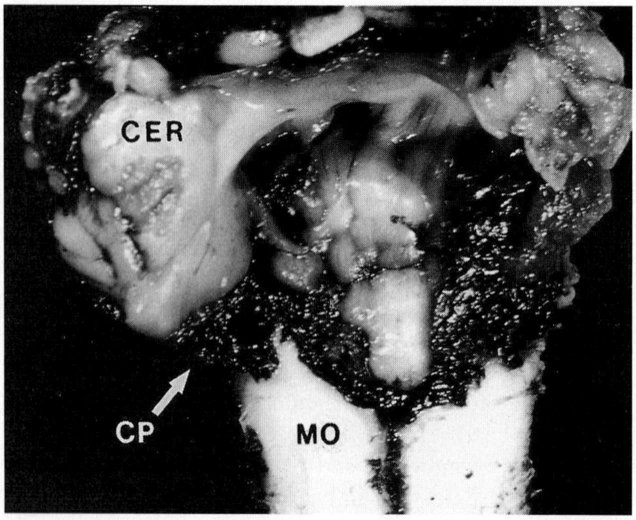

Figure 8-14 Brain, cerebellum and medulla oblongata; calf. Cerebellar hypoplasia-atrophy resulting from bovine virus diarrhea viral infection. Only a remnant of the cerebellum *(CER)* is present. Note the choroid plexus *(CP)* of the fourth ventricle, and medulla oblongata *(MO)*.

Cerebellar hypoplasia
- rat Ⓥ (parvoⓋ): rat, hamster, cat, ferret
- feline panleukopenia Ⓥ (parvoⓋ): cat, ferret
- minute Ⓥ (parvoⓋ): mice

processes. One process is typified by early necrosis of the undifferentiated cells in the external granular layer. A second process is edema of the folial white matter with focal hemorrhage in the cortex, followed by focal cavitation of the white matter and atrophy. All lesions are due to vascular impairment (ischemia) resulting from vasculitis. Leptomeningitis, characterized by accumulation of lymphocytes and plasma cells and occasionally fibroplasia, causes adhesions between adjacent cerebellar folia and focal obliteration of the subarachnoid space.

Hog cholera (swine fever) virus, also a pestivirus, can be teratogenic in the porcine fetus. The best-known neural defects resulting from fetal infection are hypomyelinogenesis (see Disorders of Myelin Formation and Maintenance) and cerebellar hypoplasia, although other lesions of the CNS (e.g., microencephaly) and nonneural tissues have been reported. The mechanism of lesion development has not been definitively determined, but a persistent infection that results in inhibition of cell division and function of selected tissues has been proposed.

Border disease viral infection (also a pestiviral infection) is capable of inducing maldevelopment in the CNS and nonneural tissues (e.g., skeleton) of lambs and goats after natural infection of the dam during pregnancy. One of the characteristic lesions in the CNS is hypomyelinogenesis (see Disorders of Myelin Formation and Maintenance). Other lesions detected in lambs include early inflammation, porencephaly-hydranencephaly, cerebellar malformation including hypoplasia, microencephaly, and reduction in diameter of the spinal cord.

Akabane viral infection (caused by a bunyavirus) occurs in cattle, sheep, and goats in Japan, Israel, and Australia. Characteristic lesions of the CNS include porencephaly-hydranencephaly, and degeneration (with loss of neurons) of the ventral horns of the spinal cord. Nonsuppurative encephalitis (typified by the accumulation of macrophages, lymphocytes, and plasma cells) also occurs. Arthrogryposis (a persistent congenital flexure or contraction of a joint) is a common lesion. The porencephalic-hydranencephalic lesion results from destruction of germinal cells during brain development, and the arthrogryposis is secondary to degeneration of lower motor neurons in the spinal cord, resulting in denervation atrophy of muscles with resultant lack of joint movement.

Bluetongue viral infection (orbiviral infection) of sheep is also known to induce porencephaly-hydranencephaly, plus cerebellar hypoplasia (all or part of the cerebellum), hypoplasia of the spinal cord, and retinopathy (retinal degeneration and dysplasia) following fetal infection during pregnancy. The mechanism involved in the development of the porencephalic-hydranencephalic lesion begins as necrosis of undifferentiated cells (including potential neuroblasts and neuroglia) in the subventricular zone that are required to form the central white matter of the cerebral hemispheres. The loss of these precursor cells

- BVD Ⓥ (pestiⓋ): calves
- hog cholera (pestiⓋ): pigs
- border disease (pestiⓋ): lambs
- bluetongue (orbiⓋ): lambs

results in cavitation (hydranencephaly/porencephaly) of the cerebral hemispheres.

Finally, two other fetal viral infections that occur in Africa are caused by **Rift Valley fever** virus (a bunyavirus) and **Wesselsbron** virus (a flavivirus). Both have been reported to cause hydranencephaly (e.g., in sheep).

Viral Effects on Differentiated Cells. Infections of neonatal laboratory animals with several viruses that include mumps virus, reovirus type I, and parainfluenza virus types I and II can induce hydrocephalus. Parainfluenza virus can also cause the lesion in the dog. Although there are some differences among the different viral infections, the basic lesion is an aqueductal stenosis (incomplete closure in the dog) that results in the development of noncommunicating hydrocephalus (see Fig. 8-9). The virus grows in and causes destruction of ependymal cells lining the ventricular system. The infection is initially accompanied by an inflammation that resolves within 2 weeks. The significant lesion results from injury of ependyma of the mesencephalic aqueduct because of its vulnerability to become occluded. The end-stage lesion is not associated with a glial response or presence of viral antigen. Instead, the original ependyma-lined aqueduct is replaced by focal aggregates of remaining ependymal cells that are separated by normal-appearing brain tissue. The final lesion is therefore more suggestive of an agenesis than a viral infection. Infection of adult laboratory animals (e.g., mice with influenza viral infection) also can induce aqueductal stenosis and hydrocephalus, but in contrast to neonatal infection, there is a persistent glial response in the area of stenosis.

Inborn Errors of Metabolism

Disturbance of Amino Acid Metabolism

Aminoacidopathy. Two diseases characterized by errors of amino acid metabolism have been described in the neonatal calf. One disease, designated **maple syrup urine disease,** occurs in young polled Hereford calves (see Disorders of Myelin Formation and Maintenance). The second disease, **bovine citrullinemia,** which was originally described in Australia, occurs in neonatal Friesian calves.

Bovine citrullinemia is a rare inborn error of metabolism of the urea cycle that results in a pronounced accumulation of citrulline in the body fluids because of a failure of the normal synthesis of arginosuccinic acid by the enzyme arginosuccinate synthetase. Grossly, the livers of affected animals are pale yellow. The brains appear normal grossly and have normal weights. Microscopic lesions in the brain are characterized by mild to moderate diffuse astroglial swelling in the cerebrocortical gray matter. Liver lesions are mild to severe hepatocellular hydropic change. The onset of the marked neurologic signs, which occur during the first week of life, is correlated with increasing concentrations of plasma ammonia. The cerebral lesions have also been suspected to result from the hyperammonemia or increased concentrations of unmetabolized excitatory aminoacids. However, the pathogenesis of the disease remains unsettled.

Lysosomal Storage Disease

Lysosomal storage generally refers to a cellular alteration in which an increased amount of material, which normally is degraded, accumulates within lysosomes, often resulting in cell death. Lysosomal storage diseases were originally thought to develop exclusively because of mutations that result in a reduction in lysosomal enzyme synthesis. More recently, however, it has become clear that other defects include synthesis of catalytically inactive proteins that resemble active normal enzymes, defects in posttranslational processing of enzyme protein destined for the lysosome, and lack of enzyme activator or protector protein. Additional defects include lack of substrate activator or protector protein, and lack of transport protein that is required for elimination of the digested material from lysosomes. Characterization of lysosomal disorders has, therefore, been broadened to include any protein that is essential for normal lysosomal function.

The best-known diseases are characterized by accumulation of the substrate or substrate precursors and sometimes even by the absence of a critical metabolic product for normal lysosomal function. As a general principle, cell swelling and cytoplasmic vacuolation occur because of the accumulation of unprocessed substrate; therefore, differences in the size and appearance of cells (i.e., neurons versus hepatocytes) depend on the availability of the substrate (i.e., carbohydrate versus lipid) in the organ system. Many lipids and glycolipids are unique to the nervous system and thus only neural cells accumulate the substrate.

An example of lysosomal storage diseases that affect human beings and animals includes the gangliosidoses (one form referred to as Tay-Sachs disease in human beings). With few exceptions, these diseases are transmitted in an autosomal recessive pattern. They are also often gene-dose dependent, and correspondingly, recessive homozygotes manifest the disease, whereas heterozygotes are phenotypically normal, but the specific enzyme activity is reduced (approximately 50% of normal). The age of onset of clinical signs, as well as the severity of the disease process, can vary among the different diseases because the deficiency of the involved enzyme is not always the same. If the gene defect is such that the mutant enzyme is not synthesized at all, there is an early onset of a severe disease. Conversely, if there is some residual synthesis of the deficient enzyme, there is later onset of a milder form of the disease since partial catabolism of the accumulated substrate permits a longer period before the loss of cell function.

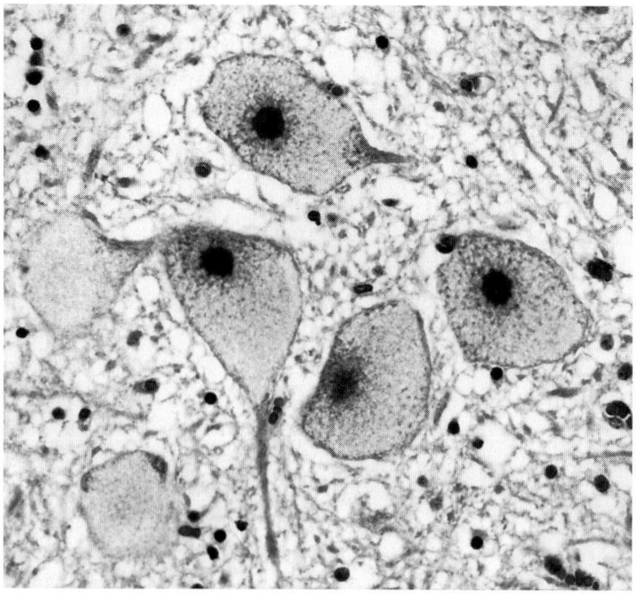

Figure 8-15 Brain, medulla oblongata, hypoglossal nucleus; pig. GM_2 gangliosidosis. The cytoplasm of swollen neuronal cell bodies (two with displaced nuclei in lower center of the photograph) appears finely vacuolated. H & E stain. *Courtesy Dr. C. H. Bridges.*

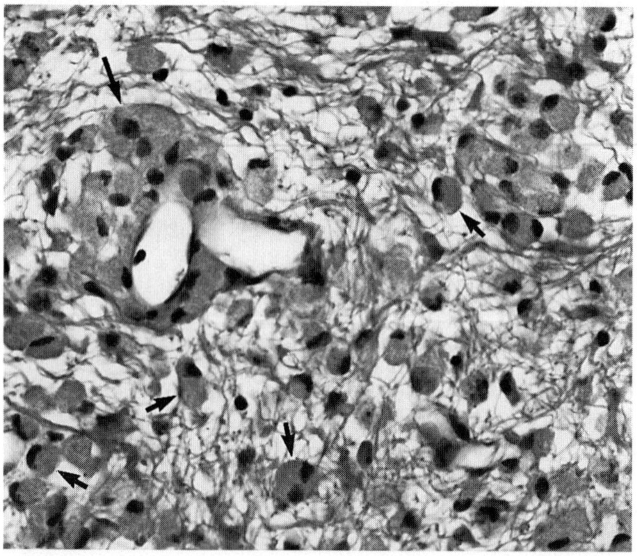

Figure 8-16 Brain, medullary white matter of cerebellum; dog. Globoid cell leukodystrophy. Globoid cells have accumulated diffusely in the cerebellar medullary white matter *(short arrows)* and perivascularly *(long arrow).* H & E stain.

Accumulation of materials in lysosomes can also be acquired. Such lysosomal storage can occur following acquired toxicities (see Plant Poisoning), accumulation of iron (e.g., as hemosiderin after erythrocytic lysis), and excess absorption and accumulation of ingested copper. One unique lysosomal storage disease, which has several forms, is **ceroid-lipofuscinosis.** Its lysosomal dysfunction

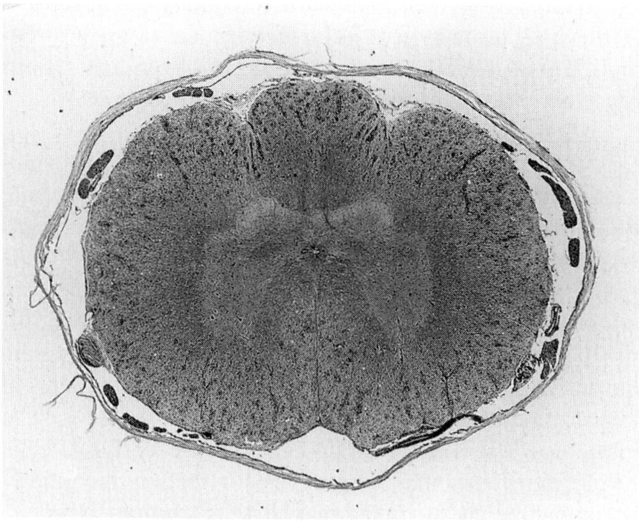

Figure 8-17 Spinal cord, thoracic level; dog. Globoid cell leukodystrophy. There is peripheral loss of myelin in all funiculi (lighter staining area). Vessels in the affected areas are prominent because of the perivascular accumulation of globoid cells. H & E stain. *Courtesy Dr. M. D. McGavin.*

has not been completely characterized. The disease resembles other lysosomal storage diseases in that it can have a recessive mode of inheritance, but is dissimilar in that it has no gene-dose effect or demonstrated lysosomal enzyme defect.

Most, but not all, lysosomal storage diseases of human beings and animals affect the CNS and cause neurologic disturbances. The lesions of the different diseases vary, but within the nervous system, neurons and occasionally other cell types (e.g., neuroglia) are generally affected. Gross lesions of the CNS vary among the different diseases. Brain atrophy occurs with globoid leukodystrophy and ceroid-lipofuscinosis in later stages of the diseases. With ceroid-lipofuscinosis, the atrophy, which most frequently involves the cerebral hemispheres (especially the cortex), but also sometimes the cerebellum, can result in a 50% reduction in brain weight. The cerebral hemispheres are increased in firmness and often have a tan color, whereas the gyri are thinned and the sulci widened (cerebral cortical atrophy).

Brain atrophy is not prominent in other lysosomal storage diseases, although brains of animals with gangliosidosis can have a firm, rubbery consistency. Microscopically, affected neurons often have a foamy (finely vacuolated) or granular cytoplasm, which is a reflection of the degree to which the stored material is removed during processing (Figs. 8-15 through 8-18). The specific features of the stored material can be best appreciated by ultrastructural examination.

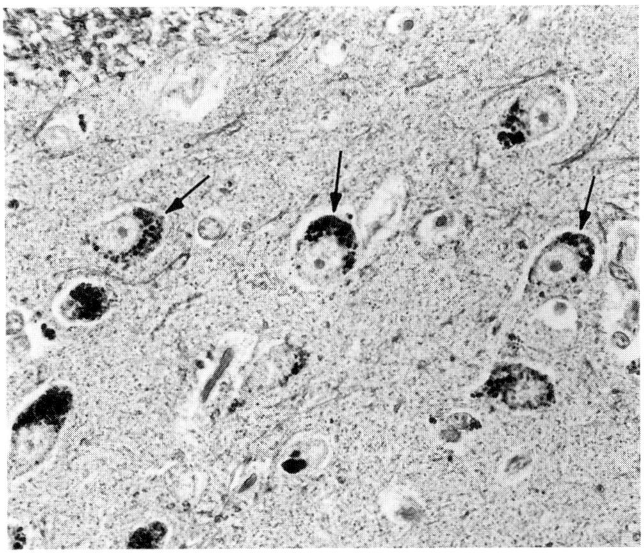

Figure 8-18 Brain, junction of frontal and parietal lobes, junction of caudate nucleus and internal capsule; Rambouillet sheep. Ceroid-lipofuscinosis. Affected neurons contain variable accumulation of granular pigment *(arrows)* that is prominent at one pole of the cell body. Sudan black stain for lipid.

One disease, **globoid cell leukodystrophy,** differs from the majority in that the primary lysosomal defect appears to involve oligodendrocytes rather than neurons. Degeneration of oligodendroglia results in the disturbance of myelin formation and maintenance and the accumulation of unprocessed myelin breakdown products (partially degraded myelin membranes, galactosylceramide, and galactocerebroside) in macrophages termed globoid cells. Globoid cells are macrophages that phagocytize the unprocessed myelin breakdown products that result from oligodendroglial destruction. It has been hypothesized that psychosine (galactosylsphingosine), which accumulates during the disease, is directly toxic to oligodendrocytes and results in direct injury to oligodendrocytes (see Disorders of Myelin Formation and Maintenance).

Features of some selected lysosomal storage diseases of animals are given in Table 8-2. For a comprehensive overview, the reader is referred to a review by Jolly and Walkley (1997).

Physical Disturbances

Factors Influencing the Susceptibility of the CNS to Trauma

In general, trauma of the central nervous system of animals occurs less frequently than in human beings. Animals are not exposed as frequently to trauma-causing situations (e.g., automobile travel) as are human beings, and there are anatomic differences that help protect the brain of animals.

Among animals, trauma of the brain is probably most frequently encountered in dogs as a result of automobile-induced injury. Trauma, particularly involving small animals, also can result from falls from significant heights (e.g., high-rise apartment buildings, balconies, roofs). Cats often have remarkably minor injury to the CNS, even after falling from considerable heights. Other examples include fracture of the spinal column or cranium of jumping horses and fractious animals (e.g., horses and ruminants) during excitement and restraint.

Predisposition to cerebral trauma is also influenced by anatomic differences. The percentage of brain mass in relation to skull size is much less in domestic animals than in primates, and in some species (e.g., bovine and porcine), the cranial cavity is additionally protected dorsally by prominent frontal sinuses. Birth trauma, which can be important in human beings, is essentially insignificant in animals because in the latter the shoulders, and particularly the pelvis, rather than the head are likely to be compressed in the birth canal. Exceptions to this generalization include brachycephalic breeds of dogs. Several factors also influence the susceptibility of the spinal cord to trauma. The amount of space between the spinal cord and the wall of the vertebral canal is very important in determining the degree of injury following swelling (e.g., edema) or compression (e.g., disk herniation). This space is greater in the cervical area (e.g., in the dog) than at the thoracolumbar level, allowing disk herniation at the latter area to often result in more severe spinal cord injury.

Functional factors also play an important role in brain injury. The brain of a freely movable head is much more susceptible to injury than a stationary, supported one. This increased susceptibility has been attributed to the ability of the cranium and its contents (the brain) to impact upon each other following trauma. This interaction can occur because the brain does not completely fill the cranial cavity, resulting in a very short distance (or space) between the brain tissue and bone. Thus, following an impact upon a stationary freely movable head, the bone will move upon the stationary brain and result in injury. In addition, the mass and velocity of the object striking the head are important. Trauma following impact of a relatively large blunt object can create marked head movement, as well as a large-impact injury, whereas a small object (e.g., bullet) moving at a high rate of speed can cause less head movement and a smaller but deeper area of tissue damage.

Factors involved in the protection of the brain include the rigidity of the cranium (dependent upon age), the round shape of the dorsum of the skull, the structure of the cranial bone (two layers of compact bone separated by spongy bone referred to as diplöe), cranial sutures, sinuses, ridges in the floor of the cranial cavity, meninges, and CSF. The spinal cord is enclosed and protected by the vertebral column, which is surrounded by soft tissues (e.g., adipose tissue and muscle). Other structures that help protect the

Table 8-2 Classification of Selected Lysosomal Storage Diseases That Involve the CNS of Animals

Disease	Storage Product	Deficient Enzyme	Species	Breed
GM_1 gangliosidosis	GM_1 ganglioside	β-galactosidase	Bovine	Holstein-Friesian
			Canine	Beagle, English Springer spaniel, Portuguese water dog
			Feline	Siamese, domestic shorthair
			Ovine	Suffolk, Coopworth-Romney
GM_2 gangliosidosis	GM_2 ganglioside	β-hexosaminidase	Canine	German shorthair pointer, Japanese spaniel
			Feline	Domestic shorthair, Korat
			Porcine	Yorkshire
Globoid-cell leukodystrophy (Krabbe's-like disease)	Galactosylceramide (galactocerebroside) and galactosylsphingosine (psychosine)	Galactosylceramidase (galactocerebroside β-galactosidase)	Canine	West Highland terrier, Cairn terrier, miniature poodle, blue tick hound, beagle, Pomeranian
			Feline	Domestic shorthair
			Ovine	Polled Dorset
α-mannosidosis	Mannose-containing oligosaccharide	α-mannosidase	Bovine	Angus, Murray gray, Galloway
			Feline	Persian, domestic shorthair
β-mannosidosis	Mannose-containing oligosaccharide	β-mannosidase	Caprine	Nubian
			Bovine	Salers
Mucopolysaccharidosis	Different glycosaminoglycans	Several different enzyme deficiencies	Canine	Plott hound (type I, Hurler's disease), miniature pinscher (type VI, Maroteaux-Lamy disease)
				Breed? (type VII, Sly disease)
			Feline	Domestic short hair (type I, Hurler's disease)
				Breed? (type VI, Maroteaux-Lamy disease)
				Domestic short hair (type VII, Sly disease)
			Caprine	Nubian (type III, Sanfilippo's disease)
Ceroid-lipofuscinosis	Subunit *c* of mitochondrial ATPase	Prelysosomal defect?	Canine	English setter, border collie, Tibetan terrier
			Ovine	South Hampshire
			Bovine	Devon
	Sphingolipid	Palmitoyl protein thioesterase	Canine	Miniature schnauzer
	Activating proteins A and D		Ovine	Swedish Landrace
	Unknown	Unknown	Canine	Chihuahua, cocker spaniel, Saluki, terrier-cross, blue heeler, Yugoslavian shepherd, Dalmatian, Australian cattle dog, golden retriever, dachshund, corgi
			Ovine	Rambouillet
			Bovine	Beefmaster
			Feline	Siamese, domestic short hair
Niemann-Pick type c disease	Primarily ganglioside in neurons	Unknown	Feline	Breed?
			Canine	Boxer

? = unknown.

spinal cord (by absorbing shock) are the intervertebral disks and the cancellous bone of the vertebrae. Vertebral ligaments maintain the alignment of the vertebral column; denticulate ligaments help to maintain the proper position of the spinal cord, and the meninges and the CSF help to cushion trauma.

Cerebral Trauma

Concussion. Concussion is a clinical designation often characterized by a temporary loss of consciousness with recovery that follows head injury. It should be noted, however, that this type of injury is only part of a spectrum that has been referred to as **diffuse brain injury.** The severity of diffuse brain injury, depending on the degree of trauma, can range from a mild, reversible concussion without loss of consciousness to severe injury that can result in a permanent neurologic deficit or even death. Diffuse brain injury involves widespread or global disruption of neurologic function. Injury of this type results primarily from rotational acceleration forces that cause shear, tensile, and compressive strains that are generated throughout the brain.

Concussive injuries of the diffuse type also occur in animals, but there are some differences between animals and human beings. For example, it is difficult to produce severe concussion in animals because the margin between a stunning blow and fatal injury is very small. The smaller the brain, the less vulnerable it is to rotational forces and the larger are the forces necessary to cause concussion. It should be noted, however, that concussion can occur more frequently than appreciated in animals. As in the human being, a movable head is much more susceptible to trauma than a fixed, supported one. Application of an appropriate concussive trauma to the mobile head of an animal results in a reversible cerebral dysfunction that lasts for a matter of seconds or, at most, a few minutes, with stronger blows causing more severe injury and even death. Long periods of coma after a single head injury of the diffuse type (referred to above as diffuse brain injury) have not been readily produced in animals. Diffuse brain injury is usually not associated with gross lesions. Microscopic lesions detected in animals have included axonal degeneration and neuronal loss, as well as regenerative processes (central chromatolysis). The more severe forms of diffuse brain injury are also associated with generalized acute brain swelling that can be followed after some time by cerebral edema. (See Brain Swelling Due to Cerebral Trauma).

Contusion. In contrast to the diffuse form of cerebral injury, contusion is characterized by **focal brain injury** that is grossly detectable, usually as hemorrhage, and can, like concussion, result in unconsciousness and even death. In fact, it would be reasonable to assume that the causative factors involved in concussion and contusion can occur together to varying degrees in the same animal. Lesions can be superficial (e.g., cerebral gyri) or more central (e.g., brain stem), and there can be associated skull fracture.

Although hemorrhage is the most common lesion, contusion of the brain results in tearing of CNS tissue. Tearing results in tissue necrosis and neuronal loss. Two designations are used to identify the location of contusive injury. A **coup contusion** is located at the impact site, and a **contrecoup contusion** at a location on the opposite side of the brain. When the two lesions occur together (e.g., coup-contrecoup or contrecoup-coup), the first term indicates the site of most severe injury (see Box 8-1 for a summary of the pathogenesis of coup-contrecoup contusion).

Many investigations have been made to determine the mechanisms involved in the development of contusive lesions, and the kinetics are complicated and still not completely resolved. Factors that have been considered to be significant include the ability of the head to move freely, the occurrence of a rotational movement of the brain over rough surfaces on the inside of the cranial vault, and the development within the cranial cavity of positive and negative pressures as well as gravitational forces. Several neuropathologic principles have been generally accepted regarding craniocerebral contusive trauma in the human being:

1. A blow to the stationary (but freely movable) head produces a cerebrocortical coup contusion beneath the point of cranial impact, but with rare exceptions causes no cerebrocortical contrecoup contusion opposite the point of cranial impact.
2. An impact of a moving head (moving before impact, as in a fall from a standing position) against a firm or unyielding surface causes a cerebrocortical contrecoup contusion opposite the point of cranial collision (often at the poles and inferior surfaces of the frontal and temporal lobes), but with rare exceptions there is no contusion beneath the point of impact.
3. Falls from great heights, as well as crushing of the head between a strong external force and unyielding surface, are generally not associated with the occurrence of contrecoup lesions.

Dawson and coworkers proposed a mechanism for both contrecoup and coup injury of the human brain that also addressed the specific deficiencies of mechanisms that have been advanced by others. An example explaining the mechanism of contrecoup injury states that when a person falls backward from a standing position due to loss of balance the gravitational torque acting on the body causes downward acceleration of the head in excess of the acceleration due to gravity. Under these circumstances the brain lags toward the trailing anterior surface of the cranium before impact (causing displacement of the CSF-protective layer between the brain and skull) and permits compressive stress to develop at this site, although impact occurs at the opposite side of the head. Because dissipation of the cerebrospinal fluid at the anterior (contrecoup) site allows compressive stress to be focal at

BOX 8-1 SUMMARY OF THE PATHOGENESIS OF COUP-CONTRECOUP CONTUSION

Conditions Involved in Coup-contrecoup Contusion

1. Head freely movable
2. Head accelerated rapidly (e.g., by being struck by a broad object, such as an automobile) or decelerated rapidly (e.g., head strikes pavement after a fall)
3. Because the brain does not fill the cranial vault, it may lag behind when the head is accelerated or decelerated rapidly
4. As a result, the brain may strike the inside of the cranial vault at the point of impact (coup injury), or there may be hemorrhage (contusions) on the opposite side (contrecoup), either from the stretching and tearing of vessels at that site or by the brain striking the inside of the cranial vault on rebound

this contrecoup site and because of the shearing stress that is generated, injury occurs. In addition, a relative rotational gliding motion between the brain and skull is produced when the impact suddenly stops the skull's motion and rotation, thus creating an additive shearing stress because the fluid lubrication necessary to facilitate gliding of the brain over the cranial surface is reduced. The concentration of this rotational shearing stress is likely to occur beneath the frontal and temporal lobes because of the rough surface of the skull that exists in this location. In contrast to contrecoup injury, coup contusions occur infrequently in this type of fall. In such situations, brain lags away from the impact site, which results in a thickening of the protective CSF layer between the brain and skull immediately beneath the point of impact, which helps explain the absence of coup injury in primates and human beings in typical moving head trauma (trauma following head movement).

Coup injury can occur when a stationary (but freely movable) head is impacted. In this type of trauma, there is neither brain lag nor disproportionate distribution of CSF before impact, which accounts for the typical absence of contrecoup contusions. With regard to falls from great heights, the dynamics involving rotation of the body about a fixed point of ground contact associated with a fall from a standing position, do not occur. Since gravity produces no torque on a freely falling object, no angular acceleration of the body is produced and, therefore, such a fall is a true free-fall state that is associated with an absence of brain lag. For this reason, contrecoup lesions occur infrequently with this type of trauma. One point should be emphasized with regard to the evaluation of coup and contrecoup cortical contusions just described. Displacement of bone associated with skull fracture can contuse the subjacent brain, regardless of the resting or moving status of the head, and such fracture-contusions have nothing to do with the coup-contrecoup mechanisms described. Also, even though the basic mechanisms discussed above apply to the human being, they should also be considered when examining cerebral contusions of domestic animals.

Hemorrhage. Although hemorrhage in animal brains can be caused by a wide variety of injuries, trauma to the head is the most common cause. (See Box 8-2 for common causes of brain hemorrhage).

Following trauma to the head, hemorrhages can develop in the epidural, subdural, and leptomeningeal (subarachnoid space and pia mater) areas and in the brain parenchyma (Fig. 8-19). Such hemorrhages can result from movement of the brain over bony ridges of the cranium with stretching and tearing of blood vessels and parenchyma, and following the cutting and penetrating action of bone fragments associated with skull fracture. Epidural hemorrhage, which is not commonly described in animals, has been reported in the horse, especially jumpers, resulting from falls while working. Epidural hemorrhage does not usually occur because the dura is tightly adhered to the inner surface of the calvarium and thus there is no epidural space. In cases of trauma associated with skull fractures and the development of slowing bleeding large vessels, the dura can become separated from the calvarium, forming a space for blood to collect.

BOX 8-2 COMMON CAUSES OF HEMORRHAGE IN ANIMAL BRAINS

1. Vasculitis (e.g., *Haemophilus somnus* infection)
2. Damage to endothelial blood vessels (e.g., by the virus of canine infectious hepatitis or by septicemia or endotoxemia)
3. Trauma
   Coup
   Contrecoup
   Contusion
   Penetrating wounds

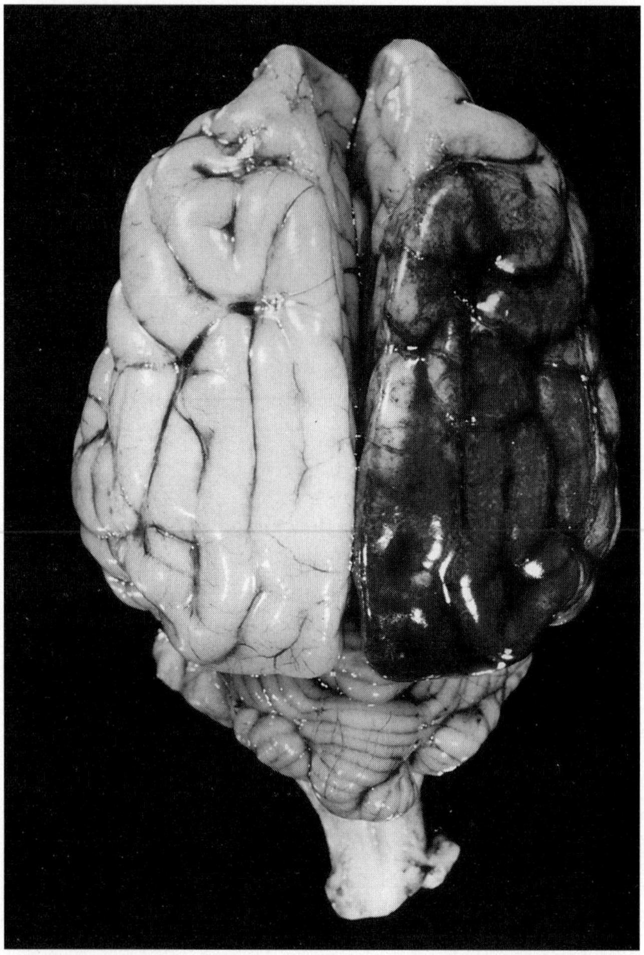

Figure 8-19 Brain, meninges of right cerebral hemisphere; dog. Leptomeningeal (subarachnoid-pial) hemorrhage over the surface of the right cerebral hemisphere.

Subdural hemorrhage, which is an accumulation of blood between the dura mater and arachnoid membrane, occurs in dogs and cats, although leptomeningal and parenchymal hemorrhage are most common in these species following head injury. Parenchymal hemorrhage can result from injury to the brain with a normal or fractured cranium by the mechanisms given above, and from penetrating objects (bullets and stab wounds).

Proposed Biochemical Mechanisms Involved in Tissue Injury Following Cerebral Trauma. CNS trauma (and its associated ischemia) can result in a number of pathophysiologic alterations that have been proposed to be important in development of CNS injury, particularly involving neurons, but also other cells of the CNS depending on the severity of ischemia. The following discussion focuses on neuronal injury.

Following trauma or ischemia, there is an early increase in energy (adenosine triphosphate [ATP])–dependent release of normally sequestered intracellular calcium ions from altered mitochondria and endoplasmic reticulum. Also during this time, neuronal depolarization potentiates the release of the neuroexcitatory neurotransmitter glutamate. Persistent activation of glutamate receptors of target cells results in a disturbance referred to as **excitotoxicity.** This altered activity leads to a significant influx of extracellular calcium into cells, causing further impairment of mitochrondrial function and the generation of reactive oxygen species (e.g., superoxide, hydrogen peroxide, hydroxy radical, and nitric oxide). These reactive oxygen species can enhance the existing excitotoxicity, cause further influx of calcium into cells as a result of membrane damage, and ultimately result in neuronal dysfunction and death. Additionally, reperfusion of ischemic tissue after the initial ischemic insult can result in generation of reactive oxygen metabolites that can be responsible for amplification of the tissue damage (see References and Circulatory Disturbances for further information).

Brain Swelling Due to Cerebral Trauma. Brain swelling, as distinguished from cerebral edema, is thought to represent, at least in part, an unregulated vasodilation following trauma, and it can cause serious brain damage (even more severe than the primary injury) if not properly controlled. This lesion therefore represents an enlargement of the brain resulting in elevated intracranial pressure due to increased diameter of the blood-containing vasculature, whereas edema results in an increased pressure following accumulation of fluid in the interstitium or intracellularly outside the circulation. Acute brain swelling can be localized (usually of lesser significance) when associated with focal lesions, or generalized (often serious) when caused by diffuse brain injury. Although rarely seen in domestic animals, one exception to the importance of focal lesions is extracerebral hemorrhage (e.g., acute subdural hematoma in human beings), which though principally involving the surface of one hemisphere, can cause more mass effect (brain swelling) in the underlying cerebral hemisphere than the hematoma itself. In such circumstances (acute subdural hematoma), the small amount of blood in the subarachnoid space is not the sole reason for the patient's neurologic state. If the hematoma is removed, the acute brain swelling can progress so rapidly that the brain protrudes (herniates) through the craniotomy site.

The more serious forms of diffuse brain injury are associated with generalized acute brain swelling. It is sometimes difficult to determine the relative importance of swelling in affected individuals because initial acute swelling (detectable as soon as 30 minutes after injury in human beings) can be followed after several hours to days by true cerebral edema (as a result of increased vascular permeability), which can be the actual deleterious lesion. Peroxidative injury to blood vessels has been one proposed cause of pathologic vasodilation in the posttraumatic CNS. For more information concerning brain swelling, see the Gennarelli reference and Circulatory Disturbances, Edema of the Nervous System for discussion of vasogenic, cytotoxic, hydrostatic, and osmotic edema.

Spinal Cord Trauma

Evaluation of spinal cord trauma should include examination not only of the spinal cord but also of the vertebral column and spinal nerve roots. Injuries to the spinal cord can involve concussion, contusion, hemorrhage, laceration, transection, and compression.

Concussion. Spinal concussion is the term applied to the immediate and temporary loss of function, that sometimes follows severe direct blows to the spinal column. Loss of function usually affects the long tracts (e.g., ventral motor tracts), but usually there is no demonstrable external change in the vertebrae or spinal cord. As with cerebral concussion, there is often only a temporary functional disability of the cord after injury, but permanent neurologic deficits can occur, depending on the degree of trauma.

Contusion. Contusion is characterized by hemorrhage, necrosis, and tears that are generally focal and grossly visible. Contusion can occur without fracture of the vertebral column, with fracture, and with fracture plus dislocation of the spinal column. The latter combination can result in tearing and transsection of the spinal cord.

Hemorrhage. The same types of hemorrhage that affect the brain (epidural [rare], subdural [rare], leptomeningeal, and parenchymal hemorrhage) also occur in the spinal cord and its meninges. Causes in this location are similar to those affecting the brain and include stretching as a result of abnormal movement and severance of blood vessels associated with vertebral fracture.

LACERATION AND TRANSECTION. Both laceration and transection can occur following vertebral fracture, laceration by penetration of bony fragments and transection by severance of the spinal cord by sharp fragments of bone associated with dislocation of the vertebrae.

COMPRESSION. Compression of the spinal cord can be due to intramedullary (within the spinal cord) or extramedullary (outside the spinal cord) pressure. Causes of intramedullary compression include intraparenchymal hemorrhages and neoplasms (e.g., nephroblastoma of the young dog). Extramedullary pressure can be caused by intervertebral disk herniation in the dog, cervical stenotic myelopathy (wobbler syndrome) in the horse and dog (see below and Chapter 10, "Diseases of Bone and Joints"), vertebral fracture and dislocation, and neoplasms of the meninges, nerve rootlets, or both.

Intervertebral disk disease occurs in the canine species, particularly dogs of the chondrodystrophic breeds typified by the dachshund and Pekingese. Intervertebral disks are present between all vertebral bodies except for the C1-2 space and the sacral vertebrae, and they act as absorbers of shock during movement. Intervertebral disks of a significant percentage of dachshunds and Pekingese begin to degenerate after approximately 1 year of age, predisposing them to sudden herniation (Hansen type I herniation) earlier than for nonchondrodystrophic breeds. Disk herniation in nonchondrodystrophic breeds (e.g., large breeds of dogs) occurs more slowly because of dorsal protrusion of a weakened, but not ruptured, disk (Hansen type II herniation). Herniation of either type occurs most frequently in the thoracolumbar and cervical areas. Intercapital (conjugal) ligaments, which extend across the floor of the vertebral canal over the dorsal aspect of each annulus fibrosus from the T1-2 through T10-11 intervertebral spaces, add support and account for the infrequent occurrence of herniation in the thoracic area. Severity of injury to the spinal cord is influenced both by the amount of space existing between the spinal cord and bone of the vertebral canal and by the speed with which herniation occurs. The space surrounding the cervical cord is greater than in the thoracolumbar area, which generally results in less compression following cervical disk herniation.

A unique and uncommon lesion in the dog, referred to as **progressive hemorrhagic myelomalacia,** can follow spinal cord injury, particularly associated with severe type I disk herniation, but can also occur following other forms of spinal trauma. This lesion, which is characterized by a softening to semiliquefaction (myelomalacia) and hemorrhage of the tissue, can develop within 12 to 24 hours after injury and can progress both cranially and caudally from the original site of trauma. The mechanism involved has not been determined, but the processes discussed above (particularly lipid peroxidation) have been considered. This lesion is to be compared with typical infarction (see Circulatory Disturbances).

Cervical stenotic myelopathy or **wobbler syndrome** is characterized by stenosis of the cervical vertebral canal that causes compressive trauma to the cervical spinal cord. It has been known for many years to affect horses, and more recently has been recognized in the dog. The disease in the horse has been referred to by several designations: the wobbler syndrome, wobbles, equine incoordination, and, more recently, cervical stenotic myelopathy. The disease has been described in many breeds. Reports indicate that the disease is not caused by a straightforward mechanism but apparently involves several factors. For example, male horses (stallions) that have rapid growth rate and large body size are reported to be at greater risk to develop the disease.

Cervical stenotic myelopathy in the horse has been divided into two syndromes, referred to as cervical static stenosis and cervical vertebral instability (dynamic stenosis).

Cervical static stenosis commonly affects horses 1 to 4 years of age. The spinal cord is compressed at C5 through C7 as the result of an acquired dorsal or dorsolateral narrowing of the spinal canal. The stenosis is due to formation of bone that requires time to develop. The compressive effect with this type of stenosis is present regardless of head position. The second form of cervical stenotic myelopathy (cervical vertebral instability–dynamic stenosis) occurs in horses ranging in age from 8 to 18 months. It is characterized by a narrowing of the spinal canal during flexion of the neck (e.g., with downward movement of the head), and primarily involves C3 through C5 vertebrae.

A disease process with many similarities to that in the horse also affects the dog. It has been known as wobbler syndrome, vertebral instability, vertebral subluxation, and cervical spondylolisthesis. The disease has been most frequently described in the Great Dane and Doberman pinscher breeds, but has also been reported in the Saint Bernard, Irish setter, fox terrier, basset hound, Rhodesian Ridgeback, and Old English sheepdog. Dogs can develop signs between 8 months and 1 year of age, with a range of 1 month to 9 years. Great Danes tend to develop lesions at a young age (e.g., 8 months to 1 year), whereas Doberman pinschers are generally older, often more than 1 year of age. The vertebral and associated spinal cord lesions in the dog have been reported to most often involve the caudal cervical area from C5 through C7 vertebrae. An exception is the basset hound in which C3 is affected. The pathogenesis appears to be similar to that in the horse.

Lesions of the CNS in cervical stenotic myelopathy are similar to the lesions in intervertebral disk herniation. The severity depends upon the speed and degree to which the compression is applied and the specific area of the cord that is involved. Central nervous tissue can tolerate a considerable degree of compression if it is applied slowly (e.g., Hansen type II disk herniation in nonchondrodystrophic breeds of dogs and possibly in equine cervical static stenosis). Rapid compression (e.g., associated with Hansen type I disk herniation in chondrodystrophic breeds of dogs, and possibly following sudden forceful compression in equine cervical vertebral instability) can lead to quickly developing hypoxia-ischemia and necrosis. Lesions detected include a spectrum of change characterized by axonal injury (Wallerian degeneration), disruption of myelin sheaths, and necrosis of the gray or white matter or both (due to ischemia secondary to interruption of the blood supply). Lesions can be visible grossly from the exterior, but more commonly on cross section.

Microscopically, after a few days, particularly at the site of injury, there is loss of architecture of the parenchyma as a result of necrosis and a beginning accumulation of macrophages (gitter cells) that have phagocytized the lipid-rich tissue debris (see Fig. 8-20 for comparable lesion). Eventually, the necrotic area is cleared and a cystic space is formed, which is surrounded by varying degrees of astrocytosis and astrogliosis. Rostral and caudal to this location, the lesion is primarily one of axonal (Wallerian) degeneration in the white matter, and the pattern of lesion development seen depends upon the level of the spinal cord that is examined relative to the site of compression. At the site of injury, all parts of the cord (white and gray matter) are affected (and often necrotic) if the compressive force is sufficient. Rostral to this site, white matter degeneration is generally limited to the ascending tracts in the dorsal funiculi and the superficial portions of the dorsolateral part of the lateral funiculi. Caudal to the area of injury, white matter degeneration tends to be limited to the descending tracts in the ventral funiculi, and the more central portions of the lateral funiculi (see p. 382 for discussion of Wallerian degeneration).

Circulatory Disturbances

The Influence of the Rate of Oxygen Deprivation on Lesion Development

The rate at which ischemia occurs in the CNS determines the degree of injury that follows. The more rapid the onset of ischemia, the more severe the lesion. If the blood flow through an artery is gradually reduced (e.g., because of arteriosclerosis), there is often sufficient time for anastomotic vessels to dilate and compensate. However, if the obstruction is sudden (e.g., caused by an embolus), much of the tissue can die before an adequate anastomotic circulation can be established. This same principle applies to compressive injury to the CNS that produces a reduction in blood flow. Such affected tissue can compensate rather remarkably if the compression is slow (e.g., slowly developing [Hansen type II] disk herniation in the dog or compression by a slowly growing neoplasm from the exterior such as meningioma in the dog), when compared with a sudden compressive injury (e.g., rapidly occurring Hansen type I disk herniation in the dog).

Susceptibility of Cells and Specific Anatomic Areas to Ischemia, Factors that Influence Ischemic Injury, and Time Required After Ischemia for Neuronal Injury

The susceptibility of cells and tissue structures of the CNS to ischemia, in decreasing order of susceptibility, are neurons, oligodendroglia, astrocytes, microglia, and blood vessels (Fig. 8-20). Neurons are not all equally susceptible to ischemia, and differences occur in relation to their location in the CNS. Susceptible neurons include those of the cerebral cortex, hippocampus, certain areas of the basal ganglia, and Purkinje cells of the cerebellar cortex. Neurons of the phylogenetically older parts of the nervous system (gray matter of the spinal cord and greater part of the brain stem) are more resistant to ischemia than the more recently developed areas such as the cerebral cortex.

Similar to the effects caused by physical disturbances discussed earlier, factors that are considered to be important in the development of ischemic neuronal injury include the mechanisms of excitatory neurotransmitter (glutamate) toxicity and generation of toxic free radicals that exert their effect (especially on lipid-rich cell membranes) through peroxidation. Other influencing factors also include the temperature of the brain at the time of ischemia, with lower temperatures (as little as 2° C decrease) having a sparing effect and higher ones (by the same amount but elevated) having an enhancing effect on neuronal injury following ischemia.

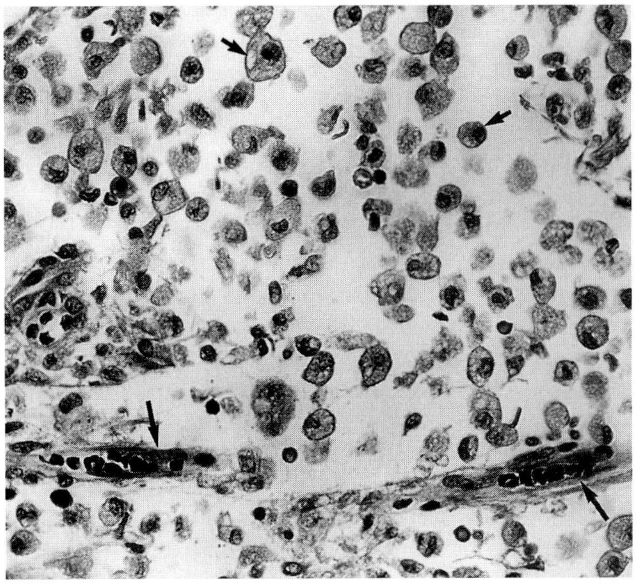

Figure 8-20 Brain, parietal lobe; dog. Infarction. The lesion has progressed to the stage of liquefaction necrosis, characterized by a predominance of vacuolated (lipid-laden) macrophages (gitter cells) *(short arrows)*. Intact blood vessels *(long arrows)*, which are more resistant to ischemia than neurons, oligodendroglia, and astrocytes, are the only tissue components remaining in the lesion. H & E stain. (See Figs. 8-25, 8-34, and 8-39 for the gross appearance of such a lesion.)

There is also evidence (demonstrated experimentally in laboratory animals) that the time required for death of neurons following ischemia need not always be the same. This difference has been associated with the severity of the ischemic insult; the more severe the ischemia, the less time required for neuronal death (ischemic cell change). Conversely, the less severe the ischemic insult, the longer the time required for neuronal death. This mechanism of injury has been referred to as **"delayed neuronal death."**

Edema of the CNS

The basis of our current understanding of cerebral edema was advanced by Klatzo in 1967 when he proposed two distinct types: the first characterized by an increased extracellular fluid resulting from increased vascular permeability (**vasogenic** type), and the second characterized by an increased intracellular fluid with normal vascular permeability (**cytotoxic** type). Other types of cerebral edema have been identified as **hydrostatic** (or interstitial) edema associated with increased hydrostatic pressure (e.g., resulting from hydrocephalus), and **osmotic edema,** which is dependent on development of abnormal osmotic forces between the blood and nervous tissue.

Vasogenic Edema. The underlying mechanism of vasogenic cerebral edema is a breakdown of the blood-brain barrier that results in movement of plasma constituents such as water, sodium, and plasma proteins into the extracellular space, particularly that of the white matter (Figs. 8-21 and 8-22). In addition to extracellular accumulation of fluid, vasogenic edema can also be accompanied by some cellular swelling (e.g., involving astrocytes). Vasogenic edema is the most common type and occurs following vascular injury. It is often adjacent to hematomas, contusions, infarcts, inflammatory foci, and neoplasms and occurs in certain toxicities.

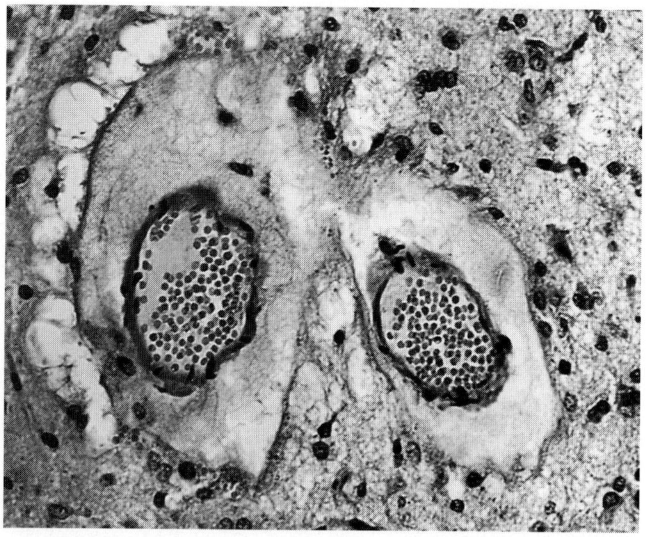

Figure 8-21 Brain, pyriform lobe; pig. Mercury toxicity. Two vessels with fibrinoid necrosis of their walls are surrounded by fibrin and vasogenic edema fluid. H & E stain. *Courtesy Dr. W. W. Carlton.*

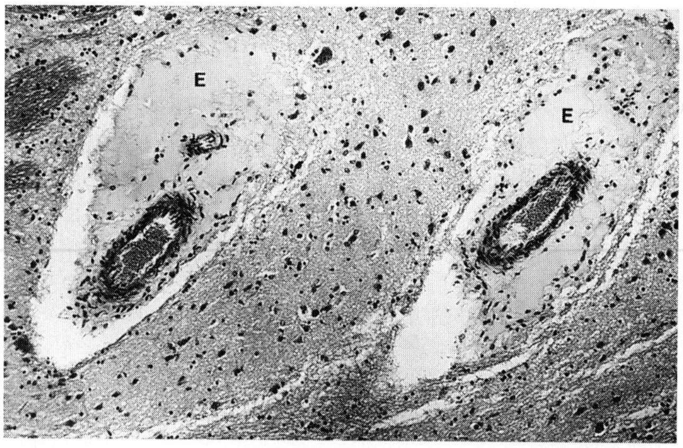

Figure 8-22 Brain, parietal lobe, level of the thalamus; feeder lamb. *Clostridium perfringens* type D enterotoxemia. Marked perivascular (vasogenic) edema fluid *(E)* surrounds each vessel. H & E stain.

Cytotoxic Edema. Cytotoxic edema is characterized by the accumulation of fluid intracellularly (e.g., in neurons, astrocytes, oligodendroglia, and endothelial cells) as a result of altered cellular metabolism, often due to ischemia. Affected cells swell within seconds of injury. The mechanism is considered to involve an energy deficit that interferes with normal function of the ATP-dependent sodium-potassium pump. Thus the cell cannot maintain homeostasis and secrete intracellular sodium. An elevated concentration of intracellular sodium is followed by an increased influx of water. The gray and white matter of the brain are both affected. The fluid taken up by the swollen cells is primarily derived from the extracellular space, which becomes reduced in size and has an increased concentration of extracellular solutes.

For this lesion to be described accurately as cerebral edema, there must be additional fluid movement into the brain and not merely a change of existing intraparenchymal fluid from extracellular to intracellular compartments. The additional fluid originates from the circulation (by way of the transcapillary fluid exchange) and from the CSF, which has extensive diffusional communication with the extracellular fluid of the brain. The blood-brain barrier remains intact during development of this type of edema, so fluid does not enter the brain by a disturbance in vascular permeability. Specific causes of this lesion include hypoxia-ischemia (particularly in the early stages); intoxication with metabolic inhibitors such as 2,4,dinitrophenol, 6-aminonicatinamide, and ouabain; and severe hypothermia.

Hydrostatic (Interstitial) Edema. Hydrostatic edema is characterized by the accumulation of a protein-free fluid in the extracellular space of the brain because of elevated ventricular hydrostatic pressure that accompanies hydrocephalus. Fluid moves across the ependyma of the ventricular wall and accumulates extracellularly in the periventricular tissue (primarily white matter). Unlike the other forms of cerebral edema that cause swelling of affected CNS tissue, hydrostatic edema causes variable degeneration and loss of the periventricular white matter. The blood-brain barrier remains intact.

Osmotic Cerebral Edema. Cerebral edema has also been associated with "water intoxication," which can result from an increased body hydration caused by (1) excessive, faulty intravenous hydration; (2) compulsive drinking caused by abnormal mental function; or (3) altered antidiuretic hormone secretion. The increased body hydration produces a hypotonic (hypoosmolar) plasma, with subsequent development of an osmotic gradient between the hypotonic plasma and the relatively hypertonic state of the normal cerebral tissue. Fluid moves from the plasma into the brain. In this type of edema, the blood-brain barrier remains intact. If it did not, the change in plasma osmolarity would soon be transmitted to the brain tissue (through vascular leakage) and would abolish the necessary osmotic gradient. Fluid accumulation occurs primarily intracellularly, but can also be present extracellularly. In addition, typically a pronounced increase occurs in the rate of formation of CSF originating from the choroid plexus and the extracellular fluid of the brain.

Sequelae of Cerebral Edema. The gross lesions that accompany cerebral edema are the result of enlargement of an organ in an enclosed, limited space; the degree of swelling obviously determines the type and extent of lesions that develop. In evaluating lesions, it is particularly important initially to examine the brain and spinal cord in the fresh state and in situ.

Because of compression against the cranium, an affected brain has flattened gyri and shallow sulci, and it can shift in position. If the edema is confined to one side, the displacement is unilateral, which can be associated with herniation of the cingulate gyrus under the falx cerebri; the extent of the unilateral intracerebral enlargement can be best appreciated following the examination of coronal (transverse) sections. Diffuse swelling usually causes a caudal shifting that can result in herniation of the brain (parahippocampal gyri of temporal lobes) beneath the tentorium cerebelli or herniation of the cerebellar vermis through the foramen magnum, resulting in "coning" of the vermis (Fig. 8-23). On cut surface, the white matter is most often affected (frequently with the vasogenic type of edema which is the most common). It is swollen and soft, has a damp appearance, and is light yellow in the fresh, unfixed state.

Microscopically, in contrast to some other tissues such as the lungs, the extracellular fluid associated with vasogenic edema fluid is often not detectable, except in

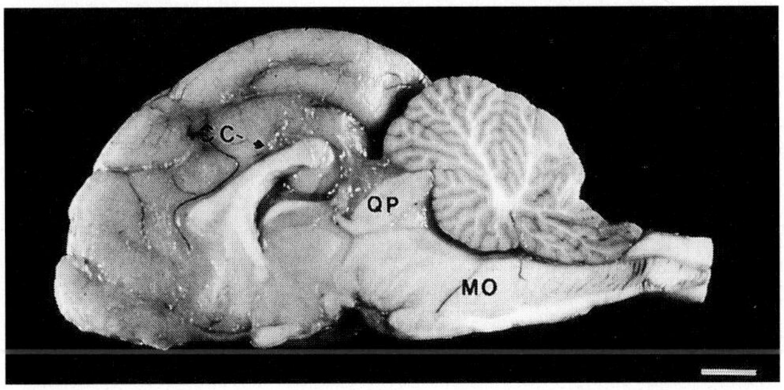

Figure 8-23 Brain, cerebellum; cat. Coning of the cerebellum (caudal displacement of the caudal cerebellar vermis through the foramen magnum with compression of the medulla oblongata *[MO]*) due to cerebral edema. Note the elevation of the corpus callosum *(CC)* and compression of the rostral cerebellar vermis by the quadrigeminal plate *(QP)*. *Courtesy Dr. D. Y. Cho International Veterinary Pathology Slide Bank.*

instances of marked vascular injury. When the extracellular space-occupying fluid cannot be identified, only its effects (separation of the parenchyma causing reduced staining intensity) can be recognized. Additionally, following prolonged vasogenic edema, the lesions include hypertrophy and hyperplasia of astrocytes, activation of microglia, and demyelination. Cytotoxic edema is characterized by cellular swelling, including swelling of astrocytes.

Infarction

Infarction means necrosis of a tissue following obstruction of its arterial blood supply. Anastomoses of the arteries that penetrate from the ventral and cortical surfaces of the brain are insufficient to prevent infarction following sudden occlusion of one or more of these arteries.

Cerebral necrosis, comparable to infarction following vascular occlusion, can also result from other causes, including cessation of cerebral circulation (e.g., caused by cardiac arrest); sudden hypotension (e.g., caused by reduced cardiac output); and reduced or absent oxygen in inspired air. Additional causes include altered function of hemoglobin (e.g., as a result of carbon monoxide poisoning), inhibition of tissue respiration (e.g., cytochrome oxidase system following cyanide poisoning), toxic substances and poisons, and nutritional deficiencies. Although resulting from different mechanisms, the necrosis that occurs has, with some variation, essentially the same gross and microscopic characteristics as that which is associated with classical infarction. Since the above causes of brain injury (excluding arterial obstruction) are not related to the blood supply of one or more specific arteries, the distribution of tissue damage will depend on the location of susceptible cells. The degree of injury, obviously, will depend upon the severity and duration of the inciting cause.

Areas of cerebral infarction differ somewhat in gross appearance from infarcts in other tissues. The abundance of lipids and enzymes, plus the relative lack of fibrous connective tissue stroma in the brain and spinal cord, results in affected areas eventually becoming soft (often referred to as malacia) because of liquefaction necrosis. The gross appearance of infarction may differ according to location. Lesions affecting the gray matter tend to be hemorrhagic (hemorrhagic infarction) (Fig. 8-24), whereas infarction of the white matter is often pale (pale infarction). This difference is probably due in part to the less dense capillary meshwork in the white matter, and in part to the fact that the vessels supplying the white matter have fewer anastomoses than those of the gray matter. Infarcted tissue goes through a characteristic sequence of changes that can permit a relatively accurate determination of the age of the infarct (Figs. 8-24 and 8-25; see also Fig. 8-20). An outline of the chronologic events that occur after an ischemic episode that lasts more than 5 to 6 minutes and is followed by resuscitation of an animal is given in Table 8-3. As can be seen, the tissue changes listed in Table 8-3 take different periods of time to develop in the living resuscitated animal after ischemia occurs. Variation in the times that specific lesions occur depends on the extent and duration of the initial ischemic event.

Recent advances have improved our understanding of the mechanisms involved in ischemic injury of the CNS. The CNS depends on blood for a continuous supply of oxygen and glucose, and interruption of this blood flow for only a few minutes results in the death of vulnerable neurons. If the cessation of flow is sustained for a longer period, all types of cells (neurons, oligodendroglia, astrocytes, and microglia) in the affected area die. It appears that death of neurons involves a process that is more complicated than just a loss of energy and that these cells can also be killed by injurious chemical mechanisms that result from disturbed neurotransmitter function.

When an artery supplying the CNS is suddenly occluded, blood supply to cells at the center of the infarcted area (the core) is rapidly stopped, and if maintained for a sufficient period, all cells die. Neurons at the border (penumbra) of this area continue to receive some blood from nonobstructed vessels. It is proposed that the axonal terminals of degenerated ischemic neurons in the core of the infarct release excessive amounts of the neurotransmitter glutamate, causing injury to still-viable neurons in the penumbra, which increases the extent of injury that can occur with infarction. This process begins following the binding of the neurotransmitter glutamate to receptors on viable neurons in the penumbra, inducing an abnormal movement of calcium ions into the recipient cells followed by an increase in intracellular calcium ion concentration. This buildup of calcium ions contributes to a multifunctional cascade that leads to neuronal death. When infarction is additionally associated with hemorrhage, the mechanical injury from the pressure, plus tissue displacement by the hemorrhage, can cause additional damage. See Table 8-3 for the reparative responses associated with the resolution of infarcts.

Vascular Disease

The incidence of cerebrovascular diseases analogous to those in human beings is low in animals, and neurologic manifestations associated with these are uncommon. Arteriosclerosis ("hardening" of arteries) can be categorized as lipid (atherosclerosis) or nonlipid arteriosclerosis; the latter encompasses arterial fibrosis, mineralization, and amyloid deposition. Additionally, vascular diseases of the CNS can result from inflammation/infection, either as a component of a systemic disease or from extension of inflammatory meningeal or parenchymal disease. Some of

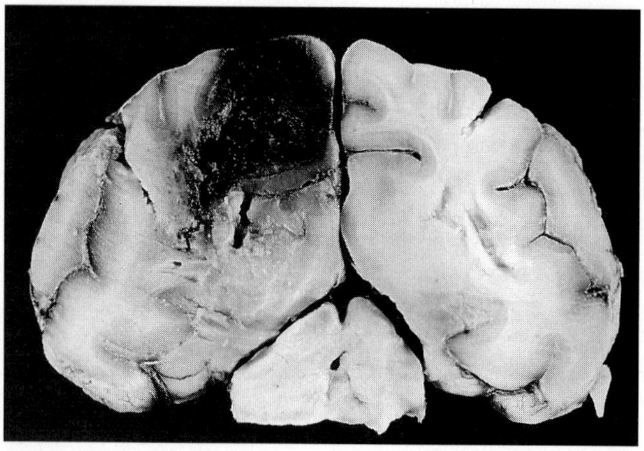

Figure 8-24 Brain, left dorsal parietal lobe; dog. Cerebral hemorrhagic infarct affecting the cortex and white matter of the endomarginal, marginal, suprasylvian, splenial, and cingulate gyri; and the centrum semiovale.

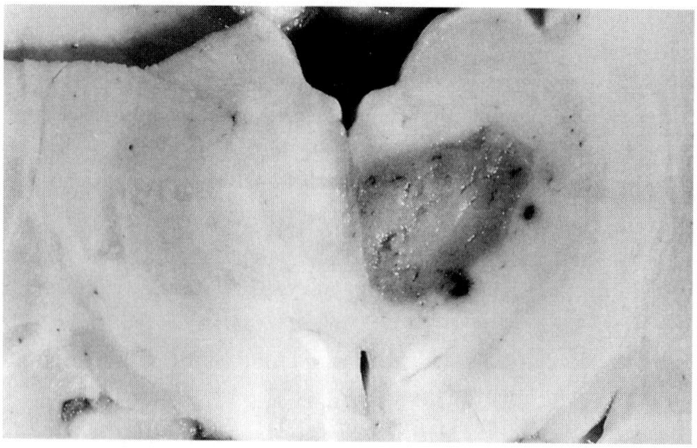

Figure 8-25 Brain, parietal lobe, thalamus; dog. There is focal malacia resulting from liquefaction necrosis in the right midcentral thalamus.

these diseases are covered later in this chapter. Thrombosis of cerebral blood vessels or venous sinuses occurs uncommonly. It can occur without evidence of overt vascular disease. Thrombosis can occur with or without evidence of a demonstrable local or systemic disease process.

Atherosclerosis. Atherosclerosis is reported in a variety of animals including nonhuman primates, pigs, dogs, and several avian species. Older pigs are most commonly and severely affected. Vessels that can be involved include aorta and its major branches, extramural coronary arteries, and meningeal arteries. Affected arteries are rigid, irregularly thickened, and white to yellow-white. Arterial lumina are narrowed or almost obliterated, but there is usually no appreciable ulceration, thrombosis, or hemorrhage. Intimal thickenings in intracranial arteries contain less lipid and have a greater tendency for fibrosclerosis than other vessels. In arteries within the brain parenchyma, there is collagenous adventitial or transmural thickening. The arterial lesions can be associated with hemorrhage or infarcts involving basal nuclei, fornix, internal and external capsules, hippocampus, and thalamus. Atherosclerosis occurs uncommonly in the dog in association with the disturbed lipid metabolism of hypothyroidism. Lesions involve meningeal arteries as well as vessels elsewhere in the body and are most severe in the intima and media (Fig. 8-26). Hemorrhage, ischemia, and infarction are uncommon but can occur.

Nonlipid Arteriosclerosis. Arterial **fibrosis** occurs more frequently in older animals and has been described in dogs and horses. In the dog, fibrosis of the intima, media, or adventitia occurs with some frequency in cerebrospinal vessels of all types and caliber. Collagenous thickening of the adventitia of small meningeal and parenchymal arteries can be accompanied by variable extension into other layers of the vessel wall. A preferential site is the choroid plexus. In old horses, a similar pattern of fibrosis occurs in vessels, but the intima may be preferentially affected. **Amyloid** deposits in meningeal and cerebral vessels are reported in older dogs and other animals. **Mineralization** (deposition of calcium or iron salts) of cerebral blood vessels occurs in

Table 8-3 Chronologic Sequence of Changes Within Infarcted Tissue (in the Living Animal) Following an Ischemic Event

Time Following Ischemic Event	Tissue Change
Immediate (seconds)	Cessation of blood flow (ischemia) and accumulation of waste products
Few minutes	Cellular injury and death; coagulation necrosis and edema; hemorrhage (especially in gray matter)
20 minutes	First microscopic evidence of neuronal injury (perfusion-fixation)
1-2 hours	First microscopic evidence of neuronal injury (immersion fixation)
2 hours	Pale staining of infarct microscopically (white matter); swelling of capillary endothelium; increase in size of astrocytic nuclei
3-5 hours	Ischemic cell change in most neurons; swelling of oligodendroglia and astroglia; beginning clasmatodendrosis of astrocytes
6-24 hours	Beginning neutrophilic infiltration; alteration of myelin (pale staining), 8-24 hours; degeneration and decrease of oligodendroglia, 8-24 hours; astrocytic swelling and retraction and fragmentation of processes (clasmatodendrosis), and degeneration*; cytoplasm of astrocytes visible, 8-24 hours*; vascular degeneration and fibrin deposition, 8-24 hours; thrombosis†, 6-24 hours; beginning endothelial proliferation at margin of infarct, 9 hours
8-24 (up to 48) hours	Initial gross detection of infarct unless hemorrhagic; infarct edematous (swollen), soft, pale, or hemorrhagic and demarcated
1-2 days	Swelling of axons and myelin sheaths; prominent neutrophilic infiltration
2 days	Prominent loss of neuroectodermal cells; continued proliferation of endothelial cells; reduced number of neutrophils; beginning increase in mononuclear cells (gitter cells)
3-5 days	Prominent number of mononuclear cells (gitter cells); disappearance of neutrophils; continued endothelial cell proliferation; number of capillaries appear increased; beginning of astrocytic proliferation (often at margin of infarct)
5-7 days	Grossly, swelling of infarct reaches maximum
8-10 days	Reduction in gross swelling of infarct; liquefaction necrosis; prominent number of mononuclear cells (gitter cells); continued endothelial cell proliferation; beginning fibroblastic activity with collagen formation, variable but most prominent in CNS tissue adjacent to the meninges; beginning increase of astroglial fiber production, 5-13 days
3 weeks-6 months	Mononuclear cells decreased; astroglial fiber density increased (especially at margin); astrocytic proliferation reduced; astrocytes return to original appearance; cystic stage of infarct, 2-4 months; vascular network may be present within cyst; endothelial cell proliferation reduced

*The degree of astrocytic injury will depend on location (e.g., central or peripheral) of the cells within the infarct.
†Obviously, thrombosis may occur earlier than 6 hours. This is the time when it may initially be prominent.

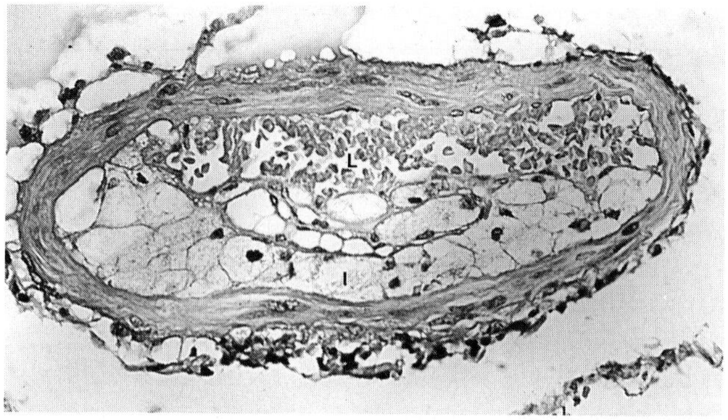

Figure 8-26 Brain, junction of parietal and frontal lobes, meningeal artery; dog. Atherosclerosis. The lumen *(L)* is narrowed because of accumulation of lipid-laden cells in the intima *(I)* on the lower side of the lumen. H & E stain.

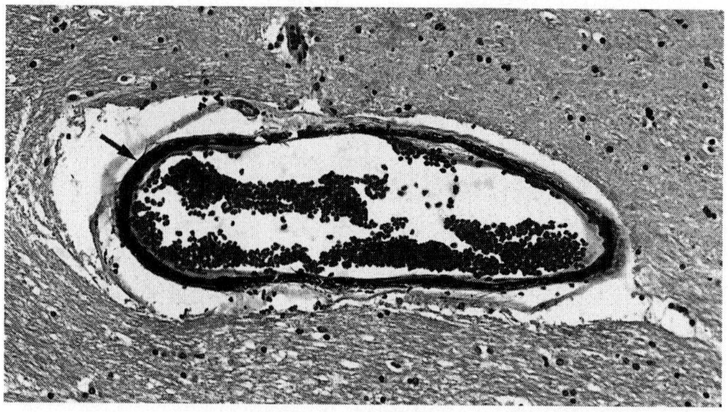

Figure 8-27 Brain, junction of parietal and frontal lobes, globus pallidus; horse. Vascular siderocalcinosis. The vessel wall *(arrow)* contains a prominent amount of dark-staining mineral. H & E stain.

the brains of several species but is especially common in adult horses (Fig. 8-27). Vessels of the internal capsule, globus pallidus, cerebellar dentate nucleus, and, infrequently, hippocampus are preferentially affected in horses, cattle, and less commonly, dogs. Meningeal vessels in old cats, old horses, and cattle, as well as vessels of the choroid plexus in old cats, are other sites of vascular mineralization. Overt ischemic damage is rarely associated with these nonlipomatous vascular lesions in any species.

Specific Diseases Associated with Circulatory Dysfunction

Vascular-mediated injury can be associated with or complicate a variety of diseases affecting the CNS. Examples of diseases caused by vascular alterations or injury and occlusive vascular disease are discussed further in the following text.

Feline Ischemic Encephalopathy. Feline ischemic encephalopathy has a peracute to acute onset and affects cats of any age. Clinical signs usually reflect unilateral cerebral involvement. The disease most often occurs in the summer months and is accompanied by signs that can include depression, mild ataxia, seizures, behavioral changes, and blindness.

The lesion is unilateral or, uncommonly, bilateral necrosis of the cerebral hemisphere, usually in the area supplied by the middle cerebral artery. The necrosis can be multifocal or involve up to two thirds of one hemisphere. Hemorrhages can occur in the parenchyma or leptomeninges. In chronic cases, cerebral atrophy, most marked adjacent to the middle cerebral artery of the affected hemisphere, can occur (Fig. 8-28). Microscopically, the lesions follow the sequence of changes in infarction listed in Table 8-3.

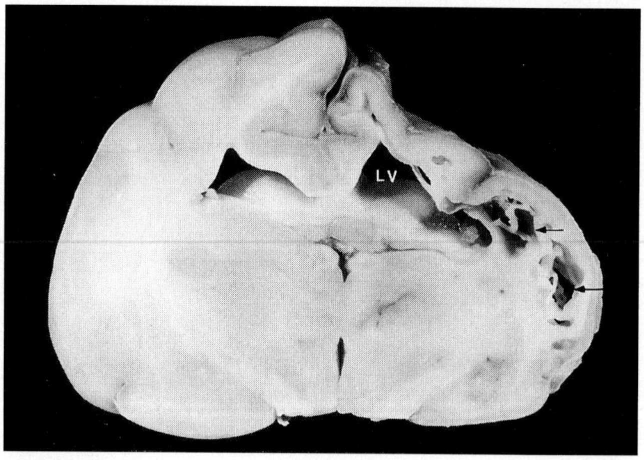

Figure 8-28 Brain, junction between parietal and occipital lobes, level of thalamus; cat. Chronic feline ischemic encephalopathy with unilateral cerebral degeneration-atrophy. The dorsolateral aspect of the right cerebral hemisphere has undergone necrosis, followed by collapse after phagocytic removal of the necrotic debris. Spaces remain *(arrows)* in place of the previously existing parenchyma and an enlarged right lateral ventricle *(LV)* that has expanded into the area of lost tissue (hydrocephalus ex vacuo).

The cause of the disease has not been established. Although specific vascular lesions (thrombosis or vasculitis) have been found in only a few cases, an ischemic mechanism is suspected and is consistent with the character of the brain damage. Recent evidence strongly supports an aberrant cerebrospinal migration of *Cuterebra*

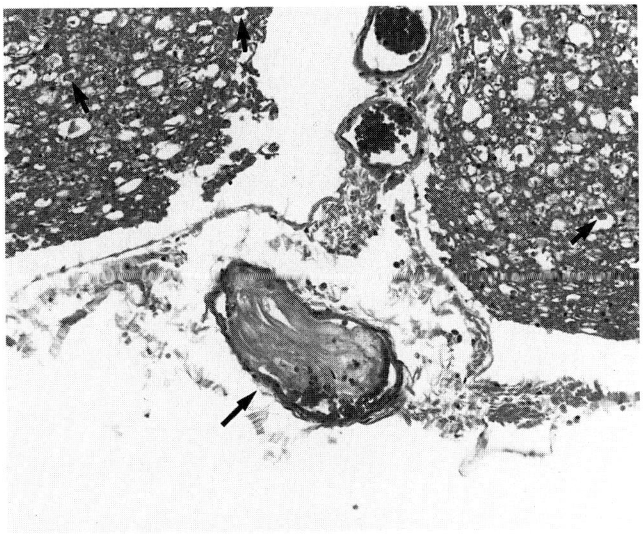

Figure 8-29 Spinal cord, lumbar level, ventral spinal vein; dog. A fibrocartilagenous embolus *(long arrow)* similar to that shown here has obstructed a ventral spinal artery or one of its branches (not illustrated) and has caused acute infarction in the central gray matter (not illustrated). A variable amount of axonal degeneration is present in the white matter *(short arrows)*. H & E stain.

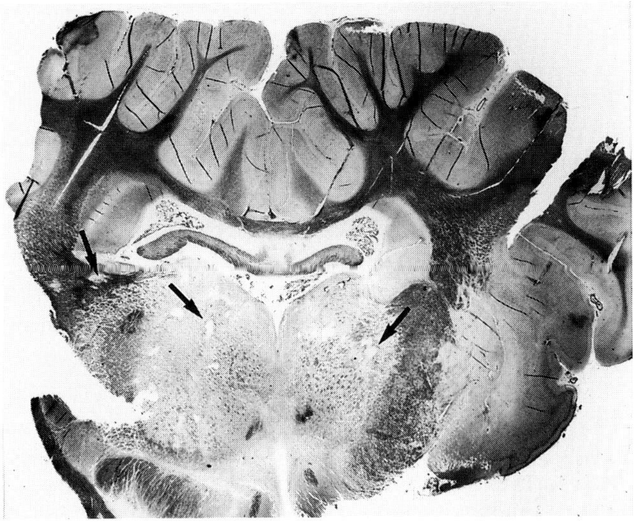

Figure 8-30 Brain, parietal lobe, level of the thalamus; feeder lamb. *Clostridium perfringens* type D enterotoxemia, acute stage of the disease process. Focal edema and necrosis *(arrows)* are present in the thalamus and adjacent white matter (internal capsule and optic radiation). H & E stain.

larva following entry into the brain via the nasal cavity. A vascular-mediated vasospasm, resulting from hemorrhage or a toxin elaborated by the parasite, has also been proposed. Possible excitotoxic effects of a parasitic toxin have also been suggested.

Ischemic Myelopathy-Encephalopathy. Ischemic (or necrotizing) myelopathy has been described in the dog, cat, horse, pig, lamb, and turkey. Clinically, there is a sudden onset of spinal cord deficits, sometimes with cerebral involvement, in certain species. In dogs, larger breeds are more commonly affected. The lesion is an acute focal infarct involving cervical or lumbar spinal cord most commonly, but any portion can be affected. Microscopically, emboli histochemically identical to the fibrocartilage of the nucleus pulposus of intervertebral disks occlude meningeal or parenchymal arteries or veins or both, in affected areas (Fig. 8-29). Herniation of degenerative disk material into the vasculature, forming occlusive emboli, is commonly accepted but the route taken by fibrocartilagenous material into the spinal (or cerebral) vessels is unproven.

Clostridium perfringens Type D Encephalopathy (Pulpy Kidney Disease, Overeating Disease). *C. perfringens* type D enterotoxemia, associated with epsilon toxin production, is a disease of sheep, goats, and cattle, but only sheep commonly exhibit the neurologic manifestations of the disease. Sheep of all ages, except newborns, are susceptible; incidence peaks between 3 and 10 weeks of age and in feeder lambs shortly after arrival at a feedlot. Resistance of newborns can be related to lack in the gut of pancreatic proteolytic enzymes necessary for activation of the epsilon toxin, as well as to trypsin inhibitors in colostrum. Lambs are typically in good condition and are found dead.

Gross lesions are absent in some peracute cases, but when present, occur in the internal capsule, basal nuclei, thalamus, hippocampus, midbrain (rostral colliculus and substantia nigra), cerebellar peduncles (especially middle), pons, and corona radiata of frontal cortex (Fig. 8-30). Lesions are focal, bilaterally symmetric, and vary from yellow-gray to red with malacia in advanced stages. Lesions in other tissues consist of pulmonary congestion and edema, serous pericardial effusion, petechiation, and soft (pulpy) kidneys.

Microscopically, the lesions in acute cases include perivascular and interstitial edema (see Fig. 8-22). The fluid in perivascular spaces is frequently protein rich and eosinophilic. Walls of arterioles can be hyalinized, and endothelial cell nuclei are swollen and vesicular. Vasogenic (interstitial) edema gives a light or pink-staining, spongy appearance to the neuropil. Both gray and white matter are affected, but changes are more severe in the latter. Pericapillary hemorrhage and acute necrosis of neurons and macroglia occur. Other changes occur with longer survival and include axonal swelling, accumulation of neutrophils and foamy macrophages, vascular prominence due to perithelial-endothelial nuclear enlargement or swelling, lymphocytic perivascular cuffing, and liquefactive necrosis.

Brain damage is due to vascular injury and breakdown of the blood-brain barrier. Binding of epsilon toxin to endothelial cell surface receptors results in opening of tight junctions, disturbed transport processes, increased vascular permeability, edema, swelling of astrocytic foot processes, and ultimately necrosis due to hypoxic-ischemic mechanisms. Some of the effects of epsilon toxin can be mediated by an adenylcyclase–cyclic adenosine monophosphate (cAMP) system.

Edema Disease (Enterotoxemic Colibacillosis) of Pigs. Edema disease is a disorder of rapidly growing, healthy feeder pigs being fed a high energy ration. Pigs are usually 4 to 8 weeks of age but younger as well as older pigs can be affected. Most affected pigs die within 24 hours. Animals that develop CNS lesions typically survive for several days (see chronologic sequence of infarction, Table 8-3).

The basic lesion is an angiopathy that leads to edematous and hypoxic-ischemic injury in a variety of tissues including the brain. Grossly, edema is present in the subcutis (often prominent in the palpebrae), gastric submucosa (cardiac region), gallbladder, colonic mesentery, mesenteric lymph nodes, larynx, and lungs, and serous effusions occur in the thoracic cavity and pericardial sac. Congestion, and sometimes hemorrhage, also occur. The characteristic gross lesions in the brain are bilaterally symmetric foci of necrosis in the terminal brain stem that can extend rostrally as far as the basal nuclei. Lesions are yellow-gray, soft, and slightly depressed. Malacia can sometimes be almost continuous from the medulla oblongata to the caudate nucleus, whereas in other pigs, the lesions involve only portions of the brain stem.

The primary microscopic lesion is a degenerative angiopathy/vasculitis noted most frequently and is most severe in the terminal brain stem to the diencephalon and in cerebral and cerebellar meninges. Cerebral, cerebellar, and spinal blood vessels are also affected. Initially, perivascular edema results from early vascular injury. Edema is followed by necrosis of medial smooth muscle cells, deposition of fibrinoid material, and accumulation of macrophages and lymphocytes in the adventitia (Fig. 8-31). Although endothelial cells and their nuclei become swollen and vesicular, this layer generally remains intact and, consequently, thrombosis is not a feature. Lesions associated with the angiopathy include pallor and spongiosis of the neuropil and necrosis of neurons and glia. An influx of macrophages can be observed with longer survival times.

The disease is associated with strains of *Escherichia coli* producing a Shiga-like toxin (similar to toxins produced by *Shigella dysenteriae*) designated Shiga-like toxin type IIe (SLT-IIe). Glycolipid cell surface receptors on endothelial cells, globotriaosylceramide or globotetraosylceramide, are binding sites for the toxin and their presence confers susceptibility to the disease. Binding of the toxin to these receptors can initiate a chain of inflammatory and immunologic reactions that lead to vascular damage.

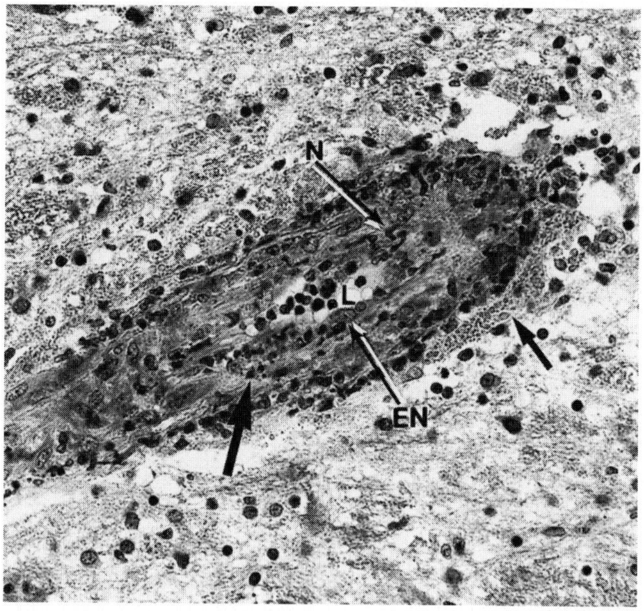

Figure 8-31 Brain, medulla oblongata; pig. Enterotoxemia (edema disease). There is cerebral vascular necrosis and inflammation with inflammatory cells, including a few neutrophils *(N)*, within and surrounding, the vessel wall. Also, note the fragmentation of cells within the vessel wall *(large arrow)* and focal accumulation of edema fluid and fragmented erythrocytes adjacent to the vessel *(small arrow)*. The lumen of the vessel *(L)* is lined by endothelial cells with enlarged nuclei *(EN)*. H & E stain.

Metabolic/Toxic Brain Injury

Osmotic Encephalopathies

Sodium Chloride (Salt) Poisoning. Sodium chloride toxicity, also known as sodium ion toxicosis or water deprivation syndrome, occurs primarily in pigs, poultry, and occasionally in ruminants. The disease is due to hypernatremia caused by excessive intake of sodium salts or severe dehydration followed by rehydration and a "rapid" hypernatremic to normonatremic or hyponatremic shift. During the initial hypernatremic phase, the brain "shrinks" because of the osmotic loss of water. An influx of sodium, potassium, and chloride ions into the brain, beginning within minutes, is an acute adaptive response to equalize the sodium imbalance. Maintenance of a normal ionic balance in the brain is critical, however, for normal function and, although a new ionic equilibrium is established, this acute response alone cannot compensate for severe or prolonged hypernatremia.

A second, more delayed adaptive response of the brain is an influx or endogenous production of organic osmolytes such as certain amino acids, polyols, and methylamines to equalize the osmotic imbalance created by hypernatremia. This response requires hours or days to establish a new osmotic equilibrium. When animals are given free access to fresh water, an acute hypernatremic to

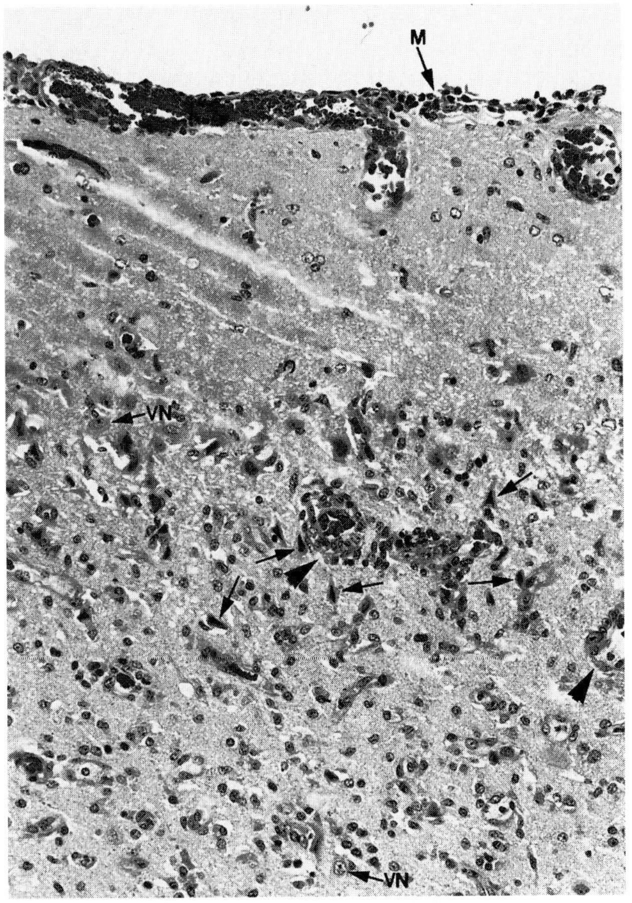

Figure 8-32 Brain, junction of parietal and frontal lobes, cerebral cortex; pig. Sodium chloride toxicity. There is a mild accumulation of mononuclear cells in the meninges *(M)*. Many neurons of the cerebral cortex have degenerated and demonstrate ischemic cell change *(arrows)*, although a few still viable neurons are also present *(VN)*. There is also increased cellularity with hypertrophy of endothelial and perithelial cells plus a few lymphocytes around blood vessels *(arrowheads)*. Tissue separation *(upper left)* has resulted from altered integrity of the cortex. H & E stain.

hyponatremic shift occurs. Within minutes, the brain attempts to offset this osmotic imbalance by eliminating sodium, potassium, and chloride ions. This early response cannot, however, offset the osmotic stress created by the increased organic osmolytes in the brain. As a result of the osmotic gradient, water enters the brain with subsequent brain swelling.

Grossly, lesions are inconstant but include cerebral and leptomeningeal congestion and edema. Zones of cerebrocortical necrosis can be detected in coronal slices of fixed brain. Microscopically, cerebrocortical neuronal necrosis, often with a laminar distribution, is accompanied by astrocytic swelling (Fig. 8-32). In pigs, leptomeninges and perivascular spaces have an infiltrate of eosinophils and, with longer survival, an influx of macrophages occurs depending on the extent of necrosis. Pallor of subcortical white matter is indicative of edema, and prominence of small cortical blood vessels is due to congestion and enlargement of endothelial cell nuclei. In ruminants, arteriolar degeneration with a transmural neutrophilic infiltrate, cerebellar Purkinje cell necrosis, and edema of basal nuclei, thalamus, and midbrain have been observed. A meningeal and perivascular infiltrate of eosinophils is an inconsistent finding.

Osmotic Demyelination Syndrome. In human beings, this syndrome is termed central or extrapontine myelinolysis. The disorder was first reported in 1959, and the majority of cases were in severely malnourished alcoholics. Since then, the disorder has been observed in a variety of clinical disease states. A major risk factor is chronic hyponatremia treated in a hospital setting by the administration of intravenous saline solution. The disease has been experimentally reproduced in dogs and laboratory rodents by inducing hyponatremia, allowing a period of stabilization (3 to 4 days is sufficient), and then administering saline-containing fluids.

Two cases of the syndrome have been reported in the veterinary literature and the authors have observed one case. In all three, there has been a clinical diagnosis of Addison's disease. Treatment consisted of intravenous administration of fluids containing normal saline solution to correct the hyponatremia typical of hypoadrenocorticism. The reported rates of correction have been 22 mmol/L in 24 hours and 16.4 mmol/L in 24 hours. In our case, serum sodium increased by 42 mmol/L in 4 days. All these rates of correction exceed the limits established for human beings and are consistent with human cases of the syndrome.

The pathogenesis is the opposite that occurs with salt poisoning. Rapid (within 24 to 48 hours) correction of chronic hyponatremia from an established equilibrium exceeds the adaptive responses of the brain, resulting in myelin destruction. The exact mechanism of demyelination is not known. Lesions occur in areas of the brain where there is a confluence or intermingling of gray and white matter. It is proposed that osmotic imbalance and water shifts between these types of tissue create stresses that result in myelin destruction.

In contrast to human beings, gross lesions in dogs are either not apparent or subtle. Slight softening and discoloration has been observed in affected brain regions. Microscopically, lesions can be limited to the reticular formation at the level of the pons or can be extensive, affecting cerebellar folia, midbrain, thalamus, basal nuclei (mainly striosomes), and at the interface of the corona radiata and cerebrocortical gray matter. In affected areas, the neuropil is pale in routine H & E–stained sections and is heavily infiltrated with foamy macrophages. Special stains (Luxol fast blue, Weil's), confirm acute myelin destruction and accumulation of myelin debris in macrophages. As is typical of strictly demyelinating lesions, axons are well preserved.

Metabolic Encephalopathy Due to Other Organ Dysfunction

Hepatic Encephalopathy. Acute and chronic liver failure, as well as hepatic atrophy associated with congenital or acquired vascular shunts, often results in clinical neurologic disease. The disorder is due to accumulation of toxic substances normally removed by the healthy liver and to disruption of normal metabolic functions in a variety of organs and tissues. Although no single toxic substance can be singled out as the cause of the neurologic deficits, buildup of ammonia and disordered neurotransmission are commonly incriminated.

In all species except the horse, lesions of hepatic encephalopathy are of two types, spongy change and formation of Alzheimer type II astrocytes. Spongy change can be present throughout the neuraxis but typically involves areas of confluence or intermingling of gray and white matter. These areas include the deep cerebrocortical gray-white matter interface, basal nuclei and adjacent internal capsule, reticular areas throughout the brain stem, and deep cerebellar nuclei. The spongy change is due to splitting and vacuolation of myelin sheaths, presumably caused by accumulation of fluid, so this change can be regarded as cytotoxic edema. Spongy change can be produced experimentally by ammonia infusion and is reversible. Alzheimer type II astrocytic change is a subtle alteration but has been reported in all domestic animals and is the only change observed in horses with hepatic failure. Alzheimer type II astrocytes are found in gray matter and have enlarged vesicular nuclei with peripheral chromatin, glycogen deposits, and demonstrable nucleoli or nucleolar-type bodies. Immunocytochemical staining for GFAP is typically weak or absent, possibly indicating a toxic effect on astrocytes.

Lesions analogous to those of hepatic encephalopathy have also been reported in animals with renal failure **(renal encephalopathy).**

Nutritional Deficiencies

Thiamine Deficiency. Thiamine (vitamin B_1) deficiency has been associated with neurologic disease in carnivores **(Chastek paralysis),** human beings **(Wernicke's encephalopathy),** and ruminants. In carnivores and human beings the association with thiamine deficiency per se is firmly established, and lesions in these species are similar. In carnivores (dog, cat, mink, fox) there is an absolute dietary requirement for the vitamin. Dietary factors (i.e., ingestion of fish containing thiaminase), dietary deficiency, or diets in which the vitamin is destroyed by other means such as heating, can all lead to thiamine deficiency. Thiamine is a critical cofactor in carbohydrate metabolism, and brain damage is related to energy failure (depletion of high-energy phosphates). Gross and microscopic lesions are bilaterally symmetric and commonly involve brain stem nuclei (especially caudal colliculi and periventricular nuclei), but cerebral cortex and cerebellum have also been affected. Lesions consist of status spongiosus, neuronal necrosis, myelin degradation, and vascular endothelial and perithelial cell nuclear prominence. Hemorrhage and an influx of macrophages also occur in some cases.

The disease in cattle, sheep, and less commonly, goats, has been termed **polioencephalomalacia** or **cerebrocortical necrosis.** The disease is seen most commonly in cattle 6 to 18 months of age fed concentrate rations. In sheep, most cases occur in younger age groups (e.g., 2 to 7 months). Rumen microbes are able to synthesize thiamine, and conclusive evidence of an absolute thiamine deficiency as the sole cause of polioencephalomalacia in ruminants has been elusive. Evidence (or theories) linking thiamine with the ruminant disorder include clinical response to thiamine injection in some individuals, decreases in ruminal thiamine, or overgrowth of thiaminase-producing microbes, ingestion of thiaminase-containing plants such as bracken fern, production of inactive thiamine analogs, and decreased absorption or increased fecal excretion of thiamine.

Polioencephalomalacia commonly occurs in cattle fed rations rich in carbohydrates with little roughage and is also associated with clinical or subclinical acidosis that may precipitate changes in rumen microflora. The disorder also occurs in association with other dietary factors including cobalt deficiency, molasses- and urea-based diets, and with diets high in sulfur (elemental sulfur as well as sulfates and sulfides), some of which are not specifically associated with thiamine deficiency.

Recently, there has been considerable interest in the relationship of high dietary sulfur to polioencephalomalacia. All sources of sulfur including formulated rations, plants rich in sulfur (e.g., *Kochia scoparia*), and concentrations of sulfur in the drinking water are additive. Total dietary intake should not exceed 0.3% to 0.4%. The exact mechanism to explain sulfur-induced polioencephalomalacia in ruminants has not been proven. Although deficiency or disordered metabolism of thiamine can be involved, it would seem not to be the sole cause or, in some instances, even a major factor in the disorder. Alternatively, polioencephalomalacia could represent a multifactoral metabolic disorder with multiple etiologies, all culminating in cerebrocortical necrosis. Any unifying hypothesis concerning the mechanism(s) of brain damage would have to reconcile all these variables.

Gross lesions, if present, are limited primarily to the cerebral cortex. Externally, the surface of the brain can be swollen as indicated by flattening of cerebrocortical gyri, and narrow sulci. In rare cases with more severe brain

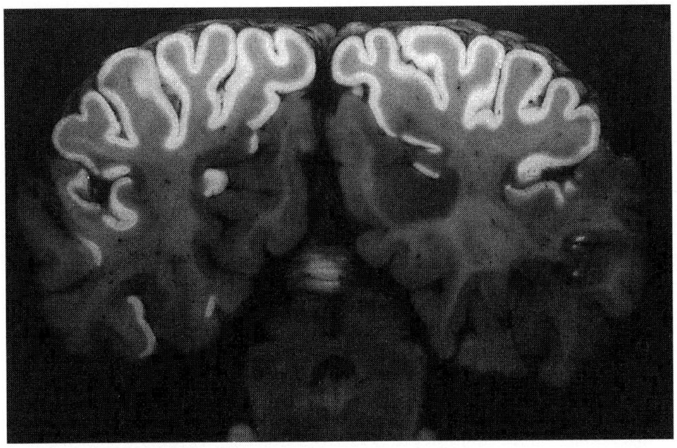

Figure 8-33 Brain, cerebral cortex of occipital lobes; steer. Bilaterally symmetric laminar pattern of autofluorescence in the cortex indicates areas of necrosis in the gray matter. Formalin-fixed tissue exposed to 365 nm ultraviolet light.

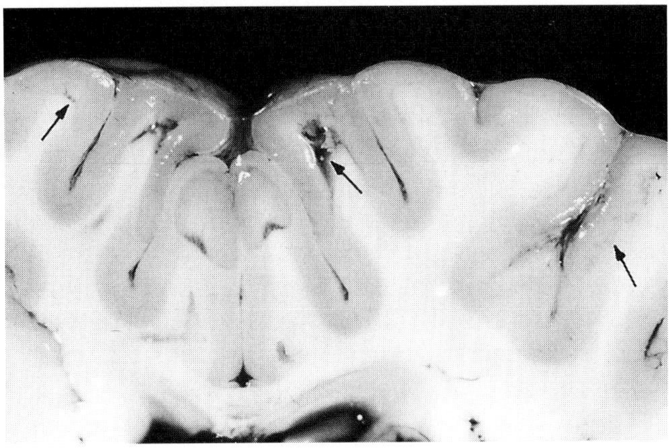

Figure 8-34 Brain, parietal lobe, level of thalamus; goat. Thiamine deficiency. Cerebrocortical malacia due to liquefaction necrosis with varying degrees of tissue separation *(arrows)*.

swelling, brain displacement with herniation of the caudal cerebrum beneath the tentorium cerebelli and the cerebellum into the foramen magnum (coning of the cerebellum) can occur. Yellow discoloration of the cerebrocortical gray matter occurs in the early stages, and it is at this time that autofluorescence is seen when the brain is examined under 375 nm ultraviolet light (Fig. 8-33). Edematous separation and necrosis involving the middle to deeper lamina or gray-white matter interface may be appreciable after 8 to 10 days (Fig. 8-34). In advanced cases with prolonged survival, areas of marked atrophy of cerebral gyri with an attenuated or absent gray matter zone are covered by meninges (Fig. 8-35).

Microscopically, the earliest changes are astrocytic swelling and neuronal necrosis (ischemic cell change) with a laminar pattern of pallor (edema). Neurons in middle to deep lamina are preferentially affected. In the early stages or mild cases, lesions can be limited to the depths of cerebrocortical sulci, but generally there is involvement of entire gyri that may be confluent over extensive areas of the cortex. After 4 to 5 days, neuronal necrosis and edema are more severe, and there is an early influx of blood monocytes that mature into tissue macrophages and become gitter cells. Macrophages and gitter cells are observed most commonly in perivascular and perineuronal spaces and in the pia arachnoid. After 8 to 10 days, necrosis and edema have resulted in laminar separation (at the gray matter–white matter interface) in which there are prominent accumulations of macrophages. Additional lesions that accompany the necrosis include vascular prominence due to endothelial cell and perithelial cell hypertrophy and hyperplasia, congestion, and a minimal influx of neutrophils. Bilaterally symmetric focal lesions of a similar nature occur in the thalamus and midbrain or colliculi and rarely in other brain stem structures. Animals

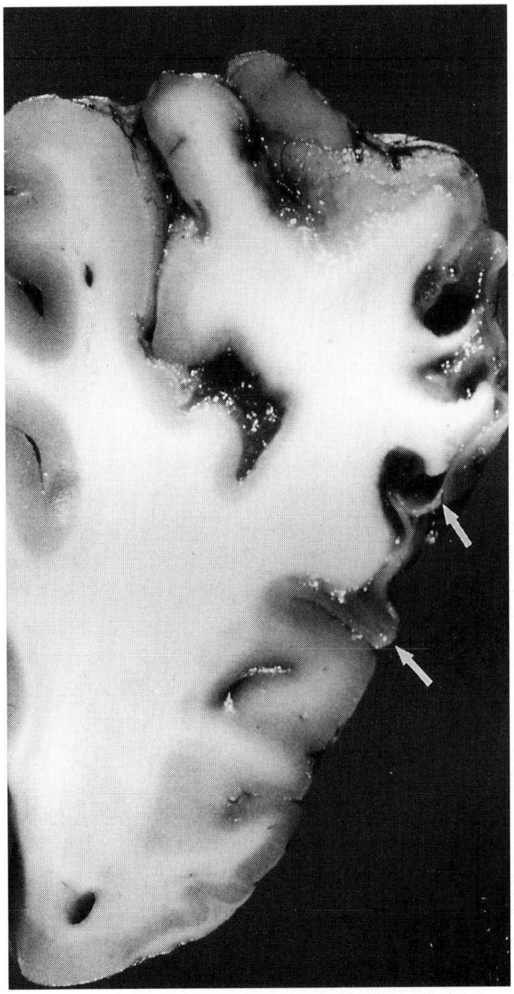

Figure 8-35 Brain, cerebral cortex of right frontal lobe; steer. Thiamine deficiency. Advanced cerebrocortical necrosis *(upper* and *middle right)* has resulted in only a remnant of outer cortex remaining *(arrows)*.

that survive can develop cerebral atrophy and hydrocephalus ex vacuo 1 to 2 years later.

Copper Deficiency. CNS disease due to copper deficiency in animals is mainly a disorder of sheep and goats and can be present at birth (**swayback** in lambs, rarely kids), or onset can be delayed up to 6 months (**enzootic ataxia** in lambs and kids). Copper is a component of several enzyme systems including cytochrome and lysyl oxidases, tyrosinase, and superoxide dismutase, as well as the protein ceruloplasmin. A deficiency of copper can affect several tissues such as skin (wool and hair growth and pigmentation), musculoskeletal development, and integrity of connective tissues. Copper deficiency can be primary (due to copper-deficient soils and inadequate intake from forage) or secondary (defective absorption due to interactions between copper, molybdenum, zinc, cadmium, or inorganic sulfates).

Approximately 50% of congenitally affected lambs and rarely kids have gross bilateral cerebrocortical lesions. Externally the cerebral cortex can be focally soft and fluctuant or collapsed. These cortical areas correspond to areas of rarefaction with a gelatinous consistency or are cystic cavities filled with clear serous fluid in the white matter of the corona radiata and centrum semiovale. Microscopically, a variable astrogliosis is associated with the degeneration of white matter, but the cavities lack a capsule of glial fibers. Myelin degradation and an influx of macrophages are minimal. Delicate neuronal and astroglial processes bisect the cavities. Neuronal necrosis in the gray matter overlying these white matter lesions is sometimes observed.

Lesions in the brain stem and spinal cord in both the congenital (swayback) and delayed-onset (enzootic ataxia) forms of copper deficiency are microscopic, similar in lambs and kids, and affect both gray and white matter. Large multipolar neurons of the brain stem (reticular formation and certain brain stem nuclei) and ventral, lateral, and, less commonly, dorsal horns of the spinal cord are affected. Neuronal cell bodies lack stainable Nissl's substance **(chromatolysis),** the cytoplasm is variably dense, pink, and homogeneous to fibrillar as a result of the accumulation of neurofilaments, and nuclei are often displaced to an eccentric position against the cell membrane (Fig. 8-36). Neuronal necrosis is variable. Lesions in the white matter of the spinal cord consist of bilateral areas of pallor in the dorsolateral aspect of the lateral funiculi (corresponding roughly to the spinocerebellar tracts) and also in the ventral funiculi adjacent to the ventral median fissure (Fig. 8-37). Involvement of the medial (septomarginal) aspect of the dorsal funiculi is infrequent. In the terminal brain stem, lesions are similar but have a somewhat scattered distribution. The spinocerebellar tracts extending into the middle cerebellar peduncles are affected. The pallor of the white matter is due to degeneration of myelinated axons. Astrogliosis is usually mild. Definitive microscopic lesions in the cerebellum as well as ventral spinal nerve rootlets and peripheral nerves are usually lacking in lambs but can occur with some frequency in kids. Changes in Purkinje cells are analogous to those already noted in neurons in other areas. Additionally, ectopic Purkinje cells and thinning of the granule cell layer occur. Bergmann's glial cell processes in the molecular layer hypertrophy. Lesions in ventral spinal nerve rootlets and peripheral nerve are due to axonal degeneration.

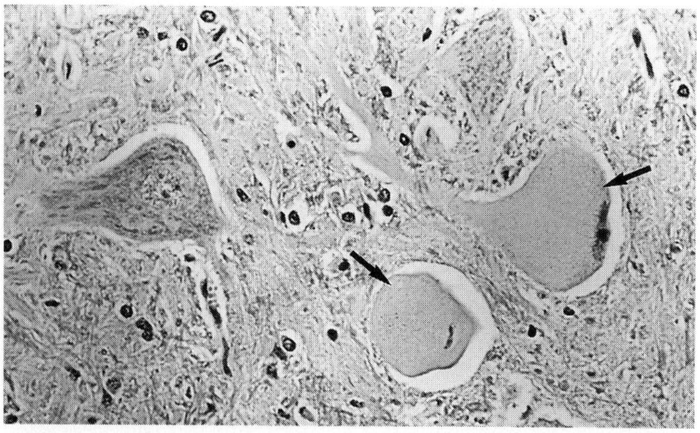

Figure 8-36 Spinal cord, cervical level; kid. Swayback-enzootic ataxia. Central chromatolysis is present in two motor neurons *(arrows)* of the ventral horn. The other neuron *(left side)* is normal. H & E stain. *Courtesy Dr. R. A. Fiske.*

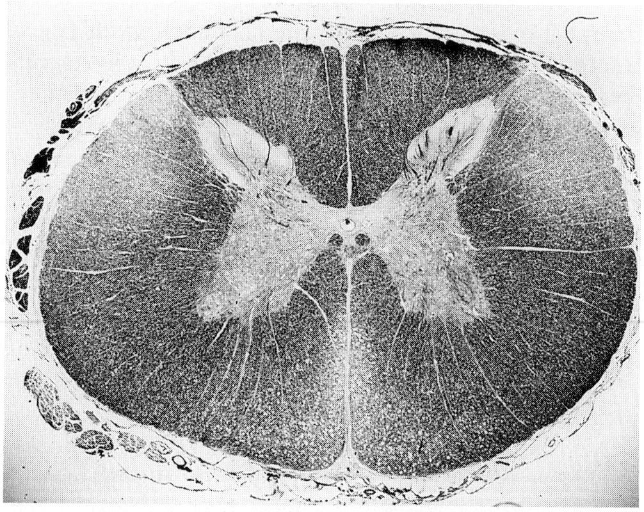

Figure 8-37 Spinal cord, cervical level; kid. Swayback-enzootic ataxia. Reduction in myelin and axonal degeneration are in the dorsal aspect of lateral funiculi and ventromedial part of the ventral funiculi. Luxol fast blue stain for myelin. *Courtesy Dr. R. A. Fiske.*

The pathogenesis of the lesions that occur in swayback and enzootic ataxia is poorly understood. It has been suggested that cerebral lesions result from loss of embryonic cells at an appropriate stage of brain development analogous to porencephaly and hydranencephaly following in utero viral infection or to dysgenesis due to biochemical disturbance. Biochemical disturbances could also account for the axonal/neuronal degeneration in the brain stem and spinal cord. Altered function of the mitochondrial enzyme cytochrome oxidase leading to energy failure could play a role in cerebral dysgenesis and axonal and ultimately neuronal degeneration. The involvement of specific brain areas, neuronal populations, and fiber tracts would require further explanation, however. More intriguing is the possible involvement of the enzyme copper-zinc superoxide dismutase. A mutation in this enzyme is present in approximately 20% of human beings with familial amyotrophic lateral sclerosis and in some individuals with the sporadic form of the disease. This human disorder, which is classified as a motor neuron disease, has a much later onset, and the mutation results in a "gain of function" of the enzyme rather than lack of function as might be present in copper deficiency. Neurofilament accumulation in brain stem and spinal ventral horn neurons and fiber tract degeneration (corticospinal in human beings versus spinocerebellar in lambs and kids) are similar; however, drawing a relevant association between these diseases of human beings and abnormal function of superoxide dismutase in swayback and enzootic ataxia in animals is premature at this time. It is also possible that the cortical white matter degeneration and brain stem or spinal lesions arise from different mechanisms.

Vitamin E Deficiency. Vitamin E (tocopherol) deficiency is associated with a variety of lesions in various tissues in different species, but with the exception of encephalomalacia in birds, a role for vitamin E deficiency in CNS disease is not firmly established. Vitamin E functions as an antioxidant, protecting cells from free radical–mediated injury. Diseases in which vitamin E might be involved are **neuraxonal dystrophy** in Morgan horses, **equine degenerative myeloencephalopathy** in a variety of purebred and mixed breed horses, and similar syndromes in Haflinger and Mongolian horses. Although these diseases might be multifactoral or even represent entirely different syndromes with overlapping clinical presentations and lesions, they are grouped here because of similarities in clinical presentation and lesions. Low vitamin E concentrations have been found in some of these diseases. Vitamin E supplementation has reduced the severity of clinical deficits and the occurrence of the disorder on certain farms that had a high incidence of degenerative myeloencephalopathy. Based on the finding of the disorder in certain breeds (Haflinger, Morgan, and Mongolian horses), the diseases could sometimes have a familial predisposition. Vitamin E deficiency associated with abetalipoproteinemia and various fat malabsorption syndromes in human beings, as well as experimentally induced deficiency, result in neurologic disorders with similarities to the equine diseases.

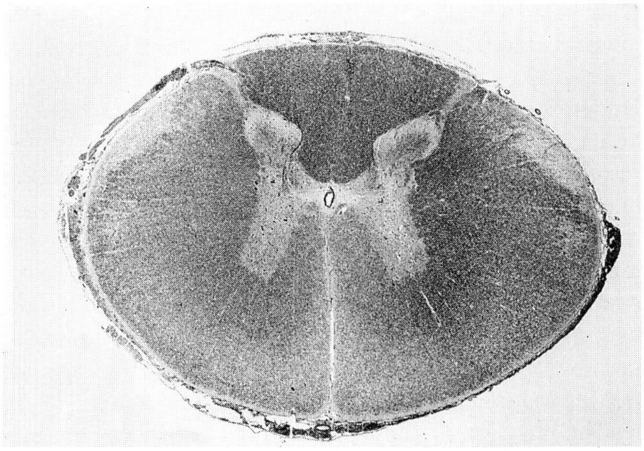

Figure 8-38 Spinal cord; thoracic level; horse. Degenerative myeloencephalopathy. There is marked loss of myelin in the dorsolateral aspect of the lateral funiculi, and less pronounced changes in the remainder of the lateral funiculi and ventromedial aspect of the ventral funiculi. Luxol fast blue stain. *Courtesy Drs. J. F. Edwards and A. DeLahunta.*

Lesions are microscopic and consist of **neuraxonal dystrophy** or **axonal spheroids** with and without other evidence of degeneration of axons and fiber tracts or, as originally described for degenerative myeloencephalopathy, axonal degeneration can be the most notable lesion (Fig. 8-38). In horses, neuraxonal dystrophy has variably been described in nucleus gracilis, medial and lateral cuneate nuclei of the terminal brain stem, and the thoracic nucleus of the spinal cord. Neuraxonal dystrophy represents a focal eosinophilic swelling in the course of an axon that can be somewhat homogeneous, laminated, or granular. The swellings are filled with amorphous debris, membranous profiles, and effete organelles. Axonal fragmentation and loss and myelin degradation in the spinal cord can have a predilection for certain tracts or can be fairly diffuse. Depending on the stage of the disease, macrophages infiltrate the white matter, and astrogliosis can be prominent.

Neuraxonal dystrophy involving the nucleus cuneatus or gracilis, unassociated with definite clinical signs, has been associated with aging in a variety of species. Also, neuraxonal dystrophies affecting young animals in other species and possibly with a hereditary basis have been observed. Some of these diseases are discussed later in the chapter.

Vitamin A Deficiency. See Chapter 14, "Pathology of the Eye and Ear."

Brain Damage Due to Seizures

Epileptic Brain Damage. Brain damage due to prolonged convulsive seizures (**status epilepticus**) is not widely recognized or even accepted in domestic animals. In human beings and experimental animals, brain damage resulting from status epilepticus is well documented. There have been isolated reports of brain damage in dogs with convulsive seizures, but one study has reported a relatively high incidence of brain lesions in dogs caused by status epilepticus. In this study, acute brain damage was widespread and corresponded well with areas of the brain prone to hypoxic-ischemic injury (i.e., cerebral cortex, pyriform cortex, basal nuclei, and hippocampus). Brain lesions consisted mainly of acute neuronal necrosis (ischemic cell change) and astrocytic swelling (see Fig. 8-6). The cause of neuronal necrosis with prolonged convulsive seizures is debatable. During seizures, cerebral blood flow and oxygen/glucose utilization increase so that the energy state remains relatively stable despite the increased metabolic demand. Furthermore, acute brain damage still occurs even with maintenance of cerebral blood flow, oxygenation, body temperature, and other metabolic parameters within normal limits in experimental animals with status epilepticus. **Excitotoxic injury** due to accumulation of neurotoxic amino acid neurotransmitters such as glutamate during the extreme neuronal activity occurring in status epilepticus is an attractive explanation. Excitotoxicity would account for both the selective vulnerability of certain brain areas and the character of the lesions. There is some evidence that the mature brain is more prone to this type of injury than the immature brain.

Chemical Intoxications

Lead. Lead poisoning has occurred in a variety of animals, but with the increased awareness of the potential for toxicity and environmental contamination and current regulations (e.g., reduced concentrations in paint and unleaded gasoline), poisoning is common primarily in cattle. The many potential sources include discarded car batteries, old flaking or peeling lead paint, emissions from smelters contaminating pastures, and some construction materials such as plumber's putty.

Lead poisoning in cattle and other species is via the oral route or, less commonly, via the respiratory system or skin (inorganic lead). Depending on the quantity absorbed, poisoning can be peracute with no gross or microscopic lesions, acute, subacute, or chronic. In peracute or acute cases, contents of the upper digestive tract could indicate the possibility for lead poisoning (e.g., fragments of battery plates or flakes of paint). Lead poisoning can affect many tissues and organs including CNS, PNS, liver, kidneys, gastrointestinal tract, bone marrow, blood vessels, and organs of the reproductive and endocrine systems. Gross lesions in the CNS are usually absent. When present, lesions include meningeal and parenchymal congestion, brain swelling with flattening of gyri, or hemorrhage. With longer survival times, there may be foci of cerebrocortical malacia and cavitation.

Microscopically, lesions in peracute cases are absent. In acute cases lesions consist of congestion, astrocytic swelling, status spongiosus, microvascular prominence due to endothelial swelling or hypertrophy, and often neuronal necrosis (ischemic cell change) characteristically confined to the tips of cerebrocortical gyri. For most cases in cattle, only a few necrotic neurons at gyral tips and minimal astrocytic swelling, vascular prominence, and congestion can be found. With longer survival times, cerebrocortical lesions progress to laminar necrosis, accumulations of macrophages, or liquefactive necrosis, the latter being rare. Lesions in dogs resemble those in cattle, but vascular damage is more obvious and consistent. Vascular lesions can progress to mural hyalinization, necrosis, and thrombosis. Other lesions include neuronal necrosis in cerebral cortex, hippocampus, cerebellum (Purkinje cells), myelin destruction in cerebrocortical white matter, and peripheral neuropathy. In horses grazing contaminated pastures, a cranial neuropathy with laryngeal and facial paralysis has been described.

Lead can damage the brain through a variety of mechanisms. Direct toxic effects on neurons, astrocytes, and cerebral endothelial cells occur by disrupting metabolic pathways. Calcium homeostasis and its roles in various biochemical reactions in the CNS including neurotransmitter action can be primary targets. Astrocytes are the principal cells in the CNS containing metallothionein. One proposed function of the protein, binding and sequestration of metals, while protecting neurons from injury, can lead to direct toxic effects on astrocytes. Accumulation of lead in astrocytes in turn could disrupt the various functions of this cell in neurotransmitter metabolism, other aspects of detoxification, and homeostasis of the neural microenvironment. Direct injury to endothelial cells and astrocytes can lead to disruption of the blood-brain barrier, edema, and subsequent CNS injury. It is likely that multiple mechanisms contribute to the brain damage. Transplacental (human beings and sheep) and neonatal lead exposure can result in delayed brain maturation and biochemical abnormalities.

Selenium. An acute paralytic syndrome termed **bilateral poliomyelomalacia** has been observed in feeder pigs associated with the inadvertent inclusion of toxic amounts of selenium in pig rations. Cutaneous manifestations of the toxicity also occur and include rough hair coats, partial alopecia, and separation and sloughing of the hoofs.

Grossly, bilateral areas of softening and yellow discoloration occur in the ventral spinal gray matter of the cervical and lumbar intumescences. Microscopically, acute lesions consist of status spongiosus and neuronal chromatolysis that with time progress to glial and neuronal necrosis and loss and microcavitation. These changes are subsequently followed by astrogliosis and the accumulation of foamy macrophages. Vascular prominence is also typical. Wallerian degeneration occurs in ventral spinal nerve rootlets. Identical lesions have been observed in the brain stem. Historically, a similar ovine bilateral symmetric poliomyelomalacia has been reported from Africa, but an association with selenium toxicity was not made.

The pathogenesis of the lesions is not proven but could involve an induced nicotinamide or **niacin** deficiency. Experimentally, **6-aminonicotinamide,** a gliotoxin and antagonist of the vitamin, causes lesions analogous to the porcine syndrome.

Arsenic. Toxicity due to ingestion or cutaneous absorption can occur with inorganic as well as organic arsenicals and can affect multiple organs including the nervous system. Inorganic compounds are predominantly herbicides or pesticides while organic arsenicals (arsanilic acid, 3-nitro-4-phenylarsonic acid) have been used as feed additives in the pig and poultry industries as growth promoters and to control enteric diseases.

Poisoning with inorganic arsenicals is an acute enteric disease with hepatic and renal manifestations but neurologic signs can occur. Probably because of the nature of the organic compounds and the manner of their use, there is greater potential for neurotoxicity. In pigs, clinical signs include blindness resulting from damage to optic nerves and tracts and incoordination, paresis, and paralysis related to spinal cord and peripheral nerve lesions. Arsanilic acid has a greater tendency to cause peripheral and optic nerve and tract damage, whereas 3-nitro compounds tend to affect the spinal cord more severely.

Gross lesions are not present. Microscopically, lesions in cranial and peripheral nerves and spinal cord consist of status spongiosus and fragmentation of myelin sheaths followed by axonal degeneration. In the spinal cord following 3-nitro poisoning, lesions are chronologically in cervical and thoracic cord followed by lesions in lumbar cord. Spinocerebellar tracts and dorsal funiculi are predominantly affected. The distribution of lesions suggests that the distal segments of long ascending fiber tracts can be preferentially injured.

Inorganic arsenicals inhibit sulfhydryl enzyme systems and disrupt cellular metabolism. The exact mode of action of organic arsenicals is unknown.

Organophosphates. Organophosphates are divided into two groups according to their use, mode of action, and type of toxicity. In the first group, typified by most organophosphate esters used as pesticides, fungicides, herbicides, or rodenticides, acute toxicity is produced by **inhibition of cholinesterase** either directly or indirectly, allowing acetylcholine to accumulate at synaptic or nerve-tissue junctions resulting in persistent depolarization. Clinical signs are variable and include hyperactivity or depression, miosis, respiratory difficulty, muscle tremors or fasciculation, and salivation. Seizures have been observed in dogs and cats, but are uncommon in cattle. Death is due primarily to respiratory failure. Gross and microscopic lesions in the nervous system are absent, and those in other tissues are nonspecific.

The second group of organophosphates is the cresyl and related compounds such as triorthocresyl phosphate used in hydraulic fluids, lubricants, flame retardants, and plasticizers. These compounds cause **delayed neurotoxicity** unrelated to cholinesterase inhibition. The triaryl phosphate group of compounds used as high-temperature lubricants is toxic for several species of animals and human beings. Signs of toxicity are delayed 1 to 2 weeks after exposure. Young animals, because of their ability to compensate for the neurologic deficits, tend to be less seriously affected, whereas recovery is slow and incomplete in adults. Susceptible animals include cats, domestic and exotic ruminants, chickens, pheasants, and ducks. Small laboratory animals, dogs, and some nonhuman primates are less sensitive. Clinical signs are those of combined sensory and motor neuropathy and spinal cord damage.

No specific gross lesions are present. Microscopically there is retrograde degeneration beginning in the distal part of axons, especially those with a larger diameter. Affected areas in the spinal cord include dorsal funiculi, spinocerebellar tracts in lateral funiculi, and ventromedial aspects of the ventral funiculi. The degeneration has been interpreted as a **dying-back neuropathy**—axonal injury extending from the periphery back toward the nerve cell body. Alterations in calcium homeostasis result in aggregation and accumulation of tubulin, neurofilaments, and neurotubules and proliferation of smooth endoplasmic reticulum. Central chromatolysis of cell bodies of affected nerves has occurred.

Organophosphorus compounds causing delayed neurotoxicity inhibit the activity of a target enzyme referred to as **neurotoxic esterase.** The function of the enzyme in the PNS and CNS is not fully understood. Phosphorylation of the enzyme by the toxic compound is proposed to interfere with its normal function, resulting in axonal injury. Other studies have shown that organophosphates causing delayed neurotoxicity interact with Ca^{2+} or calmodulin kinase II, an enzyme responsible for phosphorylation of cytoskeletal proteins (i.e., microtubules, neurofilaments, and microtubule associated protein-2), resulting in disassembly and accumulation of these proteins in the distal portions of axons, producing axonal swelling and degeneration.

Plant Poisoning

Astragalus, Oxytropis, and Swainsona Poisoning. *Astragalus*, *Oxytropis*, and *Swainsona* represent three genera of plants with species that are toxic to livestock. As many as 300 species of *Astragalus* grow in North America, and the genus is the largest of any legume family in this part of the world. Three categories of toxicity can be observed with *Astragalus*, depending on the mechanism or manner of toxicity: nitro-containing, selenium-accumulating, and poisoning of the locoweed type. Only the latter is discussed here. Locoweed poisoning or **locoism** is associated with ingestion of certain species of *Astragalus* and *Oxytropis* in North America and *Swainsona* in Australia. The toxic principles have been termed locoine and swainsonine.

Cattle, sheep, and horses are generally affected. Toxicity is usually insidious, and clinical signs are not observed until after the plants have been grazed for 14 to 60 days. There are no specific gross lesions. Microscopically lesions involve neuron cell bodies throughout the neuraxis and visceral ganglia and are analogous to the inherited lysosomal storage diseases (see following text for more detail).

Neuron cell bodies are swollen with peripherally displaced nuclei, and the cytoplasm appears foamy or finely vacuolated (see Fig. 8-15 for comparable lesion). The material that accumulates in the cytoplasm does not stain for lipid. Irregular fusiform enlargements of the proximal axon segment occur **(meganeurites)** with formation of aberrant synapses. With time lesions include distal axonal degeneration and neuronal necrosis with mineralization. Other cells in the CNS such as astrocytes are hydropic or swollen, but their appearance is less dramatic and diagnostic compared with changes in neurons. Microgliosis and neuronophagia are present but inconspicuous.

Analogous to neurons, swelling and vacuolation occur in a variety of cells throughout the body including hepatocytes, exocrine pancreas, renal tubular epithelium, endocrine organs (thyroid, parathyroid, and adrenal glands), circulating leukocytes, and cells of the mononuclear phagocyte system in liver, spleen, and lymph nodes. Ingestion of the plants of these species by females during gestation can also result in abortion or birth of weak neonates with lesions analogous to those already noted.

The mechanism of toxicity has been clarified by the isolation of the indolizidine alkaloids swainsonine and swainsonine *N*-oxide from *Astragalus lentiginosus*. Both compounds inhibit lysosomal α-mannosidase inducing an acquired α-mannosidosis that mimics the inherited disease (see Lysosomal Storage Disease). Additionally, swainsonine interferes with normal synthesis of glycoproteins containing asparagine-linked complex oligosaccharides. Swainsonine also inhibits Golgi mannosidase II, an effect not recognized in the inherited disorder.

***Centaurea* spp. Poisoning.** Horses grazing *Centaurea solstitialis* (yellow star thistle) or *Centaurea repens* (Russian knapweed) develop a disorder known as **nigropallidal encephalomalacia.** Grazing the plants for 1 month or longer during the hot summer months when other forage is dried and unpalatable can cause clinical disease. Affected horses are somnolent, have persistent chewing movements, and difficulty in prehension of feed and drinking water. Death generally is due to emaciation and starvation.

Gross brain lesions are sharply demarcated foci of yellow discoloration and malacia in the globus pallidus (pallidal) and substantia nigra (nigro). Lesions are unilateral or bilateral and varying in severity. Microscopically, necrosis with loss of neurons, axons of passage, glia, and blood vessels are accompanied by an influx of macrophages. Other brain stem nuclei are uncommonly affected. The cause of the syndrome is not proven. A sesquiterpene lactone isolated from *C. repens* termed **repin** could provide a basis for the neurotoxicity. Cytotoxicity in cell culture was associated with depletion of glutathione (a major antioxidant), an increase in reactive oxygen species, and evidence of membrane damage in PC12 cells (a pheochromocytoma cell line) and mouse astrocytes.

High concentrations of monoamine oxidase involved in dopamine metabolism normally found in the dopaminergic striatonigral tract could render these areas of the brain more susceptible to oxidative damage. The mechanism by which repin might cause an increased oxidative state with glutathione depletion and free radical production is unknown. Repin is also reported to inhibit dopamine release in the rat striatum, potentially contributing to the clinical manifestations of the disorder. Other potential toxins isolated from *C. solstitialis* include the excitotoxic amino acids aspartate and glutamate. It is unlikely that these amino acids are involved in the naturally occurring disease.

Mycotoxins

Leukoencephalomalacia of Horses. Ingestion of moldy feed, mainly corn or corn by-products, contaminated with the fungus *Fusarium moniliforme* causes an acute fatal neurologic disease in horses. Clinical signs can include depression, somnolence, head pressing, aimless wandering, or seizures. Rapid progression of these clinical signs followed by death is typical.

Gross lesions involve the white matter of the cerebral hemispheres (frontal and parietal lobes) most commonly, but cases with involvement of major white matter tracts in the brain stem and deep cerebellar white matter have occurred. As a result of the white matter damage, including edema, brain swelling is marked with flattening of cerebrocortical gyri. The lesions are often bilateral but unequal in severity and can be quite extensive. The characteristic gross lesion is yellow gelatinous malacia and liquefaction of the affected white matter (predominately breakdown of lipids) accompanied by hemorrhage (Fig. 8-39).

Microscopically, the affected white matter is coagulated or liquefied and the neuropil is disrupted by accumulation of pink-staining proteinaceous fluid with scattered neutrophils and macrophages. The lesion is surrounded by diffuse or perivascular edema, perivascular hemorrhage, and blood vessels with small leukocytic cuffs. Blood vessels are degenerate or necrotic and some are infiltrated with neutrophils, plasma cells, and eosinophils. Although not often detected, thrombosis occurs. Less characteristic

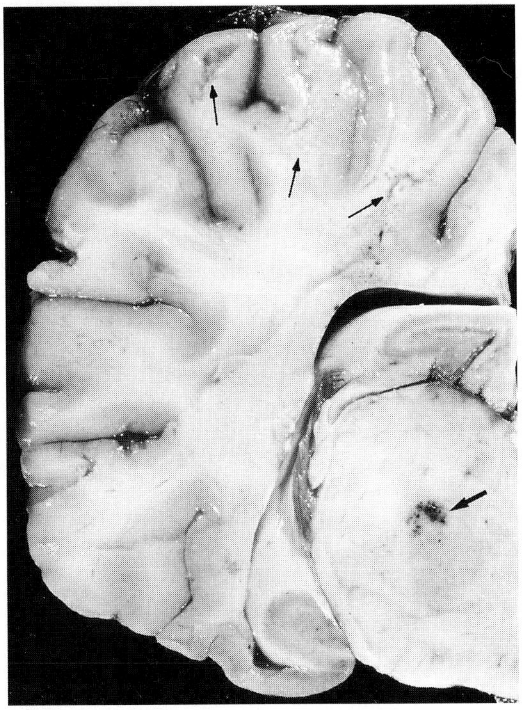

Figure 8-39 Brain, rostral occipital lobe, level of thalamus; horse. *Fusarium moniliforme*–induced encephalopathy (equine leukoencephalomalacia). There is focal malacia due to liquefaction necrosis of the cerebral white matter *(thin arrows)*. See Fig. 8-20 for illustration of microscopic lesion of a similar process. There is also focal hemorrhage in the thalamus *(thick arrow)*.

changes include edema and perivascular cuffing in the leptomeninges and neuronal necrosis in deeper layers or the entire width of the overlying gray matter. Similar lesions have been reported in the spinal cord where gray matter is preferentially affected.

This equine mycotoxicosis can be associated with hepatotoxicity, or hepatotoxicity can be the sole manifestation. Additionally, other animals including pigs and various avian species (ducks, chickens) are susceptible, but clinical disease and lesions generally reflect pulmonary, hepatic, or renal injury.

The primary toxin isolated from *F. moniliforme* has been named **fumonisin B_1,** although other fumonisins have been extracted. The exact mechanism of injury has not been fully defined. Based on the character and progression of lesions, vascular damage has been inferred as the primary injury. Although unproven, the gross lesion is thought to be an infarct by some pathologists. Fumonisins inhibit the enzyme **ceramide synthase,** interfering with the synthesis of sphingolipids. Fumonisins disrupt cellular membranes, are associated with lipid peroxidation of cells and cellular membranes, inhibit synthesis of macromolecules and DNA, and may enhance production of tumor necrosis factor-α by macrophages.

Table 8-4 Other Toxicities Involving the Nervous System

Chemicals
Heavy metals: cadmium, manganese, mercury, tin
Hexacarbons: n-hexane, others
Pesticides: carbaryl, bromethalin, chlorinated hydrocarbons
Drugs: nitrofurazones, ivermectin, levamisol, metronidazole
Plants
Cycads, *Chrysocoma tenuifolia, Helichrysum* spp., *Solanum* spp. *(dimidiatum, fastigium, kwebense),* sorghum, *Stypandra* spp.
Mycotoxins
Acremonium, Aspergillus, Claviceps, Penicillium

Other Toxicities Involving the Nervous System

Space constraints do no allow a comprehensive discussion of all toxicities affecting the nervous system. Table 8-4 is a partial listing of other poisons with potential to cause neurologic illness and CNS injury. Some of these, such as mercury, have in the past been associated with high morbidity and mortality in isolated outbreaks. An example would be the Minimata Bay incident in Japan in human beings eating fish containing high concentrations of mercury. The potential remains for serious neurologic illnesses and death from these intoxications, and the interested reader is referred to more comprehensive reference sources.

Disorders of Myelin Formation and Maintenance

Terminology

Disorders of myelin formation include **hypomyelinogenesis** (hypomyelination) and dysmyelination. Hypomyelinogenesis (hypomyelination) is a process in which there is underdevelopment of myelin. Dysmyelination refers to the abnormal formation of myelin that can be chemically defective. Demyelination,which means degeneration and loss of myelin already formed, can be divided into primary and secondary types. Primary demyelination, the type discussed in this section unless otherwise indicated, refers to a disease process in which the myelin sheath is selectively affected with the axon remaining essentially intact. Secondary demyelination, a designation criticized by some, refers to degeneration of myelin along with injury to the axon, as in Wallerian degeneration, and is not a selective injury of the myelin sheath.

Hereditary Diseases

Hypomyelinogenesis and Dysmyelination. Hypomyelinogenesis and dysmyelination most often occur in the early postnatal period and have similar clinical and pathologic features. There are some differences in the lesions and the mechanisms by which they develop. Some of these diseases in domestic animals are outlined in Table 8-5.

Table 8-5 Hypomyelinogenesis and Dysmyelination in Animals

Species	Breed	Disease Designation	Genetic Cause	Infectious Cause	Metabolic Cause
Canine	Dalmatian	Hypomyelinogenesis			
	Chow Chow	Dysmyelination	Suspected		
	Springer spaniel	Shaking pups (hypomyelination)	Sex-linked recessive		
	Samoyed	Tremor (hypomyelination)	Suspected		
	Lurcher	Tremor syndrome (hypomyelination)			
	Weimaraner	Hypomyelination	Suspected		
Bovine	All breeds	Bovine virus diarrhea (dysmyelination)		Bovine virus diarrhea (pestivirus)	
Porcine	Landrace	Congenital tremor (myelin agenesia)	Sex-linked recessive		
	Saddleback	Congenital tremor	Autosomal-recessive		
	Chester-white	Myoclonia congenita	Autosomal-recessive	Suspected	
	All breeds	Congenital tremor (dysmyelinogenesis and cerebellar hypoplasia)		Hog cholera (pestivirus)	
	All breeds	Congenital tremor (dysmyelinogenesis)		Unknown virus suspected	
	All breeds	Congenital ataxia and tremor (hypomyelinogenesis and cerebellar hypoplasia)			Trichlorfon (acaricide)
Ovine	All breeds	Border disease (hypomyelinogenesis-dysmyelination)		Border disease virus (pestivirus)	

Globoid Cell Leukodystrophy. Globoid cell leukodystrophy is unique in that it is a lysosomal storage disease with one of its primary lesions being demyelination. Brain, spinal cord, and peripheral nerves can be affected. The disease, which is inherited as an autosomal recessive, is generally seen in younger animals, often younger than 1 year. Oligodendroglia are deficient in the lysosomal enzyme galactosylceramidase (galactocerebrosidase) that normally is responsible for the degradation of galactosylceramide (galactocerebroside), galactosylsphingosine (psychosine), monogalactosyl diglyceride, and lactosylceramide. Galactosylsphingosine (psychosine) is highly toxic and causes death of oligodendroglia. Galactosylceramide, which is nontoxic and variably accumulates within oligodendroglia, is released into the extracellular space during degeneration of these cells and stimulates the accumulation of macrophages (referred to as globoid cells), which contain this storage material (see Fig. 8-16). Globoid cells, which have been proposed to originate from outside the CNS, are reported to appear in the early stage of demyelination, increase as degeneration of the white matter progresses, and tend to disappear in the late terminal stage when degeneration and astrogliosis become pronounced.

The proposed sequence of events in this disease includes (1) early myelination that progresses up to a certain stage, (2) disruption of normal myelin turnover due to deficient galactosylceramidase activity, (3) degeneration and necrosis of oligodendroglia in the CNS and Schwann cells of PNS due to accumulation of psychosine, (4) demyelination (primary type) following degeneration of these cells, (5) recruitment of intrinsic phagocytic cells (resident microglia and trafficking blood monocytes), and (6) infiltration of macrophages (which become globoid cells after phagocytosing myelin byproducts) into the nervous tissue. The latter changes occur in response to the demyelination and unmetabolized galactocerebroside.

Gross lesions of the CNS are characterized by a gray discoloration of the affected white matter (e.g., centrum semiovale of cerebral hemispheres and spinal cord). The lesion in the spinal cord tends to involve the peripheral white matter (see Fig. 8-17). Microscopically, such areas have pronounced loss of myelin. Peripheral nerves are also affected and lesions are typified by demyelination and axonal degeneration.

Spongy Degeneration. Under the heading of spongy degeneration is a group of diseases of young animals characterized by a spongy lesion (referred to here as **status spongiosus**) that primarily occurs in the white matter of the CNS but also extends into gray matter. Status spongiosus can develop by several different mechanisms that include splitting of the myelin sheath (characteristic of

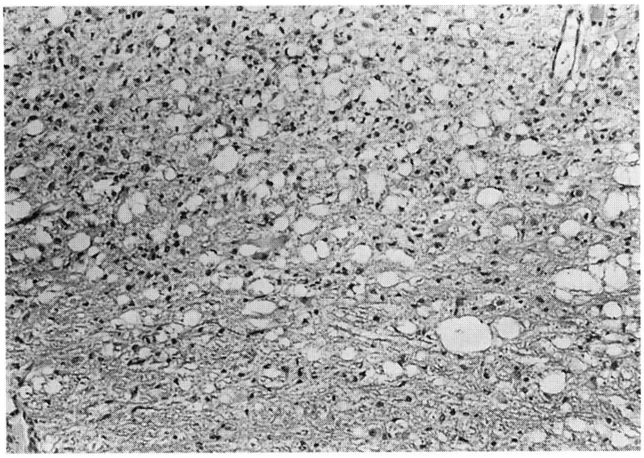

Figure 8-40 Brain, deep cerebellar white matter; dog. Noninflammatory stage of demyelination associated with canine distemper infection. A demyelinated area *(top),* typified by reduced staining intensity and status spongiosus, borders a myelinated area *(below).* Status spongiosus is present in both the demyelinated and myelinated areas. H & E stain.

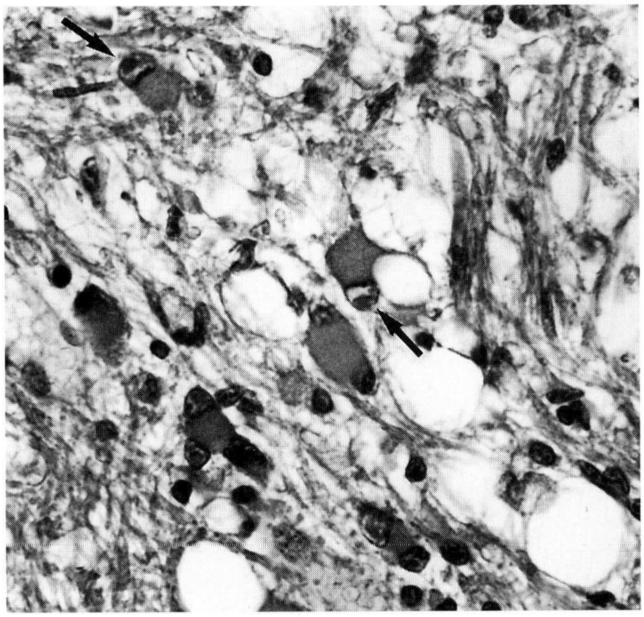

Figure 8-41 Brain, deep cerebellar white matter; dog. Noninflammatory stage of demyelination associated with canine distemper infection. Note the prominent status spongiosus and presence of gemistocytic astrocytes containing intranuclear inclusion bodies *(arrows).* H & E stain.

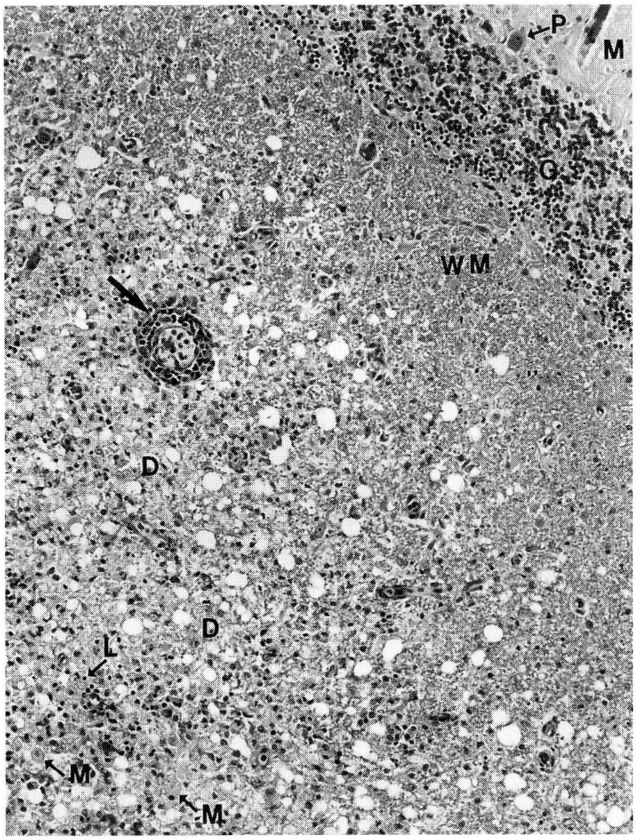

Figure 8-42 Brain, cerebellar folium; dog. Late stage of canine distemper infection. Cerebellar cortex-molecular layer *(M);* Purkinje cell layer *(P);* and granular cell layer *(G)* are at top right. Folial white matter *(WM)* is normal, except for focal status spongiosus. Perivascular cuffing *(large arrow),* demyelination *(D),* status spongiosus, focal accumulation of macrophages (gitter cells) *(↑ M),* scattered lymphocytes *(↑ L),* and loss of tissue substance are also present. H & E stain.

the diseases discussed here), accumulation of extracellular fluid, swelling of cellular (e.g., astrocytic, neuronal) processes, and axonal injury (e.g., Wallerian degeneration) when swollen axons are no longer detectable within distended spaces (see Fig. 8-4).

Gross brain lesions reported for spongy degeneration range from no gross lesions to swelling, edema, and pallor of the white matter, and dilation of the ventricles. Microscopically, the lesion is characterized by variably sized empty spaces within the white matter (see Figs. 8-40 to 8-42). Ultrastructurally, with spongy degeneration and some other disease processes characterized by status spongiosus (see following text), there is splitting or separation of the myelin sheath at the intraperiod line with the formation of large intramyelinic spaces. In some cases, myelin formation is deficient.

Some species and breeds affected include the canine (Labrador retriever, Saluki, silky terrier, Samoyed), feline (Egyptian mau), and bovine (Jersey, shorthorn, Angus-shorthorn, Hereford), and an autosomal recessive mode of transmission has been proposed for some forms of the disease. A form of the disease described in polled Hereford and Hereford calves and designated **maple syrup urine disease** is due to a branched chain ketoacid decarboxylase deficiency, resulting in an elevated concentration of the branched chain amino acids valine, isoleucine, and leucine in the serum, plasma, CSF, and urine. The unique odor associated with urine of affected animals is caused by the amino acid isoleucine. Calves are affected within 2 days of birth with a severe generalized CNS disorder characterized by dullness and weakness that progresses to recumbency and opisthotonus. A mechanism proposed for causing the characteristic status spongiosus (splitting of the myelin sheath) involves the formation of a toxic metabolite from the oxidative decarboxylation of α-keto acids.

Metabolic Diseases

Poisonings with several toxic compounds including triethyltin, hexachlorophene, isoniazid (isonicotinic acid hydrazide), and cuprizone are also characterized by the production of prominent status spongiosus within the CNS resulting from splitting of the myelin sheath at the intraperiod line. A reduction in total myelin content has also been demonstrated following administration of certain compounds (e.g., cuprizone). In addition, myelin of the peripheral nervous system can be affected by some of the above toxicities.

Circulatory and Physical Disturbances

Circulatory Disturbances. It is well known that extracellular edema (i.e., vasogenic and hydrostatic) due to inflammation, neoplasms, trauma, and hydrocephalus can cause degeneration of myelin sheaths. The underlying mechanisms for this injury are multiple and include creation of a hypoxic-anoxic environment, degeneration of oligodendroglia, and alteration in stability of the myelin sheath, permitting entrance of injurious proteolytic enzymes from the surrounding environment.

Physical Disturbances. Physical compression of CNS tissue, which can result from various causes usually chronic in nature, can also induce demyelination. Some possible mechanisms include compression on myelin sheaths and oligodendroglia, as well as interference with circulation resulting in CNS tissue ischemia.

Infectious Diseases (Confirmed or Suspected of Being Caused by Viruses)

Progressive Multifocal Leukoencephalopathy. Some viruses have the ability to induce demyelination within the CNS by directly infecting and destroying oligodendroglia. One of these diseases (progressive multifocal leukoencephalopathy), which occurs rarely in human beings and the nonhuman primate, is caused by the JC (human) or SV40 (nonhuman primate) strain of papovavirus. The disease has been associated with immunosuppression, but in some instances there is no obvious predisposing cause.

Canine Distemper. Canine distemper is one of the most important diseases of the canine species. It is caused by a morbillivirus (family Paramyxoviridae) and has a worldwide distribution. In addition to the dog, animals of the families Ailuridae (red panda), Canidae (fox, wolf), Hyaenidae (hyena), Mustelidae (ferret, mink), Procyonidae (raccoon, panda), Ursidae (bear), Viverridae (civet, mongoose), and Felidae (exotic felids including lions, tigers, and leopards) are also reported to be susceptible to canine distemper viral infection. Additionally, canine distemper has recently been reported in javelinas (collared peccaries), family Tayassuidae in the United States. Morbilliviruses other than canine distemper virus (CDV) include measles virus, rinderpest virus, peste des petits ruminants virus, phocine distemper virus of seals, and dolphin and porpoise morbilliviruses.

Lesions of the canine disease do not appear to always result from a direct viral infection with injury of susceptible cells, but to also involve other (e.g., immunologic and possibly cytotoxic) factors. The virus is pantropic and has a particular affinity for lymphoid and epithelial tissues (e.g., lung, gastrointestinal tract, urinary tract, skin) and the CNS (including the optic nerve) and eye. Lymphoid involvement (lymphoid depletion and necrosis) can result in immunosuppression affecting both the humoral and cell-mediated responses, rendering the animal less able to combat the primary viral as well as secondary bacterial infections.

Following aerogenous infection, the virus infects macrophages and monocytes located in or on the respiratory epithelium and tonsils. After a brief replication, virus spreads via lymph and blood to other lymphoid tissues, where additional replication takes place. The initial replication and spread are followed by cell-associated (monocytic) or non–cell-associated hematogenous dissemination of virus to epithelial tissues and to the CNS approximately 8 to 9 days after infection. It is at this stage of the infection that the host's immune response determines the outcome of the disease. Any one of three results can occur. First, the animal dies of an acute fulminating infection with unrestricted spread of the virus throughout the body. Death generally results from secondary bacterial infection or severe involvement of the CNS. A second type of infection is characterized by a more delayed progression of the disease accompanied by an immune response, possible subtle early signs, and variable development of later neurologic signs. Finally, some dogs recover from the infection and remain clinically normal.

Neurologic signs include convulsions, myoclonus, tremor, disturbances in voluntary movement, circling, hyperesthesia, paralysis, and blindness.

Initial natural infection of the CNS has been proposed to occur via the hematogenous route. However, more recent evidence supports entrance and spread via the CSF, presumably within infected mononuclear cells. Infection via the CSF, plus the demonstration of virus in the choroid plexus and the ependyma, also explains the typical periventricular distribution of the early demyelinating lesions that initially occur around 3 weeks after infection.

It is during this period that a pronounced immunosuppression due to CDV lymphotropism occurs. The early stage of demyelination, which is noninflammatory, coincides with the replication of CDV in the white matter, particularly in astrocytes. In addition to demyelination, there is status spongiosus, astrocytic hypertrophy and hyperplasia with focal and variable syncytial cell formation, reduced numbers of oligodendroglia, and variable neuronal degeneration (Figs. 8-40 and 8-41). Inclusion bodies (cytoplasmic, nuclear, or both) are detectable, particularly in astrocytes, which are important target cells for the distemper virus, but also in ependymal cells and occasionally in neurons (Fig. 8-41). The earliest evidence of myelin injury is a ballooning change resulting from a split in the myelin sheath, or more degenerative changes including axonal swelling. This lesion is also variably associated with astroglial and microglial proliferation. This initial injury of the myelin sheath, which has been suggested to be a result of perturbed astrocytic function following viral infection, is followed by a progressive removal of compact myelin sheaths by phagocytic microglial cells (that infiltrate the myelin lamellae) and variable axonal necrosis.

A late stage of demyelination, which is a reflection of an affected animal's improved immune status, is more pronounced and is characterized by nonsuppurative inflammation (perivascular cuffing, leptomeningitis, and choroiditis) and also can be accompanied by tissue degeneration and accumulation of **gitter cells** (macrophages) (Fig. 8-42).

Of the above-mentioned lesions affecting the white matter, status spongiosus (empty spaces in the white matter) and demyelination (uniformly pale-stained areas of the white matter) warrant special clarification. Status spongiosus can be associated with several different disease processes that are reviewed under Spongy Degeneration. Demyelination (primary demyelination) refers to a loss of the myelin sheath and is characterized microscopically by a uniform reduction in, or an absence of, myelin staining with many of the axons remaining intact. Such affected areas specifically appear pale pink following hematoxylin-eosin staining or unstained when stained with the Luxol fast blue procedure for myelin. Status spongiosus occurs within areas that are demyelinated or myelinated.

Lesions characteristically occur in the cerebellum (medullary area, folial white matter, and subpial white matter), and cerebellar peduncles (with both white and sometimes gray matter involvement of the pons). Lesions also occur in medulla oblongata (particularly in the subependymal area of the fourth ventricle), rostral medullary vellum, cerebrum (both white and gray matter), optic nerves, optic tracts, spinal cord, and meninges.

The pathogenesis of the demyelination associated with canine distemper infection is not completely understood. However, several possible mechanisms have been proposed based on investigations conducted both in vitro (e.g., in tissue culture of CNS cells) and in vivo.

There is now evidence that the acute stage of demyelination in this disease results from impairment of oligodendroglia. In contrast to astrocytes and microglial cells, which easily support CDV infection and replication, recent evidence indicates that a restricted infection of oligodendroglia occurs whereby the viral genome is transcribed (resulting in CDV messenger RNA), but is accompanied by a virtual lack of viral protein production, thus interfering with viral replication. Additionally, there is a pronounced down-regulation of myelin gene expression by oligodendrocytes in demyelinating lesions that, in part, correlates with the restricted CDV infection of these cells. This early stage of CDV infection has been recognized to develop during a period of marked viral-induced immunosuppression in the absence of inflammation. Recent findings indicate that although there is no clear morphologic evidence of inflammation (e.g., perivascular cuffing) during the acute stage of CDV infection, there is an up-regulation of T cells throughout the CNS with T cell invasion in early demyelinating lesions. Invasion of T cells is suggested to occur in response to activated microglial cytokine production. In addition, the major component of invading T cells correlates with sites of viral replication and development of an early immune response against the nucleocapsid protein of CDV. The relationship of this T cell invasion to the development of demyelination remains uncertain. It is suggested, however, that this process might facilitate the later development of a local immune response and further lesion development.

A proposed explanation for development of the late inflammatory stage of demyelination includes an interaction of macrophages with antibodies bound to the surface of CDV infected cells, resulting in release (from macrophages) of reactive oxygen radicals that destroy oligodendrocytes.

Old-Dog Encephalitis. Old-dog encephalitis is rare in mature adult dogs with clinical signs of dementia and recently has been reported to follow a long term persistent experimental infection with the CDV. Lesions are primarily in the cerebral hemispheres and brain stem. Microscopic lesions are characterized primarily by a disseminated, nonsuppurative encephalitis with variable (sometimes prominent) lymphoplasmacytic perivascular cuffing, microgliosis, astrogliosis, and variable leptomeningitis and neuronal degeneration. Nuclear and cytoplasmic inclusions, positive for distemper viral antigen, have been detected in neurons and astrocytes in the cerebral cortex, thalamus, and brain stem, but in contrast to distemper, not in the cerebellum. Demyelination also occurs but is not prominent. Although the virus has the same general polypeptide composition and contains all of the major viral proteins as the one causing conventional distemper, some differences among peptides have been reported.

The mechanisms involved in development of lesions are not known, but it has been proposed that the disease results from a persistent infection with replication of a defective form of CDV.

Visna. Visna (which means wasting) is a slowly progressive, transmissible disease of sheep. The disease is caused by a strain of the ovine maedi-visna virus (MVV) complex, one of the eight basic lenti- (slow) viruses (family Retroviridae). A different strain of the same virus causes a lymphocytic interstitial pneumonia referred to as maedi.

Viral strain differences and breed of sheep can influence the lesions that develop. For example, the visna form of the disease does not commonly occur in ovine breeds of North America, although some degree of visna-like lesions can be seen with maedi. Visna originally was described in Iceland, but sheep with similar lesions of the CNS have been detected in Europe (Netherlands), Kenya, United States, and Canada. CNS signs include an abnormal hind limb gait that progresses to incoordination and rear limb paresis over a period of weeks or months.

Early lesions primarily affect the gray and white matter subjacent to the ependyma of the ventricular system of the brain and central canal of the spinal cord. These lesions are characterized by a nonsuppurative encephalomyelitis accompanied by pleocytosis, variable edema, parenchymal necrosis, astrocytosis, choroiditis, and nonsuppurative leptomeningitis. Degeneration of myelin sheaths also occurs at this time but is often accompanied by axonal degeneration, suggesting that it could be a secondary lesion such as the one that accompanies Wallerian degeneration. Neuronal cell bodies and oligodendroglia are normal (except in areas of necrosis) during this stage of the disease. The latter cells can become infected, however, which leads to later development of demyelination (see below). Primary demyelination (particularly in the spinal cord) has been described in animals infected for prolonged periods (months to years). Such animals also have periventricular inflammation.

In addition to pneumonia, the maedi-visna viruses can also cause mastitis, arthritis (uncommonly of the carpus or hind limb joints), and a mesangial glomerulitis. Irrespective of the target organ, the lesions are to be regarded as chronic and lymphoproliferative in nature, in contrast to the well-known immunodeficiency infections caused by HIV-1, simian immunodeficiency virus (SIV), and feline immunodeficiency virus (FIV).

In recent years the understanding of the factors associated with infection, including the mechanism of lesion development, has improved. Visna is a persistent viral disease that probably results from the ability of the virus to form provirus (integration of viral and host genome). The virus can also change its antigenic characteristics (antigenic drift), which enables it to escape the effects of the host's immune response. Although the visna virus (and other lentiviruses) can infect promonocytes and monocytes in the bone marrow and blood, viral replication is restricted in these cells where it remains as provirus DNA until maturation and differentiation to macrophages, where primary replication occurs. However, the visna virus can also be present in oligodendrocytes and astrocytes located in foci of demyelination.

It has been suggested that virus gains access to these cells via close contact with infected monocytes. The primary demyelination that occurs during the late stages of the disease process (6 months to 8 years after infection) has been proposed to result from oligodendroglial cell infection. The main sources of excreted virus are the udder and lungs (as mainly cell-associated virus), and transmission occurs most readily between the dam and lamb via the milk and between confined individuals, probably via respiratory secretions. The MVV has also been detected in semen of infected rams.

It is important to emphasize that no profound immune deficiency occurs with MVV infections, as is the case for immunodeficiency lentiviral infections that infect CD4+ T lymphocytes. Nonetheless, secondary infections can still significantly accompany MVV infection.

Caprine Leukoencephalomyelitis-Arthritis (Caprine Arthritis Encephalitis). This disease was first described in the United States and has since been recognized in other parts of the world. The infection can be readily transmitted by colostrum and milk following birth, or by direct contact. A close relationship exists between the MVVs of sheep and the caprine arthritis encephalitis (CAE) virus, but genomic differences between them can be demonstrated. As with MVV infection of sheep, CAE viral infection is also a lymphoproliferative disease with a tropism for the macrophage, which acts as a carrier for the virus.

The pattern of disease in CAE is age dependent. Neurologic manifestations are usually seen in young kids 2 to 4 months of age, but unlike visna in sheep, there is a more rapid progression and signs progressing to quadriplegia develop within weeks to months. As with visna, affected goats have pleocytosis. Gross lesions in the nervous system include tan to salmon-colored foci of necrosis and inflammation that can occasionally be detected in the brain and most prominently in the spinal cord. Microscopic lesions of the nervous system are similar to those of visna (nonsuppurative encephalomyelitis), but can be more severe with CAE. Nonneural lesions include interstitial pneumonia of moderate severity in some affected kids. Such lungs fail to collapse completely and are mottled red or blue.

In adult goats, the primary target tissue is the synovium of the joints, and animals that survive the initial infection develop lymphoproliferative synovitis and arthritis. Pneumonia, lymphocytic mastitis, and encephalomyelitis also occur in adult animals.

Immune-Mediated Disorders

This category of demyelinating disease involves the development of a type IV hypersensitivity. The best-known representative of this group is an experimental model referred to as **experimental allergic encephalomyelitis (EAE).** EAE is produced by inducing a hypersensitivity to myelin or, more specifically, to myelin basic protein. If appropriate laboratory animals are inoculated with white matter or myelin basic protein (suspended in complete Freund's adjuvant), they become paralyzed after 2 to 3 weeks. Lesions are characterized by perivascular (perivenular) demyelination accompanied by accumulation of lymphocytes and macrophages. A similar process, referred to as **postvaccinal encephalomyelitis,** occurred occasionally when human rabies vaccine contained CNS tissue. The opportunity for this process to occur decreased after 1957 when duck embryo rabies vaccine came into use. A third situation in which this type of demyelination occurs follows infection with certain viruses (e.g., rubeola) in human beings. This disease, which is rare and designated **postinfectious encephalomyelitis**, is also characterized by development of lesions in the CNS comparable to those of EAE. Although such a naturally occurring process is not commonly recognized in animals, there is little reason to doubt that it can occur.

Neurodegenerative Diseases

Classification schemes for the neurodegenerative diseases are not standardized. Many of the diseases included here are those with a familial or hereditary basis and a specific, recognizable pattern of degeneration in the CNS. Others have a fairly stereotyped pattern of CNS damage, but the cause is unknown, and a familial basis is uncertain or unlikely. Table 8-6 gives an overview of neurodegenerative diseases. The classification used here, which is not meant to be all inclusive, places emphasis on the location and character of the most significant lesions.

Primary Neuronal Degenerations

Primary neuronal degenerations are those diseases with degeneration, necrosis, and loss of specific neuronal populations or affecting specific regions of the CNS in a temporally and spatially stereotyped manner. Another term used to denote some of these diseases is "abiotrophy" introduced by Gowers in 1902. The term literally means lack of ("a") a vital ("bios") nutrition ("trophy") required to sustain life of a tissue. Although these diseases in human beings and animals generally have a genetic basis, the pathogenesis for most remains to be determined.

Multisystem Neuronal Degeneration

These diseases affect connected neural systems, an example being **striatonigral** (basal nuclei and substantia nigra) and **cerebello-olivary** (cerebellar cortex and caudal olivary nucleus) **degeneration** of the **Kerry blue terrier.**

Table 8-6 Neurodegenerative Diseases in Domestic Animals

Primary neuronal degenerations
Multisystem neuronal degenerations
- Canine—Kerry blue terrier, red-haired cocker spaniel, Cairn terrier

Primary cerebellar degeneration
- Neonatal syndromes
  - Canine—Beagle, Samoyed, Irish setter
  - Ovine—Welsh mountain, Corriedale
  - Bovine—Hereford, Hereford cross, Ayrshire
- Postnatal syndromes
  - Canine—Airedale, German shepherd, Gordon setter, rough-coated collie, border collie, Finnish terrier, Bernese mountain dog, Bern running dog, Labrador retriever, golden retriever, cocker spaniel, Cairn terrier, Great Dane
  - Bovine—Holstein-Friesian, Hereford cross, Angus
  - Equine—Arabian, Arabian cross, Gotland pony
  - Ovine—Merino
  - Porcine—Yorkshire

Brain stem and spinal syndromes
- Neuraxonal dystrophy
  - Canine—Border collie, Chihuahua, Rottweiler
  - Feline—domestic
  - Equine—Morgan
  - Ovine—Suffolk
- Spinal cord—motor neuron disease
  - Canine—Brittany spaniel, Swedish Lapland, English pointer, Rottweiler, German shepherd, sheepdog, collie, pug, dachshund, fox terrier
  - Feline—Siamese
  - Bovine—Brown Swiss, Hereford (shaker calf syndrome)
  - Equine—various breeds (not believed hereditary)
  - Porcine—Hampshire, Yorkshire

Spongy degeneration (see Disorders of Myelin Formation)
Canine—Labrador retriever, Saluki, silky terrier, Samoyed
Bovine—Jersey, shorthorn, Angus-shorthorn, Hereford
Feline—Egyptian mau

Mitochondrial encephalopathy (encephalomyopathy)
Canine—English springer spaniel, Alaskan husky, Australian cattle dog
Bovine—Simmental, Limousin

Degeneration myelopathy (spinal cord—white matter)
Canine—German shepherd, Afghan hound, Kooiker, Labrador retriever, Ibizan hound, harrier, beagle, foxhound, Rottweiler, smooth fox terrier, Jack Russell terrier
Bovine—Brown Swiss, Holstein-Friesian, Murray gray
Equine—Various breeds (See vitamin E deficiency)

This hereditary disease, with onset from 5 weeks to 5½ months of age, is characterized clinically by rear limb ataxia, intention tremors, hypermetria of front and rear limbs, and atrophy of appendicular and epaxial muscles (presumably from disuse). Gross lesions are a slight reduction in size of the cerebellum and narrowing of cerebellar folia (Fig. 8-43). In more advanced stages, small foci of softening and discoloration occur in the caudal olivary nucleus and substantia nigra. Lesions in the caudate nucleus initially consist of a vague area of pallor in the body of the nucleus that progresses to marked malacia and cavitation (Fig. 8-44). There can be similar involvement of the putamen at this advanced stage. Microscopic lesions in chronologic order are degeneration and loss of cerebellar Purkinje and granule cells (Fig. 8-45), followed by neuronal loss in the caudal olivary nucleus, caudate nucleus (and putamen), and substantia nigra.

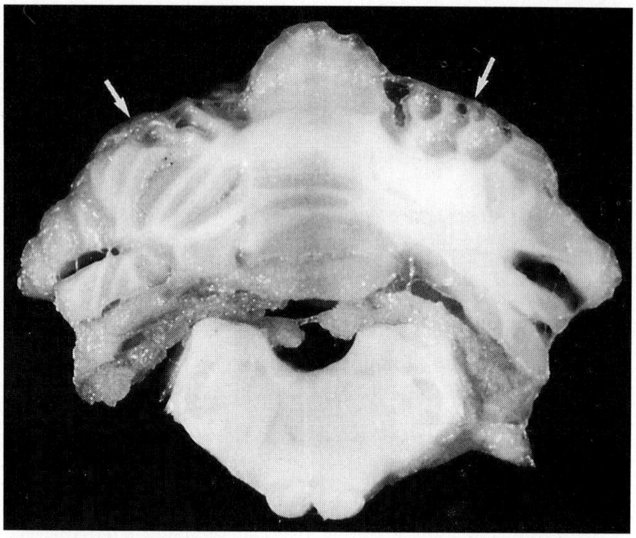

Figure 8-43 Brain, cerebellum; Kerry blue Terrier. Striatonigral and cerebello-olivary degeneration. Marked atrophy of folia of dorsal cerebellum *(arrows)* has resulted in increased width of sulci.

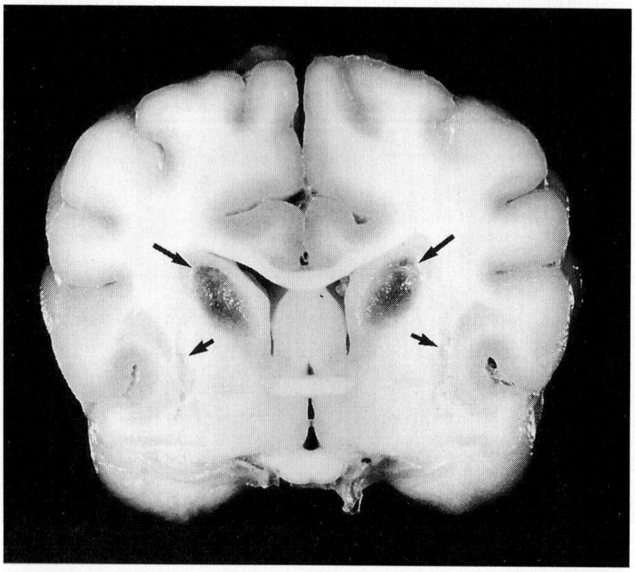

Figure 8-44 Brain, rostral parietal lobe, at level of corpus striatum; Kerry blue terrier. Striatonigral and cerebello-olivary degeneration. Note malacia due to liquefaction necrosis of caudate nuclei *(long arrows)* and putamen *(short arrows). Courtesy Vet Pathol 1983; 20:143-159.*

Astrogliosis occurs in later stages and is especially prominent in the cerebellar molecular layer. The caudate nucleus and putamen are eventually reduced to microcystic cavities bisected by a few nerve and glial fibers. The pathogenesis is unknown, but an excitotoxic mechanism associated with abnormalities in the glutaminergic corticostriatal and granule–Purkinje cell neurotransmitter systems is proposed. The cerebellar cortex and caudate nucleus are believed to be the primary sites of involvement, whereas lesions in the olivary nucleus and substantia nigra represent transsynaptic degeneration.

Multisystem neuronal degeneration of the red-haired cocker spaniel is suspected of being inherited. Clinical signs occur during the first year of life and consist of progressive ataxia and mental deterioration. Bilaterally symmetric diffuse nerve cell loss, astrogliosis, and axonal swellings occur in several nuclei including septal nuclei, globus pallidus, subthalamic nuclei, substantia nigra, tectum, medial geniculate bodies, and cerebellar as well as vestibular nuclei. Central cerebellar white matter, corpus callosum, thalamic striae, and subcortical (particularly subcallosal gyri) white matter involvement also are noted. White matter lesions consist of axonal spheroids, intense astrogliosis, subtle myelin loss, and perivascular accumulation of macrophages.

Multisystemic neuronal degeneration of the Cairn terrier has features of an inherited disorder. Between 2½ and 5 months of age, there is onset of progressive cerebellar ataxia, spastic paresis, and collapse. Widespread neuronal chromatolysis affecting multiple neuronal sys-

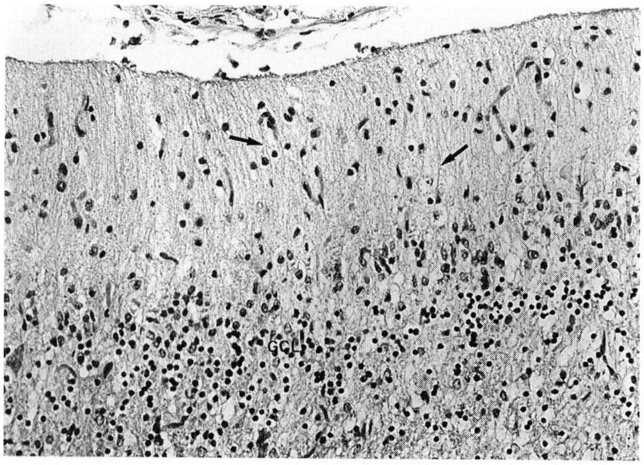

Figure 8-45 Brain, cerebellar cortex; Kerry blue terrier. Striatonigral and cerebello-olivary degeneration. Cerebellar cortex has absence of Purkinje cells, depletion of the granular cell layer (bottom third of the figure), and mild to moderate hypertrophy of vertical processes of Bergmann astroglia *(arrows)*. H & E stain.

tems is observed in the CNS and PNS. Affected areas include brain stem sensory and motor nuclei, cerebellar roof nuclei, ventral and dorsal gray columns of the spinal cord, and spinal as well as autonomic ganglia. Other lesions include degeneration in lateral and ventral spinal funiculi, necrosis of substantia gelatinosa and adjacent white matter most notable in caudal thoracic and cranial lumbar segments, and degeneration in dorsal and ventral spinal nerve rootlets and peripheral nerves.

Primary Cerebellar Degeneration

Depending on the degree of maturation of the cerebellum and related systems at the time of birth in the various species, clinical signs in animals with the **neonatal syndromes** can be manifest in the immediate postnatal period (bovine, ovine) or can be delayed until the time of ambulation (canine). Hereditary transmission is known or suspected in some instances. Lesions vary among affected species and breeds but overall include degeneration or absence of Purkinje cells, proximal swellings of Purkinje cell axons, variable loss of granule cells, cortical astrogliosis (see Fig. 8-45 for comparable lesion), and degeneration of nuclei in the cerebellar medulla.

Animals with **postnatal cerebellar syndromes** are normal at birth or at the time of ambulation. Onset of ataxia with various other clinical signs referable to cerebellar disease begins weeks or months after a period of apparently normal development. Initial clinical signs are often subtle. Progression of the signs can be slow or rapid, relentless or with static periods. Some individuals reach a stage without further progression of signs, but this is not typical of the syndrome in most animals.

Grossly, the cerebellum can be normal or reduced in size and atrophic. Microscopically, lesions are analogous to those that occur in the neonatal syndromes with loss of Purkinje cells, variable neuronal depletion in the granular layer, and astrogliosis in the molecular layer (see Fig. 8-45 for comparable lesion). Fusiform swellings of proximal Purkinje cell axons are found in the rough-coated collie and the Yorkshire pig. In the rough-coated collie and Merino sheep, lesions occur in other areas of the neuraxis. In these syndromes, degeneration and loss of neurons in the deep cerebellar and other brain stem nuclei are accompanied by axonal degeneration in the cerebellum, brain stem, and spinal cord. Loss of spinal ventral horn motor neurons has been noted in the rough-coated collie. An autosomal recessive mode of inheritance is suspected or documented in several of the diseases.

Brain Stem and Spinal Syndromes

Diseases associated with axonal swellings (axonal spheroids) in the neuraxis have been termed **neuraxonal dystrophy.** As previously noted, axonal degeneration can occur in diseases putatively included with vitamin E deficiency or have been interpreted as an aging change. Included here are diseases with a species and breed association and onset relatively early in life, generally before 1 year of age but varying between 4 weeks to 3 years. Clinical signs vary but include gait abnormalities, dysmetria or hypermetria, proprioceptive disturbance, ataxia, or other cerebellar signs. Lesions differ in severity and distribution but are characterized by prominent axonal swellings in various nuclei (often sensory) in the brain stem, cerebellum, and spinal cord. Loss of cerebellar Purkinje and granule cells have been reported in Rottweilers and cats and loss of brain stem neurons in cats. In the Morgan horse, the axonal swellings are associated with vacuolation. Dystrophic axons are also prominent in the multisystem degeneration of the red-haired cocker spaniel and in equine degenerative myeloencephalopathy, drawing some analogies between these syndromes.

Spinal Cord–Motor Neuron Disease

These diseases are characterized clinically by severe and often profound muscular weakness and widespread muscle atrophy. Onset of the diseases in the different species and breeds is typically early in life, and a hereditary basis is often suspected or proven. Sporadic cases in older adult animals also occur of unknown cause or suspected extraneous influence. Degeneration and loss of motor neurons in the ventral horns of the spinal cord and variable axonal degeneration in the ventral spinal nerve rootlets and peripheral nerves characterize the lesions. In some of the motor neuron diseases, there is prominent swelling of ventral horn neuronal cells bodies or axons, or both, associated with marked accumulation of neurofilaments. This accumulation is presumably due to posttranslational protein modification and impairment of neurofilament protein transport. Degeneration in some diseases is not strictly limited to motor neurons of the spinal cord or to motor neurons in general. Other sites of involvement are motor or sensory nuclei, or both, in the brain stem and white matter tracts in the spinal cord.

Lesions in the motor neuron disease of horses are analogous to those already described with neurofilament accumulation. The disease affects various breeds, no definitive familial association or age predilections are known, and an inherited basis is not suspected. Generalized weakness, muscle atrophy, and weight loss progress over 1 to several months.

The disease known as **shaker calf syndrome** in horned Hereford calves can only be loosely termed a motor neuron disease. The disorder occurs in newborn calves and is characterized clinically by tremulous shaking of the head, body, and tail. There is marked accumulation of neurofilaments within neurons of central, peripheral, and autonomic nervous systems. All segments of the spinal cord are severely affected. Neurons and neuronal processes in ventral horns, intermediolateral nucleus, Clarke's column, and substantia gelatinosa are swollen and

Table 8-7 Possible Mitochondrial Encephalopathies in Animals

Animal	Age of Onset	Clinical Signs	Principal Lesions
Alaskan husky	6 to 9 months	Ataxia, other motor disturbances, anxiety, blindness, hypalgesia	Spongiosis and cavitation in thalamus caudal to medulla
Cattle dog	5 to 12 months	Seizures, behavioral abnormalities followed by locomotor signs	Spongiosis and cavitation in cerebellum, brain stem nuclei, and spinal gray matter
English springer spaniel	15 to 16 months	Ataxia, disorientation, visual deficits	Status spongiosis in accessory olivary nucleus; axon loss and gliosis in optic nerve and tracts
Limousin cattle	1 to 4 months	Locomotor signs; aggressive behavior, blindness	Spongiosis, cavitation in cerebral and cerebellar white matter, brain stem nuclei, optic chiasm
Simmental cattle	5 to 12 months	Ataxia, behavioral changes	Spongiosis and necrosis in internal capsule, caudate nucleus, putamen, brain stem nuclei, spinal gray matter

distended. Wallerian degeneration occurs in ventral nerve rootlets and white matter of the spinal cord. Brain stem lesions are less prominent. Swollen cerebellar Purkinje cells and neuronal degeneration in the lateral geniculate body and frontal cortex are reported.

Spongy Degeneration

See Disorders of Myelin Formation and Maintenance.

Mitochondrial Encephalopathies

In human beings, various encephalopathic and myopathic syndromes due to point mutations in mitochondrial DNA are grouped under the acronyms **MELAS** (**m**itochondrial **e**ncephalopathy, **l**actic **a**cidosis, **s**trokelike episodes) and **MERRF** (**m**yoclonus **e**pilepsy, **r**agged **r**ed **f**ibers). The various human syndromes include Leigh's disease (subacute necrotizing encephalomyelopathy), Kearns-Sayre syndrome, Leber's hereditary optic atrophy, and others. The diseases have variable clinical presentations and lesions.

Diseases that might be classified as mitochondrial encephalopathies are not well characterized in animals. Despite this caveat, the diseases reported in Alaskan husky, Australian cattle, and English springer spaniel dogs, as well as in Limousin and Simmental cattle, could represent mitochondrial disorders. Table 8-7 summarizes the salient features of the diseases. Characteristics of these diseases in both human beings and animals are symmetric bilateral involvement of the neuraxis and lesions typified by status spongiosus with variable progression to cavitation or necrosis. In addition to the lesions outlined in the table, mitochondrial abnormalities have been noted in the brains of Australian cattle dogs, English springer spaniel dogs, and Limousin cattle, and in skeletal muscle of Simmental cattle.

Degenerative Leukomyelopathies (White Matter of Spinal Cord)

Diseases with degeneration of predominantly spinal cord white matter have been described in domestic animals. These diseases can be inherited or have familial predisposition, but not in all instances. Paresis and ataxia are the predominant clinical signs. Although there is not universal agreement, the leukomyelopathies described here are best characterized as axonal degenerations with secondary changes in myelin sheaths and myelin loss. An exception would be the necrotizing myelopathy of Afghan hounds (below) in which myelin destruction seems to predominate. Involvement of spinal gray matter and brain stem structures occurs with some of the disorders. The pathogenesis of these diseases is unknown.

Age-Related Degenerative Myelopathy (German Shepherd Myelopathy). This disease is seen most commonly in the German shepherd, but other large canine breeds can be affected. Affected dogs are usually older than 8 years, but the disease has occurred as early as 5 years of age. Lesions are most notable in the thoracic spinal cord and can be diffuse or multifocal. Dorsal aspects of the lateral and ventromedial areas of ventral funiculi can be more severely affected, but lesions can be diffuse in all funiculi. Lesions consist of ballooning and degeneration of myelin sheaths and axonal degeneration and loss. Degeneration of dorsal nerve rootlets and peripheral nerves and loss of neuron cell bodies in spinal gray matter occur as well. Altered suppressor lymphocyte activity has been noted in affected dogs, but the relevance to the CNS disease is unknown. Some investigators have reported low vitamin E concentrations (see Vitamin E Deficiency).

Inherited Necrotizing Myelopathy of Afghan Hounds. Clinical signs begin between 3 and 13 months of age and progress rapidly to paraplegia or tetraplegia within 1 to 3 weeks. Topographically, lesions in the cervical cord are in ventral and less commonly dorsal funiculi, all funiculi in thoracic cord, and ventral funiculi in lumbar areas. In well-developed lesions, there is severe destruction of the spinal white matter with an influx of macrophages and myelin degradation that progresses to microcavitation (Fig. 8-46). Neuronal cell bodies in spinal gray matter and ventral nerve rootlets are unaffected. Necrosis, perivascular accumulations of macrophages, and astrogliosis in the

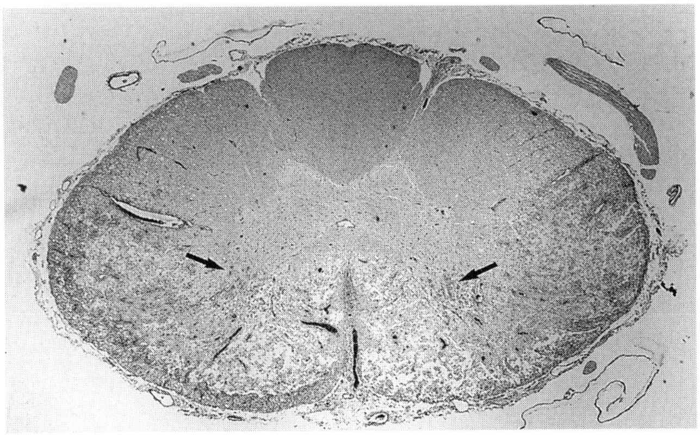

Figure 8-46 Spinal cord, caudal thoracic level (T12); dog. Afghan myelopathy. There is severe degeneration of white matter in the lateral and ventral funiculi. The neuronal cell bodies in the ventral horns *(arrows)* are intact. H & E stain.

dorsal nucleus of the trapezoid body are variable. The disease seems to have an autosomal recessive inheritance. The lesions are similar to subacute combined degeneration of the spinal cord due to vitamin B_{12} deficiency in human beings and primates, but B vitamin status in affected dogs is considered normal. A similar disease has been reported in Dutch **Kooiker** dogs, but the relative degrees of axonal degeneration versus demyelination have not been adequately described.

Axonopathy in Labrador Retrievers. In this disease, difficulty in rising and using the pelvic limbs from the onset of ambulation progress to inability to stand or walk by 3 to 5 months of age. Autosomal recessive inheritance is suspected. Bilaterally symmetric spinal cord lesions consist of axonal degeneration with formation of spheroids, loss of axons, and secondary myelin degradation involving the spinocerebellar tracts in the dorsolateral aspects of the lateral funiculi, fasciculus gracilis in the dorsal funiculus, and septomarginal white matter in the ventral funiculi. Lesions are most severe in thoracic spinal cord, tapering in severity both cranially and caudally. Lesions extend into the caudal brain stem and via caudal cerebellar peduncles to the cerebellar cortex. Neuronal chromatolysis progressing to loss of neuron cell bodies occurs in the caudal olivary nucleus. An interesting additional lesion in all affected puppies is hypoplasia or aplasia of the corpus callosum. Spina bifida also occurs in some puppies.

Degenerative Axonopathy of Ibizan Hounds. Progressive pelvic limb ataxia with an onset at or near the time of ambulation has been reported in Ibizan hounds. Lesions are bilaterally symmetric degeneration of ascending and descending tracts in all funiculi and at all levels of the spinal cord, but are most notable in thoracic segments. Large axonal spheroids containing neurofilaments are prominent. The trapezoid body is similarly affected. Dilation of myelin sheaths, formation of myelin ellipsoids, axonal degeneration, and an influx of macrophages occur in spinal nerve rootlets and peripheral nerves. Autosomal recessive inheritance is suspected.

Other Degenerative Leukomyelopathies in Dogs. Disorders that may be classified as degenerative leukomyelopathies occur in other breeds of dogs. **Hound ataxia** in harrier, beagle, and foxhounds used for hunting and fed paunch (tripe) has been described in the United Kingdom and Ireland and could represent a nutritional disorder. In 3- to 8-month-old **Rottweilers,** a syndrome characterized by widespread neuronal vacuolation in the neuraxis accompanied by axonal degeneration in spinocerebellar tracts and septomarginal areas of ventral funiculi has recently been described. In **Jack Russell** and **smooth fox terriers,** autosomal recessive diseases with axonal degeneration in dorsal parts of lateral funiculi and septomarginal areas of ventral funiculi and involvement of brain stem structures are reported from Europe.

Progressive Degenerative Myelopathy in Brown Swiss Cattle. Initial clinical signs of pelvic limb weakness, ataxia, and dysmetria occur at 5 to 8 months of age. Axonal degeneration in peripheral areas of lateral and ventral funiculi progressively diminishes centrally toward the gray matter. Involvement in dorsal funiculi is more uniform. Lesions are most severe in thoracic regions of the spinal cord and in ventromedial areas. Degeneration of axons in the medulla oblongata and Purkinje cells in the cerebellar cortex also occurs. The disease is considered to have a familial basis.

Other Degenerative Myelopathies in Cattle. Degeneration of spinal cord white matter has been described in **Australian Murray Grey** and **Holstein-Friesian** calves. Calves of both breeds are often affected at or shortly after birth. In Murray Grey cattle, there is degeneration in dorsal spinocerebellar and ventral septomarginal tracts accompanied by widespread neuronal chromatolysis in the ventral horns, thoracic nucleus, and several brain stem nuclei. Original reports suggest a primary myelinolytic disorder, but this mechanism has been questioned. The disease is inherited as an autosomal recessive trait. In Holstein-Friesian cattle, all spinal cord segments are affected and axonal degeneration with secondary myelin loss is evident in lateral and ventral funiculi, most notable peripherally. Lesions ascend into the brain stem to the level of the midbrain. An inherited basis is suspected.

Equine Degenerative Myeloencephalopathy. See Metabolic/Toxic Brain Injury, Vitamin E Deficiency.

Inflammation of the CNS

Infectious agents can spread to the CNS (1) hematogenously (most commonly) in a cell-associated (e.g. with

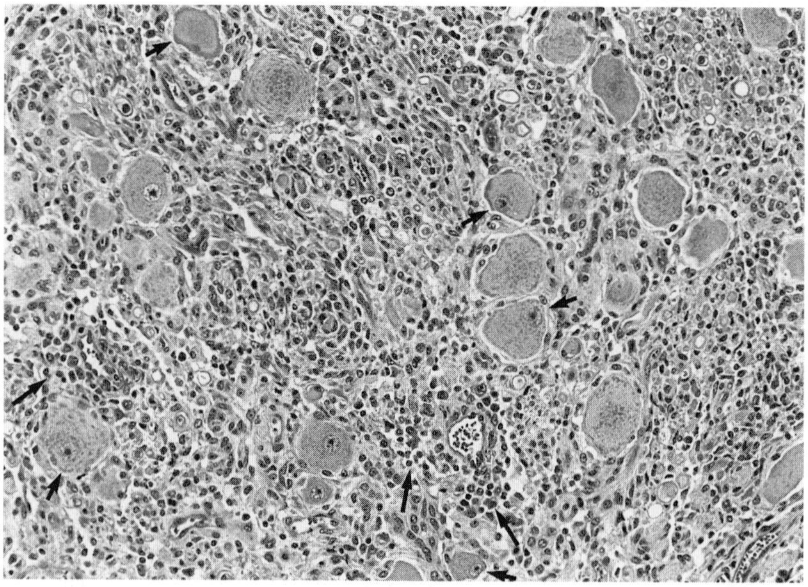

Figure 8-47 Trigeminal (gasserian) ganglion; steer. Rabies. There is mild ganglionitis with focal accumulation of mononuclear cells *(long arrows)* and varying degrees of altered neuronal cell bodies, some with peripherally positioned nuclei *(short arrows)*. H & E stain.

monocytes) or cell-unassociated state, (2) by retrograde movement within the axoplasm of peripheral axons, (3) from the olfactory mucosa that contains receptor cells whose processes synapse within the CNS and by direct spread from the nasal submucosa into the CSF via focally exposed subarachnoid space, and (4) by direct spread. Direct spread of infection can result from trauma (skull or vertebral fracture), various paracranial and paravertebral infections associated with inner ear infection, sinusitis, inflammation of the ethmoid and nasopharyngeal areas (including the guttural pouches in equidae), vertebral osteomyelitis, and following docking of lambs. Within the CNS, infectious agents can spread in the interstitium, within neurons and neuroglia, by mobile infected leukocytes that enter from the circulation, and in the CSF.

Four commonly occurring changes that typify inflammation of the CNS from many different causes include leptomeningitis, perivascular cuffing, microgliosis, and neuronal degeneration. Less common but important additional lesions include ganglioneuritis involving the peripheral nervous system (e.g., in rabies), vasculitis, necrosis (e.g., in pseudorabies of pigs), and demyelination (e.g., in canine distemper).

The type of inflammatory response can vary with the cause. A rather simplistic guideline (to which there are always exceptions) that compares the type of inflammation with different etiologic agents is as follows: suppurative or purulent response can be due to several species of bacteria; nonsuppurative (lymphocytic, monocytic [macrophage], plasmacytic) response can be due to viruses and certain other infectious agents (e.g., protozoa such as *Toxoplasma gondii*) and parasitic infestations; and granulomatous response can be due to fungi and some bacteria (e.g., *Mycobacterium* species).

Viral Infections

Rabies. Rabies virus (family Rhabdoviridae) is one of the most neurotropic of all viruses infecting mammals. Gross lesions of the infected central nervous tissue are often absent. Microscopic lesions of the CNS are typically nonsuppurative and include a variable leptomeningitis and perivascular cuffing with lymphocytes, macrophages, and plasma cells; microgliosis (which sometimes is prominent); variable (often not severe) neuronal degeneration; and ganglioneuritis (Fig. 8-47). Emphasis should be given to the fact that infected neurons often are minimally altered morphologically. Neurons can also contain intracytoplasmic inclusions (Negri bodies). Also, some species (e.g., canine) are reported to have a tendency to develop a more severe inflammatory reaction than others (e.g., bovine), in which little if any inflammation might occur. Nonneural lesions include variable nonsuppurative sialitis accompanied by necrosis and presence of Negri bodies (e.g., dog) in salivary epithelial cells.

Negri body formation within neurons of the CNS and even in the peripheral ganglia has long been the hallmark of rabies infection, although it is not detected in all cases. The inclusions are intracytoplasmic and initially develop as an aggregation of strands of viral nucleocapsid, which rather quickly transforms into an ill-defined granular matrix. Mature rabies virions, which bud from the nearby endoplasmic reticulum, can also be located around the periphery of the matrix. With time, the Negri body becomes larger and detectable by light microscopy. Classically, in H & E–stained sections, the Negri body, which is eosinophilic, has one or more small, light clear areas called inner bodies that form as a result of invagination of cytoplasmic components (that includes virions) into the matrix of the inclusion (Fig. 8-48).

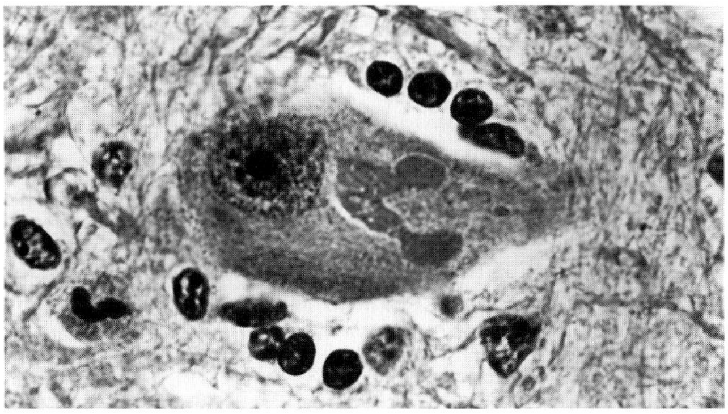

Figure 8-48 Brain, medulla oblongata; steer. Rabies. A neuron of the medulla oblongata contains a large C-shaped Negri body. The small light areas in the inclusion represent "inner bodies." H & E stain.

Inclusions that do not possess inner bodies have been referred to as Lyssa bodies, but they are actually Negri bodies without cytoplasmic indentation. It should also be noted that both fixed viruses (adapted to the CNS by passage) and street viruses (that produce the naturally occurring disease) produce the same ultrastructural features, but fixed viral strains generally cause severe neuronal degeneration that precludes the development, and thus the detection, of Negri bodies. Negri bodies also tend to occur more frequently in large neurons (e.g., pyramidal neurons of the hippocampus and large neurons of the medulla oblongata) than in smaller ones. Also, inclusions are frequently present in neurons not located in areas of inflammation.

A spongiform lesion, indistinguishable qualitatively from the lesion characteristic for several of the spongiform encephalopathies (see Prion Infections, Scrapie), was described for the first time in 1984 by Charlton. This lesion was initially detected in experimental rabies in skunks and foxes, and later in the naturally occurring disease in the skunk, fox, horse, cow, cat, and sheep. The lesion occurs in the neuropil of the gray matter (especially the thalamus and cerebral cortex), initially as intracytoplasmic membrane–bound vacuoles in neuronal dendrites (less commonly in axons and astrocytes). The vacuoles enlarge with compression of surrounding tissue and ultimately rupture with formation of a tissue space. Although the mechanism responsible for the development of this lesion has not been determined, it is thought to result from an indirect effect of the rabies virus on neural tissue (possibly involving an alteration of neurotransmitter metabolism).

Rabies is generally transmitted by a bite from an infected animal. Respiratory infection has also been uncommonly reported following exposure to virus in bat caves and from accidental human laboratory exposure. The following mechanism has been proposed for spread of rabies virus from the inoculation site (e.g., rear leg of an animal) to the CNS. The virus initially enters peripheral nerve terminals or local skeletal muscle myocytes or both at the site of inoculation. The probability is greater that virus will be taken up by both axon terminals and myocytes following a large inoculation dose. If the virus directly enters peripheral nerve terminals, the incubation period will more likely be short regardless of whether muscle cells are infected. With progressively lower doses of virus, however, there is a greater possibility that virus will enter either nerve terminals or myocytes, but not both. This situation can result in a short incubation period if virus directly enters nerve terminals as described above or could result in a more prolonged incubation period if there was initial infection and retention of virus in myocytes before its release and uptake by nerve terminals. Viral replication within infected myocytes has been suggested, but the specific degree to which this can occur remains to be clarified. Virus moves from the periphery to the CNS by axoplasmic transport (apparently via sensory or motor nerves). With sensory axons, the first cell bodies to be encountered following inoculation of a rear leg would be the sensory dorsal root ganglia or the dorsal horn of the spinal cord; for motor axons, the cell bodies of the ventral lower motor neurons or those in autonomic ganglia are the ones initially infected. It is not known whether viral infection and replication in neurons of dorsal root ganglia are essential for infection of the CNS. Virus then moves into the spinal cord and spreads to the brain.

Recent experimental results have helped clarify the mechanism by which virus spreads within the CNS. Following axoplasmic spread of virus from an inoculated rear leg to neurons of the associated segments of the spinal cord (e.g., L2 and L3), rapid spread of infection to the brain occurs via long ascending and descending fiber tracts, bypassing the gray mater of the rostral spinal cord. This early spread of virus has been suggested to explain how induction of behavioral changes occurs before there is sufficiently severe injury to cause paralysis, and allows dissemination of infection before there is time for a significant immune response. Spread of infection within neurons of the CNS recently has been proposed to occur via both anterograde and retrograde axoplasmic flow, with corresponding neuron-to-neuron spread by axosomatic-axodendritic and somatoaxonal-dendroaxonal transfer of infection. The latter type of transsynaptic spread can occur by budding of developing virions from the neuronal cytoplasm (cell body or dendrite) into a synapsing axon. Transsynaptic spread can also occur in the form of bare viral nucleocapsid (ribonucleoprotein-transcriptase complexes) in the absence of a complete virion.

As indicated, viral spread within the CNS can be quite rapid, and although neurons are the cells primarily affected, there is evidence that the occasional and slight infection can also involve the leptomeninges, ependyma, oligodendroglia, and astrocytes. During the spread of virus, there is simultaneous centrifugal movement of virus peripherally from the CNS via axons, which results in infection of various tissues including the oral cavity and salivary glands, permitting transmission of the disease in the saliva. During centrifugal spread there is also infection of neurons of dorsal root ganglia with widespread involvement of ganglia occurring terminally. Affected ganglia have a moderate to severe nonsuppurative inflammatory response that may be accompanied by neuronal degeneration (more frequently occurring than in the CNS). An additionally important feature of rabies is that infection of nervous and nonnervous tissues (i.e., limbic system and salivary glands, respectively) occur at the same time, which permits affected animals to have the required behavior plus necessary viral inoculum (in the saliva) to transmit the disease.

The clinical signs in domestic animals are similar with some differences between species. The clinical disease in the dog has been divided into three phases: prodromal, excitatory, and paralytic. In the prodromal phase, which lasts 2 to 3 days, the animal can have a subtle change in temperament. The term **furious rabies** refers to animals in which the excitatory phase is predominant and **dumb rabies** to animals in which the excitatory phase is extremely short or absent and the disease progresses quickly to the paralytic phase. Cattle generally have the furious form of rabies, and affected animals are restless and aggressive. Other somewhat unique signs of cattle with rabies include bellowing, general straining, tenesmus, and signs of sexual excitement followed by paralysis and death. Mules, sheep, and pigs usually have the excitatory form of rabies. Horses can have early signs that are atypical for a neurologic disease but terminally tend to have the furious-violent form.

When conducting a necropsy on an animal suspected of having rabies it is important to remember (1) to provide adequate protection for the prosector and (2) to collect the proper CNS tissues (cerebral hemisphere that includes hippocampus, cerebellum and medulla, and optionally the spinal cord) for examination by immunofluorescence and sometimes mouse inoculation.

Pseudorabies. Several species of domestic and wild animals are susceptible to infection with pseudorabies virus (family Herpesviridae). The disease in susceptible species other than pigs is generally fatal. Although pigs (particularly young, suckling animals) can die from infection, most mature pigs remain persistently infected and act as carriers.

Gross lesions in pigs occur in several nonneural tissues including organs of the respiratory system, lymphoid system, digestive tract, and reproductive tract. Focal tissue necrosis also occurs (e.g., liver, spleen, adrenal glands), particularly in young suckling pigs, and mortality in such animals can be high. The CNS is free of gross lesions except for leptomeningeal congestion. Microscopic lesions in pigs are characterized by a nonsuppurative meningoencephalomyelitis with ganglioneuritis. Injury to CNS tissue can be marked, with neuronal degeneration and parenchymal necrosis. Intranuclear inclusion bodies are not commonly detected in pigs but can be present in neurons, astrocytes, oligodendroglia, and endothelial cells.

The route of natural infection in pigs is intranasal (by direct contact or aerosolization), followed by reproduction of virus in the upper respiratory tract. The virus then travels to the tonsil and local lymph nodes by way of the lymph vessels. Following replication in the nasopharynx, virus invades sensory nerve endings (e.g., bipolar olfactory cells and other nerve terminals) and is then transported in axoplasm via the trigeminal ganglion and olfactory bulb to the brain. The virus has also been reported to be capable of spreading transsynaptically. Recent studies have additionally shown that some strains produce lesions in the gastrointestinal tract and myenteric plexuses, suggesting that infection might spread from the intestinal mucosa to the CNS via autonomic nerves. In latently infected pigs, the oronasal epithelium can be recurrently infected by virus spreading from the nervous system, followed by its excretion in oronasal fluid. The virus can also spread hematogenously, although in low titer, to other tissues of the body. Cellular attachment, entry, and cell-to-cell spread of the virus is mediated by glyocoprotein projections that extend from the surface of the viral particle.

Infection of secondary hosts (e.g., cattle, sheep, dogs, cats) regularly involves direct or indirect contact with pigs. Infection can occur by ingestion, inhalation, and wound infection. Dogs and cats usually become infected by ingesting organs from pigs that contain pseudorabies virus. The pathogenesis involving axonal spread to the CNS is comparable to that of pigs, with lesions that include nonsuppurative encephalomyelitis accompanied by ganglioneuritis (Fig. 8-49, see Fig. 8-47). Intranuclear inclu-

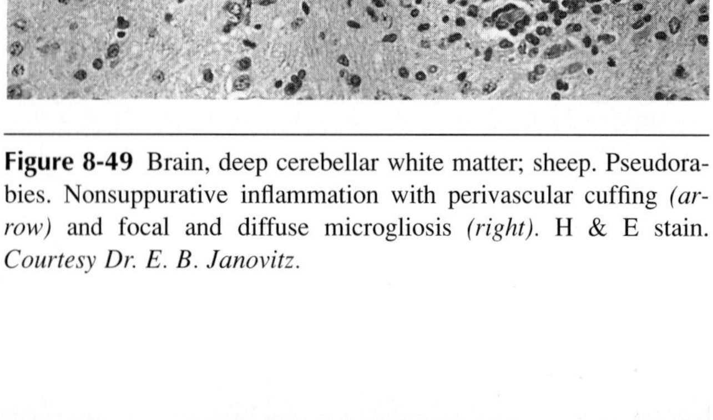

Figure 8-49 Brain, deep cerebellar white matter; sheep. Pseudorabies. Nonsuppurative inflammation with perivascular cuffing *(arrow)* and focal and diffuse microgliosis *(right)*. H & E stain. *Courtesy Dr. E. B. Janovitz.*

sion bodies, either eosinophilic or basophilic in their staining characteristics, have been described in neurons of the brain.

Equine Herpesvirus 1 Infection. Equine herpesvirus 1 (EHV-1) (an alpha-herpesvirus) is an important cause of equine abortion and perinatal foal infection and death, in addition to myeloencephalitis. EHV-1 can also cause rhinopneumonitis.

The neurologic form of EHV-1 infection has a worldwide distribution and affects other equidae including the zebra in addition to the horse, but appears to be relatively uncommon when compared with the incidence of abortion and upper respiratory tract disease caused by EHV-1. The neurologic disease may accompany or follow outbreaks of respiratory disease or abortion.

The characteristic lesion in the CNS caused by EHV-1 infection is a vasculitis (affecting arterioles, capillaries, and venules) accompanied by thrombosis and focal parenchymal necrosis (infarction). Lesions occur in both the gray and white matter of the spinal cord, medulla oblongata, mesencephalon, diencephalon, and cerebral cortex. The endothelium appears to be the site of involvement, with the subsequent occurrence of intimal and medial degeneration, hemorrhage, thrombosis, extravasation of plasma proteins into the perivascular space, neuronal degeneration (e.g., axonal swelling with ballooning of the myelin sheath and degeneration of the cell body), and variable mononuclear cellular cuffing. Other lesions include cerebrospinal ganglioneuritis and vasculitis in nonneural tissues including the endometrium, nasal cavity, lungs, uvea of the eye, hypophysis, and skeletal muscle.

The disease begins with infection of the respiratory mucosa. The neurologic disease has been experimentally reproduced by intranasal inoculation of the virus (EHV-1, subtype 1), which can replicate in the epithelium of the respiratory or intestinal tracts following infection. Intranuclear inclusions occur in the nasal mucosa. Infection of mononuclear leukocytes (predominantly, but not exclusively, T lymphocytes) then occurs and is followed by a cell-associated viremia. The virus, which is endotheliotropic, even though infection of neurons and astrocytes can occur, localizes in small arteries and capillaries of the CNS and some other tissues following direct spread from the circulating infected cells. Inflammation of the vascular wall then results in vasculitis, thrombosis, and infarction of the neural tissue supplied by the thrombosed vessel. Latent infection of the trigeminal ganglion and lymphoid tissues can also occur.

EHV-1 does not appear to be neurotropic, which is in contrast to some herpesvirus encephalitides of other species in which the virus replicates in neurons (e.g., herpes simplex viral infection in the human, infectious bovine rhinotracheitis viral infection in calves, and pseudorabies viral infection in pigs). In addition to having vasculitis as the principal lesion, the infection in the horse also differs somewhat from most other herpetic infections of the CNS in being primarily a disease of the adult (although young animals can be affected).

Bovine Malignant Catarrhal Fever. Malignant catarrhal fever is usually a sporadic highly fatal disease of cattle and other ruminants including deer, buffalo, and antelope and can involve several animals in a herd. The disease has a worldwide distribution, and the clinicopathologic features do not differ significantly from one part of the world to another. The primary target tissues are the lymphoid organs, epithelial tissues (particularly the respiratory and gastrointestinal tracts), and the vasculature, but the kidneys, liver, eyes, joints, and CNS are also affected in some cattle.

Two general types of the disease occur, the sheep-associated and wildebeest-derived forms. The causative agents involved belong to the herpesvirus subfamily Gammaherpesviridae. The disease occurring outside Africa, caused by ovine herpesvirus 2 (OHV-2), often involves close contact of presumed "carrier" sheep with susceptible ruminants. In Africa, and occasionally in wildlife facilities outside the country, the source of the infection (designated alcelaphine herpesvirus-1 or AHV-1) is the wildebeest. Two other antigenically related viruses, (that apparently do not cause natural disease) include alcelaphine herpes virus 2 (AHV-2) and hippotragine herpes virus 1 (HiHV-1), which have been isolated from African hartebeest and roan antelope, respectively.

Gross lesions of the CNS include congestion and cloudiness of the meninges. Microscopically, the lesion is a nonsuppurative meningoencephalomyelitis that can be associated with a vasculitis. Lymphocytic perivascular cuffing and varying degrees of necrotizing vasculitis occur in all parts of the brain and occasionally in the spinal cord, with the white matter most consistently involved. Other lesions in the affected CNS include variable neuronal degeneration, microgliosis, leptomeningitis, hemorrhage, choroiditis, necrosis of ependymal cells, and ganglioneuritis.

It is generally accepted that cattle and other susceptible ruminants contract the disease in nature (following respiratory or oral infection) during association with carrier sheep (presumed) and wildebeest, particularly at the time of parturition. An immune-mediated (e.g., cell-mediated) process has been proposed to be involved in lesion development.

Infectious Bovine Rhinotracheitis Virus–Induced Encephalitis in Cattle. Infectious bovine rhinotracheitis, caused by bovine herpesvirus type 1 (BHV-1), is a worldwide disease of cattle that is best known as an infection of the respiratory tract. Lesions can involve the eyes (conjunctivitis) and tissues of the reproductive, alimentary, integumentary, and nervous systems. Although BHV-1 occasionally causes a nonsuppurative meningoencephalitis, primarily in young cattle, two variants of BHV-1 isolated in Argentina and Australia (referred to as BHV-1, subtypes 3a and 3b, and recently BHV-5) have a particular tropism for the CNS and cause outbreaks of disease in young cattle ranging in age from 5 to 18 months. Infection of the respiratory and genital tracts (with abortion) also can occur.

Gross lesions are nonspecific and include meningeal congestion and petechiation in ventral areas of the brain. Microscopic lesions consist of nonsuppurative meningoencephalitis with the occasional presence of neutrophils. Other changes include vasculitis, focal malacia, neuronal degeneration, and presence of intranuclear inclusions in neurons and astrocytes.

Enterovirus-Induced Porcine Polioencephalomyelitis. Several diseases of pigs (e.g., Teschen disease, Talfan disease, and others) caused by porcine enteroviruses (family Picornaviridae) are characterized by polioencephalomyelitis. As stated, Teschen disease is caused by porcine enterovirus, and possibly by serotypes 2 and 3. Clinical signs in the different diseases vary in severity from marked and associated with death of affected animals (Teschen disease occurring sporadically in Europe and Africa) to less severe disease with signs that include fever, diarrhea, and paralysis (sometimes most severe in the hind legs) in pigs in North America and some other regions of the world.

No gross lesions are detectable. All forms of the disease are characterized microscopically by a nonsuppurative polioencephalomyelitis. The sequence of changes in degenerating neurons includes acute swelling, central chromatolysis, necrosis, neuronophagia, and variable resultant axonal degeneration. Astrocytosis, and particularly astrogliosis, also occur, especially in the later stages of the infection. Cerebral and cerebellar involvement is variable with the different forms of the disease. Ganglioneuritis, particularly of dorsal root ganglia of the spinal cord, and variable leptomeningitis of varying severity also occur.

Natural infection occurs by the oral route and is followed by viral localization and replication in the tonsil and intestinal tract (primarily ileum, large intestine, and mesenteric lymph nodes). Following replication in the intestine, virus travels hematogenously to the brain and spreads into the parenchyma.

Hemagglutinating Encephalomyelitis Viral Infection of Pigs. In 1958, a disease of nursing pigs characterized by high morbidity, vomiting, anorexia, constipation, and severe progressive emaciation was reported in Ontario, Canada. The etiologic agent is a coronavirus.

Gross lesions are limited and include cachexia and enlargement of the abdomen caused by gaseous distension of the stomach and intestines. Microscopic lesions occur in the respiratory tract, stomach, and central and peripheral nervous systems. Lesions in the CNS, which are most pronounced in the gray matter, are characterized by a nonsuppurative meningoencephalomyelitis and neuronal degeneration. The caudal brain stem (particularly the medulla and pons) and spinal cord are affected. In the peripheral ganglia, the lesions are nonsuppurative inflammation and neuronal degeneration.

Infection by the oronasal route, which has been demonstrated experimentally, is followed by viral replication in epithelial cells of the nasal mucosa, tonsils, lungs, and small intestine. After local replication, the virus spreads to the CNS by the peripheral nerves that include the trigeminal and olfactory nerves, vagus, and extensions from intestinal plexuses to the spinal cord. Neurons of peripheral ganglia also are infected. Viral antigen is restricted to the cytoplasm of neurons. The vomiting associated with the disease is presumed to result from altered function of neurons (in the vagal nucleus and its ganglion, and gastric intramural plexuses) secondary to viral infection.

Borna Disease. Borna disease, originally an equine disease named after Borna, a town in Saxony, Germany, is an encephalomyelitis caused by an unusual enveloped RNA virus that replicates in the nucleus, has no cytopathic effect, and until recently (1997) has not been visualized ultrastucturally as a recognizable virion. The disease has been recognized in Central Europe for more than 250 years. Borna disease virus has been classified as the prototype of a new virus family, Bornaviridae.

The natural infection, which tends to occur more frequently in the spring and summer, has a broad host range, having been reported in horses and sheep (the most frequently cited species) but also in cattle, goats, domestic cats (staggering disease in Sweden and Austria), dogs, rodents, rabbits, deer, alpacas, llamas, pigmy hippopotamus, sloth, ostriches, nonhuman primates, and human beings. Borna disease has an incubation period that can be relatively long, from weeks to several months.

Borna disease virus infection in horses was originally considered to result in a high mortality, up to 80% to 100% following 1 to 3 weeks of clinical illness. More recent evidence indicates that the majority of infected animals are either asymptomatic or have mild clinical disease that can be accompanied by behavioral changes, followed by recovery. The clinically severe disease in the horse is still largely confined to certain regions in Germany and Switzerland; the asymptomatic infection, which probably also occurs in other species including human beings, is considered to have a worldwide distribution.

Borna disease might also be the first infectious agent recognized to be causally significant in human biologic psychiatry. It is known that behavioral alterations can accompany Borna disease infection in animals (e.g., horses, sheep, domestic cats, and nonhuman primates), especially during the early stages, and also in human beings (schizophrenia and unipolar and bipolar psychiatric disorders particularly). A proposed mechanism for behavioral alterations involves viral protein interference with neurotransmitter function of infected neurons, particularly those located in the limbic lobe of the brain.

There are no significant gross lesions. Microscopic lesions, which are limited to the nervous system, consist of a nonsuppurative encephalomyelitis that can be severe and accompanied by neuronal degeneration. Lesions are confined largely to the gray matter, although white matter can also be affected, and are most severe in the midbrain, midbrain-diencephalon junction, and hypothalamus. Marked inflammation also occurs in the hippocampus. In addition, lesions occur in the cerebral cortex (especially laterobasal areas), olfactory bulb, caudate nucleus, and periventricular gray matter. Inflammation of the meninges and spinal cord is generally mild. A rare hemorrhagic form of the disease characterized by vascular necrosis accompanied by focal hemorrhage and tissue necrosis has also been described. Small, round to oval, eosinophilic intranuclear inclusions occur in neurons of the brain stem, hippocampus, and cerebrospinal ganglia. In the PNS, inflammation occurs in the cranial, spinal, and autonomic ganglia and in the peripheral nerves.

Experimental evidence indicates that infection of the CNS via olfactory nerves can follow intranasal viral exposure. Viral replication occurs in nuclei, although viral antigen has also been demonstrated in the neuronal perikaryon (cytoplasm). The agent is highly neurotropic, similar to the rabies virus, and is transported to the CNS from the periphery intraaxonally. Nonneuronal infection (of astrocytes, oligodendroglia, ependyma, choroid plexus epithelial cells, and Schwann cells) occurs and possibly contributes to viral replication (e.g., astrocytes and Schwann cells). The virus can also infect the retina by retrograde intraaxonal transport via the optic nerve and cause blindness under experimental conditions. After reaching the CNS, the virus spreads intraaxonally and transsynaptically (proposed) as described for rabies virus. The virus can then also spread centrifugally via the PNS, resulting in infection of various nonneural tissues that include the lacrimal and salivary glands, and endocrine tissues such as the pituitary and adrenal glands, plus other tissues. It has also been determined that peripheral blood monocytes can be infected. An additionally proposed peripheral spread of virus by autonomic transport has led to the suggestion that infection of peripheral neurons might be involved in the development of colic and other gastroenteric processes in the horse.

The specific lesions that develop in the CNS appear to depend on a viral-induced cell-mediated immune mechanism. Infected, immunosuppressed laboratory animals do not develop the disease or lesions, despite high titers of virus in the CNS. However, transfer of cells (spleen or lymph node origin) from diseased animals into immunosuppressed infected recipients can induce encephalitis and clinical disease. Antibody to Borna disease virus does not appear to play any significant role in the disease process.

Equine Encephalomyelitis. Infection of horses with Eastern, Western, or Venezuelan equine encephalomyelitis (EEE, WEE, VEE) viruses produces a range of clinical disease. The viruses are members of the family Togaviridae, genus *Alphavirus*. In addition to horses, Eastern encephalomyelitis has also been reported in cattle and pigs.

Lesions of the CNS induced by all three viruses are similar, but there are some differences. Overall, gross lesions include cerebral hyperemia, edema, petechiation, focal necrosis, and leptomeningeal edema. Microscopic lesions are most prominent in the gray matter of the brain and spinal cord and are characterized by perivascular cuffing (with lymphocytes, macrophages, and neutrophils), variable neutrophilic infiltration of the gray matter parenchyma, microgliosis, neuronal degeneration, focal parenchymal (cortical) necrosis, perivascular edema and hemorrhage, necrotizing vasculitis, thrombosis, choroiditis, and leptomeningitis.

Neutrophils are detectable during the early stages (2 days) of clinical EEE and VEE. Vasculitis, thrombosis, and cerebrocortical necrosis have been associated particularly with VEE but also with EEE. Peripheral ganglia (e.g., Gasserian or trigeminal ganglion) appear to be unaffected.

Following inoculation (by mosquito), the circulating virus initially infects several tissues hematogenously, including bone marrow, lymphoreticular tissue, muscle, and connective tissue. In some tissues (e.g., lymphoid and myeloid [bone marrow]), there may be cellular depletion, necrosis, or both. A second viremia results in hematogenous infection of the CNS. Experimental evidence suggests that the viruses replicate in endothelial cells before entering the nervous system and infecting neurons, for which it has an affinity. There is also evidence that viruses of this group (e.g., VEE virus) can be associated with alteration in the metabolism of neurotransmitters of the CNS that are responsible for certain clinical signs.

West Nile Viral Infection. West Nile virus is a cause of encephalitis in human beings and animals. The virus was first isolated from a woman in 1937 in the West Nile district of Uganda from which it received its name. In addition to Africa, the viral infection has been detected in western Asia including India and Pakistan, the Middle East including Israel, Europe, southern Russia and several adjacent countries, and recently (late summer-early fall 1999) for the first time in the eastern United States in New York City, Connecticut, and New Jersey. Also, evidence of human viral infection (presence of antibodies) has been detected in eastern Asian countries that include Borneo, China, Malaysia, the Philippines, and Thailand. West Nile virus, along with several other viruses that include

Japanese encephalitis virus and St. Louis encephalitis virus, which was initially considered to be responsible for the recent epidemic in the United States, are members of the genus *Flavivirus,* family Flaviviridae.

West Nile viral infection is best known to occur in human beings, birds, and horses, although there is evidence that infrequent infection can occur in other animal species. Although the human infection is usually not fatal, it still remains a serious threat, especially in aged individuals and those with a compromised immune system. A recent major outbreak of the infection in human beings occurred in Romania in 1996-1997 in which there were more than 500 clinical cases attributed to the disease with a death rate that approached 10%.

The virus, which has been isolated in the United States from infected human beings, birds, and horses during the recent outbreak, is most commonly transmitted via a bird-mosquito cycle. Although the infection typically does not cause clinical signs in birds, it resulted in an unusually high death rate of crows and some zoo birds in New York City. The severity of the equine infection is variable, with mortality rates as high as 44% (42 of 94 in 1996 in Morocco) reported. Reasons for the variation in severity following infection in the above-cited species should include the degree to which an exposed population has had previous contact with the virus, plus the possibility of the infecting strain having an increased virulence.

Reported clinical signs of the equine disease (originally identified as Near Eastern Equine Encephalitis in Egypt and Lourdige in France) resemble those caused by the Venezuelan, Eastern, and Western strains of equine encephalomyelitis virus, which are well known (primarily the latter two strains of virus) as a cause of equine disease in the United States. Signs of the equine West Nile viral infection include variable fever, depression, weakness to paralysis of the hind limbs, ataxia, tetraplegia, convulsions, coma, and death.

Gross lesions of West Nile viral infection in horses include hyperemia and petechiation of the brain. Microscopic lesions in birds and horses that have died of the disease are characterized by a nonsuppurative (lymphocytic/histiocytic) inflammation of the central nervous system that can vary in degree of severity.

Japanese Encephalitis. Japanese encephalitis is a particularly important disease in human beings, but infection also occurs in animals (e.g., horses, pigs, cattle, and sheep). Its geographic distribution includes India, China, and southeastern Asia. The causative virus is classified as a member of the family Flaviviridae and is transmitted by mosquitoes, mainly *Culex tritaeniorhynchus.* In nature, infection is maintained in a cycle involving vector mosquitoes, birds, and mammals (e.g., pigs)

Although young susceptible pigs can have signs, detectable illness is not a feature of viral infection in adult or pregnant pigs. However, fetal infection during pregnancy can result in mummification and stillbirth of fetuses, or the birth of weak live pigs with nervous signs accompanied by nonsuppurative encephalitis and neuronal degeneration.

Well-documented outbreaks of meningoencephalomyelitis in horses have been reported. Young or immature horses are more susceptible to infection than older animals. Lesions are limited to the nervous system. Grossly, they include mild leptomeningeal congestion, hyperemia, and occasional areas of hemorrhage within the brain and spinal cord. Microscopic lesions are characterized by an early leptomeningitis and encephalitis in which neutrophils predominate, followed by nonsuppurative inflammation, neuronal degeneration, focal hemorrhage, and focal necrosis. Neurons are the target cell. The lesions are distributed diffusely throughout the nervous system but affect the gray matter more than the white matter.

Factors involved in the pathogenesis of this viral infection include the recent finding that the susceptibility of laboratory animals (e.g., rat) to the virus is closely associated with neuronal immaturity. Such an age-dependent susceptibility of brain to viral infection has also been noted with other flaviviruses, including St. Louis encephalitis virus and yellow fever virus. The fact that fetal and neonatal pigs and young horses appear to be more susceptible than adult animals suggests that such a correlation could also exist in naturally occurring infections of animals.

Louping Ill. Louping ill (a tick-transmitted sheep encephalomyelitis) has been recognized in the British Isles for at least 200 years. It is primarily a disease of sheep but also affects cattle, horses, pigs, goats, red deer, dogs, human beings, and the red grouse. It is caused by a flavivirus (family Flaviviridae) and occurs in the British Isles and Norway. A similar disease of sheep occurs in Turkey, Greece, Bulgaria, and Spain. Some cases have been determined to be caused by similar flaviviruses, but are distinct from each other and from louping ill virus. The disease occurs in the spring and summer.

No significant gross lesions are present. Microscopic lesions are characterized by a meningoencephalomyelitis that is primarily nonsuppurative, although neutrophils can be present. Specific changes also include neuronal degeneration. The most consistent and pronounced lesions, which include inflammation and degeneration of Purkinje cells, occur in the cerebellar cortex and have been proposed to be at least partially responsible for the unique clinical signs (peculiar leaping gait) displayed by affected ataxic animals. Prominent lesions, although more variable, also occur in the medulla oblongata and spinal cord. Other areas of the CNS can additionally be affected, but less prominently. No inflammation of spinal ganglia occurs, but inflammation has been detected in peripheral (e.g., sciatic) nerves.

Following infection by the tick *Ixodes ricinus,* the virus replicates in lymphoid tissues (e.g., lymph nodes and spleen) resulting in development of a high-titered viremia. A subsequent infection of the CNS (primarily of neurons) probably occurs hematogenously. Excretion of the virus in milk of infected ewes and goats has also been reported, with the suggestion that transmission by ingestion is of possible significance in suckling kids.

Hog Cholera (Swine Fever). This disease of pigs is caused by a pestivirus and has a worldwide distribution, except for several countries (including the United States) from which it has been successfully eradicated.

Lesions of the acute disease, which primarily result from a tropism of the virus for vascular endothelium with subsequent hemorrhage, are present in many organs including the kidneys, intestinal serosa, lymph nodes, spleen, liver, bone marrow, lungs, skin, heart, stomach, gallbladder, and CNS. Microscopic lesions of the CNS are characterized by swelling, proliferation, and necrosis of endothelium; perivascular lymphocytic cuffing; infrequent hemorrhage and thrombosis; microgliosis; neuronal degeneration; choroiditis; and leptomeningitis. Lesions occur in both gray and white matter and tend to be most prominent in the brain stem (medulla oblongata, pons, colliculi) and thalamus but also occur in the cerebrum, cerebellum, and spinal cord.

Infection under natural conditions occurs by the oronasal route. The virus initially infects epithelial cells of the tonsilar crypts and surrounding lymphoid tissue and then spreads to draining lymph nodes where it replicates. Extension continues via the circulation (proposed in association with mononuclear cells, e.g., lymphocytes) to the spleen, bone marrow, visceral lymph nodes, and lymphoid tissue of the intestinal tract, where high viral titers are attained. Target cells for virus replication include endothelial cells, lymphoid cells and macrophages, and epithelial cells. Hematogenous spread of the virus throughout the infected pig (including the CNS) is usually completed in 5 to 6 days.

Feline Infectious Peritonitis. Feline infectious peritonitis (FIP), which is caused by a coronavirus and has a worldwide distribution, is mainly a disease of domestic cats, although wild felidae can be affected. It generally occurs sporadically in cats of all ages (but is most common in younger cats, e.g., ages 3 months to 3 years) and can be clinically significant, as it can result in death. The disease manifests itself in **effusive (wet)** or **noneffusive (dry)** forms.

The basic lesion of both forms of the disease is a pyogranulomatous inflammation (with a tendency to be surface oriented) that is accompanied by an initial vasculitis followed by an inconstant vascular necrosis and infarction. The **effusive form** is typified by serositis, accumulation of fluid in the abdominal and thoracic cavities, with varying degrees of inflammation of visceral tissue. Lesions of the **noneffusive form** more frequently include leptomeningitis, chorioependymitis, focal encephalomyelitis, and ophthalmitis, although involvement of other tissues (kidneys; hepatic and mesenteric lymph nodes; and less frequently, serosa and other abdominal viscera) can occur.

There are two recognized feline coronaviruses (FCoV): feline enteric coronavirus (FECV) and feline infectious peritonitis virus (FIPV) that cause FECV and FIP infections, respectively. The viruses for each infection are antigentically and morphologically indistinguishable and are currently considered to represent avirulent (FECV) and virulent (FIPV) strains of the same basic FCoV virus. Following ingestion, FECV infects and replicates in small intestinal epithelium and usually is an insignificant infection, although severe intestinal disease can occur. It has been proposed that when FECV gains the ability to replicate in macrophages (by mutation), then FIP can occur.

The FIP virus (FIPV) enters the susceptible cat primarily by ingestion following fecal contamination, although transmission by direct inoculation (cat bites, licking open wounds, etc.) and in utero (rarely) have been reported. Following infection, the virus replicates in macrophages that spread the virus to other tissues of the body (e.g., liver, visceral peritoneum and pleura, uvea, and meninges and the ependyma of the brain and spinal cord).

Following dissemination of the virus in the body, the development of disease depends on the type and degree of immunity that develops. Virus containment, with resistance to disease, occurs following development of a strong cell-mediated immunity. Humoral immunity by itself is not protective and can actually enhance development of the disease (typically the effusive form of FIP) by two proposed mechanisms. The first involves the development of virus-antibody-complement complexes that particularly accumulate in the same areas as infected macrophages (around small blood vessels), resulting in inflammation and subsequent vascular injury accompanied by effusion of large amounts of fluid. The second mechanism involves a process referred to as antibody-dependent enhancement (demonstrated to occur experimentally) that involves uptake of virus-antibody-complement complexes by macrophages followed by significant viral replication. The heavily infected macrophages, with frequent perivascular orientation, release cytokines that result in vascular impairment that leads to leakage of significant amounts of fluid.

Noneffusive FIP, in comparison, is thought to occur when partial cell-mediated immunity develops and represents an intermediate stage between nonprotective humoral immunity alone and protective cellular immunity. This mechanism is supported by the fact that cats that develop the noneffusive form of FIP following experimental infection usually have a preceding and transient bout of effusive-type disease. In addition, there is evidence to support the theory that cats recovered from FIP are immune by a process of "infection immunity" or "premunition." Once these cats no longer retain such infections, they seem to also lose protective (cell-mediated) immunity and are, in fact, more sensitive to a subsequent challenge exposure because of the presence of humoral antibody.

Prion Infections

Scrapie. Scrapie is the prototype of a group of diseases referred to as transmissible spongiform encephalopathies (TSEs). Until relatively recently, the group included the animal diseases scrapie, transmissible mink encephalopathy (scrapie infection in mink), and chronic wasting disease that affects mule deer and elk in captivity, and free-ranging mule, white-tailed and black-tailed deer, and elk. Human diseases have included kuru, Creutzfeldt-Jakob disease, and Gerstmann-Sträussler-Scheinker syndrome. More recent additions to this group include a variant form of Creutzfeld-Jakob disease and fatal familial insomnia in human beings, and bovine spongiform encephalopathy (BSE).

BSE (mad cow disease) was originally identified in Great Britain in 1986 but likely existed there as early as April 1985 (mad cow disease). This disease has subsequently been confirmed in cattle in Northern Ireland, in the Channel Isles, Isle of Man, the Republic of Ireland, Belgium, France, Luxembourg, The Netherlands, Portugal, and Switzerland. BSE has also been detected in cattle imported from the United Kingdom to Canada, Denmark, Falkland Islands, Germany, Italy, and Oman. The bovine agent has also experimentally produced disease in pigs, but only following the use of highly infectious inoculum given simultaneously by multiple routes. Finally, a BSE-like encephalopathy has been identified in Great Britain in the domestic cat (feline spongiform encephalopathy) and several zoo ruminants that include the kudu, Arabian oryx, nyala, gemsbok, and eland (exotic ungulate encephalopathy). In naturally infected cattle, the BSE agent has been identified in the brain, spinal cord, and retina; more recent reports have indicated its presence in lymphoid tissue, bone marrow, and trigeminal and dorsal root ganglia of experimentally infected calves.

Signs that accompany BSE include changes in behavior such as nervousness or aggressiveness, abnormal posture, abnormal gait, incoordination, difficulty in rising, decreased milk production, and loss of body weight despite continued appetite. Clinically affected cattle deteriorate until they either die or require euthanasia. This clinical period usually ranges from 2 weeks to 6 months. All cases of the disease in cattle have occurred in adult animals, with an age range of 3 to 11 years, but most animals develop clinical signs between 3 and 5 years of age.

Scrapie is best known as a degenerative disease that affects the CNS of sheep and was first recognized in Great Britain and other countries of Western Europe more than 250 years ago. The disease, which is currently reported throughout the world except for Australia and New Zealand, also occurs naturally in the domestic goat. The name is derived from the characteristic clinical signs of pruritus, which often results in loss of wool in sheep. The disease progresses inexorably with early signs of subtle change in behavior or temperament followed by scratching and rubbing against fixed objects (because of the pruritus). Additional signs include incoordination, weight loss (despite retention of appetite), biting of the feet and limbs, lip smacking, gait abnormalities, trembling (when suddenly stressed), recumbency, and eventually death after 1 to 6 months or longer.

Scrapie, as with the other TSEs, is quite different from other conventional viral infections. First, it is caused by a very unique agent that is still being characterized and is discussed in more detail below. Second, the disease has a variably long incubation period that depends on the species affected (e.g., from 2 months in laboratory hamsters to 2 years or more in sheep). Further, the disease lacks a typical immune response and is not accompanied by any significant inflammation within the infected CNS.

Grossly, sheep and goats have variable loss of body condition and skin lesions that result from the pruritus. Other than a reported increase in the CSF, no gross lesions of the nervous system are detectable.

Significant microscopic lesions in sheep and goats are limited to the CNS and are most commonly present in the diencephalon, brain stem, and cerebellum (cortex and deep nuclei), with variable lesions in the corpus striatum and spinal cord. Except for some minor changes, the cerebral cortex is essentially unaffected. The characteristic lesions include neuronal degeneration, astrocytosis, and variable spongiosis (generally affecting the gray matter) (Figs. 8-50 and 8-51). The type of neuronal degeneration can vary and commonly is characterized by shrinkage with increased basophilia and cytoplasmic vacuolation (Fig. 8-50), although other changes (e.g., central chromatolysis and ischemic cell change) variably occur. Astrocytosis in affected areas of the brain, including the cerebellar cortex, can be severe. There has been speculation whether the astrocytic reaction is a primary or a secondary response and recent results have helped clarify this problem. An abnormal protein (prion amyloid protein) first accumulates in astroglial cells in the brain during scrapie infection, which could mean that this cell is the primary site of replication. The spongiform change tends to affect the gray matter, and greater severity of this lesion has been associated with long incubation periods. The lesion, when it occurs in the gray matter, has been identified as resulting from dilation of neuronal processes, although other causes including vacuolation of neuronal and astroglial perikarya, swelling of astrocytic processes, dilatation of the periaxonal space, and splitting of myelin sheaths have also been reported. Another lesion that occurs variably in experi-

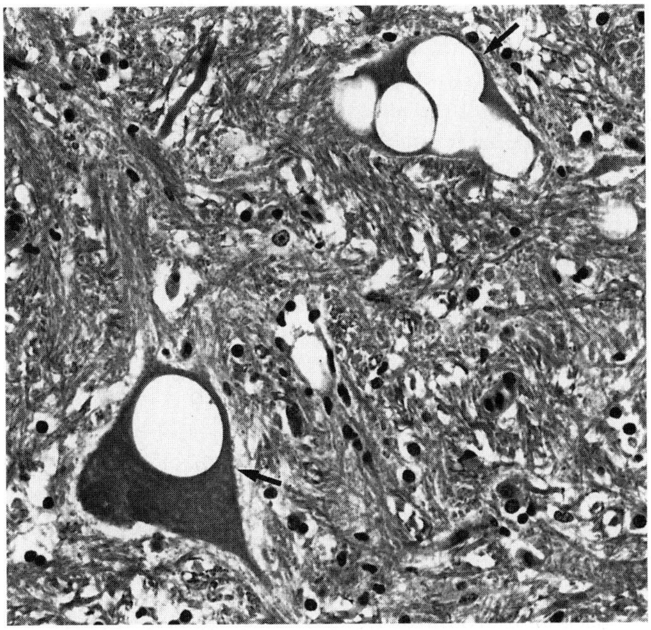

Figure 8-50 Brain, medulla oblongata; cow. Bovine spongiform encephalopathy. There is prominent vacuolation of two neuronal cell bodies *(arrows)*. H & E stain. *Courtesy Dr. A. Braniecki.*

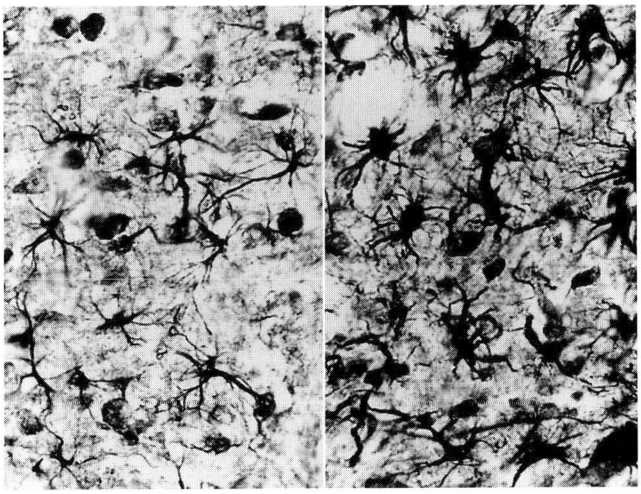

A

B

Figure 8-51 Brain, medulla oblongata; mouse. **A,** Normal brain. Compare the size, shape and density of normal astrocytes with **B,** scrapie. The pronounced hypertrophy and hyperplasia of astrocytes are characteristic of scrapie. Cajal's gold sublimate impregnation. *Courtesy Dr. W. J. Hadlow.*

mentally infected animals, and with the other TSEs, is amyloid plaque formation. Cerebrovascular amyloidosis also has been detected in scrapie-infected sheep. Microscopic lesions similar to those of scrapie occur in the gray matter of the brain stem in cattle with BSE.

A proposed pathogenesis of the natural infection in Suffolk sheep has been advanced by Hadlow and coworkers. It should be noted that Dr. Hadlow is a veterinary pathologist and diplomate of the American College of Veterinary Pathologists who first recognized and reported the similarity between scrapie and kuru of human beings. This important contribution led to the current understanding of the TSEs and a Nobel Prize for the medical scientist who originally investigated kuru in the South Pacific. Following oral infection at an early age, there is an extremely long eclipse phase (about 1 year) before the infectious agent can be detected in infected animals. At this time the agent occurs in low titers in the tonsil, suprapharyngeal (medial retropharyngeal) lymph node, and lymphoid tissue of the intestine. Infection then spreads to regional lymph nodes and eventually to other lymph nodes and the spleen. Other extraneural tissues are not significantly infected.

The agent continues to replicate in the extraintestinal and intestinal lymphoid tissues for many months, or even a year or more, before it reaches the CNS, which is the target organ. It has been proposed that the CNS in sheep is infected by hematogenous spread. However, axonal spread has also been advanced as a mechanism following study of the disease in experimental laboratory animals. The infectious agent first appears in the CNS, initially in the medulla oblongata and diencephalon, when infected sheep are clinically normal. It then spreads to other parts of the CNS and replicates to titers greater than those in nonneural tissues. Infection in nonneural tissues remains, where moderate titers persist until death of the animal. Clinical disease usually occurs when sheep are 3 to 4 years of age, when high concentrations of the agent are present in the CNS, especially in the diencephalon, brain stem, cerebellar cortex, spinal cord, and sometimes the cerebral cortex. Interestingly, the last two areas are not ones in which microscopic lesions are frequently detected. The pathogenesis of the natural disease in goats appears to be comparable to that in sheep.

With regard to the origins of BSE, epidemiologic evidence strongly suggests that this disease was caused initially (during the early 1980s) by the feeding of rations containing meat and bone meal supplements that were contaminated with the scrapie agent.

One of the most intriguing features of the TSEs concerns the uniqueness of their etiologic agents and the manner by which they can be transmitted. The TSEs represent a group of diseases that for the first time in history are caused by agents, unique for each species, that can not only be transmitted as an infectious agent by inoculation of a susceptible animal with infectious tissue (e.g., scrapie-infected brain), but can also be transmitted genetically to offspring following spontaneous mutation of the PrP (prion protein) gene in a parent. Such genetic transmissions have been documented in the human diseases Creutzfeldt-Jakob disease, Gerstmann-Sträussler-Scheinker syndrome, and fatal familial insomnia. Creutzfeldt-Jakob disease can also develop spontaneously as a sporadic disease (incidence of 1 per million) by a mechanism yet unknown, and also iatrogenically following implantation of tissues from Creutzfeldt-Jakob disease–infected donors.

Unlike conventional viruses, the agents of the TSEs have unusual resistance to inactivation by heating and ultraviolet irradiation, and no structures resembling virions can be detected ultrastructurally. Some workers have suggested that the agent is a virus whose protein(s) is coded by its nucleic acid, but morphologic and biochemical studies of purified preparations of the agent have failed to demonstrate viral particles or nucleic acids. More recently, another concept that has received the most support is that the agent is a proteinaceous infectious particle (prion) without evidence of an associated nucleic acid, and that it appears to accumulate selectively in neurons. A specific protein referred to as PrP (prion protein), a 27- to 30-kilodalton polypeptide, seems to be required for, and inseparable from, prion infectivity. It should be noted that normal cells of the body produce a normal prion protein (PrPc), which is different for each species, and whose normal function is unknown. PrPc is expressed throughout the body and is the product of a highly conserved gene found in organisms as diverse as the fruit fly and the human. An abnormal form of this prion protein (PrPsc) is present in animals and human beings that develop the characteristic spongiform encephalopathy.

Although the mechanism by which PrPsc forms has not been completely explained, a posttranslational modification of PrPc has been proposed. This mechanism proposes that PrPsc acts as a template on which PrPc undergoes a conformational change (is refolded) by a process facilitated by another protein (referred as protein X), whereby the α-helical content of PrPc diminishes and the amount of β-sheet increases, resulting in the formation of PrPsc. The features of a specific PrPsc is determined by the animal in which it is formed. When PrPsc of one species is inoculated into a different species, the recipient is less readily infected and generally has a prolonged incubation period. This resistance to infection is referred to as the "species barrier."

Chlamydial Infections

Sporadic Bovine Encephalomyelitis. *Chlamydia psittaci* and *Chlamydia pecorum* are two species that cause disease in domestic animals. Sporadic bovine encephalomyelitis is uncommon and caused by an as yet unclassified chlamydial organism. The disease was first described in the United States, but cases have since occurred in other countries. Calves younger than 6 to 12 months of age are most susceptible.

Lesions are serofibrinous polyserositis, arthritis, tenosynovitis, and nonsuppurative meningoencephalomyelitis. Gross changes in the CNS, when present, are limited to congestion and edema of the leptomeninges. Microscopic lesions extend throughout the neuraxis and consist of leptomeningeal and perivascular infiltrates of lymphocytes, plasma cells, and a few neutrophils. The basilar leptomeninges are most severely affected. Leukocytes extend into the adventitia of blood vessels accompanied by endothelial swelling and prominence, evidence of vasculitis. Additional lesions include neuronal and parenchymal necrosis and microgliosis. Necrosis presumably is secondary to vasculitis and ischemia. Immune-mediated mechanisms have also been incriminated in the genesis of the brain damage.

Protozoal Infections

Protozoal infections with CNS involvement occur in a wide variety of animals. Lesions are similar, and diagnosis of specific infections based on the light microscopic morphology of the different organisms is problematic. More careful scrutiny of these organisms by electron microscopy and characterization by immunohistochemistry has provided data to indicate that discrepancies exist in the literature regarding the etiology of various protozoal infections including those diseases caused by *Sarcocystis, Toxoplasma,* and *Neospora* spp.

Sarcocystosis. Equine protozoal encephalomyelitis is caused by *Sarcocystis neurona.* Clinical infection typically occurs in young adult horses. Lesions can occur throughout the neuraxis, but the spinal cord, particularly the cervical and lumbar intumescences, is commonly affected. When gross lesions are present, they consist of discolored necrotic foci, often with hemorrhage (Fig. 8-52). Microscopic lesions include necrosis, axonal swelling, hemorrhage, and accumulations of lymphocytes, macrophages, neutrophils, eosinophils, and a few multinucleated giant cells in perivascular areas and neuropil, or less commonly,

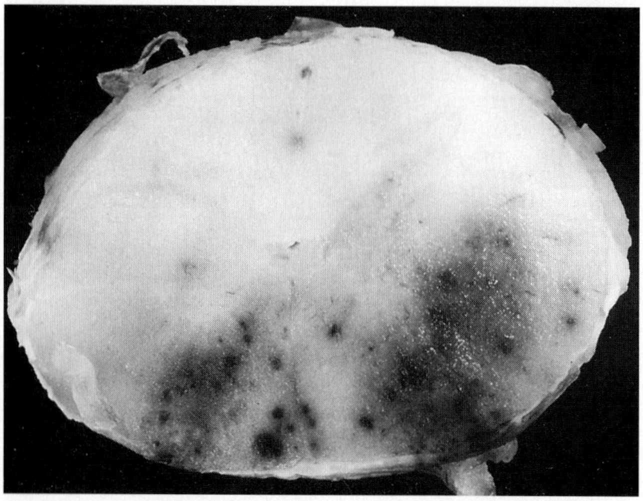

Figure 8-52 Spinal cord, lumbar level; horse. Myelitis due to *Sarcocystis neurona* infection. Prominent focal hemorrhage and necrosis are present in the right lateral funiculus, and in the right and left ventral funiculi.

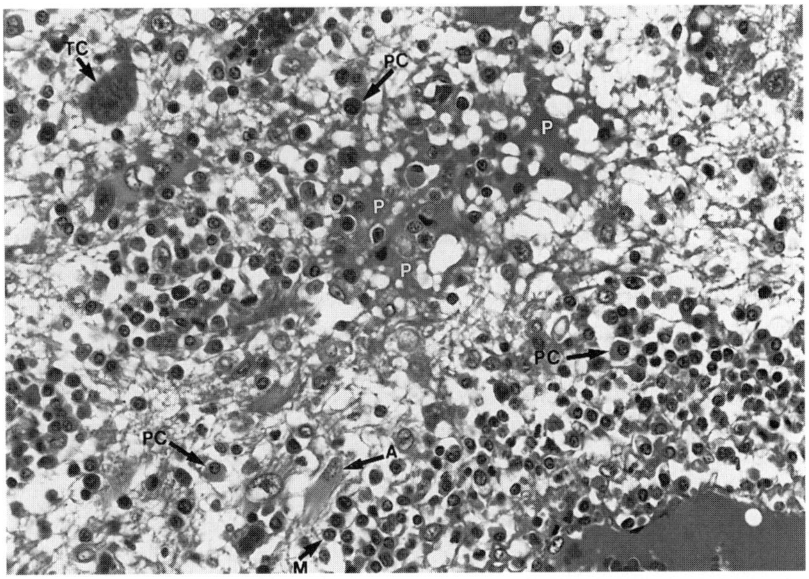

Figure 8-53 Brain; parietal lobe, dorsomedial thalamus; cat. Toxoplasmosis. Nonsuppurative encephalitis with an accumulation of macrophages *(M)* and plasma cells *(PC)*, hypertrophied astrocytes *(A)*, a *Toxoplasma* cyst *(TC)*, interstitial accumulation of plasma *(P)*, and general reduction in density of tissue due to accumulation of edema fluid *(light areas)*, are present. H & E stain.

the leptomeninges. Gemistocytic astrocytosis can be prominent. In lesions, *S. neurona* is small and crescent-shaped to round, has a well-defined nucleus, and is often arranged in aggregates or rosettes. Organisms can be difficult to detect, but occur intracellularly in a variety of cell types or occur extracellularly. *S. neurona* is not typically seen in vascular endothelial cells, a common site for other members of this genus. The typical sequence of events in the pathogenesis of the characteristic lesion is thought to be (1) focal parasitic activation and replication, (2) inflammation, (3) axonal damage, (4) axonal transection, (5) axonal swelling and degeneration, and (6) Wallerian degeneration.

S. neurona can be propagated in tissue culture where it develops in the host cell cytoplasm. It divides by endopolygeny, with development of schizonts containing merozoites arranged in rosettes around a prominent residual body. The organism differs from those of the genera *Toxoplasma, Isospora, Eimeria, Besnoitia, Hammondia,* and *Neospora,* but resembles other *Sarcocystis* spp. and *Frenkelia.* It is proposed that an opossum coccidian, *Sarcocystis falcatula,* and *S. neurona* are synonymous. Studies have suggested that the opossum represents the definitive host and avian species the intermediate host, providing a reservoir for infection of the horse.

***Sarcocytis* spp. infection in nonequine species** involves organisms similar to *S. neurona.* Such organisms have been associated with encephalomyelitis in cattle, sheep, and dogs as well as raccoons, but such infections are sporadic. Lesions and organisms have additionally been seen in the CNS of infected fetuses (e.g., bovine species).

Toxoplasmosis. *Toxoplasma gondii* can infect a wide variety of animals as intermediate hosts including fish, amphibians, reptiles, birds, human beings, and many other mammals. New World monkeys and Australian marsupials are the most susceptible, whereas Old World monkeys, rats, cattle, and horses seem highly resistant. Cats are unique in the biology of the organism, serving as both definitive and intermediate hosts.

T. gondii can parasitize a wide variety of cell types in the intermediate host and can cause lesions in such tissues as lungs, lymphoid system, liver, heart, skeletal muscle, pancreas, intestine, eyes, and nervous system. In the CNS, gross lesions include hemorrhage, hemorrhagic infarcts, ventricular dilation, and edema of sufficient severity to result in brain displacement and herniation. Early microscopic vascular degeneration and edema are followed by invasion of organisms into the parenchyma, with tissue necrosis and variable hemorrhage often striking. Perivascular cuffing with mainly mononuclear leukocytes, astrogliosis, and microgliosis; cellular necrosis involving neurons, astrocytes, and oligodendroglia; and leptomeningitis are additional lesions of the disease (Fig. 8-53). Lesions can involve any area of the neuraxis without predilection for gray or white matter, and radiculitis can occur.

Following ingestion, bradyzoites from tissue cysts or sporozoites from oocysts enter intestinal epithelia and multiply. Evidence suggests active penetration of plasma membranes by organism-secreted lytic products allowing a portal of entry rather than by uptake via phagocytosis. *T. gondii* can then spread locally, free in lymph or intracellularly in lymphocytes, macrophages, or granulocytes to Peyer's patches and regional lymph nodes. Intracellularly, organisms multiply as tachyzoites within a parasitophorus vacuole by repeated cycles of endodyogeny during the early acute stages of infection. Dissemination to distant organs is via lymph and blood, either as free organisms or intracellularly in lymphocytes, macrophages, or granulocytes. With chronicity and an increasing antibody response by the host, tachyzoites of *T. gondii* transform into slow-growing bradyzoites that replicate in tissue cysts. Infection of the CNS occurs hematogenously; neurons and astrocytes are the eventual target cells. The typical sequence of events in the pathogenesis of the characteristic lesion is similar to that in *S. neurona* infection (see previous section). In utero infections in animals and human beings can result in CNS infection. The incidence in ovine fetuses approaches 90%. In fetal brains, foci of necrosis are most common in the brain stem and are associated with a glial cell response. Additionally, bland foci of necrosis and mineralization occur in the cerebrocortical white matter and are due to fetal hypoxia and ischemia or hypotension. In older more mature individuals, *T. gondii* has been associated with immunosuppression such as occurs in concurrent canine distemper virus infection and toxoplasmosis. In some cases, this could represent activation of a latent *T. gondii* infection.

Immune-mediated mechanisms have been proposed to explain the vascular injury (type III hypersensitivity) and cellular or tissue necrosis (type IV hypersensitivity). Lysis of infected cells by primed cytotoxic, $CD8^+$ T lymphocytes also could potentially contribute to the tissue damage. Intracellular growth of tachyzoites also has been advanced as a cause of cellular necrosis. The organism does not produce a cytotoxin.

Neosporosis. Naturally occurring or experimental disease caused by *Neospora caninum* or a *Neospora*-like coccidian has been recognized in a variety of animals including the dog, cat, cattle, sheep, and horse as well as laboratory rodents. First described in 1988 as a multisystemic infection in the dog, the organism has an affinity for the nervous system. The dog has recently been identified as the definitive host for the organism but other hosts may exist. The organism has some features similar to *Toxoplasma gondii,* including division of tachyzoites by endodyogeny and having both proliferative (tachyzoites) and tissue cyst phases. However, *N. caninum* does not develop within a parasitophorous vacuole as does *T. gondii.*

Although there are morphologic differences between the organisms (i.e., *N. caninum* has a thicker cyst wall), reliable differentiation is problematic by light microscopy, and electron microscopic examination or immunohistochemistry is required. Apart from transplacental transmission proposed for a variety of species, the mechanism of infection is unknown. Organisms can infect a variety of cell types. In the CNS, neurons as well as ependymal cells, mononuclear cells in the CSF, and cells of blood vessels including endothelium, intimal connective tissue, and medial smooth muscle cells can harbor the organisms. Organisms have also been detected in spinal nerves. In all animals studied to date, the cyst form of *N. caninum* has only been seen in the CNS, whereas tachyzoites have been found in a variety of tissues.

Neurologic disease can be divided into two categories, that occurring during postnatal life and that associated with mid- to late-term abortions. Postnatal syndromes have been observed mainly in young and adult dogs but horses are also affected. In young dogs, clinical signs are an ascending paralysis due to polyradiculoneuritis and polymyositis. In adult dogs, lesions are more referable to involvement of the CNS complicated by polymyositis, myocarditis, and dermatitis. In horses, clinical signs resemble protozoal myeloencephalitis caused by *Sarcocystis neurona.* Lesions in horses include meningoencephalomyelitis, variable vasculitis and necrosis with microgliosis, and perivascular cuffing by macrophages, lymphocytes, plasma cells, or neutrophils. Multinucleated giant cells were noted in an equine case. Necrosis can be prominent with axons containing swellings located at the periphery of the lesion. Organisms can often be identified in the lesions with routine stains, but immunohistochemistry facilitates their detection and identification. The infection is systemic and lesions can occur in several other tissues. As indicated by experimental studies, administration of corticosteroids and hence, immunosuppression, increases susceptibility or exacerbates the infection or both.

Abortions due to congenital infections with *N. caninum* or *Neospora*-like organisms occur commonly only in cattle. Dairy herds are most frequently affected. Cases are reported in horses, and sheep are experimentally susceptible with lesions typical of those in cattle. Abortions can be midgestational to late term. Lesions include placentitis, myocarditis, myositis, and multiple foci of necrosis in the CNS, with peripheral gliosis. An inconsistent infiltration of leukocytes occurs throughout the neuraxis but most often in the brain stem. Additionally, bland foci of necrosis with variable mineralization occur in the centrum semiovale and corona radiata, possibly as a result of hypoxia and ischemia or hypotension related to the placentitis.

Bacterial Infections

Bacterial infections of the CNS in domestic animals occur sporadically. Infection can be hematogenous or result from penetrating injuries or fractures that disrupt the natural defenses provided by the meninges and osseous tissues. Bacteria can also spread from foci of infection in adjacent tissues such as the nasal cavity or inner ear. With one infection, listeric encephalitis, there is evidence of spread via the axons of cranial nerves.

Haemophilus somnus. *H. somnus,* a small gram-negative bacillus, causes a septicemic infection in cattle with variable clinical presentations including pneumonia, polyarthritis, myocarditis, abortion, and meningoencephalitis. The disease is most prevalent in feedlot cattle but can occur in other situations. All manifestations, particularly meningoencephalitis, tend to be sporadic with single to multiple animals in a herd affected. The CNS form of the disease has been termed **thrombotic meningoencephalitis**

(TME), but it is also commonly referred to as TEME (thromboembolic meningoencephalitis).

Gross lesions in the CNS are irregularly sized septic foci of hemorrhage and necrosis scattered randomly and visible both externally and on cut surfaces (Fig. 8-54). Lesions are most frequent in the cerebrum, commonly at the cortical-white matter junction (gray matter–white matter interface). The location of the lesion may reflect a change in the diameter of blood vessels, allowing bacteria to lodge, adhere, and replicate in these vessels. The spinal cord also has lesions. Other lesions include brain swelling due to edema and leptomeningitis with cloudiness of the CSF.

Microscopic lesions in all organs including the CNS are initially marked vasculitis and vascular necrosis that are followed by thrombosis and infarction. Septic vasculitis is the initial event followed by edema and an influx of neutrophils and macrophages in and around vessel walls and the neuropil (Fig. 8-55). Colonies of small gram-negative bacilli are frequent in thrombi, in and around affected vessels, and in areas of necrosis.

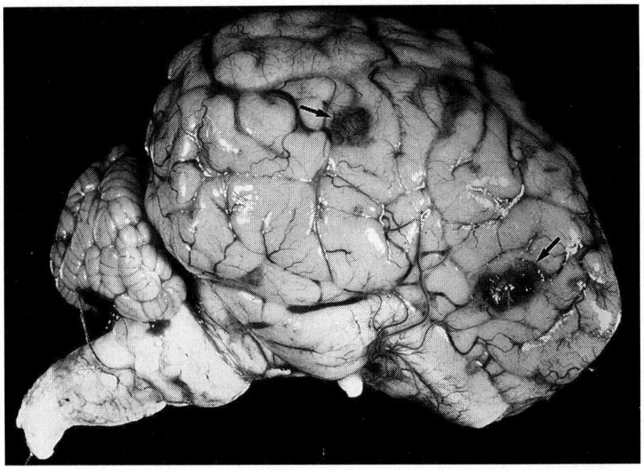

Figure 8-54 Brain; steer. *Haemophilus somnus* infection. Foci of parenchymal hemorrhage, edema, and necrosis extend to the surface of the brain *(arrows). Courtesy Dr. H. W. Leipold.*

The pathogenesis of *H. somnus* infection is not completely understood. Many cattle harbor the organism in the upper digestive tract without evidence of disease but under some circumstances, it invades to cause severe clinical infection. The mechanism(s) of invasion into the bloodstream is not definitely known, but the respiratory tract is a proposed portal of entry. Once the bacteria gain access to the circulation, the organisms adhere to endothelial cells, presumably via a receptor-mediated interaction, which results in their contraction and desquamation. Subendothelial collagen is exposed, initiating a cascade of events culminating in vasculitis, thrombosis, and tissue invasion. Lipooligosaccharide, a toxic factor produced by *H. somnus,* might protect the bacteria from host defenses. Bovine neutrophils, blood monocytes, and alveolar macrophages are incapable of killing the organism, allowing the infection to become established.

Listeria monocytogenes. Listeriosis is another bacterial infection with particular affinity to cause CNS disease, mainly in domestic ruminants. Infections in human beings also occur. Listeriosis presents in three disease forms: meningoencephalitis, abortion and stillbirth, and septicemia; the latter commonly develops in young animals, possibly from an in utero infection. The encephalitic and genital forms of the disease rarely occur together in an individual animal or in the same flock or herd.

Gross lesions are usually absent but leptomeningeal opacity, foci of necrosis in the terminal brain stem, and cloudy CSF have been noted. Microscopically, a meningo-

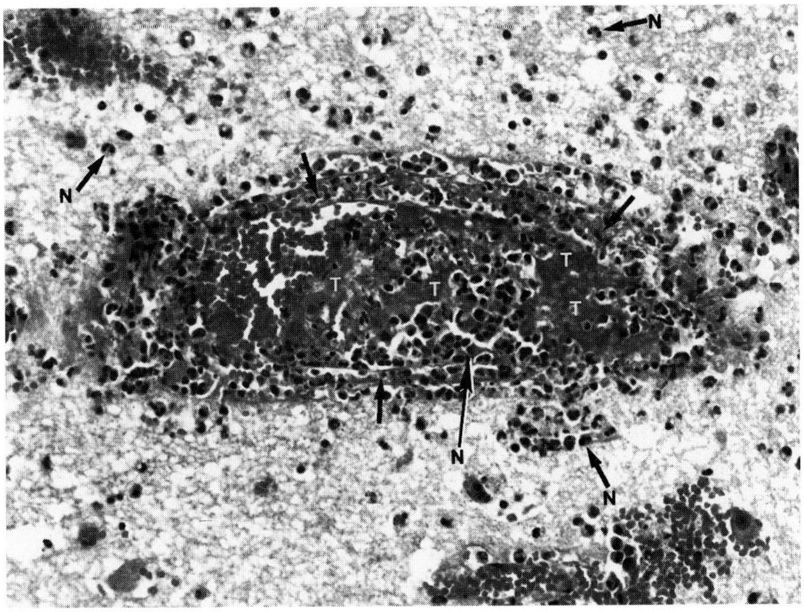

Figure 8-55 Brain, parietal lobe, centrum semiovale; steer. *Haemophilus somnus* infection. There is pronounced vasculitis of a large cerebral vessel with much of the lumen occupied by a thrombus *(T)* and neutrophils *(N)* in various stages of degeneration. Note the severe destruction of the of the vessel wall *(arrows).* Scattered neutrophils *(N)* are in the perivascular tissue with reduced density due to accumulation of edema fluid. H & E stain.

encephalitis centered about the pons and medulla and involving both gray and white matter is characteristic. The lesions, however, can extend from the diencephalon to the caudal medulla or anterior cervical spinal cord. Small early parenchymal lesions consist of loose clusters of microglia that with time enlarge and contain variable numbers of neutrophils. With progression, neutrophils dominate (Fig. 8-56), but in some foci, macrophages can be the principal cell type. Necrosis and accumulation of gitter cells can be prominent in some cases. Numerous gram-positive bacilli can be detected in some lesions. Other changes include neuronal necrosis and leptomeningitis; the latter is regularly present and is often severe with accumulation of macrophages, lymphocytes, plasma cells, and fewer neutrophils. Cranial ganglioneuritis also occurs and particularly involves the trigeminal nerve and ganglion.

There is compelling evidence that *L. monocytogenes* invades through the mucosa of the oral cavity and into branches of the trigeminal nerve. Intraaxonal migration to the trigeminal ganglion and brain (medulla) initiates central infection that spreads rostrally and caudally. The mechanism of tissue injury is not completely defined. A correlation between the degree of cell-mediated immunity and severity of brain damage suggests immunologic injury. Recent studies in a murine model, however, indicate a T lymphocyte response is only slight in early stages of fatal listeriosis. Immunization before experimental infection enhanced $CD4^+$ and $CD8^+$ T lymphocyte responses with greater survivability. Other studies have shown increased production of tumor necrosis factor-α and interleukin 10 in fatal murine infections. The former is capable of causing brain damage and augmenting other CNS immune responses, and the latter has a suppressant effect on neuroimmunologic reactions. The organism also produces a hemolysin (listeriolysin) that is a virulence factor required for intracellular multiplication.

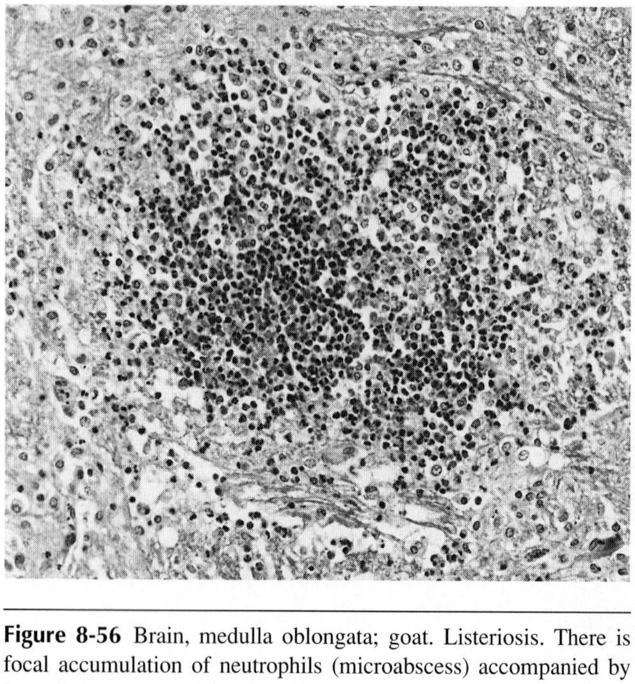

Figure 8-56 Brain, medulla oblongata; goat. Listeriosis. There is focal accumulation of neutrophils (microabscess) accompanied by loss of parenchyma. H & E stain.

Bacterial Infections of the CNS in Young Farm Animals. These infections typically involve *Escherichia coli*, *Streptococcus*, *Salmonella*, *Pasteurella*, and *Haemophilus*. Although there are differences in the diseases caused by these organisms, they tend to produce fibrinopurulent inflammation of membranous tissues of the body (neonatal septicemia). Leptomeninges, choroid plexus, and ependyma of the CNS, synovium, uvea, and the serosal lining of body cavities can be affected in various combinations (Table 8-8). Infections are often acquired perinatally, and onset is usually within a few days of birth up to 2 weeks. The portal of entry can be oral, intrauterine, umbilical, following surgical procedures (e.g., castration, ear notching), or via the respiratory system.

Gross CNS lesions are commonly present and include congestion, hemorrhage, and diffuse to focal cloudiness or opacity in the leptomeninges due to accumulation of exudate (Fig. 8-57). The ventricles contain fibrin, usually as a thin layer on the ependymal surface or as a pale coagulum in the CSF of the ventricular lumen.

Microscopic lesions vary according to the organism. With the exception of *Salmonella* spp., the lesions consist of fibrin deposition and an infiltration of mainly neutrophils in the leptomeninges, choroid plexus, and ependymal or subependymal areas of the brain (Fig. 8-58). The

Table 8-8 CNS Bacterial Infections in Young Animals

Calf

Escherichia coli—leptomeningitis, choroiditis, ependymitis and ventriculitis, synovitis, ophthalmitis and perioptic neuritis
Pasteurella spp.—leptomeningitis, ependymitis & ventriculitis
Streptococcus spp.—leptomeningitis, synovitis, ophthalmitis

Foal

E. coli—leptomeningitis, ventriculitis, polyserositis, synovitis
Streptococcus spp.—leptomeningitis, polyserositis, synovitis
Salmonella typhimurium—leptomeningitis, ependymitis and ventriculitis, choroiditis, synovitis

Lamb

E. coli—leptomeningitis, ependymitis and ventriculitis, peritonitis, synovitis
Pasteurella spp.—leptomeningitis

Pig

E. coli—leptomeningitis, ophthalmitis
Haemophilus parasuis—leptomeningitis, polyserositis, synovitis
Streptococcus suis type I and II—leptomeningitis, choroiditis, ependymitis, cranial neuritis, myelitis
Salmonella choleraesuis—leptomeningitis, ophthalmitis

epithelium of the choriod plexus and ependymal lining of the ventricles can be disrupted by cellular vacuolation, disorganization, and necrosis. The lesions can extend into the parenchyma. A vasculitis with thrombosis and hemorrhage can be associated with lesions caused by *Escherichia coli*. Lesions caused by *Salmonella* spp. are not limited to the perinatal period. CNS involvement is generally limited to foals and pigs. In contrast to the above infections, the leukocytic response tends to have a greater proportion of macrophages and lymphocytes, often to the extent that the inflammation is designated histiocytic or granulomatous. As is true in other tissues, vasculitis, thrombosis, necrosis, and hemorrhage often accompany *Salmonella* infections of the CNS.

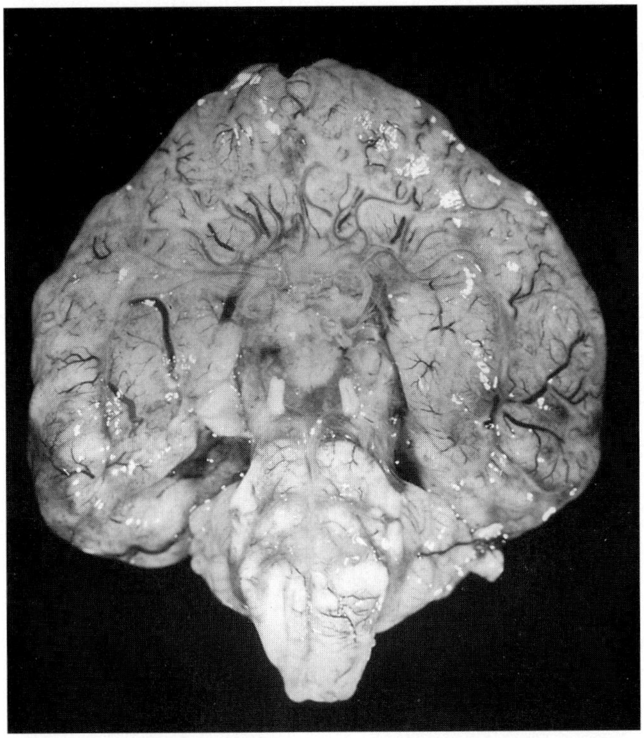

Figure 8-57 Brain, leptomeninges; calf. Purulent leptomeningitis. The meningeal opacity is due to the presence of purulent exudate in the leptomeninges (that include the subarachnoid space).

Bacterial infection with CNS and visceral involvement occurs in neonatal pigs and through the weaning period. These diseases are deserving of special mention because of the incidence and stereotyped nature of the infections. Several strains of *Streptococcus suis* are capable of causing disease. Type 1 strains generally cause disease in suckling pigs ranging in age from 1 to 6 weeks, whereas type 2 strains affect older pigs 6 to 14 weeks old. Type 2 strains are recognized as one of the more important serotypes, causing meningitis not only in pigs but in human beings, particularly those working with pigs or handling porcine tissues. Other serotypes as well as untypeable strains can also cause systemic disease and meningitis, choroiditis, and ependymitis. Extension to involve cranial nerve roots or the central canal of the cervical spinal cord occurs. The character of the inflammation is fibrinopurulent, and necrotic foci can be found in brain stem (including cerebellum) and anterior spinal cord.

Haemophilus parasuis, **Glasser's disease,** is also a frequent cause of leptomeningitis, polyserositis, and polyarthritis in 8- to 16-week-old pigs. Again, lesions are as previously noted with fibrinopurulent inflammation involving the leptomeninges, serosal linings of body cavities, and joints (see Fig. 8-58).

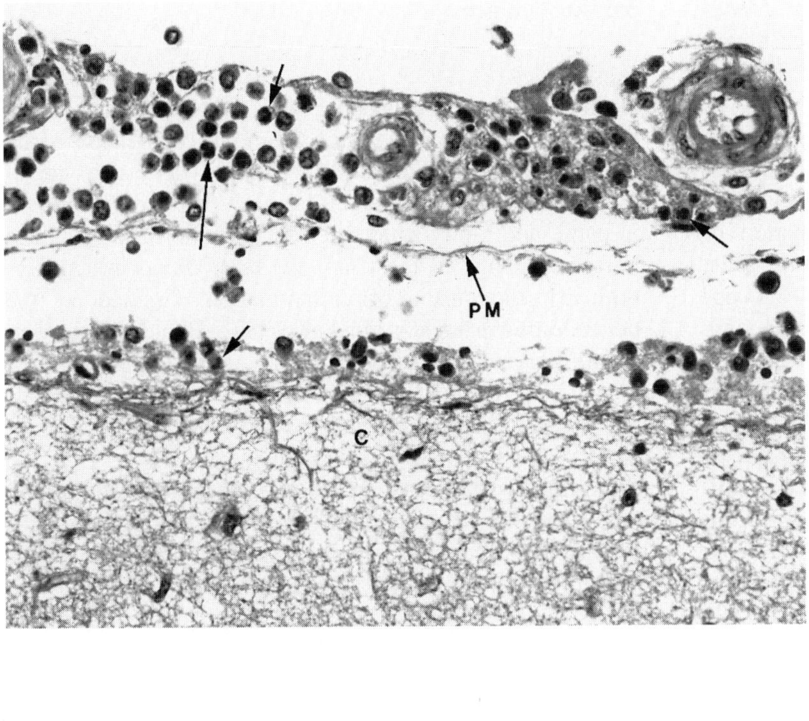

Figure 8-58 Brain, parietal lobe, leptomeninges; pig. Purulent leptomeningitis caused by *Haemophilus parasuis* infection. There is an accumulation of neutrophils *(arrows)* and scattered mononuclear cells in the leptomeninges *(top)* and the outer cerebral cortex *(C)* from which the pia mater *(PM)* has separated. H & E stain.

Brain Abscesses. Cerebral abscesses in animals are most commonly associated with penetrating wounds including fractures or spread of infection from adjacent tissues. Abscesses of the pituitary fossa occur with some frequency in cattle. Bacteria isolated from the cases include *Pasteurella multocida* and *Actinomyces pyogenes.* The abscess can result from spread of infection arising in the caudal nasal cavity or sinuses, possibly through direct extension or through the venous circulation. Incision of the pituitary fossa releases a thick viscous opaque tan to yellow exudate that can elevate the dura mater surrounding the fossa. Infection can extend via the infundibular recess of the third ventricle into the ventricular system, resulting in meningitis and empyema. Brain abscesses can also arise, most commonly in cattle and sheep, from an extension of otitis interna. These animals often present with evidence of facial nerve paralysis such as a drooping ear. The cerebellopontine angle and adjacent structures are the common locations for such abscesses. Brain abscesses may also occur in small ruminants that lack frontal sinuses from improper or misapplied dehorning procedures.

Brain abscesses are space-occupying lesions and as such can have a devastating effect on brain function. Depending on size and location, compression of vital structures and brain displacements are two common sequelae.

Mycotic Infections

Infection of the CNS by a variety of fungi and algae has been reported in domestic animals. Most reported cases are isolated occurrences and often represent opportunistic infection in immunocompromised individuals. Rare infections have involved genera such as *Aspergillus, Candida, Mucor,* dematiaceous fungi, and the blue-green algae *Prototheca.* These infections do not have a predilection for the nervous system. Of the systemic fungi, CNS infections have occurred with *Coccidioides immitis, Blastomyces dermatitidis, Histoplasma capsulatum,* and *Cryptococcus neoformans,* but only *C. neoformans* has a particular affinity for the CNS.

Cryptococcus neoformans. This infection can cause disease affecting several organs, most notably CNS, nasal passages, and lungs. Infection is initially via the respiratory route with presumably hematogenous dissemination or direct spread to other tissues. Two virulence factors have been documented. First, a thick mucopolysaccharide capsule protects the organism from host defenses. Second, virulent organisms possess a biochemical pathway that can use catecholamines and that consists of a specific transport pathway and the enzyme phenoloxidase with production of a melanin or melanin-like compound through a series of oxidation-reduction reactions. This pathway can help protect the organism from oxidative damage in the brain and presumably the adrenal glands. Both virulence factors are important for survival of the organism in the host. In addition, CSF lacks alternative pathway complement components that bind to the organism's carbohydrate capsule and facilitate phagocytosis and killing by neutrophils.

Cryptococcosis with CNS infection occurs in cats, dogs, horses, and cattle. Grossly, the leptomeninges vary from normal to cloudy, and the tissue can have a viscous appearance imparted by the mucopolysaccharide capsule of the organism. Multiple small "cysts" with a similar viscous, gelatinous appearance can be seen in the parenchyma. Microscopically, these lesions have a loosely organized, lacy appearance with often myriad cryptococcal organisms and little or no inflammation. The yeast are spherical, crescentic, or "cup-shaped," usually surrounded by a thick nonstaining (H & E stain) capsule, and reproduce by narrow-based buds.

Special stains such as periodic acid–Schiff and Gomori's methenamine silver demonstrate the organisms readily, and the capsule can be stained with mucicarmine and alcian blue. The leptomeningeal reaction can extend along the roots of cranial nerves; spread of the parenchymal infection results in ventriculitis and choroiditis. The leukocytic response can vary from sparse to granulomatous and consists of neutrophils, eosinophils, macrophages, giant cells, and small mononuclear cells, depending on the immune status of the host.

Parasitic Infestations

Lesions resulting from parasitic infestation of the CNS vary in degree and distribution. Gross lesions of hemorrhage, malacia, migratory tracts, or space-occupying cysts occur with the various parasitic stages. Microscopically, there is variable necrosis, hemorrhage, and a leukocytic response, typically with a significant infiltrate of eosinophils. The extent of the host response is often dictated by the degree of trauma and disruption created by the parasite and the level of sensitivity of the host for parasite antigens.

Insect Larvae. Among the common larvae are those of *Oestrus ovis* and *Hypoderma bovis.* The larvae of *O. ovis* develop in the nasal cavity of sheep but can penetrate into the cranial vault through the ethmoid bone. Larvae of *H. bovis* can enter the spinal canal during their migration in cattle and rarely as an aberrant parasite in the brain of horses. Damage in the CNS due to *H. bovis* in cattle is typically the result of inflammation directed at the degenerating parasites incidental with anthelmintic treatment. Larvae of *Cuterebra* spp., usually a parasite of rabbits and rodents, can invade the CNS of dogs and cats (see Feline ischemic encephalopathy).

Cestodes. *Coenurus cerebralis,* the larval form of the dog tapeworm *Multiceps multiceps,* most commonly infests sheep and occasionally other ruminants. The larval forms presumably reach the CNS hematogenously, causing some

Table 8-9 Nematodes Causing CNS Disease in Domestic Animals

Parasite	Normal Host	Aberrant Host
Nematode migration in aberrant host		
Angiostrongylus cantonensis	Rat	Dog
Baylisascaris procyonis	Raccoon	Dog
Elaphostrongylus rangifer	Reindeer	Sheep, goat
Parelaphostrongylus tenuis	Deer	Sheep, goat
Setaria digitata	Cattle	Sheep, goat, horse
Aberrant nematode migration in normal host		
Angiostrongylus vasorum	Dog (coyote)	
Dirofilaria immitis	Dog (cat)	
Stephanurus dentatus	Pig	
Strongylus spp.	Horse	

damage during migration and encysting, forming space-occupying lesions. Human beings are the definitive host of *Taenia solium,* with pigs being the intermediate host. The larval stage, *Cysticercus cellulosae,* generally develops in muscle of the pig but can also occur in the meninges and brain.

Nematodes. Nematodes cause damage in the brain either from aberrant migration in the definitive host or migration in an aberrant host (Table 8-9 and Fig. 8-59). Larval stages of the parasites are typically involved, the exception being *Dirofilaria immitis* where the adult parasite is found. Greater CNS damage is often created by the migration of the parasites in an aberrant host.

Halicephalobus (Micronema) deletrix is a free-living rhabditiform nematode that can infest nasal cavity, CNS, and kidneys of the horse. In the CNS, microscopic lesions are prominently associated with blood vessels along which the parasite apparently migrates.

Miscellaneous Disease Processes

Reticulosis

Reticulosis has been reported to occur in several species but is most common in the dog. The term reticulosis, at best a somewhat imprecise designation, is used here to give a historical perspective. The spectrum of lesions originally included three disease processes: inflammatory (granulomatous) reticulosis, neoplastic reticulosis, and microgliomatosis. Inflammatory and neoplastic forms of reticulosis have been considered by some to represent two opposing ends of a spectrum, with intermediate or transitional forms falling in between. Microgliomatosis is described as distinct from the other two types. Recently, an additional designation, **granulomatous meningoencephalomyelitis,** has been used to describe a process that is considered to be analogous, at least in some instances, to the inflammatory form of reticulosis. Ophthalmic lesions also accompany this form and involve the optic nerve, optic disk, and retina.

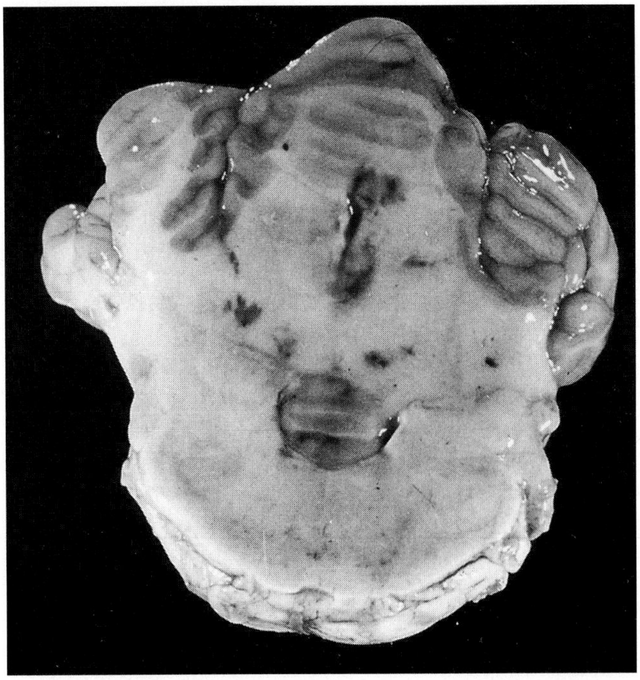

Figure 8-59 Brain, cerebellum and medulla oblongata; horse. *Strongylus vulgaris* migration. Several small foci of hemorrhage and necrosis in the cerebellar white matter are sites of larval migration.

The disease appears to occur more commonly in small breeds of dogs (e.g., poodles and terrier-type breeds). Age of affected dogs is variable and ranges from 9 months to 10 years. In three separate studies involving a total of 85 dogs with reticulosis (including all three forms), the sex distribution was 56 females and 29 males.

When present, gross lesions of the three forms are rarely discrete. They frequently are gray-white to red, expansive areas within the brain parenchyma with loss of structural detail. However, lesions can have a gelatinous or rubbery consistency with irregular, well-defined margins, or some appear granular.

Microscopically, the inflammatory form of reticulosis is characterized by perivascular accumulation of well-differentiated lymphocytes, monocytes, plasma cells, and epithelioid cells with occasional occurrence of neutrophils and giant cells, plus reticulin fibers and collagen (Fig. 8-60). Not infrequently, cells will be predominantly epithelioid. With the neoplastic form of reticulosis, cells are arranged around vessels and are also usually present in the parenchyma. The cells are less differentiated than with the inflammatory form of the disease and mitotic figures are common. Also, prominent concentrically arranged reticulin fibers are present around vessels and around cells in the parenchyma.

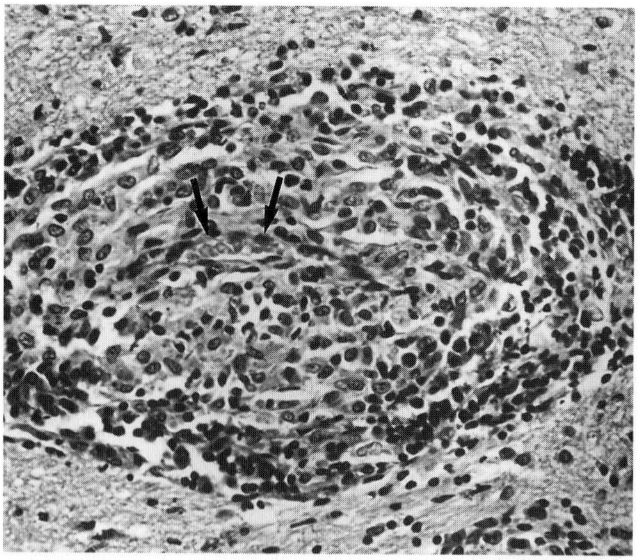

Figure 8-60 Brain, junction between parietal and occipital lobes, thalamus; dog. Inflammatory reticulosis (granulomatous meningoencephalomyelitis). Perivascular epithelioid cells are located centrally and other mononuclear cells (plasma cells, lymphocytes, and monocytes) have accumulated peripherally. *Arrows* indicate vascular lumen. H & E stain.

Microgliomatosis, which has been classified as a proliferative neoplastic disease, has some features that are quite distinct from the above-cited inflammatory and neoplastic forms of reticulosis. The cells, which infiltrate the parenchyma without topographic perivascular arrangement, resemble microglia in that their nuclei, which vary in size and shape and have prominent chromatin, are the only visible cellular component following conventional staining. Also, mitoses can be common, and there is no accompanying reticulin fiber formation as occurs with the other two forms.

The inflammatory lesion has recently been characterized as consisting primarily of $CD3^+$ T lymphocytes and activated macrophages with strong MHC class II expression, which led to the suggestion that the underlying mechanism of the disease process was a T cell–mediated delayed-type hypersensitivity of an organ-specific autoimmune disease.

Neoplasms

Neoplasms of the CNS of animals are not rare as was once believed. In fact, neoplasms occur with a frequency and variety, at least in the dog, that is similar to that in human beings. The majority of the neoplasms described have been in the dog and cat with a large portion of these in the older population.

The intention of this discussion is to present the reader with a brief overview of the more common or better-known neoplasms that occur in the CNS of animals and not to attempt to be all inclusive.

Primary Neoplasms of Neuronal Cells

Medulloblastoma. This neoplasm has characteristics similar to the less frequently occurring neuroblastoma, and both are considered to arise from cells of the neuronal lineage. The cell of origin for the medulloblastoma has not been definitely determined, but it has been proposed that the neoplasm can arise from primitive cells originating in the neuroepithelial roof of the fourth ventricle that give rise to the external granular cell layer.

In animals, the medulloblastoma has been reported in the canine and bovine species, in which young animals of both groups tend to be affected, and in the cat and pig. The neoplasm chiefly occurs in the cerebellum of puppies and calves and sometimes also in adult dogs. The neoplasm is well circumscribed, soft, gray to pink, and usually does not have hemorrhages, cysts, or necrosis. The growth can compress the fourth ventricle and cause hydrocephalus and also can infiltrate adjacent structures including the leptomeninges. It can spread (metastasize) through the CSF in the ventricular or meningeal areas. Microscopically, the neoplasm is highly cellular and consists of round to elongated nuclei that have prominent chromatin in an ill-defined cytoplasm. The cells are arranged in sheets or broad bands and also can form pseudorosettes. Mitoses can be numerous.

Primary Neoplasms of Neuroglial Cells

Neoplasms of glial cell lineage arise with some frequency in domestic animals. Increasing usage of immunohistochemical markers for glial cells and indicators of cellular proliferation will undoubtedly enhance the specificity and prognostic significance of the diagnosis of different glial cell neoplasms in animals.

Astrocytoma. Astrocytomas occur in dogs, cats, and cattle but are best recognized in the dog. It is possibly the most common neuroglial neoplasm in dogs and is described here as it occurs in the canine species. Brachycephalic breeds, Boston terrier and boxer, and dogs 5 to 11 years of age are most commonly affected. Common sites include pyriform lobe, convexity of the cerebral hemisphere, thalamus-hypothalamus, midbrain, and less frequently, the cerebellum and spinal cord.

Grossly, the affected area will be enlarged with displacement of normal tissue. A characteristic feature of less malignant forms is that there is little demarcation between neoplastic and normal tissue (Fig. 8-61). Such neoplasms are rather solid or firm and gray-white. More rapidly growing neoplasms are more readily delineated from adjacent normal tissue and are soft and friable and contain areas of necrosis, hemorrhage, edema, and cavitation. Microscopically, astrocytomas have been classified in human beings according to the degree of cytologic malignancy from grades 1 to 4, or as differentiated and undifferentiated or anaplastic. The more undifferentiated forms (grades 3 and 4) have also been

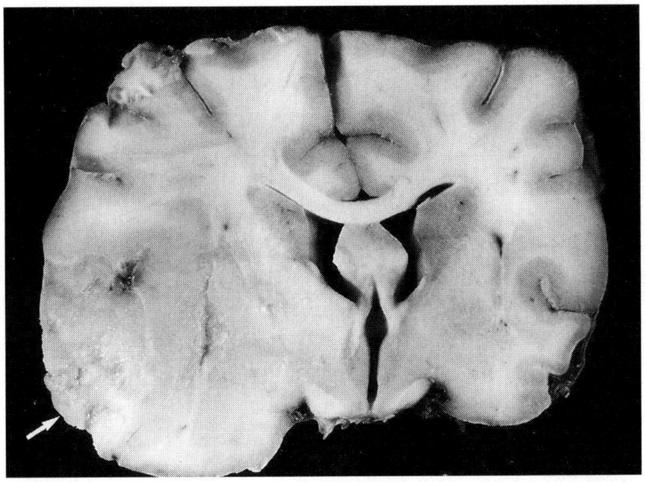

Figure 8-61 Brain, rostral parietal lobe, level of corpus striatum; dog. Astrocytoma. The neoplasm *(to right of arrow)* is characterized by a diffuse enlargement of the left pyriform lobe with lack of peripheral demarcation.

classified by some as glioblastoma or **glioblastoma multiforme.**

The more differentiated neoplasms consist of a rather uniform cell type that has a loose organization. Cell size varies, and distinct ramifying processes can be observed (Fig. 8-62). Nuclei vary in size and shape and contain more chromatin than normal astrocytes. Cells tend to be arranged around and along blood vessels, and the boundary between neoplastic and normal tissue is indistinct. Astrocytomas have been subclassified as fibrillary, protoplasmic, gemistocytic, and piloid or pilocytic based on cell morphology. The fibrillary form is the most common. Anaplastic astrocytomas and glioblastoma have been diagnosed in animals, often based on immunohistochemistry for vimentin or GFAP. Cellular pleomorphism can be extreme, and some neoplasms have giant cells.

Oligodendroglioma. Neoplasms composed of oligodendrocytes occur most commonly in the dog, but cases are reported in cats and cattle. The reported incidence varies; some reports indicate oligodendrogliomas as the most common neuroectodermal neoplasm, whereas others place it second to astroglial neoplasms. As with astrocytomas, there is a predilection for dogs of brachycephalic breeds (Boston terrier, boxer, and bulldog), and the age range is as indicated for astrocytomas. Neoplasms occur in all areas of the cerebrum, brain stem, and interventricular septum. Neoplasms tend to extend to meningeal and ventricular surfaces, but dissemination in the CSF is uncommon.

Grossly, oligodendrogliomas are relatively well demarcated from surrounding tissue. The neoplasms vary in size, are gray to pink-red, and are soft or gelatinous with areas of hemorrhage. Microscopically, the neoplasms are composed of densely packed cells. Nuclei are centrally located, hyperchromic, and surrounded by pale or non-

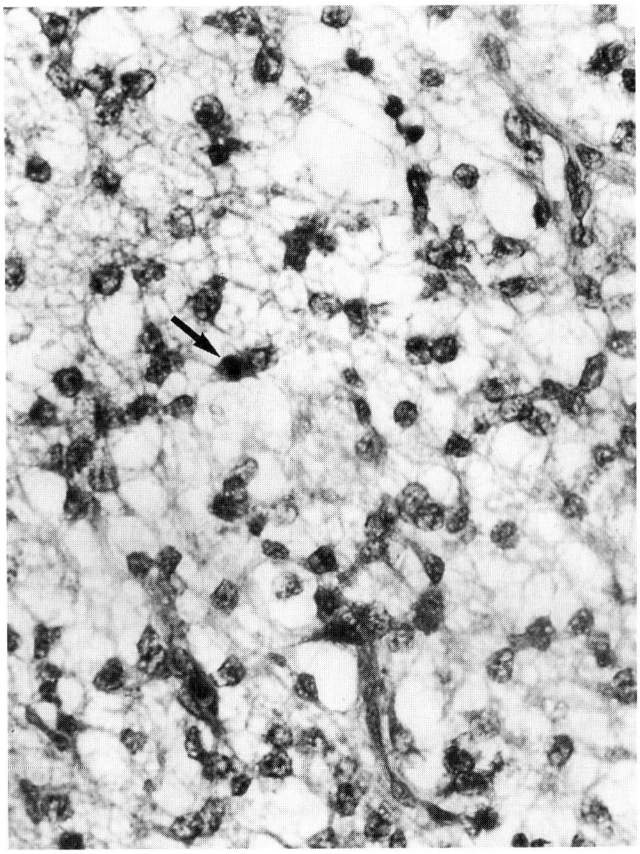

Figure 8-62 Brain, pyriform lobe; dog. Astrocytoma. The many processes of the loosely arranged cells form a fine intercellular network. Note the characteristic nuclei and occasional mitotic figure *(arrow)* in this moderately well-differentiated astrocytoma (protoplasmic type). H & E stain.

staining cytoplasm creating a perinuclear halo (Fig. 8-63). Other patterns include cells arranged in rows, especially peripherally, or in semicircles. Mitoses are generally infrequent. Regressive changes include mucoid degeneration, edema, cavitation, and rarely mineralization. Extensive necrosis is uncommon.

Ependymoma. Ependymoma is one of the less frequent neoplasms in dogs, cats, cattle, and horses. Some reports in the dog indicate a higher frequency in brachycephalic breeds. Ependymomas have continuity with the ventricular system and usually involve the lateral or, less commonly, third and fourth ventricles. They also occur in the central canal of the spinal cord. The neoplasm can spread within the ventricular system and subarachnoid space. The average age in the dog ranges from 6 to 12 years. Occurrences in a cat as young as 18 months old and in a calf 5 months old have been reported.

Grossly, the neoplasm is an expansile mass with invasive, destructive growth into adjacent tissue. The neoplasm is soft and gray-white to red depending on blood content. Regressive changes include gelatinous consis-

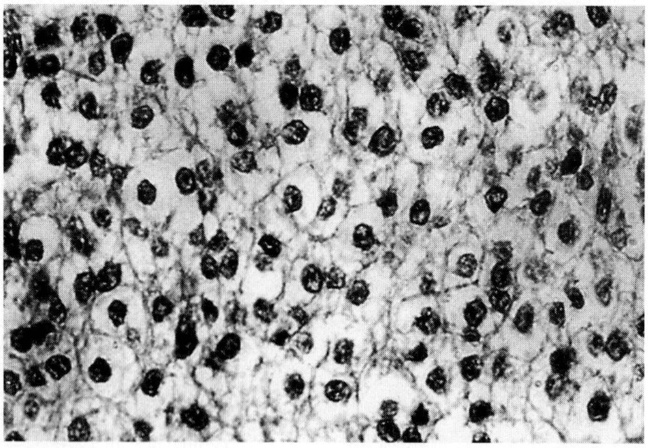

Figure 8-63 Brain, cerebral hemisphere; dog. Oligodendroglioma. The cells are densely packed and have a characteristic light zone (halo) between the hyperchromatic nucleus and plasma membrane. H & E stain.

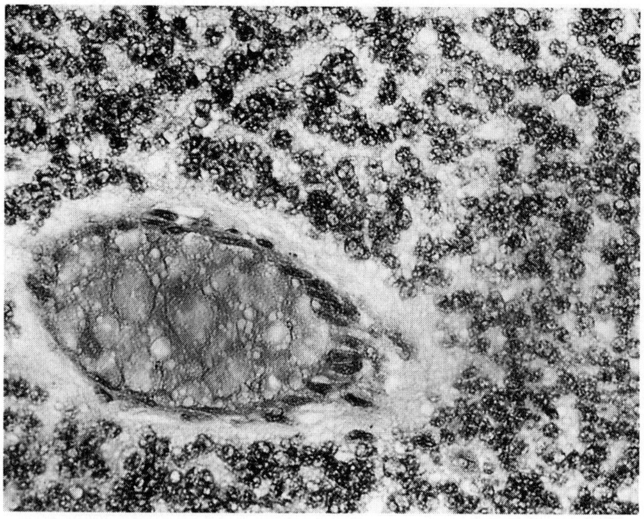

Figure 8-64 Brain, left lateral ventricle; dog. Ependymoma. Cells with moderately hyperchromatic nuclei and poorly defined cytoplasm are arranged in irregular rows and form a nuclear-free zone around a blood vessel. H & E stain.

tency and cavitation. Microscopically, ependymomas are highly cellular and well vascularized. Cells have hyperchromic, round to oval nuclei with scant or undetectable cytoplasm. Cells form perivascular rosettes with nuclear polarity away from the vessel wall (Fig. 8-64). Cells are also arranged in sheets and bands. The mitotic rate is variable. Hemorrhage, mucinous and cystic degeneration, and capillary proliferation occur. Malignancy is indicated by invasive growth, frequent mitoses, and anaplasia.

A novel intradural but extramedullary spinal mass occurring most commonly at thc thoracolumbar junction in young dogs has been previously diagnosed as ependymoma based on cell morphology and arrangement of cells. It has been proposed that these neoplasms represent a primitive nephrogenic tumor, and this concept is supported by the finding of glomeruloid and tubular structures in such neoplasms.

Embryonal or Primitive Neoplasms with Glial Differentiation. Considering the complexities of brain development and the fact that astrocytes and oligodendrocytes arise from common stem cells early in development, it should not be surprising that some neoplasms arising in the CNS have multiple lines of differentiation as indicated by immunohistochemistry. One such neoplasm is the **primitive neuroectodermal tumor.** This neoplasm has not been documented in domestic animals, but a recent report in a primate would indicate that they conceivably occur. Immunohistochemical staining for specific markers confirms multiple lines of differentiation, e.g., neuronal, astrocytic, and oligodendroglial. Typically, one cell type dominates.

Another neoplasm of uncertain histogenesis is the **rhabdoid tumor.** In human beings, this neoplasm most commonly arises in kidneys and brain and is believed to develop from embryonal stem cells. As is true of other embryonal neoplasms, young individuals are commonly affected. Rhabdoid tumors arising in the brain have cell markers of neuronal or glial differentiation. Neoplasms in the kidneys typically lack these markers. Despite their primary location, cell morphology is similar. The cells are large, round to polyhedral, and cytoplasm is eosinophilic and abundant and contains large inclusions composed of skeins of intermediate filaments. Rhabdoid tumor has recently been reported in the brain of an 18-month-old dog. Immunohistochemical staining was diffuse for vimentin, focal for neuron-specific enolase and GFAP, and negative for S-100. A novel concept is the proposal that these neoplasms arise from primordial stem cells that adopt the phenotypic characteristics of cells in the tissue of origin.

Primary Neoplasms of the Choroid Plexus

Choroid Plexus Papilloma and Carcinoma. Choroid plexus papilloma occurs most commonly in the dog but has been reported in the horse and in cattle. In contrast to the neuroglial neoplasms of the dog, there is no predilection for brachycephalic breeds. In the dog, the neoplasm occurs most frequently in the fourth ventricle, but it also can be located in the third and lateral ventricles. The age range of affected dogs in one study was 5 to 13 years, except for one that was 2 years of age.

Grossly, the neoplasm is a well-defined, expansive, granular to papillary growth that is gray-white to red and compresses the adjacent nervous tissue. Some neoplasms cause hydrocephalus. Microscopically, these neoplasms generally resemble the choroid plexus and are characterized by an arborizing vascular connective tissue stroma that is covered with a cuboidal to columnar epithelial layer. Mitoses are not present in the benign form. A more malignant variety, choroid plexus carcinoma, is characterized by invasiveness, presence of mitoses, additional occurrence of solid tumor growth, and a tendency to spread to involve the brain or spinal cord or both. Metastasis can occur within the ventricular system, or exteriorly into the subarachnoid space (through the lateral appertures), where implantation on the ependyma or meninges, respectively, occurs.

Primary Neoplasms of Mesodermal Tissue

Meningioma. Meningioma is the most common mesodermal neoplasm of the CNS of animals. It occurs most frequently in the dog and cat but has been reported in other species of domestic animals including horses, cattle, and sheep. In the dog, this neoplasm occurs in several breeds, with dolicocephalic animals being frequently represented. The majority of meningiomas in dogs occur between 7 and 14 years of age and in cats 10 years old or older. Sites of occurrence in the dog include the basal area of the brain, the area over the convexity of the cerebral hemispheres, the cerebellum-tentorium area, the lateral surface of the brain, the falx cerebri, and the surface of the spinal cord. Retrobulbar involvement (originating from the optic nerve sheath) also occurs. In the cat, the neoplasm uniquely occurs in the tela choroidea of the third ventricle but also occurs over the cerebral hemispheres, along the falx cerebri, over the cerebellum and tentorium, and rarely at the base of the brain. Occurrence in the meninges of the spinal cord is not common. Meningiomas have been reported to arise from arachnoid "cap cells," which are on the external surface of the arachnoid membrane.

Grossly, neoplasms in the dog are solitary and vary in size. The neoplasms are well defined, variable in shape (e.g., spherical, lobulated, lenticular, or plaquelike), firm, encapsulated, and gray-white. Sometimes on the cut surface there are soft, red, brown, or gray areas of hemorrhage and necrosis. The neoplasms usually grow by expansion, causing pressure atrophy of the adjacent nervous tissue. They can be invasive, and sometimes there is hyperostosis of the overlying bone. In the cat, meningiomas vary in size from barely detectable to 2 cm in diameter. Cats, and occasionally cattle, can have more than one neoplasm. Other characteristics are comparable with those described in the dog (Fig. 8-65).

Microscopically, several patterns of neoplastic cells can occur, and more than one can be present in a given neoplasm. The more common pattern is characterized by the formation of nests, islands, or laminated whorls of cells (Fig. 8-66). The cells have large cell bodies with abundant

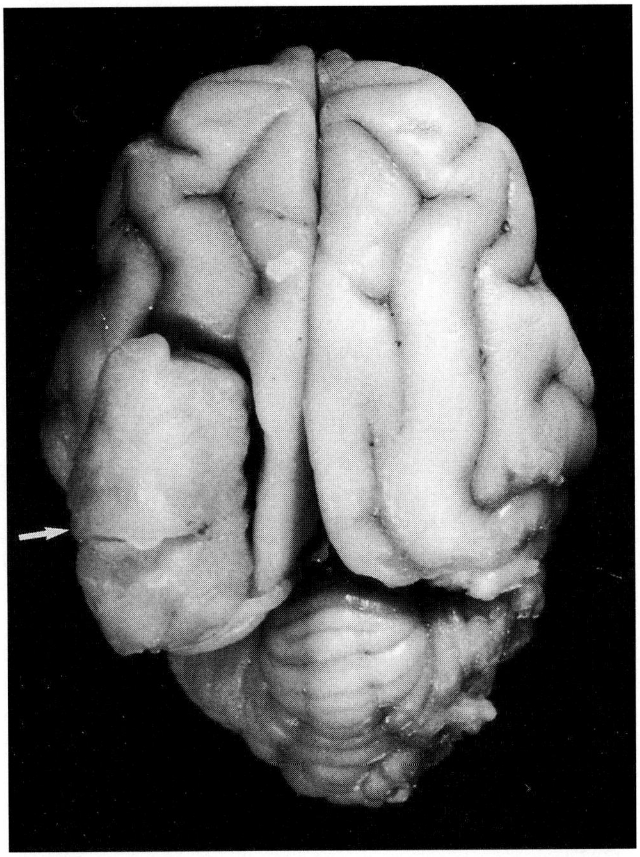

Figure 8-65 Brain, occipital and parietal lobes of left cerebral hemisphere; cat. Meningioma. The meningioma *(arrow)* has markedly compressed the left dorsal occipital and parietal lobes.

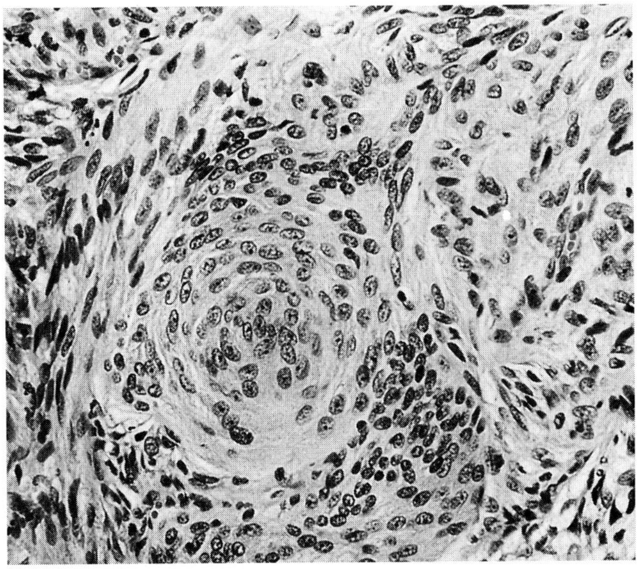

Figure 8-66 Brain, left dorsal occipital lobe; cat. Meningioma. The cells are arranged in a characteristic whorled pattern. H & E stain.

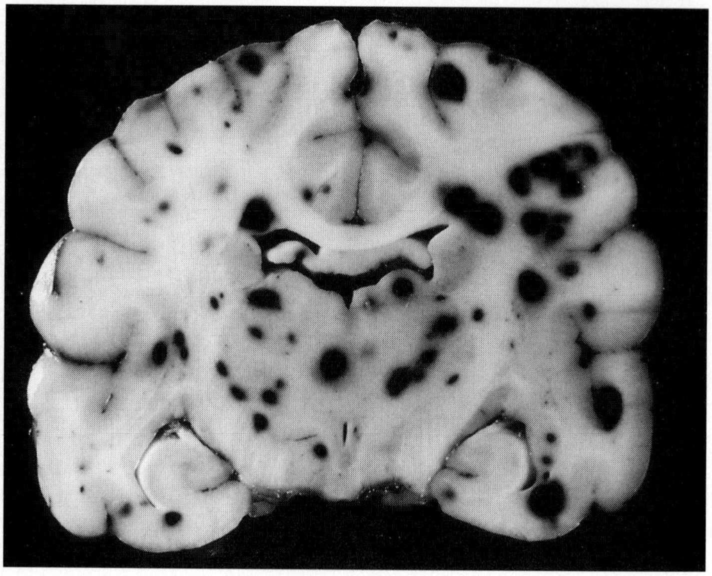

Figure 8-67 Brain, formalin-fixed, junction between parietal and occipital lobes, level of the thalamus; dog. Hemangiosarcoma. Note the prominent hematogenous metastases, which appear as black nodules of varied size distributed at random throughout the brain. In an unfixed (fresh) specimen, the nodules would appear red to dark red because of the vascular origin of the tumor. Black nodules would be consistent with metastatic melanoma in a fresh specimen. *Courtesy Dr. M. D. McGavin.*

cytoplasm, ill-defined cell boundaries, and elongated, oval, open nuclei with peripherally located chromatin. The number of cells making up a whorl can vary from a few to many, and in the center of such structures can be mineralized material (referred to as psammoma bodies). A second pattern is characterized by strands or streams of elongated cells with a rather irregular or parallel orientation. Regressive changes include hemorrhage and cavernous vascular formations. Invasive growth occurs but is less common than growth by expansion.

Secondary Neoplasms

Secondary neoplasms of the CNS can occur following growth from adjacent bone, from direct extension of adjacent neoplasms through the bone or foramina, or by hematogenous metastasis.

Benign growths include **osteomas, chondromas,** and **osteochondromas,** which can cause compressive injury to the brain and spinal cord. One neoplasm (multilobular osteoma [**chondroma rodens**]) has been described as originating from the periosteum of the canine skull. Also, malignant neoplasms adjacent to the cranium or spinal column can cause injury by direct invasion. Some examples include extracranial **osteosarcoma** and **fibrosarcoma** in the dog. Also, **malignant melanoma** of the oral cavity (soft palate) in the dog and melanoma involving the paravertebral lymph nodes in the horse can invade adjacent CNS tissue. Other examples of direct extension include **lymphosarcoma** affecting the spinal cord in the bovine species (and less frequently involving the spinal cord or brain in the dog and cat), and carcinomas of the ethmoidal area and nasal cavity.

Hematogenously metastasizing neoplasms also occur and affect the brain more often than the spinal cord. The species in which metastasis has been most commonly reported is the dog; the next most frequent is the cat. Of the metastasizing carcinomas, the **mammary gland carcinoma** in the dog has been reported to occur most frequently, although others have been described. **Hemangiosarcoma** (Fig. 8-67) is one of the most common metastasizing sarcomas in the dog; others are the mesenchymal component of the **malignant mixed mammary gland tumor,** lymphosarcoma, fibrosarcoma, and malignant melanoma. In the cat, the neoplasms that metastasize to the CNS include the mammary gland carcinoma and lymphosarcoma.

Miscellaneous Neoplastic Processes

Reticulosis. The neoplastic forms of the reticulosis group are discussed in Miscellaneous Disease Processes.

THE PERIPHERAL NERVOUS SYSTEM

Structure and Function

Separation of the nervous system into central and peripheral divisions is mainly for convenience in anatomic study. As can be readily seen, components of the peripheral nervous system (PNS) reside within the CNS (Table 8-10). The PNS can be viewed as an extension of the CNS, conveying motor impulses from and returning sensory input to the CNS. This process is accomplished by cranial, peripheral, and autonomic nerves that exit the CNS and innervate all tissues of the body.

Peripheral nerves are comprised of groups of axons, both myelinated and nonmyelinated, and of varying caliber. As with the CNS, conspicuous components of axons are neurofilaments and microtubules. Neurofilaments provide structural support; microtubules are intimately involved in bidirectional axoplasmic flow of structural components, nutrients, and trophic factors to and

Table 8-10 Components of the Peripheral Nervous System

NERVE CELL BODIES		AXONS/NERVES
Cranial nerves		
Somatic		
Motor—Nuclei of cranial nerves III, IV, V, VI, VII, XII, and nucleus ambiguus		Cranial nerves III, IV, V, VI, VII, and XII
Sensory—Olfactory mucosa, retina, brain stem nuclei		All cranial nerves
Autonomic *(parasympathetic)*		
Preganglionic	*Postganglionic*	
Nucleus of Edinger-Westphal	Ciliary ganglion	Cranial nerve III
Rostral salivatory nucleus	Pterygopalatine, sublingual, and mandibular ganglia	Cranial nerve VII
Caudal salivatory nucleus	Otic ganglion	Cranial nerve IX
Dorsal nucleus of cranial nerve X	Terminal ganglia in target organs	Cranial nerve X
Spinal nerves		
Somatic		Ventral and dorsal spinal nerve rootlets merge to form nerves containing axons of somatic and autonomic neurons
Motor—Ventral horn motor neurons/ventral nerve rootlets		
Sensory—Dorsal root ganglia/dorsal nerve rootlets		
Autonomic		
Preganglionic	*Postganglionic*	
Spinal intermediate and intermediolateral gray matter of thoracolumbar (sympathetic) and sacral (parasympathetic) spinal cord segments/ventral nerve rootlets	Para- or prevertebral ganglia (sympathetic), pelvic ganglia and terminal ganglia in target organs (parasympathetic)	

from the cell body required for maintenance of the axons and neural integrity. Transport from the neuron cell body to the distal axon (anterograde flow) occurs at fast (400 mm per day) and slow (1 and 2 to 4 mm per day) rates. Retrograde transport from the distal axon to the cell body progresses at a rate of 200 mm per day.

Schwann cells surround both myelinated and nonmyelinated axons and are responsible for formation of the myelin sheaths. Although Schwann cells appear not to play a role in axon guidance during formation of the PNS, these cells are necessary for maintenance of axons and secrete neurotrophic factors that play a role in regeneration. Axons are grouped into fascicles along with surrounding loosely organized tissue fibrils **(endoneurium)** and specialized endoneurial fibroblastic cells with phagocytic capabilities. With axonal damage, these putative endogenous phagocytic cells can be augmented by an influx of blood monocytes. Mast cells and small blood vessels also are present among the fibrils. Depending on species and anatomic location, endothelial cells of endoneurial blood vessels can be joined by tight junctions preventing free passage of some macromolecules and providing an incomplete blood-nerve barrier. Collagen bundles and modified fibroblastic cells termed perineurial cells form the **perineurium** that ensheathes individual nerve fascicles. The perineurium contributes some barrier properties by preventing the free diffusion of macromolecules into the nerve fascicles. The fibrous **epineurium** is continuous with the dura mater and encloses groups of nerve fascicles. The epineurium contains fibroblasts, mast cells, and adipocytes, the latter probably providing some protection to the nerve.

Diseases of the Peripheral Nervous System

Many disorders affecting the CNS are also manifest in lesions in the PNS, either because of damage to neuron cell bodies residing in the CNS or because the PNS is equally vulnerable to the disease. Despite this caveat, there are certain diseases that primarily affect the PNS. Diseases of the PNS can be manifest clinically as motor disturbance, sensory deprivation, or a combination of motor and sensory alterations. Space constraints do not allow an exhaustive coverage of disorders of the PNS. Many of the reported disorders seem to represent isolated occurrences in a specific breed. This section will cover the major types of PNS diseases with reference to specific disorders for illustrative purposes.

Congenital Anomalies

Agenesis and Hypoplasia. These defects are uncommon in domestic animals and are generally associated with marked anomalies in development of the musculoskeletal and central nervous systems. Colonic agangliosis or lethal white foal syndrome is a disorder involving development of the PNS and is analogous to Hirschsprung's disease in infants. Affected foals die soon after birth from functional blockage of the colon due to lack of innervation and normal gut motility. Microscopically, the myenteric and submucosal autonomic ganglia are absent. Recently, mutations in the endothelin-B receptor gene have been detected in affected horses and in some patients with Hirschsprung's disease. Both glial-derived neurotrophic factor (GDNF) and endothelin-3 (ET-3) are requisite for normal development of the enteric nervous system. It is proposed that GDNF is required for proliferation and differentiation of neuronal precursor cells destined to populate the gut. ET-3 might modulate these effects by inhibiting differentiation, allowing sufficient precursor cells to populate the gut in an anterior to posterior progression before differentiation.

Traumatic Injury

Traumatic peripheral nerve injury is relatively common in animals and can result from lacerations, violent stretching and tearing, or compression or contusion. Reaction patterns following PNS injury are analogous to those in the CNS, but peripheral nerves have a greater capacity for repair. Three patterns of lesions in the PNS have been described. Mild injury that leaves the axon intact **(neuropraxia)** can result in temporary conduction block but total recovery of function is possible. More severe damage that destroys the axon but leaves the connective tissue framework intact **(axonotmesis)** results in Wallerian degeneration distal to the point of injury, but the potential for regeneration and reinnervation is good. Severance of the nerve with destruction of the supporting framework **(neurotmesis)** results in Wallerian degeneration distal to the injury with the potential for regeneration but little chance of normal reinnervation. The pattern of Wallerian degeneration and the reaction of the neuronal cell body to damage of its axon have already been described (see Neurons, Reaction to Injury).

Disorders of Myelin Formation and Maintenance

In contrast to the CNS, disorders of myelin formation are rare. Hypomyelination has been described in golden retrievers with onset at approximately 7 weeks of age. Clinical signs include a peculiar hopping gait, depressed spinal reflexes, and circumduction of the limbs while walking. Lesions in peripheral nerves include thin myelin sheaths, increased numbers of Schwann cells, Schwann cells with abnormally increased cytoplasmic volume, and no evidence of active demyelination or effective remyelination. The lesions are believed to involve a defect in Schwann cells or abnormal axon–Schwann cell interaction. Congenital hypomyelination has also been described in a 2-month-old Dorsett lamb with tremors and incoordination.

A myelinopathic peripheral neuropathy has been described in Santa Gertrudis–Brahman cross calves with onset of clinical signs at 6 to 10 months of age. Clinical signs were dysphagia, abnormal rumination with bloat, and a weak shuffling gait. Microscopically, lesions were present in the vagus nerve and various somatic peripheral nerves. There were "sausage-shaped" thickenings of the myelin sheaths as a result of excess myelin arranged about the axons or as irregularly folded myelin sheaths not surrounding axons.

In contrast to hypomyelination or disordered myelin formation, demyelination in the PNS is common. Myelin loss occurs following axonal degeneration, compressive lesions, is frequent in inflammatory disorders, and demyelination is the primary lesion in some neuropathies. Schwann cells can proliferate to restore the myelin sheaths, often forming longitudinal columns along the course of a degenerated axon termed cell bands of Büngner. Remyelination results in internodes that are shorter than the internodes of adjacent normal myelinated axons. Another lesion that occurs with repeated episodes of demyelination is proliferation of Schwann cell processes forming concentric whirls, called **onion bulbs,** that surround the axon.

As previously noted, demyelination is the primary lesion in some neuropathies. Clinical signs in **canine inherited hypertrophic polyneuropathy,** a familial disorder in Tibetan mastiffs, begin at 7 to 10 weeks of age and include pelvic limb weakness, depressed spinal reflexes, and lack of muscle tone that progress to involve forelimbs with eventual recumbency. Microscopic lesions consist of demyelination with onion bulb formation. Accumulation of actin filaments distends Schwann cell cytoplasm. Axonal degeneration occurs but is mild. The primary defect is in the Schwann cells, but the pathogenesis is undetermined. Neuropathies with primary demyelination have also been reported in Alaskan malamutes and in beagle–basset hound crosses. A hypertrophic polyneuropathy has rarely been reported in unrelated domestic cats with onset at approximately 1 year of age.

Metabolic/Toxic Peripheral Neuropathies

A variety of metabolic disturbances can affect the PNS. These disturbances include the inherited lysosomal enzyme deficiencies (see Inborn Errors of Metabolism), endocrine disorders, and certain vitamin deficiencies. In addition to the lysosomal enzyme deficiencies, an inherited deficiency of D-glycerate dehydrogenase in domestic cats results in renal failure and predominantly motor deficits by 5 to 9 months of age. Nerve lesions include focal swelling and accumulation of neurofilaments in the axons of motor nerves and later Wallerian degeneration.

Of the endocrine disorders, hypothyroidism, hyperadrenocorticism, and diabetes mellitus can affect the PNS.

From a clinical standpoint, it may be difficult to distinguish the muscular component of the disease from the neurologic involvement. Clinical signs can reflect sensory as well as motor deficits. Lesions in these neuropathies are not well characterized and can include evidence of demyelination, remyelination, and axonal degeneration. Distal portions of the axon are commonly affected. The extent to which demyelination or axonal degeneration represents the primary lesion remains to be determined.

Nutritional neuropathies are relatively uncommon and involve vitamin A and some of the B vitamins. Vitamin A deficiency results indirectly in peripheral neuropathy by affecting bone growth and remodeling. The neuropathy is due to narrowing of the optic foramen caused by continued bone deposition with decreased resorption resulting in compression of the optic nerve, Wallerian degeneration, and blindness. B vitamin deficiencies are primarily diseases of pigs and poultry. In pigs, deficiency of pantothenic acid causes a sensory neuropathy with axonal degeneration, demyelination, and chromatolysis and neuron loss in the dorsal root ganglia, resulting in proprioceptive deficits, goose stepping, and dysmetria. Riboflavin deficiency in poultry, curly toe paralysis, is primarily a demyelinating neuropathy. Peripheral nerves are swollen because of endoneurial edema, and there is subsequent demyelination with mild axonal degeneration.

A number of toxins can affect the PNS, with or without damage in the CNS. The initial toxic effects can be at the level of the neuron cell body, the axon, or the myelin sheaths. Examples of toxins targeting neuronal cell bodies are organomercurial compounds and the cancer chemotherapeutic agent doxorubicin. In mercury poisoning, sensory neuron cell bodies are preferentially involved, whereas with doxorubicin, sensory and autonomic cell bodies are affected. Toxins targeting the axon often cause damage to the distal portions of long sensory or motor axons, giving rise to the term "dying back neuropathy." Further studies indicated that the degeneration actually affects preterminal regions of the axon, hence the terms "distal or peripheral-central distal axonopathy" to denote damage to axons in peripheral sensory and motor nerves and sensory spinal tracts, respectively. It should be noted that this pattern of damage is not solely limited to toxic injury. The pattern of distal axonopathy can be seen in the metabolic neuropathies, as well as in familial or inherited degenerative disorders. A variety of theories have been advanced to explain the increased vulnerability of the distal portions of long axons. Injury with failure of the neuron cell body to supply the basic metabolic demands of a long axon, as well as disturbances in anterograde or retrograde axoplasmic flow, have been incriminated.

Examples of toxins causing axonal degeneration are the vinca alkaloids vincristine and colchicine, both causing disassembly of microtubules and inhibiting axoplasmic flow. Of interest, taxol, an alkaloid from the western yew *(Taxus brevifolia)*, promotes the assembly of and stabilizes microtubules but also causes an axonopathy. Recently, an outbreak of distal polyneuropathy occurred in cats fed commercial diets contaminated with the ionophore salinomycin. There was acute onset of lameness and paralysis affecting the hind limbs that progressed to the forelimbs. Demyelination followed the axonal degeneration (i.e., Wallerian degeneration). Some toxins seem to cause different patterns of injury in the CNS and PNS. For instance, in the CNS, lead is noted to cause neuronal necrosis, whereas in the PNS, demyelination is prominent in some species. Another cause of primary demyelinating axonopathy is the plant coyotillo *(Karwinskia humboldtiana)* affecting mainly small ruminants in the desert southwest.

Degenerative Neuropathies

Included here are the hereditary, familial, and breed- or species-associated syndromes reported in a variety of domestic animals that result in degeneration of PNS neurons or axons or both. Primary **sensory neuropathies** have been described in **English pointers** and **longhaired dachshunds.** In pointer dogs the onset is 2 to 12 months of age with signs of self-mutilation and insensitivity to pain. Lesions consist of small dorsal root ganglia with neuronal loss and replacement by satellite cells (nodules of Nageotte), mild reduction in size of dorsal nerve rootlets, and evidence of degeneration and loss of myelinated and nonmyelinated axons with the presence of cell bands of Büngner. The sensory neuropathy in dachshunds is manifest as ataxia accompanied by urinary incontinence and evidence of digestive disturbance, suggesting an autonomic component. Clinical signs begin soon after birth. Lesions are distal axonopathy with loss of large myelinated and unmyelinated axons. Lesions also occur in the vagus nerve. A notable increase in endoneurial collagen is also present. The lesions represent a peripheral-central distal axonopathy, with axonal degeneration also present in the dorsal funiculus of the spinal cord.

A **progressive axonopathy** (also termed sensory neuropathy) occurs in **Boxer dogs** at 2 to 3 months of age with initial signs of ataxia. Signs progress to include weakness, proprioceptive deficits, and loss of muscle tone. Lesions involve brain stem nuclei, spinal cord, and peripheral nerve. Proximally in paranodal areas there are axonal swellings containing membranovesicular profiles and neurofilaments. More distally there are fewer than normal large-caliber axons. A proximal defect in neurofilament transport with atrophy of distal axons is suspected. A similar distal sensorimotor polyneuropathy has also been reported in **Rottweiler** dogs with paraparesis and tetraparesis and muscle atrophy with onset before 6 months of age.

In **German shepherds,** two distinct neuropathies are described. In one, termed **giant axonal neuropathy,** onset is at approximately 15 months of age with pelvic limb weakness and ataxia and evidence of visceral and autonomic disturbances. Microscopically, there are marked paranodal axonal swellings with neurofilament accumulations affecting distal portions of somatic and autonomic peripheral nerves, and dorsal to dorsolateral funiculi of the spinal cord. A defect in neurofilament transport is suspected. The second neuropathy has a late onset, affecting two 9-year-old littermates. Lesions were distal axonal degeneration and loss with endomysial fibrosis.

An additional suspected distal axonopathy in dogs, **dancing Doberman disease,** has also been described. Onset at 6 to 7 months of age is characterized by flexion of a rear leg progressing to alternating flexion and extension of both hind limbs. The disorder is attributed to a primary myopathy, but microscopic examination revealed evidence of a distal axonopathy.

Other degenerative axonopathies that occur in animals include **laryngeal hemiparesis** or **paralysis** in the horse, as well as multiple dog breeds including **Bouvier des Flandres, Siberian huskies** and crossbreeds, and **dalmations.** Degenerative peripheral-central distal axonopathy also occurs in **Birman cats** with axonal degeneration in brain stem, spinal cord, and peripheral nerves.

Dysautonomia is an acquired degeneration of the autonomic nervous system that has been reported in dogs, cats **(Key-Gaskell syndrome)** and horses **(grass sickness).** Clinical signs in horses are related to gastrointestinal stasis, and manifestations can range from acute to chronic. In cats and dog, clinical signs are more varied and include gastrointestinal disturbance, urinary incontinence, mydriasis, unresponsive pupils, bradycardia, and other signs associated with autonomic dysfunction. Lesions can be observed in peripheral and autonomic ganglia. Lesions vary from neuronal chromatolysis and nuclear pyknosis in more acute cases to loss of neurons and proliferation of satellite cells in cases with longer duration. Minimal to mild leukocytic infiltrates occur, but the lesions are not overtly inflammatory in nature. A toxic etiology has been postulated in the horse and cat. In horses, an association with *Clostridium botulinum* type C has been made, but its role in the disease remains unproven.

Inflammatory Neuropathies

Inflammation of the PNS can occur in conjunction with certain viral (e.g., herpesvirus and rabies) and protozoal infections of the CNS, but the latter have a particular affinity for the PNS in some cases. **Polyradiculoneuritis,** inflammation of multiple peripheral nerves and dorsal, ventral, or both dorsal and ventral, spinal nerve rootlets, and to a lesser extent **ganglionitis,** inflammation of spinal ganglia, occur in toxoplasmosis and neosporosis (see Protozoal Infections in the CNS section). Other inflammatory neuropathies of uncertain etiology occur on a sporadic basis in dogs but are rare in other species.

Acute idiopathic polyneuritis (coonhound paralysis) is an acute, fulminating polyradiculoneuritis with ascending paralysis that occurs in dogs after the bite or scratch of a raccoon. Dogs can die from respiratory paralysis. Recovery is common but can be prolonged in dogs with extensive muscular atrophy. Lesions are most severe in ventral spinal nerve rootlets and progressively diminish distally in the peripheral nerve. Involvement of dorsal spinal nerve rootlets and ganglia is inconstant and relatively minor. Lesions consist of segmental demyelination with a variable influx of neutrophils, depending on the acuteness and severity of clinical signs, along with lymphocytes, plasma cells, and macrophages. Axonal degeneration is commonly present. Evidence of remyelination with cell bands of Bünger, and axonal sprouting occur during the recovery phase, but the effectiveness of the latter to establish reinnervation of muscle is limited.

Although differences in the character of the lesions are readily apparent, coonhound paralysis has been compared with Guillain-Barré syndrome. This human syndrome typically follows a viral illness, vaccination, or some other antecedent disease. Similarities also exist between this canine disease and acute experimental allergic neuritis, the peripheral analogue of acute experimental allergic encephalomyelitis (see Disorders of Myelin Formation and Maintenance, Immune-Mediated Disorders). Coonhound paralysis and the Guillain-Barré syndrome are believed to represent an autoimmune demyelination. Despite the lack of close association of macrophages with the degenerating myelin and axons early in the development of the lesions, secretion of tumor necrosis factor-α by these cells could explain both the demyelination and axonal degeneration. Acute idiopathic polyneuritis is reported in dogs without an association with raccoons and also occurs rarely in cats, suggesting multiple factors might be involved in this type of nerve damage.

A **chronic polyradiculoneuritis** with infiltrations of lymphocytes, plasma cells, or macrophages, demyelination, and variable axonal degeneration in cranial and spinal nerve rootlets and cranial nerves is also reported in dogs and cats. With repeated episodes of demyelination, onion bulbs can be apparent. Both sensory and motor nerves can be involved with sensory disturbances and muscle atrophy.

Other inflammatory neuropathies are rare. **Brachial plexus neuritis** with primary axonal degeneration is reported in dogs and cats. Bouts of urticaria precede the neuritis suggesting an acute hypersensitivity reaction. Cranial and spinal **ganglioneuritis** with neuronal (and axonal) degeneration occurs in dogs with Siberian huskies seemingly predisposed. An immune mechanism is suspected. **Enteric (autonomic) ganglionitis** in multiple species results in neuron loss. **Neuritis of the cauda equina** in horses and dogs is primarily a demyelinating disorder. This neuritis could have an immune-mediated basis. Adenovirus type 1 has been isolated from horses, suggesting a viral antecedent.

Neoplasms of the PNS

The objective of this section is to not be all encompassing regarding neoplasms of the peripheral nervous system, but to review one of the best known examples of how neoplasia can involve this system.

Schwannoma

To fully appreciate the use of terms applied to neoplasms of the PNS in animals, it is helpful to first review such neoplasms in human beings. In human beings, the schwannoma is considered to be a neoplasm of Schwann cell origin. Microscopically, this neoplasm is characterized by having two morphologic features, known as Antoni A and B tissue, that occur in variable proportions within the neoplasm. Antoni A tissue is cellular and consists of monomorphic spindle-shaped Schwann cells, with poorly defined eosinophilic cytoplasm and pointed basophilic nuclei, that are present in a collagenous stroma of variable extent. The nuclei of these cells are commonly arranged in rows, between which are parallel arrays (stacks) of their cytoplasmic processes (Fig. 8-68). Such arrangements are referred to as Verocay bodies. Antoni B areas are also composed of Schwann cells, but their cytoplasm is inconspicuous and their nuclei appear to be suspended in a copious myxoid, often microcystic, matrix. Also, Schwannomas do not typically contain nerve fibers.

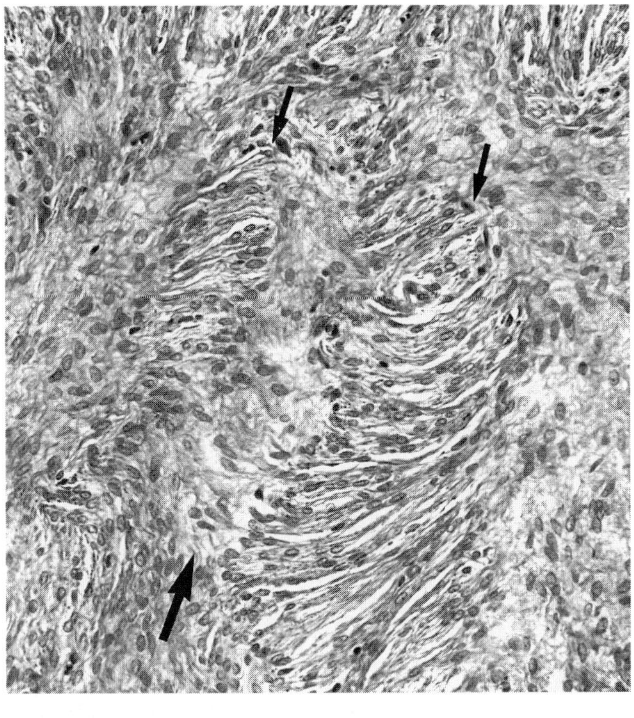

Figure 8-68 Skin, right hind limb; cat. Schwannoma. Two bundles of parallel spindle-shaped cells (with nuclei arranged in rows, *small arrows*) separated by strands of their processes *(large arrow)* indicative of Verocay body formation. H & E stain.

The human schwannoma is to be differentiated from the neurofibroma, which consists of Schwann cells, perineurial cells, and fibroblasts. Some microscopic features of the neurofibroma include elongated spindle cells with poorly defined pale eosinophilic, tapering wavy or buckled nuclei, and numerous small nerve fibers (that are not present in schwannomas). Presence of mast cells is also reported. These neoplastic components are situated in a variably prominent fibomyxoid to myxoid matrix (myxoid neurofibroma), although another variant of the neoplasm contains prominent collagen (collagenous neurofibroma).

Terminology used for neoplasms considered to be of nerve origin in animals over the years has been quite confusing. For example, the terms schwannoma, neurofibroma, and neurilemmoma have all been used at various times by different pathologists to identify the same neoplasm. More recently, it has been accepted that the majority of such neoplasms should be designated schwannomas. Although designation of the malignant variety of the neoplasm has included malignant schwannoma, the degree of differentiation in such neoplasms can prevent definitive distinction from other mesenchymal types. Veterinary pathologists have attempted to simplify the classification scheme for peripheral nerve neoplasms in animals even more by using benign peripheral nerve sheath tumor or malignant peripheral nerve sheath tumor to classify these tumors of controversial ontogeny.

Schwannomas of animals have been best recognized in the canine and bovine species, and less commonly in the cat. In the dog the neoplasm most commonly affects the cranial (fifth) or spinal nerve roots (posterior cervical-anterior thoracic roots of the brachial plexus and their extensions and roots at the thoracic and lumbar levels). Although schwannomas of the skin have been reported, there should always be careful consideration of other neoplasms (e.g., hemangiopericytoma and fibromas) that can have similar morphologic features.

The bovine neoplasm occurs most commonly in mature animals, although the lesion has also been reported in young calves, and involves the cranial eighth nerve, brachial plexus, and intercostal nerves. Additionally, autonomic nerves of the liver, heart, mediastinum, and thorax can be affected. The skin can be infrequently involved.

Grossly, schwannomas are nodular or varicose thickenings along nerve trunks, or nerve roots. They can be firm or soft (gelatinous) and white or gray in color. Schwannomas of the spinal cord nerve roots can remain inside the dura mater or extend through the vertebral foramina to the exterior.

The main microscopic characteristics described for the human being are also applicable for schwannomas of animals.

GLOSSARY OF TERMS

Astrocytosis increased numbers of astrocytes.

Astrogliosis reactive astrocytic response with increased number, length, and complexity of cell processes (astrocytic scarring). In the CNS, reparative processes following injury such as inflammation and necrosis are facilitated by astrogliosis and are analogous to fibroplasia in other organ systems.

Axonopathy, distal, of the PNS a neuropathy with axonal degeneration beginning in the peripheral, but not terminal, portions of axons of peripheral nerves.

Axonopathy, peripheral-central, distal degeneration of axons involving distal portions of peripheral nerves, as well as distal portions of long axons in the CNS (i.e., spinal cord).

Axonotmesis axonal injury of a peripheral nerve in which there is degeneration of the part distal to the site of trauma leaving the supporting framework intact, allowing for improved potential for regeneration and effective reinnervation.

Blood-brain barrier of the CNS a barrier to free movement of certain substances from cerebral capillaries into CNS tissue. Relies on tight junctions between capillary endothelial cells and selective transport systems in these cells. Endothelial cell basement membrane and foot processes of astrocytes abutting the basement membrane may also have a role in the barrier.

Blood-CSF barrier of the CNS a barrier that consists of tight junctions located between epithelial cells of the choroid plexus, and the cells of the arachnoid membrane that respectively separate fenestrated blood vessels of the choroid plexus stroma and dura mater from the CSF.

Blood-nerve barrier a barrier to free movement of certain substances from the blood to the endoneurium of peripheral nerves. Barrier properties are conferred by tight junctions between capillary endothelial cells of the endoneurium and between perineurial cells, and selective transport systems in the endothelial cells.

Brain edema increase in tissue water within the brain that results in an increase in brain volume. The fluid may be present in the intracellular or extracellular compartments or both. The term also is used to include the accumulation of plasma, especially in association with severe injury to the vasculature.

Brain swelling marked, rapidly developing, sometimes unexplained, increase in cerebral blood volume and brain volume due to relaxation (dilation) of the arterioles that occurs after brain injury.

Büngner, cell bands of a column of proliferating Schwann cells that forms within tubes (previously occupied by an axon) following Wallerian degeneration. The tubes are formed by the persisting basement membrane that surrounds Schwann cells.

Central chromatolysis dissolution of cytoplasmic Nissl substance (arrays of rough endoplasmic reticulum and polysomes) in the central part of the neuronal cell body that results from injury to the neuron (often involving the axon). The cell body is swollen, and the nucleus frequently is displaced peripherally to the cell membrane. These structural changes functionally represent regeneration with protein synthesis to produce components of the axon required for fast and slow axonal transport.

Cranium bifidum a dorsal midline cranial defect through which meningeal and brain tissue may protrude into a sac (-cele), covered by skin.

Demyelination a disease process in which demyelination (destruction of the myelin sheath) is the primary lesion. Primary demyelination is caused by injury to myelinating cells and their cell processes. Secondary demyelination occurs with axonal injury, as in Wallerian degeneration.

Dysraphism dysraphia, which literally means an abnormal seam, refers to a defective closure of the neural tube during development. This defect, which may occur at any point along the neural tube, is exemplified by anencephaly, prosencephalic hypoplasia, cranium bifidum, spina bifida, and myeloschisis.

Encephalitis inflammation of the brain.

Encephalo- a combining form that refers to the brain.

Encephalopathy a degenerative disease process of the brain.

Ganglionitis Inflammation of peripheral (sensory or autonomic or both) ganglia.

Gemistocyte reactive, hypertrophied astrocyte that develops in response to injury of the CNS. The cell body and processes of gemistocytes become visible with conventional staining (e.g., H & E stain). The cell bodies and processes of normal astrocytes are not visible with H & E staining.

Gitter cell macrophage that accumulates in areas of necrosis of CNS tissue. The cytoplasm is typically distended with abundant lipid-containing material derived from the lipid-rich nervous tissue. Gitter cell nuclei are often displaced peripherally to the cell membrane. These cells are often referred to as "foamy" macrophages.

Hydranencephaly a large, fluid-filled cavity in the area normally occupied by CNS tissue of the cerebral hemispheres resulting from abnormal development. The nervous tissue may be so reduced in thickness that the meninges form the outer part of a thin-walled sac. The lateral ventricles are variably enlarged because of their expansion into the area normally occupied by tissue.

Hydrocephalus accumulation of excess CSF resulting from obstruction within the ventricular system (noncommunicating form) associated with enlargement of any or all of the following: lateral ventricles, third ventricle, mesencephalic aqueduct, and fourth ventricle. Hydrocephalus can also occur with communication of the CSF between the ventricular system and the subarachnoid space (communicating form). Hydrocephalus ex vacuo (compensatory hydrocephalus) is characterized by an expansion of the lateral ventricle (or ventricles) caused by loss of brain tissue.

Leuko- combining form referring to white matter of the brain or spinal cord.

Leukoencephalitis inflammation of the white matter of the brain.

Macroglia a collective term referring to astrocytes and oligodendrocytes. Has also been variously used to refer solely to astrocytes or to astrocytes, oligodendrocytes, and ependymal cells of the CNS, and Müller cells of the retina.

Malacia grossly detectable (macroscopic lesion) softening of CNS tissue, usually the result of necrosis.

Meningo- combining form referring to meninges.

Meningomyelocele a form of spina bifida in which meninges and spinal cord herniate through a defect in the vertebral column into a sac (-cele) covered by skin.

Microglia resident cells of the CNS believed to arise from monocytes that populate the brain during embryonic development.

Motor neuron, lower large multipolar neurons in the brain stem and ventral horns of the spinal cord with axons extending into the PNS.

Motor neuron, upper motor neurons with axons residing solely in the CNS.

Myelitis inflammation of the spinal cord.

Myelo- combining form referring to spinal cord.

Myelopathy a degenerative disease process of the spinal cord.

Myeloschisis similar to spina bifida, except in its severe form is characterized by complete failure of the spinal neural tube to close and, therefore, a lack of development of the entire dorsal vertebral column.

Neurapraxia traumatic injury to a peripheral nerve with temporary conduction block but with no permanent axonal damage.

Neuroglial cells astrocytes, oligodenroglia, ependymal cells, and microglia of the CNS.

Neuronophagia accumulation of microglial cells around a dead neuron.

Neuropil the gray matter feltwork that consists of intermingled and interconnected processes of neurons (axons and dendrites) and their synaptic junctions, plus processes of oligodendroglia, astrocytes, and microglia.

Neurotmesis complete transection of a nerve and supporting framework with little potential for normal reinnervation.

Onion bulb concentric arrays of Schwann cell cytoplasm around an axon signifying multiple episodes of demyelination and remyelination.

Polio- combining form referring to gray matter of the CNS.

Polioencephalomalacia softening (usually the result of necrosis) of the gray matter of the brain.

Poliomyelomalacia softening (usually the result of necrosis) of the gray matter of the spinal cord.

Polioencephalomyelitis inflammation of the gray matter of the brain and spinal cord.

Porencephaly a cleft or cystic defect in the cerebral hemisphere that communicates with the subarachnoid space and also may communicate with the ventricular system. The defect may contain CSF.

Radiculoneuritis (polyradiculoneuritis) inflammation of a spinal nerve rootlet (or rootlets).

Rarefaction reduction in density of CNS tissue that may result from edema, necrosis, etc. This lesion is usually observed microscopically.

Satellitosis an accumulation of oligodendroglia around neuronal cell bodies. Although this feature can be seen in normal brains, some consider that it may also be associated with neuronal injury caused by anoxia.

Sclerosis literally means induration or hardening and, when used in describing lesions of the CNS, often refers to induration or hardening of the brain or spinal cord resulting from astrogliosis (astrocytic scar formation).

Spina bifida a dorsal midline defect involving one to several vertebrae of the spinal column due to failure of the neural tube to close, permitting exposure of the underlying meninges and spinal cord. The lesion may be associated with herniation of meninges and spinal cord tissue into a sac (-cele) covered by skin, or there may be no herniation (spina bifida occulta).

Status spongiosus an encompassing term meaning the presence of small focal, ovoid to round "clear (unstained or poorly stained [H & E stain])" spaces in the parenchyma of the CNS. The lesion can result from several different tissue alterations that include splitting of the myelin sheath; accumulation of extracellular fluid; swelling of cellular (e.g., astrocytic, neuronal) processes; and axonal injury (e.g., Wallerian degeneration) when swollen axons are no longer detectable within distended spaces.

Syringomyelia a tubular cavitation (syrinx) in the parenchyma of the spinal cord that is not lined by ependyma and may extend over several segments.

Wallerian degeneration degeneration of the distal component of an injured (compressed or severed) axon. Although the term originally referred to injury of axons in the PNS, current usage also includes the CNS. This process also results in functional and structural alterations in the cell body and proximal internode segment of the axon and in secondary demyelination.

Suggested Readings

The Central Nervous System

General References

DeFelipe J, Jones EG, eds. Cajal's Degeneration and Regeneration of the Nervous System. New York: Oxford University Press, 1991.

Fankhauser R, Luginbühl H. Zentrales Nervensystem. In: Dobberstein J, Pallaske, G, Stünzi, H, eds. Joest's Handbuch der speziellen pathologischen Anatomie der Haustiere. Vol 3. Berlin: Verlag Paul Parey, 1962:191-436.

Fenner F, Bachmann PA, Gibbs EPJ, et al. Veterinary Virology. New York: Academic Press, 1987.

Haymaker W, Adams RD, eds. Histology and Histopathology of the Nervous System. Springfield, Ill.: Charles C Thomas, 1982.

Summers BA, Cummings JF, de Lahunta A. Veterinary Neuropathology. New York: Mosby, 1995.

Sunderland S. Nerve and Nerve Injuries. London: E & S Livingstone, 1968.

Neurons and Neuroglia

Azbill RD, Xiaojun M, Annadora JB-K, et al. Impaired mitochrondrial function, oxidative stress and altered antioxidant enzyme activities following traumatic spinal cord injury. Brain Res 1997; 765:283-290.

Aschner M. Astrocytes as mediators of immune and inflammatory responses in the CNS. Neurotoxicology 1998; 19:269-282.

Braughler JM. Calcium and lipid peroxidation. In: Halliwell B, ed. Oxygen Radicals and Tissue Injury. Bethesda, Md.: Federation of American Societies of Experimental Biology, 1988:99-104.

Choi DW. Calcium-mediated neurotoxicity: Relationship to specific channel types and role in ischemic damage. Trends Neurosci 1988; 11:465-469.

David S. Reactive gliosis: Characterization of injury-induced changes in astrocytes. In: Norenberg MD, Hertz L, Schousboe A, eds. The Biochemical Pathology of Astrocytes. New York: Alan R Liss, 1988:123-134.

Fellman V, Raivio KO. Reperfusion injury as the mechanism of brain damage after perinatal asphyxia. Pediatr Res 1997; 41:599-605.

Frei K, Siepl C, Groscurth P, et al. Immunobiology of microglial cells. Ann N Y Acad Sci 1988; 540:218-227.

Hatten ME, Liem RKH, Shelanski ML, et al. Astroglia in CNS injury. Glia 1991; 4:233-243.

Jenkins LW, Povlishock JT, Lewelt W, et al. The role of post-ischemic recirculation in the development of ischemic neuronal injury following complete cerebral ischemia. Acta Neuropathol 1981; 55:205-220.

Lieberman AR. The axon reaction: A review of the principal features of perikaryal responses to axon injury. Int Rev Neurobiol 1971; 14:49-124.

Montgomery DL. Astrocytes: Form, functions, and roles in disease. Vet Pathol 1994; 31:145-167.

Moore S, Thanos S. The concept of microglia in relation to central nervous system disease and regeneration. Prog Neurobiol 1996; 48:441-460.

Neumann H, Wekerle H. Neuronal control of the immune response in the central nervous system: Linking brain immunity to neurodegeneration. J Neuropathol Exp Neurol 1998; 57:1-9.

Norenberg MD. Astrocyte responses to CNS injury. J Neuropathol Exp Neurol 1994; 53:213-220.

Perry VH, Gordon S. Macrophages and microglia in the nervous system. TINS 1988; 11:273-277.

Rabchevsky AG, Streit W. Role of microglia in postinjury repair and regeneration of the CNS. Mental Retard Develop Disabil Res Rev 1998; 4:187-192.

Raff MC. Glial cell diversification in the rat optic nerve. Science 1989; 243:1450-1455.

Rosenblum WI. Histopathologic clues to the pathways of neruonal death following ischemia/hypoxia. J Neruotrauma 1997; 14:313-326.

Siesjo BK, Bengtsson F. Calcium fluxes, calcium antagonists, and calcium-related pathology in brain ischemia, hypoglycemia, and spreading depression: A unifying hypothesis. J Cereb Blood Flow Metab 1989; 9:127-140.

Wilson JX. Antioxidant defense of the brain: a role for astrocytes. Can J Physiol Pharmacol 1997; 75:1149-1163.

Anomalies and Malformations

Brown TT, deLahunta A, Bistner SI, et al. Pathogenic studies of infection of the bovine fetus with bovine viral diarrhea virus. I. Cerebellar atrophy. Vet Pathol 1974; 11:486-505.

Greitz D, Greitz T, Hindmarsh T. A new view on the CSF-circulation with the potenital for pharmacological treatment of childhood hydrocephalus. Acta Paediatr 1997; 86:125-132.

Johnson RT. Viral Infections of the Nervous System. New York: Raven Press, 1982:203-236.

Inborn Errors of Metabolism

Jolly RD, Walkley SU. Lysosomal storage diseases of animals: An essay in comparative pathology. Vet Pathol 1997; 34:527-548.

Suzuki K. A genetic demyelinating disease globoid cell leukodystrophy: Studies with animal models. J Neuropathol Exp Neurol 1994; 53:359-363.

Physical Disturbances

Dawson SL, Hirsch CS, Lucas FV, Sebek BA. The countrecoup phenomenon. Reappraisal of a classic problem. Hum Pathol 1980; 11:155-166.

Gennarelli TA. Cerebral concussion and diffuse brain injuries. In: Cooper PR, ed. Head injury. Baltimore: Williams & Wilkins, 1982:83-97.

Lindenberg R. Trauma of meninges and brain; Bailey FW. Trauma of the spinal cord; Schwartz P. Birth injuries; Jacobson SA. Skeletal affections; and Jacobson SA. The intervertebral disk. In: Minckler J, Bailey OT, Feigin I, Jervis G, Lindenberg R, Neubuerger KT. Pathology of the Nervous System. New York: McGraw-Hill, 1971:1705-1831.

Circulatory Disturbances

Go KG. The classification of brain edema. New York: John Wiley & Sons, 1981:3-9.

Klatzo I. Presidential address. Neuropathological aspects of brain edema. J Neuropathol Exp Neurol 1967; 26:1-14.

Kornegay JN, Oliver JE, Gorgacz EJ. Clinicopathologic features of brain herniation in animals. J Am Vet Med Assoc 1983; 182:1111-1116.

Williams KJ, Summers BA, De Lahunta A. Cerebral cuterebriasis in cats and its association with feline ischemic encephalopathy. Vet Pathol 1998; 35:330-343.

Zivin JA, Choi DW. Stroke therapy. Sci Am 1991; 265:56-63.

Metabolic Disturbances

Abou-Donia MB, Lapadula DM. Mechanisms of organophosphorus ester-induced delayed neurotoxicity: Type I and Type II. Ann Rev Pharmacol Toxicol 1990; 30:405-440.

Abou-Donia MB. Biochemical toxicology of organophosphorous compounds. In: Blum K, Manzo L, eds. Neurotoxicology. New York: Marcel Dekker, 1985:423-444.

Bressler JP, Goldstein GW. Commentary: Mechanisms of lead neurotoxicity. Biochem Pharmacol 1991; 41:479-484.

Christian RG., Tryphonas L. Lead poisoning in cattle: Brain lesions and hematologic changes. Am J Vet Res 1971; 32:203-216.

Gould DH, McAllister MM, Savage JC, Hamar DW. High sulfide concentrations in rumen fluid associated with nutritionally induced polioencephalomalacia in calves. Am J Vet Res 1991; 52:1164-1169.

Holmes GL. Do seizures cause brain damage? Epilepsia 1991; 32(Suppl 5):S14-S28.

Meldrum B. Excitotoxicity and epileptic brain damage. Epilepsy Res 1991;10:55-61.

Montgomery DL, Lee AC. Brain damage in the epileptic beagle dog. Vet Pathol 1983; 20:160-169.

Olkowski AA. Neurotoxicity and secondary metabolic problems associated with low to moderate levels of exposure to excess dietary sulphur in ruminants: A review. Vet Human Toxicol 1997; 39:355-360.

Pasantes-Morales H. Volume regulation in brain cells: Cellular and molecular mechanisms. Metabol Brain Dis 1996; 11:187-204.

Robles M, et al. Cytotoxic effects of repin, a principal sesquiterpene lactone of Russian knapweed. J Neurosci Res 1997; 47:90-97.

Smith DLT. Poisoning by sodium salt—a cause of eosinophilic meningoencephalitis in swine. Am J Vet Res 1957; 18:825-850.

Soupart A, Decaux G: Therapeutic recommendations for management of severe hyponatremia: Current concepts on pathogenesis and prevention of neurologic complications. Clin Nephrol 1996; 46:149-169.

Wilson TM, Ross PF, Rice LG, et al. Fumonisin B_1 levels associated with an epizootic of equine leukoencephalomalacia. J Vet Diagn Invest 1990; 2:213-216.

Disorders of Myelin Formation and Maintenance

Appel MJG, Summers BA. Pathogenicity of morbilliviruses for terrestrial carnivors. Vet Microbiol 1995; 44:187-191.

Appel MJG, Gillespie JH. Canine distemper virus. In: Gard S, Hallauer C, Meyer KF, eds. Virology Monographs. Vol 11. New York: Springer-Verlag, 1972:1-96.

Cork LC. Differential diagnosis of viral leukoencephalomyelitis of goats. J Am Vet Med Assoc 1976; 169:1303-1306.

Griot C, Burge T, Vandevelde M, Peterhans E. Antibody-induced generation of reactive oxygen radicals by brain macrophages in canine distemper encephalitis: a mechanism for bystander demyelination. Acta Neuropathol 1989; 78:396-403.

Harper PAW, Healy PJ, Dennis JA. Maple syrup urine disease as a cause of spongiform encephalopathy in calves. Vet Rec 1986; 119:62-65.

Krakowka S, Axthelm MK, Johnson GC. Canine distemper virus. In: Olsen RG, Krakowka S, Blakeslee JR, eds. Comparative Pathology of Viral Diseases. Vol. 2. Boca Raton, Fla.: CRC Press, 1985:137-164.

Narayan O, Jolly P. Ovine-caprine lentiviruses: Infection and pathogenesis. Dev Biol Stand 1990; 72:203-205.

Raine CS. The neuropathology of myelin disease. In: Morell P, ed. Myelin. 2nd ed. New York: Plenum, 1984:259-310.

Selmaj KW, Raine CS. Tumor necrosis factor mediates myelin and oligodendrocyte damage in vitro. Ann Neurol 1988; 23:339-346.

Summers BA, Appel MJG. Demyelination in canine distemper encephalomyelitis: An ultrastructural analysis. J Neurocytol 1987; 16:871-881.

Tabira T. Cellular and molecular aspects of the pathomechanism and therapy of murine experimental allergic encephalomyelitis. Crit Rev Neurobiol 1989; 5:113-142.

Vandevelde M, Zurbriggen A. The neurobiology of canine distemper virus infection. Vet Microbiol 1995; 44:271-280.

Zurbriggen A, Schmid I, Graber HU, Vandevelde M. Oligodendroglial pathology in canine distemper. Acta Neuropathol 1998; 95:71-77.

Zink MC, Narayan O, Kennedy PGE, et al. Pathogenesis of visna/maedi and caprine arthritis-encephalitis: New leads on the mechanism of restricted virus replication and persistent inflammation. Vet Immunol Immunopathol 1987; 15:167-180.

Neurodegenerative Diseases

Brenner O, de Lahunta A, Summers BA, et al. Hereditary polioencephalomyelopathy of the Australian cattle dog. Acta Neuropathol 1997; 94:54-66.

Brenner O, de Lahunta A, Cummings JF, et al. A canine encephalomyelopathy with morphological abnormalities in mitochondria. Acta Neuropathol 1997; 94:390-397.

de Lahunta A. Comparative cerebellar disease in domestic animals. Comp Cont Educ Pract 1980; 2:8-19.

de Lahunta A. Abiotrophy in domestic animals: A review. Can J Vet Res 1990; 54:65-76.

Montgomery DL, Storts RW. Hereditary striatonigral and cerebello-olivary degeneration of the Kerry blue terrier. I. Gross and light microscopic central nervous system lesions. Vet Pathol 1983; 20:143-159.

Vandevelde M. Degenerative diseases of the spinal cord. Vet Clin North Am Small Anim Pract 1980; 10:147-154.

Inflammation of the Central Nervous System

Allen GP, Bryans JT. Molecular epizooitology, pathogenesis, and prophylaxis of equine herpesvirus-1 infections. Prog Vet Microbiol Immunol 1986; 2:78-144.

Charlton KM, Garcia MM. Spontaneous listeric encephalitis and neuritis in sheep. Vet Pathol 1977; 14:297-313.

Charlton KM. The pathogenesis of rabies. In: Campbell JB, Charlton KM, eds. Rabies: Developments in Veterinary Virology. Norwell, Mass.: Kluner Academic, 1988:100-150.

Charlton KM, Casey GA, Wandler AI, Nadin-Davis S. Early events in rabies virus infection of the central nervous system in skunks *(Mephitis mephitis)* Acta Neuropathol 1996; 91:89-98.

Charlton KM, Nadin-Davis S, Casey GA, Wandler AI. The long incubation period in rabies: Delayed progression of infection in muscle at the site of exposure Acta Neuropathol 1997; 94:73-77.

Dubey JP, Beattie CP. Toxoplasmosis of Animals and Man. Boca Raton, Fla.: CRC Press, 1988:1-220.

Dubey JP, Davis SW, Speer CA, et al. *Sarcocystis neurona* n. sp. (Protozoa: apicomplexa), the etiologic agent of equine protozoal myeloencephalitis. J Parasitol 1991; 77:212-218.

Engels M, Ackermann M. Pathogenesis of ruminant herpesvirus infections. Vet Microbiol 1996; 53:3-15.

Gronstol H. In: Gyles CL, Thoen CO, eds. Pathogenesis of Bacterial Infections in Animals. Ames, Iowa: Iowa State University Press, 1986:48-55.

Hubálek Z, Halouzka J. West Nile Fever—a reemerging mosquito-borne viral disease in Europe. Emerg Infect Dis 1999; 5:643-650.

Johnson RT. Viral Infections of the Nervous System. New York: Raven Press, 1982:203-236.

Kimberlin RH. Transmissible encephalopathies in animals. Can J Vet Res 1990; 54:30-37.

Ludwig H, Bode L. The neuropathogenesis of *Borna* disease virus infections. Intervirology. 1997; 40:185-197.

Pedersen NC. An overview of feline enteric coronavirus and infectious peritonitis virus infections. Feline Pract 1995; 23:7-20.

Polachek I. The discovery of melanin production in *Cryptococcus neoformans* and its impact on diagnosis and the study of virulence. Zentralbl Bakteriol 1991; 276:120-123.

Richt JA., Pfeuffer I, Christ M, et al. *Borna* disease virus infection in animals and humans. Emerg Infect Dis 1997; 3:343-351.

Storz J. Overview of animal diseases induced by chlamydial infections. In: Barron AL, ed. Microbiology of Chlamydia. Boca Raton, Fla.: CRC Press, 1988:167-192.

Wege H. Immunopathological aspects of coronavirus infections. Springer Seminars in Immunopathology. New York: Springer-Verlag, 1995:133-148.

Spongiform Encephalopathies (Scrapie)

Belay ED. Transmissible spongiform encephalopathies in humans. Annu Rev Microbiol 1999; 53:283-314.

Hadlow WJ. Reflections on the transmissible spongiform encephalopathies. Vet Pathol 1999; 36:523-529.

Hadlow WJ, Kennedy RC, Race RE. Natural infection of Suffolk sheep with scrapie virus. J Infect Dis 1982; 146:657-664.

Parasitic Infestations

Fankhauser R, Luginbühl H. Zentrales nervensystem. In: Dobberstein J, Pallaske G, Stünzi H, eds. Joest's Handbuch der speziellen pathologischen Anatomie der Haustiere. Vol 3. Berlin: Verlag Paul Parey, 1962:191-436.

Miscellaneous Processes

Fankhauser R, Fatzer R, Luginbühl H. Reticulosis of the central nervous system (CNS) in dogs. Adv Vet Sci Comp Med 1972; 16:35-71.

Neoplasms

Cordy DR. Tumors of the nervous system and eye. In: Tumors in Domestic Animals. 3rd ed. Berkeley: University of California Press, 1990:640-665.

Lopes MBS, VendenBerg SR. Tumors of the central nervous system. In: Fletcher CDM, ed. Diagnostic Histopathology of Tumors. Vol 2. New York: Churchill Livingstone, 1995:1221-1250.

Steele KE, Schulman FY, Mena H, et al: Rhabdoid tumor in the brain of a dog. Vet Pathol 1997; 34:359-363.

The Peripheral Nervous System

Anthony DC, Graham DG. Toxic responses of the nervous system. In: Amdur MO, Doull DG, Klaassen CD, eds. Casarett and Doull's Toxicology. 4th ed. New York: McGraw-Hill, 1991; 407-429.

Braund KG. Clinical Syndromes in Veterinary Neurology. 2nd ed. St. Louis: Mosby, 1994.

Braund KG. Degenerative causes of neuropathies in dogs and cats. Vet Med 1996; 91:722-739.

Braund KG: Endogenous causes of neuropathies in dogs and cats. Vet Med 1996; 91:740-754.

Braund KG. Idiopathic and exogenous causes of neuropathies in dogs and cats. Vet Med 1996; 91:755-769.

Charlton KM, Pierce KR. A neuropathy in goats caused by experimental coyotillo (*Karwinskia humboldtiana*) poisoning. Path Vet 1970; 7:385-407.

Cummings JF, Cooper BJ, deLahunta A, van Winkle TJ. Canine inherited hypertrophic neuropathy. Acta Neuropathol 1981; 53:137-143.

Fletcher CDM. Peripheral neuroectodermal tumors. In: Fletcher CDM, ed. Diagnostic Histopathology of Tumors. Vol 2. New York: Churchill Livingstone, 1995:1221-1250.

Furuoka H, Amanai H, Taniyama H, Matsui T. Peripheral neuropathy in German shepherd dogs. J Comp Pathol 1992; 107:169-177.

Griffiths IR, Duncan ID: Neuropathies in domestic animals. In: Cavanagh JB, ed. Recent Advances in Neuropathology. 3rd ed. New York: Churchill Livingstone, 1986:115-139.

Hearn CJ, Murphy M, Newgreen D. GDNF and ET-3 differentially modulate the numbers of avian enteric neural crest cells and enteric neurons in vitro. Develop Biol 1998; 197:93-105.

Hill BD, Prior H, Blakemore WF, Black PF. A study of the pathology of a bovine primary peripheral myelinopathy with features of tamaculous neuropathy. Acta Neuropathol 1996; 91:545-548.

Kiernan JA. Vascular permeability in the peripheral autonomic and somatic nervous systems—Controversial aspects and comparisons with the blood-brain barrier. Microsc Res Tech 1996; 35:122-136.

Longshore RC, O'Brien DP, Johnson GC, Grooters AM, Kroll RA. Dysautonomia in dogs—A retrospective study. J Vet Intern Med 1996; 10:103-109.

Pogson DM, Doxey DL, Gilmour JS, Milne EM, Chisholm HK. Autonomic neurone degeneration in equine dysautonomia (grass sickness). J Comp Pathol 1992; 107:271-283.

Poxton IR, Hunter LC, Brown R, Lough HG, Miller JK. Clostridia and equine grass sickness. Rev Med Microbiol 1997;8(Suppl 1):S49-S51.

Ropper AH. The Guillain-Barré syndrome. N Engl J Med 1993; 326:1130-1136.

Stoll G, Jung S, Jander S, van der Meide P, Hartung H-P. Tumor necrosis factor-α in immune-mediated demyelination and Wallerian degeneration of the rat peripheral nervous system. J Neuroimmunol 1993; 45:175-182.

Summers BA, Cummings JF, deLahunta A. Diseases of the peripheral system. In: Veterinary Neuropathology. St. Louis: Mosby, 1995: 402-501.

van der Linde-Shipman JS, van den Ingh TSGAM, van Nes JJ, Verhagen H, Kersten JGTM, Beynen AC, Plekkgringa R. Salinomycin-induced polyneuropathy in cats: Morphologic and epidemiologic data. Vet Pathol 1999; 36:152-156.

Yang GC, Croaker D, Zhang AL, Manglick P, Cartmill T. A dinucleotide mutation in the endothelin-B receptor gene is associated with lethal white foal syndrome (LWFS); a horse variant of Hirschsprung disease. Human Molec Gen 1998; 7:1047-1052.

CHAPTER 9

Muscle

M. Donald McGavin
Beth A. Valentine

Structural and physiologic features of skeletal muscle determine much of its response to injury. Although muscle cells are frequently called muscle **fibers** or **myofibers,** they are in fact multinucleated cells of considerable length, which in some animals may approach 1 m. This feature has a significant effect on the process of regeneration, as under favorable conditions, muscle cells are able to restore themselves after a segment has become necrotic, and segmental necrosis is a common reaction of the myofiber to a wide variety of insults. Also, the physiologic attributes of a muscle fiber—its rate of contraction, type of metabolism (oxidative, anaerobic, or mixed)—are determined not by the muscle cell itself but by the neuron responsible for its innervation, the ventral horn or the brain stem motor neurons (Fig. 9-1). This fact is significant in evaluating histologic changes in muscle fibers. It is possible to divide changes in muscle fibers into two major classes, **neuropathic** and **myopathic.** Neuropathic changes are those that are determined by the effect or the absence of the nerve supply (e.g., atrophy after denervation). However, the term "myopathy" should be reserved for those muscle diseases where the primary change takes place in the muscle cell, not in the interstitial tissue and not secondary to effects from the nerve supply. Myopathies include some types of myofiber degeneration, for example, metabolic myopathies, muscular dystrophies, myofiber necrosis, and inflammatory conditions affecting the myofiber itself, not the interstitium.

Muscle pathology has developed into a subspeciality with its own extensive literature. Inevitably, over decades, this has resulted in the development of its own terminology. Pathologists based some names on the then-current anatomic and histologic terms, but when anatomic nomenclature changed, pathologists frequently retained the older term. A good example is the term "sarcolemma." In muscle pathology, this was used for decades for the tube visible by light microscopy following removal of the contents of a muscle fiber, for example, by segmental necrosis (see Fig. 9-6, *A*). Electron microscopy reveals that the myofiber's plasmalemma is applied closely to a basal lamina, and outside of this is an interlacing network of fine reticular fibrils that form the endomysium. Exactly what constitutes the sarcolemma of light microscopy is a little unclear. It is certainly not just the basal lamina, which would not be visible by light microscopy, and most likely it includes the basal lamina and reticular fibers. Reticular fibers are a type of collagen, but do not stain with eosin or with conventional collagen stains such as trichrome stains, but only with silver reticulum stains. Over a decade ago, histologists applied the term "sarcolemma" to the myofiber's plasmalemma, thus setting the stage for confusion in the literature. The result has been that in one multiauthor textbook on muscle pathology, the word "sarcolemma" was used in three different ways: for the plasmalemma alone, for plasmalemma plus basal lamina, and for the endomysium plus basal lamina. Another convention of muscle pathology is to call those myofiber nuclei that lie at the periphery of the myofiber "sarcolemmal" nuclei, as opposed to nuclei in the center of the myofiber (a primitive state), which are called internal (or central) nuclei. Central nuclei indicate a primitive state or a myopathic change. They are normal in bird and reptile muscles.

The key structure in the "sarcolemma" of muscle pathology is the basal lamina. In myofiber necrosis, the myofiber's plasmalemma disappears, but the basal lamina remains and is the basic component of the so-called sarcolemmal tube. The basal lamina is resistant to insults that destroy the myofiber. It can be penetrated by macrophages that enter to remove necrotic debris and is responsible for orderly regeneration (see Regeneration). In this chapter, the term "sarcolemmal tube" is used for this tube formed by the basal lamina.

PHYSIOLOGIC FEATURES

Mammalian muscles are composed of muscle fibers of different contractile properties. The classification of these fibers is based on three major physiologic features: (1) rates of contraction (fast or slow), (2) rates of fatigue (fast or slow), and (3) types of metabolism (oxidative, glycolytic, or mixed). The last feature is the basis for histochemical methods that demonstrate either the concentration of myosin adenosine triphosphatase (ATPase) or mitochondrial enzymes such as succinic dehydrogenase

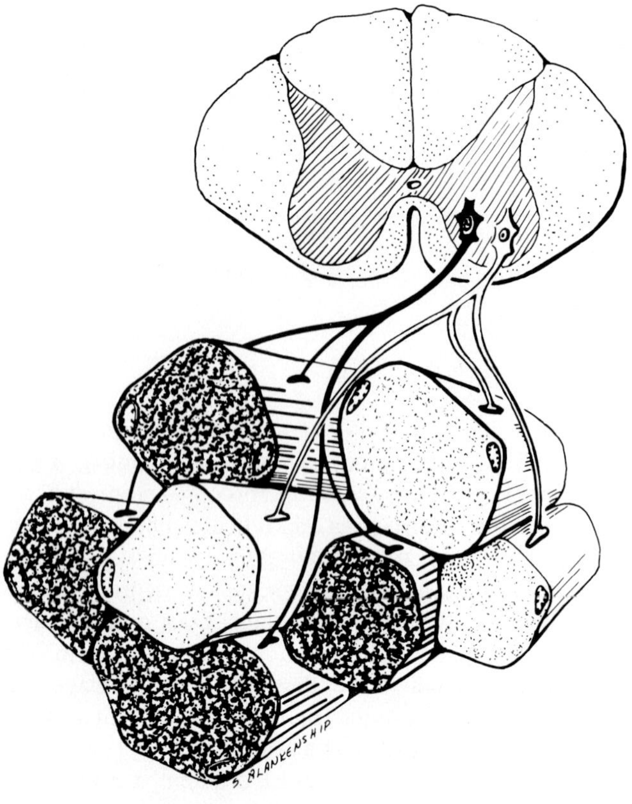

Figure 9-1 Schematic diagram of motor unit and muscle fiber types. All myofibers innervated by the one motor neuron are of the same fiber type. Thus, the motor neuron determines whether the myofibers are type I (light) or type II (dark).

and nicotinamide adenine dinucleotide–tetrazolium reductase (NADH-TR), although the latter is not confined to mitochondria. Fortunately, the physiologic and histochemical classifications are compatible, although this has not been proven for all species. In 1970, the World Federation of Neurology recommended a basic division into type I and type II fibers (Table 9-1). Type I fibers are low in myosin ATPase activity, rich in mitochondria, oxidative in metabolism, slow-contracting, and slow-fatiguing fibers. Type II fibers are rich in myosin ATPase, have fewer mitochondria, and are glycolytic, fast-contracting fibers. Type II fibers were later subdivided into type IIA and type IIB. Type IIB are the fast-contracting, fast-fatiguing, glycolytic fibers (FF) that depend on glycogen for their energy supply. Type IIA are mixed oxidative-glycolytic and, therefore, although fast contracting, are also slow fatiguing (FR). Thus, type IIA fibers are "intermediate" in the concentration of mitochondria and myosin ATPase activity between type I and type IIB, and in some classifications, are known as "intermediate" fibers.

Most muscles contain both type I and type II fibers, and these are conveniently demonstrated by the myosin ATPase reaction (see Figs. 9-8 and 9-9). The percentage of each fiber type varies from muscle to muscle and within the same muscle (Fig. 9-2). There is some correlation with function. Type I fibers (slow contracting, slow fatiguing, oxidative) are plentiful in those muscles whose main function is to maintain posture, support the weight of the animal, and slow locomotion. Muscles that contract quickly, for sprinting, contain more type IIB fibers. Muscles that contract slowly and continuously, e.g., some of the ruminants' masticatory muscles, contain a high percentage of type I fibers. Only rarely are muscles composed of only one fiber type (e.g., the ovine vastus intermedius is type I). Athletic training causes some type IIB fibers to be converted to IIA, and this is the basis of the "training affect." There are also variations within breeds and differences in the same muscle in different species; for example, the dog has no type IIB fibers.

METHODS OF EXAMINATION OF MUSCLES

Frequently, lesions in muscles can be detected and evaluated only by microscopic examination. Muscle is prone to develop artifacts, and thus successful light microscopic and electron microscopic examination of muscle tissue depend on prevention of these artifacts. Unfortunately, the most common change in muscle samples submitted for routine histopathologic examination is artifact. This problem is so severe that Harriman stated, "for many years the histopathology of skeletal muscle attracted little interest or effort. Its reactions in disease were limited, and too easily obscured by artifact. A lump of muscle hastily excised and dropped immediately into acid formalin provided a disorderly mass of hypercontracted muscle fibers, impossible to orientate."

Gross Examination of Muscle

Gross examination includes evaluation of changes in shape, color, texture, and volume (atrophy or hypertrophy). Subjective evaluation of size can be highly unreliable unless control muscles, e.g., from normal animals or from the opposite sides, are available for weighing and measuring. Colors of muscles can also be misleading. The variation in the percentage of type I and type II fibers affects the muscle's color. Type II fibers are light (so-called white fibers; e.g., the pectoral muscles of a chicken). Type I fibers are dark (so-called red fibers; e.g., the pectoral muscles of a duck). Muscles that are formed of predominantly type II fibers, such as the semimembranosus and semitendinosus (Fig. 9-2), are naturally pale. Conversely, muscles in which type I myofibers predominate, such as the canine superficial digital flexor (Fig. 9-2) and the bovine masseter, are naturally dark red. Therefore, a pale muscle is not necessarily undergoing degeneration. However, muscles undergoing necrosis are pale, and these lesions appear as distinct streaks or foci or even involve large areas of a muscle (e.g., an infarction). If necrotic areas calcify, they are glistening chalky-white foci or streaks. Muscles infiltrated by fat (e.g., steatosis) are also pale. Other discolorations detectable grossly are from pigment. The most important pigment is **lipofuscin**—

Table 9-1 Relationship Between Histochemical and Physiologic Classifications of Myofibers

Dubowitz and Brooke	Peter and Coworkers	Burke and Coworkers
Type I: low myosin ATPase activity, heavy mitochondrial staining	SO = slow twitch oxidative	S = slow contracting
Type IIA: intermediate ATPase activity, heavy mitochondrial staining	FOG = fast twitch oxidative-glycolytic	FR = fast contracting, fatigue resistant
Type IIB: high ATPase activity, light mitochondrial staining	FG = fast twitch glycolytic-glycolytic	FF = fast contracting, fast fatiguing

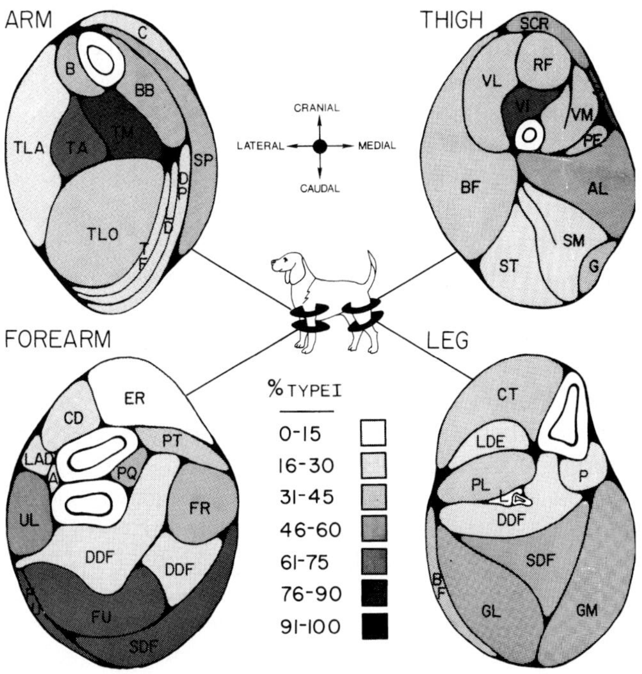

Figure 9-2 Muscles; dog. Schematic representation of the percentage of type I and type II myofibers in limb muscles in the dog. Note the wide variation from the muscle to muscle. The extensor carpi radialis has the lowest percentage of type I fibers (<5%), and the vastus intermedius the highest (91% to 100%). *Courtesy Dr. R. B. Armstrong et al. Am J Anat 1987; 163:87-98.*

the so-called wear-and-tear pigment that accumulates in secondary lysosomes that are later converted to small, compact aggregates known in electron microscopy as residual bodies. The propensity to store lipofuscin is not the same in all domestic animals. It is greatest in the skeletal muscles of cattle, particularly old high-producing dairy cattle. The masseter and diaphragm (two hardworking muscles) are the most frequently affected, although, in badly affected cows, all muscles may be discolored tan to brown. The lesion is of no clinical significance. It is most frequently seen in packing plants where it is known incorrectly as "xanthomatosis" or "xanthosis." Its significance at necropsy in muscle, as well in other organs such as myocardium, neurons, liver, kidney, and adrenal cortex, is either an indicator of old age, or of past or present episodes of cachexia or starvation. The characteristic microscopic appearance in skeletal muscle consists of rounded granules of yellow-brown to dark brown pigment at the two poles of the nucleus of the myofiber.

Occasionally **melanin** discolors the fascial sheaths and epimysium of muscles as part of the syndrome of congenital melanosis in calves, in which melanocytes are present within the fascial sheaths and epimysium. The pigment appears grossly as black foci or streaks. Muscle fibers themselves are unaffected, and the pigmentation has no clinical significance.

Myoglobin may discolor muscles after extensive muscle necrosis, known as rhabdomyolysis (see below). Damage to the myofiber's cell membrane allows myoglobin to leak into the adjacent tissues. This leakage is seen only if the muscle necrosis is extensive and sudden, as in crush injuries or in the early stages of a toxicosis (e.g., monensin poisoning in horses). It is really the result of an acute necrosis. Another cause of localized colored areas in muscle is from injections of medicaments, for example, tetracycline (yellow) and iron dextran (dark brown).

Thus a complete necropsy includes palpation of and multiple incisions into muscles. Multiple incisions should be made in the direction of the myofibers, although this is difficult or impossible to do in those muscles where the fibers do not all run in the same direction (e.g., temporalis). Incisions should be less than 1 cm apart in order not to overlook small foci, such as very early lesions of blackleg. At necropsy, a desirable procedure is to sample a mixture of muscles, including active ones (tongue, diaphragm, intercostal), inactive (psoas), proximal (biceps femoris, semimembranosus, semitendinosus, vastus lateralis, triceps brachii [lateral head]), and distal (tibialis cranialis, extensor digitorum longus). For purposes of biopsy, certain muscles are easy to sample because of their myofiber orientation. Such muscles include the triceps brachii, superficial digital flexor, vastus lateralis, biceps femoris, extensor digitorum longus, tibialis cranialis, and semimembranosus. Clinical findings should be used to determine which muscles are most likely to have lesions.

Microscopic Examination

Muscle is designed to contract when stimulated, and, if it is still irritable when placed in fixative, it will contract. This artifactual contraction of myofibers varies in severity. Contraction of a length of myofiber can result in that segment being deeply eosinophilic and round in cross section. These fibers have been confused with hyalinized fibers. In a more severe form, a short section of the myofiber contacts so violently that it disrupts the normal filaments and causes "shredding." Myofibers in the early stages of degeneration are very susceptible to artifactual contractions.

Because contraction artifacts can obscure lesions at histologic examination, their prevention at the time of fixation is important. Contraction depends on two mechanisms—an energy supply available to the myofiber to allow it to contract, and lack of restraint of the muscle sample when it is placed in fixative. If the muscle is depleted of energy (e.g., glycogen), it will not contract in the fixative. This occurs in muscles from emaciated animals, animals dying of septicemia, or diseases of long duration, if there is a long delay between death and fixation, or if rigor mortis has passed. In muscles that have energy stores and are capable of contraction, for example, muscles sampled at biopsy or at necropsy shortly after death, it is essential that the muscle sample be restrained from contracting when it is placed at fixative. This is done by several methods. One is to excise a strip of muscle approximately 5 to 10 mm wide, 3 to 5 mm thick, and several centimeters in length (the size of the sample depends on the size of the muscle) but in the direction of the fibers. This strip is placed on a wooden tongue depressor, stretched slightly, and fixed in place by ligatures or staples at each end. An optimal procedure is to clamp the strip of muscle before it is freed from the muscle belly. This can be done with a muscle biopsy clamp, or the strip of muscle can be ligated to a thin piece of wood such as an orange stick and then excised. Even these precautions will not prevent all contractions in highly irritable muscle, for example, from an athletic animal. In these cases, the only alternative is to take a second sample and reduce its energy supply before fixation. The first sample is fixed immediately to allow optimal fixation of glycogen and organelles such as mitochondria. Methods to reduce energy stores include holding the excised clamped sample wrapped in a saline solution–moistened gauze for 15 to 30 minutes at room temperature, placing the clamped muscle in physiologic saline solution for 15 to 20 minutes, or leaving the cadaver in the refrigerator at 4° C for periods up to 1 to 4 days before sampling. To produce a section optimal for histologic examination, muscle samples must not twist or contract during fixation, both of which are likely to occur in unrestrained muscle samples placed in fixative. Muscles taken during rigor will have some myofibers that have moderately to strongly contracted sarcomeres and adjacent myofibers, which are not in rigor, will be thrown into zigzag folds.

After fixation, both transverse and longitudinal sections should be cut from each muscle for histologic examination. The longitudinal section should be cut so that its muscle fibers are parallel and straight. Myofiber diameters and the percentage of abnormal myofibers are most reliably evaluated in transverse sections. However, longitudinal sections reveal the length of changes, such as segmental necrosis and the length of nuclear rows.

Enzyme Histochemistry

Histologic examination of fixed muscles is used routinely for the detection of inflammatory and degenerative changes in muscle, but for many decades, myofiber typing could be done only on frozen sections. Recently, immunohistochemical staining of myosin has been developed for demonstration of myofiber types in formalin-fixed muscle. This is a major advantage because now duplicate samples—one for formalin fixation and the other for freezing—do not have to be taken at the time of necropsy and biopsy, and myofiber typing can now be limited to those muscles in which lesions are confirmed microscopically. Fiber-type staining is absolutely essential for the complete evaluation of muscle. It is most useful in demonstrating preferential involvement of a fiber type, as in some muscular dystrophies or neuropathic changes, such as those due to denervation and reinnervation, resulting in fiber type grouping. Histochemical examination of frozen sections is still extremely useful, as in addition to staining for myosin ATPase (Fig. 9-9, *B*), it is possible to stain for mitochondrial enzyme activity such as those of NADH-TR and succinic dehydrogenase (SDH) as well as for proteins such as dystrophin (Fig. 9-28, *B*). Certain abnormal structures such as nemaline rods formed by expansion of Z bands, as seen in nemaline rod myopathy, are visible only in frozen sections stained by modified Gomori's trichrome stain or by electron microscopy. Full evaluation requires morphometric examination with calculation of the percentage of each fiber type and the mean diameter and standard deviation of each fiber type. By these means, changes in the percentage of each fiber type and atrophy or hypertrophy can be documented.

RIGOR MORTIS

Immediately after the death of an animal, the muscles are still alive biochemically. However, as energy stores are used, a sequence of changes takes place which, after a short period of relaxation, results in contraction and stiffening of muscles that fix the positions of joints. Muscles are usually affected in a specific sequence: jaws, trunk, and then extremities. Rigor passes off in the same order as onset and does not return. Classically, onset begins 2 to 6 hours after death, reaches a maximum at 24 to 48 hours, and passes off in another 48 hours—a total of approximately 4 days. However, rigor mortis is so variable in routine autopsy material as to have little value in interpretation. Variation in the rapidity and severity of rigor can be understood once the basic mechanism is defined.

According to the "sliding-filament" theory, which postulates that, in muscle contraction, actin and myosin filaments slide past each other powered by myosin heads attaching to actin-binding sites, ATP (adenosine triphosphate) is necessary for muscle relaxation after normal contraction. Rigor occurs when the majority of the myosin heads remain attached to actin-binding sites at the end of the "power stroke" because of a deficiency of ATP necessary for their release. ATP can be reconstituted from adenosine diphosphate (ADP), the energy being supplied either by glycolysis or by phosphocreatine. Factors that control the rate of onset of rigor mortis include the amount of glycogen stores, pH of muscle, and body temperature. Thus, if glycogen stores have been reduced by starvation or vigorous muscle contractions, as occurs in animals dying from tetanus, or strychnine poisoning or after being chased during hunting, onset of rigor mortis is rapid. However, in cachectic animals with little or no energy stores, rigor may be slight or in extremely emaciated cases, may not even occur at all. Rigor disappears by autolysis or putrefaction (bacterial decomposition). Thus, the basic factor in the delay in onset and the strength of rigor is the energy stores of the muscle in the form of ATP, phosphocreatine, or glycogen at the time of death. One major practical effect of rigor is to interfere with the histologic examination of muscle.

Table 9-2 Classification of Muscle Disease

Degenerative myopathies
Nutritional
Toxic
Ischemic
Muscular dystrophy
Inflammatory myopathies
Bacterial
Parasitic
Immune-mediated
Metabolic/endocrine/electrolyte-related myopathies
Inherent metabolic problems such as carbohydrate metabolic problems, mitochondrial myopathies, lipid myopathies
Endocrine
Hypothyroidism
Hypercortisolism
Electrolyte
Hypokalemia
Hyperkalemia
Other
Myotonia
Hyperthermia
Disorders of the neuromuscular junction
Myasthenia
Botulism

RESPONSE OF MUSCLE TO INJURY

The response of any organ to injury is the summation of the responses of each of the tissues or cells that compose it. Muscle is composed of myofibers surrounded by blood vessels and fibroblasts (endomysium) and penetrated by blood vessels and nerves. The primary cell to respond to injury is the myofiber. Unfortunately its range of response to insults is extremely limited, and, apart from those involving its nerve supply, the major response of the myofiber is degeneration, necrosis, and regeneration. These responses are the end result of a wide variety of insults—trauma, ischemia, infarction (e.g., bluetongue in sheep resulting from vasculitis), metabolic diseases caused by nutritional deficiencies (e.g., vitamin E, selenium), toxic myopathies (e.g., *Cassia occidentalis* poisoning), and infections such as gas gangrene. Because of this stereotyped response, it is frequently not possible to determine the cause based on gross or histologic lesions alone. Supplementary tests and clinical histories are essential. Thus, classification of muscle diseases based on lesions alone is not very satisfactory, and many classifications are based on etiology (e.g., toxic myopathy, nutritional myopathy). An example of such a classification is given in Table 9-2.

Degeneration

The term "degeneration" in general pathology implies a potentially reversible injury. In muscle pathology, it is loosely and ambiguously applied and includes reversible changes such as the vacuolar degenerations caused by hypokalemia and hyperkalemia, autophagic vacuoles, and, sometimes, even necrosis. In this chapter, the term is used for changes that may or may not lead to myofiber death, for some miscellaneous categories, such as calcification and ossification, which are included by convention, and includes the following:

1. Calcification
2. Ossification
3. "True degenerations": cloudy swelling, hydropic, vacuolar, granular, and fatty
4. Cytoarchitectural changes

Calcification

The causes of calcification are the following:

1. Calcification of necrotic muscle fibers
2. Calcification of fibers in extreme old age
3. Rare cases of macroscopic calcification of unknown cause of parts or most of a muscle
4. Segmental calcification in diseases with defects of the myofiber's plasmalemma, e.g., in canine X-linked muscular dystrophy

Calcification is the next step in the sequence of necrosis of individual myofibers (Fig. 9-3) and is prominent in some domestic animals (e.g., sheep). These deposits may be so dense as to be visible grossly as glistening, chalky-white foci or streaks. Calcification of myofibers has been a common finding in burros over 40 years of age. Macroscopic calcification of a large portion of a muscle is a rarity,

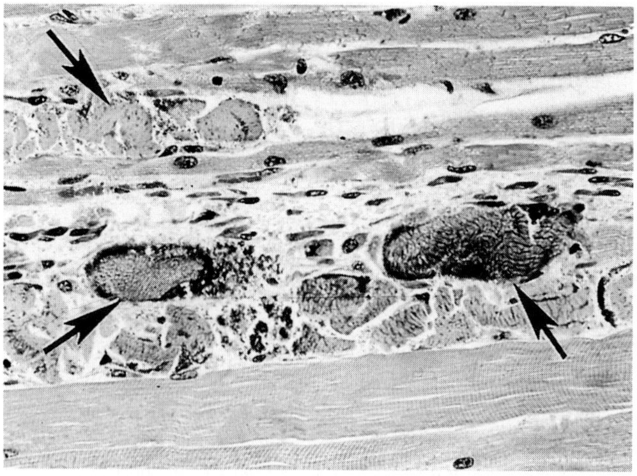

Figure 9-3 Muscle; horse. Calcification. Necrotic segments are undergoing calcification *(arrows)*. Hematoxylin-eosin (H & E) stain. ×250.

but can cause clinical stiffness. The cause is unknown. Ingestion of toxic plants that contain an active vitamin D metabolite *(Cestrum diurum, Solanum malacoxlyn)* causes widespread calcification that sometimes includes tendons and ligaments (*C. diurum* in horses) but apparently does not involve skeletal muscles.

Ossification

In the past, ossification was termed **myositis ossificans,** which in its broadest sense means the formation of nonneoplastic bone, cartilage, or both in extraosseous sites, which may or may not be in muscle. It is essentially a metaplasia to bone. The disease has been reported in horses, pigs, dogs, and cats and is subdivided into progressive and localized forms. The generalized form is better termed **fibrodysplasia ossificans progressiva,** rather than myositis ossificans progressiva, because it is a disorder of connective tissue associated with skeletal muscle, and the muscle itself is only secondarily involved. It has been described in pigs and cats. The porcine disease is inherited, but this link has not been proven in cats. Lesions may replace large portions of the muscle. The histologic appearance is of interlacing bundles of dense, fibrous connective tissue, sometimes containing dense accumulations of calcium, cartilage, and bone. The hyperplastic connective tissue compresses the adjacent skeletal muscles, which undergo atrophy. The localized form is confined to a single muscle or a single group of adjacent muscles and may or may not be associated with a history of trauma, after either single or multiple insults. This type has been seen in horses and dogs. The lesion may have zones. The central zone contains proliferating undifferentiated cells and fibroblasts; the middle one, osteoblast-depositing osteoid and immature bone; and the outer one, trabecular bone that may be being remodeled by osteoclasts.

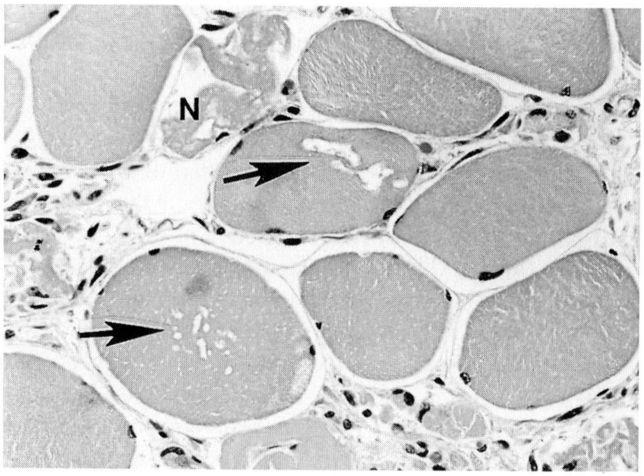

Figure 9-4 Muscle; cow. Early vacuolar degeneration *(arrows)* has already progressed to segmental necrosis *(N)* in an adjacent myofiber. H & E stain. ×250.

True Degenerations

When muscle is insulted metabolically from a wide variety of causes, the final result is frequently segmental necrosis. The muscle fiber may go through a series of degenerations before becoming frankly necrotic, or in some less severely affected fibers, the degenerations may be reversed and the fiber returned to normal. The earliest detectable change starts in the individual myofiber as extremely fine vacuoles that are barely visible by light microscopy. After hours to a day, these vacuoles become larger and are then relatively easy to detect microscopically (Fig. 9-4). If the degeneration is not reversed, the fiber or a segment of it progresses to later stages of what have been termed floccular, granular, hyaline, and Zenker's "degenerations," but all of which represent different stages of necrosis.

Vacuolar degenerations are caused by swelling of organelles or accumulation of glycogen or fat within the myofiber. Exactly which organelle is involved varies. If there is a mild damage to the myofiber, the vacuoles may be autophagic. These phagosomes are membrane-bound vacuoles in which damaged organelles undergo autodigestion by fusion with a lysosome. Glycogen vacuoles occur in Pompe's disease, a glycogen-storage disease seen in cattle. Neutral lipid droplets are present in myofibers in lipid-storage diseases (e.g., that caused by carnitine deficiency). Both hypokalemia and hyperkalemia cause vacuolar degeneration of myofibers, which can lead to overt myofiber necrosis.

Cytoarchitectural Changes

Muscle pathologists recognize a variety of "degenerations" peculiar to myofibers. These include target fibers, central cores, moth-eaten fibers, myofibrillar whorls, tubular aggregates, and nemaline rods. Some of these are visible only in histochemical preparations (e.g., target fibers in sections treated with oxidative enzyme stains), and in other cases the lesions are visible only by electron microscopy.

Necrosis

As myofibers are long, local physical insults cause necrosis of only a segment. Toxic, metabolic, and nutritional myopathies also cause segmental necrosis. Total necrosis of myofibers is rare, occurring in extensive infarcts, massive trauma, and large burns. Thus, segmental myofiber necrosis is present after many different types of insults—a type of "final common pathway." This stage of necrosis quickly merges into the stages of regeneration, described below. Necrotic portions of myofibers have several different histologic appearances. Necrotic portions of the fiber may become floccular or granular as that portion of the myofiber starts to fragment. The adjacent histologically normal portion of the myofiber can separate from the necrotic segment, forming so-called retraction caps. Early in infarction, the necrotic myofiber may fracture at Z lines, causing discoid degeneration. Occasionally, necrotic segments of myofibers are mineralized (Fig. 9-3).

Once the plasma membrane of the myofiber is damaged or a segment of the myofiber becomes necrotic, some of the contents of the muscle cell will "leak out" and be taken up into the blood. The concentrations of some of these components in serum are used as an index of the extent of myofiber damage. The most commonly used is creatine kinase (CK). Aspartate aminotransferase (AST), formerly known as serum glutamic-oxaloacetic transaminase (SGOT), is also released, but it is not as specific an indicator of muscle damage because it is also present in hepatocytes and cardiac myocytes. Because CK has a low renal threshold, it is quickly excreted in the urine. The half-life of AST in the serum is much longer, however, and serum AST concentrations remain elevated for several days following muscle injury. The term "rhabdomyolysis" was coined to replace myoglobinuria and draw attention to the fact that myoglobinuria indicates muscle damage.

Necrosis Secondary to Systemic Diseases

It is well over 100 years since Zenker described segmental hyaline degeneration (Zenker's necrosis) in the muscles of human patients dying of typhoid. Similar changes may occur in other acute infections in human beings and animals. The pathogenesis is not understood. Some may be secondary to toxemia. Experimentally, *Escherichia coli* endotoxin has been shown to cause myofiber necrosis. Lesions are usually not visible grossly and may be difficult to find histologically because they consist of scattered small segments of necrosis and regeneration. Because the necrosis leaves sarcolemmal tubes intact and the necrotic segments are small, regeneration is fast and effective. Segmental necrosis is also present in toxic and endocrine myopathies, and, in human beings, has been reported secondary to liver disease and cancer. Necrosis can be due to infarction caused by a vasculitis (e.g., equine purpura hemorrhagica), to bacterial emboli (*Haemophilus agnio* in lambs) (see Bacterial Myositides), or to ischemia as in recumbency.

Regeneration

Skeletal muscle has considerable ability to regenerate, and, under optimum conditions, a necrotic segment of a muscle fiber can be repaired so that it is indistinguishable from a normal one. However, the success of regeneration depends on the extent and nature of the injury and on whether the integrity of the supporting stroma around the muscle fiber (sarcolemmal tube) is intact. It is convenient to first consider the sequence of events that take place under optimal conditions.

If a portion of the muscle fiber is damaged by, say, a toxin, and the sarcolemmal tube is intact, the sequence of events is as follows, although it has to be recognized that some "stages" overlap with others. These are depicted schematically in Fig. 9-5.

1. In the necrotic segment, the muscle nuclei disappear, and, in hematoxylin-eosin (H & E)-stained sections, the sarcoplasm and myofibrils become hyalinized (eosinophilic, amorphous, and homogeneous), indicating the loss of normal myofibrillar structure (Fig. 9-5, *B*). The necrotic portion may separate from the adjacent viable myofiber during contraction (Figs. 9-5, *C*, and 9-6, *A*). In some species, the necrotic fiber may be mineralized (see Fig. 9-3).
2. Within 24 to 48 hours and usually between 1 and 4 days, monocytes emigrate from capillaries, become macrophages, and enter the necrotic portion of the myofiber (Figs. 9-5, *D*, and 9-6, *B*). Neutrophils may also be present initially, but they rapidly disappear as they die off. Concurrently, the satellite cells, normally located between the basal lamina and the myofiber's plasmalemma, begin to enlarge (Fig. 9-5, *C*), become vesicular with prominent nucleoli, and then undergo mitosis.
3. The proliferated satellite cells move from the peripheral location to the center of muscle fiber, among the macrophages (Figs. 9-5, *D*, 9-6, *B*, and 9-6, *C*).
4. Macrophages lyse and phagocytose necrotic debris and form a clear space in the sarcolemmal tube. At the same time the plasmalemma disappears, and the shape of the sarcolemmal tube is maintained by the basal lamina.
5. Satellite cells form myoblasts, which are embryonic cells defined as those containing myofibrillar protein such as myosin. These fuse with one another to form myotubes, which are thin, elongated muscle cells with a row of central, closely spaced nuclei. They send out cytoplasmic processes in both directions within the sarcolemmal tube (Fig. 9-5, *C*). When the

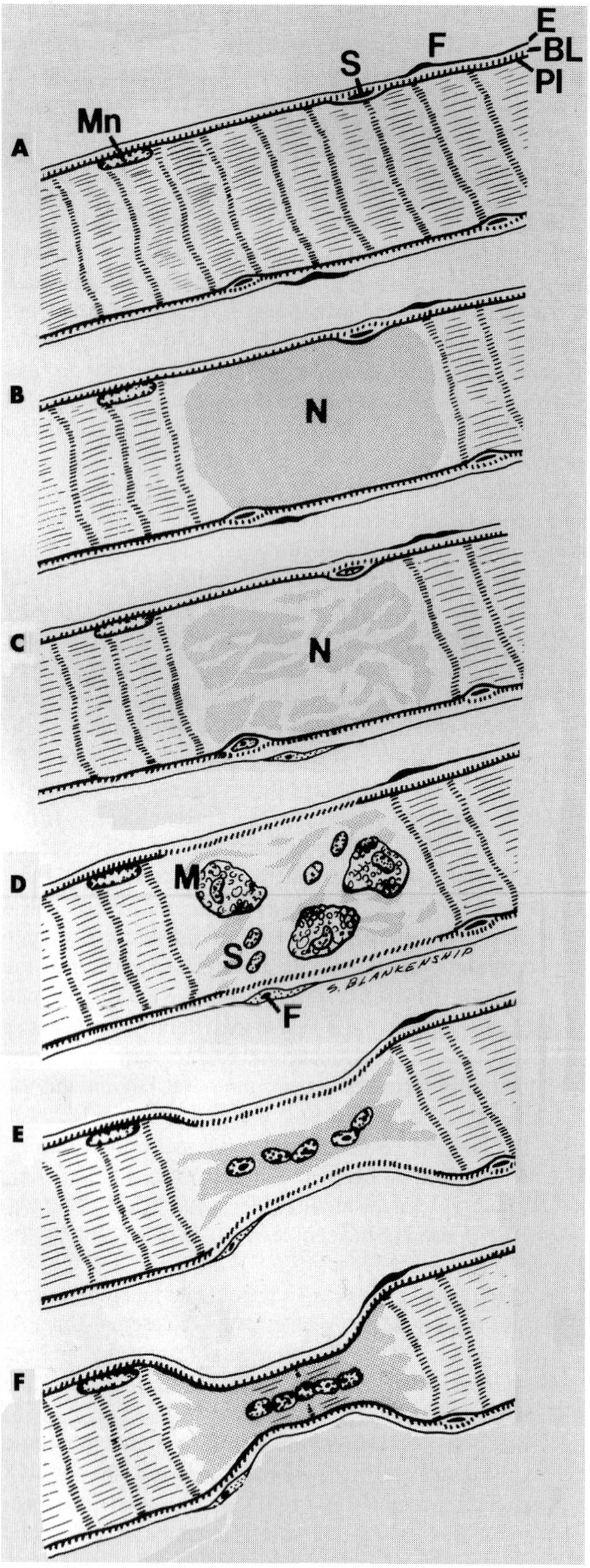

processes contact each other or a viable portion of the original muscle fiber, in most cases they fuse. At this stage, the regenerating fiber is characterized by basophilia, internal nuclei that are sometimes in rows, a lack of striations, and a narrower than normal diameter (Figs. 9-5, *F,* and 9-6, *D*).

6. The fiber grows and differentiates. Its diameter increases, and longitudinal and cross-striations appear, indicating the formation of sarcomeres.
7. Between 1 and 3 weeks after the initial injury, the muscle nuclei move to the "sarcolemmal" or peripheral position—the normal position for muscle nuclei in mature mammalian muscle, but there are species differences. Internal nuclei are retained in rodent muscle, after regeneration.

The success of regeneration depends on the following:

1. The presence of an intact basal lamina to contain and guide the proliferating myotube cells and to keep fibroblasts out.
2. The availability of viable satellite cells as a source of nuclei to undergo mitosis to form myonuclei necessary to initiate the production of sarcoplasm. Normal mature myonuclei have lost this ability. Thus, segmental necrosis in which sarcolemmal tubes are preserved, as in metabolic (nutritional and toxic) myopathies, regenerate very successfully. However, when large areas of satellite cells are killed, for example, by heat or infarction, the situation is very different. In this case, a return to normal is not possible, and healing is chiefly by fibrosis.

Regeneration by Budding

If the insult to the muscle is sufficient to disrupt the myofiber's sarcolemmal tube, as occurs in destructive lesions such as those caused by trauma, infarction, or

Figure 9-5 Schematic representation of segmental myofiber necrosis and regeneration. **A,** Longitudinal section of normal muscle fiber. *BL,* basal lamina; *E,* endomysium; *F,* fibroblast; *Pl,* plasmalemma; *Mn,* muscle nucleus; *S,* satellite cell, which lies between the basal lamina and plasmalemma. **B,** Segmental necrosis. Coagulation necrosis *(N)*. **C,** The necrotic segment of myofiber *(N)* has become floccular and detached from the adjacent viable portion of the myofiber. The satellite cells are enlarging. **D,** The necrotic segment of the myofiber has been invaded by macrophages *(M)* and satellite cells *(S)*. The latter will develop into myoblasts. The plasmalemma of the necrotic segment has disappeared. **E,** Myoblasts have formed a myotube, which has produced sarcoplasm. This extends out to meet the viable ends of the myofiber. The integrity of the myofiber is maintained by the sarcolemmal tube formed by the basal lamina and endomysium. **F,** Regenerating myofiber. Note the reduction in myofiber diameter and central rowing of nuclei. There is early formation of sarcomeres (cross-striations), and the plasmalemma has reformed. Such fibers stain basophilically with H & E.

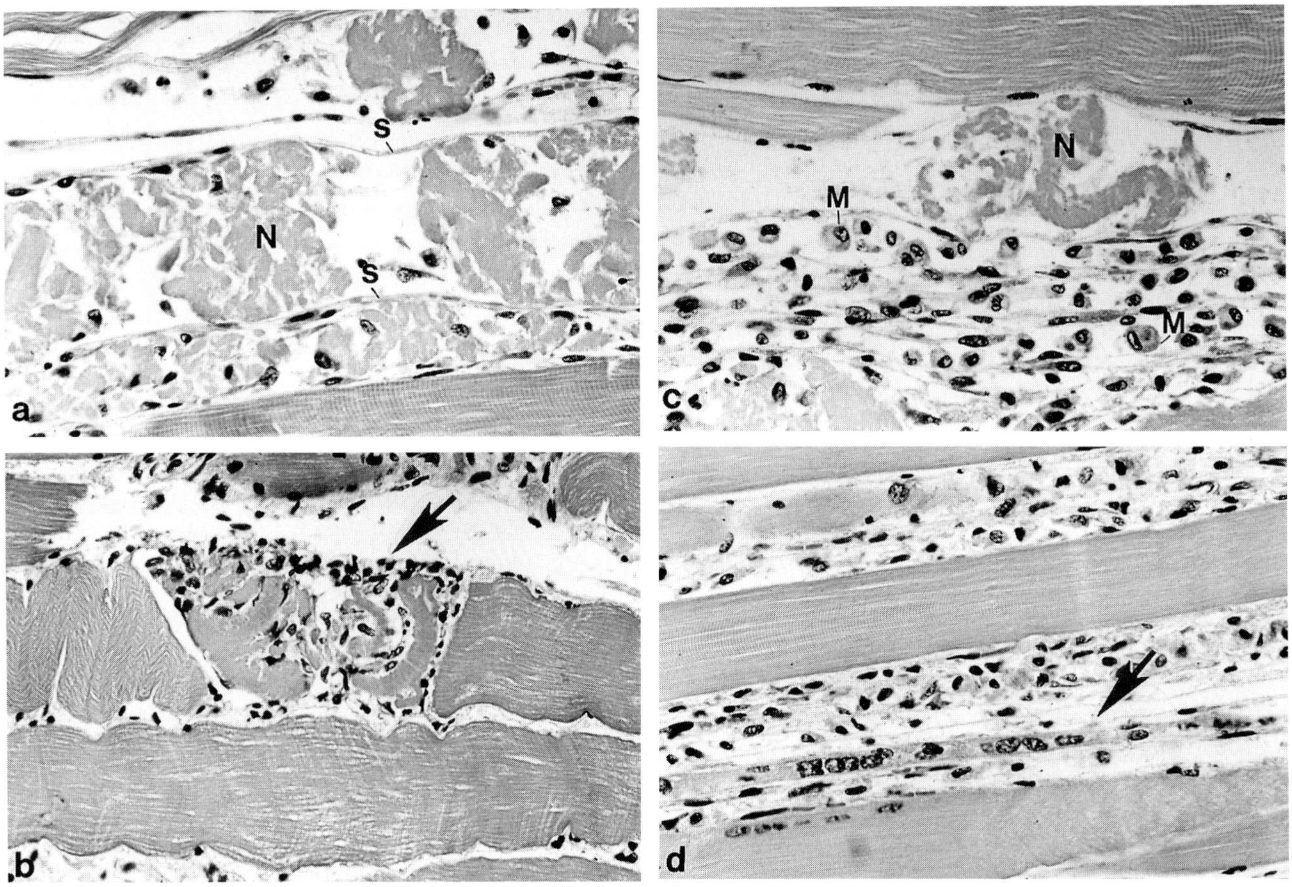

Figure 9-6 **A,** Segmental necrosis. *N,* necrotic segment undergoing "floccular" degeneration. *S,* Sarcolemma. H & E stain. ×250. **B,** Segmental necrosis. At this stage, the necrotic segment *(arrow)* is heavily infiltrated by macrophages and myoblasts, the latter formed from satellite cells. H & E stain. ×250. **C,** *N,* necrotic segment of myofiber. In the two fibers below *N,* necrotic debris has been removed by macrophages *(M).* The other mononuclear cells in the sarcolemmal tubes are satellite cells. H & E stain. ×250. **D,** Regenerating fiber *(arrow).* Note the rows of central nuclei, the narrow diameter, and the dark cytoplasm (which is due to basophilia). Above the regenerating fiber are two necrotic myofibers heavily infiltrated by macrophages and satellite cells. Between them is a normal myofiber. H & E stain. ×250.

injection of irritants, regeneration in those myofibers is by budding. As the myoblasts proliferate and extend to the end of the ruptured tube, sarcoplasm bulges from its cut end and becomes club shaped, with numerous internal nuclei forming a so-called muscle giant cell (Fig. 9-7). Similar cells can also arise from satellite cells remaining in scattered fragments of ruptured muscle fibers. Thus, the presence of muscle giant cells indicates that conditions for regeneration are not optimal. Myotubes are said to be able to bridge gaps of 2 to 4 mm, but any larger ones heal by fibrosis, which reduces the elasticity and the efficiency of contraction of the muscle.

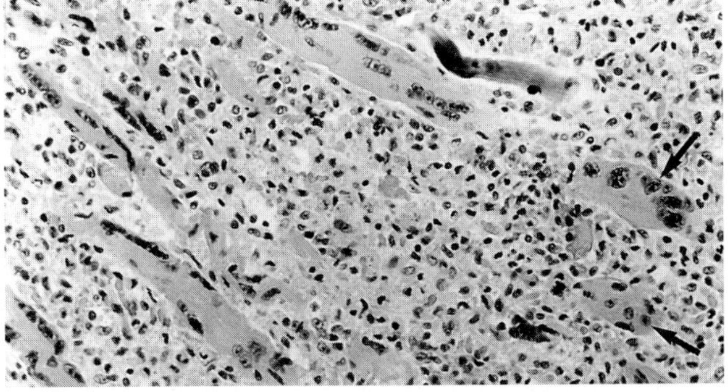

Figure 9-7 Muscle, gracilis; greyhound dog. The muscle ruptured during racing, 4 weeks before euthanasia. Note that healing is by budding (muscle giant cells) *(arrows)* and fibrosis. H & E stain.

Histopathologic Interpretation

Because segmental necrosis and regeneration are such a common result of a wide variety of insults (e.g., overexertion, vitamin E deficiency, and the effects of toxins such as monensin), a histologic diagnosis of "segmental necrosis" is often not helpful in determining the cause of the disease. However, the usefulness of this histologic diagnosis has been increased by Kakulas, who realized the significance of (1) the difference between lesions confined to one or multiple sites and of (2) whether lesions were all at one stage (e.g., segmental necrosis without macrophages) or at different stages (e.g., segmental necrosis and regeneration). As a result, he introduced the concept of **monofocal** (or focal) versus **multifocal** and **monophasic** versus **multiphasic lesions.** Monofocal lesions are those confined to one site and could be the result of a single incident of trauma, such as an intramuscular injection. Most systemic diseases cause necrosis at multiple sites. However, the concept of monophasic versus multiphasic is more useful. If there were only one insult, e.g., a single episode of overly strenuous exercise (exertional myopathy) or a toxin being fed on one occasion (e.g., a horse eating one dose of monensin), then at necropsy, all lesions would be at the same stage of necrosis or regeneration. However, if the insult were ongoing, such as occurs in vitamin E–selenium deficiency or in continuous feeding of a toxin, then new lesions (segmental necrosis) would form at the same time that regeneration was taking place; in other words, it would be a multiphasic disease. Using this approach, it is sometimes possible to rule out a diagnosis (e.g., vitamin E–selenium deficiency is usually multiphasic), but this is not an invariable rule. In cattle with borderline concentrations of vitamin E and selenium and on pasture, a sudden stress can cause a monophasic necrosis.

Changes in Myofiber Size

Under various conditions, myofibers may atrophy or hypertrophy.

Atrophy

The major types of atrophy are the following:

1. Denervation
2. Disuse
3. Malnutrition, cachexia, and senility

The term "atrophy" is used to imply either a reduction in the diameter of the muscle as a whole or in the diameter of a myofiber. In the early stages of atrophy, it may be difficult or impossible to detect loss of muscle mass by gross observation, and morphometric evaluation of myofiber diameters may be required. During growth, additional sarcomeres are added to increase length, and additional myofilaments are added to increase diameter. During atrophy, myofibrils are removed by disintegration, and this results in the sarcolemma being too large; consequently, it is thrown into redundant folds. The rate of atrophy depends not only on the lack of use but also on whether the muscle is still receiving trophic impulses from nerves.

Denervation Atrophy. This atrophy, also known by the misnomer "neurogenic atrophy," is not uncommon in veterinary medicine. Examples are so-called equine roarers, due to laryngeal hemiplegia secondary to damage to the left recurrent laryngeal nerve (Fig. 9-8, *D*). Any interference with the nerve supply to any muscle will result in its atrophy. Under some circumstances, a motor nerve supply can be reestablished, thus reversing the atrophy. Denervation atrophy is particularly rapid, and more than half the muscle mass of a completely denervated muscle can be lost in a few weeks. The histologic picture is best considered from two points of view: the sequence in the denervated myofibers and, secondarily, the changes in the muscle as a whole. The loss of a nerve fiber to a muscle results in atrophy of all myofibers innervated by that nerve. The change is even more dramatic when a whole motor unit is denervated. A motor unit consists of either ventral horn or brain motor neuron and all the myofibers innervated by it. Because the motor neuron determines the histochemical myofiber type, in this case all the atrophic myofibers will be of the same histochemical type (type I or type II) (Fig. 9-1). However, denervating diseases typically involve both type I and type II myofibers and, therefore, atrophy of both type I and type II myofibers in muscle fasciculi is the hallmark of denervation atrophy.

Following denervation, fibers become progressively smaller in diameter as peripheral myofibrils disintegrate. If an atrophic fiber is surrounded by normal fibers, it may be pressed into an angular shape, the so-called small, angular fibers (Fig. 9-8, *A, B*). However, if atrophic fibers are not compressed, they become round in cross section (Fig. 9-8, *C*). These changes are very obvious once denervation has advanced to the stage that atrophic fibers are no longer in contact with adjacent myofibers. The most striking change is the increase in the concentration of myofiber nuclei (Fig. 9-8, *C*). Although myofibrils disappear, muscle nuclei do not do so at the same rate and generally not for a year or so. Thus, the end stage of a denervated myofiber is a cell devoid of myofibrils but consisting of a row of nuclei. As the muscle fibers atrophy, the fibrous stroma of the endomysium and, particularly, the epimysium becomes more prominent because of condensation rather than proliferation. Finally, the contractile elements completely disappear, initially leaving aggregates of myofiber nuclei and, later, empty spaces surrounded by endomysium. Eventually, the endomysium compacts, and the end result is a muscle that consists completely or almost completely of fibrous tissue. Occasionally, atrophic myofibers disappear, and the space is filled by adipocytes, which can cause the muscle to become larger than normal, a condition termed **pseudohypertrophy.** In denervation atrophy, histologic examination of the intramuscular nerves is warranted, as it may reveal loss of myelinated fibers, or in the early stages, axonal degeneration.

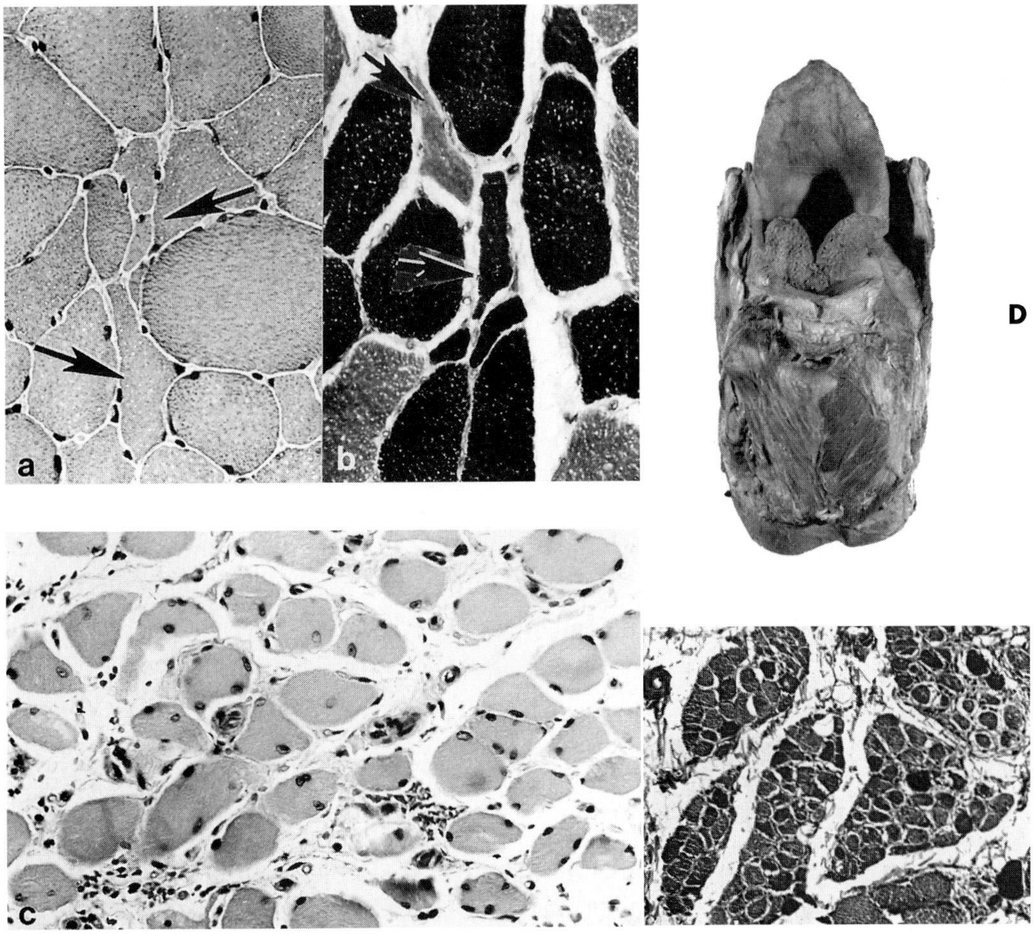

Figure 9-8 Muscle, denervation atrophy. **A,** Early denervation atrophy of several small, angular fibers *(arrows)*. H & E stain. ×250. **B,** Serial section of the same muscle stained with myosin ATPase (pH = 9.8). The atrophic angular fibers *(arrows)*, type I (light) and type II (dark) are a feature of denervation atrophy. ×250. **C,** Vocalis muscle; dog. Several months after denervation. All myofibers are atrophic, rounded, and separated from each other and have numerous muscle nuclei. H & E stain. ×250. **D** and **E,** Left cricoarytenoideus dorsalis muscle; horse with laryngeal hemiplagia. **D,** The left muscle is pale and atrophic. The right is reddish and of normal size. *Courtesy of Prof. D. F. Kelly.* **E,** Note the atrophic myofibers and atrophic fasciculi and the adjacent normal myofibers. *Courtesy of Dr. W. J. Hadlow.*

The extent of changes in the muscle fasciculi depends on how many motor units have been denervated. If all motor units are affected, then all the muscle fibers will atrophy. Such a change could be secondary to the severance of a major nerve, such as a radial nerve. However, if some of the motor units are still intact, then the muscle fasciculi will have a mixture of atrophic and normal myofibers (Fig. 9-8, *E*). If the nerve damage does not incapacitate the animal and the muscle can still be used (e.g., for locomotion), the innervated myofibers not only will retain their normal diameter but also may even become hypertrophied as a result of the increased workload. However, if the animal is incapacitated and cannot use the muscle, then the innervated motor units undergo disuse atrophy and the muscle itself has a mixture of myofibers undergoing both disuse and denervation atrophy.

If the damage is to a single motor unit (e.g., from destruction of its motor neuron or by transection of its nerve fiber), then atrophic fibers will be scattered through one or more fasciculi, depending on the number of myofibers innervated by a single neuron—the size of the motor unit (Figs. 9-1 and 9-8, *D*). Motor units of muscles that have fine motor control, such as the extrinsic muscle of the eye, are small, with as few as 10 myofibers. In large muscles of locomotion where only coarse control is necessary, a motor unit may contain hundreds or even up to 2000 myofibers. Obviously, then, the death of a single ventral horn cell innervating a gluteal muscle would cause extensive denervation atrophy of myofibers. Loss of several motor neurons innervating muscles of the same myofiber type results in a change in the normal checkerboard appearance of a myosin ATPase-stained section.

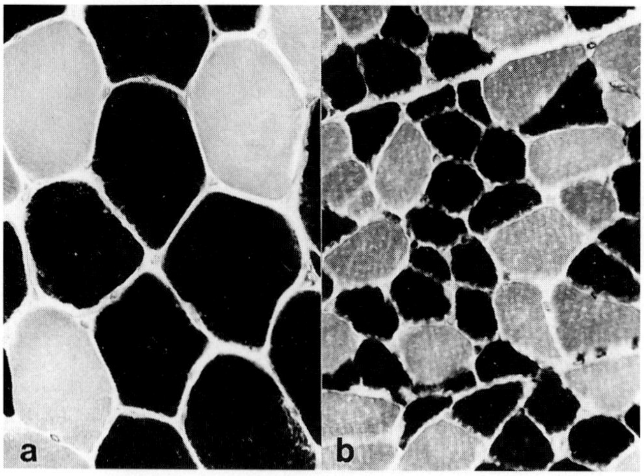

Figure 9-9 Muscle, disuse atrophy; dog. **A,** Normal biceps femoris muscle. **B,** Same muscle, 60 days after forced disuse. Both type I (light) and type II (dark) fibers are atrophic, but the type II fibers are more severely affected. Myosin ATPase (pH = 9.8). ×250.

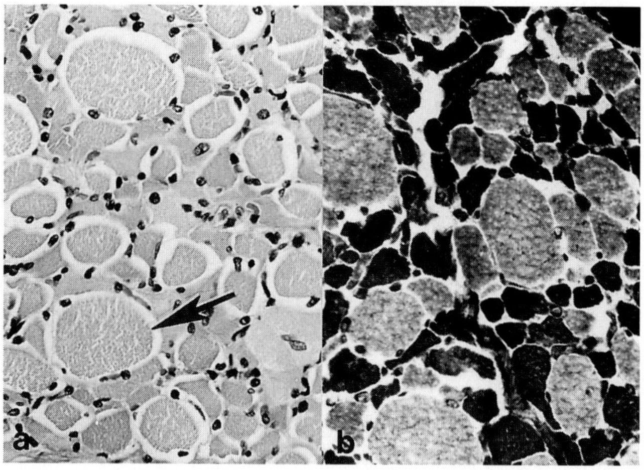

Figure 9-10 Biceps femoris muscle; dog. Emaciation. **A,** All fibers are atrophic, but some *(arrow)* are less severely affected. Note the increased concentration of muscle nuclei. H & E stain. ×250. **B,** Both types I and II fibers are atrophic, but type II (dark) are more severely affected. Some type I (light) fibers are only mildly atrophic. Myosin ATPase (pH = 9.8) stain. ×250.

However, denervated muscle fibers can be reinnervated by subterminal sprouting of fibers from adjacent normal nerves. Frequently these nerves are from a neuron that innervates a different type of myofiber, and, as muscle fiber type is a function of the motor neuron, the newly innervated myofiber will take on the fiber type determined by that neuron. This process results in a loss of the normal arrangement of type I and II myofibers, and the formation of groups of the same fiber type adjacent to each other—so-called **fiber-type grouping** (see Fig. 9-29). Typically this involves an increase in type I myofibers. This effect may be seen in both chronic neuropathic and in myopathic conditions. If the effect is widespread in a fasciculus, it can result in fiber-type predominance. **Fiber-type predominance** is the term applied to muscle in which conversion of fiber type or the loss of one fiber type results in an overall increase in the proportion of a fiber type.

Disuse Atrophy. This results in a less rapid atrophy of muscle than that due to denervation. The cause can be anything that stops the use of the muscle: fractured limbs, failure to use a painful leg, upper motor neuron damage, or recumbency. The loss of the myofibrils has similarities to that of denervation atrophy, but there are differences. Histochemical examination reveals that type II fibers atrophy faster (Fig. 9-9, *A* and *B*). In fact, this occurs so rapidly and frequently that a diffuse type II atrophy is not regarded as having any diagnostic specificity. Disuse atrophy is reversible except when atrophy has been so severe and prolonged that myofibers have been lost.

Atrophy Due to Malnutrition, Cachexia, and Senility. In starvation, muscle protein is metabolized to supply the need for nutrients. This type of muscle atrophy occurs gradually, except in cachexia occurring in some febrile diseases. All muscles of the body are not affected to the same degree (Fig. 9-10, *A*). Postural muscles are spared; type I fibers in these muscles also are spared (Fig. 9-10, *B*), and sometimes a small percentage actually hypertrophy, no doubt as the result of a compensatory hypertrophy from an increased workload. Unlike the case in muscles undergoing denervation atrophy, some muscle nuclei in muscles undergoing this type of atrophy disappear as the volume of the myofiber is reduced. On gross examination, muscles are smaller, thinner, darker, and flabbier than normal, and no fat remains. In muscles with lipofuscinosis, the brown pigment is concentrated, intensifying the brownish discoloration (see Lipofuscinosis).

Hypertrophy

This term is used in two ways: for an increase in the diameter of the muscle as a whole and for an increase in myofiber diameter even if the muscle diameter itself is not enlarged. Increase in muscle fiber diameter is basically caused by an increased workload on those fibers. Hypertrophy is subdivided into two types: **work hypertrophy** and **compensatory hypertrophy.** Work hypertrophy implies an increase in normal physiologic work, as occurs in muscles during athletic training. Compensatory hypertrophy, which is really a type of work hypertrophy by individual fibers, is in response to an increased load caused by the loss or absence of myofibers in a muscle or by denervation atrophy of adjacent myofibers in a muscle fasciculus. Thus, compensatory hypertrophy can be secondary to denervation atrophy, muscular dystrophies,

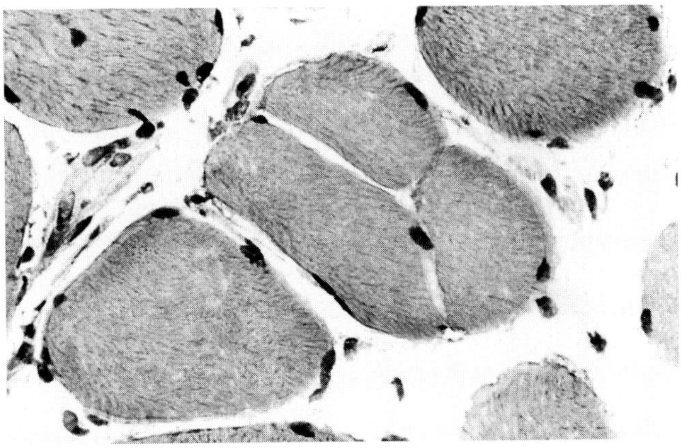

Figure 9-11 Muscle; cat. Muscular dystrophy. Longitudinal myofiber splitting. The hypertrophic myofiber has been divided into three segments, and other myofibers have marked variation in their diameters. H & E stain.

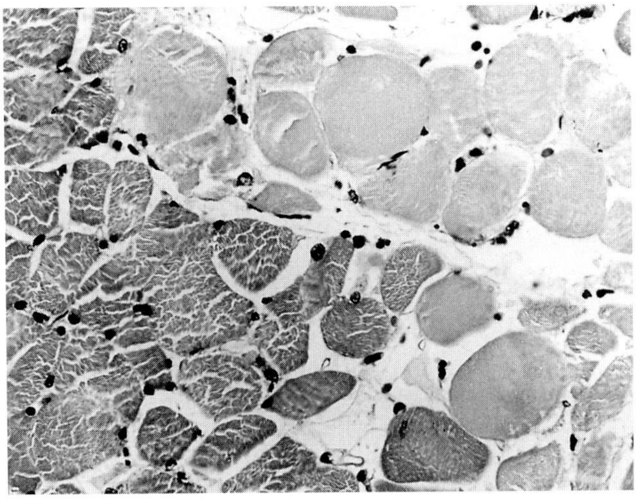

Figure 9-12 Muscle. Infarct. Note that in the infarcted area *(upper right),* all myofibers are necrotic (rounded, hyalinized), and all stromal nuclei are pyknotic, indicating necrosis. H & E stain. ×250.

cachectic atrophy, and extensive necrosis in nutritional or toxic myopathies in which muscles have lost many myofibers.

The exact mechanism modulating hypertrophy is unknown. Myofibers are increased in diameter by the addition of myofilaments. Fibers undergoing compensatory hypertrophy may enlarge to more than 100 μm in diameter. These large-diameter myofibers may undergo longitudinal fiber splitting. In histologic cross sections of muscle, these fibers have a characteristic appearance. The myofiber is divided into 2 to 4 segments that resemble the pieces of a pie (Fig. 9-11). These pieces are usually of different sizes but all still lie within the same endomysial tube. However, the split may not extend the full length of the fiber. Not all longitudinal fiber splitting is believed to be due to increased workload. Some is caused by faulty myofiber regeneration with failure of individual myoblasts to fuse completely.

DISTURBANCES OF CIRCULATION

Congestion

Passive congestion of muscles due to localized or generalized stasis results in dark red to very dark red muscles. An example is the congestion of muscles cranial to the thoracic inlet in bovine ruminal tympany—"bloat." The congestion may be so severe as to resemble hemorrhage on gross examination and presumably is due to an interference with the venous return.

Ischemia

If animals are exsanguinated at necropsy or slaughter, their muscles are pale, actually revealing their true color. Similarly, anemic animals have pale muscles. Because the relatively small energy stores of glycogen and lipid in muscle are rapidly exhausted during exercise, myofibers are well supplied with capillaries. The density of capillaries is greater for type I fibers, which depend on aerobic metabolism, than for type II fibers, which are either glycolytic or mixed oxidative-glycolytic. Athletic training also increases the density of capillaries. The basic factor in determining the effect of ischemia on muscle is the differential susceptibility of the various cells forming the muscle as a whole. Myofibers are the most sensitive, satellite cells less sensitive, and fibroblasts the least sensitive to anoxia. Thus, infarction of an area of muscle leads first to segmental necrosis, then to death of satellite cells, and, finally, to the death of all cells, including the stromal cells (Fig. 9-12). The loss of satellite cells precludes rapid regeneration. Because they are not available to form myoblasts, satellite cells have to be recruited from the edges of viable myofibers. Because all cells in the infarcted muscle die, the result is that most healing takes place by fibrosis and scar formation. Disrupted myofibers at the periphery of the lesion may attempt regeneration by budding.

The basic causes of ischemia are the following:

1. Occlusion of the vascular system
2. External pressure on a muscle
3. Swelling of a muscle in a nonexpandible compartment

Vascular Occlusion

Because of the numerous capillary anastomoses within the muscle and the well-developed collateral circulation, infarction from embolism is rare. Blockage of the iliac arteries by aortic-iliac thrombosis in the horse and of the aortic bifurcation by a "saddle" thromboembolus in the cat can cause ischemia. In the cat, the feet may be cool and cyanotic, and myofibers may undergo segmental necrosis before the collateral circulation can he established. Occasionally, in dogs, *Dirofilaria immitis* (heartworm) may cause a proliferative arteritis and thrombosis of the external and internal iliac arteries and their branches. These lesions produce thromboemboli, some of which cause scattered foci of necrosis (infarcts) in the muscles of the hind limbs. One cause of muscle infarction in sheep is vasculitis caused by the bluetongue virus. Grossly these infarcts appear as fine gray streaks, and foci or hemorrhages may be so small as not to be visible.

Equine purpura hemorrhagica is a sporadic, noncontagious disease of horses (discussed in Myopathies of the Horse). The muscle lesions are infarcts due to a vasculitis, believed to be immune mediated. The disease occurs sporadically in horses recovering from streptococcal infections such as strangles. Muscle infarction may be so extensive as to cause myoglobinuria.

The size of infarcts depends on the size of the vessel obstructed and the duration. Blockage of capillaries causes segmental necrosis, usually multifocal, and if the blockage is prolonged, multiphasic. However, when larger arteries are blocked, whole areas of muscle, including the satellite cells, are killed. Healing is by fibrosis. Intermittent obstruction to a major vessel causes two changes in muscle: (1) myofiber necrosis, and, if these fibers are not regenerated, then the result will be compensatory hypertrophy, chiefly of type I myofibers, which are responsible for bearing much of the weight of the animal; and (2) ischemia of the legs, which may cause a peripheral neuropathy. If nerves are irreversibly damaged, denervation atrophy of the muscles will result.

External Pressure on Muscle

Prolonged periods of recumbency, such as during anesthesia or in animals unable to rise, or too tightly fitting plaster casts or bandages can put external pressure on muscles. Postanesthesia myopathy is seen, particularly in horses anesthetized for long periods. The location of the lesions depends on the position of the horse during anesthesia. In dorsal recumbency the gluteals and the longissimus muscles are ischemic; in lateral recumbency in the lower leg muscles—triceps brachii, pectoralis, deltoideus, and brachiocephalicus—are ischemic. The basic mechanism is that the pressure in the muscle exceeds the perfusion pressure in the capillaries. The use of adequate padding and the maintenance of blood pressure during anesthesia has greatly reduced the incidence of postanesthetic myopathy in horses. Muscle infarction is frequently seen in "downer" cows, where the weight of the body of the animal in ventral recumbency causes ischemia of the pectoral muscles and of any muscles of the fore or hind limbs tucked under the body. Ewes in advanced pregnancy with twins or triplets develop an ischemic necrosis of the internal abdominal oblique muscle, and this can lead to rupture. The duration of ischemia determines the severity of necrosis and the success of regeneration (see Necrosis). In the case of the postanesthesia myopathy, the lesion is a monophasic, multifocal necrosis. In the downer cow, the lesions are also multifocal, but may be polyphasic if the animal has been recumbent for days to weeks.

Swelling of Muscle in a Nonexpandible Compartment

In human beings an **anterior tibial syndrome** or anterior tibial compartment syndrome sometimes follows exercise. The pathogenesis is believed to be due to swelling of the pretibial muscles, which are surrounded (cranially) by the inelastic anterior fascial sheath and (caudally) by the tibia. Swelling impedes the blood supply, and in very severe cases, unless the pressure is relieved by fasciotomy, the muscle will become infarcted. A similar mechanism causes infarction of the supracoracoid muscle of some breeds of turkeys and chickens after they flap their wings. Thus, vigorously exercised muscles enclosed in thick fascial sheaths may be susceptible to this type of infarction. It should be realized, however, that even normal myofibers may be damaged by contraction during extremely strenuous exercise. Evidence of this is the rise in the concentration of serum creatine kinase in the 24 hours following vigorous exercise.

MYOSITIS

Inflammation of muscle, termed myositis (plural: myositides), can be caused by a wide array of agents—bacteria, viruses, protozoa, and helminths—or it can be due to immune-mediated mechanisms.

The term "myositis" has been inappropriately applied to various veterinary disorders such as exertional and masseter "myositis" in the horse. These two disorders are degenerative myopathies, not inflammatory myopathies. It is vitally important to distinguish between a true myositis and a degenerative myopathy in which there is segmental necrosis. In the normal response to the necrosis, the necrotic segment is infiltrated by macrophages (Figs. 9-5 and 9-6), which "clean up" the cellular debris. Severe acute necrotizing myopathy may even be accompanied by a certain degree of infiltrating lymphocytes, plasma cells, neutrophils, and even eosinophils. Cytokines released from damaged muscle fibers are likely to recruit a variety of inflammatory cells under various circumstances, but these cells are not involved in the muscle cell damage. True myositis occurs when inflammatory cells are directly responsible for initiating and maintaining myofiber injury.

Bacterial Myositides

Bacterial infections of muscle are not numerous, but bacteria may cause suppurative (pyogenic bacteria), serohemorrhagic (clostridia), or granulomatous lesions (Table 9-3). Infection may be introduced by direct penetration (wounds or injections), hematogenously, or by spread from an adjacent cellulitis, fasciitis, tendinitis, arthritis, or osteomyelitis.

Table 9-3 Bacterial and Parasitic Myopathies

Infectious Agent	Species Affected
Clostridium sp. causing myositis	Horses, cattle, sheep, goats, pigs
Clostridium botulinum (botulism)	Horses, cattle, sheep, goats
Pyogenic bacteria	Cattle, sheep, goats, pigs
Streptococcus equi	Horses
Sarcocystis sp.	Cattle, sheep, goats
Neosporum caninum	Dogs
Trichinella spiralis	Pigs

Pyogenic bacteria introduced into a muscle usually cause a localized suppuration and myofiber necrosis. This may resolve completely or become localized to form an abscess or, in some cases, the infection may spread down the fascial planes. For example, a nonsterile intramuscular injection into the gluteal muscles may cause a myositis that extends down the fascial planes of the muscles of the femur and tibia and erupt to the surface through a sinus, proximal to the tarsus. Although the majority of inflammation is serous or seropurulent and involves fascial planes, some bacteria extend into and cause necrosis of adjacent muscle fasciculi. *Streptococcus equi* (horses), *Arcanobacterium pyogenes* (cattle and sheep), and *Corynebacterium pseudotuberculosis* (sheep and goats) are common causes of muscle abscesses. *S. equi* in horses can also cause myopathy as a result of immune-mediated vasculitis or muscle necrosis and wasting (see Myopathies of Horses). After bite wounds, cats may develop a cellulitis due to *Pasteurella multocida* that extends into the adjacent muscle. Clostridia may produce a serous or serohemorrhagic cellulitis or cellulitis and myositis.

Granulomatous Myositides

This usually takes the form of single or multiple granulomas (focal granulomatous myositis) and is relatively rare. It may be caused by *Mycobacterium bovis* (tuberculosis), usually in cattle and swine, *Actinobacillus lignieresi* (wooden tongue in cattle), *Actinomyces bovis,* and *Staphylococcus aureus* (botryomycosis in horses). Rarely, infection by *Sarcocystis* spp. may cause a granulomatous myositis of the tongue in horses.

Tuberculosis

Tuberculosis is rare in North America. Lesions are yellowish, variably sized spherical nodules with yellowish caseous contents usually enclosed in a thick fibrous capsule. Microscopically, the lesion is a granuloma with central necrosis surrounded by epithelioid and giant cells.

Actinobacillosis

Actinobacillosis (*Actinobacillis lignieresi,* wooden tongue in cattle) usually is due to the direct penetration of the tongue by the bacterium, which produces small, pale granulomas that contain "sulfa granules" composed of masses of gram-negative rods. This disease has also been reported in the tongue and the muscles of the rear limbs of a dog.

Table 9-4 Viral Myopathies

	RNA Viruses	
Disease	Family	Causal Agent
Porcine encephalomyelitis	Picornaviridae	Enterovirus
Foot-and-mouth disease	Picornaviridae	Aphthovirus
Bluetongue	Reoviridae	Orbivirus
Akabane disease	Bunyaviridae	Akabane virus

Actinomyces bovis

Actinomyces bovis produces a granulomatous osteomyelitis in the mandible or maxilla of cattle. The lesion may extend into adjacent muscles, including the masseter. Lesions have caseous to suppurative centers, surrounded by epithelioid cells and giant cells. The central exudate contains "sulfa granules" in which are gram-positive rods and branching filaments.

Botryomycosis

In horses and pigs, *Staphylococcus aureus* can cause a low-grade, persistent infection that becomes granulomatous. The disease is called botryomycosis in the horse and is usually the result of wounds. Lesions are fibrous nodules present in the muscles of the head, sternocephalicus, pectoral region and, less often, the back and thighs. In pigs, the lesions may be in castration wounds or mammary glands. The nodules are hard and have a fibrous capsule that enclosed a cavity containing yellow-brown pus and granules. Histologically, the lesions are encapsulated granulomas containing central "club" colonies in which there are demonstrable staphylococci. The granulomas can extend peripherally to involve adjacent muscles.

Fungal Granulomatous Myositis

This rare disease is mentioned here for convenience. Occasionally, *Blastomyces dermatitidis* causes lesions in the laryngeal mucosa. These may extend into the adjacent intrinsic muscles of the larynx, causing a granulomatous myositis. It has not been determined whether the infection is spread hematogenously or by direct penetration of fungi coughed up from the lungs.

Viral Myositides

Relatively few of these are recognized in veterinary medicine. Spontaneous ones are listed in Table 9-4. Gross lesions may or may not be visible and, if present, are small poorly defined foci or streaks. Muscle lesions induced by viruses are either infarcts secondary to a vasculitis, as seen in bluetongue in sheep, or multifocal necrosis, presumably because of a direct effect of the virus on the myofibers. The latter type of lesion is seen in infections by different enteroviruses (porcine encephalomyelitis, coxsackievirus, and poliovirus) and foot-and-mouth disease virus.

Porcine Encephalomyelitis

Porcine encephalomyelitis is due to a coronavirus of the *Enterovirus* genus. Besides the destruction of the neurons, which results in paralysis, the virus may also cause multifocal necrosis of myofibers, accompanied by a focal interstitial and perivascular infiltrate of lymphocytes, macrophages, and a few neutrophils.

Foot-and-Mouth Disease

The major lesions are vesicles in the skin and mucous membranes. Besides these, the heart and skeletal muscles may have yellow streaks and gray foci, which microscopically are areas of segmental myofiber necrosis accompanied by an intense lymphocytic and neutrophilic infiltration.

Akabane Virus

Akabane virus of the family Bunyaviridae can produce a nonsuppurative myositis in the bovine fetus.

Bluetongue

Bluetongue, caused by a virus of the family Reoviridae, is a noncontagious, insect-borne viral disease that causes vasculitis in a wide array of tissues, particularly the oral mucosa. Gross lesions in muscles are foci of necrosis (infarctions) and hemorrhage. Depending on the age of the lesions, necrosis, calcification, or regeneration may be present. Because of the size of the infarcts, regeneration is usually by muscle giant cells and fibrosis.

Parasitic Myositides

Parasitic infections of the skeletal muscles of domestic animals are not common. The most important ones are listed in Table 9-3. Most diseases are of little economic importance, with the exception of *Trichinella spiralis* in swine (see Myopathies of Swine).

Ancylostoma caninum Larva Migrans

The larval forms of *A. caninum* migrate somatically and, on entering the muscles of paratenic hosts, development is arrested. The larvae cause inflammation and myonecrosis. As they continue to migrate, they leave a trail of segmentally necrotic myofibers and inflammation.

Visceral Larva Migrans

This has been defined as "the invasion of, and migration through, any of the tissues of the animal body by a nematode larvae." *Toxocara canis* larvae migrate through numerous tissues of the dog. Some larvae are arrested, and granulomas form around them. These have been found in a wide array of tissues, including kidney, liver, lung, myocardium, and skeletal muscle. The lesion in muscle is a focal granulomatous myositis, with the larvae and granulomas lying between myofibers.

Dirofilaria immitis

In dogs, larvae of this nematode may be present in the external and internal iliac arteries and their branches. Thromboemboli from debris and parasites may cause multiple infarcts in the muscles of the hind limbs (see Ischemia).

Cysticercosis

A cysticercus is a larva with a solid caudal portion and a bladderlike proximal portion. It is the intermediate stage in the life cycle of several tapeworms. *Taenia solium* and *Taenia saginata,* both tapeworms of human beings, have a cysticercus stage in the pig *(Cysticercus cellulosae)* and cattle *(Cysticercus bovis),* respectively. These cysticerci preferentially lodge in the heart, masseter, and tongue, where they appear as small white or gray cysts. Histologically, there is displacement of myofibers by the cyst but little myositis; there may be a few lymphocytes, macrophages, and eosinophils around the cyst, which lies in the interstitial tissue, not in the myofiber (see Fig. 9-25). With time, the immunologic system of the host kills the cysticercus. *C. cellulosae* in pigs may become calcified. *Cysticercus ovis* in the heart and shoulder muscles of sheep and goats is the intermediate stage of *Taenia ovis,* a tapeworm of dogs.

Polymyositis

Although the word "polymyositis" etymologically simply means inflammation involving more than one muscle, the term is often reserved for those inflammatory myopathies (myositises) in which an immune-mediated mechanism is involved or believed to be involved. These are listed in Table 9-8.

CONGENITAL, NEONATAL, AND HEREDITARY DISEASES

Muscle is subject to numerous hereditary, congenital, and neonatal defects (Table 9-5). These are discussed in specific detail under the myopathies of each species of domestic animal.

Muscular Dystrophy

The term "muscular dystrophy" is highly ambiguous in veterinary literature. It was introduced in human pathology to define a group of inherited progressive muscle diseases. Unfortunately, in the 1930s the term *nutritional muscular dystrophy* was applied to nutritional myopathy due to vitamin E deficiency. This should have been termed *nutritional myopathy* or *nutritional myodegeneration.* Muscular dystrophy has been defined by Adams as a progressive, hereditary, degenerative disease of skeletal muscles. The innervation of the affected muscles is intact. The relative inadequacy of regenerative activity is a fundamental characteristic. Thus, it is presumed that the primary defect in muscular dystrophy is in the myofiber itself. The progressive nature of the disease separates it

Table 9-5 Confirmed or Suspected Inherited or Congenital Myopathies

Disorder	Species Affected	Inheritance
Myotonia	Horses	Unknown
	Goats	Autosomal dominant
	Dogs	Autosomal recessive
	Cats	Unknown
HYPP	Horses	Autosomal dominant
Glycogenoses	Horses	Unknown
	Cattle	Autosomal recessive
	Sheep	Autosomal recessive
	Cats	Autosomal recessive
	Dogs	Autosomal recessive
Muscular dystrophy	Sheep	Autosomal recessive
	Dogs, cats	X-linked recessive
Malignant hyperthermia	Horses	Unknown
	Pigs	Autosomal recessive
	Dogs	Autosomal dominant
Labrador myopathy	Dogs	Autosomal recessive
Phosphofructokinase deficiency	Dogs	Autosomal recessive
Steatosis	Cattle	Unknown
Double muscling	Cattle	Autosomal recessive
Diaphragmatic dystrophy	Cattle	Autosomal recessive
Congenital myasthenia gravis	Dogs	Autosomal recessive
	Cats	Autosomal recessive (?)

from the benign, relatively nonprogressive congenital muscle disorders, such as central core, nemaline, mitochondrial, and myotubular myopathies. Muscular dystrophies are a subgroup within the inherited diseases of muscle.

Muscular dystrophy in animals has been recognized in cattle, sheep, mice, chickens, hamsters, dogs, and cats. In human beings the disease is divided into major subtypes based on age of onset, group of muscles affected, histologic appearance, and type of inheritance. Some animal models such as the X-linked muscular dystrophy of dogs, cats, and mice have proven to be genetically homologous animal models of Duchenne dystrophy. As in human beings, muscular dystrophy in animals also preferentially involves groups of muscles (vastus intermedius in sheep, diaphragm in Meuse-Rhine-Yssel cattle), and, sometimes, a specific fiber type (type I in sheep).

Storage Diseases

There are different types of glycogen storage diseases, dependent on which enzyme is deficient. Those diseases in which glycogen accumulates in muscle have been described in horses, cattle, sheep, cats, and dogs (Table 9-5). Of these, six cause glycogen accumulation in muscle, and of the glycogenoses, only types II, III, and VII have been recognized in animals.

TRAUMA

External trauma to muscle includes bruising (crushing with hemorrhage), laceration (tearing), surgical incisions, burns, gunshot and arrow wounds, and certain injections. Some of these may result in complete or partial rupture of large muscles. Rupture is common as the result of automobile accidents. The diaphragm is frequently ruptured as a result of a sudden increase in intraabdominal pressure. A partial rupture of a muscle results in a rent in the fascial sheath, through which the muscle can herniate during contraction. In racing greyhounds, spontaneous rupture of muscles such as the longissimus, quadriceps, biceps femoris, gracilis, triceps brachii, and gastrocnemius can occur during strenuous exercise. Tearing **(myorrhexis)** of muscle fibers occurs in the adductor muscles of cattle doing the "splits" on a slippery floor.

Healing of these traumatic wounds follows the principles laid down in the section on Regeneration. Because there is often extensive interruption of sarcolemmal sheaths, most of the healing is accomplished by budding and fibrosis (see Fig. 9-7), with resultant compromise in the physiologic efficiency of the muscle. Collagen is inelastic, and thus large scars inevitably reduce the contractibility of adjacent myofibers. Cleanly transected fibers heal by scarring, and this results in essentially two separate contractile units joined by a scar whose work efficiency will be less than that of the original single myofiber. If muscle trauma is accompanied by fractures of bones, and the animal moves the limb, this may result in further trauma by the sharp bone fragments.

Thus, in muscle trauma, damage is due to direct transection of myofibers, compression of myofibers with destruction of the sarcoplasm, and secondarily from hemorrhage. The latter may increase intramuscular pressure, resulting in ischemia and further necrosis (infarction).

NEOPLASIA

Theoretically, neoplasms arising in muscle can form from any of the components of muscle: myofibers; mesenchymal tissue such as fibrous, myxomatous, or adipose tissue; blood vessels; or nerve sheaths. Actually, neoplasms of skeletal muscle—benign, malignant, or metastatic—are rare in domestic animals. The majority of benign muscle tumors, **rhabdomyomas** in the pig ox and sheep, have been cardiac, but laryngeal rhabdomyomas are recognized in the dog. Because of the granular eosinophilic cytoplasm and the large numbers of mitochondria seen by electron microscopy, these tumors were originally diagnosed as oncocytomas. Grossly, the tumors are unencapsulated and lobulated. Microscopically, they are composed of large granular cells that stain positively for myoglobin and desmin by immunoperoxidase techniques. Z-band material can be seen by electron microscopy.

Rhabdomyosarcomas are rare. Most cases have been in dogs. These tumors are usually highly malignant and metastasize either via the lymphatic or venous routes.

Thus, metastases appear in lymph nodes, lungs, and spleen, and also in heart and skeletal muscles. Grossly, they are pink unencapsulated masses. The histologic appearance of rhabdomyosarcomas varies enormously. Some have cells in which the characteristic cross-striations are found easily, whereas others are composed of undifferentiated cells with no visible striations (Fig. 9-13). Many pathologists are uncomfortable in diagnosing a rhabdomyosarcoma without seeing striations. These can be revealed most clearly in histologic sections with iron hematoxylin (Weigert's or Heidenhain's) or with Mallory's phosphotungstic acid–hematoxylin (PTAH) stains. However, searching for cross-striations in undifferentiated tumors is time consuming. A rapid, reliable method of diagnosing muscle tissue is to demonstrate the presence of myoglobin and skeletal muscle actin using the immunoperoxidase method, as only cardiac and skeletal muscle contain both these proteins.

Muscles can also be invaded locally by carcinomas and sarcomas as they proliferate and increase in size. For example, in the dog, squamous cell carcinomas of the vulva may extend into the pelvic musculature. Bovine extraocular squamous cell carcinoma may infiltrate into the adjacent orbicularis oculi muscle, and mammary adenocarcinomas and mast cell tumors occasionally extend into the adjacent cutaneous muscle.

Infiltrative lipomas are tumors of mature adipocytes in dogs. They are usually deep in the subcutis or muscles. The tumor cells tend to infiltrate along fascial planes but also extend into muscles. Grossly, muscles are soft, and muscle fasciculi are separated by yellow fat. Histologically, the mass consists of well-differentiated adipose cells. The tumor is benign, but because of the infiltrative margins, it is difficult to excise and can recur.

Rarely, skeletal muscle is invaded by local mesenchymal tumors such as hemangiosarcomas, fibrosarcomas, and myxosarcomas that have arisen either in adjacent tissue or in the muscle's stroma. Tumors metastatic to muscle are rare, but malignant lymphoma (Fig. 9-14), hemangiosarcoma, pulmonary adenocarcinoma (Fig. 9-15), and pulmonary squamous cell carcinoma have occurred in the dog.

MYOPATHIES OF THE DOMESTIC ANIMALS

These are discussed by species because this is the way diseases are considered clinically. The same disease may

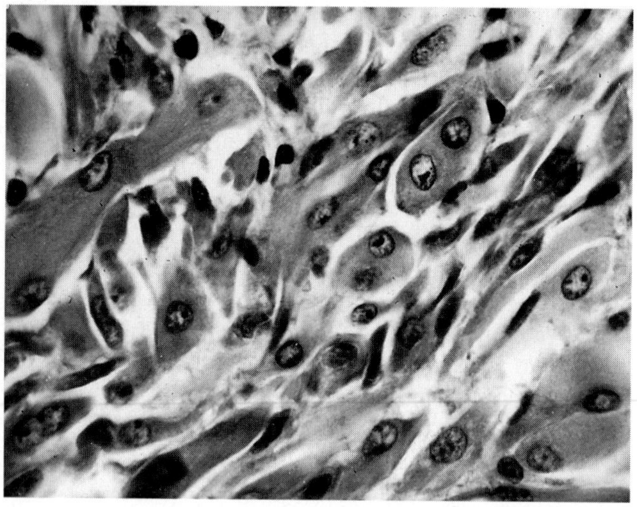

Figure 9-13 Thigh muscles; mouse. Rhabdomyosarcoma. Multinucleated pleomorphic cells. Cross-striations are not evident. H & E stain. ×475. *Courtesy Dr. W. J. Hadlow.*

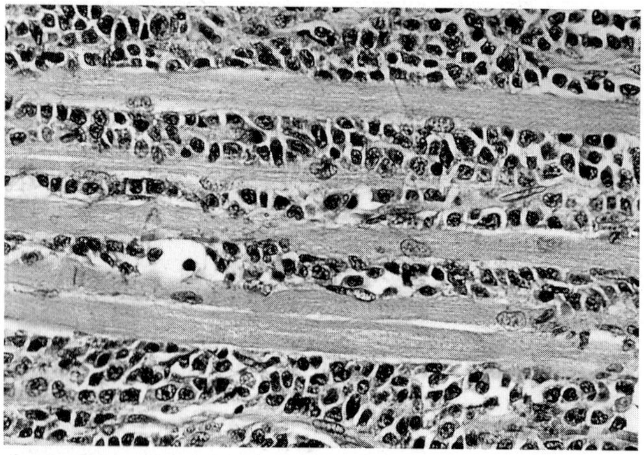

Figure 9-14 Muscle, periorbital; monkey. Malignant lymphoma. Numerous lymphoid cells lie between the myofibers, which subsequently atrophy and disappear. H & E stain.

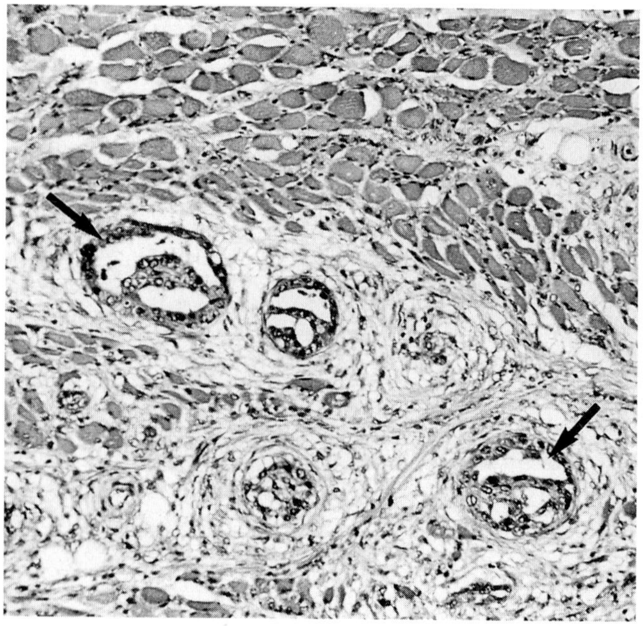

Figure 9-15 Muscle, diaphragm; dog. Bronchiogenic carcinoma *(arrows)*. The neoplasm had extended into the parietal pleural and diaphragm. H & E stain.

occur in different species. Tables 9-6 and 9-7 list the nutritional, toxic, metabolic, endocrine, and electrolyte myopathies in different species.

Myopathies of the Horse

Bacterial and Parasitic Myopathies

Clostridial Myositis ("Malignant Edema"). Clostridial myositis in the horse ("malignant edema") can be caused by infection with *Clostridium perfringens, Clostridium septicum,* or *Clostridium chauvoei,* which are large gram-positive anaerobic bacilli. Clinical signs are acute onset of heat, swelling, and pain within a muscle group and adjacent fascia, with concurrent fever, depression, dehydration, and anorexia. If sufficient muscle necrosis is present, serum CK and AST concentrations may be mildly to moderately increased. Death from toxemia/septicemia often occurs within 48 hours. *Clostridium* spp. are ubiquitous organisms that form spores within the soil and can contaminate deep, penetrating wounds, such as injections or puncture wounds. Under anaerobic conditions clostridia proliferate and produce toxins that damage blood vessels, resulting in hemorrhage and edema, and cause necrosis of adjacent muscle fibers. Affected muscle and adjacent fascia are swollen and often hemorrhagic, with edema, necrosis, and gas. Blood vessels are necrotic, but vasculitis is not seen. "Bubbles" due to gas production may be present. Gram-positive bacilli *Clostridium* spp. are generally demonstrable within affected tissue.

The diagnosis can be made with reasonable certainty based on typical historical, gross, and histopathologic findings. Cytologic examination of aspirates of affected muscle reveal gram-positive bacilli in some cases. *Clostridium* spp. may be identified by culture on anaerobic media or by fluorescent antibody testing.

Table 9-6 Nutritional and Toxic Myopathies

Disorder	Species Affected	Cause
Nutritional myopathy	Horses, cattle, sheep, goats, pigs	Selenium, or vitamin E deficiency
Ionophore toxicity	Horses, cattle, sheep, goats, pigs	Monensin, other ionophores used as feed additives
Plant toxicity	Horses, cattle, sheep, goats, pigs	*Cassia occidentalis,* other toxic plants

Table 9-7 Myopathies Due to Metabolic, Endocrine, and Electrolyte Abnormalities

Disorder	Species Affected
Hypokalemia	Cattle, cats
Hypophosphatemia	Cattle
Hypernatremia	Cats
Mitochondrial defects	Dogs, horses
Hypothyroidism	Dogs
Hypercortisolism	Dogs

***Clostridium botulinum* (Botulism).** Botulism is not due to an infection with *C. botulinum,* a gram-positive anaerobic bacillus, but rather to the effect of its toxin, which can be ingested whole or produced in the gut or rarely at the sites of wounds contaminated by *C. botulinum.* Horses are exquisitely sensitive to botulinum toxins. Profound generalized flaccid paralysis is the hallmark of botulism. Clinical signs are acute and progress rapidly, generally resulting in recumbency. Dysphagia and tongue weakness are common findings that help to distinguish botulism from other neuromuscular diseases causing recumbency. Serum concentrations of CK and AST are within normal limits (indicating the absence of damage to myofibers) or are possibly slightly increased as a result of ischemic myopathy secondary to recumbency (see below).

C. botulinum bacteria are found within the gastrointestinal tract of many mammals and their spores are in soil. Preformed toxin within contaminated feed can be ingested to cause botulism in adult horses. In foals 2 weeks to 8 months of age, ingestion of *C. botulinum* spores may lead to proliferation of toxin-producing *C. botulinum* within the intestinal tract resulting in toxicoinfectious botulism ("shaker foals"). Wound infection is an uncommon cause of botulism. Toxins produced by *C. botulinum* bind irreversibly to the presynaptic nerve terminals, preventing release of acetylcholine, thus causing flaccid paralysis. No specific gross or histopathologic lesions are present in horses dying with botulism, although aspiration pneumonia due to dysphagia can occur. Muscle fibers are intact unless recumbency has compromised their blood supply causing ischemia and regional myofiber necrosis.

Horses are exquisitely sensitive to botulinum toxin; only small concentrations of the toxin may be present in the horse. Available tests may not detect such a low concentration of toxin. Evaluation of stomach contents or contaminated feed may reveal the presence of toxin. In most equine cases, however, these analyses are unrewarding. The diagnosis is generally made based on the clinical history after elimination of other possible causes of profound muscular weakness. Affected animals should be treated with polyvalent botulinum antitoxin to prevent further binding of toxin. Recovery occurs following terminal axon sprouting and reestablishment of functional neuromuscular junctions. Vaccination with botulinum toxoid is an effective preventative measure.

***Streptococcus*-Associated Myopathy.** In this disease, the muscle damage is not caused by the direct infection of the muscles, but rather by an immune response to the streptococcus. Signs of myopathy often accompany systemic signs of poststreptococcal purpura in horses (i.e., depression, fever, dependent edema, petecchiae or ecchymoses, leukocytosis, increased serum fibrinogen, and anemia), but may be the primary presenting disease. Affected horses are weak, depressed, may have a short-strided gait or become recumbent, with myoglobinuria and marked increases in serum concentrations of CK and AST. Circulating immune complexes composed of IgA antibodies and streptococcal M antigen deposit in small vessels. This leads to vasculitis (Fig. 9-16) and vascular wall necrosis, with resultant hemorrhage and infarction of myofibers. Antibodies to streptococcal M protein may also cross-react with skeletal and cardiac muscle myosins to cause direct injury. Multiple muscles are involved (as opposed to the locally extensive lesion of clostridial myositis), containing multifocal to locally extensive hemorrhage and edema that dissect between necrotic muscle fibers, similar to that seen in clostridial myositis. Lesions are exudative and do not contain gas bubbles. Vasculitis (Fig. 9-16), the diagnostic feature, results in infarction with large areas of coagulation necrosis in muscle. Streptococcal organisms are not present within affected muscle. Diagnosis is based on a history of exposure to *Streptococcus equi,* clinical signs of purpura, signs of muscle weakness with associated marked increase in serum concentrations of CK and AST, and typical lesions of infarction secondary to vasculitis. Because this is an immune-complex disorder, bacterial cultures of affected muscle do not reveal *S. equi,* but this organism may be cultured from other affected tissues, especially lymph nodes. A high serum titer to *S. equi* is strongly supportive of this diagnosis. Horses frequently succumb to other manifestations of systemic vasculitis, such as gastrointestinal infarcts.

***Streptococcus*-Associated Muscle Atrophy.** A syndrome of profound and rapid generalized muscle atrophy has been seen in young quarter horses exposed to *S. equi*. Affected horses may not show signs of purpura hemorrhagica, and often have increased serum concentrations of CK and AST. At this time the cause is not known. Affected horses may respond to corticosteroid therapy.

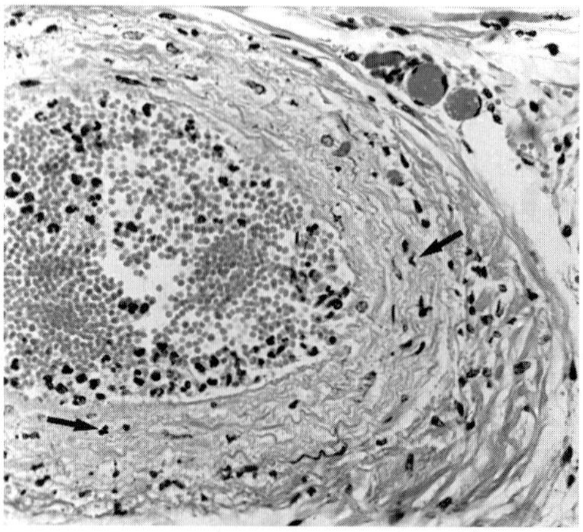

Figure 9-16 Arteriole in muscle; purpura hemorrhagica. Vasculitis. Note the numerous degenerating neutrophils *(arrows)* in the wall of the vessel. H & E stain.

Protozoal Myopathy. Protozoa (*Sarcocystis* spp.) are common incidental findings in equine skeletal and cardiac muscle. The protozoa are in cysts within the myofiber and thus are protected from the body's surveillance. Consequently there is no inflammatory response. Massive infection by *Sarcocystis fayeri* is suspected to cause a degenerative myopathy in horses, but this is rare.

Nutritional and Toxic Myopathies

Nutritional Myopathy. Foals (most commonly up to 2 weeks of age) and young adult horses are susceptible to nutritional myopathy due to a deficiency of selenium or (less commonly) vitamin E. Selenium, present in the soil, is taken up by growing plants. In many areas, however, the soil is selenium deficient, and selenium supplements to the ration must be provided. Vitamin E deficiency occurs in horses that eat marginal to poor-quality grass hay with little or no access to pasture. Affected foals show generalized weakness. This may be present at birth or become apparent soon after birth. Affected foals may become recumbent, but are generally bright and alert and often continue to suckle if bottle-fed. Their tongue and pharyngeal muscles may be weak, leading to weak suckling. Affected young adult horses often show preferential involvement of the temporal and masseter muscles ("maxillary myositis"), with swelling and stiffness of the jaw muscles and impaired mastication. Involvement of pharyngeal muscles may result in dysphagia. In more chronic cases, bilaterally symmetric atrophy of the masseter muscles may be evident. Careful examination of these horses often reveals generalized weakness, evident as a stiff, short-strided gait. Severely affected horses may have an acute onset of recumbency mimicking neurologic disease. Serum concentrations of CK and AST are generally mildly to moderately increased, although extremely high concentrations may be seen in severely affected foals and horses. Concentric needle electromyography of affected muscles results in marked abnormal spontaneous activity (positive sharp waves, fibrillations, myotonic bursts).

Oxidative injury to actively contracting muscle fibers occurs as a result of lack of selenium (a vital component of the antioxidant enzyme glutathione peroxidase) or vitamin E. Affected foals are most often those born to selenium-deficient mares. Affected young adult horses are most often stabled horses fed only hay, with clinical disease seen most commonly in the late winter or early spring.

Muscles of affected foals appear pale, often in a patchy distribution. The most severely affected muscles are those that have the highest workload (e.g., cervical muscles, proximal limb muscles, tongue, and masticatory muscles). The gross appearance depends on the extent of the necrosis and the stage. In early stages, yellow and white streaks are present, and later pale, chalk white streaks appear. Horses with impaired deglutition and swallowing may have cranioventral aspiration pneumonia. Severely selenium-deficient horses will also have pale areas of necrosis within the myocardium, especially the left ventricular wall and septum. The lesions in the muscles are those of a multifocal, multiphasic segmental necrosis. The stage of the necrosis depends on the age of the lesions. In foals with severe, acute myopathy leading to death or euthanasia, lesions are at the stage of massive muscle necrosis and mineralization with minimal macrophage infiltration (monophasic). In animals that have lived longer, e.g., in subacute cases, the lesions are multiphasic and active necrosis, macrophage infiltration, and regeneration present. If horses live long enough, fiber regeneration can restore the muscles to normal. Although type I fibers may be more sensitive to necrosis due to nutritional myopathy, in severely affected muscles almost all fiber types are affected. In cases with myocardial involvement, myocardiocyte necrosis and mineralization are present, and if the animal survives, the segmental necrotic myofibers are replaced by fibrovascular connective tissue that forms a scar.

Diagnosis of nutritional myopathy is based on typical history, increases in serum concentrations of CK and AST, deficient blood concentrations of selenium or vitamin E, and characteristic gross and histopathologic findings. This disorder in foals can be prevented by supplementing mares with selenium during gestation. Foals born in selenium-deficient areas should be given injectable vitamin E and selenium soon after birth. Young adult horses should be given sufficient dietary vitamin E and selenium. Treatment with selenium and vitamin E after the onset of clinical signs is less effective than prevention.

Toxic Myopathies—Ionophore Toxicity. Ionophores such as monensin, salinomycin, narasin, and lasalocid are often added to chicken and ruminant feeds for their antibiotic and growth-enhancing effects. Horses are exquisitely sensitive to ionophore toxicity and will succumb to very small doses. These may be present as contaminants within horse feed, or the horse may be accidentally fed ionophore-containing feeds intended for other domestic animals. Most of the available information relates to monensin toxicity. After ingestion of monensin, acute death—usually within 2 to 3 days—occurs from cardiovascular collapse and shock. Horses surviving the acute disease develop generalized weakness due to widespread necrosis of muscle. Death is often due to cardiac muscle necrosis or to recumbency and, after weeks or months, to cardiac fibrosis. Less is known about clinical signs of lasalocid and other ionophore toxicity in horses, but recumbency leading to death has been seen in lasalocid toxicity. Skeletal and cardiac muscle necrosis is associated with concurrent increases in serum concentrations of CK and AST, which may be marked. Acute cardiac failure and death due to myocardial scarring may be a later event.

These ionophores facilitate movement of cations across cell membranes, disrupting the normal ionic equilibrium, especially in excitable cells such as those of the nervous system, skeletal, and cardiac muscle. The disruption of ionic equilibrium results in calcium overload and death of skeletal and cardiac muscle. In acute monensin toxicity, no specific lesions are seen on postmortem examination within the first 48 hours, although sometimes the muscles and urine are pink from released myoglobin. In 3 to 4 days, affected skeletal and cardiac muscles may contain pale streaks. After monensin or lasalocid exposure, affected skeletal muscle fibers show similar lesions, a monophasic multifocal segmental necrosis. After 3 to 4 days there is segmental necrosis and early infiltration of macrophages. This is followed by myofiber regeneration, which can restore the muscles to normal, if the animal survives. At the same time as the myofiber necrosis, areas of cardiac myocytes are undergoing necrosis and over the next few days to weeks, these are replaced by fibrosis, as there is no significant regeneration of the myocardium. Horses dying at 14 days often have normal skeletal muscles and extensive myocardial fibrosis. A helpful diagnostic feature to differentiate between nutritional myopathy and ionophore toxicity is that in nutritional myopathy the lesions are often multifocal and multiphasic—i.e., at different stages of necrosis and regeneration. In equine ionophore toxicity, because there is a single exposure to the toxin, lesions are at the same stage of necrosis or regeneration (monophasic). Diagnosis is based on a history of ionophore exposure, with characteristic gross or histopathologic findings. Analysis of feed or stomach contents for ionophores is definitive. Treatment for ionophore-intoxicated horses is supportive, with no specific therapy.

Inherited or Congenital Myopathies

Myotonia. Congenital or early-onset myotonia is seen in Thoroughbreds, Standardbreds, and quarter horses. Various similar disorders, designated as myotonic dystrophy–like or muscular dystrophy–like, may be the same or similar disorders. Affected horses have remarkable exercise intolerance, with stiffness of posture and gait apparent at birth or soon thereafter, and often, remarkably well-defined to hypertrophied muscle groups. Clinical signs of stiffness are most apparent when the animals first begin to move, with some decrease in stiffness with exercise. Serum concentrations of CK and AST are generally normal to only slightly increased. Muscles often show prolonged dimpling after percussion. Concentric needle electromyography demonstrates characteristic waxing and waning ("dive bomber") myotonic bursts.

As with all congenital myotonias, an underlying abnormal ion channel leading to continuous abnormal muscle activity is suspected, but to date the defect, and mode of inheritance, have not been defined. No specific gross lesions are present, other than prominent muscling. Affected muscle fibers vary tremendously in size and shape, with numerous internal nuclei, altered cytoplasmic areas beneath the sarcolemma (sarcolemmal masses), and other cytoarchitectural alterations such as "ring fibers." Scattered fiber necrosis and regeneration may be seen, but is not a prominent feature. In chronic cases, affected muscles may show a varying degree of replacement of myofibers by fat, indicating a previous loss of myofibers.

The diagnosis of myotonia is based on characteristic clinical signs in a young horse, and may be confirmed by electromyography or muscle biopsy. No specific treatment is known at this time.

Hyperkalemic Periodic Paralysis (HYPP). This myotonic disorder affects quarter horses and quarter horse–related breeds whose ancestry traces to the quarter horse stallion Impressive. The disease is inherited as an autosomal dominant disease; therefore, affected horses can be either heterozygotes or homozygotes. Clinical findings are variable and are generally more severe in homozygous horses. Homozygous foals often have a distinctive laryngeal muscle dysfunction that results in laryngospasm and labored breathing. Heterozygous horses have a much more variable clinical disease. Affected horses generally have remarkably well-defined muscle groups. Episodes of muscle trembling, followed by weakness and often collapse, are the most common presenting clinical signs. These are often accompanied by increased serum potassium concentrations (hyperkalemia). Postanesthetic recumbency has also been associated with HYPP. Affected horses may appear normal for many years, may have multiple episodes of collapse, or may die acutely. Serum concentrations of CK and AST are generally normal. Concentric needle electromyography of affected horses reveals characteristic myotonic bursts.

The underlying defect in HYPP is abnormal (delayed) inactivation of sodium channel activity, resulting in membrane instability and continuous muscle fiber electrical activity. In response to increased intracellular sodium, potassium is released to the extracellular space from which it reaches the bloodstream. There are no gross pathologic findings in HYPP horses, other than prominent muscling. Affected skeletal muscle is generally histologically normal, although scattered intracytoplasmic vacuoles may be present in type II fibers (vacuolar myopathy). The characteristic pathologic finding of HYPP is only evident at the ultrastructural level, where dilated terminal cisternae of the sarcoplasmic reticulum are found.

Diagnosis may be made with reasonable certainty based on characteristic clinical signs in a horse of Impressive line breeding, especially if episodes are associated with hyperkalemia. Myotonic bursts with concentric needle electromyography are also diagnostic. The simplest and most reliable test, however, is a DNA-based test performed on peripheral white blood cells. Treatment consists of feeding a low-potassium diet, which may be successful in controlling signs in many cases. More severe cases can be treated with the diuretic acetazomide, which causes increased urinary excretion of potassium. Acute episodes can be treated by intravenous calcium and dextrose.

Polysaccharide Storage Myopathy. This myopathy is most common in quarter horses, warmblood, and draft-related breeds, although it can occur in other breeds. This disorder is thought to be inherited, although the exact mechanism of inheritance is not clear at this time. There is some evidence to suggest autosomal recessive inheritance in quarter horses. Recurrent exertional rhabdomyolysis (see below) is the most commonly recognized sign, although affected horses may also have a stiff gait, symmetric muscle atrophy, and bilateral pelvic limb or generalized weakness. In draft horses, sudden onset of recumbency and postanesthetic myopathy can occur. Serum concentrations of CK and AST are markedly increased after episodes of exertional rhabdomyolysis, but may be only mildly to moderately increased in affected horses after exercise or onset of recumbency. Concentric needle electromyography may reveal abnormal spontaneous activity (positive sharp waves and fibrillations).

Although, to date, an abnormality of the glycolytic or glycogenolytic pathways within skeletal muscle has not been identified, an underlying carbohydrate metabolic disorder is still suspected. Although clinical signs are somewhat variable, they all can be related to insufficient energy production by affected muscle fibers. In severe cases, in which horses have died or been euthanatized because of rhabdomyolysis or recumbency, muscles may be pale pink or diffusely red tinged, which may be mistaken for autolysis. Multifocal pale zones may be present. In draft horses, chronic myopathy has resulted in reduced muscle mass and pale streaks within affected muscles. The most severely affected muscles are those of the proximal thigh and paraspinal muscles of the back, although any of the large "power" muscle groups may be affected. Swollen, dark kidneys (acute pigmentary nephrosis) due to myoglobinuria may be seen in horses dying with severe rhabdomyolysis. The extent of overt fiber necrosis is extremely variable; severe acute to subacute necrosis is seen after severe rhabdomyolysis, whereas only minimal scattered fiber necrosis may be seen in recumbent horses. Fiber necrosis is rare in muscle biopsy samples taken from affected horses while they are clinically normal. The characteristic finding is aggregates of intracytoplasmic material within type II fibers (Fig. 9-17, *A*) that stains positively with periodic acid–Schiff (PAS). In some cases, PAS-positive material that resists digestion by amylase is present. This material is not simple glycogen, but is probably a complex polysaccharide (Fig.

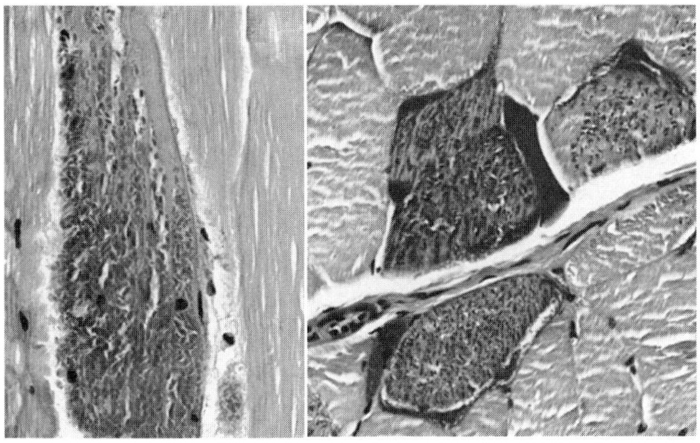

Figure 9-17 Muscle; horse. Polysaccharide storage myopathy. **A,** Longitudinal section. A myofiber contains pale staining aggregates of complex carbohydrate. H & E stain. **B,** Transverse section. These aggregates stain with the PAS reaction.

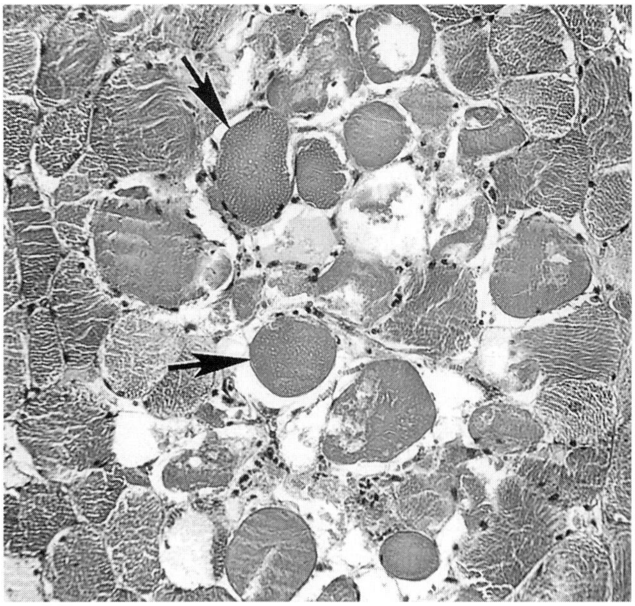

Figure 9-18 Muscle cross section; horse. Equine rhabdomyolysis. A focus of hyalinized necrotic myofibers *(arrows)* are surrounded by viable myofibers. H & E stain. ×175. *Courtesy Dr. W. J. Hadlow.*

9-17, *B*). In chronic cases, myofibers with atrophy and hypertrophy, and internal nuclei, as well as glycogen and complex polysaccharide are present. At this time, the diagnosis of polysaccharide storage myopathy depends on finding the characteristic histopathologic changes in muscle biopsy samples of gluteal, semimembranosus, or semitendinosus muscles. A presumptive diagnosis of polysaccharide storage myopathy may be made based on characteristic clinical findings in a predisposed breed. Treatment has relied on altering the diet to minimize carbohydrate intake and to provide at least 20% to 25% of total daily calories from fat, and provision of regular exercise. Grains and sweet feeds are replaced by alfalfa pellets or low-carbohydrate commercial feeds, with added fat in the form of vegetable oil, powdered animal fat, or high-fat rice bran supplements.

Glycogen Brancher Enzyme Deficiency. A congenital lack of the glycogenic enzyme known as glycogen brancher enzyme occurs in quarter horses. Affected foals present with cardiac failure at an early age. Characteristic round hyaline inclusions resembling amylopectin (polyglucosan bodies) are present in skeletal and cardiac myocytes, especially in Purkinje fibers. Inclusions are PAS positive and amylase resistant, and stain positively with iodine. As with other carbohydrate metabolic defects, a lack of energy production by affected fibers is thought to underlie cellular dysfunction. Although the mode of inheritance is not known at this time, autosomal recessive inheritance is likely.

Other Equine Myopathies

Exertional Rhabdomyolysis. Equine exertional rhabdomyolysis (tying up, azoturia, Monday morning disease) is characterized by sudden onset of stiff gait, reluctance to move, swelling of affected muscle groups (especially gluteal), sweating, and other signs of discomfort. Signs may appear during or immediately after exercise. At this time it is not clear how many horses with exertional rhabdomyolysis have underlying polysaccharide storage myopathy. Electrolyte abnormalities and selenium deficiency have also been implicated as causes of exertional rhabdomyolysis in the horse. There is some evidence to suggest that recurrent exertional rhabdomyolysis in Thoroughbreds is due to abnormal calcium homeostasis within skeletal muscle.

As muscle necrosis per se is neither painful, nor does it cause muscle swelling, it is suspected that other factors play a role in this disorder in the horse. Possible contributing factors include oxidative injury to muscle membranes and vascular injury resulting in ischemia. Gross findings are similar to those described for polysaccharide storage myopathy. Widespread or localized muscle fiber necrosis (Fig. 9-18) followed by macrophage infiltration and regeneration is seen, with concurrent increases in serum concentrations of CK and AST. Affected fibers are primarily type II fibers.

Diagnosis is based on typical clinical signs and clinicopathologic evidence of muscle injury (increased activity of CK or AST). Treatment during an acute episode includes nonsteroidal inflammatory agents and rest. Intravenous dimethyl sulfoxide (DMSO) has also proven to be useful for reduction of muscle swelling. Long-term treatment and prevention include correction of any underlying electrolyte, mineral, or vitamin deficiencies. Curiously, Thoroughbreds with recurrent exertional rhabdomyolysis due to suspected underlying calcium handling abnormalities also respond well to the high-fat and low–soluble carbohydrate diet used to treat horses with exertional rhabdomyolysis due to underlying polysaccharide storage myopathy.

Hyperthermia. A malignant hyperthermia-like syndrome occurring during general anesthesia, and development of postanesthetic hyperthermia, have been seen in horses. Some affected horses have been suspected or proven to have HYPP or polysaccharide storage myopathy, but in some cases the exact cause of these conditions is not clear. It is likely that a variety of underlying myopathies can predispose animals to anesthesia-associated hyperthermia. The extent of muscle fiber necrosis varies.

Ischemic Myopathy. A degenerative myopathy secondary to muscle hypoxia is seen in horses undergoing prolonged general anesthesia. In some cases systemic hypotension is implicated, and in others pressure produced by the weight of large muscle masses, especially when adequate padding is not provided, is suspected. Ischemic myopathy also may be seen in recumbent horses, as the result of pressure interfering with vascular perfusion. Once the horse is moved or is standing, reperfusion injury may be involved. Ischemic myopathy of the abdominal muscles may be seen after prolonged lifting of a horse with a sling. In these cases, affected muscles generally show degenerative or regenerative changes that are all at about the same stage (monophasic necrosis). Concurrent necrosis and regeneration may also be seen in horses that are recumbent or in a sling for days.

Myopathies of Cattle

Bacterial and Parasitic Myopathies

Clostridial Myositis ("Blackleg"). This disease, due to *Clostridium chauvoei,* is economically an extremely important disease that is most common in beef cattle, but it can also occur in dairy cattle. *C. chauvoei* is a spore-forming, gram-positive anaerobic bacillus. The most common presentation is acute death. Signs before death are referable to toxemia, to the heat, swelling, crepitus, and dysfunction of the affected muscle group, and to fever and anorexia. Serum concentrations of CK and AST are typically increased.

C. chauvoei spores are ubiquitous in the soil, and following ingestion are capable of crossing the intestinal mucosa, entering the bloodstream, and being carried to skeletal muscle. The spores lie dormant until localized trauma to the muscle, most often due to bruising during handling in a chute or from trauma in a crowded feedlot, results in hypoxia. The resultant anaerobic conditions allow the spores to activate, proliferate, and produce toxins. These cause capillary damage, hemorrhage, edema, and necrosis of adjacent myofibers. Locally extensive hemorrhage and edema, often with crepitus due to gas bubbles, are seen in affected muscles and in overlying fascia and subcutaneous tissue. Necrotic muscle fibers appear dark red to red-black and may be wet and exudative (early lesions) or dry (later lesions) (Fig. 9-19). Cardiac muscle may also be involved. A characteristic odor of rancid butter due to butyric acid is typically found. In other

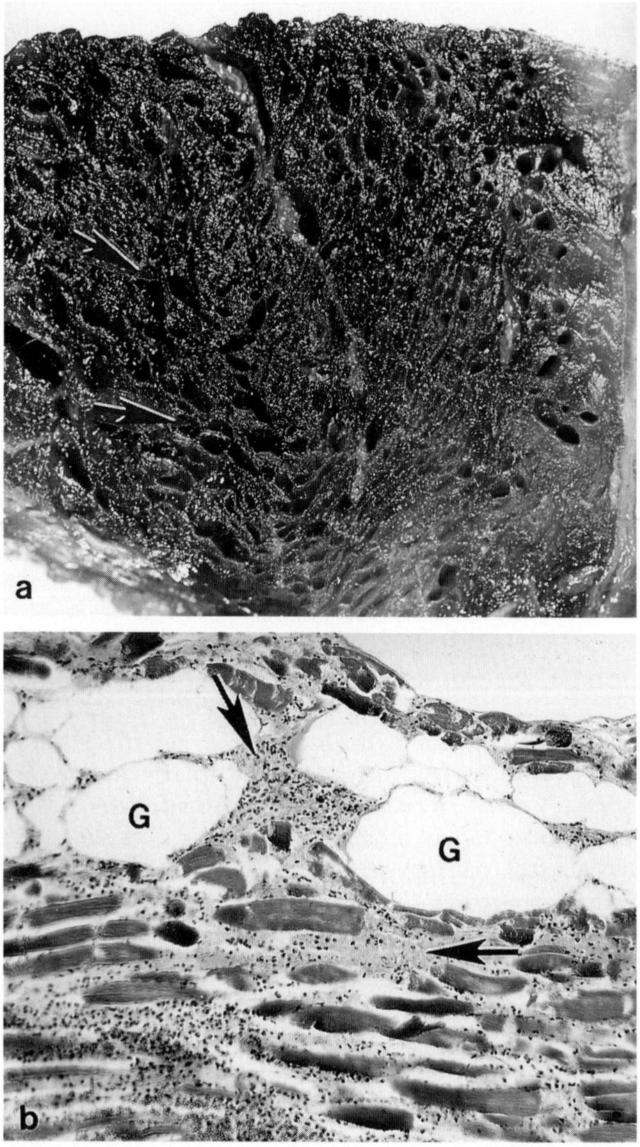

Figure 9-19 Muscle; cow. Blackleg. **A,** Cut surface of a late stage. Note the dark, dry surface with numerous gas bubbles *(arrows).* **B,** Early stage. Serohemorrhagic exudate *(arrows)* and gas bubbles *(G)* separate myofibers. H & E stain. ×85. *Courtesy Dr. W. J. Hadlow.*

parts of the body, hemorrhages and edema may be seen associated with toxemia. Because of the high fever, affected carcasses autolyze rapidly. Histologically, locally extensive areas of muscle fibers undergoing coagulation necrosis and fragmentation, and interstitial edema and hemorrhage are seen. Overt vasculitis is not seen. Gas bubbles are typical (Fig. 9-19, *B*). Gram-positive bacilli whose appearance is compatible with that of *C. chauvoei* may or may not be demonstrable within affected muscle.

Isolation of *C. chauvoei* on anaerobic media is useful for confirmation of blackleg, but only if typical gross and histopathologic findings are present, as this bacterium can be cultured from unaffected muscle that harbors dormant spores. The vaccination history and evaluation of husbandry practices are also important; unvaccinated or poorly vaccinated animals in situations in which muscle trauma is possible are most at risk. There is generally no effective treatment for cattle with blackleg, and death occurs rapidly. Prevention is the best treatment. Vaccination against clostridial toxins and maintenance of a safe environment are critical.

Clostridium botulinum (Botulism). Botulism occurs in cattle, and clinical signs and pathogenesis are similar to that in the horse. Cattle, however, are much more resistant to botulism than are horses.

Pyogenic Bacteria. Cattle are prone to develop abscesses caused by pyogenic bacteria, most commonly *Arcanobacterium (Actinomyces) pyogenes.* Abscesses in muscle occur most commonly in the hind leg. Swelling and lameness of the affected limb are seen.

A. pyogenes is a ubiquitous bacterium that can infect muscle by two routes: by direct contamination of wounds and injection sites and hematogenously. The bacterium can be found within the reproductive tract of cows and within the ruminal wall, and it has been speculated that bacteremia, occurring transiently after parturition or disruption of ruminal wall integrity, can result in colonization of damaged muscle. Lesions vary depending on the virulence of the bacteria and the age of the lesions. They vary in extent, from encapsulated intramuscular abscesses adjacent to the site of injection to a diffuse purulent cellulitis extending down the tissue planes. The cellulitis may be so severe as to extend from the muscles over the sacrum through the muscles on the lateral aspect of the thigh and over the tibia and to the hock. In some cases, there is a sinus extending through the tibial muscles, which then breaks out through the skin above the hock. Grossly, the encapsulated abscesses are filled with thick, yellow-green, foul-smelling pus. In cases of cellulitis, or really fasciitis, the same type of pus dissects along fascial planes outside the muscle and between perimysial sheaths within muscles. This inflammation extends into the adjacent myofibers resulting in myonecrosis and subsequent replacement by fibrous tissue. In the most severe forms, there may be multiple sites from multiple injections and the cellulitis may be present in the lumbar and gluteal muscles.

The color of the exudate is distinctive, and gram-positive to gram-variable coccobacilli may be seen within tissue sections. *A. pyogenes* is readily isolated on aerobic bacterial culture media.

Protozoal Myopathies. Intracytoplasmic protozoal cysts of *Sarcocystis* spp. are common incidental findings in skeletal and cardiac myofibers of cattle. Because they are intracellular, they are protected from the host's defense mechanisms and thus, there is no inflammatory response or reaction by the myocyte (Fig. 9-20). This protozoal organism is a stage of an intestinal coccidium of carnivores that uses birds, reptiles, rodents, swine, and herbivores as an intermediate host. Ingestion of oocysts by an intermediate host releases sporozoites that invade tissues, including muscle. Massive exposure may result in fever, anorexia, and progressive wasting, but this is uncommon. More often, *Sarcocystis* infection is diagnosed as an incidental finding at necropsy or during meat processing. If the cyst wall breaks down, a focus of myofiber necrosis and later granuloma formation results.

Eosinophilic Myositis. This disease of cattle is thought to be a relatively uncommon manifestation of *Sarcocystis* infection that may involve hypersensitivity. There is overt green discoloration of affected muscles caused by the massive infiltration of eosinophils (Fig. 9-21). This is accompanied by myofiber necrosis and, in chronic cases, fibrosis.

Nutritional and Toxic Myopathies

Nutritional Myopathy. Similar to horses, calves and young cattle are susceptible to nutritional myopathy due to selenium or vitamin E deficiency, except that the profound involvement of temporal and masseter muscles ("maxil-

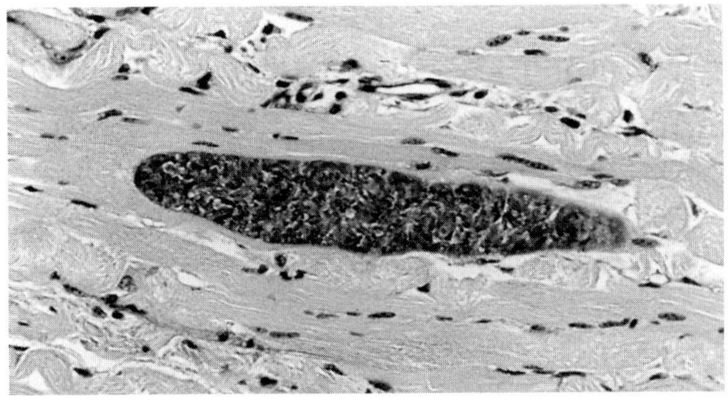

Figure 9-20 Muscle, avian; gamecock. Sarcosporidiosis. Note the elongated cyst within the myofiber and the lack of inflammation. H & E stain.

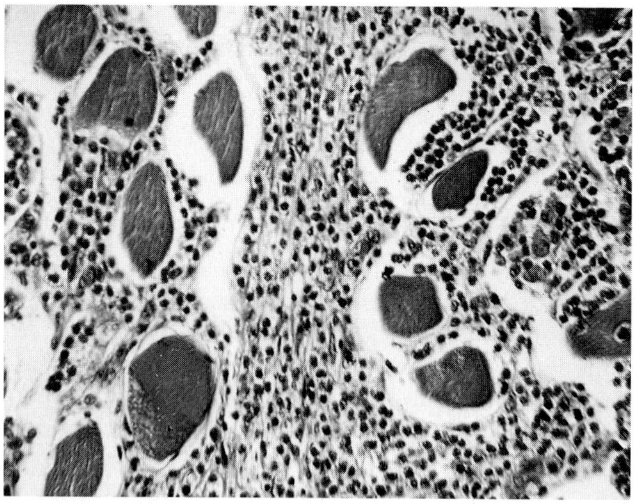

Figure 9-21 Muscle; cow. Eosinophilic myositis. Atrophic muscle fibers are separated by an exudate consisting chiefly of eosinophils. H & E stain. ×200. *Courtesy Dr. W. J. Hadlow.*

lary myositis") that can occur in horses is not seen in young cattle (Fig. 9-22).

Plant Toxicities. *Cassia occidentalis* (coffee senna, coffee weed) is the most common cause of degenerative myopathy in cattle due to plant toxicity. This plant grows throughout the southeastern United States. Pale areas within skeletal muscle, with lesser involvement of cardiac muscle, are due to fiber necrosis, with minimal to no mineralization (Fig. 9-23).

Ionophore Toxicity. Monensin toxicity in cattle is seen only with overdoses due to improper feed mixing. Anorexia, diarrhea, and weakness are the primary clinical signs. Serum concentrations of CK and AST are often extremely high. Pale areas within skeletal and cardiac muscle are due to fiber necrosis.

Congenital or Inherited Myopathies

Steatosis. This disease in cattle, sometimes called lipomatosis, is most often recognized as an incidental finding at necropsy or at slaughter. This disorder is thought to be due to defective muscle development, in which large areas of myofibers are replaced by adipocytes. Lesions are bilaterally symmetric, with the most severely affected muscles being those of the back and loin (Fig. 9-24, *A*). Severely affected muscles are composed entirely of fat, whereas less severely affected muscles may appear streaked or are partially replaced, by fat. Histologically, the space normally occupied by myofibers is filled with mature adipocytes (Fig. 9-24, *B*).

Diagnosis is readily made on gross examination, and can be confirmed by histologic examination, specifically in frozen sections stained for fat, with oil-red-O or Sudan black. Treatment is neither necessary nor possible. Although an inherited basis has not been established, it might be prudent to advise removing cattle that have produced affected calves from the breeding stock.

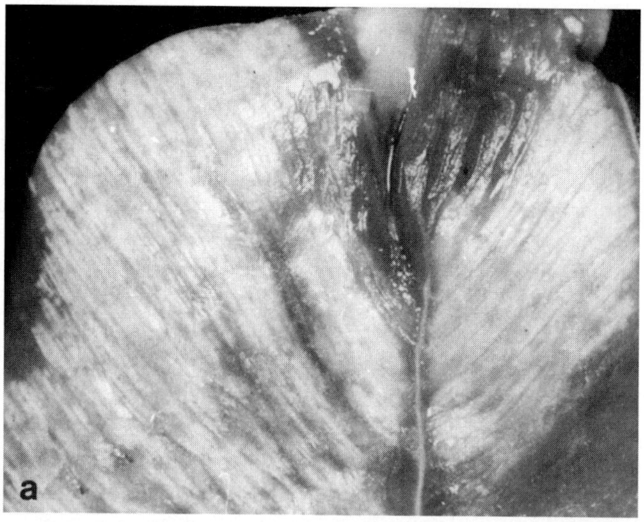

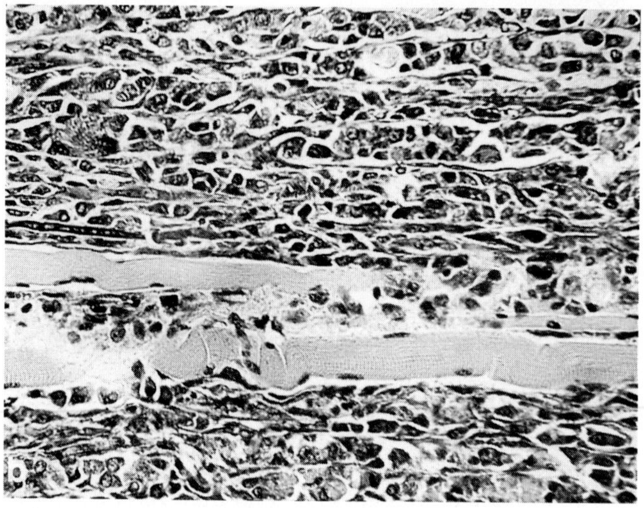

Figure 9-22 Leg muscles; lamb. **A,** Nutritional myopathy. The numerous gray and white streaks are areas of segmental necrosis and calcification. **B,** Muscle, nutritional myopathy; calf. Sarcolemmal tubes are intact and filled with myoblasts and macrophages—early regeneration. The calf, which died, also had extensive lesions in the heart. H & E stain. ×200. *Courtesy Dr. W. J. Hadlow.*

Congenital Muscular Hyperplasia ("Double Muscling"). Affected calves have large, bulky muscles of the shoulder and rump. These may cause dystocia. This disorder is inherited as an autosomal recessive trait with incomplete penetrance. The exact genetic defect is as yet unknown. Enlarged, sharply delineated bulky shoulder and rump muscles are characteristic. Body fat deposits and intramuscular fat are reduced to about 60% of normal. Although muscle fiber numbers are increased in this disorder, the

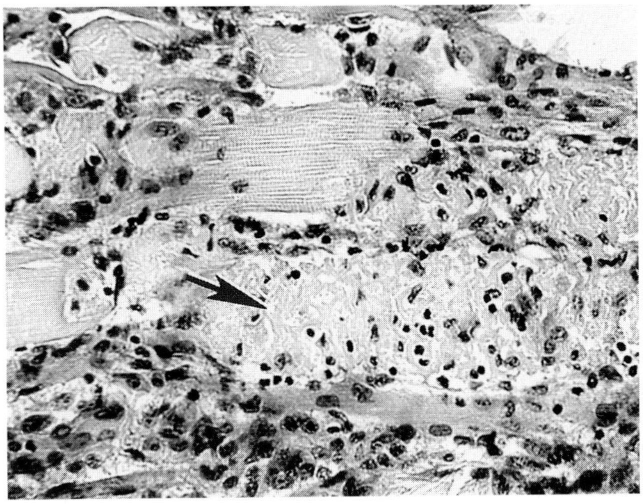

Figure 9-23 Muscle; sheep. *Cassia occidentalis*–induced segmental necrosis *(arrow)*. The necrotic segments are infiltrated by macrophages. H & E stain. ×200. *Courtesy Dr. W. J. Hadlow.*

absolute number of fibers within a muscle is difficult to determine. Characteristic histopathologic findings are hypertrophy of type II muscle fibers and decreased intramuscular adipocytes. The diagnosis of this disorder is readily made based on typical clinical findings, and can be confirmed by histopathologic examination. There is no treatment, and cattle known to produce affected calves should not be rebred.

Diaphragmatic Dystrophy. A muscular dystrophy affecting diaphragm and respiratory muscles has been recognized in Meuse-Rhine-Yssel cattle in Europe and Holstein cattle in Japan. The most common clinical sign is recurrent bloat. Examination of affected muscle indicates a progressive degenerative myopathy with marked cytoarchitectural changes. The disorder appears to be inherited as an autosomal recessive trait.

Glycogenoses. Carbohydrate metabolic defects affect skeletal muscle by interfering with muscle energy metabolism and result in abnormal storage of glycogen. Many disorders of carbohydrate metabolism have been identified in man, and an increasing number of inherited glycogenoses are being recognized in animals.

Acid maltase deficiency (glycogenosis type II; Pompe's disease). This defect has been described in Shorthorn and Brahma cattle. Affected Shorthorn cattle may show clinical signs of weakness at 3 to 7 months of age and die as a result of respiratory and cardiac failure. Affected Shorthorn cattle may also develop relatively normally until 1 to 1½ years of age, at which time weakness and neurologic deficits are evident. Affected Brahma cattle grow poorly and have muscular weakness, and neurologic disease. Electrocardiographic studies reveal abnormalities of cardiac conduction. Serum concentrations of CK and AST may be increased, with marked increases evident in severely weak animals before death.

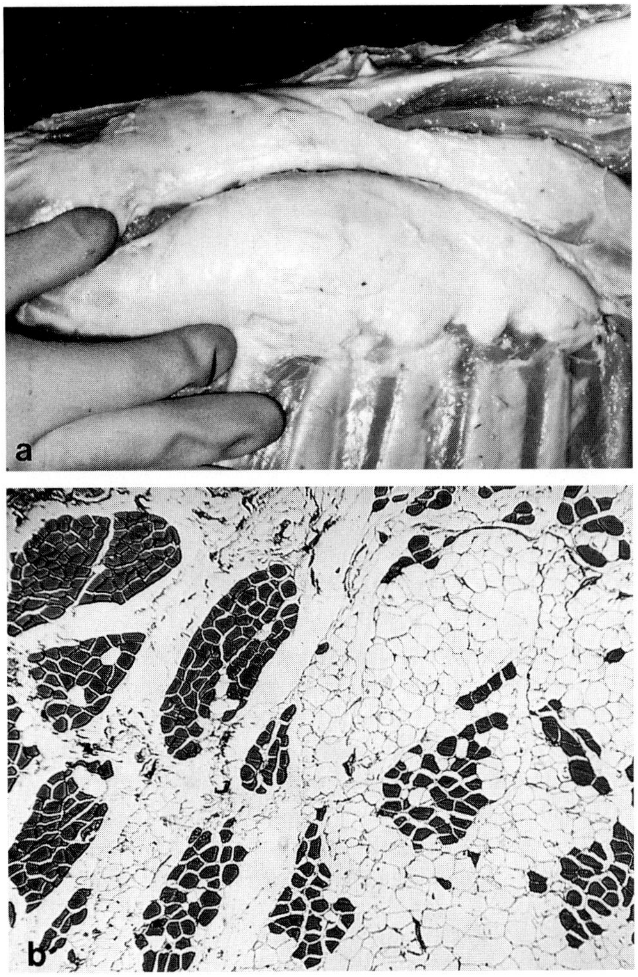

Figure 9-24 Muscle; ox. Steatosis. **A,** Longissimus muscles are enlarged and almost completely replaced by fat. **B,** Longissimus muscle. Cross section. Many myofibers in fasciculi have been replaced by fat cells. H & E stain. ×30. **B,** *Courtesy Dr. W. J. Hadlow.*

This disorder is inherited as an autosomal recessive trait. The enzyme defect results in blockage of the glycolytic metabolic pathway and in cellular dysfunction that is most evident in skeletal muscle, Purkinje cells of the heart, and neurons. Myofiber necrosis is thought to be a result of a cellular "energy crisis," that is, deprivation.

There may be no obvious changes within the skeletal and cardiac muscle, although pale streaks may be evident in those animals undergoing myofiber necrosis before death. No gross pathologic lesions are evident in the nervous system. On histopathologic examination, affected myofibers, cardiac myocytes, and neurons are filled with vacuoles containing glycogen (vacuolar myopathy and neuronopathy), which can be demonstrated by PAS staining. Glycogen accumulation in skeletal myofibers is segmental, whereas in neurons it is diffuse. Both degeneration and regeneration of skeletal muscle fibers and chronic myopathic change such as fiber atrophy, hypertrophy, and internal nuclei are present.

Diagnosis of a glycogenosis can be made based on characteristic clinical and histopathologic findings. Assay of affected muscle for glycolytic enzyme activities is necessary to determine the specific enzyme defect. There is no effective treatment of this disorder, and cattle known to produce affected calves should not be rebred.

Myophosphorylase deficiency (glycogenosis type V; McArdle's disease). This disorder has been identified in Charolais cattle. Clinical signs of exercise intolerance and inability to keep up with herdmates are recognized at a relatively early age. If forced to exercise, affected cattle become recumbent for up to 10 minutes. Serum concentrations of CK and AST are often mildly to markedly increased.

Myophosphorylase deficiency is apparently an autosomal recessive disorder similar to acid maltase deficiency, but involves only skeletal muscle. No specific findings are evident at necropsy. Histopathologic findings skeletal muscle are similar to those of acid maltase deficiency; cardiac myocytes and neurons do not store glycogen.

Diagnosis can be based on characteristic clinical and histopathologic findings. Affected animals and carriers can be detected after analysis of peripheral blood leukocyte DNA by polymerase chain reaction assay. There is no treatment, and carrier animals should not be used for breeding.

Metabolic Myopathies

Hypokalemic Myopathy. A history of ketosis occurring within a month of parturition is common. Affected cows are profoundly weak and become recumbent and unable to support the weight of their heads. Serum concentration of potassium is low, and CK and AST levels are high. Atrial fibrillation is common.

Hypokalemia can be due to anorexia. Ketosis can contribute to loss of potassium. Glucocorticoids with high mineralocorticoid activities, such as isoflupredone, used to treat ketosis or intravenously administered glucose or insulin may cause profound hypokalemia. Decreased muscle potassium interferes with normal muscle cell function, and can lead to myofiber necrosis. This can be the end result of either altered mitochondrial activity or focal ischemia secondary to vasoconstriction. Hypokalemia can also interfere with normal cardiac conduction. No specific findings are present at postmortem examination, although ischemic necrosis due to recumbency may be seen in muscles of the hind limbs (see below). Examination of muscles not involved in weight bearing reveals scattered myofiber necrosis and vacuolated myofibers.

The diagnosis is based on typical historical and clinical findings, and a low serum potassium concentration. Aggressive oral supplementation with potassium salts and supportive therapy may result in recovery in some cases, but this disorder is often fatal.

Other Metabolic Myopathies. Both hypocalcemia and hypophosphatemia can result in profound muscle weakness and recumbency in cattle. Significant changes are not seen in affected muscles, although ischemic necrosis can occur secondary to recumbency (see below). Diagnosis relies on clinical findings and identification of abnormal serum electrolyte concentrations. Treatment includes correction of the electrolyte defect by intravenous administration of the appropriate electrolyte-containing fluids, supportive care, and correction of any dietary abnormalities that may predispose to electrolyte problems.

Ischemic myopathy. Ischemic muscle necrosis due to recumbency is common in cattle and is similar to that seen in horses.

Myopathy of Gelbvieh cattle. A necrotizing myopathy of juvenile Gelbvieh cattle has been recognized. The clinical sign is neuromuscular weakness, and histopathologic change in affected muscles is a characteristic necrotizing vasculitis that results in myofiber necrosis. The pathogenesis of this disorder is not known; both vitamin E deficiency and immune-mediated disease have been suggested. Treatment with vitamin E may resolve the myopathy and neuromuscular weakness.

Myopathies of Small Ruminants

Bacterial and Parasitic Myopathies

Myositis due to *Clostridium chauvoei* (Blackleg). This disorder occurs occasionally in sheep and goats and is similar to the disease in cattle.

***Clostridium botulinum* (Botulism).** Botulism also occurs in small ruminants and is similar to the disorder in cattle.

Parasitic Myopathy. Intracytoplasmic cysts of *Sarcocystis* spp. are commonly found within skeletal and cardiac muscle fibers of sheep and goats as an incidental finding, similar to that in cattle; however, eosinophilic myositis is not recognized in sheep or goats. In goats, massive infection with *Sarcocystis* may result in lymphoid necrosis, with inflammation involving heart, skeletal muscle, lungs, liver, blood vessels, and the brain and spinal cord.

Nutritional and Toxic Myopathies

Nutritional Myopathy. Young goats, sheep, and camelids are susceptible to degenerative myopathy associated with selenium or vitamin E deficiency, and a similar disorder has been seen in young llamas. The disease in these species is similar to the disease in young cattle.

Toxic Myopathies. Sheep and goats are susceptible to plant toxicities and monensin toxicity in a manner similar to that in cattle.

Inherited or Congenital Myopathies

Myotonia in Goats. Affected goats develop severe muscle spasms in response to sudden voluntary effort, starting at about 2 weeks of age. Episodes of myotonia can last from 5 to 20 seconds and are characterized by generalized stiffness and adoption of a "sawhorse" stance. Goats often fall over. Sustained muscle dimpling occurs after percussion. Severity of signs is variable. Serum concentrations of CK and AST are normal. Concentric needle electromyography reveals the characteristic waxing and waning ("dive bomber") spontaneous activity of myotonia.

Myotonia in the goat is inherited as an autosomal dominant trait, and the variable clinical severity is attributable to increased severity in homozygotes compared with heterozygotes. The genetic defect affects the skeletal muscle chloride channel activity, resulting in decreased chloride conductance and associated ionic instability of the sarcolemma. There are no gross pathologic findings. Muscle fibers in affected goats may show moderate hypertrophy, but overt abnormalities are revealed only after ultrastructural examination in which dilated and proliferated T tubules and sarcoplasmic reticulum are seen.

Diagnosis is based on characteristic clinical signs, and can be confirmed by concentric needle electromyography. There is no treatment for this disorder, and it is rarely fatal. Although affected goats may actually be prized by collectors ("fainting goats"), it would be prudent to suggest that affected goats not be bred.

Congenital Muscular Dystrophy in Sheep. Muscular dystrophy in sheep is a progressive disorder recognized in Merino sheep in Australia. Clinical signs of neuromuscular weakness occur as early as 1 month of age and are characterized by a stiff gait and exercise intolerance. Serum concentrations of CK and AST are increased.

The underlying defect in ovine progressive muscular dystrophy is not known. The disease is inherited as an autosomal recessive trait. Because the disease affects type I myofibers, gross lesions are most easily seen in a muscle that consists only of type I myofibers (e.g., vastus intermedius). The appearance depends on the age of the animal. Initially the muscle is pale and lacks tone, but is close to normal size. In the next few years, the muscle becomes firm, more atrophic, and pale gray to almost white as the space formerly occupied by the myofibers is filled with adipocytes and fibrosis. Histologically, only type I myofibers are affected. Initially there is atrophy and hypertrophy of the myofibers and myopathic features such as internal nuclei and subsarcolemmal masses. Diagnosis is based on characteristic clinical and histopathologic findings. There is no treatment for this progressive disorder, and animals producing affected lambs should not be rebred.

Glycogenosis. A glycogen storage myopathy due to myophosphorylase deficiency has been identified in sheep in Australia, and is similar to the disease in cattle.

Myopathies of Swine

Bacterial and Parasitic Myopathies

Clostridial Myositis (Blackleg). Swine occasionally develop myositis due to *Clostridium chauvoei,* with a resulting disease similar to that seen in cattle, sheep, and goats.

Pyogenic Bacteria. Abscesses within muscle and associated fascia due to pyogenic bacteria such as *Arcanobacterium pyogenes* are common in swine and are similar to those in cattle.

Trichinosis. Infection of swine by the nematode parasite *Trichinella spiralis* is of major economic importance to the swine industry and poses a serious health hazard to human beings. No clinical disease is associated with *Trichinella* infection in swine.

The adult nematode resides in the mucosa of the small intestine. Larvae penetrate the intestinal mucosa and enter the bloodstream, from which they gain access to the muscle. Larvae invade and encyst within muscle cells. Encysted larvae are typically not visible on gross examination, although dead larvae may calcify and may be visible as 0.5- to 1-mm white nodules. Active muscles, such as the tongue, masseter, diaphragm, intercostal, laryngeal, and extraocular muscles, are preferentially affected. Focal inflammation consisting of eosinophils, neutrophils, and lymphocytes occurs associated with invasion of the muscle by *Trichinella* larvae. After cyst formation, however, inflammation is minimal to absent (Fig. 9-25).

Diagnosis is based on identification of the characteristic nematode larvae encysted within muscle fibers. In those cases in which the larvae have died and calcified, a presumptive diagnosis of trichinosis can still be made. Once encysted in the muscle, *Trichinella* larvae are basically protected from host immune response and to anthelmintic therapy.

Protozoal Myopathies. Intracytoplasmic cysts of *Sarcocystis* spp. can be found in the skeletal and cardiac muscle fibers of swine as an incidental finding.

Nutritional and Toxic Myopathies

Nutritional Myopathy. Young swine are susceptible to degenerative myopathy due to selenium or vitamin E deficiency, with a resulting disorder similar to that seen in

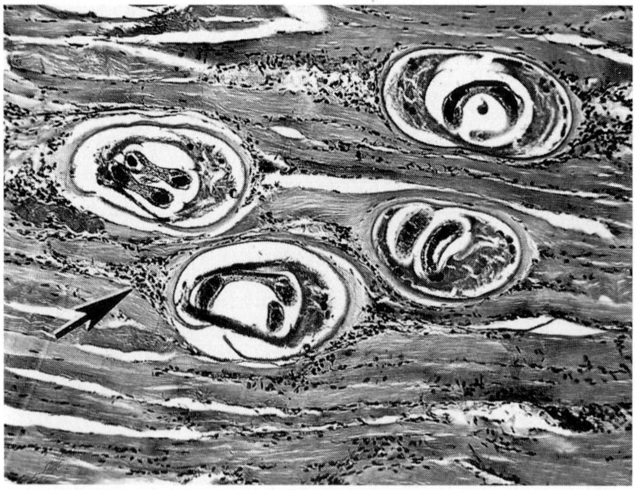

Figure 9-25 Diaphragm; rat. Trichinosis. Larvae are present within the myofibers. Note the localized mononuclear cell infiltrate *(arrow)*. H & E stain. ×100. *Courtesy Dr. W. J. Hadlow.*

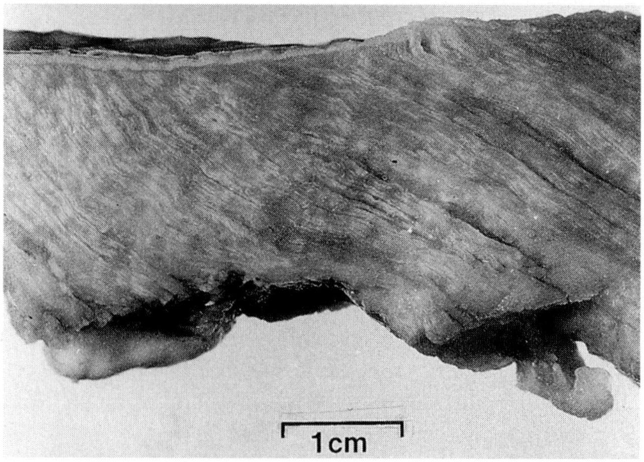

Figure 9-26 Loin muscle; pig, 4 days after a dose of monensin. The pale streaks are necrotic myofibers. *Van Vleet JF, Amstutz HE, Weirich WE, et al. Am J Vet Res 1983; 44:1460-1468.*

calves (Fig. 9-22). A distinctive clinical disorder seen in very young Vietnamese potbellied pigs, in which affected piglets have a short, stilted gait and tend to stand on their toes, is due to a degenerative myopathy thought to be associated with selenium or vitamin E deficiency. Affected piglets appear to recover spontaneously.

Toxic Myopathies. Swine are susceptible to poisoning by *Cassia occidentalis* and develop segmental necrosis of myofibers (Fig. 9-26), especially the diaphragm. Monensin toxicity results in segmental necrosis of skeletal muscle and necrosis of cardiac muscle, particularly atria.

Congenital and Inherited Myopathies

"Splayleg." This congenital disorder affects young piglets and results in splaying of the limbs to the side (abduction), and affected animals propel themselves by pushing against the ground with the pelvic limbs. This posture results in progressive flattening of the sternum. Although delayed myofibril development has been suggested, the histopathologic findings are inconclusive. Affected piglets can be treated by using a harness that holds their legs under their bodies. Encouraging locomotion while partially supporting the body allows the limb muscles to develop. Providing affected pigs with a nonslip surface is also advised.

Malignant Hyperthermia ("Porcine Stress Syndrome"). This disorder affects several strains of pigs, most commonly those with unpigmented haircoats. Incidence varies, but can be very high within certain herds. The disease in pigs is an accurate animal model of the disease in man, and is an important cause of economic losses in the pig industry. Affected pigs are clinically normal until an episode of hyperthermia is triggered by a precipitating factor such as halothane anesthesia or stress. Episodes consist of severe muscle rigidity and markedly increased body temperature and, in severe cases, progresses rapidly to death. Serum concentrations of CK and AST are markedly increased during episodes.

Susceptibility to malignant hyperthermia is inherited as an autosomal recessive trait. The genetic defect results in abnormal activity of the skeletal muscle ryanodine receptor, which is located in the T tubule and links the T tubule to the sarcoplasmic reticulum (excitation-contraction coupling). Clinical disease occurs only in pigs homozygous for the defect, although human heterozygotes may also be susceptible to hyperthermic episodes following halothane anesthesia. It is suspected that this defect originated in a common foundation animal, and has been spread by selecting animals for increased muscling and reduced body fat. In animals dying during a hyperthermic episode, affected muscles are pale, moist, swollen, and appear "cooked." Muscles of the shoulder, back, and thigh are preferentially affected. Affected fibers are either hypercontracted or, depending on time from onset of hyperthermia to death, undergoing coagulation necrosis. Histopathologic findings are not seen in susceptible pigs sampled during clinically normal periods.

This disorder is most commonly diagnosed in pigs dying acutely, and is made based on the clinical history of a precipitating stress and on characteristic gross and histopathologic findings. Given that the precise defect is known, genetic testing may allow for identification of carrier and affected animals. There is no effective treatment for severe malignant hyperthermia. Avoidance of precipitating stress factors in susceptible pigs, and removal of carrier and affected animals from the breeding stock, will reduce the incidence of this disorder.

Ischemic Myopathy

Large pigs are susceptible to ischemic myopathy secondary to recumbency, resulting in ischemic necrosis similar to that seen in horses and cattle.

Myopathies of the Dog

Parasitic

Protozoal Myopathy. The parasitic diseases affecting skeletal muscle in the dog are primarily due to protozoal organisms, of which *Neospora caninum* is the most important. Signs of progressive neuromuscular weakness, most profound in the pelvic limbs, begin in affected pups several weeks of age. Marked muscle atrophy and fixation of the pelvic limb joints occurs rapidly. Serum concentrations of CK and AST may be slightly increased. Concentric needle electromyography reveals dense, sustained spontaneous activity (fibrillations and positive sharp waves) consistent with denervation.

N. caninum is a protozoal organism, often transmitted in utero. Evidence suggests that affected bitches are chronic carriers of the organism. Both the peripheral nervous system and the skeletal muscle are invaded by organisms, which preferentially involve the ventral spinal roots, and damage to these results in denervation atrophy of muscles. Affected muscles are markedly atrophied, firm, and pale. Fixation of the pelvic limb joints persists after anesthesia or death.

Scattered foci of mixed inflammation with associated segmental myofiber necrosis are often seen within skeletal muscle, and intracytoplasmic protozoal cysts may be present. In addition, these organisms damage the ventral roots and cause denervation atrophy of affected myofibers. As nerve fibers in the ventral root that supply both type I and type II myofibers are damaged, both these myofiber types are denervated.

N. caninum infection should be suspected based on characteristic progressive neuromuscular dysfunction in a young growing pup. The finding of a mixed inflammatory-neurogenic atrophy lesion within affected skeletal muscle should prompt a search for protozoa, although these are often present in small numbers and may not be seen. Serologic tests can detect antibodies to *N. caninum,* and antibodies are available for histochemical studies of paraffin-embedded, formalin-fixed tissue. Treatment with trimethoprim-sulfadiazine may kill the organisms, but denervation atrophy and pelvic limb fixation will persist. Bitches producing affected pups may do so in subsequent litters and therefore should probably not be rebred.

Congenital or Inherited Myopathies

X-linked Muscular Dystrophy (Duchenne Type). This disorder has been confirmed or suspected in several breeds of dogs, including Irish terrier, golden retriever, Labrador retriever, miniature schnauzer, Rottweiler, Dalmatian, Shetland sheepdog, Samoyed, Pembroke Welsh corgi, and Alaskan malamute. This canine disorder is homologous to Duchenne muscular dystrophy of man. Affected dogs are always males (X-linked). Severely affected pups may develop a rapidly progressive weakness and die within the first few days of life. In less severely affected dogs, clinical signs are a stiff, short-strided gait and exercise intolerance beginning at 8 to 12 weeks of age, followed by progressive weakness and muscle atrophy. Inability to fully open the jaw often precedes signs of generalized weakness. Weakness of the tongue, jaw, and pharyngeal muscles results in difficulty with prehension and swallowing of food, and dogs often have excessive drooling as a result of pooling of saliva in the pharynx. Involvement of skeletal muscle within the esophagus can result in regurgitation and possible secondary aspiration pneumonia. Markedly increased concentrations of serum CK, AST, and alanine aminotransferase (ALT) are characteristic, even before the onset of obvious clinical disease. Concentric needle electromyography reveals remarkable spontaneous activity in the form of myotonic bursts, although rather than waxing and waning as in true myotonia, this bizarre electrical activity, stimulated by insertion or movement of the recording needle, is continuous and then ends abruptly (pseudomyotonia). Muscles do not dimple with percussion.

This disorder is inherited as an X-linked recessive trait, with inapparent disease in carrier females. It is suspected that new mutations may be relatively common, as is the case in man. The underlying defect is a lack of a cytoskeletal protein known as dystrophin, the absence of which renders skeletal muscle fibers susceptible to repeated bouts of necrosis and regeneration, especially after exercise. Necrosis of cardiac myocytes is followed by their replacement by connective tissue and this results in a progressive cardiomyopathy. Death in older animals is due either to aspiration pneumonia secondary to dysphagia or to progressive cardiac failure, although affected dogs may survive for many years.

In pups dying within the first few days of life, the strap muscles of the shoulder, neck, and pelvic limbs, and the diaphragm have pale yellow to white streaks that in severe cases involve the entire muscle. Death in these cases is thought to be due to respiratory failure related to diaphragmatic involvement. In animals with clinical disease beginning at 8 to 12 weeks, pale streaks within muscle are much less evident, although affected muscles often appear diffusely pale and may be fibrotic. The esophagus in these cases may be mildly dilated, and in all dogs 6 months of age or older, multifocal pale yellow to white zones will be present within the heart, predominantly involving the subepicardial region of the left ventricular wall, the papillary muscles, and the interventricular septum. All skeletal muscles, with the exception of the extraocular muscles, appear to be affected to varying degrees. Overt myofiber necrosis is most severe in earlier

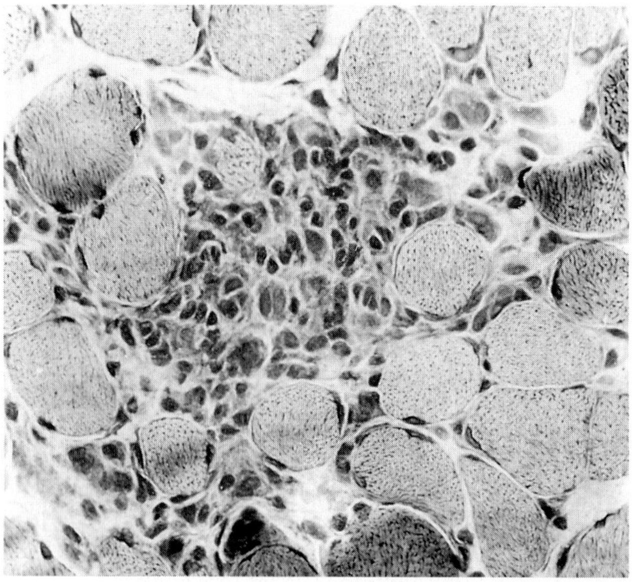

Figure 9-27 Muscle cross section; dog. X-linked muscular dystrophy. Note that some myofibers are necrotic and are infiltrated by macrophages. H & E stain. *Courtesy Dr. B. J. Cooper.*

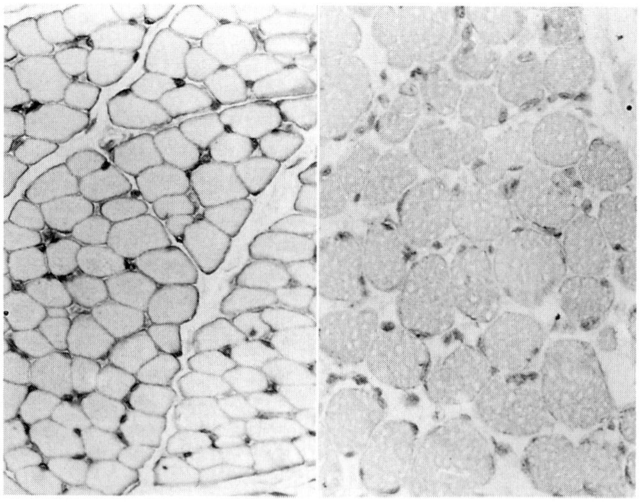

A B

Figure 9-28 Muscle cross section; dog. X-linked muscular dystrophy. **A,** Normal control. Note the dark staining of the dystrophin at the periphery of the myofibers. **B,** The lack of dystrophin in the myofibers in muscular dystrophy. Immunoperoxidase staining for dystrophin. *Courtesy Dr. B. J. Cooper.*

stages of the disorder and typically affects small clusters of contiguous fibers. Mineralization of scattered affected fibers is common. Regeneration of affected segments occurs rapidly, and characteristically both myofiber necrosis and fiber regeneration are present within the same section (Fig. 9-27). With time, ongoing necrosis and regeneration are less common, and endomysial fibrosis occurs. Chronically affected muscles can have remarkable fibrosis, and varying degrees of infiltration by adipocytes. The remaining myofibers are atrophic or hypertrophic and many contain internal nuclei. In the myocardium there are multiple foci of acute necrosis, mineralization, and progressive dissecting fibrosis.

The diagnosis may be suspected based on characteristic clinical findings in a young male dog, but must be confirmed by muscle biopsy and analysis of muscle for dystrophin. The absence of dystrophin in muscle fibers of affected dogs can be confirmed using immunohistochemical staining on frozen sections (Fig. 9-28). There is no treatment for this disorder. Carrier females should be identified either by dystrophin or DNA analysis and spayed. Any dog producing affected pups is a carrier, and approximately half of her female offspring will also be carriers.

Labrador Retriever Myopathy. Affected Labrador retrievers develop signs of neuromuscular weakness within the first 6 months of life. Exercise intolerance leads to collapse during prolonged exercise. Loss of triceps and patellar reflexes is characteristic. Affected dogs do not usually develop normal musculature. Episodes of collapse can be elicited by exposure to cold as well as by exercise. Concentric needle electromyography reveals marked abnormal spontaneous activity with normal motor nerve conduction velocities. Serum concentrations of CK and AST are often normal, although they may be mildly to moderately increased. Megaesophagus may be present.

This disorder is inherited as an autosomal recessive trait, with affected dogs occurring within the working or sporting breed lines rather than the show dog lines. Despite extensive study, the underlying defect is not known. The only specific abnormalities that may be seen at necropsy are poor muscling and possible megaesophagus. On histologic examination, affected dogs have remarkable myopathic changes characterized by clusters of atrophic myofibers, myofiber hypertrophy, internal nuclei, and rare scattered segmental necrosis and regeneration. Although the initial reports described this disorder as a type II deficiency myopathy, further studies have shown that fiber type proportions vary remarkably between muscles and between dogs, although an increase in type 1 fibers (type I myofiber predominance) is often seen. Alteration of the normal mosaic pattern of myofiber types is also seen. There is fiber type grouping, usually considered a neuropathic change, despite the absence of peripheral nerve lesions.

Based on the clinical findings, the diagnosis may be suspected, but should be confirmed by muscle biopsy. There is no treatment for the disorder, although the disease is nonprogressive after 6 months to 1 year of age, and affected animals may still be kept as pets.

Congenital Myotonia. Myotonia is most commonly seen in the chow chow dog. A similar disorder has been seen in the Staffordshire terrier. Both sexes are affected, and pups may begin to show signs of a stiff gait as early as 6 weeks of age. The signs progress for several months, and then stabilize, with variable severity. Affected dogs move with splayed, stiff thoracic limbs and often "bunny hop" in the pelvic limbs. Signs are most severe on initiation of movement and improve a little with continued exercise, but affected dogs are never clinically normal. During severe episodes, dogs may fall over, and laryngospasm may result in transient dyspnea and even cyanosis. The musculature becomes remarkably hypertrophied, and sustained muscle dimpling occurs after percussion. Characteristic waxing and waning ("dive bomber") myotonic bursts are seen with concentric needle electromyography. Serum concentrations of CK and AST are normal or mildly increased.

Available evidence supports an autosomal recessive inheritance of myotonia in the chow chow. The underlying cellular defect is not known. Hypertrophy, with prominently defined muscle groups, is the only finding on postmortem examination. In early stages of the disease, muscle appears relatively normal. With time, myofiber hypertrophy and myofiber atrophy, and rare scattered segmental necrosis or regeneration are seen. Fibrosis is mild to inapparent.

Diagnosis is based on clinical signs and can be confirmed by concentric needle electromyography or muscle biopsy. Therapeutic agents that act to stabilize excitable cell membranes, such as quinidine, procainamide, and phenytoin, can relieve some of the signs of myotonia.

Phosphofructokinase Deficiency. This is an autosomal recessive disorder that has been recognized in English springer spaniels and American cocker spaniels. Muscles from affected dogs have myopathic changes and inclusions of a PAS-positive, amylase-resistant substance classified as complex polysaccharide. Clinical signs of neuromuscular dysfunction do not occur, most likely because the skeletal muscle expresses the liver isoenzyme of phosphofructokinase. Absence of erythrocyte phosphofructokinase results in hemolysis during periods of increased respiratory activity (panting) and resultant mild respiratory alkalosis.

"Swimmer" Pups. These puppies are clinically similar to piglets with "splayleg." Affected pups cannot adduct the limbs beneath their bodies, and develop a characteristic "swimming" gait, and progressive flattening of the sternum. Although this syndrome can occur in pups with neuromuscular weakness of any sort, it is more commonly associated with overfeeding. Affected pups often recover after reduction in total daily milk intake, provision of a nonslippery surface, and development of harnesses and physical therapy to encourage them to bring their legs underneath their bodies and walk.

Endocrine Myopathies

Hypothyroidism. Signs of neuromuscular dysfunction due to hypothyroidism are extremely varied, and include generalized weakness, muscle atrophy, and megaesophagus. Electromyographic results may be normal, or have abnormal spontaneous activity and decreased motor nerve conduction velocities if there is concurrent peripheral neuropathy. Serum concentrations of CK and AST are generally normal. Other systemic manifestations of hypothyroidism may or may not be present.

Because of its role in muscle metabolism, decreased thyroid hormone results in skeletal myofiber weakness and atrophy. Hypothyroidism may also cause a peripheral neuropathy, and damage to motor nerves may cause a denervation atrophy and contribute to the neuromuscular weakness. Overall muscle atrophy may be seen. The thyroid glands may be bilaterally atrophied. Megaesophagus may be present. Symmetric alopecia (endocrine dermatopathy) may be seen. Type II myofibers are preferentially atrophied. Axonal degeneration may be seen in peripheral nerves (peripheral neuropathy), and affected muscle may also show angular atrophy of both type I and type II fibers, or fiber type grouping, all due to denervation.

Diagnosis may be suspected on the basis of clinical findings and selective type II atrophy in affected muscles but should be confirmed by evaluation of thyroid function. In many cases, replacement thyroid hormone markedly improves neuromuscular weakness.

Myopathy Due to Excessive Corticosteroids (Hypercortisolism). This disorder may be due to increased adrenocortical cortisol production or to administration of exogenous corticosteroids. Clinical findings may be very similar to those in hypothyroidism. A unique manifestation of hypercortisolism in some dogs is development of a remarkably stiff, stilted pelvic limb gait, with increased bulk and tone of proximal thigh muscles (Cushingoid pseudomyotonia). Concentric needle electromyography of these muscles reveals myotonic bursts that do not wax and wane (pseudomyotonic activity), and muscles do not dimple after percussion. Serum concentrations of CK and AST are normal. Other systemic signs of hypercortisolism such as overall muscle atrophy and alopecia may be present. The cause of Cushingoid pseudomyotonia is not known, although induction of sarcolemmal ionic instability is possible. Overall muscle atrophy may be seen. Dogs with Cushingoid pseudomyotonia have increased muscle bulk, especially in the thigh muscles. Adrenal glands may have bilateral cortical atrophy due to exogenous corticosteroid administration or may be hypertrophied because of stimulation from a pituitary tumor. Adrenal cortical neoplasia causes enlargement of the affected gland and

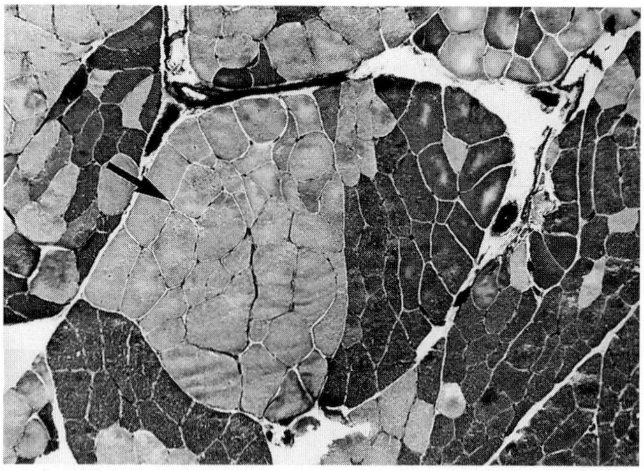

Figure 9-29 Muscle, triceps brachii; dog. Myofiber type grouping, the result of denervation and subsequent reinnervation secondary to several years of treatment with steroids. Note the loss of the "checkerboard" appearance and the groupings of type I (light) and type II fibers (dark). Myofibrillar ATPase (pH = 9.8) stain.

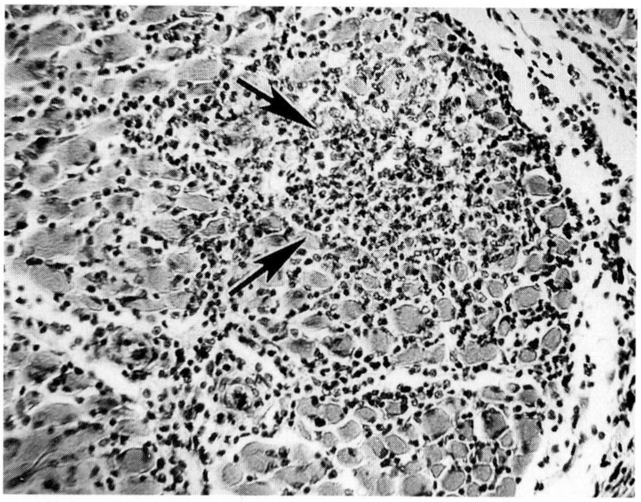

Figure 9-30 Muscle; dog. Polymyositis. Note that this affects only a portion of the fasciculus and is characterized by a lymphocytic infiltrate *(arrows)* and loss of myofibers by necrosis. H & E stain. ×200. *Courtesy Dr. W. J. Hadlow.*

Table 9-8 Myopathies Due to Immune-Mediated Disease

Disorder	Species Affected
Polymyositis	Dogs
Masticatory myositis	Dogs
Extraocular muscle myositis	Dogs
Acquired myasthenia gravis	Dogs, cats

atrophy of the contralateral gland. Findings in affected muscle and peripheral nerves are similar to those seen in hypothyroid myopathy, and include both selective type II fiber atrophy and evidence of denervation atrophy that may include fiber type grouping (Fig. 9-29).

Diagnosis may be suspected on the basis of clinical findings and selective type II fiber atrophy or evidence of denervation atrophy in affected muscle but should be confirmed by evaluation of adrenocortical function and total serum cortisol. Cessation of exogenous corticosteroids, removal of adrenal neoplasia, or chemical destruction of hyperplastic adrenal cortical tissue results in improvement in muscle mass and strength, although signs of pseudomyotonia may persist.

Immune-Mediated Myopathies

These myopathies are listed in Table 9-8.

Polymyositis. This generalized inflammatory myopathy may have an acute and rapidly progressive or an insidious onset of muscle atrophy and generalized weakness. Temporal and masseter muscle atrophy may be most obvious, and esophageal muscle involvement may result in megaesophagus. Respiratory muscle involvement can occur and, if severe, may cause respiratory distress. Pain on palpation of muscles may be present but is relatively uncommon. Serum concentrations of CK, AST, and ALT may be increased, but in chronic cases these concentrations may also be within normal limits. Concentric needle electromyography may reveal scattered foci of abnormal spontaneous activity, and motor nerve conduction velocities are normal.

Polymyositis is due to an immune-mediated inflammation that attacks components of the skeletal myofibers, and results in myofiber necrosis. The immunologic injury may be directed against skeletal muscle only or may be part of a more generalized immune-mediated disease such as systemic lupus erythematosus. Polymyositis may also occur in dogs with thymoma.

Overall muscle atrophy may be the only finding, unless megaesophagus is also present. Findings within affected muscles are extremely variable. In acute, fulminating cases, the muscle sections are filled with inflammatory cells, predominantly lymphocytes and plasma cells (Fig. 9-30), although eosinophils and neutrophils may also be present. The degree of myofiber necrosis is variable, but necrotic fibers in early stages always have either a rim of interstitial lymphocytes, or a core of invading mononuclear cells. Macrophages are also commonly seen in segmental necrosis or foci of necrotic myofibers. Regeneration is often also present (multiphasic segmental necrosis). In more chronic, insidious cases, the only lesion consists of scattered lymphocytes adjacent to myofibers. Sampling multiple muscles for histopathologic examination is recommended. Regeneration may restore myofibers

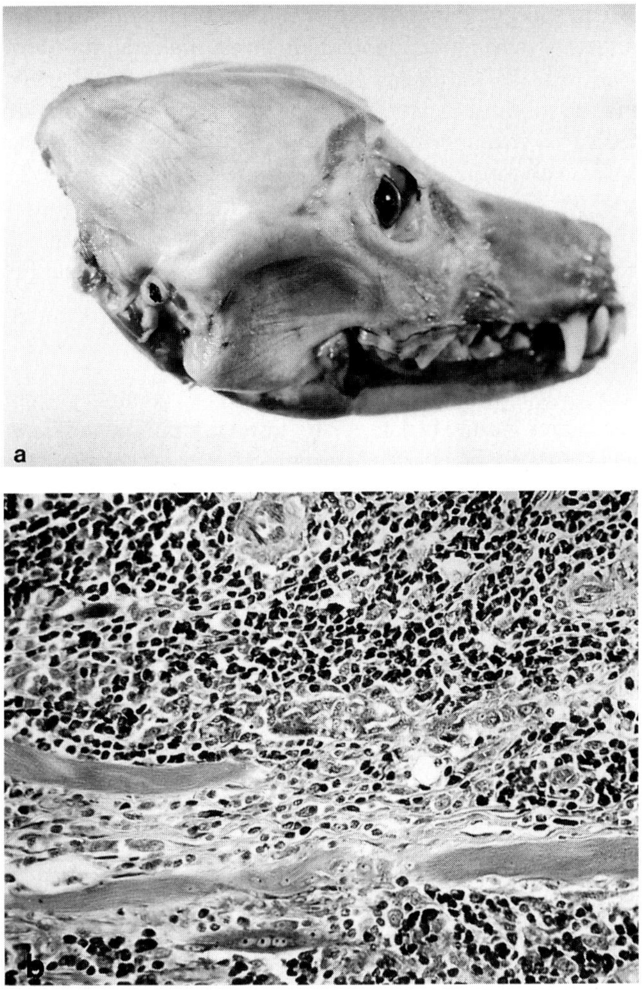

Figure 9-31 Muscle; dog. Masticatory muscle myositis. **A,** Muscle, temporalis, chronic stage, with marked atrophy. **B,** Acute stage. An extensive infiltrate of chiefly lymphocytes lies between myofibers. H & E stain. ×200. *Courtesy Dr. W. J. Hadlow.*

to normal, but in severe chronic cases, endomysial fibrosis may be evident.

Although polymyositis may be suspected based on the clinical findings, identification of characteristic changes within muscle sections is often necessary to confirm a diagnosis of polymyositis. A positive circulating antinuclear antibody titer (ANA) is useful, but is not always found. Treatment with immunosuppressive drugs such as corticosteroids may be curative, but affected animals may require lifelong therapy.

Masticatory Muscle Myositis ("Eosinophilic Myositis," "Atrophic Myositis"). Severe, acute cases have bilaterally symmetric swelling of the temporal and masseter muscles, pain, and inability to fully open the jaw. Affected dogs may have difficulty prehending food. More chronic or insidious cases have bilaterally symmetric atrophy of the temporal and masseter muscles (Fig. 9-31, *A*). This results

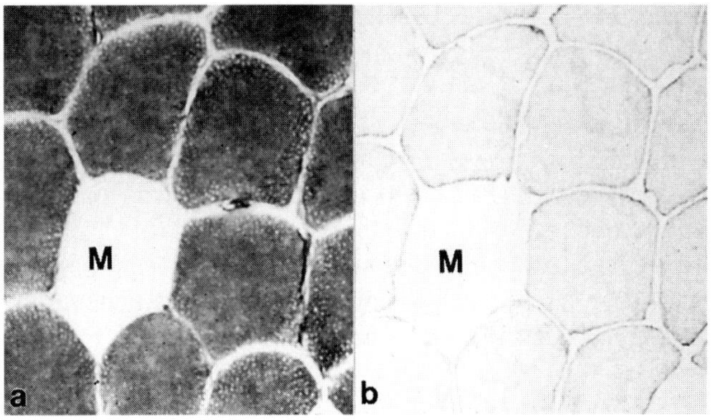

Figure 9-32 Muscle, temporalis, normal; dog. **A,** Type I myofibers are light, and the type II are dark. Myofibrillar ATPase (pH = 9.8) stain. **B,** The section was incubated with staphylococcal protein A–peroxidase conjugates (SPA-HRPO) following incubation with serum, diluted 1:50, from a dog with masticatory muscle myositis (MMM). The type I fibers *(M)* are unstained, whereas the type II fibers are positively stained, indicating their involvement in MMM. *Courtesy Dr. G. D. Shelton.*

in an inability to open the jaw fully. Pain may or may not be evident. Concentric needle EMG often reveals foci of spontaneous activity in active cases, but may be normal in more chronic cases. Serum concentrations of CK and AST are normal or only mildly increased.

The type II masticatory muscles of the dog contain a unique myosin isoform (type IIM myosin), and circulating antibodies to this myosin result in the localization of this inflammatory myopathy (Fig. 9-32). In acute cases, temporal and masseter muscles may be swollen, but in more chronic cases only atrophy is seen. Severely atrophied muscles may contain pale streaks. The degree and nature of the inflammation are variable. In acute cases infiltrates of lymphocytes and plasma cells (Fig. 9-31, *B*), sometimes with numerous eosinophils are present. Neutrophils are much less common. Inflammation is associated with myofiber necrosis. Regeneration may restore fiber integrity, but because basal laminae are often damaged, healing is by fibrosis. The presence of fibrosis is an important prognostic indicator, as fibrosis is an irreversible change.

The diagnosis may be suspected on the basis of characteristic clinical findings, but masticatory muscle myositis should be differentiated from polymyositis involving the temporal and masseter muscles. Serologic testing to detect anti–type IIM myosin antibodies specific to masticatory muscle myositis is available. Electromyography and evaluation of multiple muscle biopsy samples may also help to differentiate these two disorders. Treatment with immunosuppressive doses of corticosteroids generally alleviates pain and results in increased mobility of the jaw and increase in muscle mass. Some degree of atrophy and loss of complete jaw mobility may persist. A single course of corticosteroids may be curative; however, some cases may require more extended therapy.

Idiopathic Masticatory Muscle Atrophy. Dogs may develop a progressive atrophy of temporal and masseter muscles that is not associated with pain or difficulty opening the jaw or prehending food. Examination of affected muscle from these dogs reveals mild generalized atrophy of myofibers, but no evidence of inflammation, degeneration, fibrosis, or denervation. There is no treatment for this disorder.

Extraocular Muscle Myositis. Acute onset of bilateral exophthalmos is seen. Affected dogs are usually less than 2 years of age, and golden retriever dogs appear to be predisposed. Serum concentrations of CK and AST are generally normal.

An immune-mediated attack directed specifically at extraocular muscles is suspected. The extraocular muscles, with the exception of the retractor bulbi muscle, are swollen and pale yellow. A predominantly lymphocytic inflammation with associated myofiber necrosis and regeneration are seen. Because the extraocular muscles are difficult to biopsy, diagnosis generally is based on typical clinical findings. Corticosteroid therapy is effective, but episodes may recur.

Disorders of the Neuromuscular Junction

Myasthenia Gravis. Typical signs are episodic collapses in an adult dog, and normal gait and strength after rest. Clinical signs can, however, be variable. Megaesophagus may be the only presenting sign. In some cases, mild weakness persists between episodes. Repetitive motor nerve stimulation reveals a sharp decremental response, followed by relatively uniform amplitude potentials. Serum concentrations of CK and AST are normal. A congenital form of myasthenia gravis, inherited as an autosomal recessive trait, occurs in Jack Russell terriers, smooth fox terriers, and springer spaniels. Clinical signs of congenital myasthenia gravis appear at an early age (6 to 8 weeks of age) and are typically quite severe.

In most cases, myasthenia gravis is an acquired disease, with circulating antibodies directed at the acetylcholine receptors of the neuromuscular junction. In some cases, onset of myasthenia gravis may occur associated with thymoma or, less commonly, thymic hyperplasia. Congenital myasthenia gravis is due to abnormal development of the neuromuscular junction and is inherited as an autosomal recessive trait. No findings are evident at postmortem examination unless megaesophagus is present, and no abnormalities in muscle are seen on light microscopic examination. Ultrastructural examination reveals characteristic abnormalities of the neuromuscular junction.

Diagnosis may be suspected on the basis of typical clinical findings. Intravenous edrophonium (Tensilon), which prolongs the active life of acetylcholine at the neuromuscular junction, results in a marked, transient improvement in muscle strength. Serologic testing for antibodies to acetylcholine receptors is often the test of choice for diagnosis of acquired myasthenia gravis. Thymic abnormalities should be ruled out, as removal of a thymoma or of a hyperplastic thymus results in resolution of clinical signs. In other cases, corticosteroid therapy is often beneficial. There is no effective treatment for congenital myasthenia gravis.

Other Canine Myopathies

Exertional Rhabdomyolysis. Massive acute rhabdomyolysis associated with exertion occurs in racing greyhounds and sled dogs. Predisposing factors are not clear, but in sled dogs a change to a very high fat diet has resulted in decreased exercise-induced muscle injury.

Malignant Hyperthermia. There are sporadic reports of a malignant hyperthermia–like condition in dogs, and breeding studies indicate an autosomal dominant inheritance. There are many similarities to this condition in pigs.

Dermatomyositis. A condition involving skin and muscle disease has been described in collies and Shetland sheepdogs. Although the dermatopathologic changes are distinctive, the muscle involvement is much less well documented, and may reflect extension of inflammation from overlying affected skin.

Breed-Specific Myopathies. A number of breed specific myopathies have been reported in the dog, including mitochondrial myopathy in Old English sheepdogs and myopathy of Bouvier des Flandres dogs and Clumber spaniels.

Myopathies of the Cat

Inherited or Congenital Myopathies

X-Linked Muscular Dystrophy (Duchenne-Type Muscular Dystrophy). Affected cats develop a progressive, persistent stiff gait associated with marked muscular hypertrophy. Age of onset is from a few months to 21 months of age. Affected cats have difficulty grooming, jumping, and lying down. Concentric needle EMG reveals dense and sustained abnormal spontaneous activity, similar to findings in the dystrophic dog. Serum concentrations of CK, AST, and ALT are elevated, typically to very high levels. Affected cats may die under anesthesia.

Dystrophic cats lack the muscle cytoskeletal protein dystrophin, which is also the cause of Duchenne dystrophy in boys and X-linked muscle dystrophy in the dog. The cause of the remarkable muscular hypertrophy in affected cats, as opposed to the muscle atrophy seen in the dog and man and the pseudohypertrophy due to fat infiltration that can occur in man, is not known.

Marked muscular hypertrophy, often very prominent in the diaphragm, is found. Affected muscles may contain pale areas. Focal pale or chalky areas within the myocardium are typically found. Histologically, affected muscles show a range of changes. Concurrent segmental myonecrosis and myofiber regeneration (multiphasic necrosis) are characteristic. Chronic myopathic changes, found in older animals, include myofiber atrophy, hypertrophy (Fig. 9-11), internal nuclei, and mild to moderate endomysial fibrosis. Myocardial lesions consist of multifocal necrosis and mineralization of cardiac myofibers and fibrosis, primarily in the left ventricular free wall, papillary muscles, and septum.

The diagnosis may be suspected on the basis of characteristic clinical and histopathologic findings in a young male cat. Confirmation relies on assay of muscle samples for dystrophin or on immunohistochemical testing for dystrophin in frozen sections.

Congenital Myotonia. Cats with congenital myotonia present with signs similar to those of dystrophic cats, but the muscular hypertrophy is less remarkable. Serum concentrations of CK and AST are normal or slightly increased. A stiff gait is most obvious. Concentric needle electromyography reveals waxing and waning ("dive bomber") potentials characteristic of myotonia.

The pathogenesis of feline congenital myotonia is not known at this time, although a skeletal muscle ion channel defect is suspected. Other than mild muscular hypertrophy, there are no findings at necropsy. Significant myofiber hypertrophy and increased variation in myofiber diameters are the only histopathologic finding.

The diagnosis of congenital feline myotonia is based on characteristic clinical findings. At this time, no type of treatment has been attempted.

Glycogenosis in Norwegian Forest Cats. Affected cats may be stillborn or die within a few hours of birth. Those that survive lack energy and develop muscle tremors, and a bunny-hopping pelvic limb gait at about 5 months of age. The disease is progressive, resulting in severe muscle atrophy and tetraplegia. Concentric needle EMG reveals abnormal spontaneous activity with normal motor nerve conduction velocities. Serum concentrations of CK and AST are mildly to moderately increased.

This disorder is due to decreased activity of branching enzyme, resulting in defective carbohydrate metabolism and a generalized glycogen storage disease. The disorder is inherited as an autosomal recessive trait. Muscle atrophy and fibrosis of severely affected pelvic limb muscles in cats surviving 1 year or longer is evident. There is severe storage of PAS-positive, amylase-resistant material forming "lakes" within skeletal muscle fibers and prominent myofiber atrophy. Myofiber necrosis and regeneration are seen. Cardiac myocytes have similar inclusions, myocyte necrosis, and replacement by fibrosis. Abnormal glycogen storage is also seen within smooth muscle and neurons in the central nervous system.

Diagnosis can be suspected on the basis of characteristic clinical and histopathologic findings. Confirmation is based on assay of glycogen branching enzyme in blood leukocytes. There is no treatment for this disorder.

Myopathies Due to Electrolyte Abnormalities

Similar to cattle, cats with severe electrolyte abnormalities may show signs of neuromuscular weakness that may be associated with degenerative myopathy. Although degenerative myopathy has been reported secondary to increased blood sodium concentrations (hypernatremia), hypokalemic myopathy occurs far more frequently.

Hypokalemic and Hypernatremic Myopathy. Affected cats show severe generalized weakness, with ventriflexion of the neck. Concentric needle electromyography may demonstrate foci of abnormal spontaneous activity. Serum concentrations of CK, AST, and ALT are often increased, sometimes markedly. Blood concentrations of potassium are low in hypokalemia and blood concentrations of sodium are high in hypernatremia.

The cause of the weakness and myofiber necrosis is complex and involves abnormal skeletal muscle energy metabolism and possible ischemia due to vasoconstriction. Hypokalemia may be due to decreased dietary intake or increased urinary excretion of potassium and in cats is often a consequence of chronic renal disease. It may also occur secondary to gastrointestinal disease or inappropriate fluid therapy. Hyperthyroidism has been associated with development of hypokalemic myopathy in cats. Hypernatremic myopathy has been reported in a 7-month-old cat with hydrocephalus and transient hypopituitarism.

No specific gross pathologic findings are present except in cats with hypokalemia due to chronic renal disease, in which the kidneys are small and fibrotic, or in cats with hydrocephalus and hypernatremia. In hypokalemic myopathy, myofiber necrosis and regeneration of variable severity are present concurrently (multiphasic). If renal disease is present, chronic interstitial nephritis is most commonly seen. No abnormalities were detected in a muscle biopsy from the cat with hypernatremic myopathy, although the mildly increased serum concentration of creatine kinase and abnormal electromyography suggest mild and perhaps transient myofiber necrosis and regeneration.

The diagnosis is based on characteristic clinical findings of weakness, and hypokalemia or hypernatremia. Treatment of affected cats has been very successful. Immediate fluid therapy is used to correct the electrolyte abnormality, followed by diet change to maintain normal electrolyte concentrations. If there is an underlying hyperthyroidism, this should be treated.

Disorders of the Neuromuscular Junction

Myasthenia Gravis. Feline acquired and congenital myasthenia gravis are similar to those disorders in the dog, but occur less commonly.

Other Feline Myopathies

Nemaline myopathy is a congenital disorder described in domestic short-haired cats. These have a characteristic progressive abnormal gait and muscle atrophy at an early age. The characteristic pathologic finding of expanded Z line material (nemaline rods) within skeletal muscle fibers is only apparent in frozen sections or ultrastructurally. A congenital myopathy resulting in spasticity has also been described in Devon Rex cats. The inheritance of these disorders is unclear.

Suggested Readings

Adams RD. Diseases of muscle 3rd ed. Hagerstown, Md: Harper & Row; 1975.

Armstrong RB, Saubert CW IV, Seeherman HJ, Taylor CR. Distribution of fiber types in locomotory muscles of dogs. Am J Anat 1982; 163:87-98.

Bradley R, Fell BF. Myopathies in animals. In: Walton J, ed. Disorders of Voluntary Muscle. 4th ed. Edinburgh: Churchill Livingstone, 1981:824-872.

Burke RE, Levine DN, Zajac FE III, Tsairis P, Engle WK. Mammalian motor units: Physiological-histochemical correlations in three types in cat gastrocnemius. Science 1971; 174:709-712.

Carpenter JL, Schmidt CM, Moore FM, Albert DM, Abrams KL, Elner VM. Canine bilateral extraocular polymyositis. Vet Pathol 1989; 26:510-512.

de Lahunta A. Lower motor neuron–general somatic efferent system. In: Veterinary Neuroanatomy and Clinical Neurology. 2nd ed. Philadelphia: WB Saunders, 1983:53-129.

Dubowitz V. Muscle biopsy: A practical approach. 2nd ed. London: Baillière, 1985.

Hadlow WJ. Myopathies in animals. In: Pearson CM, Mostofi FK, eds. The Striated Muscle. Baltimore: Williams & Wilkins. 1973; 3640.

Harriman DGF. Muscle. In: Adams JH, Corsellis JAN, Duchan LW, eds. Greenfield's Neuropathology. 4th ed. New York: Wiley, 1985; 1026.

Hulland TJ. Muscle and tendon. In: Jubb KVF, Kennedy PC, Palmer N, eds. Pathology of Domestic Animals. 4th ed. New York: Academic Press, 1993:183-265.

Kakulas BA, Cooper BJ. Experimental and animal models of human neuromuscular disease. In: Walton J, Karpati G, Hilton-Jones D, eds. Disorders of Voluntary Muscle. 6th ed. New York: Churchill Livingstone, 1994:437-496.

Orvis JS, Cardinet GH III. Canine muscle fiber types and susceptibility of masticatory muscles to myositis. Muscle Nerve 1981; 4:354-359.

Peter JB, Barnard RJ, Edgerton VR, et al. Metabolic profiles of three fiber types of skeletal muscles in guinea pigs and rabbits. Biochemistry 1972; 11:2627-2634.

Selected neurologic and muscular diseases. Veterinary Clinics: Equine Practice. Vol. 13, no. 1. Philadelphia: WB Saunders, 1997.

Shelton GD, Cardinet GH III. Pathophysiologic basis of canine muscle disorders. J Vet Intern Med 1987; 1(1):36-44.

Valentine BA, Winand NJ, Pradhan D, Moise NS, de Lahunta A, Kornegay JN, Cooper BJ: Canine X-linked muscular dystrophy as an animal model of Duchenne muscular dystrophy: A review. Am J Med Genet 1992; 42:352-356.

Van Vleet JF, Amstutz HE, Weirich WE, et al. Acute monensin toxicosis in swine: Effect of graded doses of monensin and protection of swine by pretreatment with selenium–vitamin E. Am J Vet Res 1983; 44:1460-1468.

Van Vleet JF, Ferrans VJ, Herman E. Cardiovascular and skeletal muscle system. In: Haschek-Hock WM, Rousseaux CG, eds. Handbook of Toxicologic Pathology. Orlando, Fla.: Academic Press, 1991; 539-624.

CHAPTER 10

Bone and Joints

STEVEN E. WEISBRODE
CECIL E. DOIGE†

DISEASES OF BONE
Normal Structure and Function
Bone at the Cellular Level

Structure and function can be discussed at the organ, tissue, and cellular levels. In this section, normal structure and function are briefly reviewed beginning at the cellular level and include bone matrix and mineral. Cells directly involved with the structural integrity of bone include osteoblasts, osteocytes, and osteoclasts.

Osteoblasts are mesenchymal cells that arise from bone marrow stromal stem cells under the influence of paracrine and endocrine stimuli. Osteoblasts cover bone-forming surfaces and are responsible for production of bone matrix (osteoid; see page 501) and initiation of matrix mineralization. When active, osteoblasts are plump, cuboidal cells (Fig. 10-1) with abundant basophilic cytoplasm (rich in rough endoplasmic reticulum). Inactive osteoblasts are diskshaped with little cytoplasm because of the reduction in amount of rough endoplasmic reticulum and golgi involved with matrix synthesis and secretion. Osteoblasts send thin, tortuous, cytoplasmic processes into the matrix, and some of these make contact with similar cytoplasmic extensions of osteocytes. This interconnecting network of osteoblasts and osteocytes forms a functional membrane that separates the extracellular fluid bathing bone surfaces from the general extracellular fluid and regulates the flow of calcium and phosphate ions to and from the bone fluid compartment (Fig. 10-2). For calcium to get into bone, it is postulated that calcium passes between osteoblasts. To get out of bone, it is speculated that an intracellular pump (within osteoblasts) moves calcium outward across the cell membrane to the general extracellular fluid compartment. Osteoblast membranes are rich in alkaline phosphatase; an indirect estimate of osteoblast synthetic activity can be determined by measuring the concentration in blood of the bone isoenzyme of alkaline phosphatase. The function of this enzyme in the osteoblast is uncertain, but it could play a role in mineralization and in pumping calcium across cellular membranes. Osteoblasts have receptors for parathyroid hormone (PTH), and activation of these receptors increases the activity of the osteoblast calcium pump and, by paracrine factor(s), initiates bone resorption by osteoclasts (see page 500).

Osteocytes are osteoblasts that have been surrounded by mineralized bone matrix. They occupy small spaces in the bone called lacunae (singular: lacuna) and make contact with osteoblasts and other osteocytes by means of long cytoplasmic processes that pass through thin tunnels (canaliculi; singular: canaliculus) in mineralized bone matrix (Fig. 10-3). Osteocytes likely have a role in regulating the composition of the fluid in the bone fluid compartment and might be capable of removing bone mineral ions from perilacunar bone. Because of the large surface area of perilacunar and canalicular bone available for rapid ion exchange, it is possible that significant amounts of calcium could be made available to the bone fluid compartment and, eventually, the extracellular fluid compartment without structural changes within the bone. Thus, using an osteoblast-osteocyte calcium pump system, significant amounts of calcium from bone could be made available to the blood without osteoclastic resorption of bone. Under conditions of extreme stress to calcium homeostasis, osteocytes might have the ability to resorb perilacunar mineral and matrix, thus enlarging the lacuna (osteocytic osteolysis). This process apparently is rare and likely does not contribute significantly to development of osseous lesions. Osteocytes also retain a limited capacity for bone formation. The role of osteocytes in maintenance of mature bone is uncertain because dead cortical bone can persist for long periods without losing structural integrity.

Osteoclasts are multinucleated cells responsible for bone resorption (Fig. 10-4). They are derived from hematopoietic stem cells, of the granulocyte-monocyte series. They have abundant eosinophilic cytoplasm, which has a specialized brush border that is adjacent to a bone surface undergoing resorption (Fig. 10-5). Osteoclasts resorb bone in two stages. First, the mineral is dissolved by secretion of hydrogen ions through a proton pump located in the brush border. These hydrogen ions are derived from carbonic acid produced within the osteoclast from water and carbon dioxide by the enzyme carbonic anhydrase.

†Deceased.

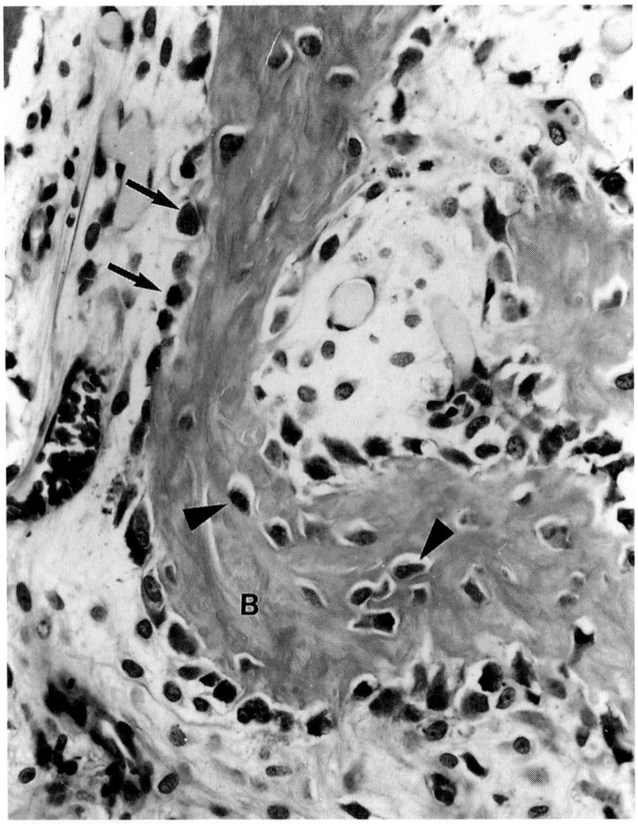

Figure 10-1 Bone. Reactive (repair) woven bone *(B)* at a fracture site. Bone surfaces are covered by plump osteoblasts *(arrows);* large irregularly arranged osteocytes *(arrowheads)* are located in lacunae and are surrounded by osteoid with coarsely bundled collagen. Hematoxylin and eosin (H & E) stain.

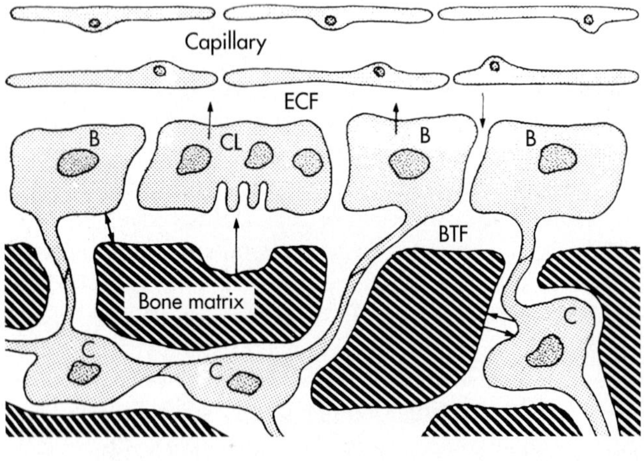

Figure 10-2 Diagram of hypothesized calcium movement *(arrows)* and relationships of osteoblasts *(B)*, osteocytes *(C)*, and osteoclasts *(CL)* to blood vessels, extracellular fluid *(ECF)*, and bone tissue fluid *(BTF)* compartment. *Redrawn from Matthews JL, Vander Wiel C, Talmage RV. Bone lining cells and the bone fluid compartment, an ultrastructural study. Adv Exp Med Biol 1978; 103:456.*

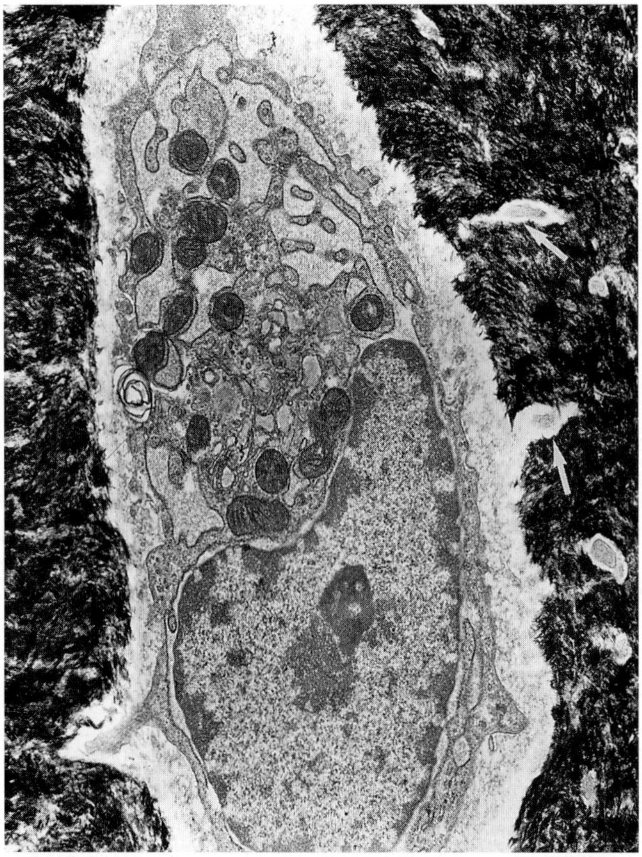

Figure 10-3 Bone, tibia, rodent. Transmission electron photomicrograph. A recently embedded osteocyte has residual rough endoplasmic reticulum and Golgi apparatus used during its osteoblastic period. Cell processes are extending into the mineralized matrix *(black)* through tunnels called "canaliculi" *(arrows)*. Uranyl acetate and lead citrate stain.

Second, the collagen of the matrix is cleaved into polypeptide fragments by proteinases released from the numerous lysosomes in the osteoclast and secreted through the brush border. The concavity in the bone created by the resorption is called a Howship's lacuna.

PTH is a potent systemic stimulator of osteoclastic bone resorption. In response to PTH, osteoclasts increase in number, and their brush borders become more abundant. Most investigations, however, have found that osteoclasts do not have receptors for PTH and that osteoblasts, which do have receptors for PTH, actually initiate the resorption process by signaling to osteoclast precursors and preparing the bone surface for osteoclast attachment. In response to PTH, osteoblasts contract and expose bone surfaces to which the osteoclasts can attach. The activated osteoblasts secrete or activate collagenases that remove a thin layer of normal unmineralized collagen fibers that remains on bone surfaces.

Removal of this layer allows the osteoclast to attach to a fully mineralized surface. Osteoclasts are unable to attach to unmineralized matrix (osteoid). In addition, osteoblasts release paracrine cytokines that attract and stimulate osteoclast precursors in the local environment. Calcitonin is a systemic inhibitor of osteoclasts. Osteoclasts have receptors for calcitonin and respond to this hormone by involuting their brush border and detaching from the bone surface. The stimuli for osteoclastic bone resorption in local disease processes are under the influence of cytokines (e.g., interleukin 1 [IL-1], IL-6, tumor necrosis factor [TNF]) and prostaglandins released not only from inflammatory cells such as the macrophage but, likely also, from a great variety of hyperplastic, neoplastic, and degenerated tissues.

Bone at the Matrix and Mineral Level

Interstitium of bone is what provides the organ's strength. It consists of a mineralized matrix. **Bone matrix** consists of type I collagen and "ground substance" (e.g., water, proteoglycans, glycosaminoglycans, noncollagenous proteins, and lipids, discussed below). Type I collagen polymers are secreted by osteoblasts and assembled into fibrils that are embedded in the ground substance and then mineralized. The type I collagen molecule is composed of three intertwined amino acid chains. Unique to these chains is the hydroxylated form of the amino acid proline

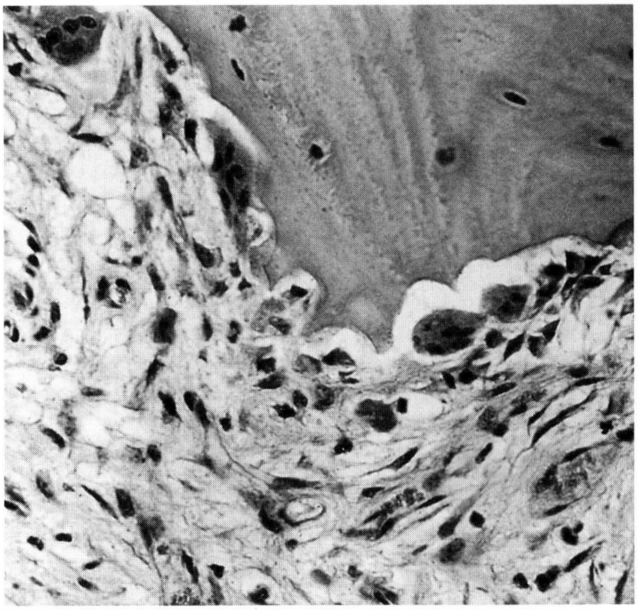

Figure 10-4 Bone, in region of necrosis undergoing osteoclastic resorption. The activity of multinucleated osteoclasts results in an irregular (resorbed) bone surface. The resorption cavities are called Howship's lacunae.

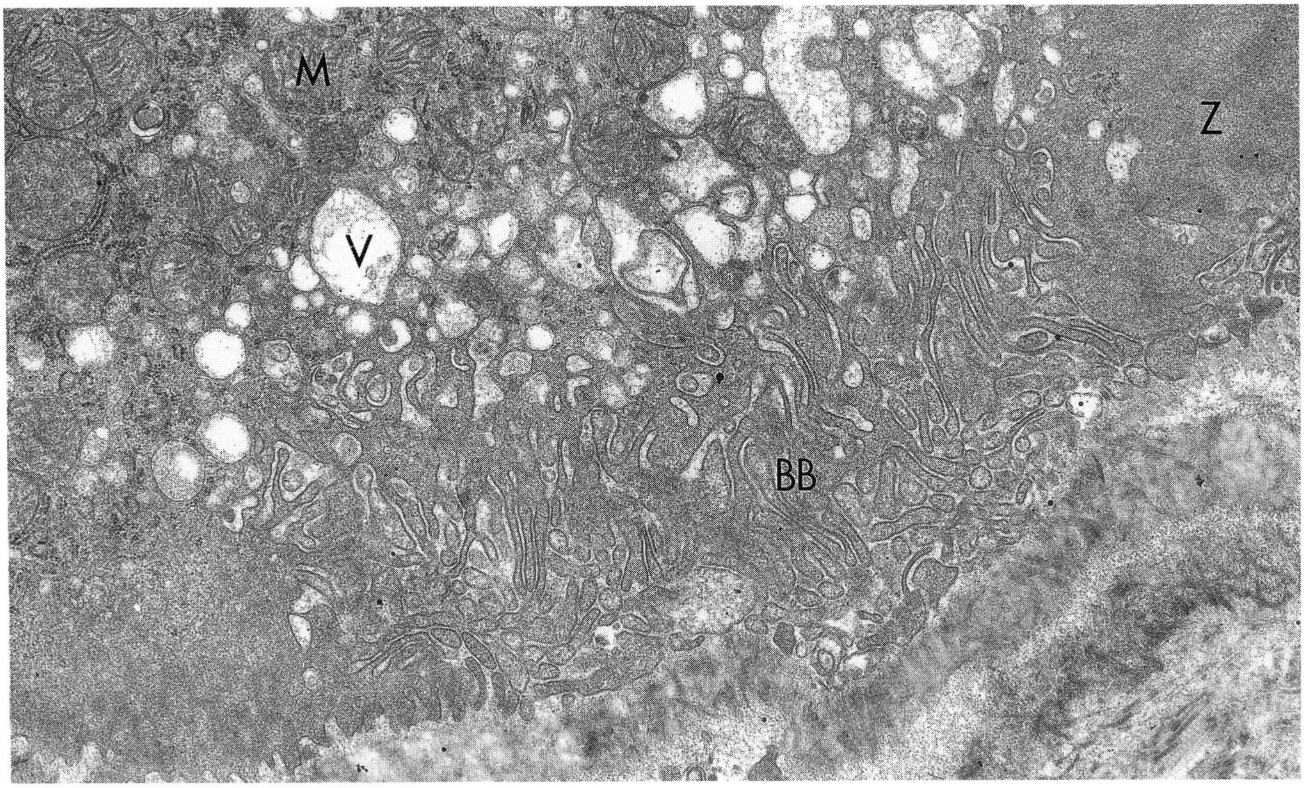

Figure 10-5 Bone, tibia, rodent. Transmission electron photomicrograph. Brush border *(BB)* of an osteoclast. Receptors in the dense zone *(Z)* adjacent to the brush border bind to ligands in the bone matrix attaching the osteoclast to the bone surface and preventing diffusion of acids and enzymes needed to dissolve the underlying mineral and matrix. Mitochondria *(M)* and numerous vesicles *(V)* containing lysosomal enzymes are present. Uranyl acetate and lead citrate stain.

(hydroxyproline). Type I collagen molecules have extensive crosslinkages among the amino acid chains within the molecule and between adjacent molecules. Within the collagen, molecules are deposited in rows with a gap between each molecule and with the rows staggered so that the molecules overlap by one fourth of their length. This specific packing of the collagen molecules and the cross-linkages contribute to the strength and insolubility of the fibrous component of the bone matrix. Other than in rapidly deposited reactive bone (woven bone, discussed on pages 503 and 507), primary trabeculae, and bone of early fetal development, collagen fibers are arranged in lamellae (singular: lamella). The orientation of the collagen fibers in each lamella is slightly different, giving a herringbone-like pattern. In Haversian (osteonal) bone, lamellae are arranged in concentric layers. In trabecular bone, the lamellae usually are arranged parallel with the surface. The collagen content of bone and its lamellar arrangement give bone its strength. The mineral content gives bone its hardness. The ground substance of bone, also synthesized by osteoblasts, consists of noncollagenous proteins, proteoglycans, and lipids. Many of the noncollagenous proteins are cytokines capable of influencing bone cell activity. These cytokines, such as **transforming growth factor-beta,** may play pivotal roles in controlling the extent of bone formation and resorption in normal remodeling and in disease. Also, among the noncollagenous proteins are enzymes that can function in degradation of collagen (e.g., collagenases) in bone resorption and can destroy inhibitors of mineralization (e.g., pyrophosphatases). Other noncollagenous proteins in the matrix can function as adhesion molecules and help bind cells to cells, cells to matrix, and mineral to matrix. Examples are osteonectin and osteocalcin. The role of proteoglycans in bone matrix is uncertain. They could play a role in inhibiting mineralization and promoting cell matrix interactions. Lipids can assist in binding calcium to cell membranes and in promoting calcification.

Bone mineral in fully mineralized bone is approximately 65% of the bone by weight and consists, in part, of calcium, phosphorus, carbonate, magnesium, sodium, manganese, zinc, copper, and fluoride. The production of osteoid (unmineralized organic matrix) by osteoblasts is followed by a period of maturation, after which mineral is deposited at the exchange of water. The process of mineralization is gradual and might not be complete, at least in reactive bone, for several months. Mineralization in woven bone is initiated within cytoplasmic blebs (matrix vesicles) of osteoblasts in the osteoid (Fig. 10-6), and these matrix vesicles have phospholipids and enzymes such as alkaline phosphatase and adenosine triphosphatase in their membranes. These enzymes can act to destroy inhibitors of mineralization, such as inorganic pyrophosphates, that are present in the osteoid and, along with the membrane phospholipids, concentrate calcium and phosphorus within the matrix vesicle. Initially this mineral is amorphous but after reaching critical mass, becomes crystalline. The crystalline hydroxyapatite pierces the lipid membrane of the matrix vesicle and extends to the gaps (holes) between collagen molecules. It is within these holes that the mineral crystals are first deposited in collagen. Once the gaps are filled with mineral, the process continues so that eventually the surfaces of collagen fibers as well as spaces between collagen fibers are mineralized. Initiation of mineralization in lamellar bone might not require matrix vesicles. Glycoproteins such as sialoprotein and osteonectin can act as the nidus for the mineralization process.

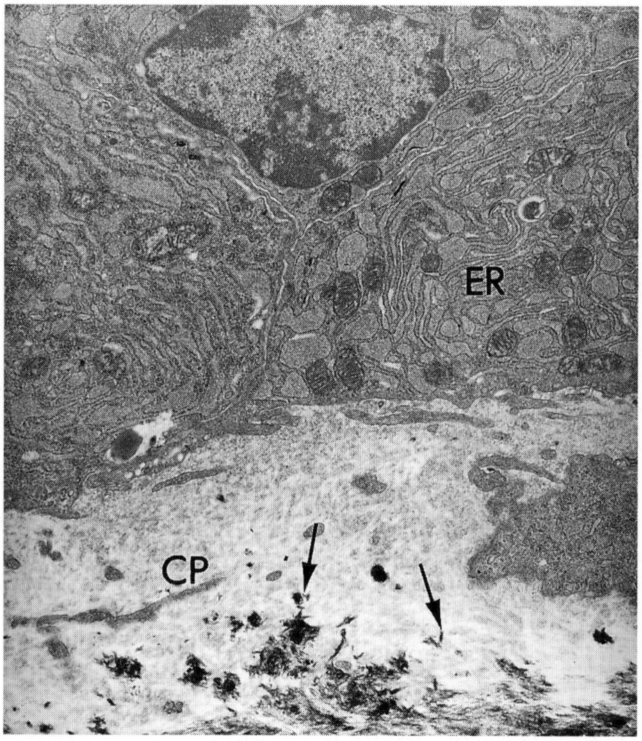

Figure 10-6 Bone, tibia, rodent. Transmission electron photomicrograph. Osteoblasts with abundant endoplasmic reticulum *(ER)* on an actively mineralizing surface. Cell processes *(CP)* of the osteoblasts extend out into the osteoid. Mineralization *(black spicules)* is initiated within matrix vesicles *(arrows)* then grows onto the adjacent collagen. Uranyl acetate and lead citrate stain.

Bone as a Tissue

Bone is organized into osteons or Haversian systems in the compact bone of the cortex and in subchondral bone of larger animals. In cortical bone, osteons are longitudinally orientated cylinders of concentric layers of lamellae that contain centrally located vessels and nerves. Haversian or compact bone is made up of numerous osteons (Fig. 10-7). Bone between the osteons is called interstitial lamellae. Layers of bone oriented circumferentially beneath the endosteal and periosteal surfaces are called circumferential

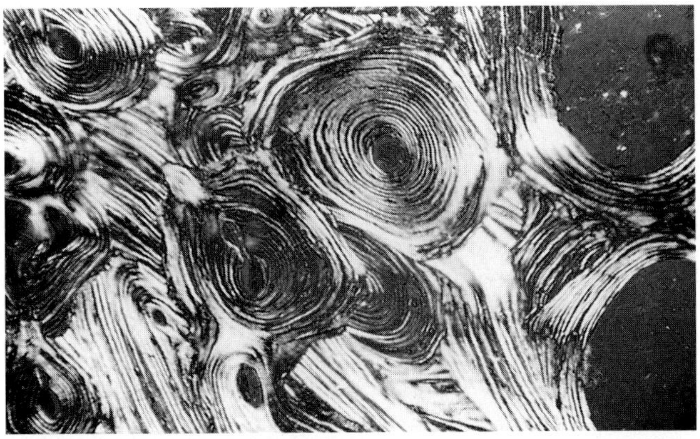

Figure 10-7 Bone. Polarized light micrograph. Endocortical surface of bone has undergone extensive osteonal remodeling. Collagen fibers are birefringent when viewed in appropriate plane with polarized light. Usually alternate lamellae polarize when viewed in the same plane. This alternating pattern of birefringence demonstrates the parallel arrangement of collagen layers in lamellar bone. All of the bone present is lamellar. Much of the cortex has been remodeled into osteonal bone (concentric layers), but there are areas of cortex that remain unosteonized. The endosteal surface to the right is forming a trabecula extending into the marrow space. Unstained and fully mineralized.

lamellae. The osteonal system provides channels for the vascular supply to thick bone of the cortex and also acts as tightly bound cables, giving the cortical bone strength yet limited flexibility. This osteonal system also might be important in limiting propagation of microcracks in bone by diverting cracks along cement lines.

In contrast to the dense compact bone of the cortex and the subchondral bone plates, the bone in the medullary cavity is in the form of anastomosing plates or rods and is called cancellous, trabecular, or spongy bone. The orientation of the trabeculae usually reflects adaptation (modeling) to mechanical stresses applied to the bone.The lamellae within a trabecula usually are arranged parallel with the surface of the trabecula. They are not arranged into tubes or osteons, as in cortical bone. The basophilic lines apparent in histologic tissue sections are called cement lines. These lines are mineral rich and collagen poor.

Bone rapidly produced in response to injury, inflammation, or neoplasia and the bone of the primary trabeculae and early fetus is called woven bone and often is referred to as reactive bone formation. Other than these exceptions, bone is deposited in lamellae and called lamellar bone. In woven bone, the collagen fibers are haphazardly arranged, and this bone is of inferior strength when compared with lamellar bone (see Fig. 10-12).

In most species, bone undergoes constant replacement called remodeling: old bone is resorbed and replaced by new. This turnover of old bone to new bone allows for the repair of accumulated microscopic injury in the bone (microfractures). In normal bone remodeling the negative net change in bone mass is slight (slightly less bone is replaced than removed, which is one of the causes of reduced bone mass in aged animals). In disease states such as hyperparathyroidism, resorption is often increased and formation decreased leaving a significant net negative bone balance. Not all species undergo bone remodeling; in small, short-lived animals such as the mouse and rat cortical bone is not remodeled. Not all areas of bone in larger species undergo remodeling. It is common to find unremodeled cortical bone in aged small dogs and cats. These unremodeled regions likely have been spared hard mechanical use (stress) and did not experience strain (deformation in structure) sufficient to initiate remodeling. The remodeling unit of cortical bone is called the osteon, and, for trabecular bone, it is called the basic structural unit. The shape of the osteon is cylindrical. The basic structural unit has the contour of a shallow bowl filled with parallel layers of lamellae.

The term "modeling" is used to describe change of the shape or contour of a bone in response to normal growth, altered mechanical use, or disease. In modeling, bone surfaces can undergo formation or resorption exclusively depending on the stimulus. This process allows the shape or size of bone to change and enables the medullary cavity to enlarge and the overall shape of the bone to be maintained while the bone is growing. Modeling is in contrast to normal remodeling in which resorption must precede formation to keep bone mass and shape constant. Both modeling and remodeling are under programmed genetic control but can be markedly altered by disease and changes in use of the bone. The adaptation of the shape and size of bone to accommodate altered use through modeling is known as Wolff's law. Changes in modeling and remodeling secondary to changes in mechanical use might be mediated by mechanical effects on osteocytes, stretch receptors on bone cells, streaming potentials, and piezoelectrical activity. Streaming potentials and piezoelectrical activity refers to electrical currents induced in bone due to fluid fluxes in the bone extracellular fluid and when collagen fibers and mineral crystals are deformed by mechanical forces respectively. Electrical currents can affect cell function (bone formation and resorption) and thus influence bone modeling (bone mass and orientation of osteons and trabeculae).

Bone as an Organ

Individual bones of the skeleton vary in their manner of formation, growth, structure, and function. Flat bones of the skull develop by the process of intramembranous ossification, in which mesenchymal cells differentiate into osteoblasts and produce bone directly. Cartilage precursors are not involved. Most bones develop from cartilaginous models by the process of endochondral ossification.

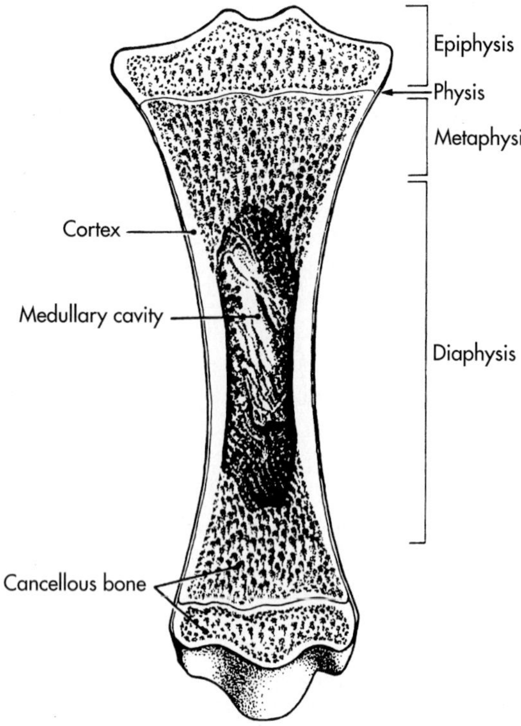

Figure 10-8 Diagram showing the anatomic components of a long bone.

Cartilaginous models are invaded by vessels, and primary (diaphyseal) and secondary (epiphyseal) centers of ossification develop and provide for further growth and increasing strength.

The long appendicular bones and the vertebral bodies are divided anatomically into epiphyses, metaphyseal growth plates (physes), metaphyses, and diaphyses (Fig. 10-8). The epiphysis is cartilaginous in the fetus, with ossification beginning centrally (secondary center of ossification). Growth of the epiphysis also contributes to the overall length of the bone and is accomplished by endochondral ossification at the articular-epiphyseal cartilage complex (the zone of endochondral ossification beneath the articular cartilage in animals that have not completed ossification of the epiphysis).

The metaphyseal growth plate, or physis, consists of hyaline cartilage. The chondroosseous junction in the metaphysis is a fragile lattice of bone-covered spicules of calcified cartilage. Cartilage of the metaphyseal growth plate is divided into a reserve or resting zone, a proliferative zone, and a hypertrophic zone (Fig. 10-9). The hypertrophic zone is sometimes further subdivided into zones of maturation, degeneration (really apoptosis), and calcification. The resting or reserve zone serves as a source of cells for the proliferating zone where cells multiply, accumulate glycogen, produce matrix, and become arranged in longitudinal columns. This replication of cells results in the overall lengthening of the bone. In the hypertrophic zone, chondrocytes secrete macromolecules that modify the matrix to allow capillary invasion, initiate matrix mineralization, and eventually these chondrocytes undergo apoptosis. Calcification begins in the longitudinal septa of cartilaginous matrix between columns of chondrocytes. Matrix vesicles derived from chondrocytes (analogous to those described above for mineralization of bone) form in the hypertrophic zone and initiate the mineralization process as previously described for bone.

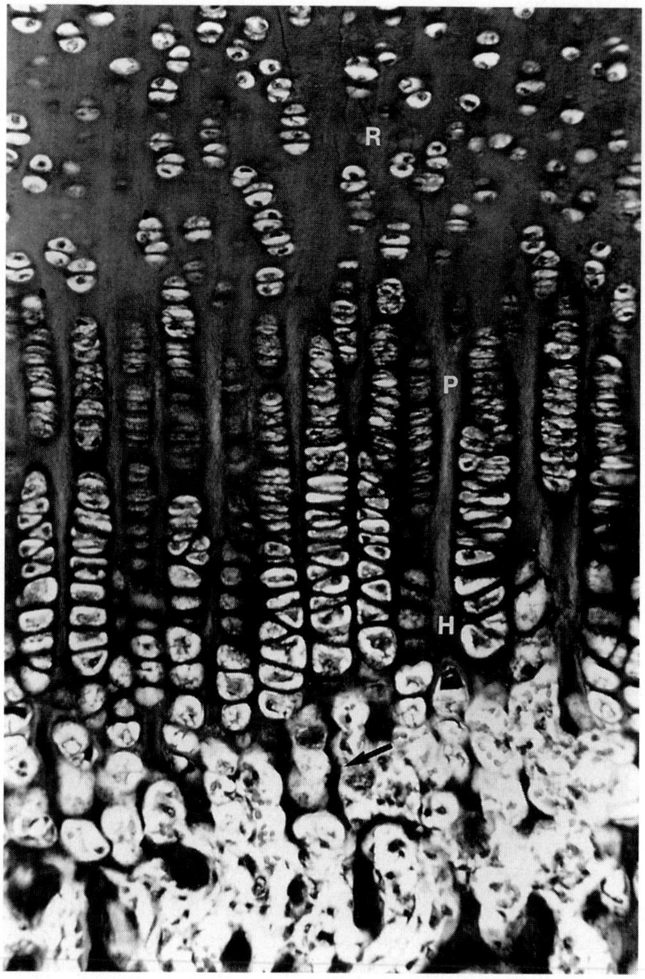

Figure 10-9 Bone; growth plate; dog. Resting *(R)*, proliferating *(P)*, and hypertrophic *(H)* zones of the growth plate are visible. Apoptotic chondrocytes are released from their lacunae by invading vessels and chondroclasts leaving only the longitudinal septa *(arrow)* as a basis of the primary trabeculae. H & E stain.

Growth plates are thickest when growth is most rapid; as growth slows, the plate becomes thin and "closes" (it is entirely replaced by bone) at skeletal maturity. Androgens and estrogens play a major role in determining the time of growth plate closure.

One end of the metaphysis is bordered by the calcified cartilage of the physis and the other by the diaphysis (central shaft of the bone). The periosteum covering the physis is called the perichondrial ring. The perichondrial ring adds new cartilage to the periphery of the physis, enabling the physis to expand in width as the animal grows. Primary trabeculae in the metaphysis consist of mineralized spicules of cartilage ("cartilage cores," the original longitudinal cartilage septa of the growth plate) covered by osteoid. Secondary and tertiary trabeculae are wider, branched, and often contain residual fragments of cartilage. The metaphyseal cortex beneath the perichondral ring is normally very thin in the growing bone, as its surfaces are the sites of very active osteoclastic bone resorption. Structurally, this area is the weakest part of the bone. The diaphysis or shaft of the bone has a thick cortex. In adult animals, the medullary cavity of the diaphysis has few trabeculae and contains mostly fatty marrow.

Except for articular surfaces (including the ends of the vertebral bodies), the surfaces of bones are covered by periosteum. This covering is a thin membrane that is loosely attached to underlying bone except at heavy fascial attachments on bony prominences and at tendon insertions, where its attachments are strong and are associated with large vessels penetrating the underlying bone. Microscopically, the periosteum is composed of an outer fibrous layer that provides structural support and an inner osteogenic or cambium layer capable of forming normal lamellar appositional bone on the cortex of growing bones and abnormal woven bone formation in response to injury. The periosteum is well supplied with lymph vessels and with fine myelinated and nonmyelinated nerve fibers that explain the intense pain when the periosteum is injured.

Blood Supply to Bone

Arterial blood from the systemic circulation enters bones through nutrient, metaphyseal, and periosteal arteries (Fig. 10-10). Nutrient arteries penetrate the diaphyseal cortex under strong, protective fascial attachments; once within the medulla, these arteries divide into proximal and distal intramedullary branches. The proximal and distal metaphyseal arteries are smaller and more numerous and penetrate the cortex and anastomose with the terminal branches of the nutrient arteries in the medullary cavity. These anastomoses protect against infarction if a nutrient artery is obstructed.

Small periosteal arteries also pass through the diaphyseal cortex at sites of fascial attachment, and can supply one quarter to one third of the outer cortex. The remainder of the cortex is supplied by the nutrient artery and its anastomotic branches. This blood flow is centrifugal (from medulla to periosteum), owing to greater pressures in the intramedullary vessels. The chondrocytes of the physis nearest the epiphysis are supplied by epiphyseal arteries. The chondrocytes of the physis nearest the metaphysis are supplied by branches of metaphyseal and nutrient arteries. As capillaries from these vessels approach the metaphyseal side of the physis, they make abrupt turns (loops). These loops are sites predisposed for bacterial embolization in neonatal sepsis.

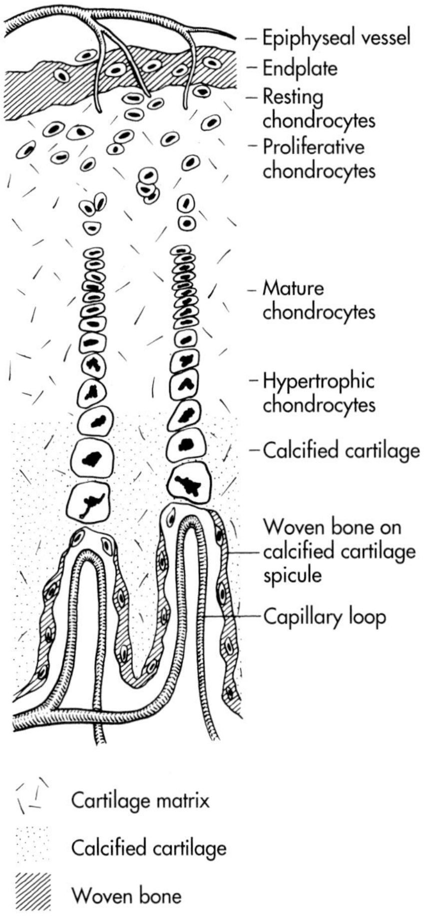

Figure 10-10 Diagram of the major blood supply to the physis. Branches of the epiphyseal artery supply the resting zones of the growth plate. Branches of the metaphyseal artery form capillary loops at the metaphyseal end of the physis undergoing endochondral ossification. *From Banks WJ. Applied veterinary histology. 3rd ed. St Louis: Mosby, 1993.*

Postmortem Examination and Evaluation of Bones

The entire skeleton is rarely examined at necropsy. Rather, the extent of the examination is dictated by the clinical history. Antemortem clinical and radiographic findings are invaluable and should be in hand before the postmortem examination is begun, especially for cases suspected of having relatively small localized lesions. It should be remembered that a lesion responsible for lameness may involve the skeletal, muscular, or nervous systems.

Pathologists should routinely examine certain areas of the skeleton. This procedure provides completeness to the necropsy and leads to familiarity with normal osseous structures. At least one long bone (preferably the femur) should be cut longitudinally and examined at necropsy. This examination should include an assessment of marrow for fat cell stores and hemopoietic activity, thickness of cortical bone, amount and distribution of cancellous bone, thickness and uniformity of metaphyseal growth plates, articular surfaces, and tendon insertions. Bony tissues are more readily seen if bone marrow contents are flushed out with a jet of water.

Postmortem changes do not usually pose major problems in the evaluation of the skeleton at necropsy. Postmortem bacterial invasion is less rapid than in most other tissues, and bone marrow cultures can be useful in detecting bacteremia. Bones can be fractured at euthanasia and by postmortem transport and handling.

Reactions of Bone to Injury

Bone, like other tissues exposed to injury, has predictable reactions and mechanisms of repair. Bone tissue consists mostly of mineral and collagen, which are extracellular and, other than having the ability to fracture, cannot respond to injury without being altered by changes in the activity of bone cells. As with cells in any organs, those in bone can undergo atrophy, hypertrophy, hyperplasia, metaplasia, neoplasia, degeneration, and necrosis. The amount of inorganic bone material present is a direct effect of the net activity of these cells. For example, bone resorption and bone formation can be increased at the periosteum, but, if the hyperplasia, hypertrophy, and functional activity of osteoclasts exceed that of osteoblasts, the net effect will be a loss of cortical bone. Changes in bone cell number, size, and activity can alter the modeling and remodeling of bone, as well as cause focal lytic or proliferative lesions.

Response to Physical Injury and Changes in Mechanical Use

Direct physical injury to the periosteum either by surgery or due to separation by underlying hemorrhage, edema, inflammation, or neoplasia, is usually accompanied by pain and lifting of the periosteum. This is followed by formation of new bone by activation and proliferation of osteoblasts of the osteogenic (cambium) layer of the periosteum. Such periosteal reactive bone formation is called an exostosis and can remodel and regress, or it can persist. In adult animals, removal of the periosteum at surgery is not harmful, if areas of heavy fascial attachment or muscles that carry intramedullary vessels are left opposed to the bone. Mechanical disruption of the perichondral ring can lead to peripheral extension of physeal cartilage with formation of osteocartilaginous nodules. These nodules resemble multiple cartilaginous exostoses in dogs, especially as they become more distant from the physis with subsequent normal growth.

Tension and compression (weightbearing) are important mechanical factors that affect bone mass. Normal mechanical use is required for maintenance of the structure of the skeleton. For example, in the adult skeleton, normal mechanical use causes a suppression of bone resorption. Decreased mechanical use reduces this inhibition as well as suppresses bone formation. The net effect of decreased mechanical use, therefore, is less bone due to increased resorption and decreased formation (Fig. 10-11). It is not known how bone cells sense altered mechanical use, but mechanical stretch receptors on cells and response to bioelectric potentials from piezoelectric forces (generated by physical forces distorting collagen) and streaming potentials (generated by fluid flow through the canalicular system) are likely mediators.

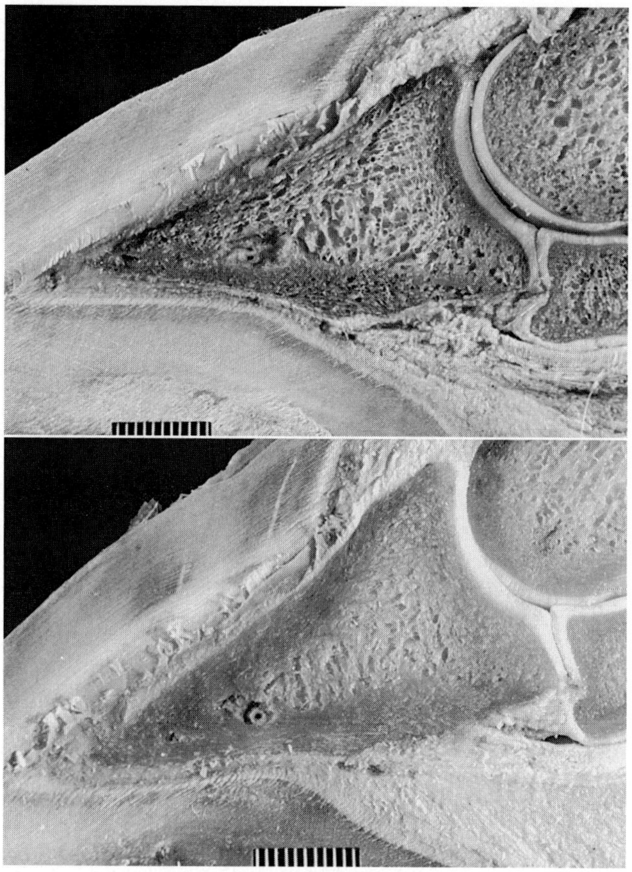

Figure 10-11 Bone; third phalanx; foal. Left rear leg was in cast for 2 months to repair avulsion of muscles from their insertions. There is marked disuse osteopenia (atrophy) of the left third phalanx *(upper specimen)* compared with the right. The increase in resorption and decrease in formation associated with disuse has resulted in marked porosity of the cortical and subchondral bone. The cortex now has the appearance of cancellous bone (cancellization of the cortex). (Scale is in millimeters.)

Fracture Repair

Broken bones are a common occurrence. It is important to understand how and why fractures heal, and, more important, why they do not. Fractures can be classified as traumatic (normal bone broken by excessive force) or pathologic (an abnormal bone broken by minimal trauma

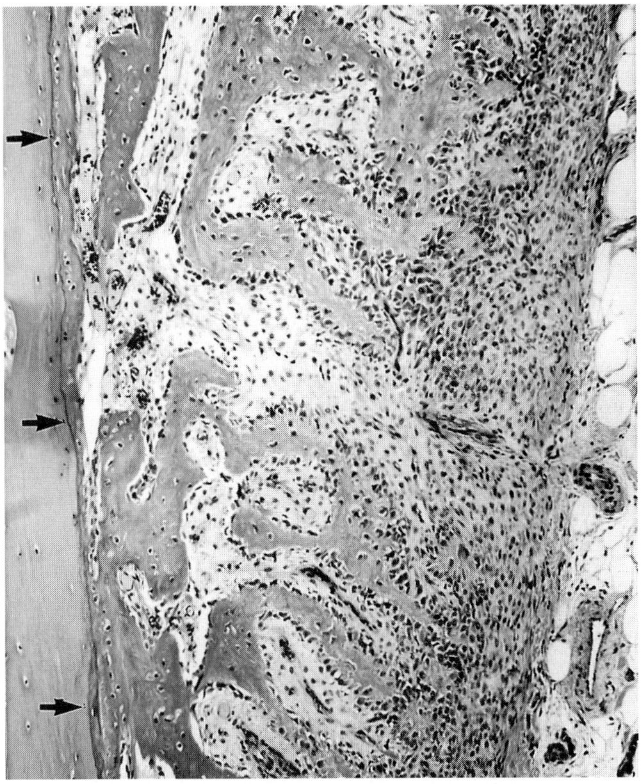

Figure 10-12 Bone. External (periosteal) callus. Arrows indicate demarcation between the preexisting lamellar cortical bone and the callus, which is composed of course trabeculae of woven bone covered with a hypercellular cambium layer of the periosteum. H & E stain.

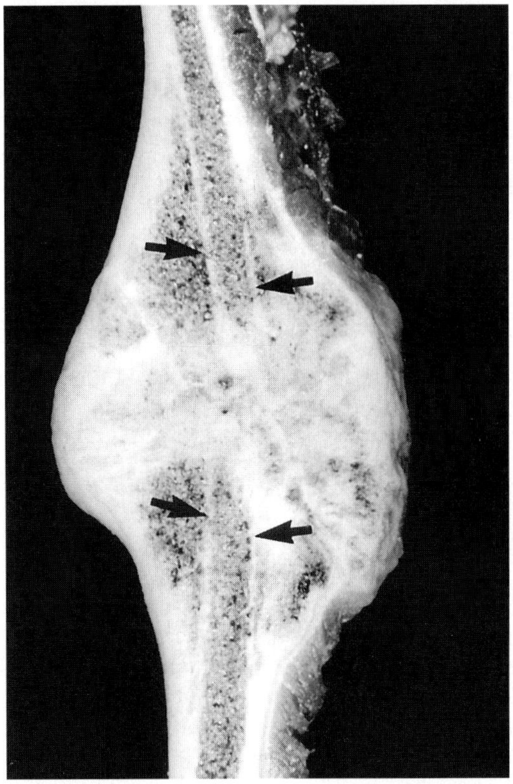

Figure 10-13 Bone, rib; horse. Fracture of unknown duration. There is abundant external callus; the original cortex *(arrows)* is visible.

or by normal weightbearing). Osteomalacia, osteomyelitis, and bone neoplasms are examples of lesions that can weaken a bone and predispose it to pathologic fracture. Fractures can be classified in many other ways: closed or simple, if the skin is unbroken; open or compound, if the skin is broken and the bone is exposed to the external environment; comminuted, if the bone has been shattered into several small fragments; avulsed, if the fracture was caused by the pull of a ligament at its insertion into bone; greenstick, if one side of the bone is broken and the other side is only bent so that there is no separation or displacement; transverse or spiral, depending on the orientation of the fracture line; and infractions when there is fracturing of trabeculae without external deformation of the cortex.

The events that normally occur in the healing of a closed fracture of a long bone are summarized below. The reader should understand that this description represents a summary of a complex process that is subject to a great deal of variation. At the time of fracture, the periosteum is torn, the fragments are displaced, soft tissue is traumatized, and bleeding occurs forming a hematoma. Due to impaired blood flow and isolated bone fragments, bone at the broken ends and marrow tissue can undergo necrosis. The hematoma and tissue necrosis can be important in subsequent callus formation. Growth factors are released by macrophages and platelets in the blood clot. Growth factors also are released from the dead bone by the lysis and acidification of the matrix. These growth factors are important in stimulating proliferation of repair tissue (woven bone). Mesenchymal cells with osteogenic potential that can be derived from the periosteum, endosteum, medullary cavity, and, possibly, from metaplasia of endothelial cells proliferate in the hematoma to form a loose collagenous tissue. These cells mature into osteoblasts and, later, produce woven bone. The term "callus" refers to an unorganized meshwork of woven bone that forms after a fracture (Fig. 10-12). It can be external (that formed by the periosteum) or internal (that formed between the ends of the fragments and in the medullary cavity). This "primary" callus should bridge the gap, encircle the fracture site, and stabilize the area (Fig. 10-13). In time, woven bone at the fracture site is replaced by stronger, mature lamellar bone (secondary callus).

Depending on the mechanical forces acting at the site, the callus can eventually be reduced in size by osteoclasts until the normal shape of the bone is restored. This process, however, might take years to complete.

Callus can contain hyaline cartilage. The amount of cartilage present in the callus reflects the adequacy of the blood supply. Less than optimal oxygen supply promotes mesenchymal stem cell to differentiate into chondroblasts rather than osteoblasts. Cartilage does not provide as strong a callus as woven bone. However, it will eventually undergo endochondral ossification and, therefore, ultimately contribute to the formation of the bony callus. In addition to an adequate blood supply, stability of the bone fragments is of prime importance in fracture repair. Mechanical tension and compression at the fracture site influence the reparative process. Minimal movement of the bone edges in contact with one another (slight compression) and a good blood supply favor direct bone formation with minimal periosteal callus. Excessive movement and tension favor the development of fibrous tissue. Mature fibrous tissue is not wanted in the callus because it does not stabilize the fracture and, unlike cartilage, will not act as a template for bone formation. Excessive fibrous tissue between bone ends in a fracture might result in a nonunion. With time the bony ends of the nonunion can become smooth and move in a pocket of fibrous tissue and cartilage to form a false joint or pseudoarthrosis. Other factors that can interfere with the normal repair process include malnutrition, bacterial osteomyelitis, and the interposition of large fragments of necrotic bone, muscle, or other soft tissue that might lead to delayed union or nonunion. Fixation devices that cause rigid immobilization of the fractured segments can alter the repair process, and external callus might be minimal with direct bone formation between bone ends.

Metallic implants used in fracture stabilization can have a number of different effects on the skeleton. Metallic devices that are too large deprive the bone of normal mechanical forces (stress shielding) and result in bone loss (disuse atrophy). Intramedullary fixation devices have the potential to damage the blood supply. Implanted material (metal, plastics, and bone cement) often is separated from the surrounding bone by a thin layer of fibrous tissue, sometimes with metaplastic cartilage that forms in response to operative trauma, implant mobility, or corrosion of the implant. Microscopic particulate debris from implanted fixation materials ("wear debris") can elicit a macrophage or giant cell response. These inflammatory cells can release cytokines and growth factors that result in bone resorption and deterioration at the bone-implant surface. Neoplasia thought to be induced by metallic fracture fixation devices has been reported rarely in the veterinary literature and is usually associated with chronic osteomyelitis.

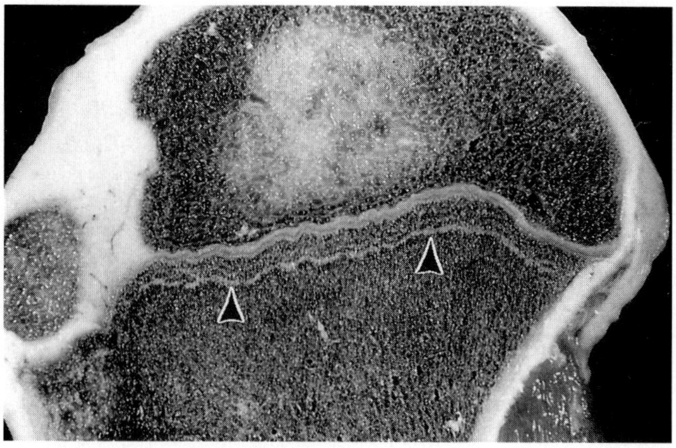

Figure 10-14 Bone, proximal humerus; calf (newborn). Arrest lines *(arrowheads)* parallel to the physis indicate previous temporary cessation of longitudinal growth in utero.

Abnormalities of Growth and Development

Given the complexity of the development and growth of bone, it is not surprising that a vast array of errors occur during the maturation of the skeleton. In this section, several acquired and genetic growth disturbances are presented. Additional nutritional and hormone-mediated disturbances of growth are presented under "Metabolic Diseases."

The physis (growth plate) is a fragile structure whose activity and shape are affected by its blood supply and by applied mechanical forces. In the case of multiple nutrient deficiencies, such as occur in debilitating disease or general malnutrition, the growth plate becomes narrow (growth is impaired) and the metaphyseal face of the plate can be sealed by a layer of bone due to transverse trabeculation (trabecular bone forming parallel with the growth plate) (Fig. 10-14). If growth resumes, this layer of bone is carried into the metaphysis. It is called a growth arrest line and is visible grossly and radiographically as a linear bony density parallel with the growth plate.

Acquired impairment of osteoclastic activity within the primary trabeculae can result in the retention of primary trabeculae that fail to model into secondary and tertiary trabeculae. These trabeculae continue to elongate as long as production by the growth plate continues. The retention of the primary trabeculae results in a dense band beneath the growth plate; this band is called a growth retardation lattice (Fig. 10-15). The band is apparent because normally most of the primary trabeculae are removed in the process of modeling. The persistence of the primary trabeculae results in a dense collection of thin, mineralized spicules that are apparent grossly and in radiographs. Diseases that cause growth retardation lattices include canine distemper and bovine viral diarrhea. In addition, toxic damage to osteoclasts, such as with lead poisoning, can cause a growth retardation lattice (lead line). The name, growth

· osteosclerosis
· metaphyseal sclerosis

retardation lattice, is perpetuated here because it is in common use, but it is important to understand that the lesion is in modeling of the trabeculae rather than a reduction in longitudinal growth. Abnormal retention of primary trabeculae also can be seen with congenital defects in function of osteoclasts (see "Osteopetrosis").

Weakening or destruction of the matrix of the physeal cartilage as occurs in animals with hypervitaminosis A and with manganese deficiency can lead to premature closure of growth plates. If the entire plate is affected, no further longitudinal growth is possible. If closure is focal, as can be seen subsequent to localized inflammation, epiphyseal-metaphyseal bony bridges act as anchors to retard longitudinal growth and because the closure is focal, angular deformities can develop due to uneven longitudinal growth.

The response of the physis to specific nutritional deficiencies is highly variable. Thickening (due to failure of removal) of physeal cartilage or cartilage of the articular-epiphyseal complex can occur because of failure of mineralization or maturation of cartilage or failure of vascular penetration into the growth plate. Rickets and osteochondrosis are examples of diffuse and multifocal, respectively, failure of mineralization and are discussed later. Metaphyseal osteomyelitis due to infection, idiopathic sterile inflammation as in canine hypertrophic osteodystrophy, or infraction of primary trabeculae due to trauma can result in obstruction of vessels that are needed to bring in osteoclasts and osteoblasts from the medullary cavity for endochondral ossification. Conversely, obstruction of the blood supply to the epiphyseal side of the physis leads to narrowing and premature closure of the physis.

Congenital malformations are primary structural defects due to localized errors in the embryonic period; **deformities** are alterations in shape or structure of a previously normally formed part, and they usually arise late in fetal life. Although the cause is often not apparent, teratogenic substances, such as thalidomide, chromosomal abnormalities, and poorly understood in utero factors can be responsible. Some lesions, such as syndactyly (fusion of adjacent digits) in cattle, are inherited.

A number of generalized abnormalities in development are characterized by defective cartilage development and are classified as **chondrodysplasias.** Affected animals are short-legged, and the disproportionate dwarfism is variable in severity. The bones of the calvarium might be of normal size since these arise from membranous bone rather than endochondral bone.

Osteopetrosis

This is an osteosclerotic (increased bone mass) disease that occurs in dogs, sheep, horses, cattle, and several strains of mice and is described by some as a metaphyseal dysplasia. The basis for the disease is failure of osteoclasts

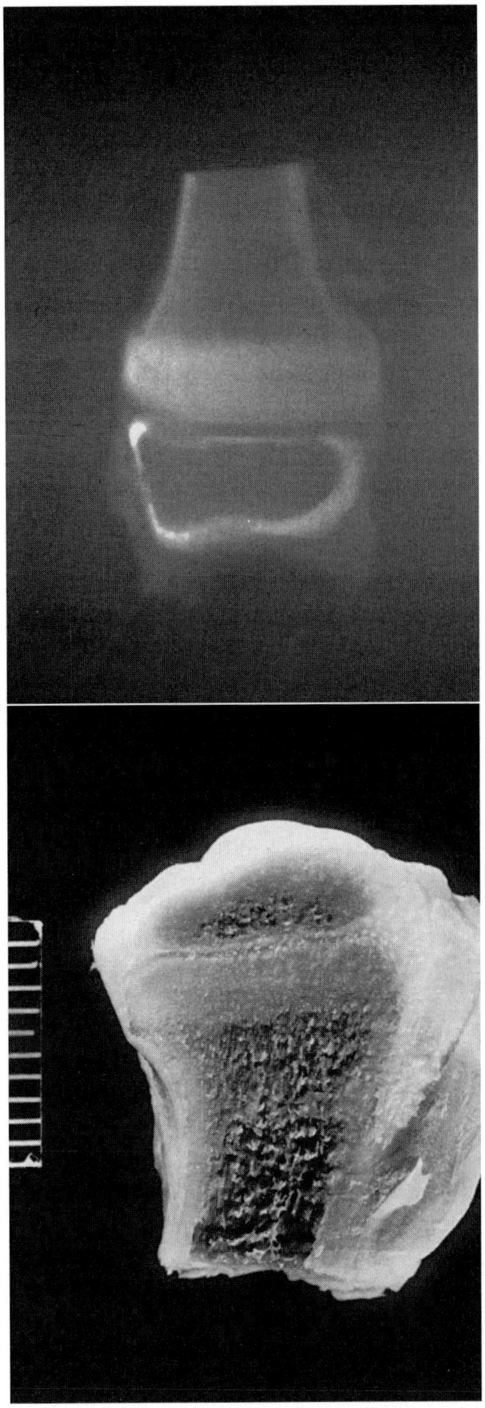

A

B

Figure 10-15 Bones, dog. Growth retardation lattice due to canine distemper virus. **A,** Radiograph. A band of increased bony density (osteosclerosis) is present in the metaphysis due to decreased resorption of trabeculae. The "cut-back zone" of the metaphyseal periosteal is widened (flared) due to impaired resorption. **B,** Primary trabeculae are retained due to impaired function of osteoclasts infected with the canine distemper virus. (Scale in **B** is in millimeters.)

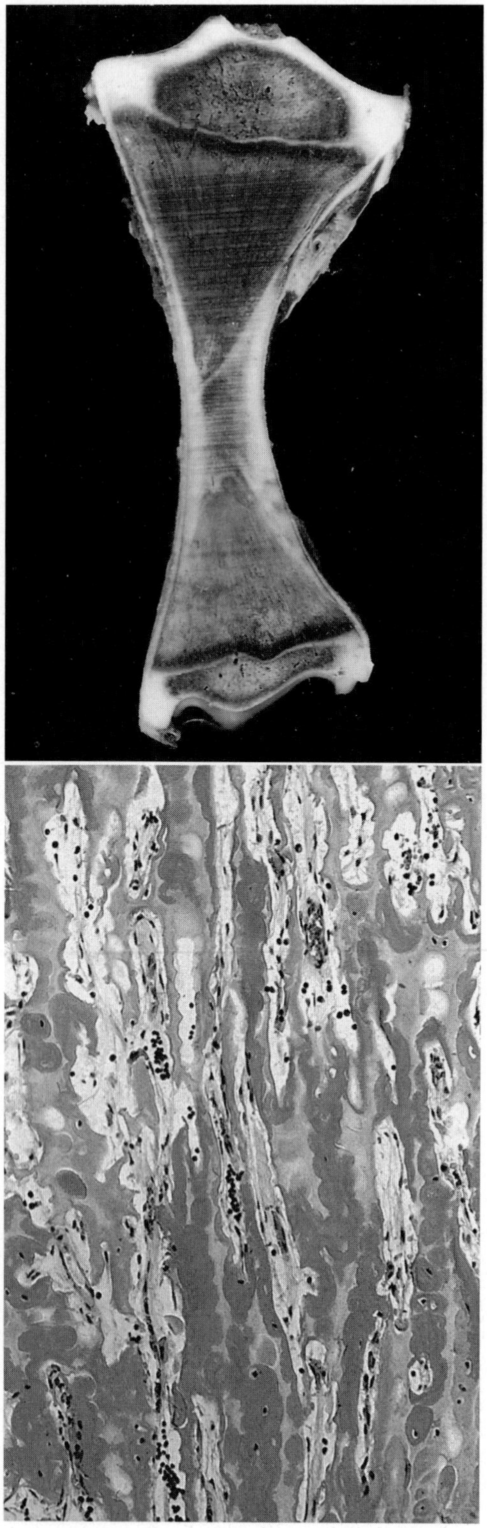

Figure 10-16 Bone, tibia; calf (Aberdeen Angus). **A,** Osteopetrosis with retained primary trabeculae filling the entire medullary cavity. **B,** Retained straight unmodeled trabeculae with cartilage cores filling marrow cavity. H & E stain.

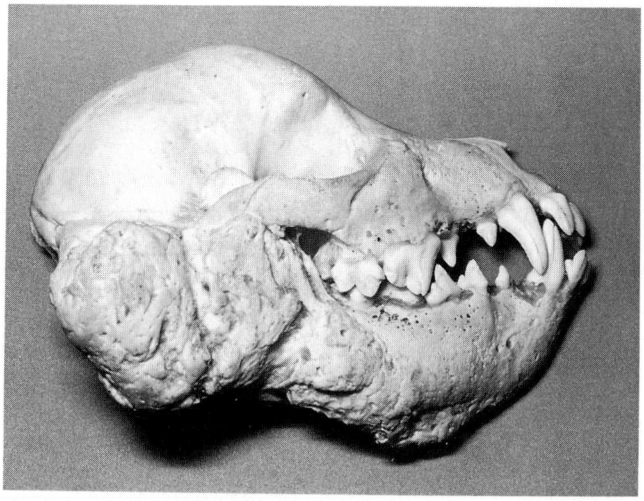

Figure 10-17 Bone, head; dog (West Highland White terrier). Craniomandibular osteopathy. Extensive periosteal new bone formation with bony bridging of the craniomandibular joint. Macerated and bleached. *Specimen courtesy of Dr. Wayne Riser.*

to resorb and shape (model) the primary trabeculae. As a result, spicules of bone with central cores of calcified cartilage fill the medullary cavity. This process affects all bones that develop in a cartilaginous model (elongate by endochondral ossification from a growth plate). Affected bones are dense and have no medullary cavity (Fig. 10-16). The defect in Angus cattle is inherited as an autosomal recessive trait. Affected calves are typically stillborn a few weeks premature and also have brachygnathia inferior, impacted molar teeth, and deformed cranial vaults. The nature of the osteoclast failure has been defined in several strains of mice. This has not yet been done in domestic animals with osteopetrosis.

Congenital Cortical Hyperostosis

This disease of newborn pigs (an example of diaphyseal dysplasia) is characterized by new periosteal bone formation on major long bones. Lesions can be a consequence of disorganization of the perichondral ossification groove. Affected limbs (one or several) are visibly thickened by edema and by radiating spicules of bone that form on the periosteal surfaces of the metaphysis and diaphysis. Piglets are stillborn or die shortly after birth because of other defects. The pathophysiology of the bone lesions is not understood.

Craniomandibular Osteopathy

Craniomandibular osteopathy (also known as "lion jaw") typically occurs in West Highland white or Scottish terrier dogs. Lesions are bilaterally symmetric and are the results of new periosteal bone and irregular resorption resulting in overall irregular thickening of the mandibles, the occipital and temporal bones, and, occasionally, other bones of the skull (Fig. 10-17). The tympanic bullae are often severely affected. Less commonly, new periosteal bone occurs on the bones of the limbs. Numerous, thin, irregular basophilic cement lines (reversal lines) indicating sites where resorption had stopped and subsequent bone formation had occurred give affected bone a characteristic mosaic appearance at microscopic examination. The disease often becomes apparent at 4 to 7 months of age and can regress. For affected dogs, mastication is painful and difficult, and the muscles of the skull become atrophic from disuse. The etiopathogenesis of this disease is unknown.

Osteogenesis Imperfecta

This is an osteopenic disease described in calves, lambs, and puppies; it involves bone, dentin, and tendons. Clinically, affected animals might have multiple fractures, joint laxity, and defective dentin. The basis of the lesion is a functional defect in osteoblastic production of type I collagen and, in some cases, decreased synthesis of certain noncollagenous proteins (i.e., osteonectin).

Angular Limb Deformity

This term refers to lateral deviation of the distal portion of a limb. These deformities can occur in any species, but are most common in foals. The deviation has originated at various locations, such as the distal radial physis, the carpus, or the distal metatarsal physis. It can be present at birth or can be acquired later in life. Causative factors vary greatly; malpositioning of the fetus in utero, excessive joint laxity, hypothyroidism, trauma, poor conformation, overnutrition (consumption of excess proteins and calorie), and defective endochondral ossification of epiphyses of carpal, tarsal, and long bones have all been implicated. Angular limb deformities also can develop because of unequal growth across an epiphysis, such as the distal radius. This lesion can be due to trauma and focal disruption of the blood supply to either the epiphyseal side of the physis or the articular-epiphyseal complex. For example, disruption of the blood supply to the lateral portion of the epiphyseal aspect of the physis would cause decreased longitudinal growth on the lateral side and lateral deviation of the limb due to continued growth from the medial side. In a similar manner, disruption (retardation) of growth on one aspect of the articular-epiphyseal cartilage complex can lead to malformation of the epiphysis and, eventually, to angular limb deformity.

Metabolic Bone Diseases

These systemic skeletal diseases are generally of nutritional, endocrine, or toxic origin. Structural abnormalities occur in both growing and adult skeletons during normal modeling and remodeling. Metabolic bone disease are often called osteodystrophies. The term "osteodystrophy" is a general one and implies defective bone formation. The classical metabolic osteodystrophies are osteoporosis, fibrous osteodystrophy, rickets, and osteomalacia. These terms imply specific pathologic changes but do not necessarily imply a specific cause. For example, osteoporosis can be due to a calcium deficiency, glucocorticoid therapy, or physical inactivity. Different osteodystrophies can coexist in the same skeleton. For example, the skeleton of an animal with a severe calcium deficiency accompanied by excess dietary phosphorus might have features of both osteoporosis and fibrous osteodystrophy. In practice, most nutritional deficiencies in domestic animals do not involve a single element; more often, deficiencies are multiple, not severe, and not the "classic" lesions produced under experimental conditions.

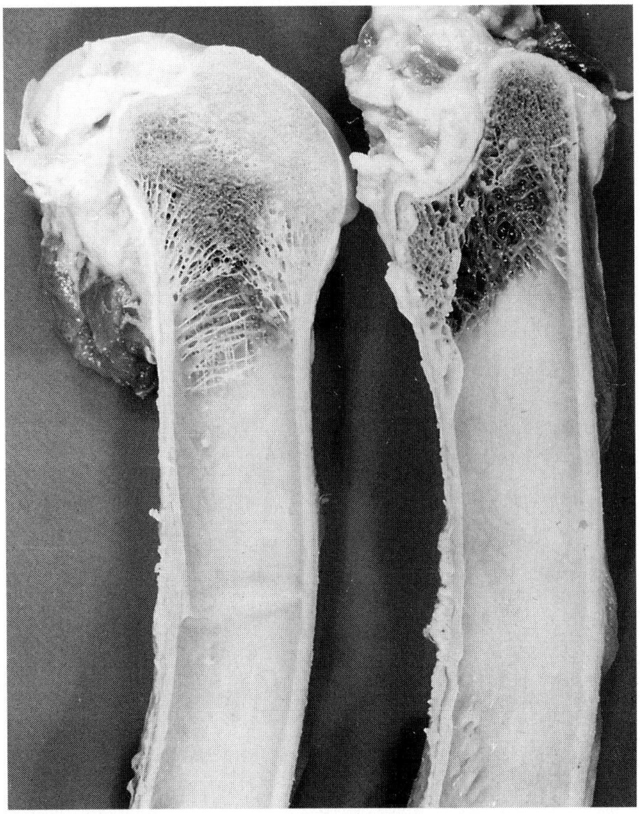

Figure 10-18 Bone, femur; sheep (ewe). Osteoporosis associated with cachexia of chronic disease. Note the reduced amounts of cortical and trabecular bone. The marrow has been flushed from the specimen.

Osteoporosis

Osteoporosis refers to the clinical disease of bone pain and fracture due to a reduction of bone density/mass. The bone remaining is normally mineralized. When there is reduced bone mass but no clinical disease, the term osteopenia is used. In both osteoporosis and osteopenia, the cortical bone is reduced in thickness and increased in porosity (see Figs. 10-11 and 10-18). Trabeculae become thinner, fewer in number, and develop perforations within the plates. The medullary cavity becomes enlarged due to endosteal resorption of cortical bone. The end result is a bone that lacks strength and is more easily fractured. In senile osteoporosis in human beings, in addition to decreased bone density, the turnover rate is reduced allowing microcracks (small cracks in the bone visible only microscopically) to accumulate. These microcracks superimposed on the reduced bone mass make bones more brittle than would be predicted from the reduced mass alone. In growing animals, osteoporosis is potentially reversible. In adults, however, once trabecular bone is lost, it cannot be reformed. Some of the causes include calcium deficiency, starvation, physical inactivity, and the administration of glucocorticoids. A calcium deficiency can result in hypocalcemia, which is compensated for by increased PTH output and increased bone resorption. It is not clear why calcium deficiency does not result in fibrous osteodystrophy, as described on page 513. Starvation and malnutrition can result in arrested growth and osteoporosis, largely due to reduced bone formation because of deficiencies of protein and mineral. Reduced physical activity (disuse or immobilization osteoporosis) causes increased bone resorption and decreased bone formation. This disuse loss of bone might be mediated through changes in piezoelectrical activity, streaming potentials, and stretch receptors. Loss of bone mass associated with long-term paralysis or immobilization is not necessarily progressive; rather, the skeleton stabilizes at a new (reduced) level. Postmenopausal osteoporosis is a common and important disease in women; it often results in vertebral deformity or collapse and pathologic fractures of the femoral neck. Declining concentrations of estrogens, physical inactivity, reduced muscle tone, and inadequate calcium intake are factors that can modify this disease. Interestingly, ovariohysterectomy in the bitch is not associated with clinical osteoporosis. In experimental studies a transient osteopenia has been found in ovariectomized dogs; these studies confirm years of veterinary clinical observations that spayed dogs are not at risk to develop osteoporosis. Osteopenia associated with reduced estrogens from ovarian atrophy or ovariectomy appears to be greatest in animals with estrous cycles that extend throughout the year (e.g., rat, pig, and primate).

Rickets and Osteomalacia

These diseases of the immature and mature skeleton, respectively, are characterized by failure of mineralization, with subsequent bone deformities and fractures. In the growing animal, rickets is a disease of bone and cartilage undergoing endochondral ossification. In the adult, osteomalacia is a disease only of bone, most commonly caused by deficiency of vitamin D or phosphorus. However, failure of mineralization and osteomalacia can occur in chronic renal disease and in chronic fluorosis. Phosphorus-deficient animals often have reduced feed intake, are unthrifty, and have impaired reproductive performance. The microscopic lesions of rickets reflect the generalized failure of mineralization of growth plate cartilage and bone, as well as poorly understood disorganization of chondrocytes in the growth plate. Endochondral ossification requires an orderly sequence of events culminating in mineralization of the physis, apoptosis of chondrocytes, and vascular invasion of cartilage from the subjacent bone. If any one of these events does not occur, the cartilage is not removed and replaced by bone. In rickets, the growth plates are thickened due to failure to mineralize (Fig. 10-19). In mammals, when mineralization of the cartilage matrix does not occur, blood vessels with accompanying chondroclasts do not invade the physis. Since the ability of the chondrocytes to proliferate and hypertrophy is at least partially retained in rickets, the growth plate thickens because production of cartilage is normal but removal is reduced. It is uncertain if the disorganization of chondrocytes in vitamin D–deficiency rickets is due to a primary affect of vitamin D metabolites (specifically, 24,25-

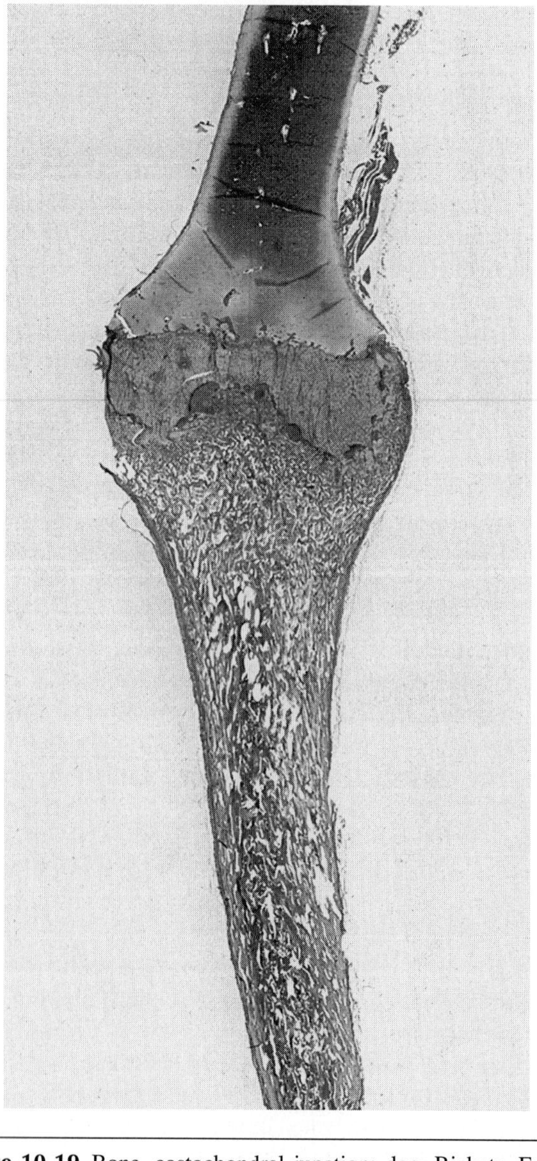

Figure 10-19 Bone, costochondral junction; dog. Rickets. Failure of endochondral ossification results in irregular retention (thickening) of the growth plate. H & E stain.

dihydroxyvitamin D) or a mechanical consequence of the failure of endochondral ossification. Metaphyses have excess osteoid (unmineralized matrix), islands of surviving chondrocytes, and fibrous tissue. Osteoclasts are not able to adhere to osteoid. Therefore, because osteoid cannot be resorbed, it accumulates and abnormally wide seams of osteoid occur on bone-forming surfaces. Hypocalcemia can develop in a vitamin D deficiency, and lesions of secondary hyperparathyroidism (fibrous osteodystrophy), also can develop. Grossly, bones of the rachitic skeleton are deformed, break easily because of reduced mineralization, and are enlarged or "flared" at the metaphyses of the long bones and ribs. The flared metaphyses reflect the thickening of the physis and failure of the normal modeling of the metaphysis (cut-back zone) because the poorly mineralized matrix cannot be resorbed.

Osteomalacia is the disease in the mature skeleton. It develops over time in the new bone formed in the process of skeletal remodeling. The disease is similar to rickets, but because the physes are absent, there are no physeal lesions in the adult skeleton. Microscopically, wide seams of unmineralized osteoid are formed. Clinically, affected animals have bone pain, pathologic fractures, and deformities such as kyphosis and scoliosis.

Fibrous Osteodystrophy

This term describes the skeletal lesions that are the result of increased widespread osteoclastic resorption of bone and its replacement by fibrous tissue that occur in primary, secondary and pseudohyperparathyroidism. Weakening of bones leads to lameness, pathologic fractures, and deformities. In domestic animals, primary hyperparathyroidism, as in cases of functional parathyroid adenoma, parathyroid carcinoma, or idiopathic bilateral parathyroid hyperplasia, is rare. Secondary hyperparathyroidism is more common and can be either nutritional or renal in origin (nutritional or renal fibrous osteodystrophy). Nutritional hyperparathyroidism is caused by dietary factors that tend to decrease the concentration of serum ionized calcium to which the parathyroid glands respond by increased output of PTH. It is most common in young, growing animals that are fed rations deficient in calcium and have a relative excess of phosphorus. Unsupplemented cereal grain rations fed to swine, all-meat diets fed to dogs and cats, and bran fed to horses are examples of low-calcium–high-phosphorus diets that can cause secondary hyperparathyroidism and, eventually, fibrous osteodystrophy. Increased concentrations of dietary phosphorus are important in the evolution of fibrous osteodystrophy, perhaps by interfering with the intestinal absorption of calcium.

The lesions of fibrous osteodystrophy begin with osteoclastic resorption of cancellous and endocortical bone, together with the proliferation of fibrous tissue within the marrow space especially near endosteal and trabecular surfaces. In advanced disease, entire cortices can be replaced by reactive woven bone and fibrous tissue. These lesions are in response to increased concentrations of PTH rather than to the direct effect of altered serum electrolytes. Sometimes, the proliferation of fibrous tissue is exuberant and associated with increased external dimension of the bone. This process is more common in the maxilla and mandible and might reflect the response of the weakened bone to the intense mechanical stress of mastication. Bones affected with fibrous osteodystrophy can fracture, their articular surfaces collapse, and some such as the vertebrae and ribs are deformed (Figs. 10-20 and 10-21). Clinical signs vary from a mild lameness to

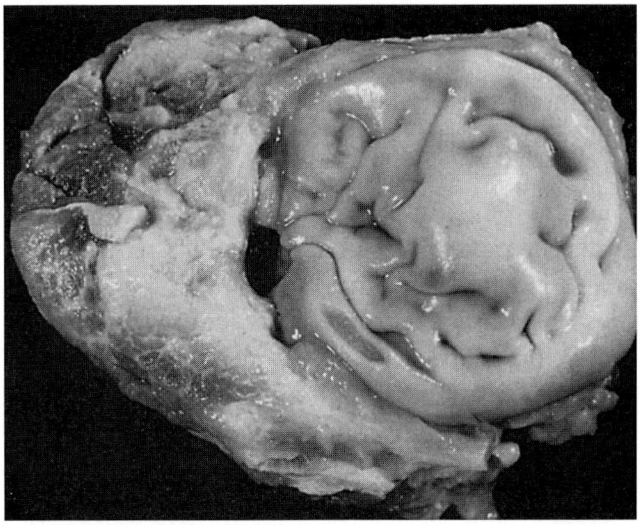

Figure 10-20 Bone, humerus; pig. Nutritional fibrous osteodystrophy. The cartilage of the humeral head is creased and collapsed due to loss of supporting subchondral bone.

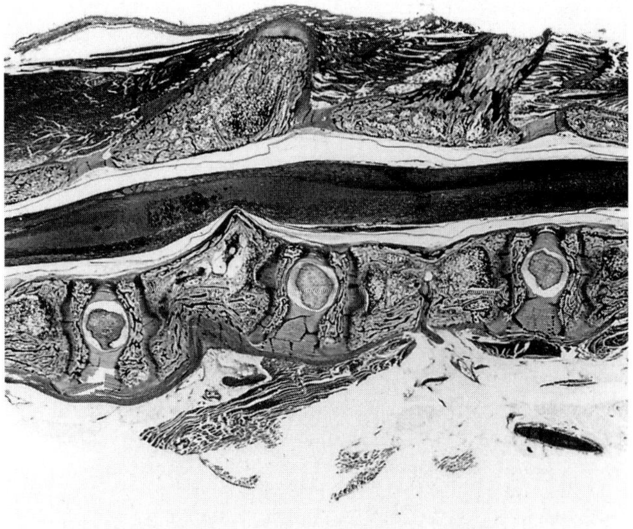

Figure 10-21 Bone, vertebral column; cat. Nutritional fibrous osteodystrophy. A pathologic folding fracture of one vertebra is compressing the spinal cord. H & E stain. *Specimen courtesy of Dr. Wayne Riser.*

multiple fractures resulting in an inability to stand. Growth plates are normal in fibrous osteodystrophy unless there is an accompanying vitamin D deficiency, in which case young animals have superimposed lesions of rickets.

Renal Fibrous Osteodystrophy

This is a general term that refers to the skeletal lesions (Fig. 10-22) that develop secondary to chronic, severe renal disease. Osteomalacia and fibrous osteodystrophy can occur as separate diseases or in combination as a result of chronic renal disease in human beings. Fibrous osteodystrophy, which is sometimes complicated by osteomalacia, occurs in the dog, the animal most commonly affected with renal osteodystrophy. Dogs can have bone pain (lameness) and loss of teeth and deformity of the maxilla or mandible due to the osteoclastic resorption of bone and replacement by fibrous tissue. The pathogenesis of the renal osteodystrophies is complex and, likely, varies depending on the extent and nature of the renal disease and the availability of dietary vitamin D. Loss of glomerular function, inability to excrete phosphate, inadequate production of 1,25-dihydroxyvitamin D by the kidneys, and acidosis are central to the development of renal osteodystrophy. Phosphate retention because of decreased renal excretion leads to hyperphosphatemia. As the calcium and phosphorus product exceeds solubility, calcium is precipitated in soft tissue resulting in hypocalcemia. This hypocalcemia stimulates PTH output with subsequent fibrous osteodystrophy. The reduced production of 1,25-dihydroxyvitamin D by the diseased kidneys together with impaired mineralization due to the acidosis of uremia explain the development of osteomalacia.

A

B

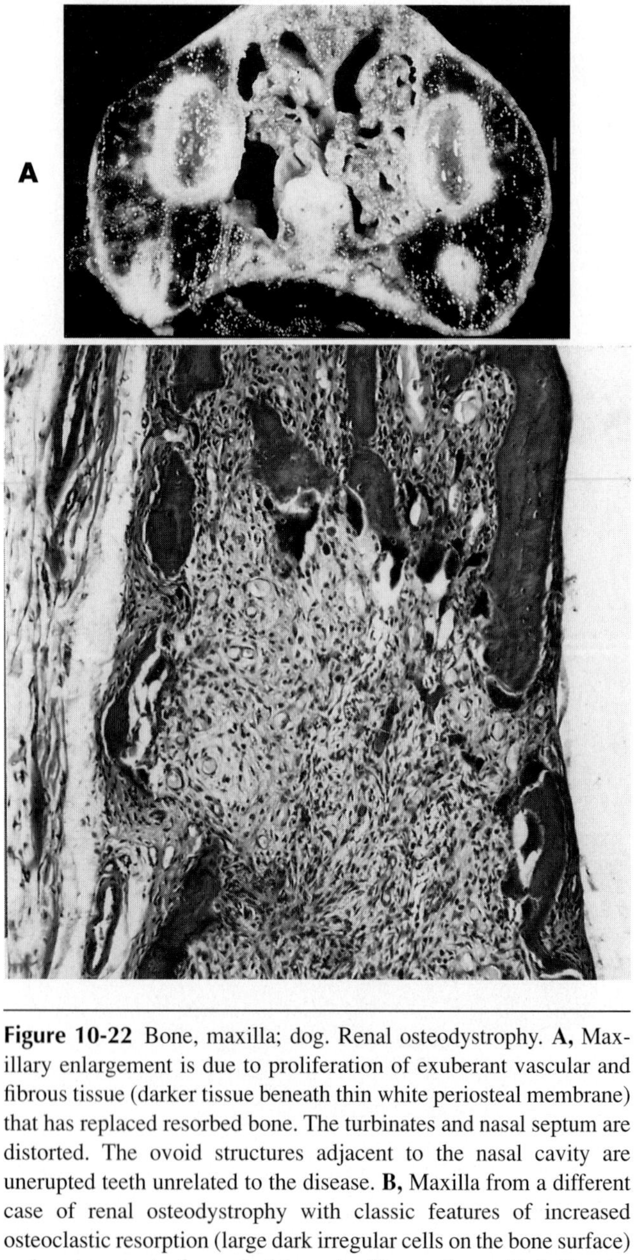

Figure 10-22 Bone, maxilla; dog. Renal osteodystrophy. **A,** Maxillary enlargement is due to proliferation of exuberant vascular and fibrous tissue (darker tissue beneath thin white periosteal membrane) that has replaced resorbed bone. The turbinates and nasal septum are distorted. The ovoid structures adjacent to the nasal cavity are unerupted teeth unrelated to the disease. **B,** Maxilla from a different case of renal osteodystrophy with classic features of increased osteoclastic resorption (large dark irregular cells on the bone surface) and replacement of resorbed bone by fibrous tissue. H & E stain.

Toxic Osteodystrophies

A number of different substances are toxic to bone and/or growth cartilage. Lesions that develop are described as toxic osteodystrophies. A portion of ingested **lead** can be bound to the mineral of bone and physeal cartilage undergoing mineralization, and in young animals, after exposure to a bolus dose, this region of lead deposition can be seen radiographically as a transverse band of increased density in the metaphysis parallel to the physis. This "lead line" (a growth retardation lattice, as described above) is not due to lead itself, which is present in very small amounts, but to lead-induced malfunction of osteoclasts. Osteoclasts in the area can contain acid-fast inclusion bodies.

Chronic **hypervitaminosis D** can produce bone lesions of osteosclerosis. In acute, massive exposures, death is due to hypercalcemia and widespread soft tissue mineralization; bone lesions are not apparent. In long-term intake of smaller doses, such as is seen in ruminants ingesting plants (e.g., *Cestrum diurnum* in the southern United States), containing water-soluble glycosides of 1,25-dihydroxyvitamin D, the persistent hypercalcemia causes chronic lowering of PTH and elevation of calcitonin. This combination effectively stops bone resorption. In addition, vitamin D apparently has a direct stimulatory effect on osteoblasts. The inhibition of bone resorption and stimulation of bone formation result in a denser skeleton. The matrix produced in hypervitaminosis D is usually abnormal. In decalcified histologic sections, the matrix is woven and stains variably basophilic indicating rapid deposition and formation of abnormal ground substance, respectively. Paradoxically, mineralization of the bone can be incomplete, possibly a consequence of the abnormal ground substance.

Aseptic Necrosis of Bone

Aseptic necrosis of bone in human beings occurs in a variety of clinical conditions, including occlusive vascular disease (bone infarction), hyperadrenocorticism, fat embolism, nitrogenous embolism, sickle cell anemia, and intramedullary neoplasms. In domestic animals, aseptic necrosis of bone has been associated with intramedullary neoplasms and various nonneoplastic lesions. Decreased venous outflow from the bone and increased bone marrow pressure are important factors in the pathogenesis of ischemic or aseptic necrosis of bone. The gross appearance of necrotic bone varies with its extent and the response to it. Large areas of necrotic cortical bone has a dry, chalky appearance, and the periosteum can be removed easily. Microscopically, the hallmark of bone necrosis is cell death and loss of osteocytes from their lacunae.

Following an episode of ischemia leading to infarction, the cellular elements of the marrow lose their differential staining, and circular spaces (pooled lipid) develop within a few days. If the region of dead bone remains avascular, the coagulated tissue and mineralized matrix can persist for some time. Large areas of necrotic cortical bone can remain for years. Dead osteocytes elicit little reaction; their nuclei become pyknotic, but their disappearance from lacunae is slow and might not be complete for 2 to 4 weeks.

Reaction to and repair of necrotic bone requires revascularization that is associated with infiltration of macrophages and invasion by fibrous tissue that advances from the margins of the lesion (Fig. 10-23). The bone marrow might eventually regenerate entirely, or a scar might form and remain. The necrotic matrix remains fully mineralized and might even "hypermineralize" due to calcification of the dead osteocytes and their lacunae. This mineralization is only possible with some vascularization that brings additional calcium to the region. Dead bone is slowly removed by osteoclasts. In necrotic trabecular bone, that portion which is not removed by osteoclasis often is surrounded by new woven bone (Fig. 10-24). This sandwich of central dead bone covered by woven bone can

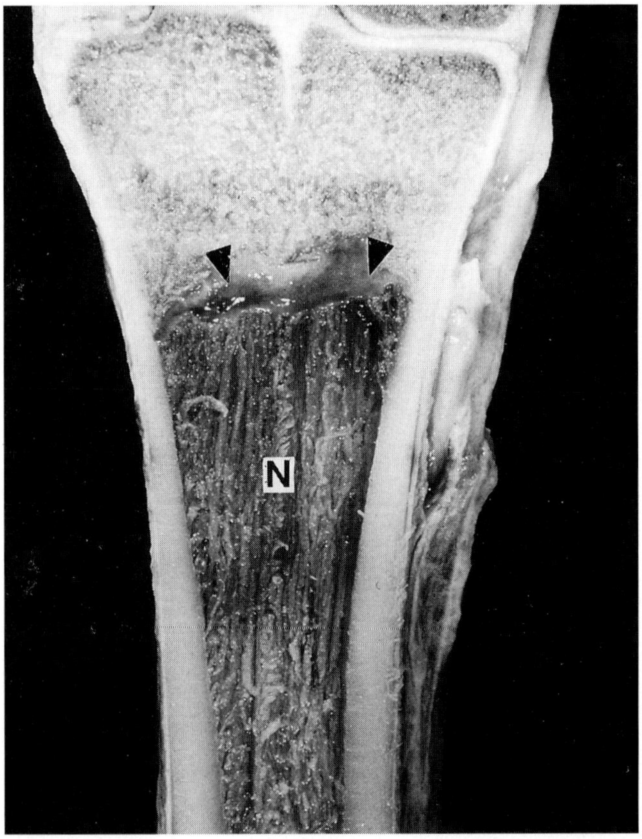

Figure 10-23 Bone, proximal metacarpus; calf. Ischemic necrosis *(N)* of the distal portion of the bone caused by external pressure of a tightly fitted cast. A reactive zone of fibrous tissue and inflammatory cells is at the margin *(arrowheads)* of viable tissue.

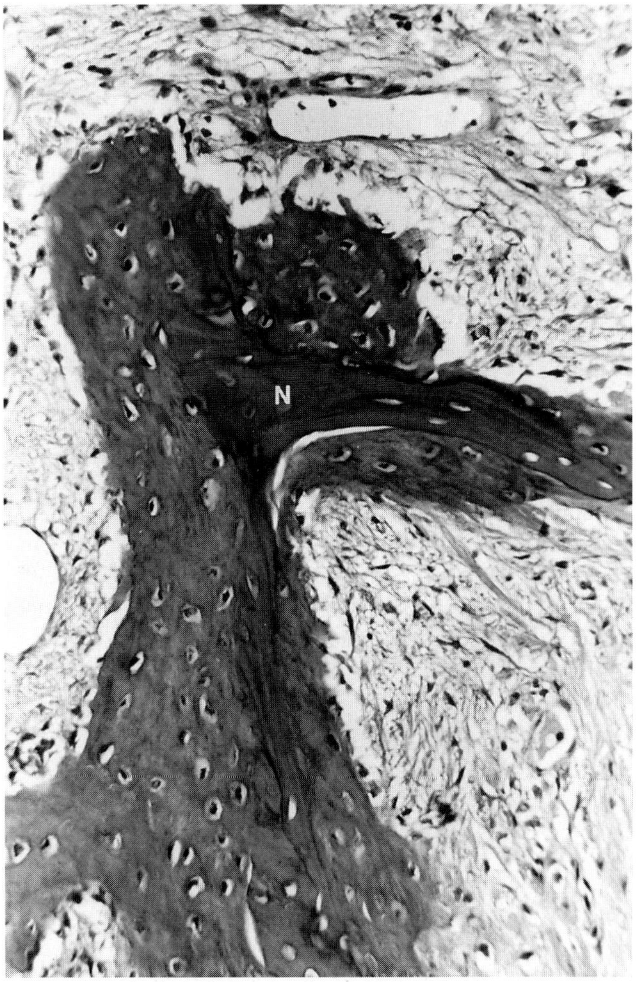

Figure 10-24 Bone, femoral head; pig. Necrosis produced experimentally by ligature around the femoral neck. Woven bone with peripheral fibrosis of the marrow surrounding a spicule of necrotic bone *(N)* with many empty osteocytic lacunae. H & E stain.

persist for months and give (along with osteocyte mineralization described above) the necrotic region a radiodense appearance. The resorption of necrotic bone with simultaneous replacement by new bone is termed "creeping substitution." The process is slow and often incomplete. Small areas of bone necrosis might not be detected clinically or radiographically.

In the femoral heads of young, small, and miniature breed dogs, aseptic necrosis is associated with clinical signs because of the collapse of the articular cartilage due to resorption of the necrotic subchondral bone (Legg-Calvé-Perthe's disease) that occurs late in the course of the disease. Apparently, the initial infarction is asymptomatic. The cause of the infarction is usually not determined but might be due to venous compression or increased pressure within the joint capsule. Such intracapsular pressure has resulted in increased intraosseous pressure and bone necrosis. Although the long-term use of steroids in human beings has been associated with necrosis of the femoral head, steroids do not appear to induce osteonecrosis in domestic animals.

Inflammation of Bone

Osteitis

Inflammation of bone is designated osteitis: **periostitis** if the periosteum is involved and **osteomyelitis** if the medullary cavity of the bone is involved. These are common, sometimes life-threatening, lesions that require early diagnosis and vigorous treatment. Osteomyelitis is often a chronic, disfiguring process caused by necrosis and removal of bone and by the compensatory production of new bone; the two processes often proceed simultaneously over a prolonged period. Osteitis is often a painful process leading to debilitation of the affected animal. Osteitis and its extensions in animals are usually caused by bacteria, although viral, fungal, and protozoal agents can be involved. *Actinomyces pyogenes* and other pyogenic bacteria are common causes of suppurative osteomyelitis in farm animals. *Staphylococcus intermedius* is the most common cause of osteomyelitis in the dog.

Bacteria can be introduced by a variety of routes directly into bone at the time of a compound fracture, infection extending directly from surrounding tissues, as in sinusitis, periodontitis, or otitis media, or more commonly, osteomyelitis develops as an extension from suppurative arthritis. Suppurative arthritis can progress to the stage of destruction of articular cartilage, which allows direct extension of the inflammation into subchondral bone. Alternatively, the inflammation can penetrate the thin metaphyseal-epiphyseal cortex in the area of insertion of the joint capsule.

In theory, hematogenous osteomyelitis can begin in any capillary bed in bone where bacteria lodge and survive. In practice, it occurs most commonly in young animals and is localized typically in the metaphyseal area of long bones and vertebrae where capillaries make sharp bends to join medullary veins. Here bacterial localization is apparently facilitated by slow flow and turbulence of blood in the larger descending limbs, a lower phagocytic capacity, and discontinuous endothelial cells. No vascular anastomoses are located in this region, and thrombosis of these capillaries results in bone infarction that is a predisposing factor for bacterial localization. It is likely that ligand-receptor binding between bacteria and endothelial cells plays a role. Thrombosis of vessels and local tissue infarction are important in the evolution of bacterial osteomyelitis. The composition of the exudate in metaphyseal osteomyelitis is determined by the infectious agent, but, in bacterial infection in domestic animals, it is typically purulent (Fig. 10-25). Exudate accumulates in the medullary cavity and spreads; the increased intramedullary pressure compresses vessels causing thrombosis and infarction of intramedullary fat, bone marrow, and bone. In areas of inflammation, bone resorption is mediated mostly by osteoclasts stimulated by prostaglandins and cytokines released by local tissue and inflammatory cells. Reduced blood flow through large vessels also promotes osteoclastic bone resorption, possibly by altering electrostatic charges in bone. In addition, proteolytic enzymes released by inflammatory cells and activation of matrix metalloproteinases by the acid environment of inflammation assist in resorbing matrix. Lack of drainage and persistence of the offending agent in areas of necrotic bone account for the chronicity of the process. Bacteria can persist for years in cavities and areas of necrosis. Inflammation can spread in the medullary cavity, penetrate into and through cortical bone, and undermine the periosteum where it further disrupts the blood supply to the bone. Chronic periostitis is characterized by multiple spreading pockets of exudate and areas of irregular periosteal new bone formation. Additional sequelae to osteomyelitis include extension of inflammation to adjacent bone, hematogenous spread to other bones and soft tissues, pathologic fractures, and development of sinus tracts that penetrate cortical bone and drain to the exterior (Fig. 10-26).

Occasionally, fragments of dead bone become isolated from their blood supply and surrounded by a pool of exudate (bone sequestrum). Sequestra can form when bone fragments are contaminated at the site of a compound fracture, when the fragments at a fracture site become infected hematogenously, or when fragments of necrotic bone become isolated and thus avascular in osteomyelitis. These isolated fragments of bone (sequestra) and associated exudate can become surrounded by a dense collar of reactive bone (the involucrum). Sequestra can persist for long periods and interfere with repair. They often become pale and chalky and lack the glistening appearance of normal bone (Fig. 10-27).

A

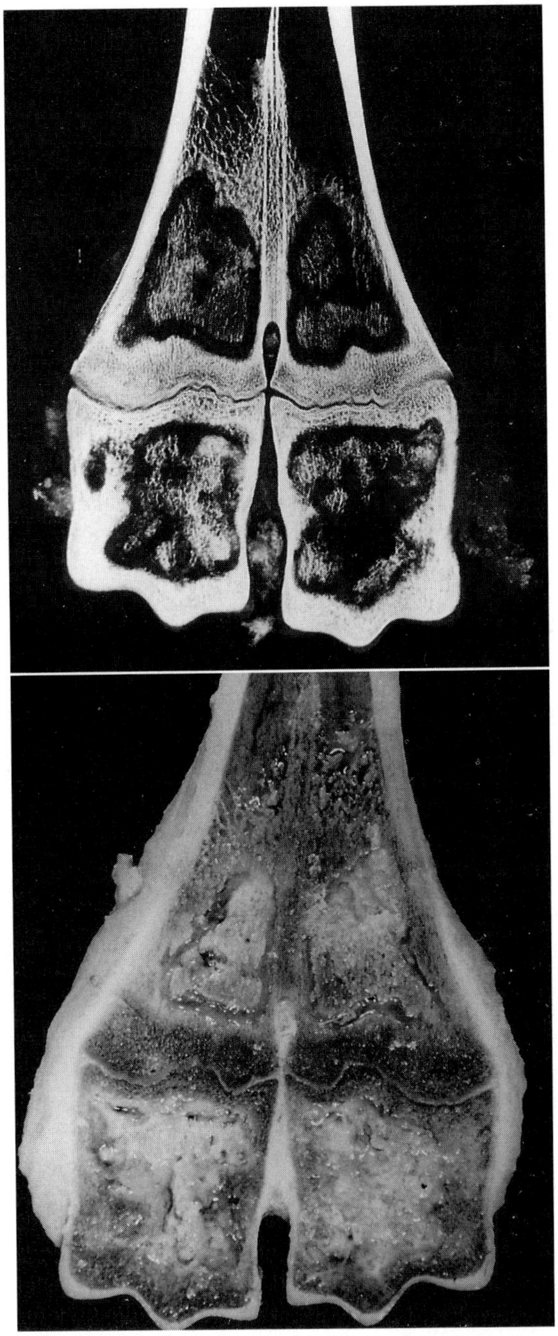

B

Figure 10-25 Bone, metacarpus; calf. **A,** Radiograph. Marked lysis of metaphyses and epiphyses. **B,** Purulent hematogenous bacterial osteomyelitis is present in the regions of lysis.

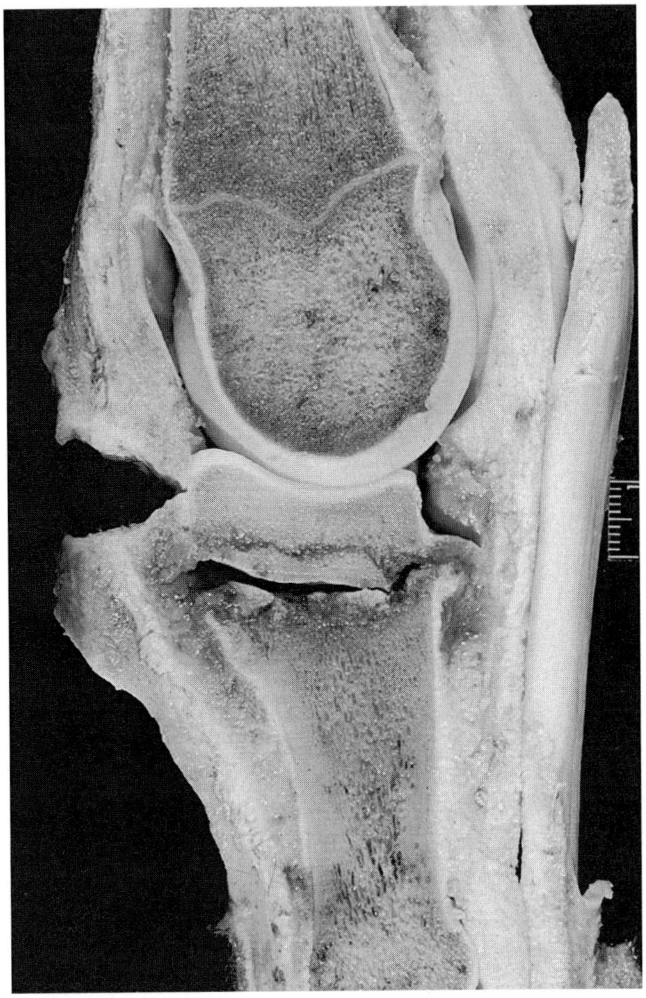

Figure 10-26 Joint, metacarpal-phalangeal, equine. Metaphyseal bacterial osteomyelitis and periostitis of the proximal first phalanx. The inflammation has destroyed the physis and extended through the metaphyseal cortex. (Scale is in millimeters.)

Hematogenous bacterial osteomyelitis is uncommon in dogs and cats, but it is common in farm animals. As an example, hematogenous vertebral osteomyelitis caused by *Actinomyces pyogenes* is a common cause of posterior weakness or paralysis in pigs, and the bacteremia is secondary to bacterial infections of sites of trauma to the skin, particularly of the tail and feet. These primary lesions are often healed by the time vertebral osteomyelitis becomes clinically apparent. As in the long bones, localization of bacteria (in vertebrae) is often in the metaphyses, with subsequent bone necrosis and cavitation leading to pathologic fractures, displacement of the vertebral body, and compression or laceration of the spinal cord (Fig. 10-28). Occasionally, the periosteum of the vertebral canal is elevated by the exudate, causing compression of the spinal cord; in other areas, the inflammatory process extends outward to cause large paravertebral abscesses.

In growing animals, articular cartilage can be lysed by extension of osteomyelitis from the subjacent articular-epiphyseal complex. Epiphyseal cartilage (cartilage of the epiphysis that has yet to undergo endochondral ossification) and physeal cartilage also can be eroded by invasion of osteomyelitis from adjacent bone. In addition, these cartilages can be the sites of direct bacterial embolization

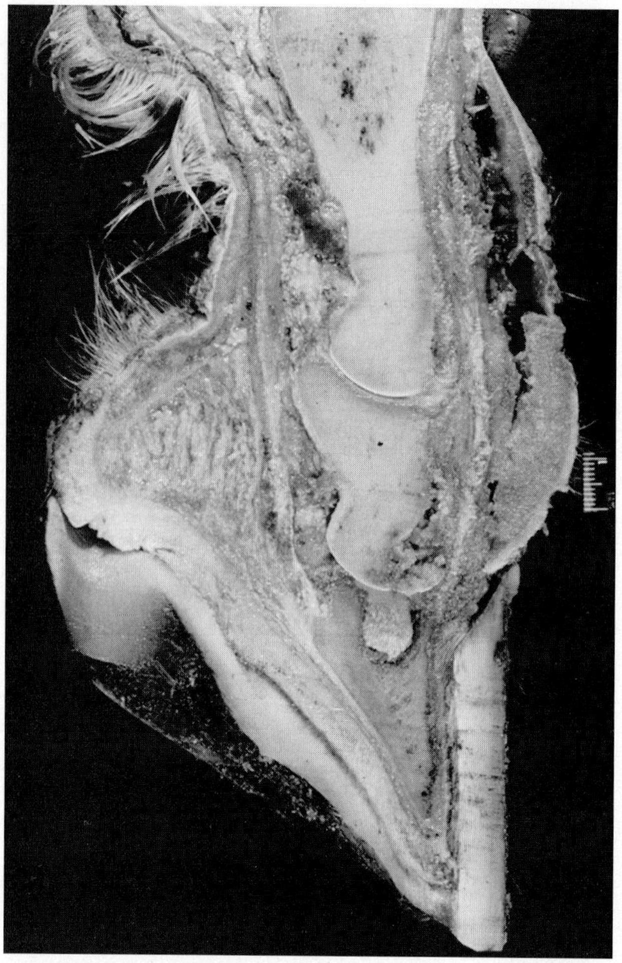

Figure 10-27 Forefoot, horse. Periostitis, osteomyelitis and sequestrum formation due to trauma and bacteria. Inflammation has caused lysis of the anterior surface of the first and second phalanges with sequestrum formation (lighter region) in proximal third phalanges. (Scale is in millimeters.)

since these cartilages are vascularized (compared with avascular articular cartilage). In contrast to cartilage lysis, it is possible for growth cartilage to appear thickened secondary to osteomyelitis due to disruption of endochondral ossification by the inflammatory process and failure to replace cartilage with bone.

Mandibular Osteomyelitis and Periostitis

This disease, caused by *Actinomyces bovis,* occurs in cattle (Fig. 10-29). *A. bovis* is a soil-borne, gram-positive filamentous bacterium. Trauma to oral mucosa and eruption of teeth allow the organism to enter the osseous tissues of the mandible, where chronic pyogranulomatous inflammation develops. Necrosis and loss of bone, marked reactive periosteal new bone formation, scar tissue, formation of numerous small abscesses, and multiple draining fistulae characterize the disease. The affected mandible is irregularly enlarged; teeth can loosen and fall out.

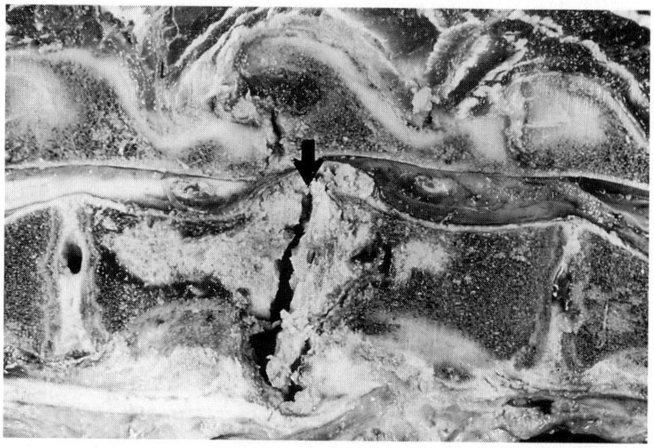

Figure 10-28 Bone, vertebral column, pig. Osteomyelitis due to hematogenous embolization of bacteria to the veterbra on the left with extension of the inflammation through the intervertebral disk and into the adjacent vertebra. Note the exudate, lysis of vertebral body and intervertebral disk, pathologic fracture, and compression of the spinal cord *(arrow).*

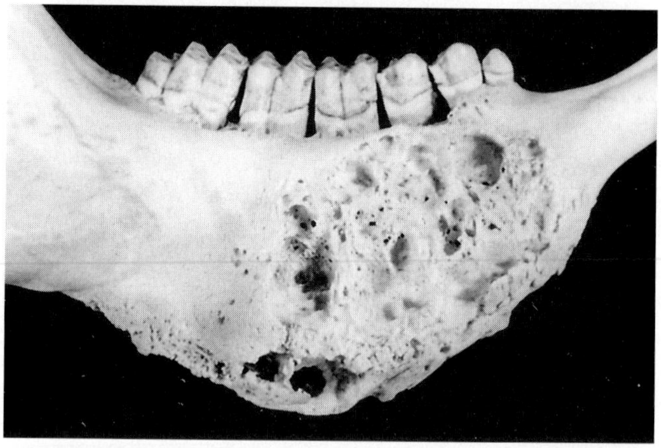

Figure 10-29 Bone, mandible; cow. Osteomyelitis due to *Actinomyces bovis.* The cavities within the reactive bone indicate the location of pockets of pyogranulomatous exudate surrounding colonies of bacteria. Macerated and bleached specimen.

Fungi and viruses also can cause disease in bone. Mycotic agents such as *Coccidioides immitis* and *Blastomyces dermatitidis* frequently spread hematogenously to bone to produce granulomatous or pyogranulomatous osteomyelitis with bone lysis and irregular new bone formation. Various viral agents also localize in bone. The viruses of hog cholera and infectious canine hepatitis can cause endothelial damage, resulting in metaphyseal hemorrhage and necrosis, and acute inflammation. Osseous localization of the distemper virus injures osteoclasts disrupting metaphyseal modeling and producing a growth retardation lattice as described earlier; the feline leukemia virus has been associated with myelosclerosis (increased density of medullary bone) in cats. These latter two viruses do not cause an inflammation of bone.

Hypertrophic Osteodystrophy

Also termed metaphyseal osteopathy, this is a disease of young, growing dogs of the large and giant breeds. These names are unfortunate because they are misleading. The initial lesions are those of a suppurative and fibrinous osteomyelitis of the metaphysis. The cause and pathogenesis are unknown; infectious agents have not been isolated. Clinically, it is characterized by lameness, fever, and swollen, painful metaphyses in multiple long bones. Radiographically, metaphyseal zones of increased lucency and increased density are adjacent and parallel to the physes. Prominent metaphyseal periosteal new bone formation develops in chronic cases. Lesions are usually bilaterally symmetric. Microscopic findings include widespread suppurative and fibrinous inflammation and necrosis of the metaphyseal marrow and bone. The death of osteoclasts and osteoblasts results in persistence of long, thin primary trabeculae that are not reinforced by apposition of bone matrix. These trabeculae collapse and fracture without external distortion of the bone (infractions). Inflammation might also be present in the periosteum of the metaphysis. Most animals recover spontaneously.

Eosinophilic panosteitis is another canine bone disease with an unfortunate name. The lesion is neither inflammatory nor eosinophilic. It is a proliferative disease characterized by idiopathic formation of endosteal and periosteal woven bone. It occurs in growing dogs, is painful, and self-limiting. Morphologic studies are few because the disease is easily recognized clinically and resolves spontaneously so that biopsy evaluation is rarely needed.

Proliferative and Neoplastic Lesions

Surprisingly, bone, as a tissue, offers little resistance to an expanding or invading neoplasm, and many skeletal neoplasms are accompanied by both bone resorption and new bone formation (Fig. 10-30). Pain, hypercalcemia, increased serum alkaline phosphatase activity, pathologic fracture, and distant metastases are other possible manifestations of a skeletal neoplasm. New bone formation occurs, at least in part, in response to stress on a weakened cortex and is prominent in neoplasms that have a marked fibrous stroma, whereas it is minimal in neoplasms with little stroma, such as plasma cell myeloma and lymphosarcoma, even though bone lysis can be marked. Tumor-associated bone destruction is largely accomplished by osteoclasts. Prostaglandins, cytokines, acid metabolic by-products, and lytic enzymes released by inflammatory or neoplastic cells might be responsible for local bone resorption and formation in response to a neoplasm. Hypercalcemia, due in part to bone resorption induced by release of bone-resorbing factors from extraskeletal neoplasms, is well documented (humoral hypercalcemia of malignancy). In

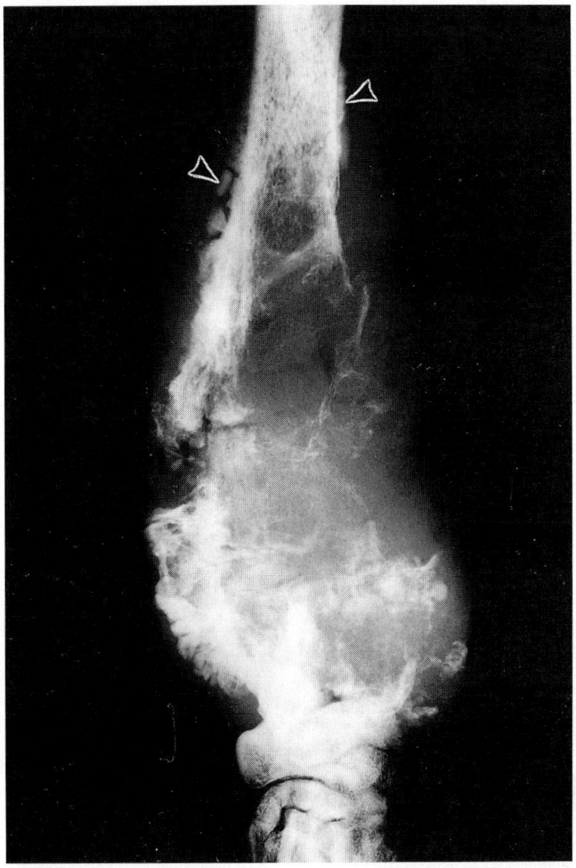

Figure 10-30 Bone, distal radius; dog. Radiograph. Osteosarcoma with extensive destruction of preexisting bone and some new bone formation on the periosteal surface *(arrowheads)*.

animals, the most common example is adenocarcinoma of the apocrine glands of the anal sac in the dog. This neoplasm produces PTH-related protein and metastasizes widely, but rarely to bone.

Nonneoplastic Proliferative and Cystic Lesions

Lesions considered here vary widely in their cause, structure, and ultimate effect on the host. New (reactive) bone formation (often excessive) also occurs in fracture repair, in chronic osteomyelitis, and in degenerative joint disease in the form of periarticular osteophytes. The term **exostosis** or **osteophyte** refers to a usually nodular, benign, bony growth projecting outward from the surface of a bone. An **enthesophyte** is an osteophyte at the insertion of a ligament or tendon. In addition to bone, these proliferations can have variable amounts of cartilage. Hyperostosis is used to indicate that the dimension of the bone has increased and, usually, implies more uniform thickening on the periosteal surface rather than the nodular appearance of an osteophyte. An **enostosis** is a bony growth within the medullary cavity, usually originating from the cortical-endosteal surface, and can result in obliteration of the marrow cavity. All the above are nonneoplastic proliferative lesions in which growth is seldom continuous. Some exostoses can remodel and some regress. Nonneoplastic proliferative lesions can be mistaken for skeletal neoplasia in some biopsy specimens. Conversely, small superficial biopsies might contain only nonneoplastic reactive bone overlying a malignancy. These statements serve to highlight the problem of making a morphologic diagnosis from a small biopsy specimen without benefit of a clinical history, radiographic findings, and other laboratory data. One must also remember that more than one process might be active at any one site; e.g., osteosarcoma might be complicated by fracture repair or by osteomyelitis.

Hypertrophic osteopathy (hypertrophic pulmonary osteopathy) occurs in human beings and in domestic animals, with the dog the most commonly affected. The disease is characterized by progressive, bilateral, periosteal, new bone formation in the diaphyseal regions of the distal limbs (Fig. 10-31). The word "pulmonary" is included because most cases have intrathoracic neoplasms or inflammation. Other, less commonly associated lesions or agents are endocarditis, heartworms, and rhabdomyosarcoma of the urinary bladder in young giant breed dogs and ovarian neoplasms in the horse. Although the association between the pulmonary lesions and the proliferation of new periosteal bone on the extremities is not clear, it has been postulated that pulmonary lesions lead to reflex vasomotor changes (mediated by the vagus nerve) and to increased blood flow to the extremities. New bone formation with thickening of the limbs can occur very rapidly but can regress if the primary lesion is removed. Regression of the bone lesions also occurs after vagotomy. Increased arterial pressure, hyperemia, and edema of the periosteum lead to thickening of the periosteum both by fibrous tissue and, later, by new bone formation. Lesions can be reproduced in dogs by creating shunts that allow blood to bypass the pulmonary circulation, thereby increasing the stroke volume of the left heart and increasing the blood flow to peripheral tissues.

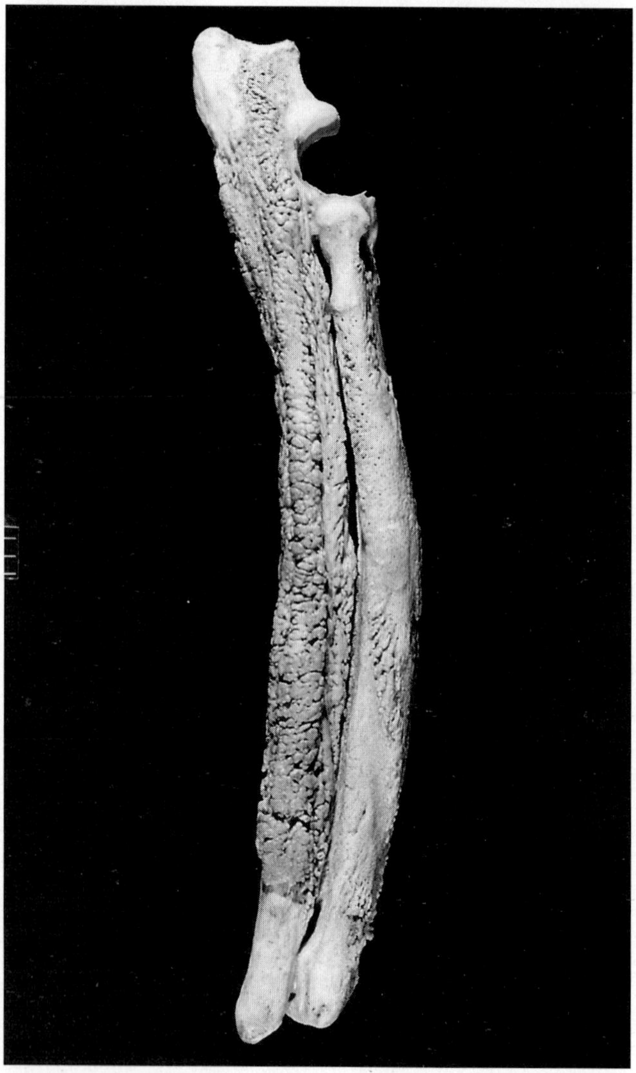

Figure 10-31 Bone, radius and ulna; dog. Hypertrophic pulmonary osteopathy. Marked periosteal proliferation of woven bone causes roughened irregular surface. Macerated and bleached. (Scale is in millimeters.)

Osteochondromas (multiple cartilaginous exostoses) occur in dogs and horses and reflect a defect in skeletal development rather than a true neoplasm. This lesion is inherited and lesions appear shortly after birth. Osteochondromas project from bony surfaces as eccentric masses that are located adjacent to physes (Fig. 10-32). They arise from long bones, ribs, vertebrae, scapulas, and bone of the pelvis and can be numerous. Microscopically, they have an outer cap of hyaline cartilage that undergoes orderly endochondral ossification to give rise to trabecular bone that forms the base of the lesion. Trabecular bone and bone marrow are continuous with those of the adjacent bone. Normally, growth ceases at skeletal maturity when the cartilage cap is replaced by bone. Although the origin of osteochondromas is not clear, some arise secondary to a defect in the perichondral ring as peripheral pieces of physeal cartilage are pinched off and carried away from the growth plate by longitudinal growth. Clinically, their importance is threefold. They might interfere mechanically with the action of tendons or ligaments; they can act as space-occupying masses that protrude into the vertebral canal and cause spinal cord compression; and they can undergo malignant transformation and give rise to chondrosarcomas. Osteochondromas in cats are different in that they develop in mature animals, less commonly affect long bones, do not have orderly endochondral ossification, and might have a viral origin. Osteochondromas in cats, like those in horses and dogs, can undergo malignant neoplastic transformation.

Fibrous dysplasia is an uncommon lesion that has been found at various sites (skull, mandible and long bones) in young animals. It could be a developmental defect, and can be single or multiple. Typically, preexisting bone is replaced by an expanding mass of fibroosseous tissue that can weaken the cortex and enlarge the external contour of the bone. The lesion is firm, often has mineralization when sectioned, and can have multiple cysts filled with sanguinous fluid. Microscopically, well-differentiated fibrous tissue has trabeculae of woven bone. Osteoblasts are not recognizable on trabecular surfaces, a feature that helps to distinguish this lesion from ossifying fibroma.

Bone cysts are classified as subchondral, simple, or aneurysmal. Radiographically, all appear as lucent areas without evidence of aggressive growth. Subchondral cysts are sequelae to osteochondrosis and degenerative joint disease. Subchondral bone cysts due to osteochondrosis represent failure of endochondral ossification with subsequent necrosis of retained growth cartilage. Bone never was present in such lesions. Subchondral cysts secondary to degenerative joint disease represent herniation of synovial fluid into the subchondral bone through fissures in the articular cartilage. These herniations become lined by a synovial cell-like membrane. The cause of this herniation of fluid is not known but could be related to increased pressure within the joint. Bone lysis is by osteoclasis secondary to either pressure or cytokines released from the expanding cyst. The category of simple bone cysts can overlap substantially with that of fibrous dysplasias; a clear distinction between them can be difficult to make.

Simple bone cysts can contain clear, colorless, serum-like fluid, or the contents can be markedly serosanguinous. The wall of the cyst is composed of variably dense fibrous tissue and woven to lamellar bone. Bone peripheral to this has undergone modeling to accommodate the expansile growth of the cyst. Aneurysmal bone cysts consist of spaces filled with blood or serosanguinous fluid. Tissue adjacent to the spaces can vary from well-differentiated fibrous or fibroosseous tissue to marked proliferation of undifferentiated mesenchymal cells admixed with osteoclastlike multinucleated giant cells. Hemorrhage and hemosiderosis are frequent. An endothelial cell lining is usually not present. The cause of simple and aneurysmal bone cysts is unknown. They could be consequences of ischemic necrosis, hemorrhage, or congenital or acquired vascular malformations. Caution should be exercised in the interpretation of microscopic lesions in biopsy specimens of cysts, and these lesions should be correlated with the radiographic appearance to rule out cystic cavitation in a neoplasm.

Primary Neoplasms of Bone

Benign neoplasms arising in the connective tissue of bone are not common in animals.

Ossifying fibromas are uncommon and occur as large, often heavily mineralized nodules of the maxillae and mandibles of horses and cattle. Although these neoplasms

A

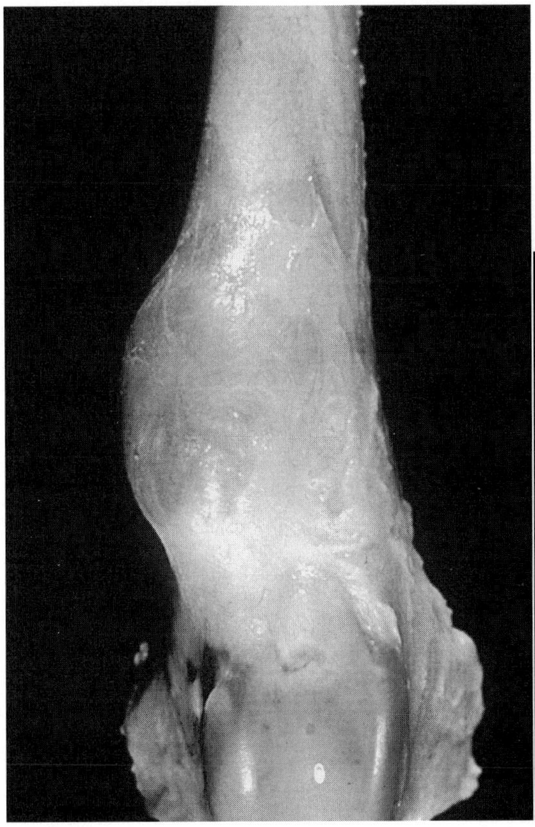

B

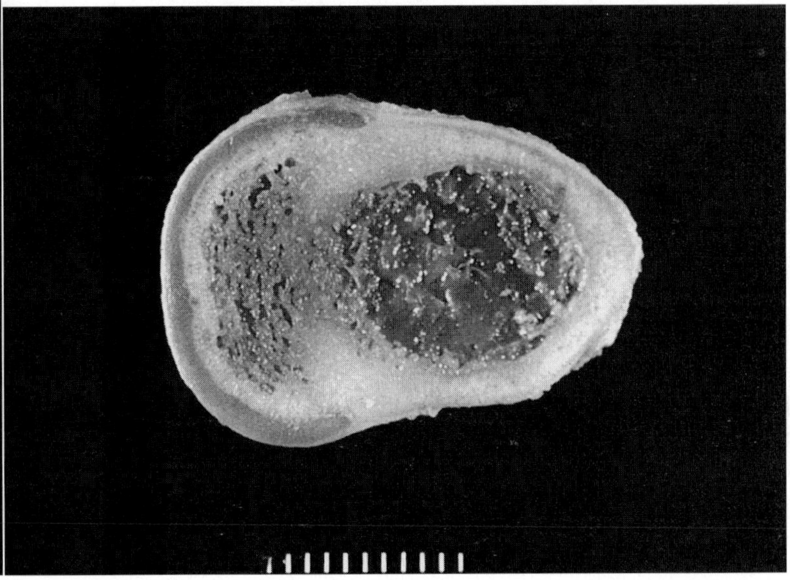

Figure 10-32 Bone, distal femur, dog. **A,** Cartilage-capped exostosis (osteoma chondroma) has formed a fusiform enlargement in the metaphysis. **B,** Horizontal section through the lesion reveals a well-organized cartilage cap with subjacent endochondral bone formation. H & E stain. (Scale in **B** is in millimeters.)

are considered benign, they destroy adjacent cortical and trabecular bone by expansile growth. Microscopically, they are composed of well-differentiated fibrous tissue with scattered spicules of woven bone covered by osteoblasts (Fig. 10-33). Bone content increases with time, and, ultimately, the histologic appearance approaches that of an osteoma.

Fibrosarcomas are malignancies of fibroblasts that produce collagenous connective tissue but not bone or cartilage. Cells can be arranged in a whirling or interlacing pattern. Central fibrosarcomas arise from fibrous tissue within the medullary cavity, whereas periosteal fibrosarcomas arise from periosteal connective tissue. Central fibrosarcomas must be distinguished grossly and microscopically from osteosarcoma. In general, central fibrosarcomas grow more slowly, are accompanied by less formation of reactive new bone, are slower to metastasize, and produce a smaller tissue mass than osteosarcomas. Grossly, fibrosarcomas are gray-white, fill part of the medullary cavity, and replace cancellous and cortical bone.

Chondromas are benign neoplasms of hyaline cartilage. They are uncommon neoplasms of dogs, cats, and sheep and often arise from flat bones. Cartilage neoplasms in the skeleton do not arise from articular cartilage and are usually in adult animals that do not have growth cartilage. Chondromas are multilobulated and have a blue-white cut surface. They tend to slowly but progressively enlarge and can cause thinning of underlying bone. Microscopically, they are composed of multiple lobules of well-differentiated hyaline cartilage. Endochondral ossification of the neoplastic cartilage is possible. They are difficult to distinguish from low-grade, well-differentiated chondrosarcomas. Chondromas that arise in the medullary cavity are called enchondromas.

Chondrosarcomas are malignant neoplasms in which the neoplastic cells produce cartilaginous matrix but never osteoid or bone. They are most common in mature dogs of the large breeds and in sheep. In sheep, they arise from the ribs and sternum; in dogs, the major sites of origin are the nasal bones, ribs, and pelvis. In general, chondrosarcomas most frequently arise in the flat bones of the skeleton. Chondrosarcomas can evolve from multiple cartilaginous exostoses in dogs and in human beings. Most arise in the medullary cavity and destroy preexisting bone. Given time, they become large, lobulated neoplasms with a gray or blue-white cut surface. Some neoplasms are gelatinous on sectioning, and some have large areas of hemorrhage and necrosis. Microscopically, the range of differentiation of neoplastic cells is wide: some neoplasms are well differentiated and are difficult to distinguish from chondroma; other neoplasms are composed of highly anaplastic cells and have only a few areas in which differentiation into chondrocytes and chondroid matrix is apparent. Nonneoplastic bone can be present because of endochondral ossification of the malignant cartilage. Chondrosarcomas have a longer clinical course, grow more slowly, and develop metastases later than osteosarcomas.

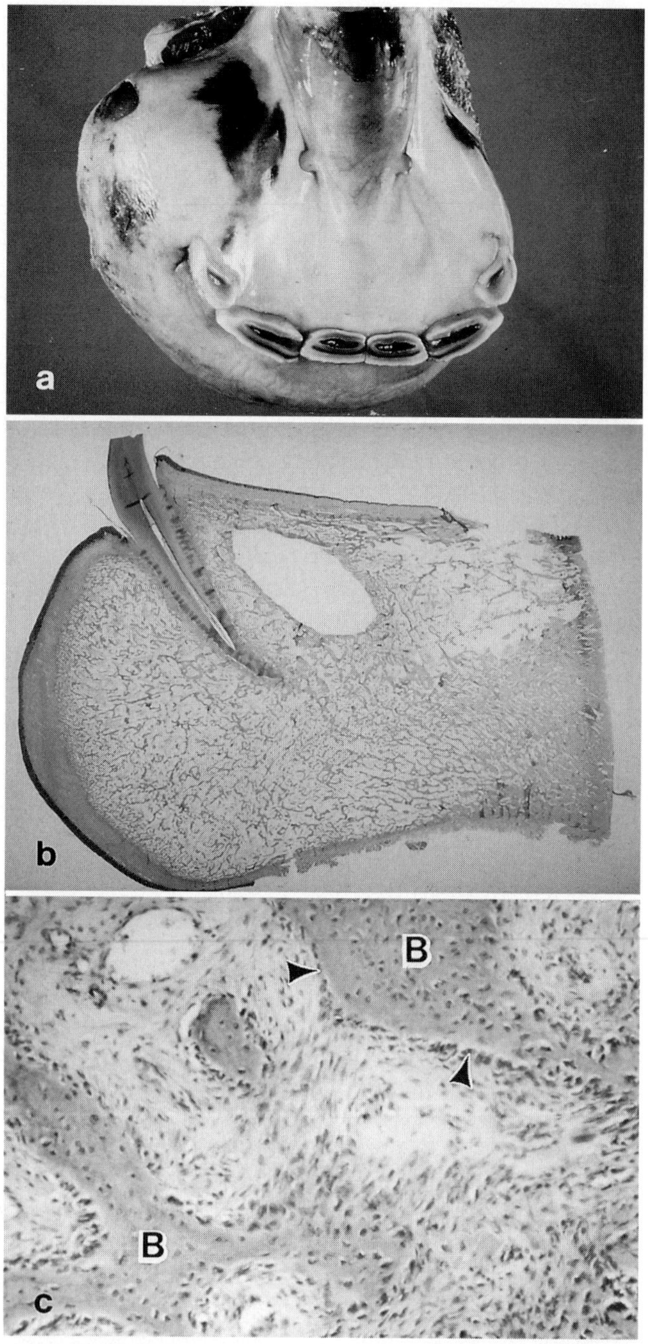

Figure 10-33 Bone, mandible; horse. Ossifying fibroma. **A,** Distortion of the mandible. **B,** Low magnification. Sagittal section. The mass consists mostly of fine bony trabeculae. **C,** High magnification. Active osteoblasts *(arrowheads)* line the trabeculae *(B)*. H & E stain. *Courtesy of Dr. J.C. Woodard.*

Osteomas are uncommon benign neoplasms that usually arise from bones of the head. They occur as a single, dense mass that projects from the surface of the bone. They do not invade or destroy adjacent bone; their growth is slow and progressive but not necessarily continuous. Microscopically, osteomas are covered by periosteum and are composed of cancellous bone that becomes more dense with time. Trabeculae are lined by well-differentiated osteoblasts and osteoclasts. The intertrabecular spaces contain delicate fibrous tissue, adipocytes, and hemopoietic tissue.

Osteosarcomas are malignant neoplasms in which neoplastic cells form bone, osteoid, or both. They can be classified as simple (bone formed in a collagenous matrix), compound (both bone and cartilage are present), or pleomorphic (anaplastic, with only small islands of osteoid present). Classification has also been based on cell type and activity (osteoblastic, chondroblastic, or fibroblastic), radiographic appearance (lytic, sclerotic, or mixed), or origin (central, juxtacortical, or periosteal). An uncommon form of osteosarcoma is the telangiectatic type that grossly resembles hemangiosarcoma. Microscopically, these neoplasms are composed of osteoblasts, osteoid, and large cystic, blood-filled cavities lined by malignant osteoblasts. Osteosarcomas are common neoplasms, comprising approximately 80% of all the primary bone neoplasms in the dog. They arise most commonly at metaphyses (distal radius, distal tibia, and proximal humerus are the most usual sites). However, osteosarcomas can occur in ribs, vertebrae, bones of the head, and various other parts of the skeleton. Rarely, they arise in soft tissues. Typically, these neoplasms occur in mature dogs of the large and giant breeds. Growth of the neoplasm is often rapid and painful. Grossly, central or intraosseous osteosarcomas have a gray-white appearance and contain variable amounts of mineralized bone. Large pale areas surrounded by zones of hemorrhage (areas of infarction) and irregular areas of hemorrhage are common in rapidly growing intramedullary neoplasms. Neoplastic tissue tends to fill the medullary cavity locally and can extend proximally and distally but, typically, does not penetrate articular cartilage or metaphyseal growth plates. Therefore, osteosarcomas do not invade into the joint space. Cortical bone is usually destroyed (see Fig. 10-30), and neoplastic cells penetrate and undermine the periosteum and can extend outwardly as an irregular lobulated mass (Fig. 10-34). Destruction of cortical bone is accompanied by varying amounts of new reactive periosteal bone. Microscopically, variable amounts of woven bone or osteoid are produced by the neoplastic osteoblasts. Bone formation can be abundant and widespread, or it can be minimal, as in anaplastic or fibroblastic osteosarcomas that are composed of sheets of poorly differentiated mesenchymal cells or fibroblastic tissue respectively.

In terms of biologic behavior, osteosarcomas in the dog are characterized by aggressive local invasion and, except for those arising in bones of the head, early hematogenous pulmonary metastasis. Although pulmonary metastasis is common and occurs early, metastasis can be widespread and can involve both soft tissues and other bones.

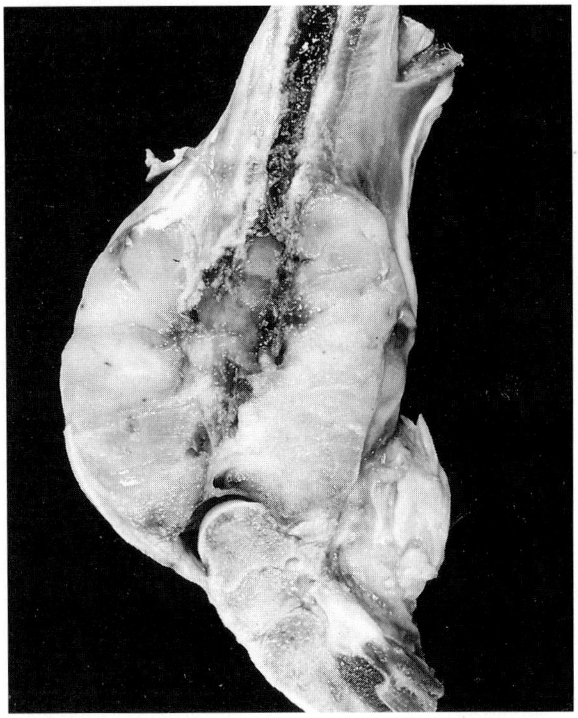

Figure 10-34 Bone, radius; dog. An osteosarcoma has destroyed the cortices but has not bridged the joint space.

The above description relates to central or intraosseous neoplasms. Rarely osteosarcomas are also juxtacortical (parosteal) in origin. These neoplasms arise on the external surface of a bone and form an expansive mass that adheres to and surrounds the underlying cortex. Invasion of the shaft or metastasis is a late event, so early en-bloc excision might effect a cure. It is important to distinguish these neoplasms from central osteosarcomas because parosteal osteosarcomas have a more favorable prognosis.

Multiple skeletal osteosarcomas that occur in human beings and dogs could represent a primary neoplasm that has metastasized to bone. The lesions have a random distribution, and pulmonary metastases are likely to be present. Alternatively, multiple skeletal osteosarcomas could have a multicentric origin.

Although the cause of naturally occurring osteosarcomas in human beings and domestic animals is largely unknown, osteosarcomas can develop in association with other disease. Osteosarcomas have been associated with bone infarctions, previous fractures, and the use of metallic fixation devices in human beings and domestic animals. Osteosarcomas of viral origin are reported in mice.

A unique form of skeletal malignancy occurs in the skull of the dog and is awkwardly called a **multilobular tumor of bone.** These are single, nodular, smooth-contoured, immovable masses on the flat bones of the

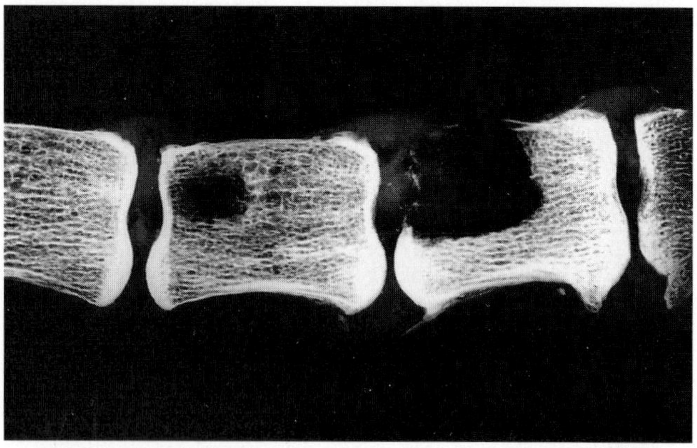

Figure 10-35 Bone, lumbar vertebrae; dog. High-detail radiograph. Multiple foci of osteolysis due to metastatic osteosarcoma.

skull. Neoplastic tissue is firm, the cut surface being composed of multiple, gray, partially mineralized lobules set in a background of fibrous tissue. These neoplasms are slow growing, locally invasive, and can compress and invade the brain. They metastasize to the lungs late in the clinical course, and the metastases are frequently small and clinically silent. The microscopic appearance consists of multiple lobules, each having centrally located cartilage or bone surrounded by plump mesenchymal cells that blend into well-differentiated interlobular fibrous tissue.

Various other neoplasms such as liposarcomas, giant cell tumors, and hemangiosarcomas can arise in bone, and neoplasms such as lymphosarcomas and plasma cell myeloma can involve the bone marrow and surrounding bone.

Secondary Neoplasms of Bone

At autopsy, 60% of (human) cancer patients have skeletal metastases. These are predominantly in red bone marrow, where the vascular sinusoidal system is apparently predisposed to trap circulating malignant cells. The true incidence of skeletal metastasis in animals is unknown and might be low because early euthanasia shortens the course of the disease. However, bone scanning techniques and detailed necropsies might establish that skeletal metastases are more common than presently estimated. Metastatic neoplasms can be associated with pain, hypercalcemia, lysis of bone, pathologic fracture, and reactive new bone formation. Rib shafts, vertebral bodies (Fig. 10-35), and humeral and femoral metaphyses are common sites of metastatic neoplasms in dogs. In cats, skeletal metastases are rare, but the distal extremities appear to be predisposed sites.

DISEASES OF JOINTS

Normal Structure and Function

Joints (articulations) join skeletal structures, provide for movement, and, in some cases, have shock-absorbing functions. Most of the material in this section is confined to the synovial joints.

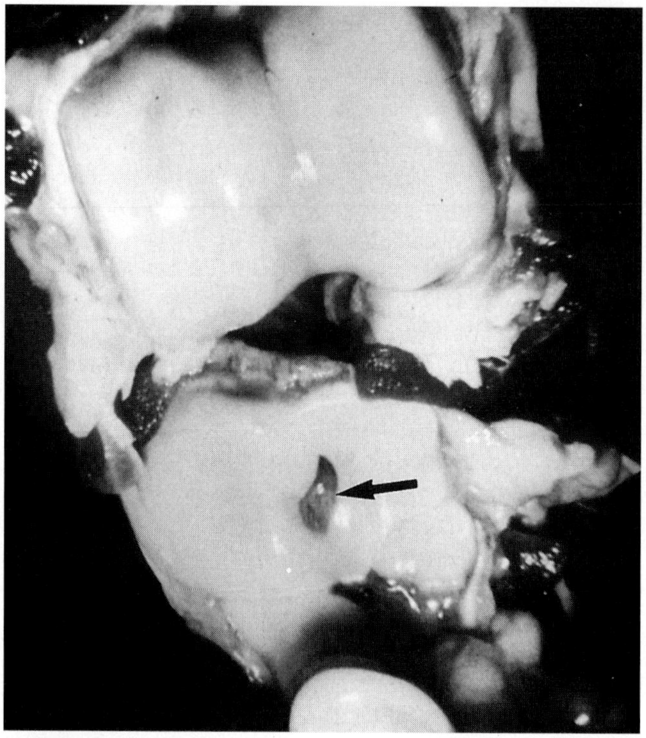

Figure 10-36 Joint, elbow; pig. The depression in the proximal articular surface of the radius is a normal structure called a synovial fossa *(arrow)*.

Synovial joints occur in both the axial and appendicular skeleton. Such joints allow for a variable degree of movement and, anatomically, are composed of two bone ends bound together by a fibrous capsule and ligaments. The inner surface of the joint capsule is lined by a synovial membrane, and the bone ends are covered by articular cartilage. The joint space contains synovial fluid, and fibrocartilaginous menisci are present at some sites. Synovial joints operate with very low coefficients of friction and are self-lubricating, self-sustaining units. Articular cartilage serves as the bearing substance and subchondral bone as the supporting material. Articular cartilage functions to minimize friction created by movement, to transmit mechanical forces to underlying bone, and to maximize the contact area of the joint under load. Joints receive and absorb energy of impact. Both articular cartilage and subchondral bone deform under pressure, but it is the subchondral bone that has the most significant force-attenuating properties.

Articular (hyaline) cartilage is normally a white to blue-white material with a smooth, moist surface. Cartilage thickness is greatest in the young and at sites of maximum weightbearing. Thinning and yellow discoloration occur in old age. At its margins, articular cartilage merges with the periosteum and the insertion of the joint capsule. Depressions known as synovial fossae are present on non-weightbearing surfaces and are often present on the articular surfaces (Fig. 10-36). These depressions are normal, bilaterally symmetric structures of uncertain function present in the larger joints of the horse, pig, and ruminants and are easily mistaken for lesions. Articular cartilage contains no nerves or blood or lymph vessels, and its nutrition is obtained by diffusion from synovial fluid and, to a lesser extent, from subchondral vessels. In the immature skeleton, articular cartilage overlies the still growing cartilage of the epiphysis (epiphyseal cartilage). The epiphyseal cartilage contains blood vessels and will undergo endochondral ossification and, thereby, contributes to the growth of the epiphysis. Defects at the junction of the articular cartilage and epiphyseal cartilage (the articular epiphyseal complex) occur in osteochondrosis. At skeletal maturity, the epiphyseal cartilage has been replaced by a bony subchondral plate. The deeper regions of the articular cartilage mineralize and remain, as they are not removed by endochondral ossification. The junction between the unmineralized articular cartilage and the deeper mineralized cartilage is called the tidemark. The mineralized cartilage serves to anchor articular cartilage to subchondral bone and limits the diffusion of substances between bone and cartilage. Articular cartilage is 70% to 80% water by weight. It is a viscoelastic, hydrated fiber-reinforced gel that contains chondrocytes, type II collagen fibers, and proteoglycan aggregates. Chondrocytes are responsible for the production, maintenance, and turnover of intercellular substances. Normal turnover is enzymatic and is balanced by enzyme inhibitors. Disease occurs if there is increased destruction or decreased synthesis of components of the matrix. It is important to remember that compared with bone, which normally renews itself by remodeling, in cartilage only the proteoglycans turn over. The cells and collagen of cartilage are infrequently, if ever, replaced. Chondrocytic mitotic activity is minimal in adult animals and cellularity of articular cartilage declines with age. Collagen fibers provide tensile strength and are arranged in arcades so that the tops of the arcades are parallel to the articular surface and the sides are perpendicular to the surface and parallel with the radial or intermediate zone of chondrocytes. Proteoglycan aggregates are macromolecules composed of hyaluronic acid with radiating protein cores to which glycosaminoglycan molecules of keratan and chondroitin sulfate are attached. By binding water, proteoglycans provide stiffness to resist compression and impede the outflow of water when cartilage is under weightbearing load. Functionally, the superficial zone of articular cartilage resists shearing forces, the middle zone functions in shock absorption, and the base serves to attach articular cartilage to the bone. In scanning electron micrographs, the surface of articular cartilage is not smooth but rather has numerous depressions that can serve as reservoirs for synovial fluid.

Joint lubrication depends on the microscopic roughness, elasticity, and hydration of articular cartilage and on the presence of mucin (hyaluronate and glycoprotein) in synovial fluid. Lubrication of the synovial membrane itself is hyaluronate-mediated boundary lubrication. Lubrication of articular cartilage is accomplished by the complementary action of weeping (squeeze-film) and boundary lubrication. In weeping lubrication, the loaded articular surface is supplied with pressurized fluid that carries most of the load. The fluid is water released from underlying cartilage subsequent to pressure of weightbearing. When non-weightbearing, the water returns to the cartilage due to the hydrophilic properties of proteoglycans. This flushing of water in and out of the articular cartilage enables nutrients to enter cartilage from the synovial fluid and waste products to be removed. Only a small part is carried by cartilage-to-cartilage surface contact, which is lubricated by a glycoprotein-facilitated boundary system. Boundary lubrication implies that a substance sticks to the surface and minimizes contact. Joint stiffness is often due to inability of periarticular soft tissues to lengthen, rather than to intraarticular friction.

The joint capsule consists of outer fibrous and inner synovial tissue layers. The outer layer is a heavy sheath that contributes to joint stability and attaches to bone at its insertion at the margins of the joint and, thereby, encloses a segment of bone of variable length within the joint cavity. It is well supplied with blood vessels and nerve endings. The synovial membrane covers all the inner surfaces of the joints except for that of the surface of the articular cartilage. The synovial membrane is normally very thin and barely visible grossly. Tiny surface projections (villi) are normally present and are more prominent in some areas than in others. Synovial intimal or lining cells, one to four cells thick, form a discontinuous surface layer. They are designated as "A" cells (phagocytic cells that produce hyaluronate); "B" cells (fibroblastlike cells, rich in rough endoplasmic reticulum), which may produce glycoprotein; and "intermediate" cells, which have some of the characteristics of both. A cells are of bone marrow origin and could be part of the monocyte-macrophage cell system. The synovial subintima can be classified according to the type of predominant tissue (areolar, adipose, or fibrous). It contains blood and lymph vessels that supply and drain the intraarticular structures. Adipose tissue sometimes accumulates within the synovium, forming fat pads that serve as soft cushions in joint cavities.

Synovial fluid is a dialysate of plasma supplemented with proteoglycans from the synovial intima that nourishes and lubricates intraarticular structures. Normally, it is a clear, colorless to pale yellow, viscous fluid.

Postmortem Examination and Evaluation

Several large synovial joints should be opened and examined routinely at necropsy. Joints should be disarticulated so that articular surfaces, synovial fluid, and all associated structures are clearly visible. Consideration should be given to aspirating synovial fluid before disarticulation to obtain a sample free of contamination and suitable for culture and analysis that includes viscosity (mucin precipitation), cell count, and cytology. Articular cartilage must be examined as soon as the joint is opened, because dehydration of cartilage occurs rapidly on exposure to air. Fine fingerlike proliferations of synovium (villous hypertrophy) are best evaluated if the specimen is submerged in water. Microscopic examination of synovium might be required to confirm the presence of synovitis. Thin, longitudinal, sagittal slabs of tissue that contain articular cartilage, subchondral bone, the joint capsule, and its insertion should be collected for microscopic examination.

Reactions to Injury

Although articular cartilage contains metabolically active cells, it has a limited response to injury and minimal capacity for repair. Superficial cartilage defects that do not penetrate into subchondral bone persist for long periods. Clusters or clones of chondrocytes (evidence of local chondrocyte replication in response to injury) are present but are ineffective in filling the defect. Some flow or spreading of cartilaginous matrix into the defect might also occur. This phenomenon of matrix flow is likely facilitated by loadbearing and joint movement. In short, superficial injuries to articular cartilage neither heal nor necessarily progress, although progression can occur when there is stiffened (sclerosis of) subchondral bone. However, if a cartilaginous defect extends into subchondral bone, the defect is quickly filled with vascular fibrous tissue that often undergoes metaplasia to fibrocartilage. Repair by the formation of hyaline cartilage is infrequent. Formation of fibrocartilage can be hastened in full-thickness cartilaginous defects by exercise or prolonged passive motion. Injury to articular cartilage is not painful unless the synovium or subchondral bone is involved. Having no blood supply, articular cartilage does not participate in the inflammatory response, although it can be injured by inflammation in nearby synovial tissue. Given that the alternate compression and release of normal weightbearing facilitates the diffusion of fluid with nutrients into and fluid with metabolic waste products out of articular cartilage, it follows that constant compression or lack of weightbearing leads to thinning (atrophy) of articular cartilage.

Sterile injury to cartilage can be a consequence of trauma, joint instability, or lubrication failure because of changes in synovial fluid and synovial membrane. Destruction of articular cartilage in response to sterile injury and infectious inflammation is mediated by a combination of enzymatic digestion of matrix and failure of matrix production by degenerated or necrotic chondrocytes. These changes can be initiated by damage to the cartilage directly or indirectly by lesions in the synovium. Lysosomal enzymes (collagenase, cathepsins, elastase, arylsulfatase) and neutral proteases, which are capable of degrading proteoglycans or collagen, can be derived from inflammatory cells, synovial lining cells, and chondrocytes. Matrix metalloproteinases (gelatinases, collagenases, and stromalysins) capable of matrix digestion are present in the matrix in inactive form. They can be activated by products of degenerating or reactive chondrocytes and inflammatory cells. Intraarticular prostaglandin and nitric oxide concentrations are increased in degenerative and inflammatory joint disease.

Prostaglandins and nitric oxide inhibit proteoglycan synthesis in synovium and chondrocytes; this reduction in proteoglycan content can lead to degeneration and loss of the cartilage (see below). Interleukin 1 (IL-1) is a cytokine secreted by activated macrophages (synovial type A cells or subintimal macrophages); it promotes secretion of prostaglandins, nitric oxide, and neutral proteases from synovial fibroblasts and chondrocytes. Release of TNF from macrophages in joints has effects similar to IL-1: increasing concentrations of agents that will decrease matrix synthesis and increase matrix destruction. Cytokines and growth factors that can be anabolic to cartilage include IL-6, tranforming growth factor-beta, and insulin-like growth factor. In addition, to act as a control on the destructive effects of activated metalloproteinases, tissue inhibitors of metalloproteinases (TIMPS) are present in the matrix.

The loss of proteoglycans from cartilage alters the hydraulic permeability of the cartilage, thereby interfering with joint lubrication and leading to further mechanically induced injury to the cartilage. The loss of proteoglycans, with subsequent inadequate lubrication of the articular surface, leads to disruption of collagen fibers on the surface of articular cartilage. Affected areas of cartilage are yellow-brown and have a dull, slightly roughened appearance. As more proteoglycans are lost, the collagen fibers condense, and fraying of surface collagen fibers extends along the sides of the arcades as multiple vertical

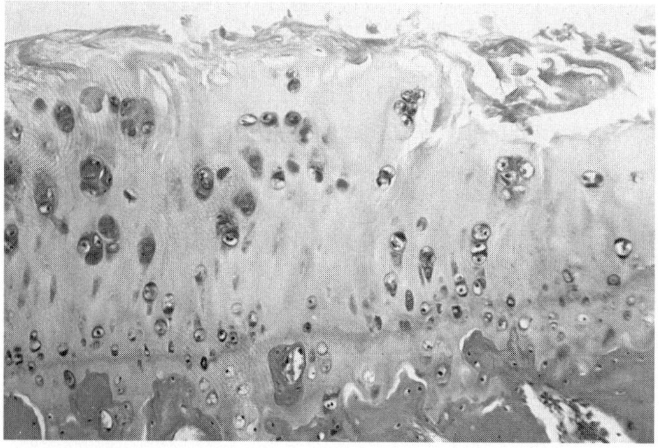

Figure 10-37 Joint, stifle (tibia), guinea pig. Degenerative joint disease. Hypocellular, fibrillated, eroded cartilage with clusters of reactive chondrocytes. H & E stain.

clefts (fibrillation). Fibrillation is accompanied by loss of surface cartilage (erosion) and eventual thinning of the articular cartilage. Subsequent to fibrillation and erosion, necrosis of individual chondrocytes occurs in the radial zone and making cartilage hypocellular. In response to the fibrillation, erosion, and necrosis of chondrocytes, remaining chondrocytes can undergo regenerative hyperplasia (cluster or clone formation) (Fig. 10-37), but the ability of chondrocytes in the adult to divide is limited and the regenerative attempt is almost always ineffective. Loss of articular cartilage can become complete with exposure of subchondral bone (ulceration) (Fig. 10-38). Continued rubbing on subchondral bone causes it to become dense, polished, and ivory-like (eburnation) (Fig. 10-39).

Degenerative changes in articular cartilage are often accompanied by the formation of periarticular osteophytes and by some degree of secondary synovial inflammation and hyperplasia. The synovitis is characterized by the presence of variable numbers of plasma cells, lymphocytes, and macrophages in the synovial subintima (beneath the layers of synoviocytes) and by hyperplasia and hypertrophy of synovial lining cells. Osteophytes form as multiple bony or cartilaginous outgrowths arising at or near the junctional zone—the zone on the surface of the bone where articular cartilage, periosteum, and the insertion of the joint capsule merge. Osteophytes do not grow continuously, but once formed, they persist as multiple periarticular spurs of bone that cause joint enlargement (see Figs. 10-45 and 10-48). Osteophytes can result from mechanical instability within the joint causing stretching or tearing of the insertions of the joint capsule or ligaments, or they can form from stimulation by cytokines such as transforming growth factor-beta released from reactive or degenerating mesenchymal cells within the joint.

The synovial membrane commonly responds to injury by villous hypertrophy and hyperplasia, hypertrophy and hyperplasia of synoviocytes, and pannus formation. Pannus is a fibrovascular and histiocytic tissue that arises from the synovial membrane and spreads over adjacent cartilage as a velvety membrane. Pannus is usually formed only as a response of synovium to inflammation and is rare in degenerative joint disease even with secondary inflammation. Villous hypertrophy (Fig. 10-40) occurs with and without synovitis. The proportions of A and B cells in the synovium also can change in various disease processes. Fragments of articular cartilage can adhere to the synovium, where they are surrounded by macrophages and giant cells. Larger pieces of detached cartilage (as in osteochondrosis) can float free and survive as "joint mice" that continue to be nurtured and remain viable by synovial fluid. Inflammatory cell infiltrates in the synovial

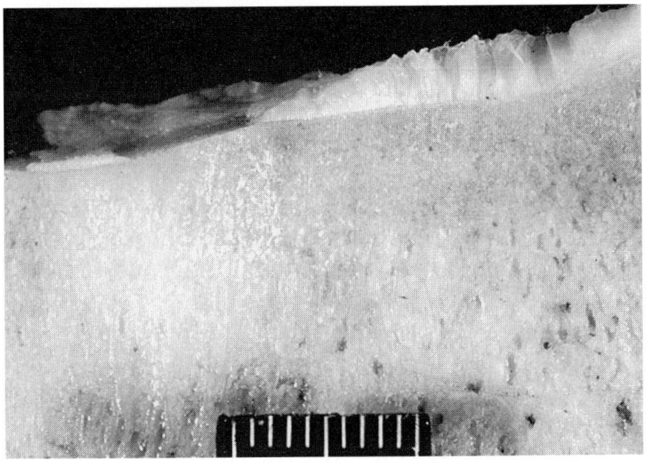

Figure 10-38 Joint, stifle (femur), bull. Degenerative joint disease. Fibrillation, erosion, and ulceration of cartilage. (Scale is in millimeters.)

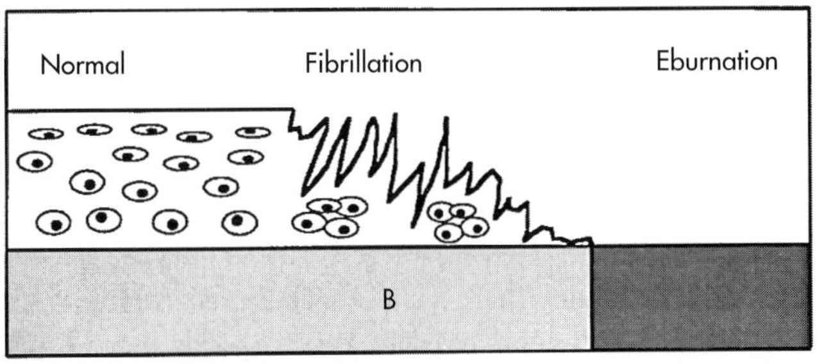

Figure 10-39 Diagram showing the structural changes that characterize fibrillation and eburnation of articular cartilage. Subchondral bone *(B)* has increased density in the area of eburnation, and the overlying cartilage is ulcerated.

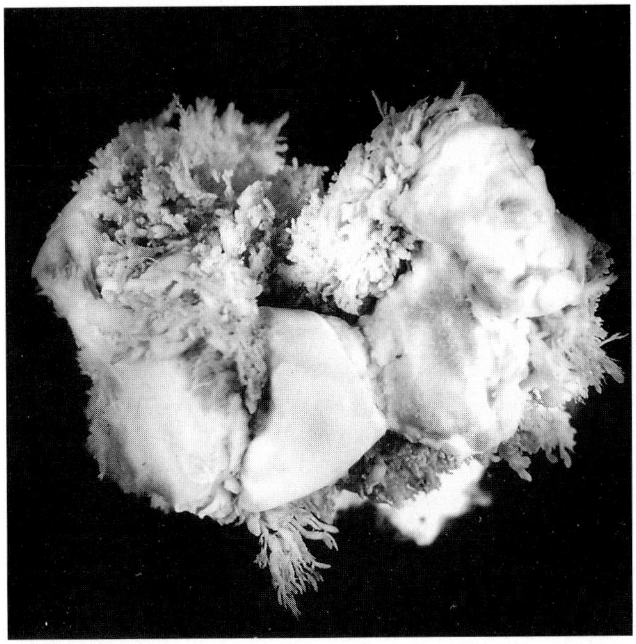

Figure 10-40 Joint, elbow (humerus); dog. Synovial hyperplasia and hypertrophy. Numerous reactive villouslike projections of synovial membrane extend into the joint space. Photographed submerged in water.

membrane can impair fluid drainage from the joint, and joint fluid can lose some of its lubricating properties because hyaluronic acid can be degraded by the superoxide-generating systems of neutrophils.

Pannus can develop in association with chronic infectious nonsuppurative synovitis and with some immune-mediated diseases, such as rheumatoid arthritis. In the pannus, tissue histiocytes and monocytes of bone marrow origin transform into macrophages, and, they, along with the collagenases from fibroblasts, cause lysis of cartilage. As the pannus spreads, the underlying cartilage is destroyed. In time, if both opposing cartilaginous surfaces are involved, the fibrous tissue can unite the surfaces, causing fibrous ankylosis (immobilization) of the joint. In some cases of immune-mediated arthritis, inflammation is present in the subchondral bone marrow as well as in the synovium. Pannus can develop in marrow from subchondral bone and penetrate into the overlying articular cartilage.

Because of their antiinflammatory effect, glucocorticoids are injected into joints. Sometimes a rapid progression of degenerative changes takes place within the joint and is designated "steroid arthropathy." These degenerative changes relate to the antianabolic effects of glucocorticoids on chondrocytes. They reduce the synthesis of cartilaginous matrix, lead to proteoglycan depletion, retard repair, and reduce the mechanical strength of cartilage.

Abnormalities of Growth and Development

A number of congenital neuromuscular disorders that are characterized by restricted articular movement occur in animals. In many cases, this restriction can be relieved by sectioning tendons or the joint capsule. Congenital malformation of articular surfaces or fusion of joints is uncommon; the former can be secondary to restricted articular movement. Restricted or reduced articular movement can be mild and self-correcting or can be severe and crippling. The term "arthrogryposis" implies persistent congenital flexure or contraction of a joint. It has been associated with inactivity or paralysis of the fetus in utero. This paralysis or paresis can be secondary to damage to the central nervous system such as with intrauterine viral infections (Akabane virus and bluetongue virus) in cattle and sheep or can be caused by maternal ingestion of poisonous plants (lupine poisoning in cattle, poison hemlock in swine). Alkaloids in poison hemlock (coniine) and lupine plants (anagyrine) are believed to cause sustained contraction of uterine muscle, and fetal deformity might be due to external compression and reduced fetal movement. Arthrogryposis in cattle can be associated with other lesions such as scoliosis, torticollis, and cleft palate.

Hip dysplasia occurs in dogs and in cattle. In the dog, it is a major inherited (polygenic) orthopedic problem and is most common in large and giant breeds. Many different

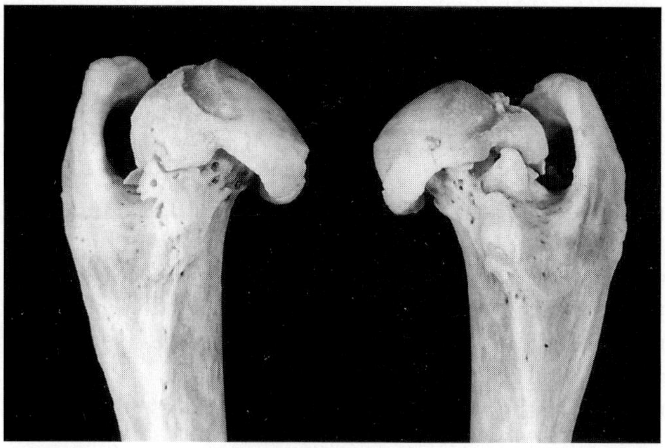

Figure 10-41 Joint, hip (femur); dog. Hip dysplasia. Both femoral heads are markedly flattened and have prominent osteophyte formation at the periphery resulting in bony "lipping." Macerated and bleached.

theories regarding the etiopathogenesis have been advanced, but most agree that it is a biomechanical disease in which inadequate muscle mass leads to joint laxity of the hip (instability) and, eventually, to degenerative joint disease. The lesions are not present at birth, but can be well advanced by 1 year of age. The severity of the lesions varies but can be reduced by restricting the rate of skeletal growth. Joint laxity leads to subluxation and subsequent abnormal modeling of the acetabulum. The dorsal rim of the acetabulum flattens and becomes shallow and wide. In time, the lesions consist of erosion and ulceration of articular cartilage, eburnation of underlying bone, malformation of articular surfaces, and formation of periarticular osteophytes (Fig. 10-41). The joint capsule is stretched and thickened, and areas of osseous and cartilaginous metaplasia can develop within it. The round ligament of the femoral head can rupture, and luxation can occur. Hip dysplasia, which might be inherited, also occurs in bulls of some beef breeds. Affected animals have shallow acetabula, joint laxity, and instability, which lead to degenerative joint disease early in life.

Inflammatory Lesions

The term **arthritis** implies inflammation of intraarticular structures, while the term **synovitis** is restricted to inflammation of the synovium. Arthritis is characterized by the presence of inflammatory cells in the synovial membrane, but the nature of the inflammatory process is often reflected best in the volume and character of the exudate in the joint fluid. Joint diseases are classified as inflammatory or noninflammatory. The problem with this classification becomes apparent when striking secondary lymphoplasmacytic and histiocytic synovitis is found in "noninflammatory" diseases such as degenerative joint disease. Arthritis can be classified as to cause, duration, and

Arthrogryposis
· Akabane (V)
· bluetongue (V)
· lupine poisoning - cattle
· poison hemlock - swine

the nature of the exudate produced (serous, fibrinous, purulent, lymphoplasmacytic). The term "arthropathy" is all-encompassing and refers to any joint disease. Like osteomyelitis, arthritis can be a serious threat to the well-being of an animal. It is painful and can lead to permanent deformity and crippling. Synovitis can be due to infectious agents, to the presence of foreign material such as urates in gout, or to trauma to intraarticular structures; or it can be partially or entirely immune mediated. Chronicity can be due to an inability of the animal to remove the causative agent or substance, repeated trauma, persistence of bacterial cell wall material, or ongoing autoimmune-mediated inflammation. Injury to intraarticular structure can be directly due to the offending agent or substance, to the inflammatory process, to proteolytic enzymes released from cells of cartilage or synovial tissues, activation of latent matrix metalloproteinases, or failure of degenerating or necrotic chondrocytes to maintain the proteoglycan content of the matrix. Substances associated with inflammation that contribute to joint injury include prostaglandins, cytokines, leukotrienes, lysosomal enzymes, free radicals, nitric oxide, neuropeptides, and products of the activated coagulation, kinin, complement, and fibrinolytic systems in synovial fluid.

Bacterial arthritis is uncommon in dogs and cats but is common in cattle, swine, and sheep, where it is often of hematogenous origin and polyarticular. Neonatal bacteremia secondary to omphalitis or oral-intestinal entry commonly leads to polyarthritis in lambs, calves, piglets, and foals. Bacteria can also reach the joint by direct inoculation, as in a puncture wound, by direct extension from periarticular soft tissues, or by extension from adjacent bone. Bacterial osteomyelitis can extend through the metaphyseal cortex into the joint, or epiphyseal osteomyelitis can lyse directly through articular cartilage. The duration of bacterial arthritis is variable. Some organisms are rapidly removed and synovitis is short-lived. In other instances, bacteria can persist, and the inflammatory process can become chronic. In some cases, it is postulated that the initial bacterial synovitis can lead to chronic immune-mediated arthritis because of cross-reactivity between antigens in the breakdown products of bacterial cell walls and normal antigens within the joint. In addition, some cross-reactivity (molecular mimicry) likely occurs between bacterial heat-shock proteins and articular glycosaminoglycans. These concepts are significant for they explain how an arthritis that begins as an infectious process might persist as a sterile immune-mediated one and how an infection elsewhere in the body can result in sterile immune-mediated arthritis through antigenic molecular mimicry (reactive arthritis).

The extent and mechanism of cartilaginous destruction differ somewhat in fibrinous and purulent arthritis. Acute fibrinous arthritis is characterized by deposition of fibrin within the synovial membrane and on the surface of intraarticular structures (Fig. 10-42). The process can resolve early with complete fibrinolysis and repair without residual defects. However, if deposits of fibrin are extensive, they can be invaded and replaced by fibrous tissue, leading to restricted articular movement. Fibrinous arthritis of long duration is often accompanied by marked villous hypertrophy, lymphoplasmacytic synovial inflammation, pannus formation, and progressive destruction of cartilage. In summary, articular cartilage can remain intact in fibrinous arthritis unless destroyed by pannus.

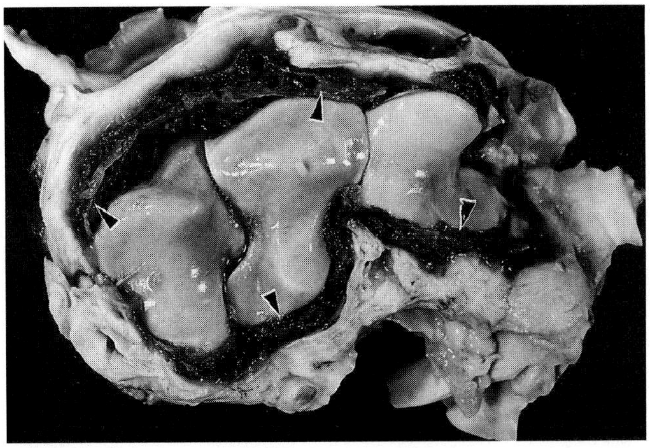

Figure 10-42 Joint, carpus; cow. Fibrinous synovitis. Fibrin *(arrowheads)* limited to the synovium at the periphery of the joint.

An example of chronic fibrinous arthritis is that caused in swine by *Erysipelothrix rhusiopathiae* septicemia. Survivors can have lesions secondary to localization of *E. rhusiopathiae* in the skin, synovial joints, valvular endocardium, or intervertebral disks. Chronic painful polyarthritis is a common sequela. Initially, the arthritis is fibrinous, and, later, it is lymphoplasmacytic with marked villous hypertrophy of the synovial membrane (Fig. 10-43). Pannus formation, accompanied by destruction of articular cartilage, and fibrous ankylosis of joints can occur. Localization of the organism in the terminal vessels of the annulus fibrosus of the intervertebral disks is common and leads to inflammation and destruction of the vertebral disks, followed by fibrous replacement of the vertebral disks and surrounding structures (discospondylitis).

In contrast, purulent arthritis is accompanied by progressive and often extensive lysis (necrosis) of articular cartilage, with the process commonly extending into adjacent subchondral bone. Proteolytic enzymes derived from large numbers of neutrophils present in the joint are likely responsible. *Arcanobacterium pyogenes* is a common cause of purulent arthritis in cattle and pigs.

Many different infectious agents cause arthritis in animals. For example, *Escherichia coli* and streptococci cause septicemia in neonatal calves and piglets and localize in joints, meninges, and, sometimes, serosal

Arthritis
: Erysipelothrix rhusiopathiae
Arcanobacterium pyogenes
E. coli
Streptococci
Hemophilus parasuis
Mycoplasma hyorhinis
Mycoplasma hyosynoviae

Cattle: Arcanobacterium pyogenes
E. coli:
Streptococci
Histophilus somni

Goat: CAE

Dog: Rheumatoid
SLE
pyometra
otitis externa

Bird/reptile: Gout

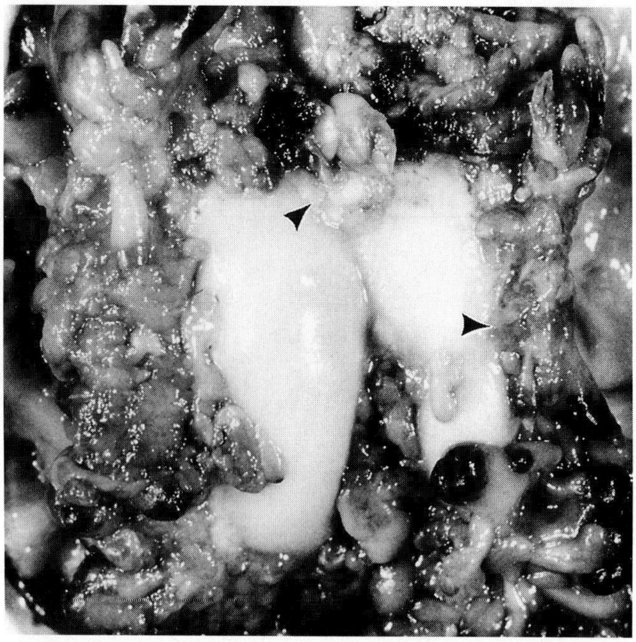

Figure 10-43 Joint, stifle (femur) pig. Erysipelas. Chronic fibrinous synovitis due to *Erysipelothrix rhusiopathiae* has villous hypertrophy of the synovial membrane and pannus formation *(arrowheads)*. The tips of some villi are hemorrhagic and necrotic. *Courtesy of Dr. K. Johnston.*

surfaces. Often synovitis is acutely serofibrinous and often becomes more purulent with time. *Haemophilus parasuis* causes Glasser's disease in swine 8 to 16 weeks of age. Lesions consist of fibrinous polyserositis, polyarthritis, and meningitis. Acute serofibrinous polyarthritis is seen frequently in cattle dying of thromboembolic meningoencephalitis caused by *Haemophilus somnus. Mycoplasma bovis* causes fibrinous polyarthritis in feedlot cattle, and the disease is characterized by lameness and swelling of the large synovial joints of the limbs that can contain large volumes of serofibrinous exudate. *Mycoplasma hyorhinis* causes fibrinous polyarthritis and polyserositis in weanling pigs. Chronic cases can form pannus and synovial villous hypertrophy. *Mycoplasma hyosynoviae* causes polyarthritis in older swine (more than 3 months old). The caprine arthritis-encephalitis virus (a retrovirus) causes chronic arthritis in older goats. The disease is characterized by debilitating lameness, carpal hygromas, and distension of the larger synovial joints. Advanced cases have marked synovial villous hypertrophy with necrosis and mineralization and mononuclear cell infiltration, pannus formation, and destruction of articular cartilage.

Arthritis in the dog is often classified as erosive or nonerosive. Rheumatoid arthritis in the dog is an uncommon, chronic, erosive polyarthritis that resembles the disease in human beings. In human beings and dogs, the cause is unknown, although it is clear that the process is immune mediated (involves humoral and cell-mediated immunity). Antibodies (rheumatoid factor) of the IgG or IgM classes are produced in response to an unknown stimulus. Alterations in the stearic configuration of IgG, persistent bacterial cell wall components that cross-react with normal proteoglycans, anticollagen antibodies, and defective suppressor T cell activity are factors that might be involved. Immune complexes are ingested by neutrophils. These cells release lysosomal enzymes, which sustain the inflammatory reaction and injure intraarticular structures. The pathogenesis of joint destruction in rheumatoid arthritis is described above in reaction to injury of joints to inflammation. In addition to inflammatory mediators and their effects on synovium and cartilage, rheumatoid arthritis characteristically has exuberant pannus formation. Fibroblasts in pannus can enzymatically degrade cartilage and pannus can act as a physical barrier between the synovial fluid and the cartilage preventing nutrition of the chondrocytes. Antibodies against normal and altered collagen from articular cartilage are present in human cases of rheumatoid arthritis and might be important mediators of the ongoing joint inflammation and injury that occur in this disease. In dogs, rheumatoid arthritis is characterized by progressive lameness involving the peripheral joints of the limbs. Grossly, the lesions consist of marked villous hypertrophy of the synovial membrane, erosion of cartilage, pannus formation, formation of periarticular osteophytes, and, when severe, fibrous ankylosis of affected joints. Microscopically, the alterations in the joint are hyperplasia of synovial lining cells and infiltration of large numbers of plasma cells and lymphocytes into the synovium. Additionally in the synovium, necrotic foci, fibrinous exudate, and infiltrating neutrophils can be present. Large numbers of neutrophils are present in the joint fluid.

Chronic nonerosive arthritis occurs in dogs with systemic lupus erythematosus, and such dogs can have anemia, thrombocytopenia, polymyositis, or glomerulonephritis. Nonerosive polyarthritis also occurs in dogs in association with chronic disease processes such as pyometra or otitis externa. Immune complexes can localize in synovium and lead to synovitis. In these diseases, villous hypertrophy is minimal, pannus formation does not occur, and destruction of articular cartilage is not to be expected. The exudate in the synovial fluid in chronic nonerosive arthritis is neutrophilic, with only a mild lymphoplasmacytic inflammation present in the synovium.

Crystal-induced synovitis and degeneration of articular cartilage occur in gout when urate crystals are deposited in and around joints in which they incite an acute or chronic inflammatory reaction. Gout occurs in species that do not have the enzyme uricase (human beings, birds, reptiles). Deposits of urate, called tophi, are white, caseous, and periarticular and can be large enough to be visible grossly (Fig. 10-44). Periarticular and synovial deposits of

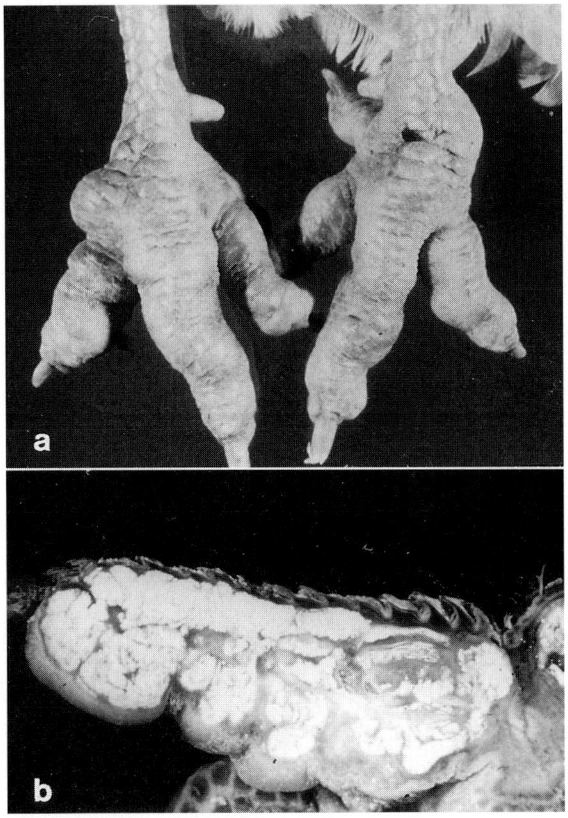

Figure 10-44 Bone, digits; bird. Gout. **A,** The joints are irregularly swollen. **B,** Cross section. White pasty uric acid deposits are present.

calcium pyrophosphate (pseudogout or calcium pyrophosphate deposition disease) and calcium phosphate (calcium phosphate deposition disease) have been reported as a cause of synovitis and lameness in dogs and nonhuman primates. Single or multiple joints can be involved.

Degenerative Joint Disease

Degenerative joint disease (osteoarthritis, osteoarthrosis) is an ancient disease of synovial joints that occurs in all animals with a bony skeleton. It is a destructive disease of articular cartilage characterized by a sequence of changes starting with fibrillation and progressing to erosion and ulceration of articular cartilage, formation of periarticular osteophytes, sclerosis of subchondral bone, and osteochondral modeling. It can be monoarticular or polyarticular, can occur in immature or mature animals, and can be symptomatic or represent an incidental finding. Affected animals have variable degrees of joint enlargement and deformity, pain, and articular malfunction. The etiopathogenesis of degenerative joint disease is incompletely understood, and it is likely that the term encompasses a variety of diseases that have a common end stage. Initial changes can be due to traumatic injury to articular cartilage, inflammation of the synovium, or increased stiffness of the subchondral bone. Degenerative joint disease often progresses to sclerosis of subchondral bone, but some investigators consider stiffness (sclerosis) of subchondral bone as the initial lesion and this stiffness predisposes the cartilage to mechanical damage. The initial biochemical change in articular cartilage is loss of proteoglycan aggregates, which leads to improper binding of water and a net increase in the water content of the cartilage. The increased water and its improper binding lead to softening (chondromalacia). Core proteins of proteoglycan aggregates are susceptible to the action of neutral proteoglycanases, which are increased in early degenerative joint disease. In electron micrographs, the findings include focal loss of the amorphous layer covering the surface of the articular cartilage and fraying of the superficial collagen fibers. Continued proteoglycan loss interferes with joint lubrication and allows collagen fibers that were previously separated by a hydrated gel (proteoglycans and water) to collapse on each other along lines perpendicular to the joint surface. Weightbearing on these collapsed/condensed fibers causes fissuring (fibrillation). This fibrillated surface with its reduced proteoglycan content is subject to physical wear and progressive loss (erosion) of cartilage. Eventually, complete cartilage loss (ulceration) exposes the underlying subchondral bone (Fig. 10-38). With use of the joint, the subchondral bone becomes smooth and hard (eburnation and sclerosis). Subchondral bone cysts (see previous discussion under "Cysts") can develop in degenerative joint disease, but these are less common in animals than in human beings. Marginal (periarticular) osteophytes (Figs. 10-45 and 10-48) are a prominent feature, and synovitis characterized by villous hypertrophy, hyperplasia of synoviocytes, and infiltration of lymphocytes, plasma cells, and macrophages are usually present.

Synovitis in degenerative joint disease is secondary to release of inflammatory mediators by injured chondrocytes and from synovial macrophages that have phagocytized cartilaginous breakdown products. Proteases and cytokines released by cells of the inflamed synovium cause additional joint damage in responses of cartilage to injury. Grossly, degenerated cartilage initially has a matte finish associated with focal softening and fibrillation and often is yellow or yellow-brown (Fig. 10-46). Lesions can be diffuse but often are focal; in hinge-type joints, they can occur as linear grooves (Fig. 10-47). The pathogenesis of these grooves is uncertain but might represent damage done by jetties of synovial fluid secondary to incongruities of the joint surfaces. Advanced lesions can have marked loss of cartilage and modeling of the subchondral and metaphyseal bone (Fig. 10-48). Joint fusion (ankylosis) might occur.

Age-related degeneration of articular cartilage is common in all species and can be of minimal clinical significance. Lesions are of greatest importance when they occur at an early age and progress rapidly. Some of the

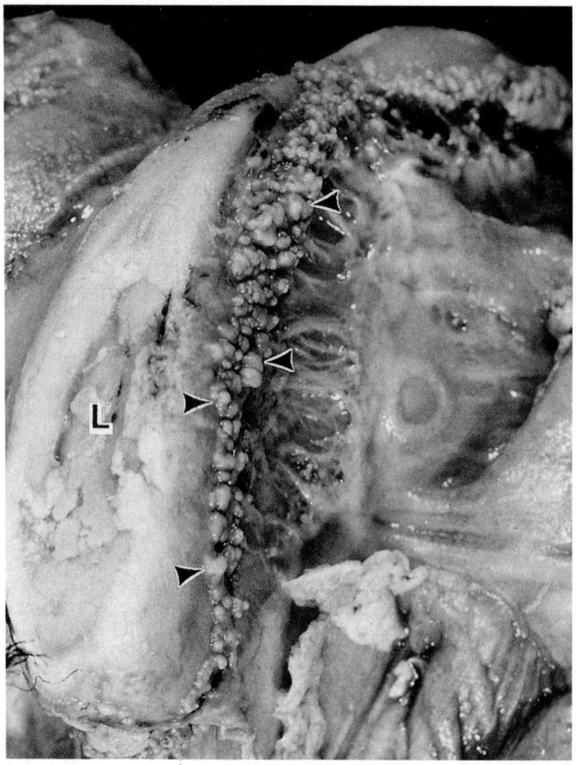

Figure 10-45 Femur. Distal articular stifle (femur); bull. Degenerative joint disease of the lateral trochlear ridge. Cartilage loss *(L)* is extensive. There are numerous small periarticular osteophytes *(arrowheads)*.

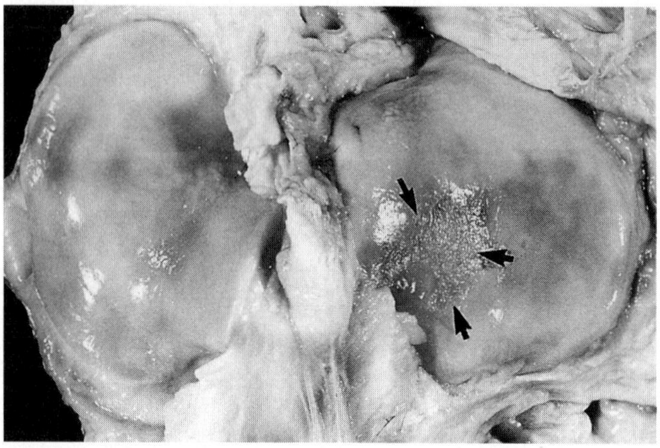

Figure 10-46 Tibia, proximal articular surface; horse. Degenerative joint disease. Articular cartilage has areas of chondromalacia, discoloration, and fibrillation (outlined by *arrows*).

causative factors that have been implicated in the evolution of degenerative joint disease include repeated trauma to articular cartilage, abnormalities in conformation, joint instability, and joint incongruence. In addition, degeneration of cartilage occurs secondary to inflammatory arthritis and diseases such as osteochondritis dissecans that disrupt the articular surface.

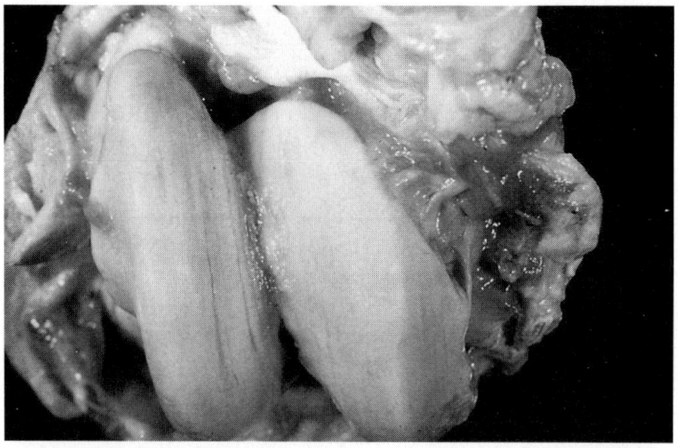

Figure 10-47 Joint, hock (tibial tarsal bone); horse. Degenerative joint disease. Linear erosions are present in the articular surface.

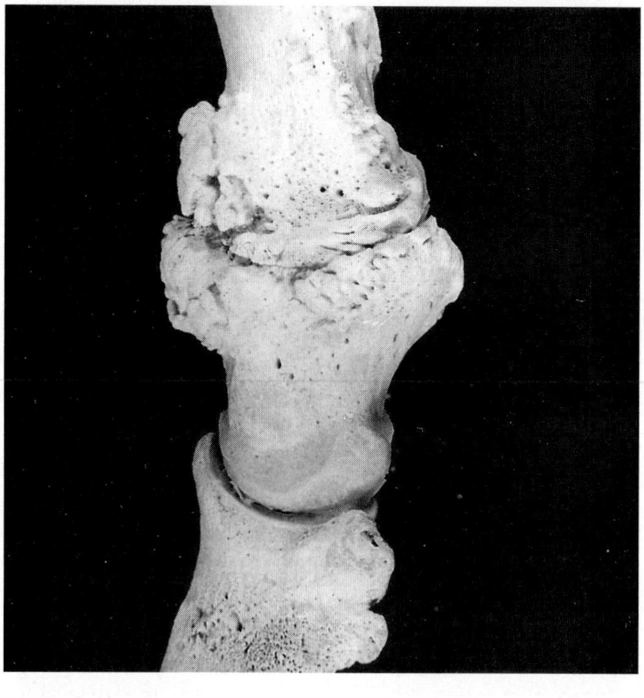

Figure 10-48 Joints, digit; horse. Degenerative joint disease. Extensive modeling of subchondral bone with osteophyte formation of the proximal interphalangeal joint ("high ring-bone"). Macerated and bleached.

Osteochondrosis

The osteochondroses consist of a heterogeneous group of lesions in growth cartilage of young animals and are characterized by focal or multifocal failure (or delay) of endochondral ossification. As such, osteochondrosis involves the metaphyseal growth plate and the articular-epiphyseal cartilage complex. The lesions are common and represent an important orthopedic entity that has a number of different clinical manifestations in pigs, dogs, horses, cattle, poultry, and rats. Interestingly, the disease is not recognized in cats. Many investigators have made the point that the term "osteochondrosis," which implies degeneration of cartilage and bone, is inappropriate because the lesions are initially in the cartilage. The hallmark of the uncomplicated gross lesions of osteochondrosis is retention of growth cartilage due to its failure to become mineralized and replaced by bone (a failure of endochondral ossification). Grossly, the retained cartilage is usually a white, firm (similar to hyaline cartilage) wedge at the articular epiphyseal complex or physis. The term dysplasia has been used for these wedges of intact retained cartilage. Variations in this gross appearance might reflect stages of resolution or secondary necrosis (Fig. 10-49). Hemorrhage and mineralized debris can occur at the junction of the dysplasia and adjacent bone. Often small dysplastic areas produce no clinical signs. Such dysplasias are common especially in the distal femurs of pigs, the distal femur, distal tibia and vertebral articular facets of horses, the proximal humerus of dogs, and the proximal tibia of rapidly growing birds. Microscopically, these areas are composed of hypertrophic, sometimes poorly aligned chondrocytes without evidence of mineralization or vascular invasion. Dysplasias can progress or spontaneously resolve by endochondral ossification. Those dysplasias that progress can become cartilaginous flaps of osteochondritis dissecans at the A-E complex or bone cysts at the physis.

In progressive dysplasias, clefts can develop in the regions of retained cartilage. These clefts can be linear and form by necrosis of cartilage, possibly induced by pressure or failure of nutrient diffusion, or they may follow acellular streaks within the cartilage. These streaks appear microscopically as eosinophilic lines, sometimes with central fissures, and are of variable contour and direction (Fig. 10-50). They are composed of densely packed collagen fibers with minimal proteoglycans and can be remains of cartilage vascular canals or zones of "physiologic" necrosis of chondrocytes. These streaks are found in normal cartilage, but they can appear exaggerated in some cases of osteochondrosis. Cleft formation can cause mechanical instability and lead to separation within cartilage or of cartilage from the underlying bone. Clefts that arise in the articular epiphyseal complex can cause loosening of the dysplastic cartilage from the adjacent epiphyseal bone. Trauma can cause the cleft to extend through the overlying articular cartilage and a flap is formed. This lesion of dysplastic cartilage with flap formation is called **osteochondritis dissecans** (OCD) (Fig. 10-49). Should this flap fracture off and become free in the joint space, it is called a "joint mouse." OCD can be

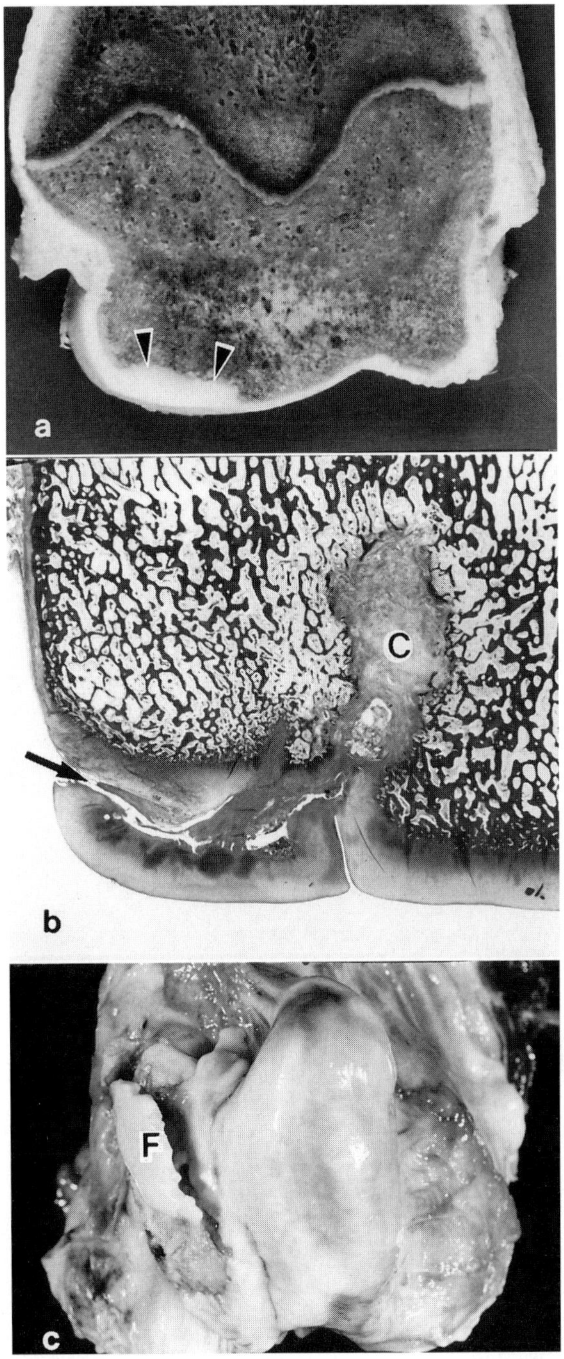

Figure 10-49 Joint. Osteochondrosis. **A,** Distal radius. A dysplasia is present at the articular epiphyseal complex *(arrowheads)* **B,** Femoral condyle. A cleft *(arrow)* in the deeper regions of retained cartilage has formed a flap characteristic of osteochondritis dissecans. A "cyst" *(C)* is present in the subchondral bone because of focal failure of normal bone formation resulting from osteochondrosis and degeneration of the retained cartilage. H & E stain. **C,** Femur. Osteochondritis dissecans with a cartilaginous flap *(F)* in the lateral trochlear ridge of the femur. *Courtesy of Dr. Wayne Riser.*

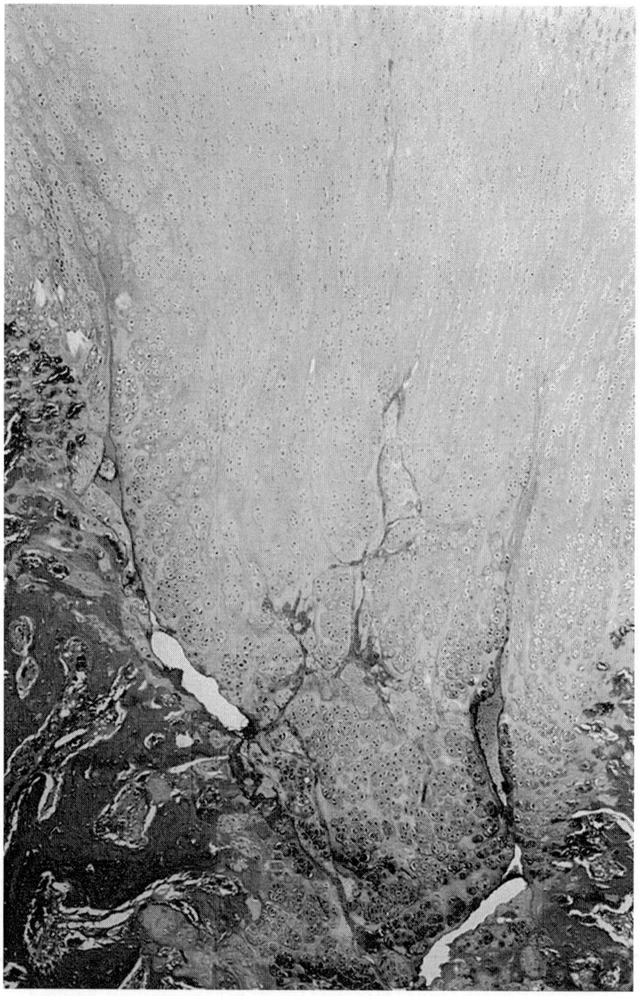

Figure 10-50 Joint, horse. Osteochondrosis. Dysplasia at articular epiphyseal complex with numerous eosinophilic streaks and cavities, likely remnants of previous cartilage canals that had contained blood vessels. H & E stain.

accompanied by pain, joint effusion, and nonspecific secondary lymphoplasmacytic synovitis. Free-floating "joint mice" occasionally interfere with mechanical movement of the joint. The lesions of OCD develop in various synovial joints, including those of the facets of the vertebral column. Common sites of OCD are the humeral head in the dog, the anterior aspect of the intermediate ridge of the distal tibia in horses, and the medial condyles of the distal femur and distal humerus in pigs. The disease is a significant cause of lameness in young breeding pigs. It is clear that the lesions of OCD can be slow to heal, are accompanied by synovitis, and, in time, lead to degenerative joint disease.

If the retained cartilage in a dysplasia undergoes liquefactive necrosis, a bone cyst can develop. This could be the pathogenesis of some subchondral bone cysts.

Epiphysiolysis is often listed as a lesion of osteochondrosis, but it is not associated with dysplasia (retention of cartilage). Epiphysiolysis represents separation of the epiphysis from the metaphyseal bone and, likely, involves some degree of trauma acting on regions of degeneration/necrosis in the metaphyseal growth plate. The femoral head can be involved in market-weight pigs and in young gilts. In young sows, separation of the ischial tuberosity at its growth plate is a common cause of posterior weakness and inability to stand. In dogs, the process of epiphysiolysis can be the basis for an ununited anconeal process. Necrosis without dysplasia appears to be common at the articular epiphyseal complex of the cervical intervertebral facets in horses.

The cause of osteochondrosis is unknown. The fact that there is a high incidence in species bred and fed to achieve maximal body weight at a young age suggests that it might be a mechanical complication superimposed on "normal" multifocal defects of endochondral ossification. Presumably, uneven patterns of endochondral ossification are common, and most go undetected. Only in animals selected for rapid weight gain might these develop into clinically significant lesions. Little evidence is available to indicate that the lesions of osteochondrosis result from a specific nutritional deficiency. However, copper deficiency, perhaps conditioned by excess dietary zinc, in thoroughbred suckling foals has produced lysis of the articular-epiphyseal complex and formation of thin flaps of cartilage. Also, lesions of cartilage retention are less frequent in foals from mares fed increased dietary copper. Osteochondrosis-like lesions have been reported at greater incidence in growing dogs fed high-calcium diets.

Not only are the causes of osteochondrosis not known, but the nature of the initial lesion in areas of dysplasia is still under debate. Much emphasis has been placed on necrosis of cartilage in the resting zones, likely secondary to ischemia from thrombosis of cartilage vessels in this zone of cartilage, as the initial lesion. Subsequent studies have produced inconsistencies, and results indicate that the initial lesion is the result of abnormal matrix that resists mineralization and vascular invasion. The most recent studies have examined the role of apoptosis in the development of osteochondrosis in poultry but the findings have been contradictory.

Wedges of retained mineralized cartilage are not considered lesions of osteochondrosis but likely occur secondary to trauma and infractions of the primary trabeculae that produce a physical barrier to vascular invasion.

Degeneration of Intervertebral Disks

Degeneration of the intervertebral disks is often an age-related phenomenon in many species. In general, loss

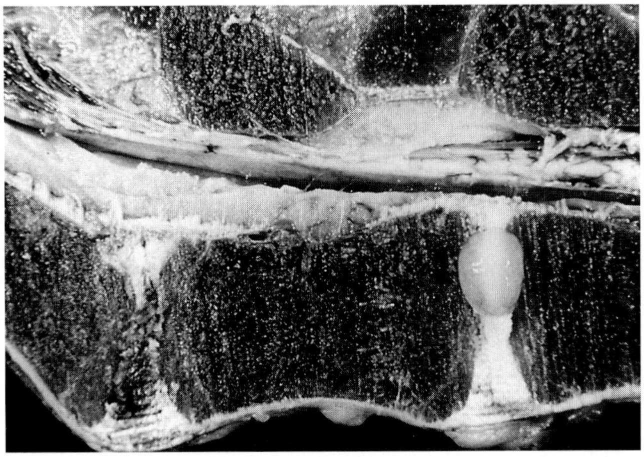

Figure 10-51 Joint, intervertebral disk (lumbosacral); pig. Degenerate intervertebral disk disease. The nucleus pulposus in the disk on the left is degenerate and lysed as compared with the normal disk on the right, which is white and bulging from cut surface.

of water and proteoglycans, reduced cellularity, and an increase in collagen content of the nucleus pulposus occur, so that the distinction between the nucleus pulposus and the annulus fibrosus is obscured. The central part of the disk is yellow-brown and is composed of friable fibrocartilaginous material (Fig. 10-51). These degenerative changes are likely caused by various metabolic and mechanical insults that lead to breakdown of proteoglycan aggregates in the nucleus pulposus and to degenerative changes in the annulus fibrosus. Both rotational and compressive types of movement injure the annulus fibrosus. Changes in structure of the nucleus pulposus, together with a weakened annulus, often lead to concentric and radial tears or fissures in the annulus that allow bulging or herniation of the nucleus pulposus material (Fig. 10-52). Herniation is usually dorsal in domestic animals. In human beings (rarely in domestic animals), disk material can be extruded through the end-plate into the vertebral body, producing a lesion known as Schmorl's node.

In chondrodystrophic breeds of dogs such as the dachshund, chondroid metaplasia of the nucleus pulposus is followed by calcification during the first year of life. These alterations can result in disk prolapse, with total rupture of the annulus fibrosus and extrusion of disk material into the vertebral canal at sites of mechanical stress, such as the cervical and thoracolumbar vertebrae.

Senile degenerative disk disease is independent of breed in the dog and also occurs in human beings, pigs, and horses. These lesions are characterized by progressive dehydration and collagenization of the nucleus pulposus and degeneration of the annulus fibrosus. The lesions develop slowly, and calcification is rare. Prolapse of the disk is secondary to partial rupture of the annulus fibrosus

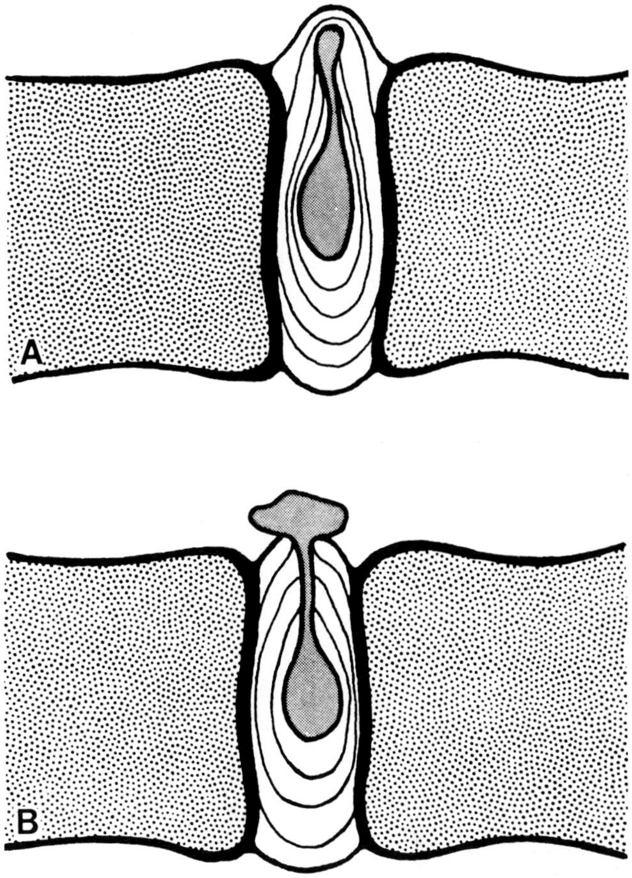

Figure 10-52 Prolapse of the nucleus pulposus may be secondary to partial rupture of the annulus fibrosus **(A)**; total rupture of the annulus fibrosus allows extrusion of nucleus pulposus material into the vertebral canal **(B)**.

and is characterized by bulging of the dorsal surface of the disk into the vertebral canal. An important consequence of degeneration of intervertebral disks is prolapse of the disk. Prolapse or herniation can be dorsal (spinal cord compression) or lateral (spinal nerve compression and entrapment). Because each intervertebral joint is a three-joint complex (intevertebral joint and two facet joints), the reduced disk thickness that follows degeneration and dehydration allows overriding of articular facets and some degree of joint instability. These changes contribute to the evolution of degenerative disease and enlargement of articular facets. Enlargement of the facets can cause impingement on spinal nerves and even compression of the spinal canal through intervertebral foramen. Degeneration of intervertebral disks and the ensuing intervertebral joint instability can result in the development of osteophytes on vertebrae at intervertebral spaces (spondylosis) in many species, such as dogs, cattle, pigs, and horses. Vertebral osteophytes are usually ventral and lateral; if dorsal, they can cause stenosis of the vertebral canal.

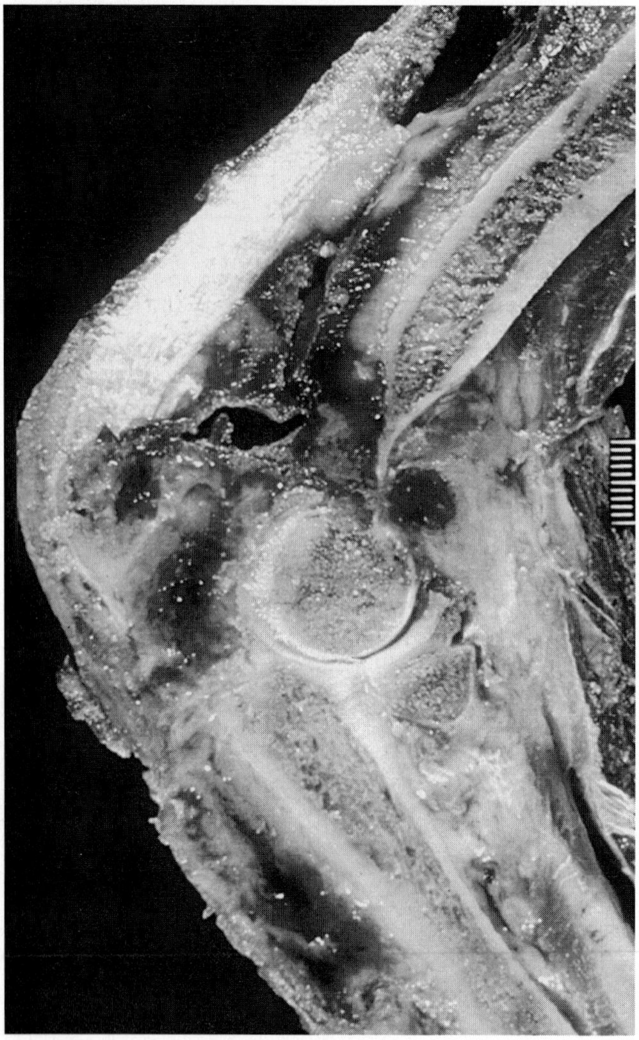

Figure 10-53 Joint, elbow, dog. Synovial cell sarcoma. Mass is within the joint space and invading bone (but not cartilage) on either side of the joint. (Scale is in millimeters.)

Neoplasms of Joints

Synovial cell sarcoma is the term given to a malignancy of synovial origin. A benign counterpart is not recognized. Synovial cell sarcomas are relatively rare and found mostly in dogs. The neoplasm arises within the joint space and erodes bone on both sides of the joint by invading bone at the perichondral margin (Fig. 10-53). Microscopically the neoplasm can have both fibroblastic and epithelioid features. Poorly differentiated synovial cell sarcomas can metastasize.

Suggested Readings

Bullough PG. Atlas of orthopedic pathology with clinical and radiographic correlations. Philadelphia: JB Lippincott, 1992.

Bullough PG. Bullough and Vigorita's orthopedic pathology. 3rd ed. London: Mosby-Wolfe, 1997.

Jones TC, Mohr U, Hunt RD. Monographs on pathology of laboratory animals. Cardiovascular and musculoskeletal systems. Boston: Kluwer Academic, 1990.

Palmer N. Bones and joints. In: Jubb KVF, Kennedy PC, Palmer N, eds. Pathology of Domestic Animals. 4th ed. San Diego: Academic Press, 1992.

Pool RR. Tumors and tumor-like lesions of joints and adjacent soft tissues. In: Moulton JE, ed. Tumors in Domestic Animals. Berkeley: University of California Press, 1990.

Woodard JC. Skeletal system. In: Jones TC, Hunt RD, King NW, eds. Veterinary Pathology. 6th ed. Baltimore: Williams & Wilkins, 1997.

Woodard JC, Jee WSS. Skeletal system. In: Haschek WM, Rousseaux CG, eds. Handbook of Toxicologic Pathology. San Diego: Academic Press, 1991.

CHAPTER 11

Integumentary System

ANN M. HARGIS
PAMELA E. GINN

GENERAL CONSIDERATIONS

Overview

The study of the skin bridges the disciplines of clinical medicine and pathology. The gross evaluation of the skin is synonymous with a clinical or dermatologic evaluation of the skin. Many small animals are brought to their veterinarian for skin disorders. Because the skin is one of the largest organs in the body, it is adversely affected by numerous internal and external factors, and skin lesions are easily seen by owners. Horse owners are also concerned about the esthetic appearance of their animal's skin. The skin, therefore, has economic importance in veterinary practice because of the number of cases evaluated. The skin also has economic importance in food animal practice. For instance, some cutaneous parasites blemish hides; decrease production of meat, wool, and milk; predispose animals to secondary bacterial infections; and cause downgrading at market.

Functions

The skin participates in temperature and blood pressure regulation, protects against fluid and electrolyte loss, serves as a barrier to physical, chemical, and microbiologic agents, produces vitamin D, is a sensory organ, and stores fat, water, vitamins, carbohydrates, protein, and other nutrients. Although absorption is not a primary function, many substances can be absorbed by the skin. In addition, the epidermal keratinocyte, a major source of cytokines, is now considered to be an integral part of the immune system. Cytokines produced by keratinocytes include some interleukins (ILs), colony-stimulating factors (CSFs), tumor necrosis factor (TNF), and growth factors. These cytokines comprise an interactive network and play a significant role in mediating inflammation and immune responses of the skin. The production of cytokines by keratinocytes is regulated to maintain homeostasis, and malfunction of cytokine production or release may result in cutaneous disease.

ANATOMY AND HISTOLOGY OF THE SKIN

General

The skin, a large and complex organ that has haired and hairless portions (Figs. 11-1 and 11-2), consists of epidermis, dermis, hair follicles, digital appendages, and sebaceous, sweat, and other glands. Histologic structure varies greatly among different sites and among different species of animals. The haired skin is thickest over the dorsal aspect of the body and on the lateral aspect of the limbs, and is thinnest on the ventral aspect of the body and the medial aspect of the thighs. The skin of large animals is generally thicker than those of small animals. The subcutis, lobules of adipose tissue and fascia, connects epidermis and dermis with the underlying fascia and musculature.

Epidermis

Haired skin has a thinner epidermis, whereas nonhaired skin of the nose and footpads has a thicker epidermis (Figs. 11-1 and 11-2). The epidermis of haired skin consists of four basic layers, whereas that of hairless skin consists of five layers. The cells that form keratin are referred to as keratinocytes. The outermost layer of the epidermis is the stratum corneum, which consists of many sheets of flattened, keratinized cells. Keratin is an intracellular fibrous protein that is in part responsible for the toughness of the epidermis, enabling the epidermis to form a protective barrier. The next layer is the stratum granulosum, which consists of effete cells with basophilic keratohyalin granules. In nonhaired skin, the stratum corneum and stratum granulosum are separated by an additional layer of compacted, fully keratinized cells, the stratum lucidum, best seen on the footpad. Deep to the stratum granulosum is the stratum spinosum, a layer of polyhedral-shaped cells attached to one another by desmosomes. During processing for microscopic examination, the cells of the stratum spinosum contract, except for the desmosomal attachments. These attachment sites create the appearance of "spines" or intercellular bridges,

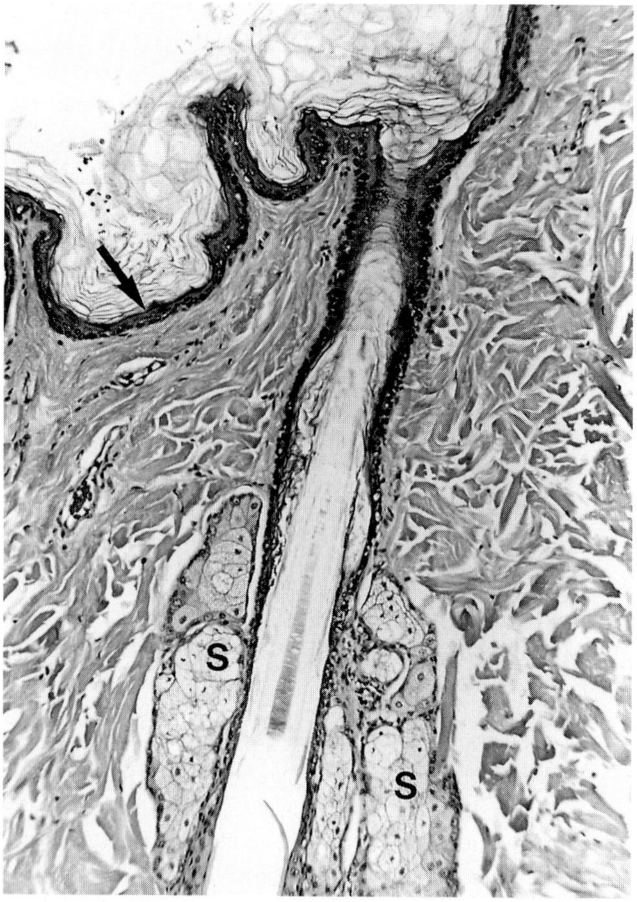

Figure 11-1 Skin, haired; dog. Normal. The epidermis *(arrow)* is thinner in haired than hairless skin, and hair follicles and sebaceous glands *(S)* are present. Hematoxylin-eosin (H & E) stain.

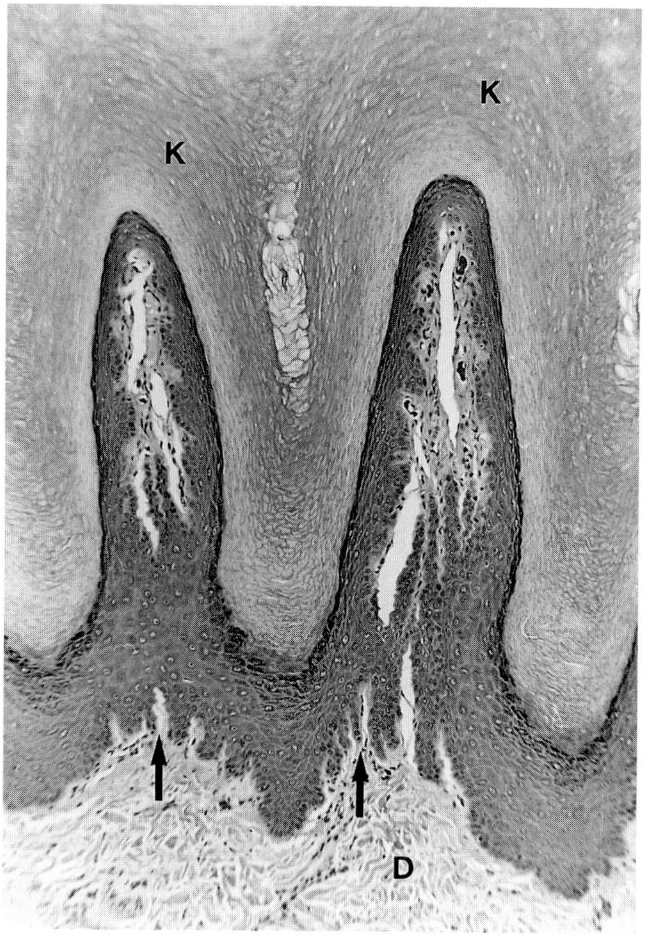

Figure 11-2 Skin, hairless; dog. Normal. The epidermis is thick and interdigitates *(arrows)* with the dermis *(D)*. Note dense zone of keratin *(K)* comprising the stratum corneum. H & E stain.

leading to the naming of this layer. The stratum spinosum in haired areas is thinner in dogs and cats and is thicker in cattle, horses, and pigs. The innermost layer of the epidermis is the germinal layer or stratum basale, which consists of a single layer of cuboidal cells resting on a basement membrane.

Intermixed within the basal cell layer are melanocytes, Langerhans' cells, and Merkel's cells. Melanocytes, derived from the neural crest, are also present in lower layers of the stratum spinosum and produce melanin pigment giving color to skin and hair. Melanocytic granules, transferred to keratinocytes and distributed as a caplike cluster of granules above each nucleus, help protect the nuclei from ultraviolet light. Langerhans' cells are bone marrow–derived cells of monocyte-macrophage lineage that process and present antigen to sensitized T cells, thereby modulating immunologic responses of the skin. Merkel's cells, neuroendocrine cells of the basal layer, function as slowly adapting mechanoreceptors, and, by a paracrine role, regulate the function of adjacent epidermal and adnexal structures. Intraepidermal lymphocytes, known to be T cells in the human and mouse, are few in number and are part of the skin-associated immune system.

The epidermis and dermis are separated by a basement membrane. In hairless areas such as the footpads and nasal planum, this junction is irregular due to epidermal projections that interdigitate with dermal papillae, thus strengthening the epidermal-dermal attachment by providing resistance to shearing. In densely haired areas, the junction is smooth and the anchoring function is provided by hair follicles. The more sparsely haired skin of pigs has more epidermal-dermal interdigitations (rete ridges) and fewer hair follicles.

Dermis

The dermis (corium), consisting of collagen and elastic fibers in a glycosaminoglycan ground substance, supports hair follicles, glands, vessels, and nerves. The superficial dermis is comprised of fine collagen fibers and is wider in the skin of cattle and horses than in skin of dogs and cats. The deep dermis is comprised of larger collagen bundles than the superficial dermis. Skeletal muscle fibers from the cutaneous muscle extend into the dermis and are responsible for voluntary skin movement. Fibroblasts, mast cells, lymphocytes, plasma cells, macrophages, and, rarely, eosinophils and neutrophils can be found in normal dermis.

Vessels and Nerves

Cutaneous arteries give rise to three vascular plexuses: deep, middle, and superficial. The deep plexus supplies the subcutis and deep portions of follicles and apocrine glands; the middle plexus supplies the sebaceous glands, mid portion of follicles, and arrector pili muscles; and the superficial plexus supplies the superficial portions of follicles and epidermis. Lymph capillaries arise in the superficial dermis and connect with a subcutaneous plexus. The lymph vessels then converge to form larger channels that eventually reach peripheral lymph nodes.

Nerve supply to the skin consists of motor and sensory fibers. Visceral efferent sympathetic nerves supply the smooth muscle of blood vessels, the arrector pili muscles, and myoepithelial cells of glands. The rich supply of nerves to the epidermis and dermis is mostly general somatic, afferent, myelinated, and nonmyelinated fibers. A dermatome is the area of skin supplied by the branches of one spinal nerve.

Hypodermis (Subcutis, Panniculus)

The hypodermis attaches the dermis to subjacent muscle or bone and consists of adipose tissue and collagenous and elastic fibers, which provide flexibility. Adipose tissue can insulate against temperature variation and, in the case of footpads, serve in shock absorption.

Adnexa

Hair Follicles

Growth of hair is seasonal in animals, with the time of growth and mitotic activity termed the anagen phase. A transitional phase, during which cellular proliferation ceases, is the catagen phase. The follicle then enters a resting state, the telogen phase, after which mitotic activity and new hair production resumes and old hair is shed. The duration of the hair cycle is controlled by number of daylight hours, environmental temperature, genetic factors, and a complex interaction of growth factors and neuropeptides.

Forms of hair follicles vary in different animals. Cattle and horses have evenly distributed simple follicles with one large (primary) follicle usually with sebaceous and sweat glands and arrector pili muscles. Pigs have simple follicles grouped in clusters. Goats, dogs, and cats have compound follicles that consist of primary follicles associated with smaller secondary follicles. Sheep have simple follicles in hair-growing areas and compound follicles in wool-growing areas. Primary follicles have the hair bulb rooted more deeply in the dermis than secondary follicles. The depth of the hair bulbs varies with species. In dogs and cats the anagen hair bulbs of primary follicles are at the dermal-subcutaneous junction, whereas in horses and cattle the anagen hair bulbs are in the mid dermis. In all species, the bases of telogen follicles are more superficially located than the bases of anagen follicles. Typically, primary and secondary hair shafts emerge through a common follicular opening. Tactile hairs include sinus and tylotrich hairs. Sinus hairs, also termed vibrissae, are simple follicles with a sinus containing blood located between the inner and outer layers of the dermal sheath. Sinus hairs generally occur on the muzzle, above the eyes, on lips, throat, and the palmar aspect of the carpus of cats. Sinus hairs function as mechanoreceptors (touch receptors). Tylotrich hairs also function as mechanoreceptors and are scattered among the regular body hairs.

The arrector pili muscles extend from the connective tissue sheath of the hair follicles and attach to the superficial dermis. Arrector pili smooth muscles are well developed on the back of animals, especially dogs. Muscle contraction causes erection of hairs and expression of the contents of sebaceous glands.

Sweat Glands

Apocrine glands (epitrichial glands), located throughout haired areas of skin in domestic animals, are tubular or saccular coiled glands lined by secretory cuboidal to low columnar epithelium surrounded by contractile myoepithelial cells. The ducts of the apocrine glands open in the superficial portion of the hair follicle. Apocrine gland activity is grossly visible in horses as they sweat after exercise or during high temperature, but in other domestic species apocrine gland secretion is rarely grossly visible. Other apocrine glands include the interdigital glands of small ruminants, glands of the external ear canal and eyelids of domestic animals, anal sac glands of dogs and cats, and the mental organ of pigs. Eccrine glands (atrichial glands) are merocrine in secretion and, in contrast to ducts of apocrine glands, the ducts open directly onto the surface of the epidermis. They are tubular glands lined by cuboidal epithelium surrounded by myoepithelium, are confined mainly to footpads of dogs and cats, frog region of ungulates, carpus of pigs, and nasolabial region of ruminants and pigs.

Sebaceous Glands

Sebaceous glands are simple, branched, or compound alveolar glands that undergo holocrine secretion, with ducts opening into hair follicles except at some mucocutaneous junctions where the glands open on the surface of the skin. Well-developed sebaceous glands are found in the supracaudal gland of dogs and cats; infraorbital, inguinal, and interdigital regions of sheep; the base of the horn of goats; the anal sac glands of cats; the preputial glands of horses; and the submental organ of cats.

Specialized Structures

Some specialized cutaneous structures such as the anal sacs are especially prone to develop lesions. These bilateral diverticula, located between internal and external sphincter muscles of the anus in dogs and cats, have ducts that open onto the anus at the level of the anocutaneous junction. Ducts and sacs are lined by stratified squamous epithelium; in cats, the sac wall has sebaceous and apocrine glands, but in dogs the wall has only apocrine glands.

Circumanal (hepatoid, perianal) glands occur most commonly near the anus and are also present in skin near the prepuce, tail, flank, and groin. These glands have nonpatent ducts and are composed of peripheral reserve cells that surround lobules of differentiated cells resembling hepatocytes, thus the synonym "hepatoid glands."

The claws shield the third phalanx and consist of a wall (dorsal and lateral sides) and sole (ventral side), both of which are stratified squamous keratinizing epithelium. The wall consists of hard keratin and the sole of softer keratin. The dermis of the claw consists of dense collagen, elastic tissue, and blood vessels that can bleed profusely if the claw is trimmed too short. The dermis is continuous with the ungual crest of the third phalanx and extends distally as the periosteum of the phalanx. The claw fold is a fold of skin that covers the wall laterally and dorsally for a short distance. Hooves consist of the wall, sole, and frog in solipeds; and a wall, sole, and prominent bulb in ruminants and pigs. The hoof wall comprises three structurally distinct layers (stratum externum, stratum medium, and stratum internum), which are formed by the proliferation and downward movement of epidermal cells arising from a specialized junction of the epidermis and dermis, a region known as the coronary band. The stratum internum interdigitates with the dermis anchoring the hoof to the dermis. In general, the deeper portion of the dermis blends with the periosteum of the third phalanx.

RESPONSE TO INJURY

Numerous endogenous and exogenous factors can potentialy cause significant cutaneous alterations (Fig. 11-3). Determining a definitive diagnosis depends on obtaining a complete history including age, breed, and sex of animal; conducting a thorough physical examination paying particular attention to the distribution of skin lesions; and performing additional diagnostic tests. Cutaneous biopsy samples are often indicated and, although the skin has a limited range of responses to injury, the distribution and types of inflammatory cells often represent a recognizable pattern that can be used to formulate a list of specific etiologic agents to be considered or suggest categories of disease with a common pathogenesis. Systems have been developed for the recognition of histopathologic patterns to facilitate diagnosis in veterinary dermatopathology (Table 11-1). Recognition of patterns, both clinically and histologically, may facilitate differential diagnoses (Table 11-2). Responses to injury are illustrated by changes in the epidermis, dermis, adnexa, and panniculus.

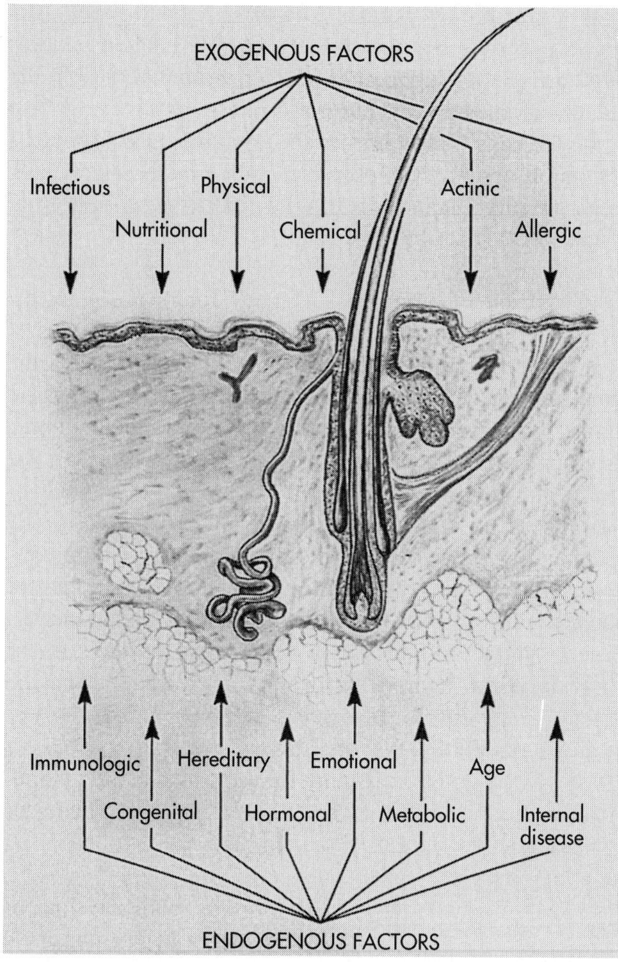

Figure 11-3 Skin diagram. A myriad of exogenous factors and endogenous factors influence the gross and microscopic appearance of the skin. Because the skin can respond to these factors in a limited number of ways, different skin disorders may have a similar appearance. Identification of the cause of a skin disorder therefore often requires not only histopathologic evaluation, but clinical history including clinical lesion distribution and appearance.

Epidermis

Alterations in Epidermal Growth or Differentiation

Basal cells, in their postmitotic state, migrate outward from the basal layer, eventually forming the cornified layers of the epidermis. In the normal epidermis, balance is established between the proliferation of the basal cells and the loss of differentiated cells from the surface, resulting in an epidermis of constant thickness. The orderly proliferation,

Table 11-1 Histopathologic Diagnosis by Use of Lesion Morphology (Pattern)*

Pattern	Brief Features	Few Examples
Diseases of the epidermis		
I. Pustular diseases	Superficial epidermal pustules	Impetigo, pemphigus foliaceus, superficial bacterial infection
II. Bullous and vesicular diseases	Vesicles/clefts in deep epidermis or dermal-epidermal junction	Pemphigus vulgaris, lupus erythematosus, bullous pemphigoid, epidermolysis bullosa, viral diseases
III. Necrotizing diseases	Individual keratinocyte necrosis or confluent necrosis	Burns, superficial necrolytic dermatopathy, erythema multiforme, toxic epidermal necrolysis
IV. Spongiotic diseases	Intercellular edema and vesicles	Allergic contact dermatitis, eosinophilic plaque
V. Exudative and ulcerative diseases	Erosion or ulceration with cell migration and crusts	Miliary dermatitis, indolent ulcer, pyotraumatic dermatitis
VI. Hyperplastic diseases	Proliferation of epidermis	Acral lick dermatitis, actinic dermatitis, acanthosis nigricans
VII. Hyperkeratotic diseases	Increase in epidermal and follicular keratin	Primary idiopathic seborrhea, ichthyosis, zinc-responsive dermatosis, ear margin seborrhea
Diseases of the dermis		
VIII. Perivascular diseases	Inflammation oriented around vessels	Hypersensitivity reactions, parasitic dermatosis
IX. Vascular diseases	Inflammation or degeneration of vessel walls	Immune-mediated vasculitis, septic vasculitis
X. Lichenoid and interface diseases	Lichenoid (dense band of inflammation parallel to epidermis that may obscure epidermal dermal junction) Interface (mild dermal inflammation oriented intimately with and often obscuring epidermal dermal interface and associated with vacuolar or apoptotic basal cells)	Mucocutaneous pyoderma, lupus erythematosus, uveodermatologic syndrome (VKH-like disease), idiopathic lichenoid dermatosis, lupoid onychodystrophy, epitheliotropic lymphoma
XI. Infectious nodular and diffuse diseases	Macrophages and neutrophils in granulomas or diffuse (with organisms)	Feline leprosy, blastomycosis, mycetoma, pythiosis, habronemiasis
XII. Noninfectious nodular and diffuse diseases	Macrophages and neutrophils in granulomas or diffuse (without organisms)	Foreign body reactions, histiocytosis, juvenile sterile granulomatous dermatitis and lymphadenitis
XIII. Nodular and diffuse diseases with eosinophils or plasma cells	Nodular and diffuse inflammation with eosinophils or plasma cells	Plasma cell pododermatitis, eosinophilic granuloma
XIV. Dysplastic or depositional diseases	Increased dermal substance or substance not normally found	Calcinosis cutis, calcinosis circumscripta, amyloidosis, mucinosis, collagen dysplasia
Diseases of adnexal appendages		
XV. Pustular and nodular diseases without follicular disruption	Variable inflammation in and around follicles and adnexa	Superficial bacterial folliculitis, dermatophytosis, sebaceous adenitis
XVI. Pustular and nodular diseases with follicular disruption	Severe inflammation in and around follicles and adnexa with disruption of follicles	Folliculitis and furunculosis, acne, callus pyoderma, deep bacterial pyoderma
XVII. Atrophic diseases of follicles	Hair cycle arrest with or without inflammation	Endocrine alopecia, telogen effluvium
XVIII. Dysplastic diseases of hair follicles	Abnormal growth or development of hair follicles	Color mutant alopecia, black hair follicular dysplasia
Diseases of the panniculus		
XIX. Diseases of the panniculus	Inflammation: lobular or septal or diffuse with variable types of cells	Post-rabies-vaccine alopecia, idiopathic sterile nodular panniculitis, feline pansteatitis

*Information for this table was adapted with permission from Gross TL, Ihrke PJ, Walder EJ. Veterinary dermatopathology: A macroscopic and microscopic evaluation of canine and feline skin diseases. St. Louis: Mosby–Year Book, 1992.

Table 11-2 Differential Diagnoses of Selected Patterns That Can Be Recognized Clinically as Well as Histologically*

Pattern	Pustules or Crusts	Vesicles or Bullae	Necrosis or Ulceration	Scaling or Other Hyperkeratotic Lesions	Nodules ± Draining Tracts	Alopecia
Disorders	Superficial bacterial infection Impetigo Pemphigus foliaceus and erythematosus Dermatophilosis Exudative epidermitis Subcorneal pustular dermatosis Footpads† Pemphigus foliaceus Superficial necrolytic dermatitis Lupus erythematosus	Pemphigus vulgaris Lupus erythematosus Bullous pemphigoid Epidermolysis bullosa Dermatomyositis Chemical and thermal burns Photosensitization Viral diseases Herpesvirus Poxvirus Calicivirus Picornavirus Rhabdovirus Drug reactions	Vasculitis with or without infarction Chemical and thermal burns Superficial necrolytic dermatitis Erythema multiforme Toxic epidermal necrolysis Ergot or fescue grass toxicity Frostbite Feline indolent ulcer Feline ulcerative dermatosis syndrome Ulcerative dermatosis of the collie and sheltie Self-trauma	Primary idiopathic seborrhea Ichthyosis Zinc-responsive dermatosis Sebaceous adenitis Ear margin seborrhea Vitamin A–responsive dermatosis Callus Cutaneous horn Actinic dermatitis Nasodigital hyperkeratosis Idiopathic canine distemper Familial digital hyperkeratosis Superficial necrolytic dermatitis	Masses caused by deep infections with bacteria, fungi, algae, pythium, migratory parasites (e.g., actinomycosis, feline leprosy, mycetoma, blastomycosis, pythiosis, habronemiasis) Sterile inflammatory lesions (e.g., foreign body reactions, histiocytosis, juvenile sterile granulomatous dermatitis and lymphadenitis, xanthogranuloma venomous bites) Panniculitis Neoplastic lesions	Follicular inflammation Infectious Noninfectious Postinflammatory and posttraumatic alopecia Endocrine alopecia Idiopathic flank alopecia Telogen effluvium Anagen defluxion Postclipping alopecia Follicular dysplasia Color mutant Black hair follicular Pattern alopecia of dachshund and other toy breeds Other congenital alopecias Feline psychogenic alopecia Poor nutrition with protein deficiency Feline paraneoplastic alopecia

*Some of these disorders could be placed in different patterns. For instance, disorders characterized by vesicles or bullae may develop into an ulcerative pattern after the vesicles or bullae rupture.
†Hyperkeratotic disorders may also affect footpads (e.g., canine distemper, idiopathic nasodigital hyperkeratosis, zinc responsive dermatosis).

differentiation, and cornification of epidermal cells is regulated by such factors as cytokines, vitamins, and minerals such as zinc and copper, fatty acids, and hormones. The regulatory cytokines are produced by a variety of cell types (endothelial cells, leukocytes, fibroblasts, and other cell types including keratinocytes). Keratinocytes thereby play a self-regulatory role, and inflammatory cells, among others, can influence keratinocyte growth and differentiation. Disorders of cornification may be primary such as in primary idiopathic seborrhea of the cocker spaniel or schnauzer comedone syndrome, but more often are secondary to a variety of factors such as inflammation, trauma, or metabolic or nutritional disorders.

Hyperkeratosis is an increase in the thickness of the stratum corneum and occurs in two forms. In orthokeratotic hyperkeratosis (also referred to as hyperkeratosis), the cells are anuclear, and in parakeratotic hyperkeratosis (also referred to as parakeratosis), the cells have nuclei. Subtypes of hyperkeratosis include basket weave, compact, and lamellar. Both parakeratosis and hyperkeratosis are common nonspecific responses to chronic stimuli (e.g., superficial trauma, inflammation), and also occur specifically in certain diseases. Hyperkeratosis is a feature of the primary cornification disorder of the cocker spaniel (Fig. 11-4), ichthyosis, and vitamin A deficiency. Diffuse parakeratosis is a feature of zinc-responsive dermatosis and superficial necrolytic dermatopathy (hepatocutaneous syndrome) (Fig. 11-5). Hyperkeratosis and parakeratosis may be accompanied by alterations in the thickness of the granular cell layer. Generally, hyperkeratosis is associated with an increased thickness of the granular cell layer (hypergranulosis), and parakeratosis is associated with a decreased thickness of the granular cell layer (hypogranulosis).

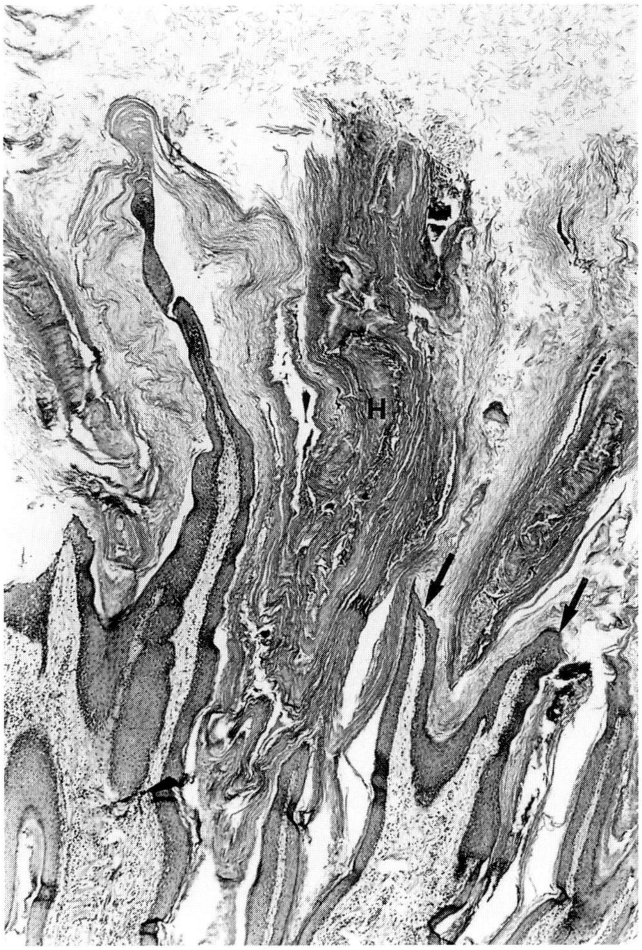

Figure 11-4 Skin, haired; dog. Idiopathic seborrhea. Note the marked orthokeratotic hyperkeratosis *(H)*. The keratin distends follicular openings *(arrows)* creating a papillomatous appearance in the epidermis. H & E stain.

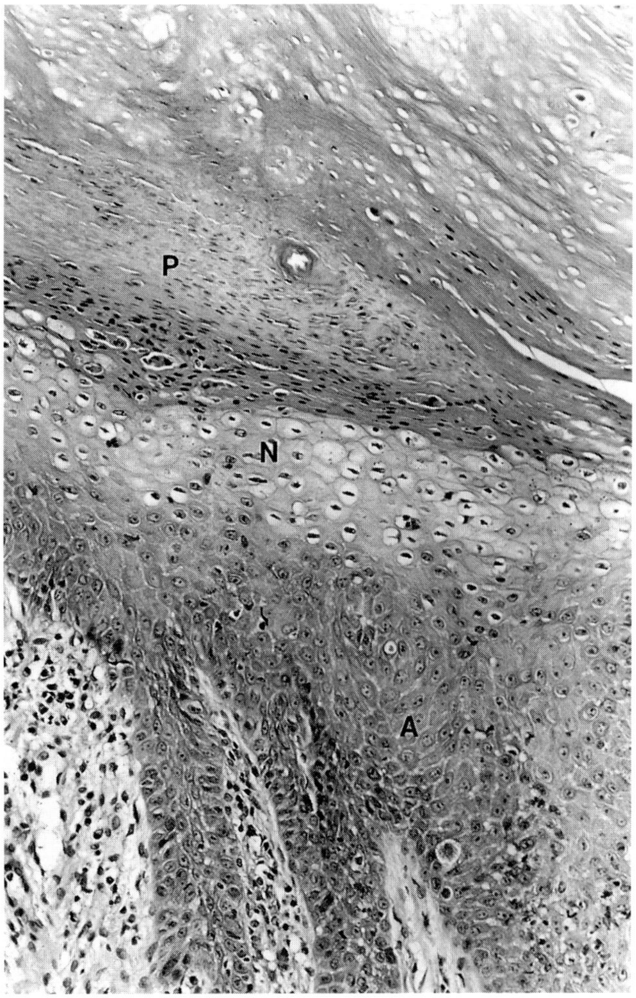

Figure 11-5 Skin; dog. Superficial necrolytic dermatitis. Nuclear retention is present in the stratum corneum (parakeratotic hyperkeratosis [parakeratosis]). The epidermis has a trilaminar pattern created by the parakeratotic zone *(P)*, subparakeratotic edema/necrolytic zone *(N)*, and acanthotic zone *(A)*. H & E stain.

Hyperplasia of the epidermis is an increase in the cells within the epidermis, most often within the stratum spinosum, and is referred to as **acanthosis.** Hyperplasia is a response common to a variety of chronic stimuli and occurs in a variety of types including, psoriasiform, papillated, and pseudocarcinomatous (pseudoepitheliomatous). In psoriasiform hyperplasia, the epidermis forms numerous ridges of uniform length and width that extend down into the dermis and give this type of hyperplasia a very regular or uniform histologic appearance. This type of hyperplasia is a feature of psoriasiform lichenoid dermatitis of the springer spaniel and porcine juvenile pustular psoriasiform dermatitis (pityriasis rosea). In papillated epidermal hyperplasia, the epidermis has fingerlike (papillary) projections above the skin surface. This hyperplasia is a feature of some papillomas, nevi, and calluses. Pseudocarcinomatous hyperplasia refers to marked hyperplasia of the epidermis, resulting in many branching and anastomosing epidermal ridges reaching down into the dermis. Mitotic figures may be numerous, but in contrast to squamous cell carcinoma, the keratinocytes maintain normal polarity, are not atypical, and are restricted to the confines of the basement membrane (Fig. 11-6). Pseudocarcinomatous hyperplasia is often seen in lesions such as in skin damaged by chronic actinic radiation before the development of squamous cell carcinoma or, at the edges of nonhealing ulcers.

Dyskeratosis refers to the premature keratinization of cells in the viable layers of the epidermis. Dyskeratotic keratinocytes are shrunken and separated from adjacent cells and have a pyknotic nucleus and brightly eosinophilic cytoplasm due to the accumulation of keratin filaments. Dyskeratosis occurs when epidermal maturation is deranged such as in zinc-responsive dermatosis. Dyskeratosis is also a feature of epidermal dysplasia seen as a premalignant change in the development of a squamous cell carcinoma.

Apoptosis refers to programmed cell death. Apoptotic keratinocytes have morphologic features similar to dyskeratotic cells. In apoptosis the eosinophilia is due to cytoplasmic organelle condensation. Apoptotic cells are phagocytosed by adjacent keratinocytes. Phagocytosis before cellular disintegration prevents the development of an acute inflammatory response that would be elicited by the liberated cellular constituents. Thus, the process of apoptosis is significantly different from necrosis, in which cell lysis occurs releasing cellular contents into the extracellular space. Apoptosis is seen with diseases such as lupus erythematosus and erythema multiforme (Fig. 11-7).

Necrosis refers to death of cells and is characterized by nuclear pyknosis, karyorrhexis, or karyolysis, organelle swelling, plasma membrane rupture, and release of cytoplasmic elements into the extracellular space accompanied by acute inflammatory response. Causes of epidermal necrosis include physical injury (lacerations,

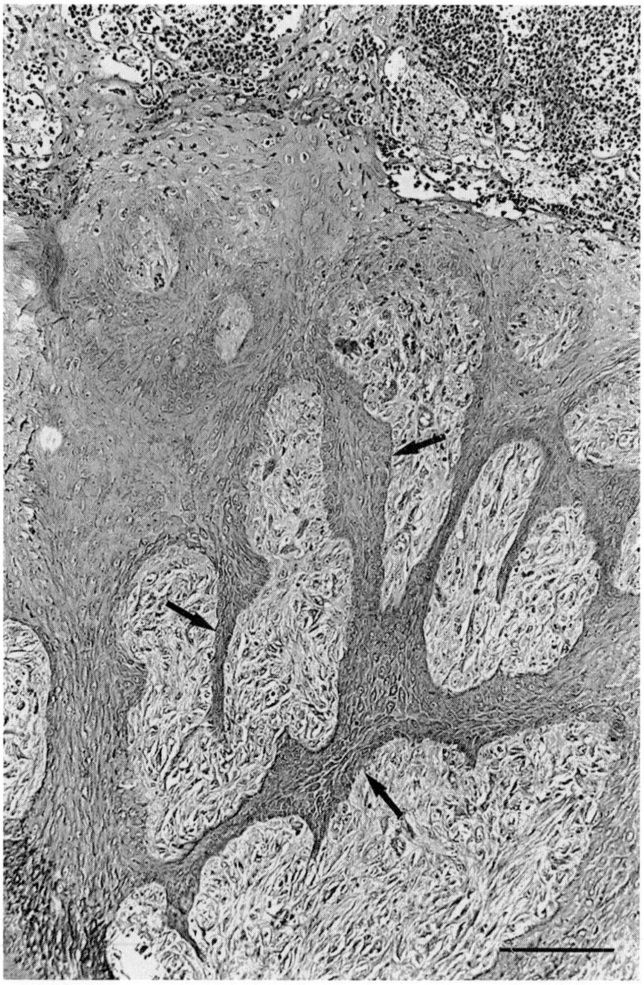

Figure 11-6 Skin, penile sheath; bovine. Fibropapilloma. Epidermal hyperplasia consisting of acanthosis and pseudocarcinomatous hyperplasia *(arrows)*. Pseudocarcinomatous hyperplasia refers to marked hyperplasia of the epidermis resulting in branching and anastomosing epidermal ridges reaching down into the dermis. The keratinocytes do not invade through the basement membrane. H & E stain. Bar = 100 μm.

thermal burns), chemical injury (irritant contact dermatitis), and ischemic injury (vasculitis, thromboembolism).

Atrophy is a decrease in the number and size of the cells within the epidermis and occurs as a consequence of sublethal cell injury. Cutaneous atrophy occurs in response to hormonal imbalances such as hyperadrenocorticism in dogs and cats, partial ischemia, and severe malnutrition.

Alterations in Epidermal Cell Adhesion

Edema may occur intercellularly or intracellularly. Intercellular edema is called spongiosis because, as the intercellular spaces widen with fluid, the epidermis develops a "spongy" appearance. Severe intercellular edema results in the formation of spongiotic vesicles and is common in inflammatory dermatoses. Intracellular

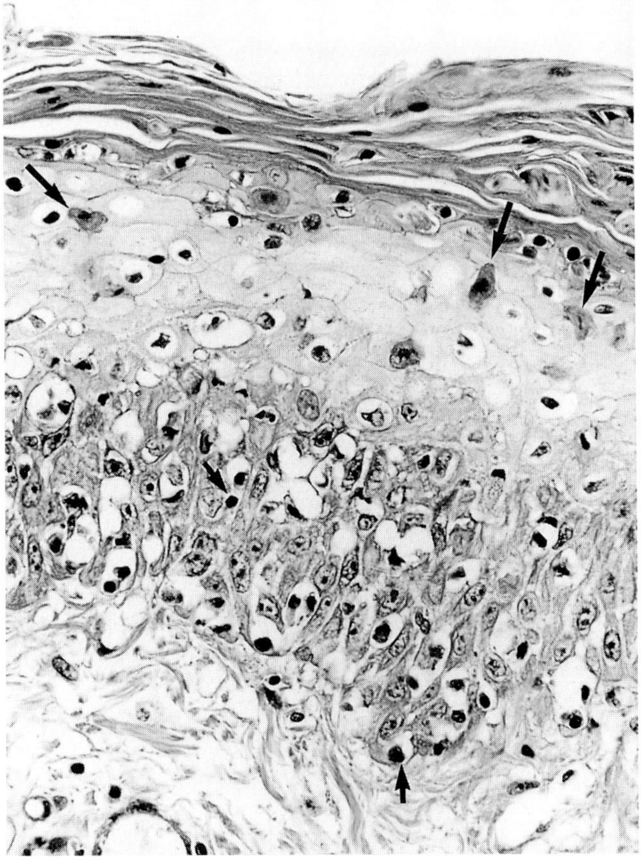

Figure 11-7 Skin; dog. Erythema multiforme. Apoptotic keratinocytes *(long arrows)* and lymphocytes *(short arrows)* are present in the epidermis. The increased staining density of apoptotic keratinocytes is due to cytoplasmic organelle condensation. H & E stain.

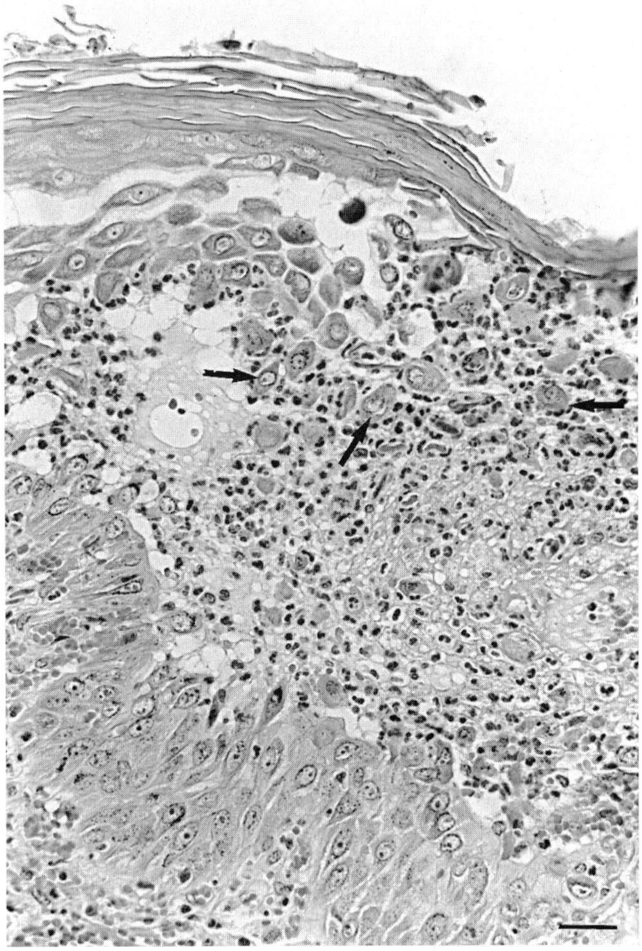

Figure 11-8 Skin; horse. Pemphigus foliaceus. The subcorneal pustule contains acantholytic cells *(arrows)*, epidermal cells separated from each other due to the breakdown of intercellular bridges. The roof of the pustule is formed by the stratum corneum, and the base of the pustule is formed by the stratum spinosum. Clipping or scrubbing the surface of the pustule can lead to rupture and make the sample nondiagnostic. H & E stain. Bar = 25 μm.

edema results in cellular swelling, and if the swelling is severe, the swollen cells may burst, forming microvesicles supported by the cell walls of the ruptured cells. This type of epidermal damage is termed "reticular degeneration." Intracellular edema limited to the basal layer of the epidermis is termed hydropic or vacuolar degeneration and may result in the formation of intrabasilar vesicles. **Hydropic degeneration** is a consequence of damage to basal keratinocytes where the basal keratinocytes cannot maintain normal homeostasis and fluid accumulates within the cells. Examples of diseases commonly resulting in hydropic degeneration include lupus erythematosus, dermatomyositis, and drug eruptions. **Ballooning degeneration,** a form of intracellular edema of cells in more superficial layers of the epidermis, is characterized by swollen cells losing their intercellular attachments and the possible formation of a vesicle. Viruses that infect the epidermis, such as the pox viruses, cause lysis of cytoplasmic keratin and a buildup of excessive fluid resulting in ballooning degeneration.

Acantholysis refers to the loss of cohesion between keratinocytes due to the breakdown of intercellular bridges via immune destruction such as in pemphigus (type II cytotoxic hypersensitivity) or due to neutrophilic enzymatic destruction as seen in superficial pyoderma. The microscopic lesions vary with the location of acantholysis. In pemphigus foliaceus, acantholysis occurs in the subcorneal epidermis, resulting in release of free-floating keratinocytes in subcorneal vesicles and pustules (Fig. 11-8). In pemphigus vulgaris, acantholysis occurs in the epidermis, just above the basal layer, resulting in the separation of the upper epidermis from the basal cells (often referred to as a row of tombstones) attached to the basal lamina (Fig. 11-9). Fluid accumulating between the separated layers forms a vesicle.

Vesicles are fluid-filled cavities within or beneath the epidermis (Fig. 11-10). Vesicles are generally 5 mm or smaller, and **bullae** are greater than 5 mm. These lesions develop in any layer of the epidermis or beneath the epidermis. Vesicles may form through acantholysis, epidermal or dermal edema, degeneration of basal cells and keratinocytes, or other processes such as frictional trauma and burns that cause a lack of cohesion between the epidermal cells or between the epidermis and dermis, resulting in the accumulation of fluid within a cavity. The level of vesicles or bullae formation within the epidermis is suggestive of certain diseases. For instance, intraepidermal vesicles may occur in viral infections, suprabasilar vesicles in pemphigus vulgaris (see Fig. 11-9), intrabasilar vesicles in lupus erythematosus, and subepidermal vesicles in bullous pemphigoid or thermal burns.

Inflammatory Lesions of the Epidermis

Exocytosis is the migration of leukocytes into the epidermis. Exocytosis of leukocytes is common in inflammation and is usually accompanied by spongiosis (intercellular edema). The type of leukocyte in the epidermis is influenced by complex interactions of cytokines and may indicate the disease process present. For instance, eosinophils may be numerous in ectoparasitism. Lymphocytic infiltrates into the epidermis are often seen with immune-mediated diseases such as lupus erythematosus. Malignant lymphoma affecting the skin may also be characterized by intraepidermal lymphocytes. Erythrocytes may also be present in the epidermis, usually associated with trauma, circulatory disturbances such as marked vasodilation, and vasculitis.

Pustules (microabscesses) are vesicles filled with inflammatory cells (see Fig. 11-8) and vary in inflammatory cell content and location in the epidermis. The pustules of superficial bacterial infections generally contain degenerate neutrophils and coccoid bacteria and are often located beneath the stratum corneum (subcor-

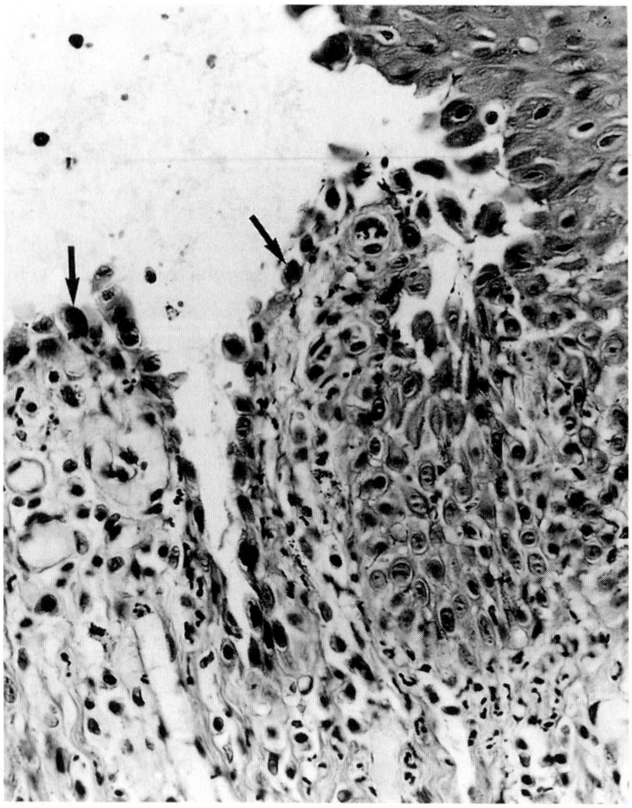

Figure 11-9 Skin; dog. Pemphigus vulgaris. Suprabasilar clefting has left a row of basal cells *(arrows)* attached to the dermis. The single row of basal cells is fragile and easily damaged and can lead to formation of ulcers, with subsequent fluid loss and secondary bacterial infection. H & E stain.

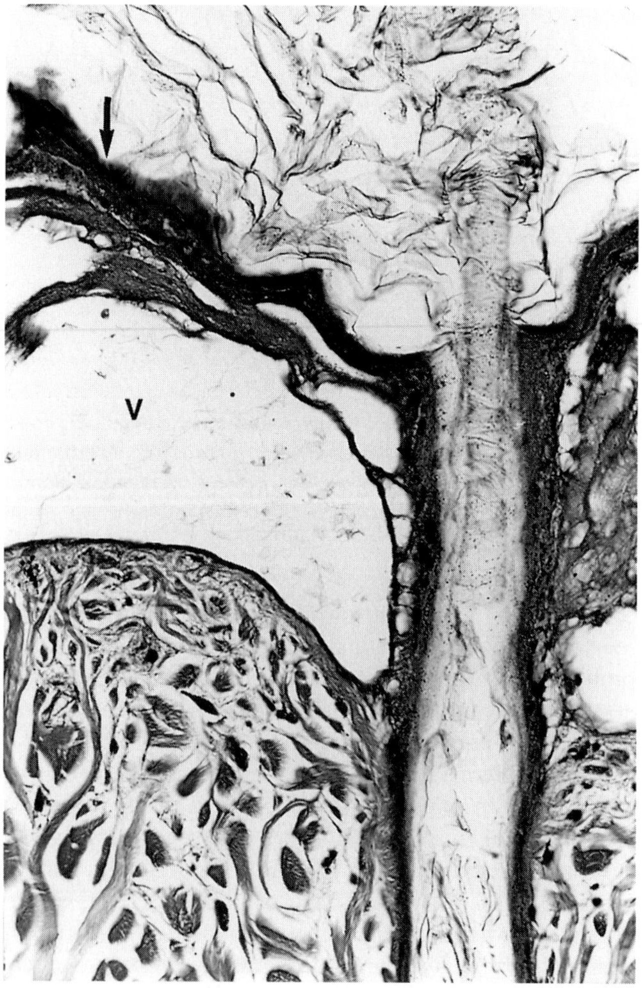

Figure 11-10 Skin, haired; dog. Thermal burn. There is necrosis of epidermis *(arrow)* and follicular epithelium. Fluid from increased capillary permeability has accumulated between the dermis and necrotic epidermis forming a vesicle *(V)*. H & E stain.

neal). In ectoparasitic hypersensitivity, pemphigus foliaceus, and feline eosinophilic plaque, the pustules may be filled with eosinophils. Vesicles containing neoplastic lymphocytes are found in epitheliotropic lymphoma.

Crusts, dried exudate on the epidermal surface, are indicative of a previous exudative process. Crusts are not specifically diagnostic but may hold the key to diagnosis in some diseases. For example, in dermatophilosis, the most diagnostic portion of the skin is the crust, which is multilaminated and contains the gram-positive, branching, and coccoid organism, *Dermatophilus congolensis.* Similarly, crusts formed through aging of pustules in pemphigus foliaceus are multilaminated and, frequently, contain numerous acantholytic cells. Crusts may also contain hair shafts infected with spores and hyphae of dermatophytes.

Alterations in Epidermal Pigmentation

Pigmentary alterations include hyperpigmentation, hypopigmentation, and pigmentary incontinence. Melanin is produced by melanocytes located in the stratum basale of the epidermis, the external root sheath and hair matrix of follicles, and, perivascularly, in the dermis. Melanocytes have surface receptors for hormones, such as melanocyte-stimulating hormone, and these hormones regulate melanogenesis. Other factors that influence the amount of melanin pigment in skin and hair are genes, age, temperature, and inflammation.

Hyperpigmentation results from an increased production of melanin from existing melanocytes or an increase in the number of melanocytes. Most hyperpigmentation of the epidermis results from increased production of melanin from existing melanocytes; possible mechanisms include increases in rate of production of melanosomes, in melanosome size, in melanosome transfer to keratinocytes, and increased survival of melanosomes in keratinocytes. Examples of epidermal hyperpigmentation by increased production of melanin include chronic inflammatory diseases and some of the endocrine dermatoses. An example of hyperpigmentation due to increased number of melanocytes is a lentigo, a rare localized nonneoplastic proliferation of melanocytes confined to the epidermis and resulting in formation of a black macular circumscribed lesion that is usually less than 1 cm in diameter.

Hypopigmentation may be congenital or hereditary and develops because of a lack of melanocytes, failure of melanocytes to produce melanin, or failure of transfer of melanin to epidermal cells. Hypopigmentation may also be acquired via a loss of existing melanin or melanocytes (depigmentation). Because copper is a component of tyrosinase, production of melanin pigment is dependent on copper, and copper deficiency may result in reduced pigmentation. **Pigmentary incontinence** refers to the loss of melanin pigment from the basal layer of the epidermis due to damage to the cells of the basal layer and the accumulation of the pigment in macrophages in the upper dermis. Pigmentary incontinence may be a nonspecific lesion associated with inflammation; however, it is also seen with diseases that specifically damage the stratum basale such as lupus erythematosus. Leukotrichia (Fig. 11-11) and leukoderma refer to decreased pigmentation of hair and skin, respectively.

Dermis

Alterations in Growth or Development

Atrophy, a decrease in the quantity of collagen fibrils and fibroblasts, results in a decrease in the thickness of the dermis noted clinically by thin, translucent skin with more visible vasculature. The principal causes of atrophy are catabolic diseases associated with protein degradation, such as hyperadrenocorticism in dogs and cats, and starvation. In cats with hyperadrenocorticism, collagen loss is sufficient to increase fragility of the skin, which tears with normal handling.

Fibroplasia develops in response to various injuries, particularly ulceration. It consists of proliferation of fibroblasts and newly formed collagen fibrils which, in granulation tissue, are parallel to the surface of the skin and oriented perpendicular to proliferating vessels, histologically providing a "lattice-work" appearance to the proliferative tissue. Grossly, the small capillary buds seen on the surface produce a "granular" appearance, thus the name "granulation tissue." Fibrosis refers to the gradual deposition and maturation of collagen to form a scar. During fibrosis, the collagen production increases and the fibroblasts and vessels decrease resulting in less cellular, dense collagen bundles (e.g., a scar), which grossly appears white and glistening.

Collagen dysplasia is generally an inherited abnormality of collagen resulting in decreased tensile strength and increased stretchability. The skin tears with minor trauma

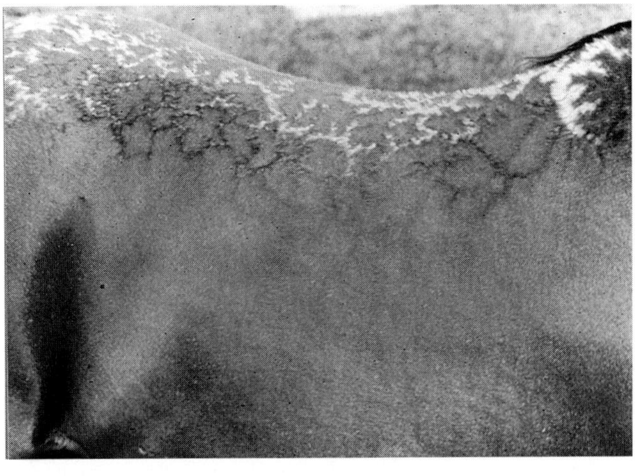

Figure 11-11 Skin; horse. Leukotrichia (depigmentation of hair shafts). Leukotrichia is best evaluated grossly. This horse has acquired leukotrichia in a reticulated pattern over the dorsum of the trunk. Histologically, the white hair shafts are devoid of melanin pigment. *Courtesy of Dr. H. Power.*

Dermatosporaxis
Dog – collagen packing defect
Cat – collagen packing defect
– procollagen peptidase def. – Himalayan
Cattle – amino terminal procollagen peptidase def.

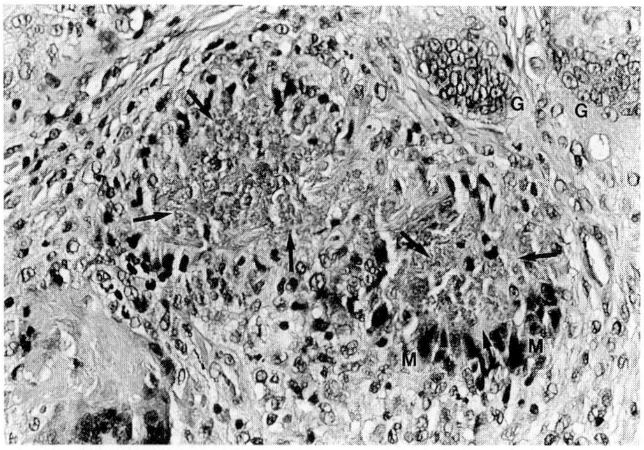

Figure 11-12 Skin; cat. Eosinophilic granuloma. Fragmented collagen *(arrows)* is bordered by a row of macrophages *(M)*, multinucleated giant cells *(G)*, and degranulated eosinophils (eosinophilic and granulomatous inflammation). H & E stain.

and heals by formation of scars. Microscopic features vary among the collagen dysplasia disorders, and in some cases the skin has no microscopic alterations. Collagen bundles may vary in size and shape and consist of tangled fibers with an abnormal organizational pattern.

Solar elastosis is caused by chronic exposure of the skin to the ultraviolet light rays of sunlight. Solar elastosis, most prominent in the horse, consists of increased numbers of thick, interwoven, basophilic fibers in the dermis of sun-damaged areas. In human beings, it has been shown that the altered elastic tissue is newly formed as a result of altered function of fibroblasts, not a degeneration product of preexisting elastic fibers.

Degenerative Disorders of the Dermis

Collagen degeneration, characterized by increased granularity and eosinophilic staining intensity, develops in disorders associated with infiltrates of eosinophils and subsequent eosinophil degranulation, such as reactions to insect bites, mast cell tumors, and eosinophilic granulomas (collagenolytic granulomas) (Fig. 11-12).

Collagen lysis is dissolution of collagen fibrils and develops subsequent to ischemia and in microbial and parasitic infections.

Disorders Characterized by Deposits in the Dermis

Amyloid is a protein that may be deposited in the dermis either as a primary event of unknown cause or secondary to chronic infections, tissue destruction, or plasma cell neoplasms. Microscopically, amyloid, consists of amorphous eosinophilic material.

Mucin, a normal component of the ground substance of the dermis, consists of protein bound to hyaluronic acid and may be deposited in increased quantity in focal areas or diffusely. Because hyaluronic acid has a great affinity for binding water, the skin in cases of **mucinosis** has a thick, puffy appearance. In cases of severe mucinosis, the skin, when pricked with a needle, may exude mucin (a stringy fluid material). In histologic sections, much of the water is lost and mucin appears as fine amphophilic granules or fibrils that separate dermal collagen. Examples of disorders with dermal mucin deposition are termed myxedema in hypothyroidism and mucinosis in the Chinese Shar Pei dog.

Calcium deposits in the dermis may be due to alteration in dermal collagen (dystrophic calcification). They may also develop in association with abnormal metabolism of calcium, phosphorus, and vitamin D (metastatic calcification) or for unknown reasons (idiopathic calcification). Calcification may involve individual or groups of collagen fibers resulting in increased basophilia in stained sections and fragmentation of the fibers during sectioning. Calcium may also be deposited as amorphous nodular aggregates. Calcium deposits elicit a granulomatous inflammatory response, a foreign body reaction to the deposits.

Inflammatory Disorders of the Dermis

Dermatitis, inflammation of the dermis, begins with hyperemia, edema, and migration of leukocytes. The inflammatory response to different stimuli can be quite similar. However, the distribution and types of leukocytes often evolve into recognizable patterns that suggest a pathogenesis. Patterns include perivascular (Fig. 11-13), interface (mild inflammation affecting the basilar epidermis and superficial dermis that often obscures the epidermal dermal interface), nodular, or diffuse. The types of cells in the inflammatory infiltrate also vary. Perivascular and eosinophilic dermatitis is suggestive of hypersensitivity; interface and lymphocytic dermatitis is suggestive of lupus erythematosus; and nodular and granulomatous dermatitis indicate a prolonged cell-mediated response often associated with persistent infection with acid-fast bacteria or fungi. Thus, patterns of inflammation and cellular composition of infiltrates are useful in microscopic diagnosis.

Adnexa

Adnexa refers to appendages or adjunct parts, which in the skin includes hair follicles and glands.

Alterations in Growth and Development of Adnexa

Atrophy refers to gradual reduction (involution) in size and may be physiologic or pathologic. Physiologic atrophy is related to the normal cyclic changes of the hair follicle. Pathologic atrophy is greater than that expected for a given stage of the hair cycle. Causes include hormonal abnormalities, nutritional abnormalities, inadequacy of blood supply, inflammation, and general state of health including stressful events or systemic illness. Some types of pathologic atrophy can be reversed when the underlying cause is corrected. Damage to germinal epithelium can

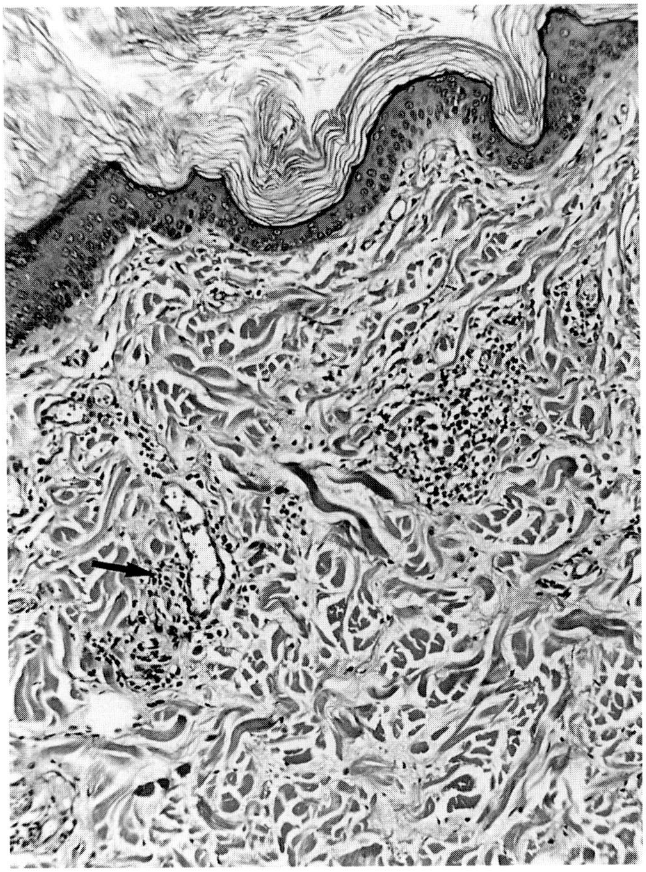

Figure 11-13 Skin; dog. Perivascular inflammation. Vessels of superficial dermis are dilated and are bordered by leukocytes that have migrated through vessel walls into the surrounding perivascular dermis *(arrow)*. H & E stain.

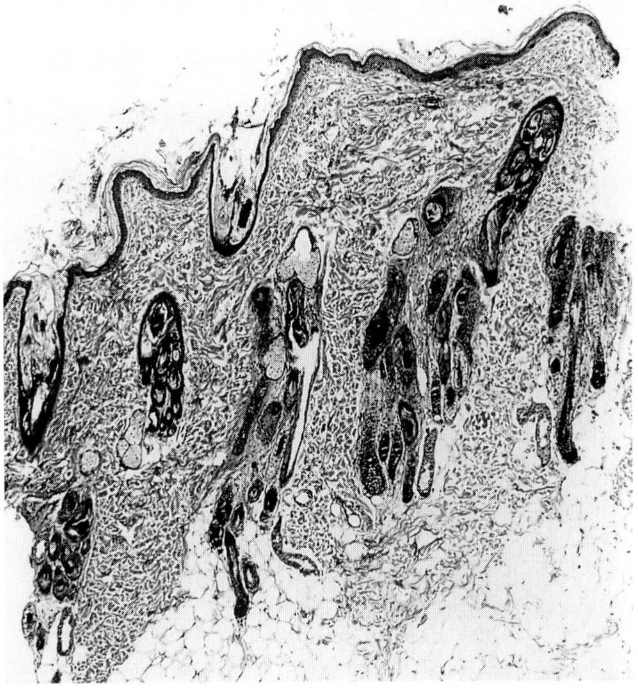

Figure 11-14 Skin, haired; dog. Black hair follicular dysplasia. The follicles are irregular (wavy) and distorted. H & E stain.

result in destruction or total loss of the adnexa with replacement by a scar. Examples include severe inflammation, thermal burns, thrombosis causing infarction, and severe physical trauma.

Hypertrophy is an increase in the unit size of a structure or an individual cell. Follicular hypertrophy, follicles that are longer and wider than normal for the site, occurs secondary to repeated surface trauma in acral lick dermatitis. **Hyperplasia** is an increase in the number of cells in a structure. Enlargement of adnexa, a common response to injury, usually involves both hypertrophy and hyperplasia, and is observed in sebaceous and apocrine gland hyperplasia associated with chronic allergic dermatitis.

Follicular dysplasia refers to incomplete or abnormal development of follicles and hair shafts. Different types of follicular dysplasia are described, but most are poorly characterized. Microscopic features vary, but include an abnormally formed follicle, which produces an abnormal hair shaft, resulting clinically in a reduced or absent hair coat. The follicular dysplasia conditions that are the most easily recognized microscopically are color associated, and include color mutant alopecia and black hair follicular dysplasia (see Fig. 11-14) where melanin pigment abnormalities serve as a marker for the dysplasia.

Inflammatory Disorders of the Adnexa, Vessels, and Panniculus

Folliculitis is inflammation of a hair follicle. Folliculitis can be subdivided histologically according to the anatomic segment of the hair follicle affected and the types of leukocytes present. These two histologic features of folliculitis can be used to determine a more specific cause of the follicular inflammation. The major subclassifications of folliculitis include perifolliculitis, mural folliculitis, bulbitis, and luminal folliculitis. **Perifolliculitis** refers to inflammation around, but not involving, the hair follicle. Leukocytes arrive via the perifollicular vessels. Perifolliculitis is not specific for any category of disease and may precede or coincide with other types of folliculitis. **Mural folliculitis** refers to inflammation limited to the wall of the follicle. The leukocytes migrate from perifollicular vessels into the follicular wall. Mural folliculitis is further characterized by the types of leukocytes present. For example, necrotizing eosinophilic mural folliculitis is

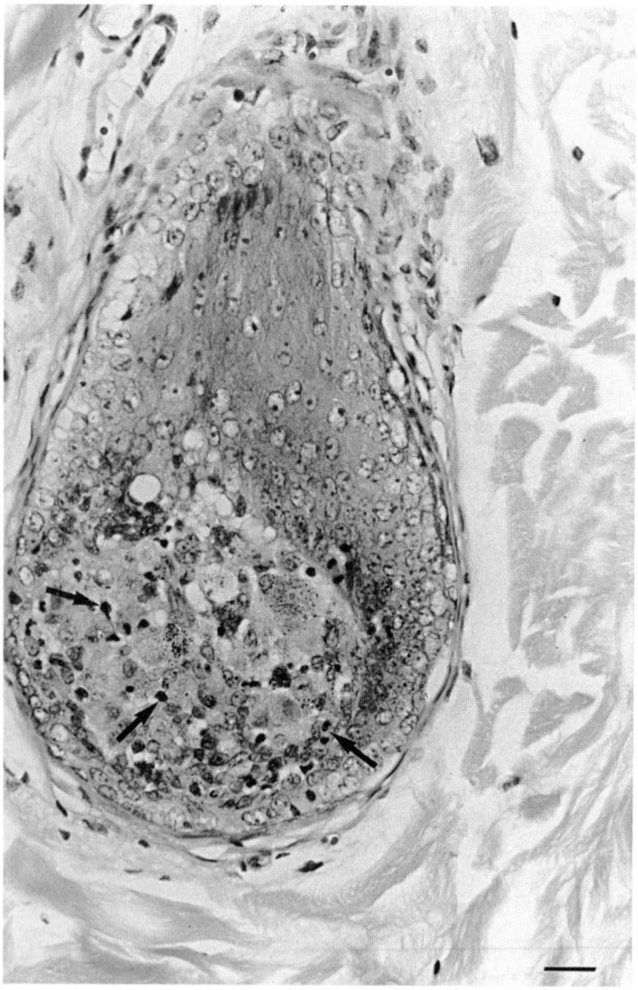

Figure 11-15 Skin, haired; horse. Alopecia areata. This anagen hair has an intrabulbar infiltrate primarily composed of lymphocytes *(arrows)* and fewer granulocytes. H & E stain. Bar = 25 μm.

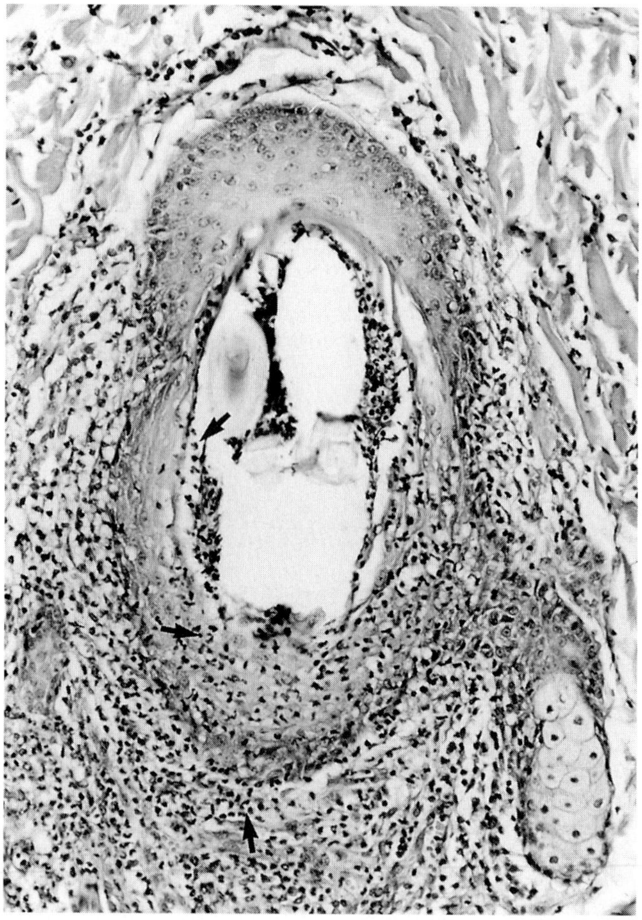

Figure 11-16 Skin, haired; dog. Luminal folliculitis. Neutrophils *(arrows)* are present in the follicular lumen and wall, and perifollicular dermis. H & E stain.

often seen in mosquito bite hypersensitivity in the cat and *Culicoides* hypersensitivity in the horse. **Bulbitis** refers to inflammation directed at the deepest portion of the hair follicle, the bulb. Alopecia areata is a specific example of bulbitis occurring in horses, dogs, and cats, and is characterized by lymphocytic infiltrates of the bulb of anagen hairs (Fig. 11-15) resulting in alopecia. In dogs, antifollicular cell-mediated and humoral immunologic responses have been documented in alopecia areata. The damage to hair matrix cells within the hair bulb results in formation of dystrophic (abnormal) hair shafts. **Luminal folliculitis** refers to inflammation involving the lumen and usually the wall of hair follicles (Fig. 11-16) and is most often indicative of parasites *(Demodex, Pelodera),* bacteria (staphylococci), or dermatophytes *(Microsporum, Trichophyton).* Luminal folliculitis can weaken the follicular wall leading to rupture, known as furunculosis (Fig. 11-17), and exposure of follicular contents to the components of the dermis. The presence of hair fragments, keratin, sebum, and possible infectious agents in the dermis leads to a suppurative inflammatory response that progresses to more long-standing pyogranulomatous and scarring inflammation. Perifolliculitis, luminal folliculitis, and furunculosis often follow in sequence. The inflammation may resolve with appropriate treatment or extend into the deep dermis and panniculus and form sinuses that drain to the surface and are difficult to resolve. Severe inflammation can lead to complete destruction of adnexal units and replacement by scar tissue.

Sebaceous adenitis is a specific inflammatory reaction targeting sebaceous glands; it occurs in dogs (Fig. 11-18) and rarely cats. Early lesions are characterized by accumulations of lymphocytes around sebaceous ducts. Fully developed lesions consist of lymphocytes, neutrophils, and macrophages that replace sebaceous glands. Chronic lesions have total loss of sebaceous glands,

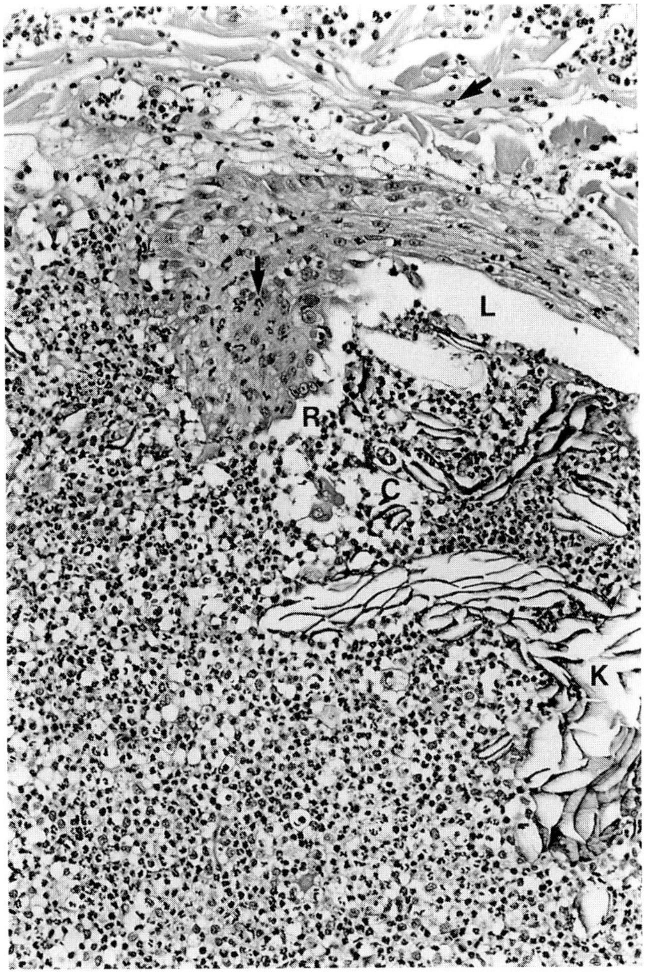

Figure 11-17 Skin, haired; dog. Folliculitis and furunculosis. Note rupture *(R)* in the follicular wall, inflammatory cells *(C)*, and keratin *(K)* in the follicular lumen *(L)*, and neutrophils *(arrows)* in the follicular wall and perifollicular dermis. H & E stain.

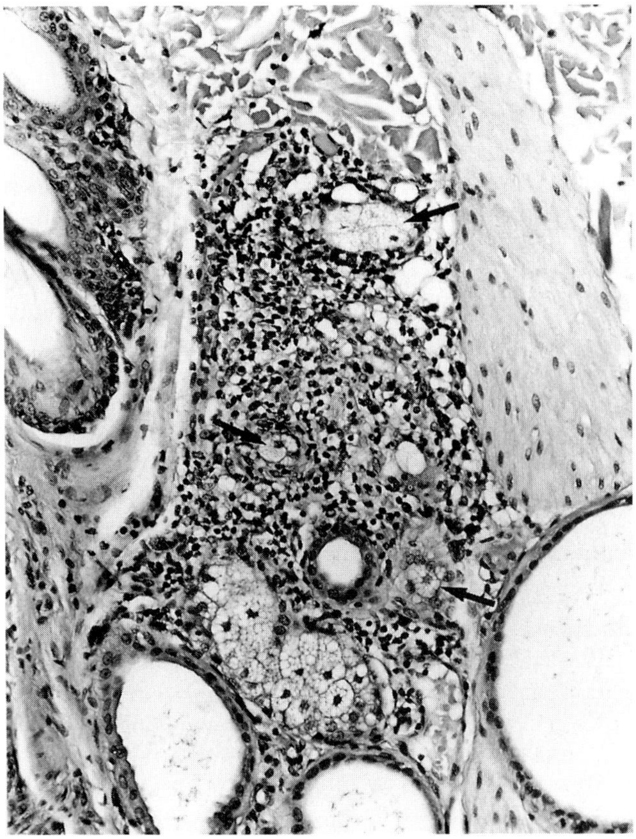

Figure 11-18 Skin, haired; dog. Sebaceous adenitis. Inflammation is beginning to efface the sebaceous glands. A few clusters of sebaceous gland cells *(arrows)* are visible within the area of inflammation. H & E stain.

scarring, and epidermal and follicular hyperkeratosis. Sebaceous gland inflammation may occur secondary to folliculitis, demodicosis, uveodermatologic syndrome, or leishmaniasis.

Hidradenitis, inflammation of apocrine glands, is seen in suppurative and granulomatous inflammation.

Vasculitis, inflammation of vessels where the vessels are the primary target of injury, may be the result of infectious agents, immunologic injury, toxins, disseminated intravascular coagulation, or may be idiopathic. The species most commonly presenting with vasculitis are the horse and the dog. Most cases are idiopathic in that a specific cause cannot be determined. Histologic lesions include damage to the vessel wall such as the presence of few necrotic cells or foci of fibrinoid necrosis, mural infiltrates of leukocytes, and intramural or perivascular edema, hemorrhage, or fibrin exudation. Vascular injury leads to the clinical lesions of edema and hemorrhage, and if severe, may include ischemic necrosis and infarction. Ulceration with or without sloughing of the skin and distal extremities may occur. Classic examples include immune complex deposition in vessel walls (systemic lupus erythematosus), infection with an endotheliotropic organism *(Rickettsia rickettsii),* and septicemia with bacterial embolism in pigs *(Erysipelothrix rhusiopathiae).*

Panniculitis, inflammation targeting the subcutaneous adipose tissue, can be caused by infectious agents (bacteria, fungi), immune-mediated disorders (systemic lupus erythematosus), physical injury (trauma, injection of irritant material, foreign bodies), nutritional disorders (vitamin E deficiency), pancreatic disease (pancreatitis, pancreatic carcinoma), or may be of undetermined cause (idiopathic). Panniculitis may be primary or secondary. In primary panniculitis, the subcutaneous adipose tissue is the target of the disease process. An example of primary panniculitis reported in cats is pansteatitis, which occurs in animals fed diets high in polyunsaturated fats and low in antioxidants such as vitamin E. Lack of vitamin E leads to oxidation of lipids of the subcutaneous adipose tissue inciting a pyogranulomatous inflammatory response. In secondary panniculitis, the subcutis is affected by a process primarily involving the contiguous dermis that extends down into the subcutis. A deep bacterial folliculitis with furunculosis can lead to a secondary panniculitis. Clinically, cases of panniculitis present with palpable nodules that may ulcerate and drain an oily material. Lesions are most often on the trunk and proximal limbs and may be solitary or multifocal. Solitary lesions may be cured by excision, whereas multiple lesions may resolve with specific therapy or result in scar formation. Microscopically, inflammation may be concentrated in the fat lobules (lobular panniculitis), interlobular septa (septal panniculitis), or involve both areas.

Pathologic Reactions of the Entire Cutaneous Unit

Responses of the skin to injury often involve multiple cutaneous components. Lesions evolve through different stages, and some lesions may resolve. Therefore, biopsy samples taken from multiple areas of a lesion often have different stages of inflammation involving multiple components and creating different reaction patterns. Interpretation of a biopsy sample may not lead to a specific diagnosis; however, the pattern of changes often suggests categories of disease (Table 11-2). The reactions of the various components of the skin can be illustrated by a poxvirus infection. When a poxvirus invades the epidermis, the virus replicates in the cells of the stratum spinosum and causes cytoplasmic swelling (ballooning degeneration) and rupture (reticular degeneration) of some of the epidermal cells. Cytoplasmic viral inclusions form in some cells. Cellular constituents released from damaged epidermal cells are chemotactic for leukocytes. The chemotactic factors increase blood flow to the site of viral invasion by dilation of vessels, cause margination of leukocytes along dermal vessel walls, and increase vascular permeability (dermal edema), causing formation of erythematous macular lesions. Chemotactic factors also cause migration of leukocytes out of the vessels into tissues. Initially, a perivascular dermatitis consists of lymphocytes and a variable number of neutrophils. The early epidermal degeneration, dermal edema, and inflammation form papular lesions. Ballooning and reticular degeneration of keratinocytes progress and result in the formation of intraepidermal vesicles. Leukocytes in perivascular sites under the influence of inflammatory mediators from the epidermis migrate to the epidermis, and leukocytes enter the vesicle to form pustules. Some poxviruses also cause epidermal hyperplasia by stimulating host cell DNA synthesis, presumably by a viral gene product similar to epidermal growth factor, resulting in pseudoepitheliomatous hyperplasia. The pustule enlarges and eventually ruptures, releasing the exudate onto the skin surface; the exudate dries and forms a crust (scab). The primary lesions of vesicles and pustules are fragile and often transient, lasting only hours, and so are difficult to identify and biopsy. The secondary lesions of crusting and scarring are longer standing. In this way, multiple components of the skin participate in the development and resolution of the lesions and are responsible for the clinical stages of macule, papule, vesicle, pustule, crust, and scar.

BIOPSY TECHNIQUE

Biopsy Site Selection

Multiple cutaneous sites representative of the range of lesions should be selected for biopsy. Fully developed nontreated primary lesions such as macules, papules, pustules, nodules, neoplasms, vesicles, and wheals are often the most useful for diagnosis. However, primary lesions may not be present; secondary lesions (scales, crusts, ulcers, comedones, fissures, excoriations, lichenification, pigmentary abnormalities, and scars) then need to be sampled and evaluated. These secondary lesions may be diagnostic or contribute substantially to the diagnosis when multiple cutaneous sites are selected for biopsy. One of the most useful secondary lesions is the crust, because acantholytic cells from drying pustules in pemphigus foliaceus and organisms such as *Dermatophilus congolensis* or dermatophytes may be identified in crusts. Also, the margin of a chronic ulcer may represent a squamous cell carcinoma, or the scale at the edge of an epidermal collarette (peripheral expanding ring of scaling) may represent superficial spreading pyoderma.

Biopsy Technique

Excisional biopsy samples (entire lesions) are recommended for large pustules or vesicles that may be damaged by use of a smaller punch biopsy instrument. Deeper excisional biopsy samples are generally necessary for diagnosis of lesions, such as panniculitis, that are deep to the skin. Digital amputation may be required, particularly in dogs for the diagnosis of nail bed lesions. Electrocautery should not be used for small biopsy samples as the samples are damaged and rendered nondiagnostic. Tissue forceps should grasp, if at all, only one nonaffected margin, preferably in the subcutis.

Biopsy Site Preparation

Generally, the skin at a punch biopsy site should not be surgically prepared because the procedure may remove the diagnostic portion of the sample (see Fig. 11-8). Gentle clipping of hair is acceptable. For an excisional biopsy of lesions deep to the epidermis, surgical preparation of the skin is acceptable.

Fixation

Punch biopsy specimens should be placed in 10 times the volume of 10% neutral buffered formalin (NBF). To avoid warping in the fixative, thin excisional biopsy specimens should be gently attached to a flat object, such as a piece of tongue depressor, and allowed to dry for 20 to 30 seconds to adhere to the object, then immersed in formalin. In cold climates during winter months, adding 1 part alcohol to 9 parts 10% NBF reduces chances of freezing of the specimens during transport. For immunofluorescence evaluation, specimens should be placed in Michel's medium, which better preserves immunoglobulin and complement. Immunoperoxidase staining can be performed on formalin-fixed samples, provided the samples are not in formalin longer than 48 hours. Prolonged fixation in formalin results in cross-linking of protein.

History

The diagnosis by a pathologist after histopathologic evaluation often requires knowledge of the gross features of the lesions. Therefore, it is essential to include with the biopsy samples the following information: age, breed, sex of the animal, location, gross appearance, duration of lesions, and the presence or absence of symmetry and pruritus. Clinical information including results of clinical laboratory evaluations, current medications, and response to therapy should be included along with a list of clinical differential diagnoses. History can be critical to reaching a diagnosis. For instance, presence of luminal and mural folliculitis with no apparent follicular infectious agents in hematoxylin and eosin (H&E)–stained sections in conjunction with the history of lack of response to appropriate antibiotic therapy would stimulate the application of a fungal stain to the sections to evaluate for occult dermatophyte infection. Without the history of lack of response to appropriate antibiotic therapy, the folliculitis could easily be presumed to be of bacterial origin, and the fungal infection missed.

CONGENITAL AND HEREDITARY DISEASES

The terms "congenital" and "hereditary" are not synonymous. Congenital lesions develop in the fetus (in utero), are present at birth, and have a variety of causes. An example is hypotrichosis in the fetus associated with maternal dietary iodine deficiency. Inherited conditions are transmitted genetically and are not always manifested phenotypically in utero or at birth, but may develop later in life. An example is familial canine dermatomyositis, which may not develop until 8 weeks of age or later.

Acanthosis Nigricans

Primary idiopathic acanthosis nigricans is considered a genodermatosis (genetically determined skin disorder) of young dachshunds. The disease is manifested by bilateral axillary hyperpigmentation, lichenification, and alopecia, which may involve large areas and include secondary seborrhea and pyoderma. Microscopically, the epidermis is thickened principally by acanthosis. Hyperkeratosis and focal parakeratosis are accompanied by increased melanin pigment in the epidermis. The term "acanthosis nigricans" has also been used to encompass a variety of disorders that in their chronic form are manifested by axillary or more diffuse lichenification, alopecia, and hyperpigmentation.

Alopecia and Hypotrichosis

Alopecia or atrichia (absence of hair from skin where hair is usually present) and hypotrichosis (less than the normal amount of hair) have been reported in most species of domestic animals. In some animals, the alopecia or hypotrichosis has been recognized as standard for the breed (e.g., Mexican hairless dog, Sphinx cat, and Ulster pig). Degree, location, and age of onset of hairlessness vary. In some instances, the alopecia or hypotrichosis is not due to an absence or reduction of the number of hair follicles, but a failure of hair growth or failure to maintain hair within follicles caused by an abnormality of the hair follicles (follicular dysplasia) (see Fig. 11-14).

Collagen Dysplasia

Collagen dysplasia (hyperelastosis cutis, dermatosparaxis, cutaneous asthenia) occurs in most domestic animals and comprises a clinically, genetically, and biochemically heterogeneous group of diseases. In each, the skin tears easily, is hyperextensible, and loose, but the severity of these lesions varies among species. Specific enzyme defects of collagen synthesis or processing are the causes of some collagen dysplasia syndromes, but the cause of others has not been established. Grossly, cutaneous hyperextensibility and laxity (Fig. 11-19) are associated

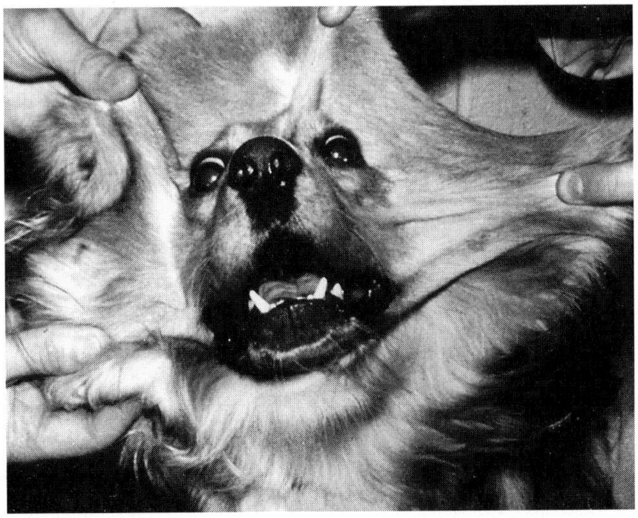

Figure 11-19 Skin; dog. Collagen dysplasia. The skin is hyperextensible. In this dog the skin can be stretched more than the skin of a normal dog. *Courtesy of Dr. B. Baker.*

with numerous scars. Microscopic features vary among the disorders of collagen dysplasia and in some cases the skin is histologically normal. If microscopic lesions are present, the histologic pattern is dysplastic; i.e., collagen bundles may vary in size and shape and have an abnormal organizational pattern. In some cases, electron microscopy or biochemical analysis are required to make a more definitive diagnosis.

Epidermolysis Bullosa (Red Foot Disease)

Epidermolysis bullosa refers to a group of mechanobullous diseases resulting in development of cutaneous blisters (bullae). The diseases vary in mode of inheritance, clinical manifestations, and anatomic location of the blisters. Animals affected with the diseases usually die because of their inability to obtain nourishment, loss of fluid and protein, and secondary infection leading to bacteremia. Epidermolysis bullosa has been reported in some breeds of sheep, horses, cattle, and dogs. Lesions may be present at birth or develop shortly thereafter and are located where epithelial surfaces are subjected to minor mechanical trauma such as oral mucosa, lips, and extremities including the coronary band. Shearing forces that normally cause no problem are sufficient to cause injury in these animals. Microscopic lesions are those of an epidermal vesicular disease in which vesicles form in different locations (subepidermal, epidermal-dermal junction, intraepidermal) depending on the specific disease. As healing occurs, the reepithelization causes external displacement of the vesicles, and with secondary infection the vesicles become pustules.

Epitheliogenesis Imperfecta (Aplasia Cutis)

Epitheliogenesis imperfecta results from the failure of the squamous epithelium of skin, adnexa, and oral mucosa to develop completely. The disease varies in severity and has been reported in most domestic species. It is inherited in some species, but inheritance is not proven in other species. Grossly, lesions consist of sharply demarcated areas of ulceration located most often on the face, extremities, or mucous membranes, and may be small (1 cm) or involve extensive regions such as the entire distal limb (Fig. 11-20). Without the protective covering of the squamous epithelium, the underlying tissue is easily traumatized, may become infected, and bacteremia may develop. Small lesions may heal with scarring and not interfere with life. With extensive involvement, the entire skin may be affected, including hooves, ears, lips, and eyelids, and may result in abortion of the affected fetus.

Hypertrichosis

Excessive growth of hair may be congenital or hereditary. Abnormally hairy fleece at birth develops subsequent to in utero border disease virus infection of fine- and medium-wooled fetal lambs. In addition to abnormal fleece, affected sheep have defective myelination of the brain and spinal cord, abnormalities of body conformation, poor growth, and reduced viability. Microscopically, primary follicles and wool fibers are enlarged and the number of the secondary follicles and wool fibers is reduced. After fetal infection prior to 90 days of gestation, there is an initial phase of retardation of follicular growth followed by an extended period of rapid growth of primary follicles, resulting in production of larger more heavily medulated primary wool fibers. The exact mechanism controlling the exaggerated growth of primary follicles is unknown. It has been speculated that reduction in number of the later developing secondary fibers could be indirectly due to impaired nutrition associated with placentitis. Hypertrichosis in lambs also has been associated with maternal hyperthermia.

Ichthyosis

Ichthyosis is an inherited cutaneous disease seen principally in dogs and cattle. It has also been reported in llamas and pigs. The skin is thickened by marked hyperkeratosis and may crack into plates resembling fish scales, thus the origin of the name. The basic defect is increased adherence of keratinocytes, which prevents normal desquamation. In

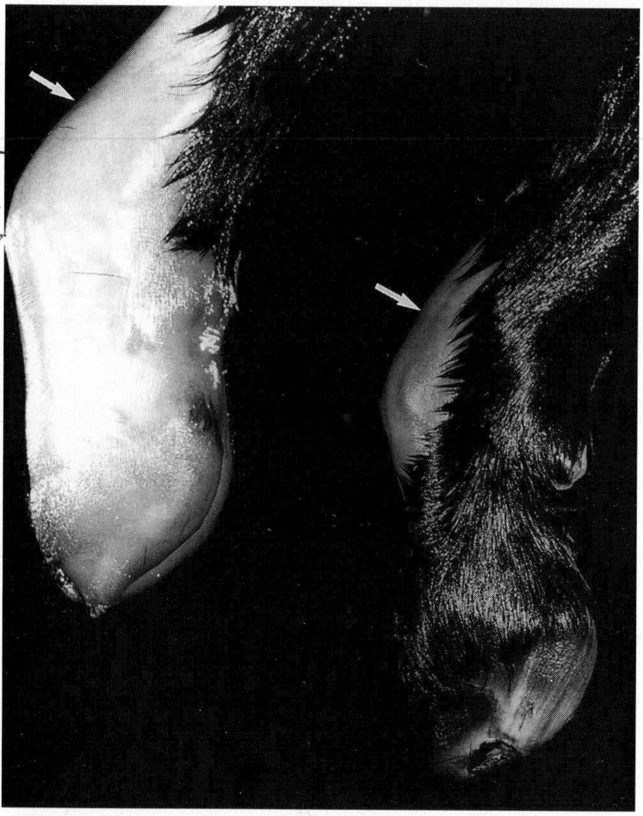

Figure 11-20 Skin; calf. Epitheliogenesis imperfecta. Epidermis over the extremities is multifocally absent *(arrows). Courtesy of Dr. M. D. McGavin.*

cattle, two forms of the disease have been described. One (ichthyosis fetalis) is lethal, and most calves are stillborn or die within days of birth. Grossly and microscopically the skin is alopecic and covered by thick keratinized plaques separated by fissures. Fissuring of the skin leads to exudation of protein and fluids with common secondary bacterial and fungal infection often leading to death or euthanasia. In the second and less severe form (ichthyosis congenita), lesions in some calves are mild at birth and progress with age. The skin becomes thickened, folded, and covered by scale, and partial alopecia develops. More severe lesions are seen where hair is shorter, particularly on the limbs, abdomen, and muzzle. In dogs, ichthyosis is rare and present at birth (Fig. 11-21). Grossly, there are scales adherent to the epidermis, which shed in sheets remaining attached to hair shafts. There may be marked thickening of nasal and digital pads with fronds of keratin accumulating. Alopecia may be seen. In addition to marked epidermal and follicular hyperkeratosis, hypergranulosis, keratinocyte vacuolation, and reticular degeneration are seen in the skin of some affected animals.

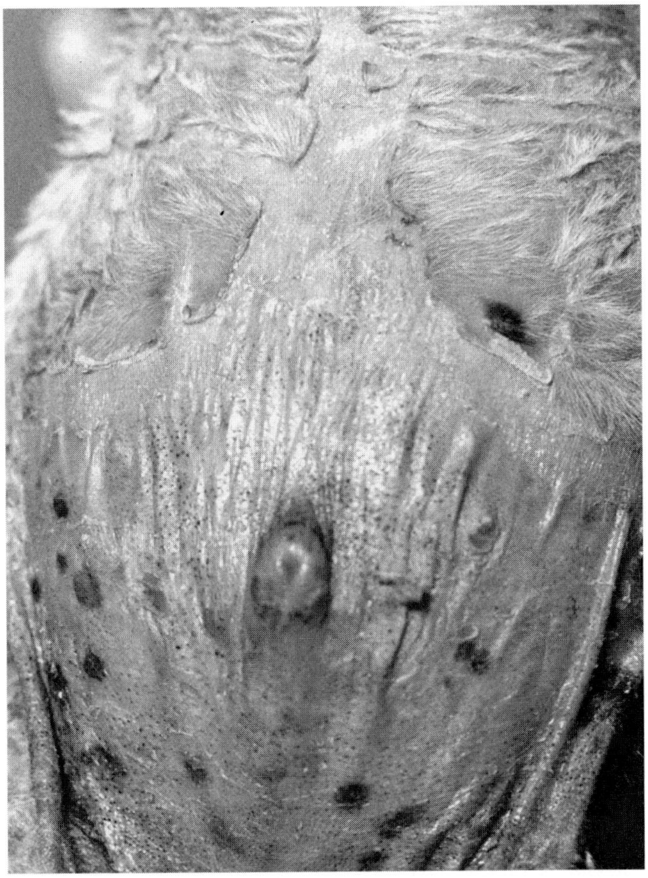

Figure 11-21 Skin, abdomen; dog. Ichthyosis. The skin has adherent plates of scale (excessive keratin), and the skin surface is wrinkled. *Courtesy of Dr. D. Lewis.*

Porcine Juvenile Pustular Psoriasiform Dermatitis (Pityriasis Rosea)

This disorder of suckling and young pigs may be inherited. Lesions are symmetric and develop on the abdomen, groin, and medial thigh and begin as small papules covered by brown crusts. The lesions coalesce and spread and develop into umbilicated plaques with white centers and erythematous, scaly borders. Lesions resemble those of dermatophytosis, but otherwise are of no significance. Microscopically, lesions are psoriasiform epidermal hyperplasia (epidermal hyperplasia with epidermal ridges of uniform length and width), parakeratosis, and epidermal pustules with superficial perivascular dermatitis.

Lethal Acrodermatitis of Bull Terriers

Lethal acrodermatitis is an autosomal recessive inherited disease of defective zinc metabolism in white bull terriers. Lesions generally begin between 6 and 10 weeks of age. Most affected dogs are dead by 15 months of age, usually due to bronchopneumonia. Cutaneous lesions begin between the digits and on footpads and progress to involve mucocutaneous areas, especially of the face. Severe interdigital pyoderma, paronychia (inflammation of the skin around the nails), and villous thickening and fissuring of footpad keratin ensue. Exfoliative dermatitis may also develop on pinnae, muzzle, elbows, hocks, and, in some dogs, can become more generalized, with crusting, ulceration, and secondary pyoderma. Microscopically, the principal lesion is extensive diffuse parakeratotic hyperkeratosis with accompanying acanthosis. Lesions of secondary infection consist of epidermal pustular dermatitis and folliculitis. Dogs do not respond to oral or parenteral zinc supplementation.

ENVIRONMENTALLY RELATED DISEASES

Actinic Rays

Sunlight is composed of visible (400 to 700 nm), ultraviolet (100 to 400 nm), and infrared (700 to 20,000 nm) light rays. The portion of the ultraviolet (UV) light most damaging to the skin is ultraviolet B (UVB) and is in the range of 290- to 320-nm wavelength. However, photodynamic chemicals, if present in the skin, can chemically react with longer wavelengths creating cutaneous damage (photosensitization, phototoxicity). The amount of light reaching the skin is dependent on a variety of environmental and host factors such as quantity of ozone, smog, and cloud cover, which tend to absorb and scatter some of the UV rays. Altitude and latitude are also very important. The atmosphere at high altitude has less particulate matter to absorb and scatter the UV rays. At latitudes farther from the equator, because of the oblique angle of entry into the atmosphere, the path of sunlight through the ozone layer is longer than at latitudes closer to the equator, so more of the harmful UV light is absorbed by the ozone. The path of sunlight through the ozone layer is also one of the reasons that sunlight has more damaging UV rays in summer months and at midday. Host factors include quantity of hair, degree of pigmentation, and thickness of the stratum corneum. Therefore, solar damage is more prevalent at high altitude and at latitudes close to the equator, and in animals spending most of their time outdoors. Lesions generally develop in poorly haired or lightly pigmented sites.

Solar Dermatosis and Neoplasia

The damage to skin by UV light can be acute (sunburn) or chronic (solar dermatosis, neoplasia). An early transient erythema may be due to the heating effect of the light rays, and, possibly, to photochemical changes. The later developing erythema is called "sunburn erythema" and is associated with warmth, tenderness, and swelling. The pathogenesis of sunburn erythema may involve diffusion of inflammatory mediators, such as cytokines, from radiation-damaged keratinocytes, or from direct damage to endothelial cells by UV light. One of the more influential alterations caused by exposure to UV light rays is the formation of thymidine dimers between pyrimidine bases of DNA. The damage can be easily and accurately repaired before the cell undergoes mitosis by an enzyme system that removes the damaged area and synthesizes a new strand of DNA. However, if the cell undergoes mitosis before the damage is repaired, a gap in the DNA strand is left at the location of the thymidine dimer. The gap is repaired by a postreplication repair method that is thought to be error-prone and may lead to mutations and the development of neoplasms. Factors that irritate the skin and increase the rate of cell division increase the number of cells repaired by the postreplication repair method, and, therefore, may enhance development of neoplasms. UV radiation may also alter immunologic reactivity by inducing suppresser T cells, which favor growth of neoplastic cells. Preneoplastic and neoplastic lesions are common alterations in chronically solar-damaged skin in domestic animals.

Solar Dermatitis

The lesions of sunburn occur in all domestic animals. In cats, gross lesions occur where there is little or no hair and little pigment—on external ear tips, eyelids, nose and lips, and are most severe in white cats. Dogs have lesions most commonly in nonpigmented, sparsely haired skin of ventral abdominal, inguinal, and perianal areas. Lightly pigmented younger pigs are more susceptible, and the pinnae and tip of the tail may slough if injury is severe. In lightly colored dairy goats, lesions may develop on the lateral aspects of the udder and teats. Grossly, lesions begin as erythema, scaling, and crusting. After years of exposure, the skin becomes wrinkled and thickened and squamous cell carcinomas may develop. Hemangiomas and hemangiosarcomas have developed in the nonpigmented conjunctiva of dogs and horses and in the skin of dogs and cats. The difference in type of neoplasm may be due in part to thickness of the epithelium, which influences the depth of penetration of the UV rays. UV light may also play a role in the development of melanomas in goats.

Microscopically, in early UV-induced injury, the number of apoptotic cells (sunburn cells) scattered in the epidermis may be so numerous as to form a band of these cells along with intercellular edema, vacuolation of keratinocytes, and loss of granular cell layer. By 72 hours, hyperkeratosis, parakeratosis, and acanthosis are present along with dermal lesions of hyperemia, edema, perivascular mononuclear infiltrates, endothelial swelling, and hemorrhage. Hyperkeratosis, parakeratosis, and acanthosis may persist, and pseudocarcinomatous hyperplasia (marked hyperplasia of the epidermis resulting in many branching and anastomosing epidermal ridges reaching down into the dermis) and dermal fibrosis may develop. Comedones (hair follicles dilated with keratin and sebum) may develop in some dogs. In some animals and in some anatomic locations, elastic tissue and collagen are damaged by solar radiation.

Photosensitization

Photosensitization occurs when long-wavelength UV, or less frequently visible light, is absorbed by a photodynamic chemical in the skin, or by a complex of photodynamic molecule and a biologic substrate, which results in the activation of the photodynamic substance. The photodynamic substances activated by light of the appropriate wavelength cause direct tissue damage by production of radical oxygen products and inflammatory mediators. The photodynamic agent may enter the dermis via the systemic circulation or via direct contact.

Photosensitization can occur in several forms. The first, **primary photosensitization,** is often due to ingestion of preformed photodynamic substances contained in a variety of plants such as *Hypericum perforatum* and *Fagopyrum sagittatum* (buckwheat), or fungal-contaminated plants. Administration of phenothiazine, tetracycline, thiazides, or sulfonamides also may cause primary photosensitization. Photosensitization may also develop because of **abnormal porphyrin metabolism.** These diseases usually are inherited as an enzyme deficiency resulting in abnormal synthesis of photodynamic agents including uroporphyrin and coproporphyrin. Examples include bovine congenital porphyria and bovine erythropoietic (hematopoietic) protoporphyria. **Hepatogenous (secondary) photosensitization** is due to hepatic disease that impairs excretion of phylloerythrin, a product of chlorophyll formed in the alimentary tract. Hepatogenous photosensitization can occur secondary to inherited hepatic defects, biliary obstruction, or as a result of hepatic injury from a variety of sources.

Grossly, in photosensitization, lesions are located on areas of the body with nonpigmented skin and hair, and on parts of the body exposed to the sun, such as the blaze, muzzle, coronary band, cannon, and pastern in horses. In cattle, lesions occur in white-haired areas and on the teats, udder, perineum, and muzzle. In sheep with heavy fleeces, lesions occur on the pinnae, eyelids, face, muzzle, and coronary bands, but, in shorn sheep, lesions may occur on the back. Sheep may have extensive edema of the head resulting in the synonyms of "swelled head" and "facial eczema." Lesions initially include erythema and edema, followed by blisters, exudation, necrosis, and sloughing of necrotic tissues. The microscopic lesions consist of necrotic keratinocytes, epidermal degeneration, and subepidermal vesiculation associated with marked vascular degeneration, which results in edema, subsequent necrosis with infarction, sloughing, and secondary bacterial infection.

Photoenhanced Dermatoses

Immune-mediated cutaneous disorders that are aggravated by exposure to UV radiation include lupus erythematosus, dermatomyositis, and pemphigus erythematosus. Cytokines liberated from keratinocytes may play a role in photoenhancement. Photoactivated vasculitis in the white-haired extremities of horses is a poorly understood disorder thought to be associated with exposure to the sun, but which may not resolve with removal from sun exposure. Lesions initially consist of well-demarcated erythematous, moist, crusted lesions, and later hyperkeratotic plaques. Microscopically, lesions occur in small, thin-walled vessels of superficial dermal papillae. There is vascular dilation, endothelial degeneration, mild hyalinization of vessel walls, thrombosis, and perivascular edema and mild hemorrhage without significant inflammation. More chronic lesions have epidermal acanthosis, hyperkeratosis, and crusting.

Chemical Injury

Chemical injuries of the skin are due to local application to the skin and from absorption of chemicals from the gastrointestinal tract and distribution to the skin. For a chemical to cause injury via local application, it must penetrate the hair and protective epidermal layers. Penetration is enhanced by physical damage to the stratum corneum, especially that caused by excessive moisture. Chemical injuries of the skin include contact irritant dermatitis (local application), systemically distributed chemicals such as arsenic, mercury, thallium, iodine, and organochlorines and organobromines, and poisonings by plants, fungal-contaminated plants, and plants containing selenium, mimosine, and tricothecenes.

Contact Dermatitis

Of the two forms of contact dermatitis, one is immunologically mediated (see allergic contact dermatitis, p. 578), and the other is due to direct damage by the irritant substances. Most cases of contact dermatitis are nonimmunologic and are due to direct contact with substances such as body or wound secretions; to application of drugs; and to the accidental exposure to irritants such as acids, alkalies, soaps, detergents, and irritant plants. In dogs and cats, lesions of irritant contact dermatitis develop on the glabrous (sparsely haired) skin of the abdomen, axillae, flanks, interdigital spaces, perianal area, ventral tail, ventral chest, legs, eyelids, and feet. Horses develop lesions on the muzzle, ventrum, lower limbs, and where riding tack contacts the body, and on the perineum and caudal aspect of the rear legs. Grossly, erythemic patches and papules and, rarely, vesicles develop, but self-inflicted trauma may lead to ulcers and crusts. Microscopically, lesions consist of spongiotic dermatitis, neutrophilic vesicopustules, and superficial perivascular neutrophilic inflammation. Chronic lesions consist of epidermal hyperplasia, hyperkeratosis, and superficial perivascular inflammation. Lesions may be obscured by self-inflicted trauma making histologic diagnosis difficult. Corrosive substances (strong acids or alkalies) may cause epidermal necrosis.

- ingestion of grass/grain contaminated by fungus Claviceps purpurea → toxic alkaloid ergotamine → arteriolar vasoconstriction & capillary endothelial damage → PV edema & thrombosis → tissue ischemia (infarction)

Ergot

Ergot poisoning occurs when animals ingest seed heads of grasses and grains that have been infected by the fungus, *Claviceps purpurea*, which has produced toxic alkaloids. The alkaloids, particularly ergotamine, cause arteriolar vasoconstriction and damage capillary endothelium, leading to perivascular edema and thrombosis resulting in tissue ischemia (infarction). Cold temperatures increase the severity of the lesions. The species most commonly poisoned are cattle fed contaminated grain and grazing pastures infected with the alkaloid-producing fungus. Lesions develop after about 1 week of consumption, beginning as swelling and redness of extremities, particularly of the hind legs. Tips of pinnae and tail are affected with dry gangrene (infarction) and may slough.

Fescue

Fescue poisoning due to excessive consumption of *Festuca arudinacea* develops after about 2 weeks of ingestion of the plant and consists of necrosis (dry gangrene) of distal extremities with lesions identical to those of ergot poisoning.

Selenium

Selenium toxicity occurs worldwide, but poisoning is more frequent in Nebraska, Wyoming, and the Dakotas in the United States and portions of Western Canada. Selenium poisoning develops after ingestion of plants that have accumulated toxic concentrations of selenium, or with overdosage of a selenium supplement. Some plants selectively accumulate selenium, regardless of soil selenium content. These selective accumulators (obligate accumulators, e.g., *Astragalus, Stanleya*) require selenium for growth, generally are not palatable, and are eaten only when other plants are unavailable. Many other plants (facultative accumulators, i.e., *Aster, Atriplex*) do not require selenium for growth, but will accumulate toxic concentrations of selenium if grown in soil with high selenium concentration. These facultative accumulator plants are commonly eaten by livestock and more often are the cause of poisoning. Acute or chronic selenium poisoning has developed in most domestic animals, although susceptibility to selenium poisoning varies with species, dosage, diet, and other factors. In acute poisonings, signs relate to involvement of multiple organ systems. Animals with chronic selenium intoxication are emaciated, have poor-quality hair coat, and partial alopecia. Horses lose the long hair of the mane and tail, develop hoof deformities, and shed the hooves. The mechanism of action is not completely understood and is probably multifactorial. Replacement by selenium of sulfur in various molecules is a possible mechanism of toxicity.

Physical Injury

Acral Lick Dermatitis

Acral lick dermatitis (lick granuloma, neurodermatitis) is a relatively common psychogenic dermatitis usually of an extremity (acral = extremity) in dogs due to persistent licking and chewing (Fig. 11-22). Usually, a single lesion occurs in carpal, metacarpal, metatarsal, tibial, or radial areas. Grossly, lesions are circumscribed, hairless, and, sometimes, ulcerated. Microscopically, the hyperkeratosis is compact, and marked hyperplasia involves the epidermal and follicular epithelium. Ulcers may be present with marginal epidermis thickened by acanthosis. The dermis is thickened by collagenous fibers oriented parallel with the hair follicles (vertical streaking) and contains perivascular and periadnexal plasma cell accumulations and hyperplastic sebaceous glands. Some cases are complicated by secondary bacterial folliculitis and furunculosis. A mild sensory polyneuropathy may be associated with lesion development.

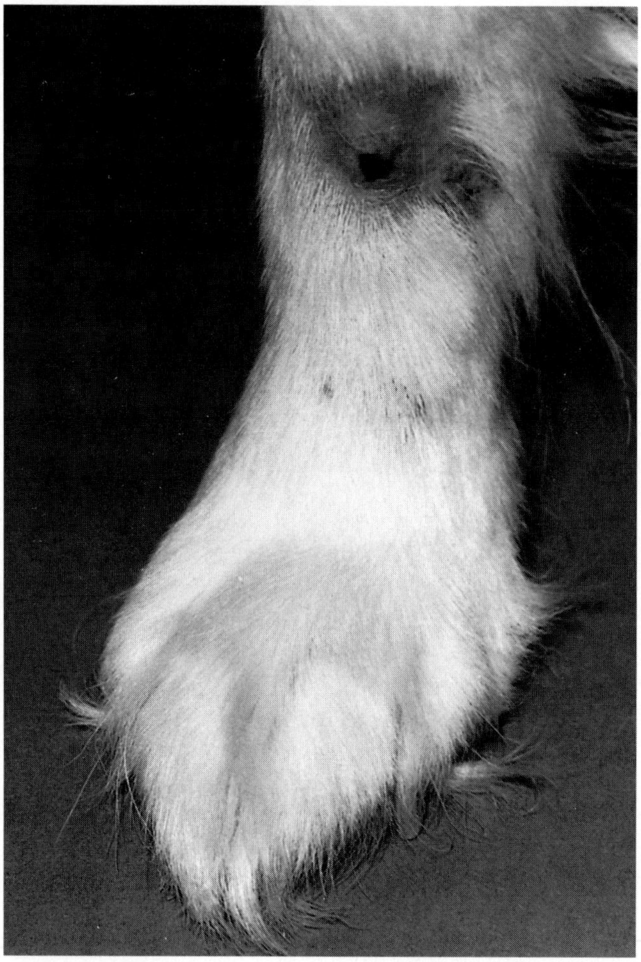

Figure 11-22 Skin, leg; dog. Acral lick dermatitis. Chronic licking has resulted in an area of alopecia. A small dark ulcer is present in the alopecic area.

Feline Psychogenic Alopecia

Psychogenic alopecia occurs in cats of the more emotional breeds and is multifactorial. A partial alopecia is due to the breaking of hairs from gentle, but persistent, licking. Linear or symmetric areas of alopecia are found along the dorsal midline or in the perineal, genital, caudomedial thigh, and abdominal areas. Microscopically, the skin is generally normal, but telogen follicles may be increased. The principal differential diagnosis is alopecia associated with persistent licking due to hypersensitivity. Endocrine associated alopecia is rare in the cat.

Callus

A callus is a raised, irregular, plaquelike area of cutaneous thickening that develops due to friction, usually over pressure points on bony prominences or on the sternum. Callosities can develop in all domestic animals, but are particularly common in giant breed dogs and in pigs kept on concrete or other hard flooring without adequate bedding. Secondary folliculitis, furunculosis, and ulceration may develop. Microscopically, the epidermis and follicular epithelium are thickened by hyperkeratosis and acanthosis, and comedones (follicles dilated with keratin and sebum) are present in some lesions. The follicular openings may be widened by excessive keratin. Dilated follicles may rupture (furunculosis) releasing bacteria, keratin, and sebum resulting in secondary pyoderma and a foreign body inflammatory response.

Injection Site Reactions

Injections of vaccines or therapeutic drugs into the subcutis can result in granulomatous nodules in the panniculus. These granulomas have central foreign and necrotic material bordered by macrophages and multinucleated giant cells and surrounded by a zone of granulation tissue, eosinophils, and perivascular lymphocytes, which

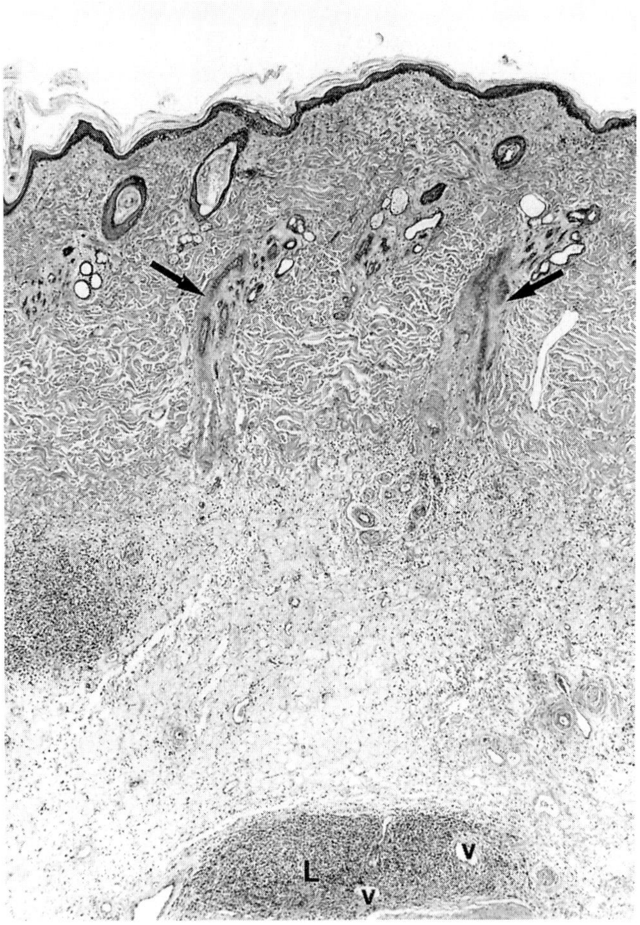

Figure 11-23 Skin, haired; dog. Note injection site reaction with small, atrophic follicles *(arrows)* in the dermis. There are lymphocytic aggregates *(L)* around vessels *(V)*. Mild vasculitis is a feature of this type of injection site reaction. H & E stain.

with time form lymphoid follicles. In small breeds of dogs, especially poodles, injection of killed rabies vaccine has resulted in localized lymphoplasmacytic panniculitis and perivasculitis, mild vasculitis, and severe follicular atrophy (Fig. 11-23).

In cats, a causal relationship between vaccination and development of fibrosarcomas, osteosarcomas, rhabdomyosarcomas, malignant fibrous histiocytomas, and chondrosarcomas has been established. The antigen load and degree of inflammation caused by subcutaneous vaccine administration are thought to be important factors predisposing to tumor development. Vaccine administration in cats results in a local granulomatous inflammatory response that can, in a small number of cats, proceed over months to years to a marked fibroblastic response and eventual neoplastic transformation of mesenchymal cells.

Intertrigo (Skin Fold Dermatitis)

Intertrigo and bacterial growth develop secondary to irritation from skin friction and moisture from tears, saliva,

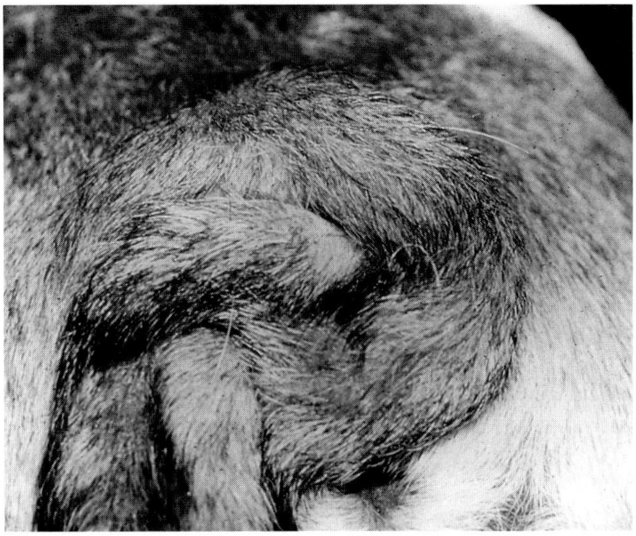

Figure 11-24 Skin, tail; dog, English bulldog. "Screw tail." Excessive skin folds are present around the tail. *Courtesy of Dr. A. Werner.*

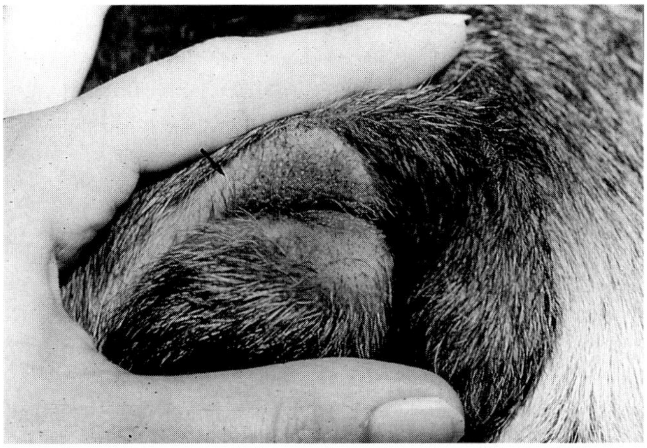

Figure 11-25 Skin, tail; dog, English bulldog. Intertriginous pyoderma. The lesion is present in the skin fold *(arrow)* of the dog depicted in Fig. 11-24. The skin folds have been separated to expose the lesion. *Courtesy of Dr. A. Werner.*

cutaneous glandular secretions, or urine. Locations of intertrigo include the facial fold (brachycephalic breeds), lip fold (breeds with large lips such as Saint Bernard), body fold (Shar Pei breed), vulvar fold (obese female dogs with a small vulva), and tail fold (dogs with corkscrew tails such as English bulldogs) (Figs. 11-24 and 11-25). Intertrigo between the udder and medial thigh (udder-thigh dermatitis) develops principally in cows with large, pendulous udders. Gross lesions of intertriginous dermatitis consist of erythema, edema, crusting. Severe cases of udder-thigh dermatitis in cows may have sloughing of the skin and subcutis. Microscopically there is inflammation of the superficial dermis, sparing the epidermal dermal junction, consisting of plasma cells and fewer lymphocytes, neutrophils, and macrophages. Epidermal pustules may be present. Ulceration may be seen.

Pyotraumatic Dermatitis (Acute Moist Dermatitis, "Hot Spots")

Pyotraumatic dermatitis, especially common in dogs, is secondary to irritation and is, principally, the result of self-inflicted trauma of biting or scratching because of pain and itching. Primary irritants include allergies, parasites, matted hair, and irritant chemicals. Dogs with long hair and dense undercoats are predisposed, and lesions develop more commonly in hot humid weather. Flea bite dermatitis is a common predisposing cause, and lesions may coalesce to involve large portions of dorsal lumbar and thigh skin. Grossly, the lesions are hairless, red, moist, exude fluid, and have red and circumscribed edges. Microscopically, these dogs have either superficial erosive to ulcerative exudative dermatitis or a deeper suppurative folliculitis (pyotraumatic folliculitis, deep pyoderma). Biopsy is required to differentiate the more superficial pyotraumatic dermatitis from the deeper suppurative folliculitis.

Radiation

Highly proliferative cells, such as those of the anagen hair matrix, are most susceptible to radiation-induced damage, but epidermal basal cells and vascular endothelial cells are also affected by radiation injury. The earliest lesion is erythema. Edema, epidermal blistering, ulceration, and hair loss may ensue. Chronic changes include pigmentary alterations (hyperpigmentation with lower doses and hypopigmentation with higher doses), leukotrichia (depigmentation of hair shafts due to loss of follicular melanocytes), dermal scarring, epidermal atrophy, and ulceration. Lesions may resolve or become permanent depending on the degree of damage sustained. Squamous cell carcinomas may develop in some sites of severe radiation damage.

Temperature Extremes

Extremes in temperature such as excessive and prolonged cold can cause injury by osmotic effects due to increased intracellular salt concentration, which develops when ice crystals form and dissolve in cells, and by endothelial injury. Slow chilling may produce vasoconstriction, some cellular damage, and secondary vasodilation with increased permeability followed by edema. Exposure to more severe and persistent cold temperatures causes vasoconstriction, increased blood viscosity, and tissue anoxia. Lesions due to cold temperatures are uncommon in well-nourished healthy animals, but may develop in an animal recently moved from a warm to a cold climate and in neonates that are hypoglycemic or inadequately dried after birth. Lesions are located in the extremities such as the ear tips of cats, the scrotum of dogs and bulls, and ear tips, tail, and teats of cattle. Grossly, lesions consist of gangrene and sloughing of necrotic tissue.

Lesions due to excessive heat (local hyperthermia, burns) occur from exposure to liquids, flames, friction, electricity, heating pads, and lightning. Burns are categorized as partial- or full-thickness, or first-, second-, and third-degree burns. In full-thickness burns, destruction of the entire skin and dermal appendages is total. Therefore, wounds must be repaired by grafting; scarring may develop; and the lesions may be life threatening. Partial-thickness burns have preservation of some part of the epidermis or dermal appendages from which epithelial regeneration may develop. These lesions are less severe, lower temperatures are usually involved, and damage is due to accelerated cellular metabolism, inactivation of enzymes, and vessel injury. Grossly, the lesions are erythema due to capillary dilation, edema due to increased capillary permeability, and vesicle formation due to fluid accumulation at the dermal-epidermal junction (burn blister) (see Fig. 11-10). Microscopically, partial-thickness burns have coagulation necrosis of the epidermis, subepidermal vesicles due to accumulation of fluid from superficial capillaries, necrosis of superficial portions of follicles and sebaceous glands, and degeneration of the subepidermal collagen. In more severe burns the necrosis may extend to the panniculus. Due to coagulation of blood vessels, exudation may not develop, but cellular and vascular lesions including vasculitis and thrombosis will develop at the junction of viable and necrotic tissue. Secondary infection is manifested by accumulations of large numbers of neutrophils also at the junction of viable and necrotic tissue.

Snake and Spider Bites

The families Elapidae (coral snake) and Viperidae (rattle snake, water moccasin, and copperhead) contain the majority of the poisonous snakes in the United States. The genera *Latrodectus* (e.g., black widow) and *Loxosceles* (e.g., brown recluse) are the most common venomous spiders associated with cutaneous injury. Snake bites are most common on the extremities of large animals and cause swelling, erythema, and edema that may be followed by necrosis and sloughing of tissue and death of the animal. Spider bites are found on the face and legs; the severity of lesions is dependent on the type of spider, with some bites characterized by erythema and swelling followed, in severe cases, by necrosis and ulceration. Microscopic lesions of more severe spider bites include an exudative, ulcerative dermatitis, dermal necrosis, neutrophilic and histiocytic infiltrates of the dermis and panniculus, and vasculitis.

INFECTIOUS CAUSES OF SKIN DISEASE

Cutaneous infections develop when there is disruption in the defense mechanisms of the skin. Defense mechanisms include a physical barrier (hair coat, pigment, and stratum corneum), a chemical barrier (fatty acids, complement, immunoglobulin, and others), and a microbial barrier (resident microbial flora such as *Micrococcus* sp., coagulase-negative staphylococci, and others). Predisposing factors to skin infections include those factors that compromise the epidermal integrity such as friction, trauma, excessive moisture, dirt, matted hair, chemical irritants, freezing and burning, irradiation, and parasitic infestation. Factors that comprise host immune function such as inadequate nutrition may also contribute.

Poxviruses

Poxviruses are DNA epitheliotropic viruses that infect most domestic, wild, and laboratory animals and birds. Dogs and cats are rarely infected with poxviruses, although infection with contagious ecthyma (parapoxvirus) has been reported in dogs, and cutaneous infection caused by a poxvirus of the orthopoxvirus genus has been reported in cats in Europe. Poxviruses have major differences in the range of species they will infect, with some being species specific and others zoonotic. Many poxviruses of animals can cause skin lesions in human beings. Lesions develop secondary to pox viral invasion of epithelium, by ischemic necrosis due to vascular injury, and by stimulation of host cell DNA resulting in the formation of epidermal hyperplasia. The severity of poxviral infection is variable in part due to the localized or systemic nature of the infection and in some instances to secondary infections. Cutaneous poxviral sequential lesions consist of macule, papule, vesicle (variably severe), umbilicated pustule, crust, and scar. Sheeppox and goatpox are the most pathogenic poxviruses; infection causes significant mortality, especially in young animals due to systemic disease, but these diseases do not occur in the United States or Canada.

Contagious ecthyma (contagious pustular dermatitis, orf, sore mouth) is a common localized infection of young sheep and goats caused by a parapoxvirus with worldwide distribution. Less commonly, human beings, cattle, wild ungulates, and dogs are infected. Morbidity in lambs is usually great and, although mortality is usually low, it can approach 15% in lambs. Lesions are initiated by abrasions from pasture grasses or forage, begin at the commissures of the mouth, and spread to the lips, oral mucosa, eyelids, and feet. Lambs may infect the teats of ewes, and the lesions may spread to the skin of the udder (Fig. 11-26). Contagious ecthyma is of economic importance due to weight loss in lambs that are reluctant to eat because of oral and perioral lesions. Gross and microscopic features are consistent with the typical poxvirus lesions except that the vesicle stage is very brief, the ulcer and crust stages are clinically prominent, and lesions are especially proliferative. Inclusion bodies are only briefly detectable.

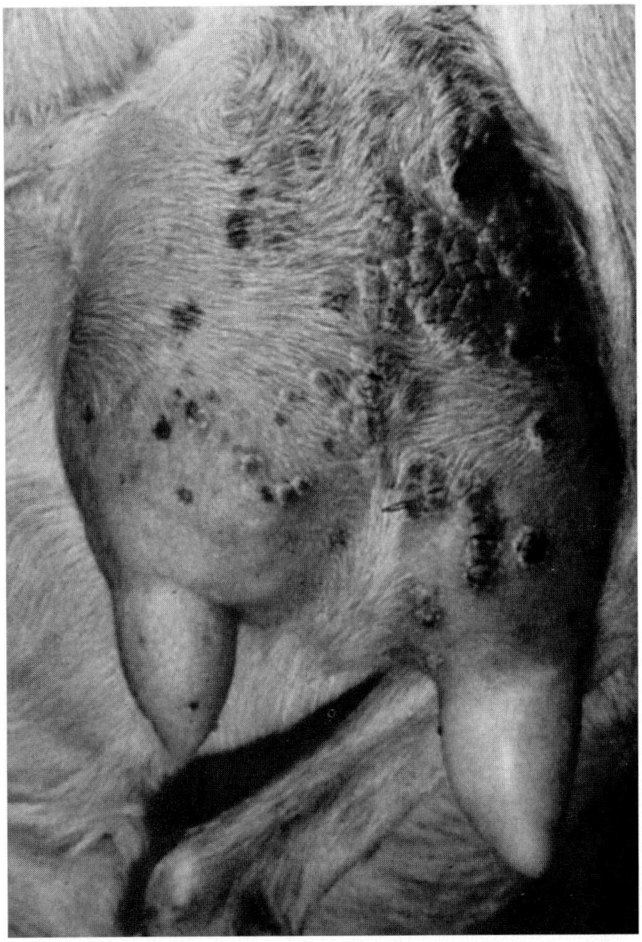

Figure 11-26 Skin, udder; goat. Contagious ecthyma. The lesions consist of pustules and crusts. Pustules are transient and rapidly develop into crusts. *Courtesy of Dr. C. Buergelt.*

Herpesviruses

Herpesviruses are DNA viruses that are uncommonly associated with cutaneous lesions. Cutaneous lesions may develop in association with nondermatotropic herpesviruses such as infectious bovine rhinotracheitis (bovine herpesvirus-1) and equine coital exanthema (equine herpesvirus-3). Cutaneous lesions have rarely been reported in cats with feline herpesvirus-1 infection. Two dermatotropic herpesvirus infections with economic importance are bovine herpesvirus-2 and bovine herpesvirus-4. Herpesviruses may be latent, and lesions can recur at times of stress. Gross lesions consist of vesicles that rupture to form ulcers that are covered by crusts. Microscopic lesions in herpesvirus infections depend on the stage, but early degenerative changes include ballooning and reticular degeneration, the sequelae to degeneration of epidermal cells and acantholysis. Syncytial cells may be seen. Intranuclear inclusions develop, but because of rapidly developing necrosis, may not be found except at the margins of ulcers.

Bovine Herpes Mammillitis Virus

Bovine herpesvirus-2, a dermatotropic virus (Allerton virus), may cause a more generalized disease (pseudo–lumpy skin disease) or, as seen in the United States, a localized infection of the teat (mammillitis is inflammation of the nipple), termed bovine herpes mammillitis. Localized infection occurs more commonly in lactating dairy cows, but may develop in beef cows, pregnant heifers, and suckling calves. Trauma is implicated in the pathogenesis as normal skin is resistant to viral penetration. Bovine herpes mammillitis is of economic importance due to decreased milk production and secondary bacterial mastitis. Lesions develop on the teats and skin of the nearby udder or, occasionally, the perineum. Suckling calves may develop lesions on the muzzle.

Bovine Herpes Mammary Pustular Dermatitis

Bovine herpesvirus-4 causes a similar but milder disease than the localized form of bovine herpesvirus-2.

Feline Ulcerative Facial Dermatitis and Stomatitis

Ulcerative, often persistent, facial dermatitis associated with necrosis, prominent eosinophilic inflammation, and herpesvirus inclusion bodies within epithelial cells has been reported in cats. Feline herpesvirus-1 was identified in lesions by polymerase chain reaction methodology. Previous glucocorticoid therapy or stress from overcrowding may play a role in lesion development. Most cases developed under circumstances suggesting reactivation of latent herpesvirus infection. The cases were different from those previously reported in domestic cats in that lesions persisted, were limited to the skin of the face, and often were accompanied by dramatic eosinophilic dermatitis.

Other Viruses

Cutaneous lesions are seen with foot-and-mouth disease (picornavirus), vesicular stomatitis (rhabdovirus), swine vesicular disease (picornavirus), and vesicular exanthema (calicivirus). Feline leukemia virus is associated with the development of lymphoma and fibrosarcoma. A few cats with feline leukemia virus infection have developed cutaneous horns of the footpads and dermatitis characterized by epidermal and follicular acanthosis with epidermal giant cells, dyskeratosis, necrosis, and ulceration (Fig. 11-27). In immunoperoxidase-stained sections the hyperplastic epidermis in cases with epidermal giant cells is strongly positive for feline leukemia virus. Both feline leukemia virus and feline immunodeficiency virus, because of their immunosuppressive capabilities, can predispose to chronic skin infections including abscesses, paronychia, and demodicosis. Rarely, feline calicivirus has been implicated as a cause of cutaneous lesions.

Rickettsial Infection

The most important rickettsial disease associated with cutaneous lesions is canine Rocky Mountain spotted fever.

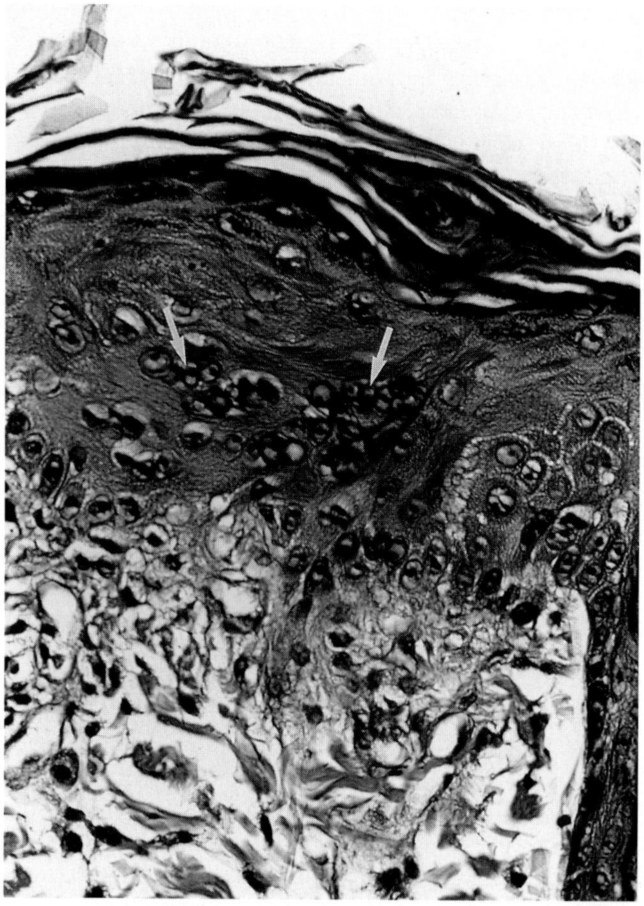

Figure 11-27 Skin; cat. Cutaneous feline leukemia virus infection. Epidermal hyperplasia (acanthosis) with epidermal multinucleated giant cells *(arrows)* present. H & E stain.

This disease is caused by *Rickettsia rickettsii,* and is transmitted by ticks, including *Dermacentor andersoni* in the western United States, *Dermacentor variabilis* in the eastern United States, and *Amblyomma americanum* in the southern United States. The disease is seasonal, corresponding with the increased activity of ticks and contact with ticks. In addition to systemic signs, affected dogs have cutaneous, ocular, genital, and oral erythema with petechiae, edema, necrosis, and ulceration as a result of the vasculitis caused by the rickettsia.

Bacterial Infection

Cutaneous bacterial infections are frequently referred to as **pyodermas** and are generally classified as superficial or deep. Pyodermas are among the most common lesions of the skin of dogs, but are uncommon in cats and other domestic animals.

Superficial Bacterial Infections (Superficial Pyodermas)

These infections involve the epidermis including that of the upper infundibulum of hair follicles, usually heal without scarring, and, generally, the regional lymph nodes

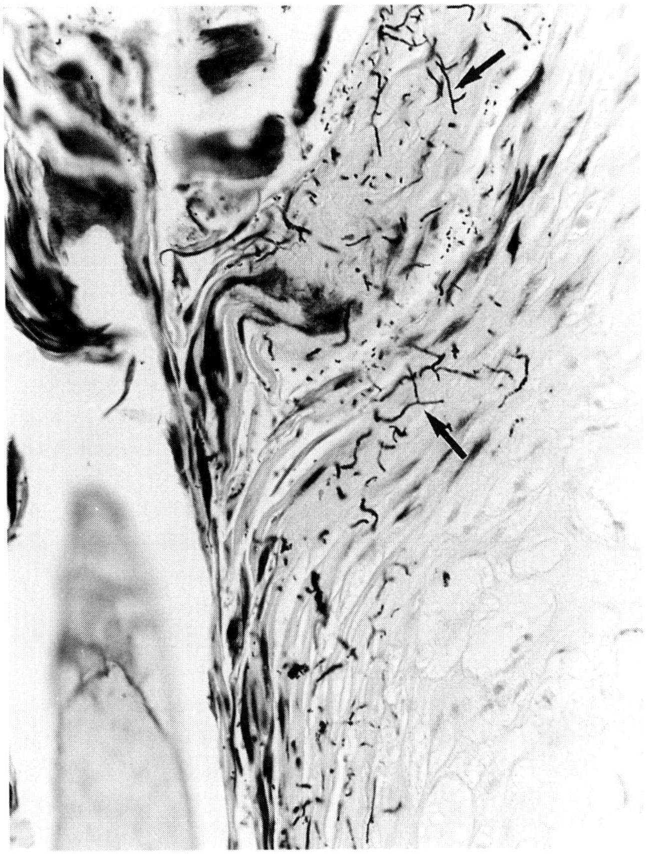

Figure 11-28 Skin, haired; cow. *Dermatophilus* species infection. The stratum corneum contains filamentous bacteria *(arrows)*. The bacteria subdivide longitudinally and transversely. H & E stain.

are not affected. Grossly, the lesions are erythema, alopecia, papules and pustules, crusts, and epidermal collarettes (peripheral expanding rings of scaling) centered on the openings of hair follicles. Microscopically, the patterns include intraepidermal pustular dermatitis and superficial suppurative luminal folliculitis. Although bacteria are the cause of the lesions, they are not always microscopically demonstrable.

Superficial Pustular Dermatitis (Impetigo)

This infection is observed in dogs, cats, piglets, cows, does, and ewes and is caused by coagulase-positive *Staphylococcus* sp. in association with such predisposing factors as cutaneous abrasions, viral infections, increased moisture, and poor nutrition. Older dogs with immunosuppression, usually due to hyperadrenocorticism, may develop a bullous impetigo. In cows, does, and ewes, lesions are predominantly on the udder. In kittens the dorsum of the neck and shoulders are affected because of overzealous "mouthing" by the queen; *Streptococcus* sp. and *Pasteurella* sp. are the more common bacterial

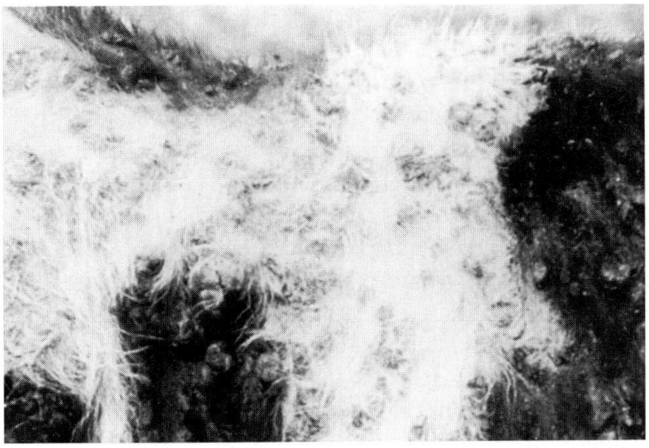

Figure 11-29 Skin, haired; cow. *Dermatophilus* species infection. The hair is matted by crusts composed of dried exudate, keratin, and bacteria. *Courtesy of Dr. F. Lozano-Alarcon.*

isolates. Gross lesions consist of pustules that develop into crusts, principally (except in kittens) in nonhaired skin. The microscopic lesion is a nonfollicular neutrophilic subcorneal pustule.

Dermatophilosis (streptothricosis) caused by *Dermatophilus congolensis* is characterized by cutaneous lesions in cattle, sheep, and horses more often than dogs, cats, pigs, and goats. The bacterium is transmitted by carrier animals and is more common in tropical and subtropical countries and during wet weather. Lesions tend to develop on the dorsum of the back and distal extremities, and after epidermal irritation from ectoparasites, trauma, or prolonged wetting of the skin, hair, or wool, which allows for penetration of the damaged epidermis by the *Dermatophilus* "zoospore." Proliferation of the bacterium in the outer root sheath of the hair follicle and superficial epidermis results in the development of gram-positive filamentous branching organisms that subdivide longitudinally and transversely (Fig. 11-28). These bacteria stimulate an acute inflammatory response in which neutrophils migrate from superficial vessels into the dermis and through the epidermis to form microabscesses. The inflammation inhibits further penetration of the bacterium. The epidermis regenerates and the newly regenerated epidermis is reinvaded by residual bacterial organisms. Repeated cycles of bacterial growth, inflammation, and epidermal regeneration result in the formation of the multilaminated pustular crusts. Grossly, lesions consist of papules, pustules, and thick crusts that may coalesce and mat the hair or wool (Fig. 11-29). The microscopic lesions are those of a hyperplastic superficial perivascular dermatitis with multilaminated crusts of alternating layers of keratin and inflammatory cells.

Exudative epidermitis of pigs (greasy pig disease) caused by *Staphylococcus hyicus* is an acute, often fatal, dermatitis of neonatal piglets and a mild disease in older piglets. Predisposing factors include cutaneous lacerations, poor nutrition, and viral infections. In the course of the disease a staphylococcal exotoxin called "exfoliatin" is produced, and the bacterial toxin binds to filaggrin in the keratohyalin granules of the stratum granulosum. This reaction may be responsible for the lesions of focal erosion of the stratum corneum. Dermatitis and brownish exudate develop around the eyes, pinnae, snout, chin, medial legs, and spreads to the ventral thorax and abdomen. The lesions rapidly coalesce and become generalized resulting in a greasy, malodorous exudate covering an erythematous skin surface (Fig. 11-30). If piglets survive, the exudate hardens and cracks with the formation of fissures. Subacute disease develops gradually in older piglets, and lesions are generally localized to the skin of the face, pinnae, and periocular regions. Grossly, the epidermis is thickened with scaling. The early histopathologic lesion is subcorneal pustular dermatitis with extension to the hair follicle, resulting in superficial suppurative folliculitis. In the fully developed lesion, the epidermis is hyperplastic and has thick crusts of keratin, microabscesses, and cocci. The dermis is congested and edematous with superficial perivascular neutrophilic to eosinophilic dermatitis in early stages and mononuclear perivascular infiltrate in later stages.

Other superficial pyodermas include ovine fleece rot (due to excessive moisture and *Pseudomonas*), and equine pastern folliculitis (grease heel), a secondary pyoderma of the caudal pastern and/or fetlock. Ovine fleece rot is important economically because it predisposes sheep to myiasis and reduces the value of affected wool.

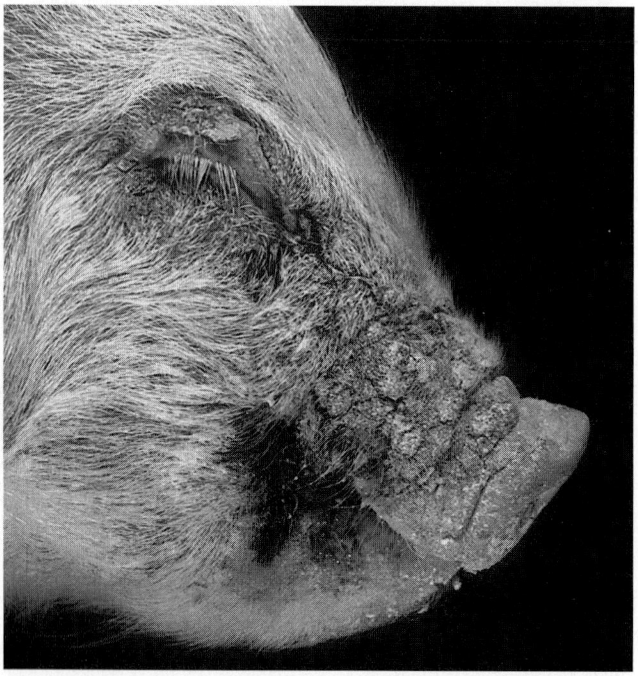

Figure 11-30 Skin; piglet. Exudative epidermitis. The skin around nose and eye is lichenified and has fissures. Foci of greasy exudate are adherent to hair and surface of skin. *Courtesy of Dr. M. D. McGavin.*

Deep Bacterial Infections (Deep Pyodermas)

These infections are less common than superficial infections and develop most frequently in dogs. Deep bacterial infections cause folliculitis that involves the entire infundibulum and deeper portions of the follicle, and may develop into furunculosis involving the surrounding dermis and subcutis. Deep bacterial infections often heal with scarring and generally involve regional lymph nodes. These diseases are often secondary to immune suppression, demodicosis (dogs), or disorders associated with follicular hyperkeratosis (chin acne, elbow callus). Deep pyodermas may originate as a sequela to superficial bacterial folliculitis. Grossly, the lesions depend on age and stage, and include follicular crusted papules, pustules, alopecia, nodules, abscesses, ulcers, fistulas, and hemorrhagic bullae. Deep pyoderma, especially on the face of some large breed dogs, may resemble superficial pyotraumatic dermatitis (acute moist dermatitis). The microscopic patterns include pyogranulomatous folliculitis and furunculosis, nodular to diffuse dermatitis, and panniculitis. Draining sinuses may develop, often in association with a foreign body response to extruded follicular contents (e.g., hair, keratin, mites). Chronic lesions associated with significant scarring may replace hair follicles and adnexal glands. Bacteria isolated include *Staphylococcus* sp., *Streptococcus* sp., *Corynebacterium pseudotuberculosis, Pasteurella* sp., *Proteus* sp., *Pseudomonas* sp., and *Escherichia coli. Staphylococcus intermedius* is the primary pathogen of canine skin.

Staphylococcal folliculitis and furunculosis develop most commonly in the dog (see Fig. 11-17), frequently affect the horse, goat, sheep, but are uncommon in cow, cat, and pig. In dogs, lesions are localized or generalized and develop on the muzzle, bridge of the nose, pressure points, interdigital areas, and chin. Deep pyoderma of adult German shepherd dogs (German shepherd folliculitis, furunculosis, and cellulitis) is a unique deep pyoderma with an apparent genetic predisposition. Lesions are located on the dorsal lumbosacral, ventral abdominal, and thigh areas. Hypersensitivity to fleas or alterations in immune or neutrophil function have been proposed as predisposing causes, but most have been discounted. In horses, lesions develop most commonly in association with tack, especially in the saddle area, or on the caudal aspect of the pastern or tail. In goats, the face, pinnae, distal limbs, and glabrous areas of the udder, ventral abdomen, medial thighs, and perineum, are most commonly affected. In adult sheep, lesions develop on the face, limbs, and teats, whereas in lambs the lips and perineum have lesions. Microscopic lesions include suppurative luminal folliculitis, possibly in conjunction with furunculosis. Pyogranulomatous and scarring inflammation may efface dermal architecture and extend into the deep dermis and panniculus and form sinuses that drain to the surface.

Subcutaneous abscesses are localized collections of purulent exudate located within the dermis and subcutis. Abscesses are common in cats due to the frequency of bacterial contamination of puncture wounds. The exudate may be surrounded by a wall of collagen and fibroblasts. Bacteria involved are frequently inhabitants of the mouth and include *Pasteurella multocida, Fusobacterium* sp., β-hemolytic streptococci, *Peptostreptococcus anaerobius,* and *Bacteroides* sp.

Bacterial granulomatous dermatitis is associated with traumatic implantation of bacteria that generally are saprophytes of low virulence. Grossly, lesions are diffuse or nodular and may ulcerate and drain to the skin surface by fistulas (Fig. 11-31). Microscopically, collections of macrophages with or without giant cells are present. Caseous necrosis and neutrophils are present in some lesions. Etiologic agents may be seen in the macrophages, exudate, or in vacuolar spaces within tissue, but may be present in low number and difficult to identify in histologic sections.

Mycobacterial organisms produce granulomatous to pyogranulomatous lesions in many species including cattle, pigs, dogs, and cats. Cutaneous lesions are usually caused by *Mycobacterium lepraemurium* (feline leprosy) or saprophytic opportunistic mycobacterial organisms including *M. fortuitum, M. smegmatis, M. chelonei, M. phlei,* and other species (so-called atypical mycobacterial infections). These organisms are inhabitants of soil or water and contaminate wounds in several species. Cutaneous infections with *M. tuberculosis, M. bovis,* or *M. avium* are rare. Feline leprosy occurs in cats living along the Pacific coast of North America and develops in cats without age, breed, or sex predilection. Lesions develop commonly on the head, neck, and limbs but may occur anywhere (Figs. 11-32 and 11-33). The saprophytic atypical mycobacterial infections also occur most often in the cat and are characterized by recurrent, draining nodules or fistulas frequently located in the dermis and subcutis of the inguinal area. The acid-fast organisms, especially with the saprophytic opportunistic mycobacterial agents, may be rare in histologic specimens.

Botryomycosis is used as a diagnostic term for a granulomatous dermatitis caused by nonfilamentous bacteria (usually *Staphylococcus aureus*) that form small yellow "sulfur" granules. The granules consist centrally of bacterial colonies surrounded by radiating club-shaped

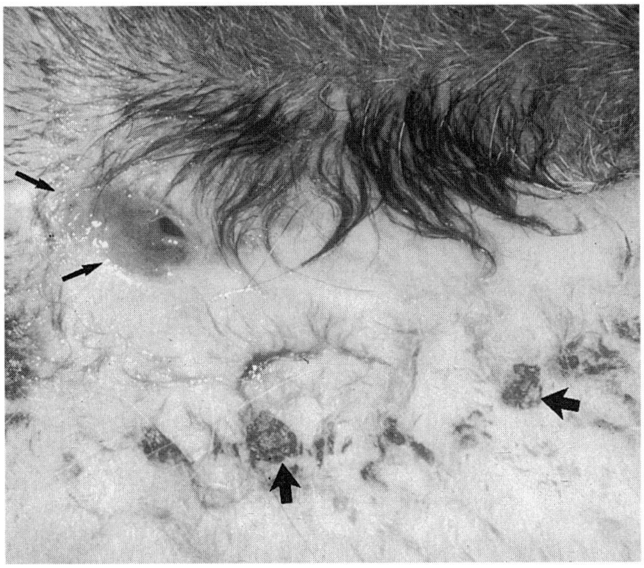

Figure 11-31 Skin, abdomen; cat. Nodular granulomatous dermatitis due to infection by *Mycobacterium fortuitum.* The skin of the abdomen has multiple nodules *(broad arrows).* One nodule is ulcerated and draining *(thin arrows). Courtesy of Dr. R. Marsella.*

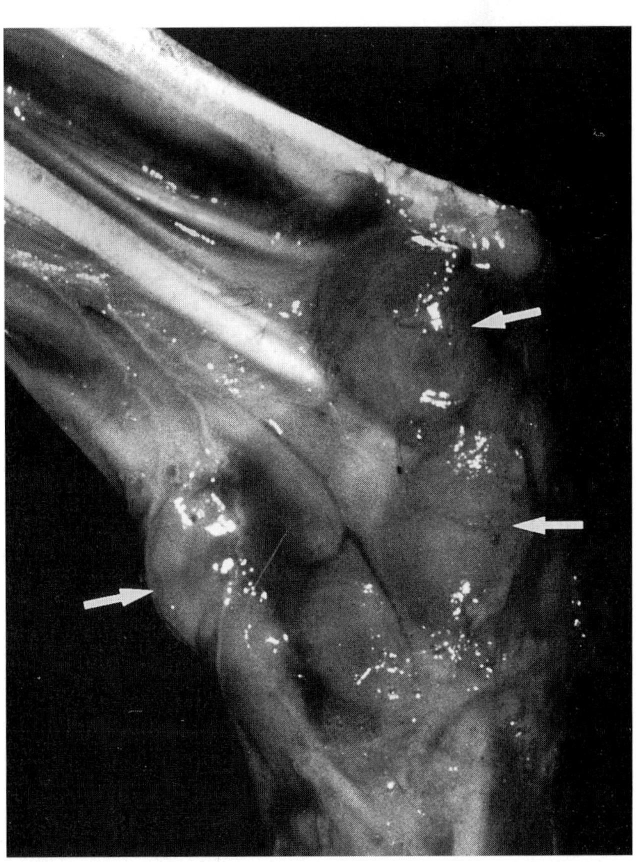

Figure 11-32 Skin, leg; cat. Feline leprosy. Multiple nodules in the subcutis and adjacent muscles *(arrows)* consisting of granulomatous inflammation are present. (The epidermis and dermis have been removed.) *Courtesy of Dr. C. Leathers.*

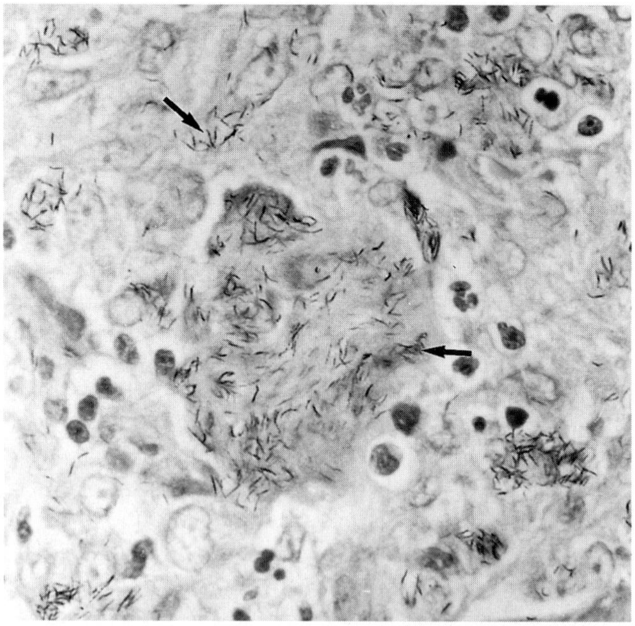

Figure 11-33 Skin, dermis; cat. Feline leprosy. Macrophages contain numerous mycobacteria *(arrows).* Ziehl-Neelsen stain.

bodies of homogeneous eosinophilic material. The material, considered antigen-antibody complexes, is termed Splendore-Hoeppli material. Filamentous bacteria may form similar granules in tissue and can be differentiated from staphylococcal infections by gram-staining and culture. These organisms include various species of *Actinomyces, Actinobacillus,* and *Nocardia. Nocardia asteroides* generally does not form granules. *Borrelia suilla* is a spirochete that causes ulcerative dermatitis (ulcerative granuloma, necrotic ulcer, porcine spirochetosis) in pigs that are kept under unsanitary conditions.

Digital Infections of Ruminants (Bacterial Pododermatitis)

Infections of the digits of cattle and sheep are usually mixed bacterial infections sometimes separated into two basic groups, "contagious footrot" and "necrobacillosis of the foot," based on the contagious nature of the infection and the type of bacteria principally responsible for infection. Contagious footrot is caused principally by *Bacteroides nodosus* acting synergistically with *Fusobacterium necrophorum* with other bacteria. Necrobacillosis of the foot is caused principally by *F. necrophorum* with other bacteria, including *Bacteroides melaninogenicus* in cattle.

Contagious footrot in sheep develops when predisposing factors such as moisture and trauma damage the interdigital epidermis and allow colonization by a variety of microorganisms from skin or feces, including *F. necrophorum.* If the sheep harbors the obligate anaerobic bacteria, *B. nodosus,* in interdigital skin, footrot will develop. Contagious footrot is a synergistic bacterial infection principally involving *B. nodosus* (elaborates proteases and growth-enhancing factors, which aid bacterial penetration of the epidermis and bacterial growth) and *F. necrophorum* (responsible for most of the necrosis and inflammation). Contagious footrot in sheep occurs in virulent and benign forms. The virulent form is due to more virulent *B. nodosus* that produces significantly more proteolytic enzymes, allowing more bacterial penetration of the epidermis. Early lesions of virulent footrot are interdigital, affect both digits, and consist of red, moist, and swollen eroded skin. The inflammation spreads to the epidermal matrix of the hoof and results in separation of the horn by a malodorous exudate. The germinal epithelium is not destroyed and regeneration is attempted, but the new horn is destroyed. In chronic infections, hooves may become long and misshapen. Benign footrot (scald) is mild, confined to interdigital skin, may have slight separation of the horn of the heel, and the hoof may overgrow. Footrot in cattle is similar to benign footrot in sheep.

Necrobacillosis of the foot of sheep includes ovine interdigital dermatitis and foot abscesses. Ovine interdigital dermatitis is an acute necrotizing dermatitis that clinically is similar to benign footrot. Ovine interdigital dermatitis is differentiated from footrot by the failure to demonstrate *B. nodosus* in smears or cultures of exudate. Foot abscesses include heel abscesses (infective bulbar necrosis) and toe abscesses (lamellar abscesses). Foot abscesses are more common in wet seasons and in heavy adult sheep. In addition to *F. necrophorum, Arcanobacterium pyogenes (Actinomyces pyogenes)* may be isolated from the lesions.

Necrobacillosis (foul in the foot) of cattle occurs secondary to trauma and is caused by *F. necrophorum* and *B. melaninogenicus.* The condition is associated with lameness and is characterized by an interdigital dermatitis and cellulitis with fissures and necrosis that may extend into joint spaces.

Systemic Bacterial Infections

Septicemic salmonellosis may cause cyanosis of the external ears and abdomen due to capillary dilation and congestion. In addition, thrombosis may cause necrosis of distal extremities. Cutaneous lesions associated with *Erysipelothrix rhusiopathiae* (erysipelas) in pigs consist of square to rhomboidal, firm, raised, pink to dark purple areas (Fig. 11-34) and are due to vasculitis, thrombosis, and ischemia (infarction). Bacterial infections may also develop from direct extension of bacterial infections of deeper tissues such as clostridial myositis and cellulitis. *Clostridium novyi* may cause severe cellulitis, toxemia, and death in young rams whose heads have been traumatized by butting during the breeding season. Spores

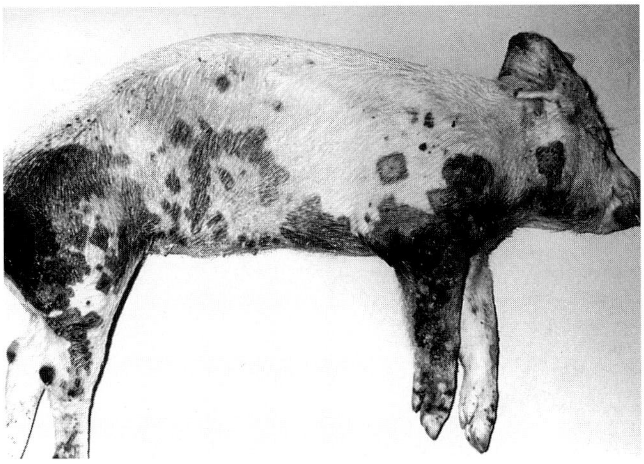

Figure 11-34 Skin; pig. Erysipelas. Rhomboidal lesions are present in the skin. The lesions are due to vasculitis, which has caused infarction. *Courtesy of Dr. M. D. McGavin.*

in the soil gain entrance through cutaneous lacerations at the base of the horns, germinate, produce toxins, and result in cellulitis and toxemia. Swelling of the head and neck result in the common term "big head" or "swelled head." In horses the purpura developing occasionally as a sequela to *Streptococcus equi* may be due to immune complex vasculitis. Clinically, horses present with petechial hemorrhages of the skin and mucous membranes and edema with serum exudation of distal extremities. Microscopic lesions consist of vascular wall disruption by neutrophils, perivascular edema, hemorrhage, and fibrin exudation.

Fungal (Mycotic) Infection

Mycotic infections have been classified into four basic categories: superficial, cutaneous, subcutaneous, and systemic. Mycotic infections tend to occur more often in animals with compromised resistance due to debilitating systemic diseases such as diabetes mellitus or neoplasia, or in animals treated with immunosuppressive agents or long-term, broad-spectrum antibiotics.

Superficial Mycoses

Superficial mycoses are infections restricted to the stratum corneum or hair with minimal or no tissue reaction. Piedra, caused by *Trichosporon beigelii,* has minute swellings of the hair shaft.

Cutaneous Mycoses

Cutaneous mycoses (also included as superficial mycoses by some authors) are infections of keratinized tissues including hair, feathers, nails, and epidermis. The fungi are usually restricted to the keratinized layer, but tissue destruction and host response may be extensive. Infections in animals include dermatophytosis, cutaneous candidiasis, and malassezia dermatitis.

Dermatophytoses are fungal infections of the skin, hair, and nails of animals caused by taxonomically related fungi known as dermatophytes. Pathogenic genera include *Epidermophyton, Microsporum,* and *Trichophyton.* Dermatophytosis occurs worldwide, is the most important cutaneous (superficial) mycosis, and is common in human beings and animals, especially in cats. Dermatophytoses are more contagious than other fungal infections, are more common in hot, humid environments, and young animals are more susceptible than adults. Animals kept in overcrowded, dirty, or damp areas and those with inadequate nutrition are also more susceptible. Species that more commonly infect domestic animals are included in genera *Microsporum* and *Trichophyton. Epidermophyton* is adapted to human beings (anthropophilic) and rarely infects animals. Zoophilic dermatophytes (e.g., *Microsporum canis*) are animal pathogens. *M. canis* is so well adapted, especially in long-haired, purebred cats, that inapparent infections occur. Geophilic dermatophytes (i.e., *M. gypseum*) occur in soil as saprophytes but under favorable condition may infect human beings and animals.

Dermatophytes invade keratinized tissues (stratum corneum, hair shafts, and nails) by producing proteolytic enzymes, which help penetrate the surface lipid coat. The fungal hyphae invade the keratin, and the hyphae break up into chains of arthrospores. The products elaborated by the dermatophytes cause dermal irritation and damage to the epidermis. The fungal products and cytokines released from damaged keratinocytes result in epidermal hyperplasia (hyperkeratosis, parakeratosis, acanthosis) and inflammation. Inflammatory cells arrive via the superficial vessels (superficial perivascular dermatitis) and, subsequently, migrate through the epidermal layers (exocytosis) to the invaded keratinized layers, forming intracorneal microabscesses. Exocytosis of inflammatory cells into follicular walls results in folliculitis, and, if the follicular wall is destroyed, in furunculosis. Bacterial infection increases the severity of the folliculitis and furunculosis. Gross and microscopic lesions may be highly variable and range from an asymptomatic lesionless infection to a nodular eruptive lesion (kerion), to a granulomatous nodular lesion with distorted fungal hyphae (pseudomycetoma), to discolored, malformed, friable, broken or sloughed nails (onychomycosis). Gross lesions in haired skin are often circular or irregularly shaped, scaly to crusty patches of alopecia (Fig. 11-35) that may coalesce to involve large portions of the body. Areas of hair loss are due to broken hair shafts and loss of hairs from inflamed follicles. Follicular papules and pustules may be present. Fungi tend to die in areas of inflammation in the center of lesions and are viable peripherally, giving rise to the peripheral red ring and the term "ringworm." Microscopic patterns include perifolliculitis, luminal folliculitis, or furunculosis, as well as epidermal hyperplasia with intracorneal microabscesses. In many cases, septate

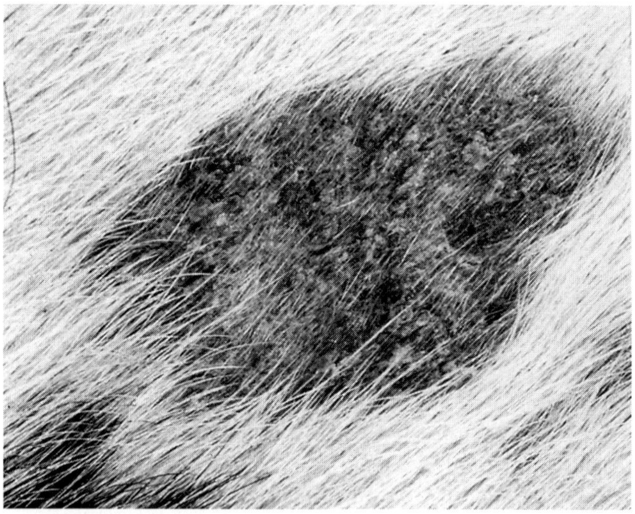

Figure 11-35 Skin, haired; cow. Dermatophytosis. Note hairless encrusted area. *Courtesy of Dr. H. D. Liggitt.*

hyphae or spores are present in hair shafts and in epidermal or follicular keratin (Fig. 11-36).

Candidiasis is caused by *Candida* sp. that are normal inhabitants of the skin and gastrointestinal tract. Infection occurs when host resistance is compromised. Infections with *Candida* sp. are rare in domestic animals and tend to occur on mucous membranes and at mucocutaneous junctions. Exudative, papular, pustular to ulcerative dermatitis of the lips (cheilitis), stomatitis, and otitis externa may develop. Microscopically, lesions are in the epidermis and consist of spongiotic neutrophilic pustular inflammation with parakeratosis and ulceration with organisms present in the superficial exudate.

Malassezia dermatitis is caused by *Malassezia pachydermatis (Pityrosporum canis),* a yeast isolated from normal external ear canal and skin. This yeast proliferates when the microclimate or host defenses are altered and may cause clinical disease. Lesions may be regional (interdigital, muzzle, otic, perianal, or intertriginous) or more generalized. Grossly, the lesions are erythematous, often hyperpigmented, lichenified, alopecic, and scaly. Microscopic lesions consist of hyperkeratosis, focal parakeratosis, variable spongiotic pustular dermatitis, acanthosis, and the presence of *M. pachydermatis.* Because *Malassezia* organisms may be present in low number in animals without cutaneous lesions, identification of at least 3 to 5 yeasts per high-power field is considered necessary to implicate the yeast in lesion development (Fig. 11-37).

Subcutaneous Mycoses

Subcutaneous mycoses are caused by fungi that invade cutaneous and subcutaneous tissues after traumatic implantation. Some infections remain localized, but others

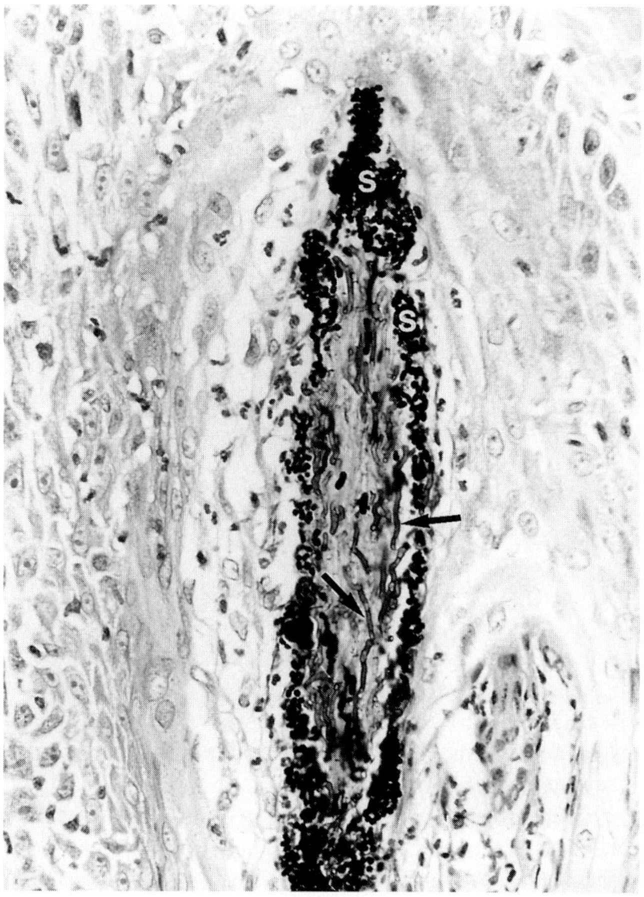

Figure 11-36 Skin, haired; dog. Dermatophyte infection involving hair follicle. Note spores *(S)* along periphery and hyphae *(arrows)* within hair shaft. The hair loss is due to breakage of hair shafts and loss of hair shafts from inflamed follicles. Gomori methenamine-silver (GMS)–H & E counterstain.

spread to the lymph vessels. Diseases in this general category include eumycotic mycetomas, subcutaneous phaeohyphomycosis, sporotrichosis, subcutaneous zygomycosis, and pythiosis (not a true fungus). The gross appearance of subcutaneous mycoses and deep granulomatous infections caused by bacteria are similar; usually one or more nodular areas ulcerate and have draining fistulas (Fig. 11-38). Microscopically, the subcutaneous mycoses consist of nodular to coalescing, suppurative, pyogranulomatous, or granulomatous inflammation.

Eumycotic mycetomas occur most often in horses and dogs and are rare fungal infections resulting in tumorlike enlargements that consist of granulomatous inflammation. *Curvularia geniculata* is the most commonly isolated fungus in animals; other fungal genera include *Madurella* and *Acremonium.* The exudate of mycetomas has granules that vary in size, shape, color, and texture. Microscopically, the hyphae are septate, branching, and may be located within an acellular matrix.

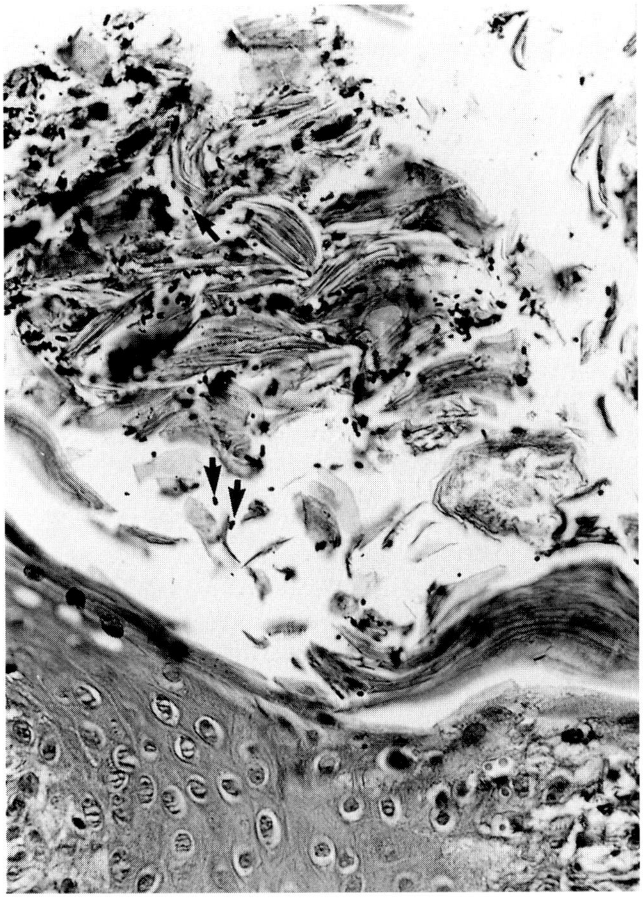

Figure 11-37 Skin, haired; dog. *Malassezia*-associated dermatitis. Stratum corneum with numerous *M. pachydermatis* organisms. The *Malassezia* are bilobed ("peanut"-shaped *[arrows]*). GMS stain.

Dermatophytic pseudomycetoma is a rare deep dermal and subcutaneous infection by *Microsporum canis* that develops predominantly in Persian cats, suggesting the possibility of a specific genetic deficit in natural or specific immunity in this breed. Gross lesions are similar to other subcutaneous mycoses. Microscopically, aggregates of fungal hyphae with irregular dilations are found within the subfollicular dermis or subcutis associated with a granulomatous inflammatory response. Hair shafts within adjacent follicles contain *Microsporum* hyphae and spores.

Phaeohyphomycosis is a mycotic infection caused by species of pigmented fungi (dematiaceous) of a variety of genera that have dark-walled, septate hyphae. Genera include *Alternaria, Drechslera, Exophiala,* and *Phialophora.* Subcutaneous phaeohyphomycosis occurs in cats (see Fig. 11-38), cattle, horses, and, rarely, dogs.

Sporotrichosis, caused by *Sporothrix schenckii,* is an uncommon mycosis that occurs in cutaneous, cutaneous–lymph vessel, and disseminated forms in horses, mules, cattle, cats, and dogs. Cutaneous nodules ulcerate and fistulae may develop at the site of traumatic implantation and along lymph vessels (lymphangitis), but visceral dissemination is uncommon. Organisms occur as ovoid to elongate (cigar-shaped) bodies and are often sparsely distributed and difficult to find, except in cats, where organisms are numerous. The exudate containing organisms is infectious to human beings if introduced into cutaneous wounds.

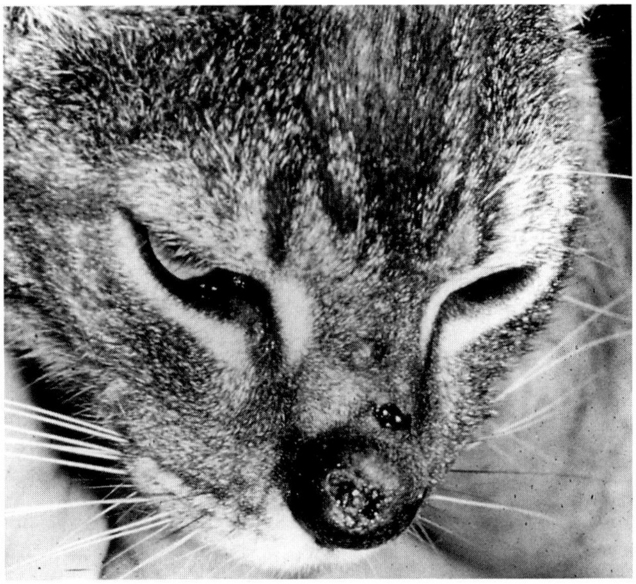

Figure 11-38 Skin, nose; cat. Phaeohyphomycosis infection of nasal planum and dorsum of muzzle. Swelling and ulcerated areas are present. Exudate may drain from ulcerated areas. *Courtesy of Dr. A. Werner.*

Zygomycosis (phycomycosis) and **oomycosis (pythiosis)** are cutaneous infections with hyphae or hyphal-like structures caused by two classes of organisms, the Zygomycetes (kingdom Fungi) and the Oomycetes (kingdom Protista). Infection with both classes of organisms is more common in tropical or subtropical climates, including the Gulf Coast of the United States. These infections are characterized clinically by proliferative, sometimes destructive, erythematous nodular lesions that ulcerate and drain (Fig. 11-39). A unique gross feature is yellow, friable, fragments of necrotic tissue and hyphae that can be dislodged from the lesions. Histologically, hyphae or hyphal-like structures are in areas of eosinophilic to pyogranulomatous inflammation, but may not be readily visible in H & E–stained sections; special stains such as Gomori's methenamine silver stain may be required to demonstrate the organisms. Differentiation between zygomycosis and pythiosis requires culture, and is therapeutically important as infections with Zygomycetes (true fungi) may be responsive to antifungal treatment, whereas infections with Oomycetes are not.

Zygomycosis refers to dermal and subcutaneous infections caused by *Basidiobolus* sp. and *Conidiobolus* sp., saprophytic fungi that gain entry to the body by inhalation or traumatic implantation by wounds or insects. Most *Basidiobolus* sp. infections have been seen in the horse; infections with *Conidiobolus* sp. have been seen in dogs, llamas, sheep, and horses. Systemic dissemination of *Conidiobolus* sp. has developed in the dog and sheep. Oomycosis refers to dermal and subcutaneous infection by *Pythium insidiosum,* which most often affects the skin of the limbs and trunk of dogs, horses, cattle, and cats. Pythiosis in the dog is a rapidly progressive, debilitating, and often fatal disease seen most often in young, large-breed dogs. Many cases of pythiosis are seen in conjunction to exposure to freestanding water.

Systemic Mycoses

The lungs are almost invariably the primary portal of entry and infection in the systemic mycoses, but cutaneous and subcutaneous infections can occur as part of the disseminated disease or by direct implantation of fungi by trauma.

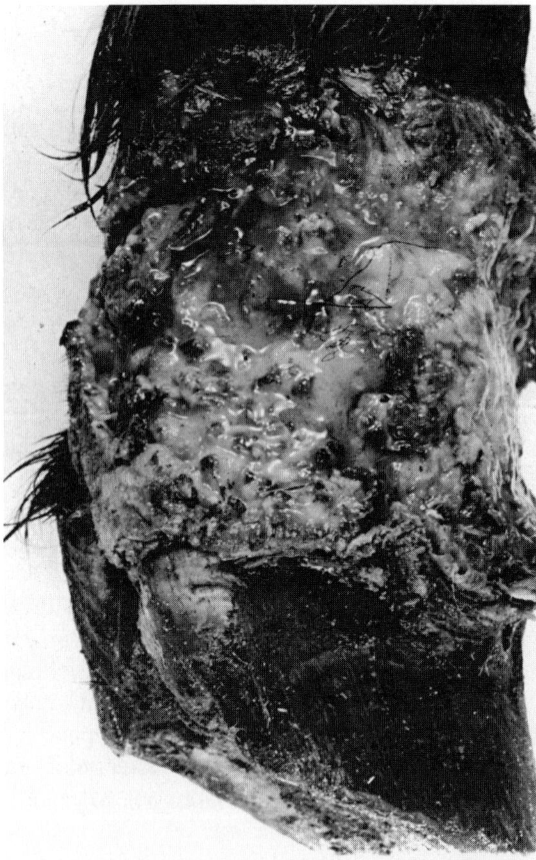

Figure 11-39 Skin, distal leg; horse. Pythiosis. Ulcerative, proliferative, destructive, draining lesion containing necrotic material. *Courtesy of University of Florida Clinical Dermatology Service.*

Systemic mycoses include blastomycosis, coccidioidomycosis, cryptococcosis, and histoplasmosis. Infections with these fungi may occur in hosts with apparently normal immune function. Grossly, one or more nodular areas may ulcerate and have draining fistulas. Histopathologically, the lesions are granulomas or pyogranulomas. Cryptococcosis may have a granulomatous response, but generally the inflammation is less severe than with the other fungi. The cryptococcal organisms have a mucinous capsule that does not stain with H & E. When inflammation is mild, the capsules of the numerous organisms in a lesion give the tissues a multicystic appearance microscopically. Cytology or microscopy are required for diagnosis. The morphologic features of the organisms (including mucicarmine-positive capsule) are sufficient for diagnosis.

Algal Infections

Protothecosis is a rare infection of animals caused by achloric (colorless) alga of the genus *Prototheca.* Grossly, the lesions are nodular, and the microscopic pattern is nodular to diffuse granulomatous dermatitis and panniculitis. The organisms can be identified in tissues by the characteristic endospores especially when stained with Gomori's methenamine silver stain, or by immunohistochemistry or culture.

Parasitic Infections

Ectoparasites include mites and ticks (which have eight legs), and lice, fleas, and flies (which have six legs). The presence of these ectoparasites is called an infestation. Endoparasites causing cutaneous lesions include nematodes, trematodes, and protozoa, and their presence is called an infection. Parasites cause a number of untoward effects including damage to hides and predisposition to secondary infection. Arthropod parasites (jointed limbs) also serve as vectors of bacterial, spirochetal, helminthic, rickettsial, protozoal, and viral infections. Cutaneous reaction to parasites varies with parasite number, location, feeding habits, and host immune response. The cutaneous reaction is often mediated in part by immune mechanisms (hypersensitivity).

Mites

Mite infestations cause serious cutaneous lesions in domestic animals and may cause economic loss in food animals. Sheep in the United States are free of mite infestation except for *Demodex* sp. and *Psoroptes* sp. Cattle, however, can be infested with mites of *Sarcoptes, Psoroptes,* and *Chorioptes* genera, which are reportable diseases. Mite infestations can also cause serious cutaneous diseases in dogs, cats, and pigs. In *Sarcoptes scabiei* infestation, mites may be difficult to find, except for infestation of the external ears of pigs. *Demodex* sp. mites are normally inhabitants of hair follicles and sebaceous glands of all domestic species. Identification of large numbers of adult mites or an increased number of immature mites is required for diagnosis of demodicosis.

Demodicosis is caused by host-specific mites; it is a major problem in dogs but is uncommon in other animals. Most species of *Demodex* mites live in the lumens of hair follicles or sebaceous glands. Transmission from dams to offspring occurs during nursing. Canine demodicosis is caused by *D. canis* and occurs in two clinical forms, localized and generalized, both of which are more common in juvenile dogs.

Purebred dogs of many breeds are predisposed to infestation, suggesting an inherited basis for the disease related to a primary deficit in cell-mediated immunity. Secondary immunodeficiency due to T-cell suppression is also associated with demodicosis. The secondary immunodeficiency improves as the demodicosis resolves. Results of studies conflict as to whether this immunodeficiency is due to the accompanying bacterial infection or to the mites. Demodicosis occurs in adult animals with underlying metabolic disorders (hypothyroidism, hyperadrenocorticism) or given therapeutic regimens (glucocorticoids or cytotoxic drugs) that may compromise the immune system. Idiopathic cases also occur.

Grossly, localized demodicosis consists of one to several small scaly, erythematous, alopecic, areas on the face or forelegs (Fig. 11-40). Generalized demodicosis usually involves large areas of the body; lesions consist of larger coalescing patches of erythema, alopecia, scales, and crusts. The microscopic lesions include epidermal hyperkeratosis, lymphoplasmacytic perifolliculitis (Fig. 11-41), focal mild degeneration of follicular basal cells, follicular pigmentary incontinence, and intraluminal mites. Sebaceous gland inflammation may also occur. Perifollicular granulomas with portions of mites are often seen. Staphylococcal folliculitis and furunculosis may complicate demodicosis and, in severe cases, cellulitis with lymphadenitis and septicemia may develop.

In cats, demodicosis is rare and caused by two species of mites, one *(Demodex cati)* lives in follicles and sebaceous glands, and the other (as yet unnamed) resides on the skin surface. Lesions associated with *D. cati* are usually localized unless the immune response is compromised as in feline retroviral infections. The most common sign associated with the presence of the unnamed species of *Demodex* mite is pruritus resulting in symmetric alopecia. The unnamed species is contagious between cats, and there is an asymptomatic carrier state. Demodicosis in cattle and goats is of little clinical significance, but extensive infection can damage hides by development of multifocal nodules in the skin of shoulders, neck, and face, or in a more generalized distribution.

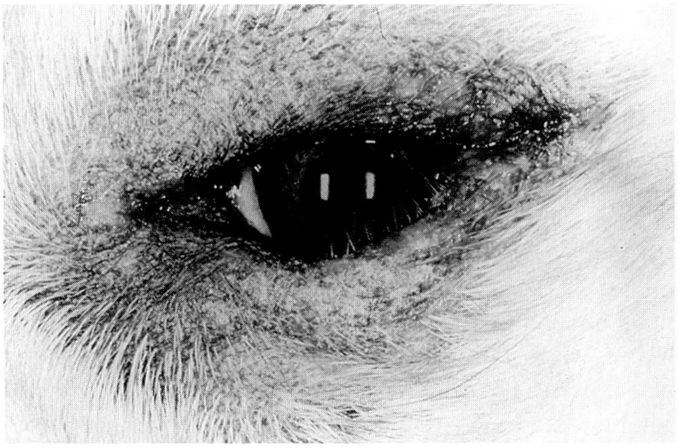

Figure 11-40 Skin, periocular; dog. Localized demodicosis. Skin is alopecic, swollen, lichenified, and hyperpigmented.

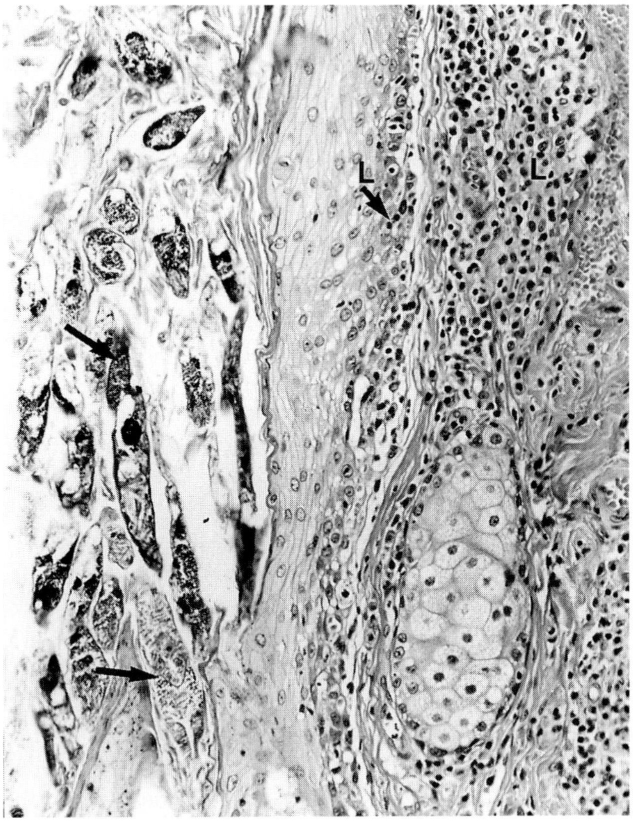

Figure 11-41 Skin, haired; dog. Localized demodicosis. Lymphocytic perifolliculitis is present (lymphocytes *short arrow [L]* are in the follicular wall and perifollicular dermis), and elongated *Demodex canis* mites *(long arrows)* are in the follicular lumen. H & E stain.

Scabies is caused by *Sarcoptes scabiei.* This highly contagious mite is the most important ectoparasite of pigs, is common in dogs, and is uncommon to rare in horses, cattle, sheep, goats, and cats. The mites burrow in tunnels in the stratum corneum and cause intense pruritus due principally to hypersensitivity reactions, although irritation from secretions also plays a role. Lesions begin on the external ears, head, and neck, and may become generalized. Gross lesions include erythematous macules, papules, crusts, and excoriations. Chronic lesions are scaly, lichenified, and hairless. Microscopically, early lesions consist of superficial perivascular dermatitis with eosinophils, mast cells, and lymphocytes. Mild focal spongiosis may be seen. Small parakeratotic crusts may develop as spongiotic lesions age. Chronic lesions are associated with epidermal acanthosis, compact hyperkeratosis, parakeratosis, crusting, and perivascular dermatitis with eosinophils, mast cells, and lymphocytes. In areas of excoriation, neutrophils and dermal scarring may be evident. Mites, mite eggs, or feces may be found in tunnels in the stratum corneum, but are not commonly seen in tissue sections due to small numbers of mites.

Notoedric mite infestation, caused by *Notoedres cati,* the sarcoptiform mite of cats, is a rare but highly contagious, pruritic disease characterized initially by an erythematous papular rash followed by scales, crusts, and alopecia with lichenification when chronic. Lesions begin on the neck and pinnae and extend to the head, face, and paws and may become generalized. Microscopic lesions consist of epidermal hyperplasia, mild spongiosis, crusts, and superficial perivascular dermatitis with eosinophils.

Otodectic mite infestation caused by *Otodectes cynotis* occurs in the external ear canals of carnivores and occasionally may be present on other parts of the body. Hence, it is important to differentiate *Otodectes* from *Sarcoptes* and *Notoedres* mites.

Psoroptic mite infestation in sheep, cattle, horses, goats, rabbits, and other animals is caused by several species of host specific mites. *Psoroptes cuniculi* infests the external ear canals of rabbits, horses, goats, and sheep. *Psoroptes equi* infests the base of the mane and tail and skin under the forelock of horses. *Psoroptes ovis* causes serious disease in cattle and sheep, producing parasitic lesions of thickened skin and dry scales and crusts that begin on the withers and spread because of persistent self-inflicted trauma. In sheep, psoroptic mite infestation is called "sheep scab." Lesions develop on the withers and sides. The wooled areas are chiefly involved with crusts that become adherent to the matted fleece and in time expand and coalesce. Damage is due to self-inflicted trauma, resulting from the pruritus associated with irritant and hypersensitivity reactions. The microscopic lesion is a spongiotic, hyperplastic, or exudative superficial perivascular dermatitis with eosinophils.

Chorioptic mite infestation, caused by host-specific mites, develop in cattle, horses, goats, and, in some countries, sheep. Mites on the skin surface produce gross lesions of erythematous, papular, crusted, scaly, hairless, thickened skin on the lower hind limbs, scrotum, tail, perineum, udder, and thigh of cattle; lower limbs of horses; scrotum and lower hind limbs of sheep; and lower limbs, hindquarters, and abdomen of goats.

Cheyletiellosis, caused by infestation with *Cheyletiella* sp., occurs in dogs, cats, rabbits, wild animals, and human beings. In dogs and cats, lesions consist of hyperkeratosis manifested as dry, white, scaly dandruff along the back. Some infestations are asymptomatic. Cats may have focal, multifocal, to generalized red papules or crusts, characterized microscopically by a superficial perivascular dermatitis with eosinophils.

Psorergatic mite infestation, caused by *Psorergates ovis,* occurs in sheep in Australia, New Zealand, South Africa, and Argentina. Sheep in the United States have been free of *Psorergates* sp. mites since 1973. Suspected cases of psorergatic mange should be reported to the state veterinarian. The infestation initially results in papules and scales along the trunk. Over time, the fleece becomes ragged as severe pruritus leads to secondary crusts, lichenification, and hyperpigmentation with alopecia.

Trombiculidiasis, is infestation by harvest mites (chiggers). The larvae tunnel into the epidermis and inject saliva that gels to form a characteristic stylostome used to obtain digested tissue fluids. Grossly, small red papules or crusts containing several orange to red larvae develop on parts of the skin in close contact with plants or the ground. Lesions are intensely pruritic. The microscopic lesions are a hyperplastic, superficial perivascular dermatitis with eosinophils, mast cells, and intraepidermal mites. The microscopic identification of a stylostome is pathognomonic.

Ticks

Ticks, both soft (argasid) and hard (ixodid), cause injury by loss of blood (producing anemia), by irritation due to bites, by hypersensitivity reactions, by acting as vectors of other diseases, by causing tick paralysis and toxicosis, and by predisposing to secondary bacterial disease and myiasis. Local cutaneous reactions vary in severity with the tick and its secretions, and host resistance. Gross lesions consist of focal erosions, erythema, and crusted ulcers with alopecia and nodules in some individuals. Microscopic lesions include epidermal and dermal necrosis, and perivascular to diffuse inflammation at the margins of the necrotic area; the exudate is composed of eosinophils, macrophages, and lymphocytes. In a section of skin parallel to hair shafts, lesions are triangular in shape with the apex at the panniculus. Some lesions are granulomas (arthropod bite granuloma) in which the inflammatory cells efface the tissue architecture and are

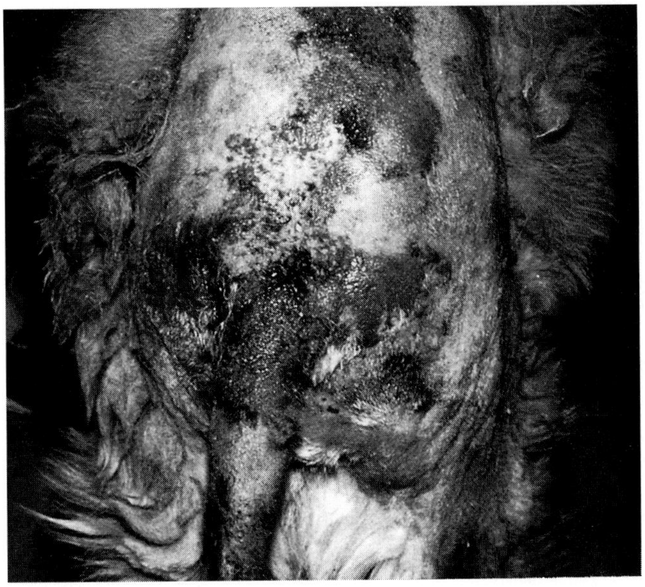

Figure 11-42 Skin, haired; dog. Pyotraumatic dermatitis (acute moist dermatitis). Erosion, moist exudate, and crusting are present over rump of a dog with flea bite hypersensitivity (hair has been clipped). *Courtesy of Dr. B. Baker.*

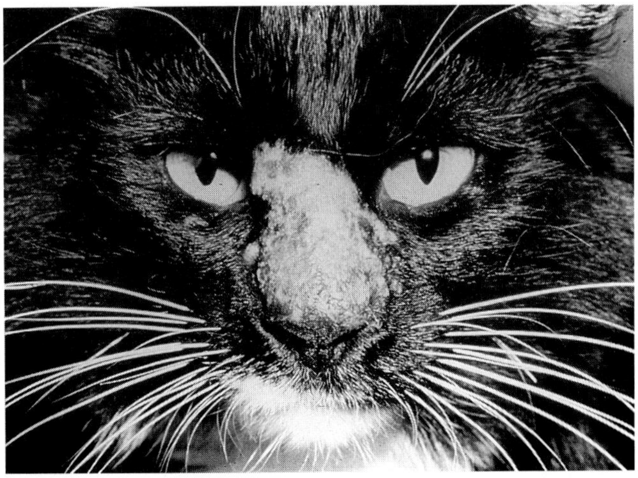

Figure 11-43 Skin, face; cat. Mosquito bite hypersensitivity. Alopecia, depigmentation, and swelling are present in skin of the dorsum of muzzle. *Courtesy of Dr. A. Werner.*

interspersed among collagenous fibers and lymphoid follicles. Cutaneous basophil hypersensitivity likely contributes to the reactions induced by tick bites.

Lice

Pediculosis, or infestation with lice, causes anemia, weakness, damage to hair and wool, and discomfort. Biting lice, feeding more on epithelial cellular debris and less on blood, cause less severe systemic signs than sucking lice. Pediculosis occurs more commonly in winter when temperatures are cooler, the wool or hair coat is longer, animals are congregated, and the plane of nutrition is lower. Infestations are relatively host specific, are spread by direct contact, and are relatively easy to control because the life cycle takes place entirely on the host. Pediculosis in swine is an economically important disease as the lice transmit *Eperythrozoon suis,* and the viruses of swinepox and African swine fever. Primary lesions caused by lice are few, and most are secondary to scratching. Gross lesions consist of papules, crusts, and secondary excoriations with lice and eggs visible in the lesions. Animals infested with sucking lice may be anemic.

Fleas

Flea infestation is principally a problem in dogs and cats. Fleas can cause severe skin irritation due to frequent biting and release of enzymes, anticoagulants, and histamine-like substances, hypersensitivity reactions to saliva, and secondary host-inflicted trauma from scratching and biting (Fig. 11-42). Severe infestations may cause blood loss (anemia) especially in puppies, kittens, or small debilitated adults. Lesions occur over the dorsal lumbosacral region, caudomedial thighs, ventral abdomen, flanks, and, in cats the neck area, and consist of multiple red papules and secondary excoriations. *Ctenocephalides felis* is the most common flea causing infestation in dogs and cats, and it also transmits *Dipylidium caninum.*

Flies

Cutaneous reactions due to fly bites may be minor to severe and are due to bites by adult flies and to myiasis by larvae. Reactions to the bites of flies vary and include irritation, anemia, direct toxicity, and hypersensitivity. Biting flies include *Haematobia irritans* (horn fly), *Stomoxys calcitrans* (stable fly), and horse flies, deer flies, black flies, biting gnats, and mosquitoes. The sheep ked *(Melophagus ovinus)* is another common ectoparasite that sucks blood. Lesions of biting flies are due to local irritation and include wheals and papules centered around a puncture wound that may bleed. Such lesions may persist with hair loss, scales, hemorrhagic crusts, erythema, and secondary excoriations due to self-inflicted trauma, especially if the animals are hypersensitive to the bites. Such hypersensitivity occurs with *Culicoides* sp. in horses (Queensland itch, sweet itch), and mosquitoes in cats (Fig. 11-43). Microscopic lesions associated with fly bites vary depending on the fly involved. Dermal hemorrhage and edema with a central area of epidermal necrosis ("nibble mark") are early lesions seen with bites of some flies. Hemorrhagic crust covers areas of necrosis, and perivascular neutrophilic, eosinophilic, and mixed mononuclear inflammation may be seen. Intraepidermal eosinophils including eosinophilic pustules may be identified, and eosinophilic folliculitis and furunculosis may be present in reactions to mosquito bites. Epidermal hyperplasia, hyperkeratosis, parakeratosis, and crusting are associated with self-trauma.

Myiasis is infestation of tissues by the larvae of dipterous flies (flies with two wings or winglike appendages) and is a disease of neglect occurring in moist areas of the body soiled by urine, feces, or bodily secretions. Flies are attracted by the odor of such areas. Sheep (ovine fleece rot) are most commonly affected. In myiasis due to blow flies (calliphorids) and flesh flies (sarcophagids), eggs are deposited on soiled hair or wool or in wounds. Grossly, matted hair or wool and multiple irregular cutaneous holes or ulcers with an offensive odor are observed. Lesions may become extensive due to the secretion of proteolytic enzymes by larvae. Death may occur and is due to septicemia or toxemia.

In **cuterebra myiasis,** *Cuterebra* sp. eggs are deposited on stones or vegetation and young animals (rabbits, rodents, and, less often, cats and dogs) become infested by contact with the eggs. Nodules containing larvae are located in the subcutis and are associated with an opening in the skin for respiration by the larvae.

In **hypoderma myiasis,** larvae of *Hypoderma lineatum* and *H. bovis* penetrate the skin of the legs of cattle and less frequently horses and bison and migrate proximally in the subcutis of the leg. The larvae may be found in many areas of the body. After weeks to months, first-stage larvae reach the esophagus *(H. lineatum)* or vertebral canal *(H. bovis)* where they grow to become second-stage larvae, and then migrate to the subcutis of the back where they become established in subcutaneous nodules (Fig. 11-44), similar to those of *Cuterebra* sp. with an opening for respiration, and mature to third-stage larvae. Microscopically, these larvae are located in a cavity filled with fibrin and a few eosinophils and bordered by granulation tissue containing clusters of eosinophils.

Screwworm myiasis, caused by *Cochliomyia* sp. and *Chrysomyia* sp., is an important disease in domestic and wild animals. The disease occurs in Africa, Asia, Central and South America, and Mexico, but has been eradicated in the United States and nearly so in Mexico. Screwworm flies deposit larvae in wounds or near mucocutaneous junctions of living animals. The larvae penetrate and feed on tissues liquefied by secretions of proteolytic enzymes. Grossly, malodorous wounds contain larvae and shreds of tissue. Death may occur in untreated animals. When it is necessary to differentiate screwworm myiasis from cutaneous myiasis caused by other flies, larvae can be preserved in 70% alcohol and submitted for identification. Screwworm myiasis is a reportable disease in some countries, including the United States.

Helminths

Cutaneous infections with helminths are generally not life threatening but may be unsightly and irritating in companion animals and cause hide damage in food animals. Infections are due to migration of helminth larvae that as adults live in noncutaneous sites, or by filarial infections (filarial dermatitis) in which adults or microfilaria spend some time in the skin or subcutis. Rarely, such adult helminths as *Dracunculus insignis* and *Anatrichosoma cutaneum* parasitize the skin.

Hookworm dermatitis is due to *Ancylostoma* or *Uncinaria* larvae. Red papules that coalesce and develop into lichenified alopecic areas, occur on the feet of dogs and, less frequently, on other areas in contact with an unsanitary environment contaminated by hookworm larvae. Footpads may become soft, the keratinized portion may separate, and secondary bacterial dermatitis and

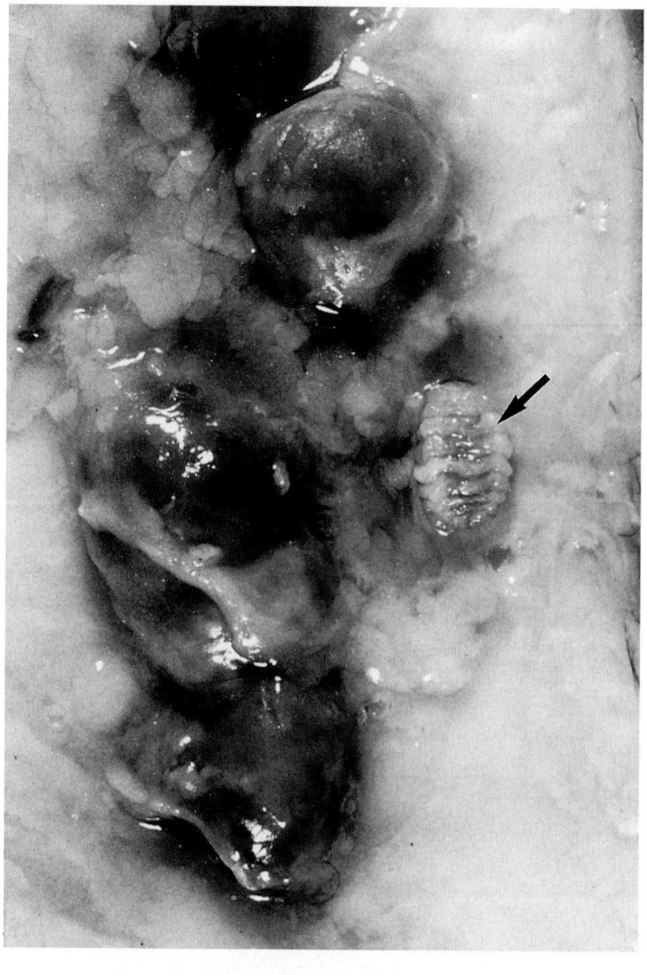

Figure 11-44 Skin, subcutis; cow. *Hypoderma* species larvae. Multiple nodules each containing a single larva are present. One nodule is incised, exposing a larva *(arrow)*.

paronychia may develop. Hyperplastic spongiotic perivascular dermatitis with eosinophils, serocellular crusts, and migration tracks are the principal lesions. Parasitologic evaluation of fresh tissue may allow larval identification.

Cutaneous habronemiasis (summer sores) occurs in horses and is caused by infection with the larvae of *Habronema* sp. or *Draschia* sp. deposited on the skin by house or stable flies. Larval deposition and lesions occur on parts of the body where the skin is either traumatized, such as the legs, or moist and soft, such as the medial canthus of the eye (Fig. 11-45) and prepuce. Larvae are unable to penetrate normal skin, but the fly bites cause sufficient damage to allow larval penetration. Grossly, single or multiple, proliferative, ulcerated red to brown, tumorous masses are present that on section have small, yellow to white, gritty foci. The microscopic lesion is a nodular dermatitis with eosinophils, epithelioid macrophages, and, sometimes, giant cells bordering larvae or necrotic debris. Granulation tissue infiltrated by neutrophils is present on the ulcerated surface.

Other helminth parasites associated with cutaneous larval migration include *Pelodera, Necator, Strongyloides, Gnathostoma,* and *Bunostomum*. Schistosome cercariae, especially of birds, can cause similar lesions.

Onchocerciasis is a filarial dermatitis principally affecting horses. The prevalence of the disease has been reduced by the use of a new class of antiparasitic agents, the avermectins. Microfilaria, transmitted by intermediate hosts such as the Simuliidae (black flies, gnats) and Ceratopogonidae (biting midges), may be present without significant dermal inflammation. Differences in lesion severity may reflect different degrees of hypersensitivity to microfilaria or hypersensitivity to the bites of the intermediate hosts. Adult parasites are located in nodules in connective tissue, and microfilaria are located in the dermis, particularly of the ventral midline. In equine onchocerciasis, lesions develop on the head, neck, medial forelimbs, ventral thorax, and abdomen. Gross lesions consist of patchy to diffuse alopecia, erythema, scaling, crusting, and pigmentary changes. Some horses have a characteristic, variably pigmented, circular area of dermatitis on the forehead. Keratitis, conjunctivitis, and uveitis are observed in some horses. Microscopic cutaneous lesions vary from none to a superficial and deep perivascular dermatitis with eosinophils, lymphocytes, and microfilariae.

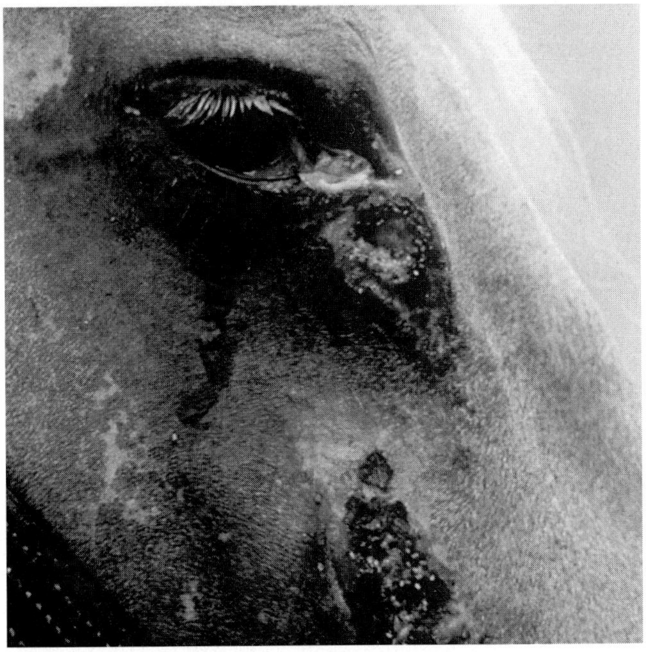

Figure 11-45 Skin, face, horse. Cutaneous habronemiasis. Ulcerated, nodular, draining lesions involve the medial canthus of the eye and the skin ventral to the eye. Fly bites have damaged the soft tissue near the eye and allowed larval penetration in the damaged skin. *Courtesy Dr. Valerie Fadok.*

Stephanofilariasis, a filarial dermatitis of cattle, buffalo, and goats, is transmitted by flies and caused by six species of parasites of the genus *Stephanofilaria*. Each species causes lesions in a different body location. *Stephanofilaria stilesi* occurs in cattle in the United States and causes lesions along the ventral midline that consist initially of small (1 cm) circular patches with moist erect hairs, foci of epidermal hemorrhage, and serum exudation. Such foci expand and coalesce into a large area covered by crusts, which upon healing, consist of thickened hairless plaques as large as 25 cm in diameter. Microscopic lesions are a superficial and deep perivascular dermatitis with eosinophils, epidermal hyperkeratosis, parakeratosis, acanthosis with spongiosis, eosinophilic microabscesses, and crust. Adult parasites and microfilaria may be seen. Lesions are caused by a reaction to the parasites free in the dermis, to the bites of the flies serving as the vector, and in some cases, self-inflicted trauma. Other causes of filarial dermatitis include *Elaeophora* sp., *Parafilaria* sp., *Suifilaria* sp., and rarely *Dirofilaria* sp. *Parafilaria bovicola* infection in cattle has increased in Europe; lesions consist of hemorrhagic nodules in the subcutis containing adult parasites. These may rupture and bleed.

Protozoa

In the United States, cutaneous protozoal infections may develop as part of systemic infections, principally with *Leishmania*. Leishmaniasis is caused by a variety of species of the family Trypanosomatidae. The disease, which can occur in cutaneous, mucocutaneous, or visceral forms, is rare in animals in the United States except in endemic areas in Oklahoma and Texas. It is endemic in Mediterranean countries and some other parts of the world. Infections in dogs, cats, and horses have been reported. Many cases in the United States have been associated with foreign travel of people and their animals. Sandflies serve as the vector for infection of animals; dogs, cats, and rodents serve as reservoirs of infection for human beings. *Leishmania* organisms are found principally in monocytes and macrophages of the spleen, bone marrow, less often the liver, and rarely cells in peripheral blood. Cutaneous lesions in dogs consist of generalized alopecia with silvery white scales, or more severe lesions of nodules and ulcers. Lesions occur chiefly in anatomic areas where sandflies feed—around the muzzle, ears, and eyes. Microscopically, lesions include hyperkeratosis, parakeratosis, crusts, and granulomatous nodules in the periadnexal dermis. Accumulations of macrophages along with fewer lymphocytes and plasma cells may efface sebaceous glands. Organisms may be intracellular or extracellular.

IMMUNOLOGIC SKIN DISEASES

General

Immunologic diseases are classified as either hypersensitivity (allergic) or autoimmune. Hypersensitivity is a mild to severe reaction that develops in response to normally harmless foreign compounds including antiserum, hormones, pollen, and insect venoms. Autoimmune diseases develop when antibodies or T cells react against self-antigens, rather than against foreign antigens. "Autoimmune disease" in this section is a general term referring to a spectrum of diseases in which autoimmune mechanisms appear to participate in lesion production. Four basic immune reactions, types I, II, III, and IV, mediate the tissue damage in hypersensitivity and autoimmune diseases. Another reaction, cutaneous basophil hypersensitivity, is less well characterized, but may be operative in some hypersensitivity reactions such as flea allergy in dogs. Most cutaneous hypersensitivity reactions are mediated either by type I or type IV reactions, or by a combination of one or more of the four reactions. Autoimmune mechanisms tend to be mediated by type II or III reactions, although more than one mechanism may be involved. Hypersensitivity reactions are common in dogs and horses, less common in cats, and are uncommon in food animals. Autoimmune diseases with cutaneous manifestations are uncommon in domestic animals, accounting for 1% to 2% of dermatoses in most species. Of the cutaneous autoimmune disorders, pemphigus foliaceus is the most prevalent, followed in incidence by discoid and systemic lupus erythematosus. In domestic animals, certain breeds of dogs, horses, and cats seem to be predisposed to develop particular autoimmune diseases.

Mechanisms of Tissue Damage

Type I Reactions

These inflammatory reactions are mediated by preformed or newly synthesized pharmacologically active substances that are released by mast cells and basophils following reaction between antigen and specific antibody (usually IgE) bound to receptors on the membrane of the mast cells or basophils. Preformed substances released from mast cells include histamine, factors chemotactic for eosinophils and neutrophils, prostaglandins, serine esterases, and TNF-α. Substances synthesized upon mast cell stimulation include leukotrienes, cytokines, and platelet-activating factor. Type I hypersensitivity can be systemic (anaphylaxis) or local or both and in the skin may result in pruritic, circumscribed wheals with raised, erythematous borders. The reaction occurs in two phases, immediate (15 to 30 minutes) and late (6 to 12 hours), and is generally referred to as an immediate hypersensitivity reaction. The eosinophil products, major basic protein and eosinophil cationic protein, are toxic to epithelial cells and contribute to tissue damage in the late-phase reaction. The production of IgE is genetically controlled, and therefore, inherited predispositions to type I hypersensitivity occur. Cutaneous type I hypersensitivity reactions include atopic dermatitis (most common), urticaria, and angioedema, and hypersensitivity associated with bites of flies such as *Culicoides* sp., with mites such as *Sarcoptes* sp., with gastrointestinal parasites, and with ingestion of dietary components (proteins, grains, preservatives, and so on). This type of reaction is characterized microscopically by capillary dilation, edema, mast cell degranulation, and infiltrates of eosinophils.

Type II Reactions

Type II hypersensitivity reactions are dependent on IgG or IgM antibodies formed against either normal or altered cell membrane antigens. Cell damage occurs by either complement fixation, antibody-dependent cell-mediated cytotoxicity, or antibody-directed cellular dysfunction. The first two mechanisms are most common in type II reactions affecting the skin. Type II reactions involving the skin may be caused by deposition of autoantibody to desmosomal or hemidesmosomal proteins and are present in pemphigus (uncommon) and bullous pemphigoid (rare). The lesions vary with the location of the target antigen; in pemphigus and pemphigoid, vesicles develop either within the epidermis or subepidermally.

Type III Reactions

These reactions are mediated by immune complexes formed in the circulation or in tissues. Immune complexes are often deposited in vessel walls and result in complement fixation and in the generation of cytokines and leukotactic factors, leading to vasculitis. Tissue damage results from lysosomal enzymes released from neutrophils, activation of complement and coagulation systems, platelet aggregation, and free oxygen radicals. Immune complex vasculitis may be responsible for the purpura seen in infections with *Streptococcus equi*. Lesions of systemic lupus erythematosus are due to immune complex deposition. The lesions of familial canine dermatomyositis may be associated with immune complexes.

Type IV Reactions

Type IV reactions are mediated by sensitized $CD4^+$ (helper) T cells in the case of delayed-type hypersensitivity or by $CD8^+$ (cytotoxic) T cells in the case of cellular cytotoxicity. The delayed-type reaction is mediated by sensitized T cells which, after contacting a specific antigen, release lymphokines (cytokines) and/or recruit other lymphocytes and macrophages. The reaction is largely dependent on IL-2 and interferon-γ. Interferon-γ activates macrophages that work to eliminate the targeted antigen. In the cytotoxic reaction, the $CD8^+$ T cells kill the targeted host cell directly. These reactions take many hours to develop and are initiated by antigens bound to host cell major histocompatibility molecules. Type IV hypersensitivity reactions are used in the diagnosis of diseases such as tuberculosis, histoplasmosis, and coccidioidomycosis. The skin reaction typically develops 24 to 48 hours after exposure to the specific antigen and consists of perivascular mononuclear cell accumulations and dermal edema.

Combination Reactions

The strict categorization of hypersensitivity reactions is an oversimplification. Categories and lesions may overlap, and there are species differences. Hypersensitivity to fleas, ticks, *Staphylococcus* sp., hormones, and drugs are mediated by a combination of types I, II, III, or IV reactions. Therefore, histopathologic examination may provide the general category of inflammatory reaction pattern and rule out other disease processes but may not lead to a diagnosis of the specific hypersensitivity present.

Hypersensitivity Reactions

Atopy

In atopy (atopic dermatitis, allergic inhalant dermatitis), an example of a type I hypersensitivity reaction, the skin is the major target organ in dogs, cats, and horses. The route of allergen exposure has been considered to be respiratory, but percutaneous absorption may also occur, at least in dogs. Atopy is the second most common hypersensitivity dermatitis in dogs and accounts for 8% to 10% of canine skin disorders. In atopic dermatitis, T cells and cytokines interact to initiate lesions, for instance, T helper type 2 (T_{H2}) cells produce IL-4 and express IL-1 receptors. IL-4 enhances T lymphocyte and mast cell multiplication. IL-3 is synergistic, particularly in the facilitation of mast cell differentiation and development. IL-4 also stimulates B lymphocytes to switch production from IgM to IgE. IgE activates mast cells. IL-1, produced by keratinocytes, is required for proliferation of T_{H2} cells. *Staphylococcus aureus* in human skin may enhance the production from keratinocytes of sufficient IL-1 to allow T_{H2} cells to become activated and produce the lesions of atopic dermatitis. In dogs, IgE and subclasses of IgG are thought to play a role. The predominant clinical sign of atopy is pruritus and, in dogs, is often manifested as face rubbing and foot licking. Clinical signs of feline atopy are varied and include those associated with facial, pinnal, or generalized pruritus, miliary dermatitis, eosinophilic granuloma complex, and symmetric alopecia. Horses may have pruritus of the head, pinnae, ventrum, legs, and tailhead or recurrent urticaria. Primary skin lesions may not be seen, and those present may be mostly the result of self-inflicted trauma. Dogs may have secondary pyoderma or seborrhea. Microscopically there is a hyperplastic superficial perivascular dermatitis with mixed populations of mast cells, nonmetachromatic mononuclear cells, and variable numbers of eosinophils. Some animals, particularly horses, have deep perivascular inflammation as well. Eosinophils are seen less frequently in dogs than other species and are the predominant inflammatory cell in horses and cats, which may also develop eosinophilic folliculitis. Diagnosis of atopy is based on clinical signs, physical examination, intradermal skin testing, and the use of the radioallergosorbent test (RAST) and the enzyme-linked immunosorbent assay (ELISA) for elevated allergen-specific IgE.

Flea Bite Hypersensitivity

The most common hypersensitivity dermatitis in dogs and cats results from flea bites and includes type I and type IV reactions and cutaneous basophil hypersensitivity. Flea bite hypersensitivity is pruritic, and cutaneous lesions occur principally along the dorsal lumbosacral area (see Fig. 11-42), ventral abdomen, caudomedial aspects of the thighs, flanks, and, in cats, around the neck, but may be generalized in highly sensitive animals. Secondary lesions are due to self-inflicted trauma. Grossly, there is a papular dermatitis with secondary excoriations, and some dogs with chronic disease have multiple firm alopecic nodules (fibropruritic nodules) in the dorsal lumbosacral area. Microscopically, flea bite hypersensitivity is characterized by hyperplastic superficial perivascular dermatitis with edema, mast cells, basophils, lymphocytes, histiocytes, and eosinophils. Intraepithelial eosinophils or nibble marks may be seen. Eosinophilic folliculitis and furunculosis may be seen in cats. In dogs, fibropruritic nodules consist of a core of coarse thick collagen bundles covered by a hyperplastic epidermis.

Culicoides Hypersensitivity

This is a common worldwide pruritic dermatitis in horses, caused principally by type I and type IV hypersensitivity reactions to salivary antigens from bites of *Culicoides* sp. Signs and lesions may be seasonal or nonseasonal depending on climate, usually develop in horses over 2 years of age, and arise in geographic areas in which the species of *Culicoides* involved feeds. Gross lesions depend on the age of the lesions and severity of pruritus. Initially lesions are papules. Pustules and nodules may develop. With self-trauma, crusts, alopecia, excoriations, and lichenification evolve. Common sites are the tail base, withers, and head. Microscopic lesions include superficial and deep perivascular dermatitis with numerous eosinophils. Some horses will have eosinophilic folliculitis, intraepidermal pustules, and eosinophilic granulomas. Older lesions have epidermal hyperplasia, hyperkeratosis, crusts, and dermal fibrosis.

Allergic Contact Dermatitis

Allergic contact dermatitis, an example of a type IV hypersensitivity reaction, is due primarily to contact with chemicals such as aniline dyes in carpets, plant resins, chemicals in shampoo, and historically to plastics in food dishes. The lesions are pruritic, resulting in self-inflicted trauma, are variable in severity, and are located in regions in contact with the antigen, typically in glabrous areas unless the antigen is a liquid or aerosol. Grossly, erythema, papules with or without vesicles, and exudation develop into crusts. Chronic lesions are lichenified, hyperpigmented, and alopecic. Microscopic lesions include spongiotic superficial perivascular dermatitis with mononuclear cells, and, when chronic, epidermal hyperplasia. Some cases have many eosinophils including eosinophilic epidermal pustules.

Hypersensitivity Reactions to Drugs

Hypersensitivity reactions to drugs are uncommon in dogs and cats, are rare in other domestic animals, and may result from any of the four types of hypersensitivity reactions. The drugs most commonly associated with hypersensitivity reactions include penicillins and trimethoprim-potentiated sulfonamides, but many drugs may cause a hypersensitivity reaction. Gross and microscopic lesions are highly varied. Microscopic lesions include different histopathologic patterns: perivascular dermatitis, lichenoid or interface dermatitis, vasculitis, vesiculopustular dermatitis, necrotizing dermatitis, panniculitis, or perforating folliculitis.

Autoimmune Reactions

Diseases Characterized by Vesicles or Bullae as the Primary Lesion

Pemphigus. This group of diseases is caused by production of autoantibodies directed against proteins responsible for keratinocyte cell-to-cell adhesion (desmosomes) or cell-to-substrate adhesion (hemidesmosomes). Desmosomes are more numerous in the more superficial layers of the epidermis and vary in protein subunit composition. Hemidesmosomes are found on the basal surface of the basal layer of the epidermis. Vesicles or bullae form within varying levels of the epidermis or at the basement membrane zone according to the location of the target antigen. Severity of clinical disease is related to the depth of bullae formation, with the more severe signs associated with separations deep within or below the epidermis. Antigen-antibody binding may result in a type II immune reaction or promote proinflammatory cytokine release from keratinocytes.

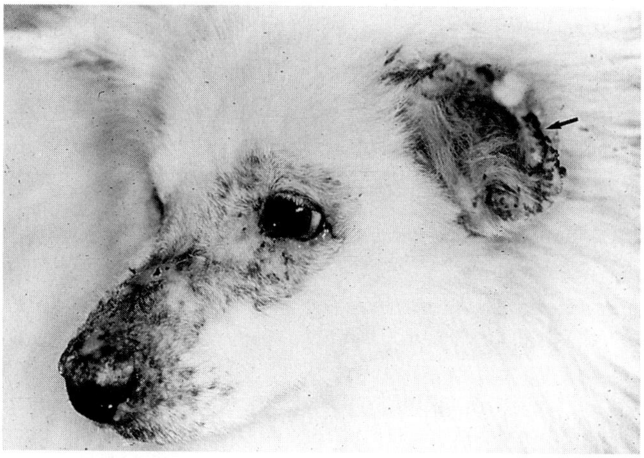

Figure 11-46 Skin, face; dog. Pemphigus foliaceus. Alopecia, focal ulcers, crusts, and depigmented areas are present on medial aspects of both pinnae *(arrow)*, periocular areas, and dorsum of muzzle including the nasal planum. These lesions are also erythematous (not evident in black and white photograph).

Pemphigus foliaceus is the most common and more mild form of pemphigus; it occurs in domestic animals and has been reported in the dog, cat, horse, and goat. Autoantibodies are formed against protein components of the desmosomes. Tissue damage leading to separation of keratinocytes (acantholysis) therefore occurs in the superficial layers of the epidermis. In the dog the desmosomal protein component, desmoglein 1, is the target of autoantibodies. The primary lesions of vesicles and pustules may be localized (muzzle, pinnae, periocular skin, footpads, nailbed, coronary band) or generalized and symmetric. The vesicles and pustules are in the superficial epidermis, covered by only a small amount of keratin or a few epidermal cells. The vesicles are therefore fragile, quickly rupture with minor mechanical pressure on the surface, and lead to secondary crusts, scales, alopecia, and superficial erosions (Figs. 11-46 and 11-47). Microscopically, subcorneal or intragranular pustules with acantholytic cells are observed in the horse (Fig. 11-8), but in the dog pustules often are in the stratum spinosum. Crusts should be included in the biopsy sample, especially if well-developed pustules or vesicles are no longer present, as laminated crusts with acantholytic cells may help establish the histologic diagnosis. Eosinophils are the predominant inflammatory cell in about one third of the canine and equine cases. **Pemphigus erythematous** is thought to be a mild form of pemphigus foliaceus with lesions restricted to the face and pinnae.

Pemphigus vulgaris is a very severe form of pemphigus and has been reported in the dog, cat, horse, and llama. In the dog, autoantibodies are formed against

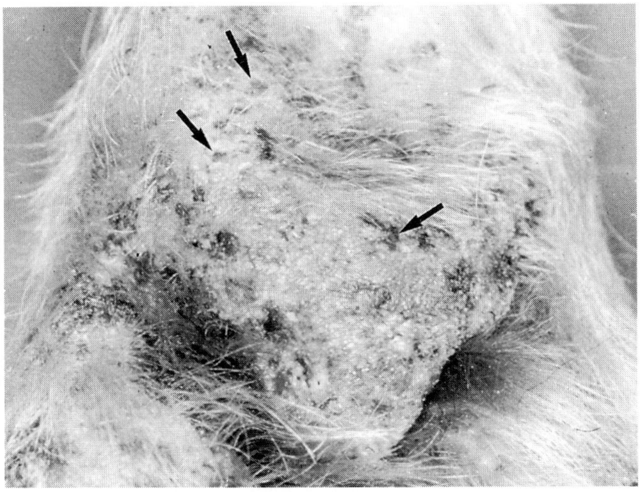

Figure 11-47 Skin, foot pad; dog (same dog as in Fig. 11-46). Pemphigus foliaceus. Erosions *(arrows)* and depigmentation are present. Crusts are also a feature of this disease, but are not present on this foot pad.

desmoglein 3, one of the prominent desmosomal proteins of basal epithelial cells. Microscopic lesions consist of a suprabasilar vesicle leaving a row of basal cells attached to the basement membrane ("row of tombstones") (see Fig. 11-9) and a superficial perivascular to interface dermatitis. Vesicles or secondary erosions and ulcers are found in the oral cavity, at mucocutaneous junctions, and skin subject to mechanical stress such as in the axilla or groin. Although there is reference to **pemphigus vegetans** in the veterinary literature, more recent studies evaluating autoantibodies to desmosomes and hemidesmosomes have not definitively documented pemphigus vegetans in animals.

Paraneoplastic pemphigus is a unique form of pemphigus documented to occur in human beings with a variety of neoplasms, in the dog in association with malignant lymphoma, and in the horse with hemangiosarcoma. This type of pemphigus is unique in that immunologic studies reveal the deposition of IgG at keratinocyte intercellular bridges and the presence of serum antibodies to a unique set of epithelial cell surface proteins. Antibodies to one particular 190-kDa epithelial cell surface protein are considered to be a marker for paraneoplastic pemphigus. Paraneoplastic pemphigus is refractory to immunosuppressive therapy, may involve both cutaneous and mucocutaneous sites, and histologically may display changes typical of erythema multiforme, the various forms of pemphigus or bullous pemphigoid. In addition, death may occur as a consequence of the cutaneous lesions before development of clinical signs directly attributed to the neoplasm.

Bullous pemphigoid (BP) is characterized by autoantibodies directed against the hemidesmosomal proteins, BPAG I and BPAGII, and more rarely to desmoplakin. The location and character of clinical lesions are similar to pemphigus vulgaris. BP has been reported in the dog and horse (Fig. 11-48). Separation of layers of the basement membrane leads to the microscopic lesions of vesicles and bullae with a roof lined by basal cells and a floor formed by the basement membrane. The bullae may contain fibrin, eosinophils, or neutrophils. A superficial perivascular to lichenoid dermatitis may also be present, particularly if ulceration has occurred.

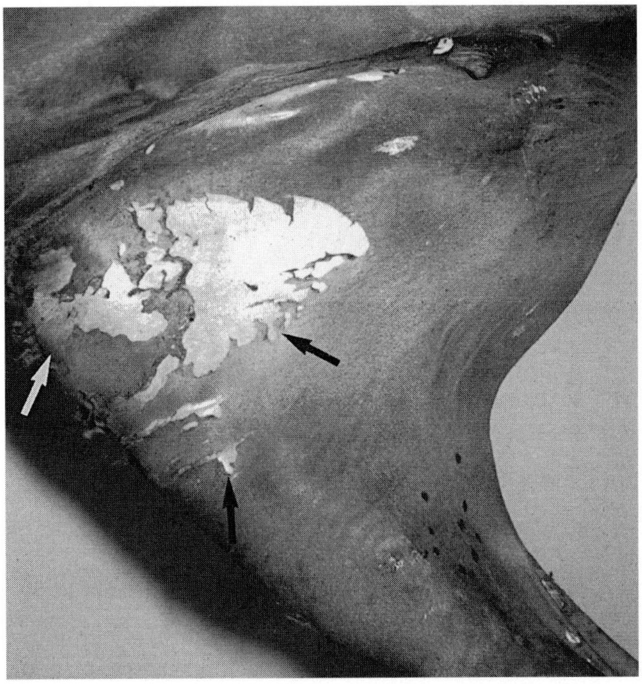

Figure 11-48 Skin, medial thigh; horse. Bullous pemphigoid–like dermatitis. The epidermis is easily separated from the underlying dermis, leading to the formation of vesicles, bullae, and large areas of ulceration. The epidermis is separating from the dermis *(arrows)*. *Courtesy of Dr. S. Terrell.*

Lupus erythematosus is recognized in two forms: systemic lupus erythematosus (SLE) and discoid lupus erythematosus (DLE). **Systemic lupus erythematosus** is a multiorgan disease of dogs and rarely cats and horses. Factors involved in development include a genetic predisposition, viral infections, hormones, and UV light. SLE is a disease of immune dysregulation, which includes defective T cell suppresser function and cytokine dysregulation. The defective T cell suppression function may be due to anti–T cell antibodies or a primary suppresser T cell deficiency. B cell hyperactivity results in the formation of autoantibodies to a variety of cells (e.g., erythrocytes, leukocytes, platelets) and to nucleic acids. Immune complexes form by antigen-antibody binding and are deposited in a variety of tissues, including skin, and result in a type III hypersensitivity response. Cutaneous lesions may be localized or generalized, commonly involve the face, pinnae, oral mucosae and distal extremities, and consist of erythema, depigmentation, alopecia, scaling, crusting, ulceration, and sometimes stomatitis or panniculitis. Microscopic lesions include a lymphohistiocytic interface dermatitis with basal cell degeneration and pigmentary incontinence. The basal cell degeneration progresses to subepidermal vesicles which progress to ulcers and crusts. Basement membrane thickening and immune complex vasculitis may also be seen.

Discoid lupus erythematosus is relatively common and is a mild variant of SLE in which there is no involvement of other organs and the antinuclear antibody titer is negative. Lesions consisting of depigmentation, erythema, scaling, erosion, ulceration, and crusting generally occur in the skin of the nasal planum, dorsum of the muzzle, and less commonly, the pinnae, lips, and periocular region, and in the oral mucosae. DLE can be exacerbated by sunlight. Microscopic lesions are lichenoid interface dermatitis often with many lymphocytes, plasma cells, basal cell degeneration, and pigmentary incontinence. As with SLE, the basal cell degeneration may lead to subepidermal vesicles, loss of the epidermis, and ulceration and crusting.

Dermatomyositis, an inherited disease with variable expressivity, occurs in juvenile and adult onset forms in collies and Shetland sheepdogs (Fig. 11-49). Other breeds are occasionally affected. Dermatomyositis may develop in puppies as early as 8 weeks of age, with lesions of a vesicular dermatitis of face, lips, and external ears, and progresses to involve the distal extremities, especially over bony prominences and the tip of the tail. Myositis and atrophy of muscles of mastication, distal extremities, and, sometimes, esophagus develop after the dermatitis. The myositis is multifocal, variably severe, and composed of lymphocytes, plasma cells, histiocytes, and fewer neutrophils or eosinophils that replace necrotic myofibers. Perifascicular myofiber atrophy (atrophy at the periphery of muscle bundles) occurs occasionally. Ultrastructurally, endothelial cells in capillaries in muscle contain inclusion bodies that resemble those produced by picorna viruses (Fig. 11-50); immune complexes seem to play a role in lesion development. The disease severity varies. Mild lesions heal without scarring, and moderate lesions heal with permanent foci of alopecia and hyperpigmentation. Lesions in biopsy samples include interface dermatitis with basal cell degeneration of the epidermis and follicular wall, variable epidermal vesicles and pustules, follicular atrophy, and dermal scarring. A cell-poor vasculitis, a significant feature of dermatomyositis is not always identified in small biopsy samples. The rostral and most superficial portion of the temporalis muscle is the biopsy site of choice to confirm the myositis.

Erythema multiforme (EM) and toxic epidermal necrolysis (TEN) are two uncommon to rare diseases affecting the skin and possibly mucous membranes. Both conditions occur as adverse drug reactions, in association with systemic infections, neoplasia, or may be idiopathic. EM has been seen in dogs, cats, horses, and cattle and is characterized clinically initially by circular areas of erythema. The erythema disappears from the center of the lesions, producing targetlike lesions that are most common on the trunk and groin. Papules, vesicles, ulcers, erosions, and serpiginous erythematous lesions also may be seen. Histologically, individual keratinocytes in all layers of the epidermis undergo apoptosis (see Fig. 11-7) and are surrounded by lymphocytes. The condition may be self-limiting. TEN is seen principally in dogs and cats and

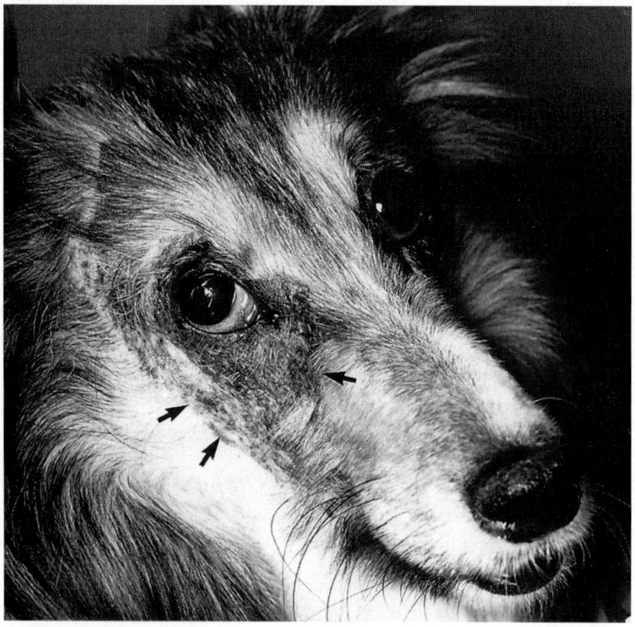

Figure 11-49 Skin, face; dog. Dermatomyositis. Hair loss and hyperpigmentation are present in the skin around the eye and on the face *(arrows)*.

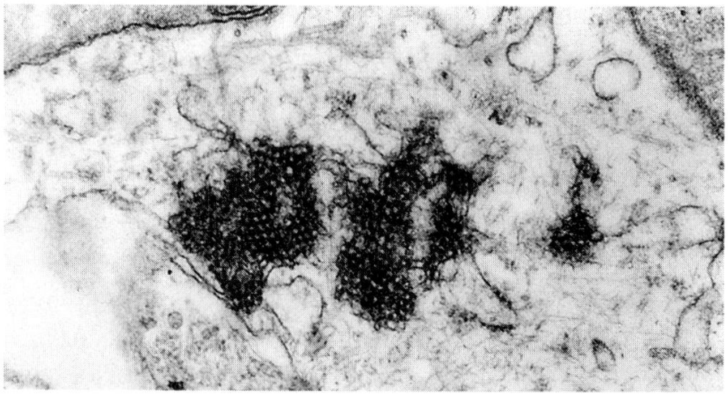

Figure 11-50 Transmission electron micrograph. Muscle, endothelial cell; dog. Viral-like inclusion. Note clusters of small rounded bodies in endothelial cell within muscle of a dog with dermatomyositis. Uranyl acetate–lead citrate stain.

is often considered a more severe form of EM. TEN is characterized clinically by vesicles, bullae, and epidermal detachment starting on the face and becoming generalized. Histologically there is full-thickness necrosis of the epidermis with separation of the epidermis from the dermis. TEN is life threatening.

Other uncommon to rare autoimmune or immune-mediated diseases with cutaneous lesions include cold agglutinin disease, cutaneous vasculitis, linear IgA dermatosis, alopecia areata, ulcerative dermatosis of the collie and Shetland sheepdog, and uveodermatologic syndrome (Vogt-Koyanagi-Harada–like syndrome [VKH]).

Diagnosis of Autoimmune Skin Disorders

The diagnosis is based on distribution and appearance of gross and microscopic lesions. Other diagnostic tools include the demonstration of immunoglobulin (IgG, IgM, or IgA) with or without complement in intercellular areas (pemphigus vulgaris, foliaceus, and erythematosus), at the basement membrane (pemphigus erythematosus, BP, SLE, DLE, and linear IgA dermatosis), or in vessels (cutaneous vasculitis), and the results of clinical immunologic tests such as antinuclear antibody titers and Coombs' test.

METABOLIC SKIN DISEASES

General

Cutaneous endocrine disorders are due to imbalances in hormones and generally are manifested as nonpruritic, bilaterally symmetric alopecia. The hair in the remainder of the coat is dull, dry, easily epilated, and fails to regrow after clipping. Hyperpigmentation may develop in the epidermis. These lesions are referred to as "endocrine alopecia." In disorders associated with alterations in sex hormones, the alopecia often begins in the perineal and genital areas and may extend cranially. However, it is not uncommon for a cutaneous endocrine disorder to have asymmetric alopecia and epidermal hyperpigmentation along with secondary pyoderma or seborrhea. Microscopically, uncomplicated endocrine disorders of the skin consist of hyperkeratosis of superficial epidermis and of hair follicles; normal, atrophic, or hyperplastic epithelium; follicular dilation; increased numbers of catagen or telogen hair follicles; lack of hair shafts in follicles; and increased epidermal pigmentation. These general features support the diagnosis of an endocrine disease, but often are not sufficiently specific to be diagnostic for an individual endocrine disorder. Also, inflammation due to secondary seborrhea or pyoderma frequently complicates the diagnosis. Selected clinical and histologic features of individual endocrine disorders (e.g., clinical evidence of cutaneous and muscle atrophy and histologic evidence of mineral deposition in the case of hyperglucocorticoidism) in conjunction with clinical testing are used to establish a more definitive diagnosis. Cutaneous endocrine disorders are more common in dogs than in cats, food animals, or horses.

Hypothyroidism

Deficiency of thyroid hormone is the most common endocrine disorder in dogs and is caused by idiopathic thyroid atrophy and lymphocytic thyroiditis. A variety of systemic and cutaneous signs and lesions result from thyroid hormone deficiency. Gross lesions consist of endocrine alopecia that develops, in most dogs, over the trunk and neck. Microscopic lesions include those listed above for endocrine alopecias. However, acanthosis of epidermis and follicular infundibular epithelium may be seen, and in some animals there is an increase in dermal mucin (myxedema), which results in dermal thickening. Secondary pyoderma is a common complication.

Congenital iodine deficiency develops in fetuses due to maternal ingestion of diets deficient in iodine or containing substances that interfere with production of thyroid hormones (goitrogens). Congenital iodine deficiency can occur in any domestic animal but usually occurs in large animals; it is associated with the birth of dead fetuses or weak neonates. These neonates may have alopecia, and thyroid glands are usually enlarged.

Hyperadrenocorticism (Hyperglucocorticoidism)

Hyperadrenocorticism results in cutaneous lesions principally in dogs and cats because of bilateral adrenal cortical hyperplasia secondary to a pituitary neoplasm, a functional adrenal cortical neoplasm, or the administration of exogenous glucocorticoids. In dogs, cutaneous lesions include endocrine alopecia that generally spares the head and extremities, thinning of the skin, comedones, increased bruising, poor wound healing, and increased susceptibility to infection (Fig. 11-51). Dystrophic calcification of the dermis of the back, inguinal, and axillary areas may occur in dogs, particularly in cases of iatrogenic

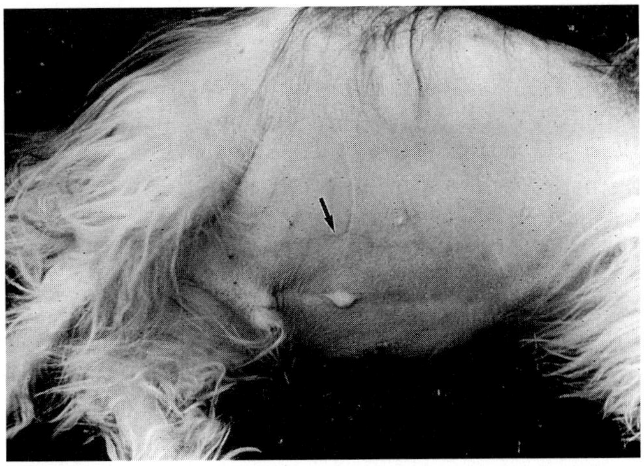

Figure 11-51 Skin; dog. Hyperadrenocorticism. Truncal alopecia, distended abdomen, and thin skin are present. Blood vessels are faintly visible *(arrow)*. The distended abdomen and visibility of blood vessels are due to protein catabolism and loss of dermal collagen and muscle. *Courtesy of Dr. A. Mundell.*

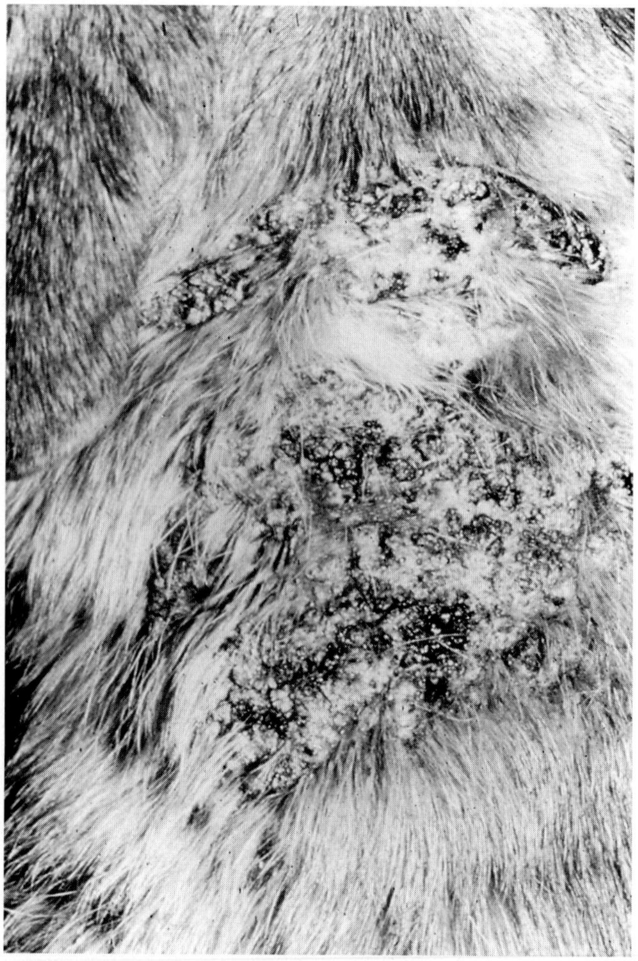

Figure 11-52 Skin, dorsal neck; dog. Hyperadrenocorticism and calcinosis cutis. The skin is alopecic, thickened, ulcerated, and crusted. The inflammation is due to a foreign body response to the calcium deposits. *Courtesy of Dr. A. Mundell.*

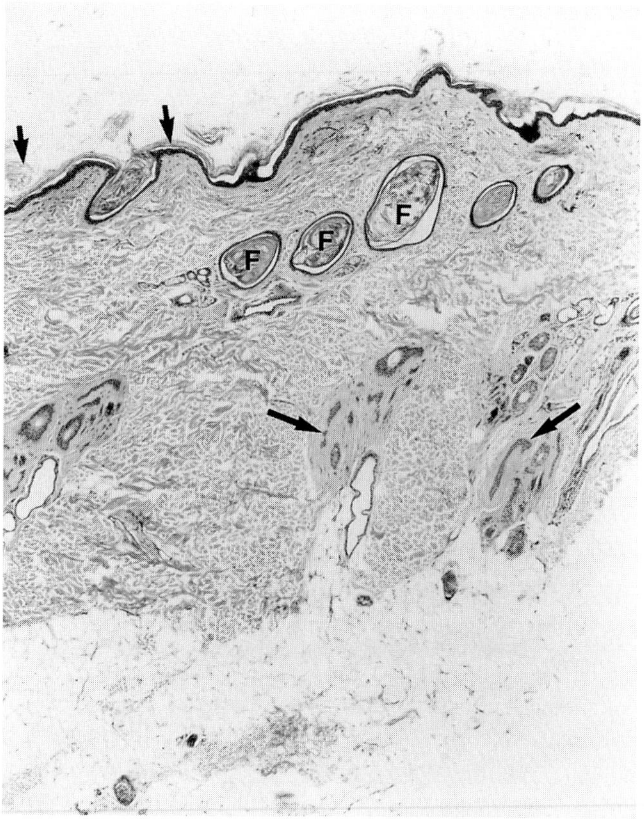

Figure 11-53 Skin; dog. Hyperestrogenism. Male dog with iatrogenic hyperestrogenism from diethylstilbestrol therapy. Note epidermal orthokeratotic hyperkeratosis *(small arrows)*, follicles dilated with keratin *(F)*, and small atrophic follicles *(large arrows)*. H & E stain.

hyperadrenocorticism (calcinosis cutis) (Fig. 11-52). Grossly, lesions of calcinosis cutis are firm, thickened, sometimes gritty, often ulcerated and alopecic, crusted plaques or nodules. In cats, the dermal collagen fibers may be markedly thin and atrophic, resulting in extremely fragile skin that may tear with normal handling. Microscopically, the lesions of hyperadrenocorticism include epidermal, dermal, and follicular atrophy, follicles dilated with keratin, and calcinosis cutis (dogs). There is little or no inflammatory reaction to calcium deposits when glucocorticoid concentration is high, but a foreign body reaction (granulomatous inflammation) and draining sinuses may occur when the concentration is lowered.

Hyperestrogenism

Hyperestrogenism may develop in male and female dogs. In females, estrogen may be secreted by ovarian cysts, rarely an ovarian neoplasm, or be due to estrogen administration. In males, elevated serum concentrations of estrogen are usually derived from a functional testicular Sertoli cell tumor. Iatrogenic estrogen administration has also caused hyperestrogenism in male dogs. In addition to endocrine alopecia, female dogs have an enlarged vulva and abnormalities of the estrus cycle. Male dogs may have gynecomastia, pendulous prepuce, or an enlarged prostate due to squamous metaplasia of prostatic ducts. Cutaneous microscopic lesions include orthokeratotic hyperkeratosis, follicular dilation with keratin, and telogen follicles (Fig. 11-53).

Castration/Growth Hormone–Responsive Dermatosis (Alopecia X of Nordic Breeds, Adrenal Sex Hormone Alopecia)

This condition is seen most often in Nordic breeds of dogs (e.g., Pomeranian, chow chow, Samoyed, Keeshond, Siberian husky, Alaskan malamute, Norwegian elkhound, Finnish spitz, American Eskimo, and others). Poodles, and sporadically other breeds of dogs, may also be affected.

Dogs with this condition (or conditions) are grouped together by having in common (1) plush hair coats in the normal state, (2) alopecia sparing head and distal extremities, (3) normal thyroid and glucocorticoid levels, and (4) skin biopsy samples with telogen follicles and often prominent flame follicles (follicles with prominent tricholemmal keratin that forms spikes into the follicular stratum spinosum). The alopecia often develops at 1 or 2 years of age in otherwise healthy dogs of either sex. The alopecia is symmetric and involves the perineum, caudal thighs, ventral abdomen and thorax, neck, and trunk; the head and distal extremities are spared. Hyperpigmentation is usually present. Thyroid function testing, ACTH (adrenocorticotropic hormone) response test, low-dose dexamethasone suppression test, and serum chemistry results are normal. Abnormalities in a number of hormones have been detected, but most work has involved the evaluation of 21-hydroxylase enzyme and other adrenocortical enzymes necessary for adrenal steroidogenesis. In the Pomeranian dog, partial deficiency of 21-hydroxylase enzyme has been detected and results in dysregulation of adrenal hormone synthesis, decreased cortisol levels, and in hyperprogestinism and hyperandrogenism (similar to late-onset, nonclassic congenital adrenal hyperplasia in people). Castration may provide a temporary response to the alopecia by removing testicular hormones. Microscopic lesions include follicular inactivity (telogen-stage follicles) and flame follicles (Fig. 11-54), which are prevalent in some breeds. Hyperpigmentation and dermal atrophy are variable.

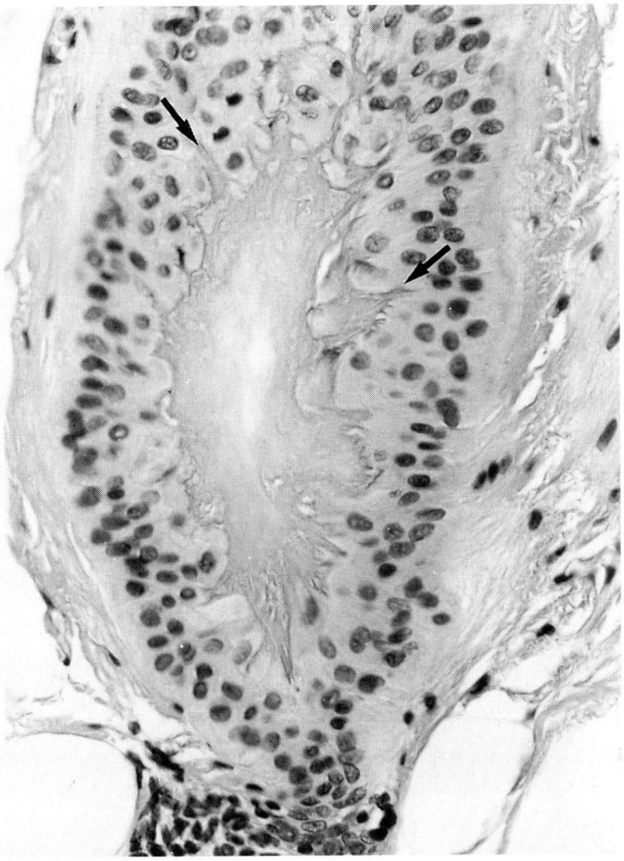

Figure 11-54 Skin, haired; dog. Flame follicle. The hair follicle has excessive tricholemmal keratinization resembling the spikes *(arrows)* of a flame and consistent with a "flame follicle." H & E stain.

Hypersomatotropism

This syndrome due to excess production of growth hormone is rare in adult dogs and has cutaneous lesions of thick, folded skin over the head, neck, and extremities. Hypertrichosis may develop. Microscopic lesions consist of hyperplasia of the epidermis, dermal fibrosis, and mucinous degeneration of the dermis.

Hyposomatotropism

Deficiency of growth hormone in dogs younger than 3 months of age is usually due to cysts that have destroyed the pituitary gland. Deficiencies of thyroid, adrenal, and gonadal hormones are frequent accompanying problems. Pituitary deficiency results in failure to grow, retention of the puppy hair coat, and development of endocrine alopecia.

Seasonal Flank Alopecia

Seasonal flank alopecia develops more commonly in dogs living in northern latitudes. Many breeds are affected, but English bulldogs, boxers, and Airedale terriers are among the more commonly affected breeds. Alopecia develops seasonally or cyclically in the skin of the flank, usually bilaterally. Histologically, follicles are atrophic and keratin markedly dilates primary follicle lumens. The keratin also dilates the openings of secondary follicles as they enter the primary follicle, giving the follicles the appearance of an upside-down "footprint" (Fig. 11-55). The cause of seasonal flank alopecia is not known, but an abnormal response of the skin to changes in the photoperiod has been suggested.

Conditions Resembling Endocrine Disorders

Alopecia resembling endocrine alopecia may be seen in nonendocrine diseases such as feline symmetric alopecia (excessive licking), postclipping alopecia (clipping hair in selected breeds of dogs with failure of hair to regrow), telogen effluvium (stress or systemic illness), anagen effluvium (chemotherapeutic drugs), and follicular dysplasia syndromes (abnormal follicle development).

NUTRITIONAL SKIN DISEASES

Malnutrition may be primary (dietary deficiency of proteins, fats, carbohydrates, vitamins, minerals, amino acids, or fatty acids) or secondary (diet is adequate, but malnutrition results from nutrient malabsorption, impaired nutrient use, increased nutrient loss, or increased nutrient needs such as pregnancy, neonatal growth, disease states, or cold weather). Inadequate diets may involve imbalances between dietary nutrients (e.g., copper deficiency and molybdenum excess, and vitamin E deficiency and excess dietary fatty acids). Diets inadequate in one nutrient may be inadequate in multiple nutrients, or there may be a greater deficiency in one nutrient relative to the others (e.g., starvation, the diet may be inadequate in protein, fats, and carbohydrates, as well as vitamins and minerals, or there may be a greater deficiency in protein relative to other nutrients). A variety of nutritional deficiencies result in similar cutaneous lesions; the lesions heal when the animal is fed a balanced diet. Deficiencies affecting the skin include protein-energy malnutrition (starvation), fatty acid deficiency, vitamin deficiencies (A, C, E), and deficiencies of riboflavin, pantothenic acid, biotin, niacin, iodine, cobalt, copper, and zinc. A few selected deficiency conditions are described.

Protein-Calorie Malnutrition (Starvation)

Protein-calorie malnutrition is a range of clinical syndromes that result from inadequate dietary intake of protein and calories to meet the needs of the body. Often diets are deficient in multiple components including protein, carbohydrates, and fats, which supply overall caloric intake. Deficiency of calories per se results in weight loss (adults) or retarded growth (young growing animals) and reduced subcutaneous fat and muscle, providing a thin, emaciated appearance. Increased energy demands such as pregnancy or cold weather can worsen the severity of the malnutrition, leading to ketosis in pregnant sheep, birth of weak neonates or dead fetuses, lack of estrus cycles, and death. A greater deficiency of protein relative to calories also results in malnutrition, referred to herein as "protein deficiency." In early stages the malnutrition associated with protein deficiency resembles that associated with deficiency of calories and results in weight loss and reduced production (e.g., milk) in adults and reduced growth in young animals. In addition, prolonged protein deficiency also results in peripheral edema due to the reduction in the quantity of the serum protein, albumin. Owing to the requirement of protein for the production of hair coat, the hair coat of malnourished animals (protein-calorie malnutrition as well as protein deficiency) is thin and dull with failure to shed or to complete the normal hair cycle. The epidermis and dermis may be atrophic with reduced subcutaneous fat and muscle, and surface scales (hyperkeratosis) may be present. In cases of long-standing severe protein deficiency, subcutaneous and dermal edema are present.

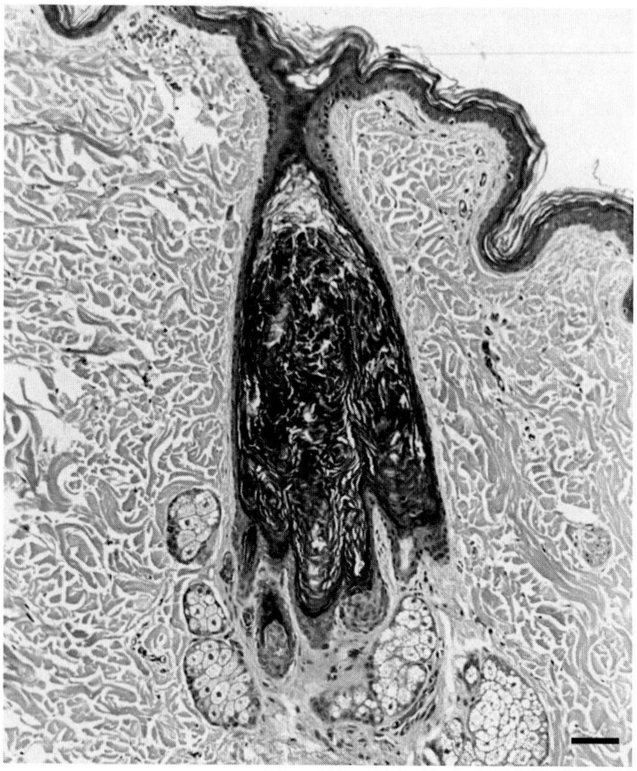

Figure 11-55 Skin, haired; dog. Seasonal flank alopecia. Note dilated distorted follicle with dilations at the base. The follicle resembles a footprint with toes to the bottom. H & E stain. Bar = 150 μm.

Zinc Deficiency

Zinc deficiency occurs chiefly in pigs and dogs and is of less importance in ruminants. It results from diets containing high concentration of phytic acid (binds zinc), low concentration of zinc, or high concentration of calcium, or inherited absorptive or metabolic abnormalities. Zinc deficiency, although once common in pigs, occurs infrequently today because of dietary supplementation. The lesions are circumscribed, reddened papules and plaques, scales, and thick crusts and fissures along the ventral abdomen and medial thighs. Some pigs have generalized symmetric lesions, especially involving the lower limbs, periocular areas, pinnae, snout, scrotum, and tail. Microscopically, the lesions are parakeratosis, hypergranulosis, acanthosis, and pseudoepitheliomatous hyperplasia. Secondary bacterial invasion results in pustular dermatitis and folliculitis.

Canine Zinc Responsive Dermatosis

This dermatosis occurs in two forms. One form occurs principally in Siberian huskies and Alaskan malamutes, but other large-breed dogs may be affected. Alaskan malamutes have an inherited reduced ability to absorb zinc from the intestine. Scaling and crusting develop in the skin around the mouth, chin, eyes (Fig. 11-56), external ears, pressure points, and footpads. The second form of zinc deficiency occurs in rapidly growing pups of large-breeds fed diets low in zinc or high in calcium or phytates, which may interfere with zinc absorption, and is characterized by scaly plaques on the skin subjected to repeated trauma, footpads, and planum nasale. Microscopically, there is marked diffuse parakeratosis that extends into the hair follicles. Parakeratosis is accompanied by a superficial perivascular lymphocytic dermatitis. Eosinophils may be the present.

Zinc Deficiency in Ruminants

Zinc deficiency has been reported in cattle, sheep, and goats. Cutaneous lesions include alopecia, scaling, and crusting of the skin of the face, neck, distal extremities, and mucocutaneous junctions. Microscopically, the lesions consist of parakeratosis and, in some cases, hyperkeratosis. An autosomal recessive inherited form of zinc deficiency has also been reported in young calves. The cutaneous lesions in the calves resolve with zinc supplementation.

Generic Dog Food Dermatosis

Some dogs fed generic dog foods for 1 to 2 months develop bilaterally symmetric scaling and crusting involving the skin of the bridge of the nose, mucocutaneous junctions, pressure points, and distal extremities. Lesions include hyperpigmentation and lichenification, focal erosions, papules, pustules, and alopecia. Microscopically, the lesions are parakeratosis, dyskeratosis, laminar epidermal edema and spongiosis, and mixed cellular infiltrate in the dermis. The cause may be due partially to zinc deficiency. Deficiency of multiple trace minerals, vitamins, or amino acids also may be involved.

Copper Deficiency

Copper is an essential component of tyrosinase, and deficient animals develop depigmented hair or wool. Black sheep may develop bands of more lightly and darkly pigmented wool corresponding to variations in dietary intakes of copper. Cattle may develop depigmented hair around the eyes providing the appearance of "spectacles" (eyeglasses). The coat color also may change from black to reddish brown. In sheep, the wool becomes straight (loss of crimp) and is less desirable for commercial use due to imperfect oxidation of sulfhydryl groups in prekeratin, a process that requires copper.

Vitamin E Deficiency

Cats with vitamin E deficiency or fed diets with an excess of dietary fatty acids may develop steatitis. Grossly, the subcutaneous tissue contains firm, nodular, yellow to orange masses. Microscopic lesions are lobular to diffuse panniculitis with early lesions of fat necrosis, edema, and infiltrates of neutrophils. Granulomatous inflammation follows rapidly and is composed of macrophages and multinucleated giant cells with ceroid pigment.

Vitamin A Deficiency

Vitamin A–responsive dermatosis is a rare disorder primarily occurring in cocker spaniels. Gross lesions are most prominent in ventrolateral thoracic and abdominal skin; they consist of generalized scaling with fronds of keratin extending from follicular openings. Microscopic lesions are marked dilation of follicles with keratin.

DISORDERS OF EPIDERMAL GROWTH OR DIFFERENTIATION

Primary Idiopathic Seborrhea

Primary idiopathic seborrhea is a disorder of cornification with the epidermal turnover time reduced by about one third (e.g., 22 days to 8 days in the cocker spaniel). In seborrhea, there are increased quantities of free fatty acids and cholesterol and reduced quantities of diester waxes in surface lipids, and a change from nonpathogenic resident bacteria to pathogenic, coagulase-positive staphylococci. Seborrhea occurs most commonly in dogs and less commonly in horses and cats. Clinically, two forms of seborrhea have been described, a dry form (seborrhea sicca) with dry skin and white to gray scales that exfoliate (Fig. 11-57), or a greasy form (seborrhea oleosa) with scaling and excessive brown to yellow lipids that adhere to the skin and hair. An animal may have seborrhea sicca in

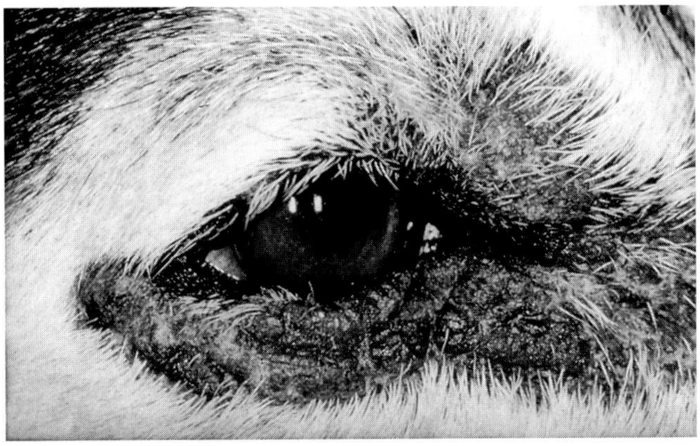

Figure 11-56 Skin, periocular; dog, Siberian husky. Zinc-responsive dermatitis. Periocular skin is thickened, alopecic, pigmented, and covered by tightly adherent scales.

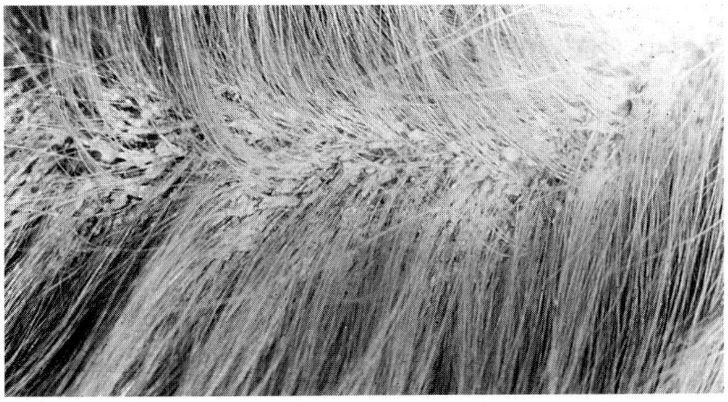

Figure 11-57 Skin, haired; dog. Idiopathic seborrhea. Hair is parted to reveal excessive scaling.

some areas of the body and seborrhea oleosa in others. Microscopic lesions include disproportionate hyperkeratosis of the epidermis and follicular epithelium. The epidermis has a papillary appearance due to widening of follicular ostia by the keratin (see Fig. 11-4). At the edges of follicular ostia, foci of parakeratosis form over a spongiotic epidermis containing a few scattered leukocytes. The dermal papillae are edematous and congested.

Secondary Seborrhea

Secondary seborrhea is not a primary disorder of cornification; however, it clinically resembles the primary cornification disorders (dry exfoliative or greasy adherent scales) and thus needs to be differentiated from them. The lesions of secondary seborrhea resolve completely if the underlying disease can be eliminated. Secondary seborrhea is common and is caused by a variety of unrelated cutaneous disorders such as allergy, ectoparasitism, fungal infection, dietary deficiency, endocrine disease, and internal diseases. Microscopic changes include epidermal and follicular hyperkeratosis with or without parakeratosis plus the lesions associated with the underlying disease.

Sebaceous Adenitis

Sebaceous adenitis, inflammation of sebaceous glands, is probably immune-mediated. Sebaceous adenitis occurs most commonly in dogs. Lesions are diffuse in the longer-haired breeds and multifocal, annular, and serpiginous in short-haired breeds. Microscopic lesions include inflammation of the sebaceous glands (see Fig. 11-18), and in some cases, extensive orthokeratotic hyperkeratosis. Chronic cases have no remaining sebaceous glands and mild residual inflammation and fibrosis in the perifollicular dermis near the isthmus (site normally occupied by sebaceous glands).

DISORDERS OF PIGMENTATION

Hypopigmentation

Disorders associated with reduced pigment may be inherited or acquired, involve skin or hair, be generalized or localized, idiopathic, or associated with other diseases. Terms used for these disorders include leukoderma and vitiligo for loss of pigment in the skin, leukotrichia for loss of pigment of the hair (see Fig. 11-11), hypopigmentation or incomplete albinism for generalized less than normal amount of pigment in the skin or hair, albinism for a hereditary lack of pigment, and dilution for reduced pigmentation. Examples of some of the disorders include Chediak-Higashi syndrome, color mutant (dilution) alopecia, the Maltese dilution of cats, leukoderma and/or leukotrichia of Doberman pinchers and Rottweilers, periocular leukotrichia in Siamese cats, and Arabian fading syndrome. Immune-mediated disorders associated with depigmentation include discoid lupus erythematosus and uveodermatologic syndrome (VKH-like disease).

Hyperpigmentation

Hyperpigmentation may result from inflammation, irritation, and metabolic disorders; consequently hyperpigmentation is seen in all species with epidermal melanin pigment. Hyperpigmentation also is a feature of benign and malignant masses (lentigines, melanocytic tumors, and pigmented basal cell tumors). Lentigines are rare, nonneoplastic, well-circumscribed, macular to slightly raised plaques characterized by irregular epidermal hyperplasia, hyperpigmentation, and increased numbers of pigmented melanocytes. Lentigines are often multifocal and have been described in dogs and cats.

DISORDERS OF UNKNOWN PATHOGENESIS (IDIOPATHIC DISORDERS)

Disorders Characterized by Infiltrates of Eosinophils

Eosinophilic Plaques

These common lesions of the skin of cats occur on the abdomen and medial thigh and are thought to be associated with hypersensitivity reactions. Lesions consist of raised, variably sized erythematous, pruritic, and eroded to ulcerated plaques. Microscopically, epidermal lesions include acanthosis, variable spongiosis, erosion, and ulceration, accompanied by superficial and deep, perivascular to diffuse predominantly, eosinophilic dermatitis. Foci of collagen degeneration may be observed.

Eosinophilic Granulomas (Collagenolytic Granulomas)

Eosinophilic and granulomatous lesions with collagen degeneration (collagenolysis) occur in cats, dogs, and horses. The causes of these syndromes are poorly understood, but collagen degeneration may develop in any lesion with associated eosinophil degranulation such as reactions to parasites, foreign bodies (including hair), or in mast cell tumors. Gross lesions include papules, nodules, plaques (sometimes linear), and ulcers in the skin (Fig. 11-58), and nodular or ulcerated lesions in the oral mucosae of dogs and cats, and footpads of cats. Microscopically, nodular dermatitis (or stomatitis) consists of fragmented degenerate collagen fibers bordered by degranulated eosinophils and macrophages. Some indolent ulcers (rodent ulcers) on the upper lip of cats have areas of collagen degeneration and eosinophilic and granulomatous inflammation and are considered to be eosinophilic granulomas.

Multisystemic Eosinophilic Epitheliotropic Disease in the Horse

A generalized, exfoliative dermatitis characterized histologically by a hyperplastic perivascular, eosinophilic to lymphoplasmacytic dermatitis occurs in the horse. The dermatitis is accompanied by eosinophilic, lymphoplasmacytic, and sometimes granulomatous inflammation and fibrosis in other organs including the alimentary tract, pancreas, liver, uterus, and bronchial epithelium. Clini-

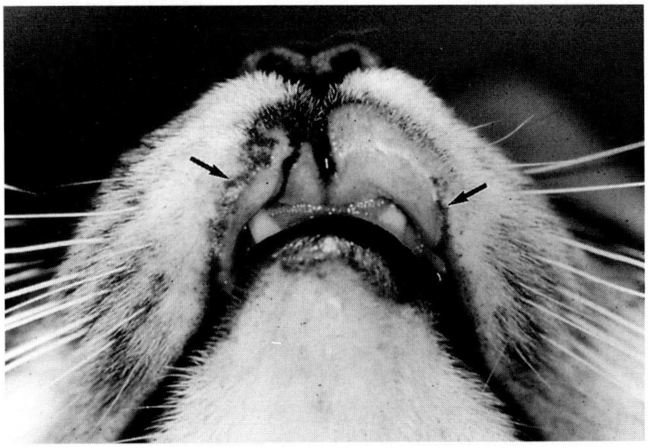

Figure 11-58 Skin, lips; cat. Eosinophilic granulomas. Bilateral ulceration *(arrows)* of upper lip is present. One side is more severely affected.

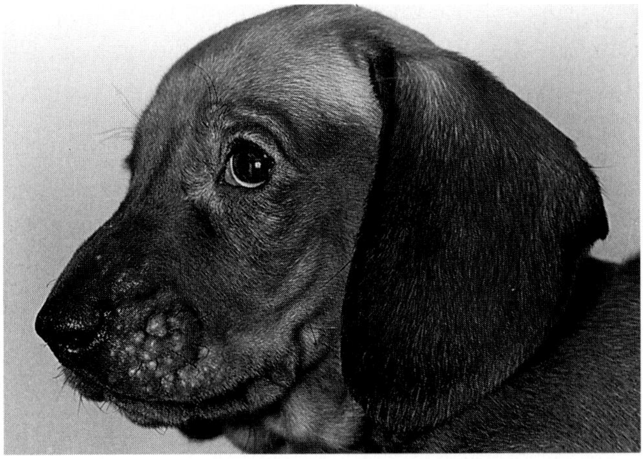

Figure 11-59 Skin; dog. Dachshund puppy. Juvenile sterile granulomatous dermatitis and lymphadenitis (juvenile pyoderma). Note pustular lesions of 1 day duration on muzzle. *Courtesy of Dr. D. Prieur.*

cally, the horses lose weight and become progressively debilitated. Initial cutaneous lesions include dry scales and serous exudate of the epithelium of the skin of the head, coronets, and oral cavity. The lesions progress to generalized excoriations with ulcerations and alopecia. Secondary infections are common. The etiology of the condition is unknown; however, one case documents the coexistence of an intestinal T cell lymphoma and postulates tumor cell overproduction of IL-5, a powerful eosinophilopoietin.

Sterile Granulomatous Disorders

Juvenile Sterile Granulomatous Dermatitis and Lymphadenitis (Juvenile Pyoderma, Juvenile Cellulitis, Puppy Strangles)

This disorder of unknown cause occurs in pups younger than 4 months (Figs. 11-59 and 11-60), with one or more of the pups of a litter having pustular and nodular dermatitis and edema of the face, ears, and mucocutaneous junctions. Microscopically, lesions are those of granulomatous or pyogranulomatous perifolliculitis, dermatitis, and panniculitis.

Other Sterile Granulomatous and Pyogranulomatous Disorders

These disorders develop in the skin of dogs and cats and include sterile granuloma and pyogranuloma syndrome, cutaneous xanthoma (xanthogranuloma), and idiopathic nodular panniculitis. These lesions are characterized grossly by single or multifocal papules, plaques, or nodules and, microscopically, by discrete, coalescing, or diffuse accumulations of populations of a mixture of cells including, but not limited to, macrophages (histiocytes) and neutrophils. The lesions must be differentiated from those of the infectious granulomatous disorders and the

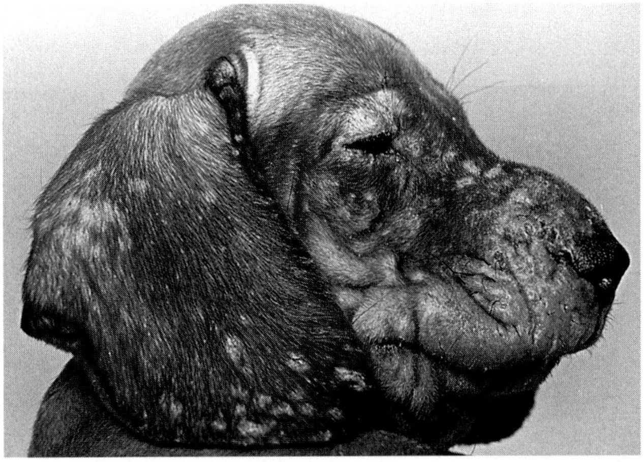

Figure 11-60 Skin; dog (same as in Fig. 11-59). Juvenile sterile granulomatous dermatitis and lymphadenitis (juvenile pyoderma). The lesions, of 12 days' duration, have progressed to include alopecia, edema, and crusting. *Courtesy of Dr. D. Prieur.*

reactive histiocytic disorders recognized in dogs (cutaneous and systemic histiocytosis; see Table 11-3).

Equine Generalized Granulomatous Disease (Sarcoidosis)

This uncommon disorder of horses has cutaneous lesions and more widespread systemic involvement, resulting in anorexia and weight loss. Cutaneous lesions include generalized alopecia, scales, crusts, and, occasionally, nodules or tumorlike masses. Microscopic lesions are multifocal granulomas with multinucleated giant cells. The disease has been termed "sarcoidosis" because of its

Text continued on p. 595

Table 11-3 Selected Cutaneous Neoplastic and Neoplastic-like Lesions of Domestic Animals

Lesion	Cause	Species, Age, Breed, Sex	Location	Gross Pathology	Histopathology	Biologic Behavior	Unique Features
Cutaneous papilloma (wart) (verruca)	Often caused by papilloma virus	Common in horses, cattle Infrequent in dogs, goats, sheep Rare in cats Often young age Congenital in foals	Horse: about the nose, lips, inner aspect of ears (aural plaques) Any location, often the head	Flattened to papillary mass, single or multiple, on narrow or broad base Inverted variety occurs	Papillary projections of epithelium over collagen core Epithelium thickened by hyperkeratosis and acanthosis	Most benign and will regress Occasional transformation to squamous cell carcinoma	May have viral inclusion bodies May have koilocytes (keratinocytes with swollen clear or gray cytoplasm)
Fibroepithelial polyp (skin tag)		Dogs	Any location	Raised smooth polyp	Epidermis covering collagen core	Benign	More collagen than squamous papilloma
Fibropapilloma	Bovine papilloma virus 2	Young bulls, cows	Glans penis of bulls Vulva and vagina of cows	Irregular mass attached to glans penis; less papillary than cutaneous papilloma	Proliferative epithelium and whorls and fascicles of fibroblasts and collagen	Look aggressive histologically and may recur after excision but do not metastasize	Location Viral cause
Cutaneous cysts Follicular Sebaceous duct Dermoid Apocrine Ciliated	Follicular and apocrine (occluded follicles or ducts) Dermoid (genetic) Ciliated (developmental anomaly)	Any species, often dogs and cats	Anywhere on skin Dermoid: dorsal midline of Rhodesian ridgeback Ciliated: neck of cats	Cyst filled with soft, tan, greasy keratin and sebum (follicular and sebaceous); hair (dermoid); or clear fluid (apocrine and ciliated)	Cystic structure with the wall composed of epidermal or adnexal epithelium Ciliated: from thyroglossal duct or respiratory epithelium	Nonneoplastic	Rupture and foreign body inflammation may develop
Cutaneous horn	Associated with benign or malignant epithelial tumors FeLV cat footpads *Dermatophilus* associated Papilloma virus	All domestic species	Any location Footpads of cats Areas of *Dermatophilus* infection in ruminants	Hard, conical, hornlike growth Greater height than diameter	Horn consists of laminations of compact keratin Base may be a hyperplastic, neoplastic, or inflammatory lesion	Both neoplastic and nonneoplastic varieties Depends on nature of underlying lesion	Gross appearance

Hair follicle tumors Trichoepithelioma Tricholemmoma Pilomatricoma Trichoblastoma (hair follicle tumor of basal cells)	Genetic (breed predilections) May be multicentric in predisposed breeds	Dogs, occasionally cats Pilomatricoma Kerry blue terrier Trichoepithelioma Basset hound	Any location	Firm and discrete tumors Some cystic Some ulcerate Some mineralize	Variable, depending on tumor Resemble portion of follicle from which arise	Most tumors of follicular origin are benign Malignant varieties of trichoepithelioma and pilomatricoma have been described	May mineralize May result in foreign body response if cystic tumor ruptures
Infundibular keratinizing acanthoma (intracutaneous cornifying epithelioma)	Genetic (breed predilection)	Norwegian elkhound; may be multicentric	Often back and tail when multicentric	Dermal or subcutaneous mass, often with pore opening onto skin surface	Invaginated cyst with wall composed of lobules of stratified squamous epithelium	Benign	Resembles squamous cell carcinoma histologically
Malignant trichoepithelioma (matrical carcinoma) Malignant pilomatricoma	Unknown	Dogs	Any location skin	Large, dermal or subcutaneous mass Poorly circumscribed; invade subcutis	Not usually connected with epidermis Similar to benign, but greater nuclear pleomorphism and mitotic activity	Malignant variety Trichoepithelioma: Frequent metastasis to lymph nodes or lungs. Recurrence also reported. Pilomatricoma: may metastasize	Matrical keratinization Pilomatricoma has no trichohyalin granules; often has calcification or ossification
Benign basal cell tumor* Basal cell carcinoma	Unknown	Benign basal cell tumor of epidermal origin (cats) Carcinoma (dogs and cats) Rare in other domestic animals	Often head, neck, and cranial trunk	Generally solitary firm nodules or plaques that may ulcerate Carcinoma: may be multicentric	Benign: resemble basal cells Carcinoma: ragged margins, solid, clear cell, and keratinizing types	Benign Carcinoma locally aggressive with low potential for metastasis	Lack intercellular bridges May contain melanin pigment and can be confused with melanoma May be contiguous with epidermis

*Classification and terminology of benign basal cell tumors varies with authors. Differences appear largely related to epidermal versus follicular origin and therefore histologic appearance of the tumors.

Continued

Table 11-3 Selected Cutaneous Neoplastic and Neoplastic-like Lesions of Domestic Animals—cont'd

Lesion	Cause	Species, Age, Breed, Sex	Location	Gross Pathology	Histopathology	Biologic Behavior	Unique Features
Squamous cell carcinoma (In situ carcinoma termed "Bowen's disease" in cats develops in haired skin, multicentrically)	Solar radiation Trauma Carcinogens Papilloma virus in Bowen's disease Some unknown	All species, especially white cats, Hereford cattle, light colored horses, white or partly white dogs Less in pigs Adults to aged	Non or lightly pigmented and sparsely haired skin Nail bed (dogs, cats) Penis or prepuce (horses)	Variable: nodular, proliferative, crusty, ulcerative Cutaneous horn may be present	Cords and islands of squamous cells Keratin pearls Dyskeratosis Intercellular bridges Basement membrane disrupted	May recur Metastasis to lymph nodes and beyond may develop Those of equine penis and feline nail bed are more aggressive Solar-associated are slow to metastasize	Keratin pearls, intercellular bridges Spindle cell and pseudoglandular varieties occur
Nail bed tumors Inclusion cyst Papilloma Keratoacanthoma Squamous cell carcinoma Melanoma	Unknown Trauma	Dogs; large breeds, black-haired, predisposed to multiple squamous cell carcinomas Cats	Nail bed May be multiple	Variable Swelling of nail bed Loss of nail Deformed nail	Depends on type of lesion or tumor	Malignant melanoma of dogs and squamous cell carcinoma of cats can be aggressive	Differentiate from pulmonary carcinoma in cat that may metastasize to multiple digits
Apocrine adenoma: simple, complex, mixed, and ductal Apocrine adenocarcinoma: simple, complex, mixed, and ductal	Unknown	Older dogs and cats	Any location; glands present Older female dogs: bilateral adenocarcinomas may develop from apocrine glands of anal sacs	Adenoma: small, slow growing, cystic, circumscribed Carcinomas: firm, fibrous, infiltrative	Benign: variable appearance; resemble glandular or ductal epithelium Mixed type has myoepithelium, cartilage, or bone Carcinomas of anal sac usually solid	Adenomas: benign Carcinomas: aggressive; may metastasize early	Carcinomas may resemble exudative dermatitis Anal sac carcinomas are often associated with hypercalcemia
Sebaceous gland adenoma Sebaceous gland epithelioma Sebaceous gland carcinoma	Unknown	Adenoma common in adult dogs: cocker spaniel, poodle Less cats Rare other animals	Head, neck, anywhere	Adenoma: gray-tan, greasy, lobulated, raised Epithelioma: discrete, firm, may ulcerate Carcinoma: often ulcerates	Adenoma: similar to sebaceous gland Epithelioma: more basal cells and mitoses Carcinoma: less fat in cells; less differentiated	Adenomas benign Epitheliomas may recur Carcinomas locally invasive; rarely metastasize	Eyelid meibomian gland tumors are similar Nodular hyperplastic lesions of sebaceous glands also common

Perianal gland adenoma (hepatoid gland adenoma) Perianal gland epithelioma Perianal gland carcinoma	Hormonal influence	Older dogs 90% male	Skin near anus, base of tail, prepuce, vulva; less elsewhere	One or more raised nodules often ulcerated, circumscribed, orangish tan and greasy on cut surface	Adenoma: similar to perianal gland Epithelioma: more basal cells and mitoses Carcinoma: infiltrative, less differentiated, and has more mitoses	Most are adenomas, which are benign In males, castration or estrogen therapy may cause regression of adenomas Carcinomas: low-grade malignancy	Location and hormonal sensitivity
Canine cutaneous histiocytoma	Unknown Langerhans cell of origin	Dogs: more than half of tumors develop before dog is 2 years of age Purebred dogs predisposed	Head, especially pinna, distal forelegs, and feet	Usually single Dome-shaped Circumscribed Often ulcerated	Sheets of large, round cells (histiocytes) replace adnexa and collagen Frequent mitoses Later necrosis and lymphocytic inflammation	Rapid growth followed by regression Rarely recur No metastasis	Young dogs Rapid growth Regression
Canine reactive histiocytosis (cutaneous and systemic)	Unknown Langerhans cell of origin	Adult dogs Systemic: Bernese mountain dogs and few other breeds	Cutaneous: multiple cutaneous sites Systemic: skin and other organs	Multiple cutaneous and subcutaneous plaques and nodules with or without systemic lesions	Histiocytic cells and variable mix of lymphocytes, plasma cells, and neutrophils	Remissions, relapses Prolonged course Slowly progressive	Recurrent May have nasal lesion or systemic involvement
Histiocytic sarcoma (disseminated) also known as malignant histiocytosis)	Unknown	Bernese mountain dog Retriever (golden, Labrador) Rottweiler, others	Skin and subcutis are rarely affected Multisystemic involvement	Multinodular, invasive, destructive	Anaplastic large, round or plump spindle cells, other leukocytes	Aggressive Usually fatal disease	Breed predisposition Multisystemic masses Anaplastic cell populations
Cutaneous lymphoma Dermal form Epidermal form T cell type (mycosis fungoides) Angiocentric form T cell type (lymphomatoid granulomatosus)	Unknown	Dogs; less in cats and horses Age variable	Skin or oral Dermis or epidermis	Variable: 1. Red scaly skin 2. Mucocutaneous ulceration or depigmentation 3. Single or multiple cutaneous masses 4. Infiltrative and ulcerative mucosae with or without systemic lesions	Dermal: sheets of lymphocytes in dermis Epidermal: lymphocytes in epidermis and adnexal epithelium Angiocentric: lymphohistiocytic dermal masses with angiocentric pattern	Ultimately terminate fatally Lymphomatoid granulomatosus is aggressive, has angiocentric pattern, and may invade vessels and cause infarction	Epidermal form may mimic dermatitis, autoimmune disease, or stomatitis Equine lymphosarcoma is pleocellular and can be confused with inflammation

Continued

Table 11-3 Selected Cutaneous Neoplastic and Neoplastic-like Lesions of Domestic Animals—cont'd

Lesion	Cause	Species, Age, Breed, Sex	Location	Gross Pathology	Histopathology	Biologic Behavior	Unique Features
Merkel cell tumor	Neuroendocrine origin	Dog, rare tumor	Skin or oral	Nodular mass	Nests of round cells with collagen septa	Usually benign	200 nm granules seen ultrastructurally
Cutaneous plasmacytoma (extramedullary plasmacytoma)	Unknown	Dog, rarely cat Aged adult Both sexes	Ear, lip, digit, and other mucocutaneous and cutaneous sites	Usually solitary, raised, reddish, discrete nodule	Densely cellular Single or multiple, variably sized nuclei; many mitoses Resemble plasma cells; may have amyloid	Usually do not recur Subcutaneous or those with amyloid may be aggressive and recurrent Rare association with multiple myeloma	Cytoplasmic immunoglobulin present May have amyloid deposits
Mast cell tumor (mastocytoma)	Unknown Genetic influence Cats: FIV associated?	Common tumor of dogs, especially boxers; less other species Siamese cats have histiocytic variety Generally adults; less neonates	Dog: often legs, trunk Feline: head	Solitary or multiple nodules Poorly circumscribed edematous swellings May ulcerate early	Sheets of large round cells with bluish granular cytoplasm Not encapsulated Many eosinophils in dogs especially Vasculitis Collagen degeneration	Canine: behavior may correspond to histologic grade May disseminate Feline histiocytic type may spontaneously regress Equine generally benign	Metachromatic granules, eosinophils Other lesions: vasculitis, collagen degeneration, gastrointestinal ulceration Prolonged coagulation time
Melanoma Benign (melanocytoma), junctional dermal compound Malignant melanoma	Genetic factors Unknown Ultraviolet light in Angora goats	Common: dogs and horses, and some strains of pigs and Angora goats Uncommon: cats Rare: other species	Dogs: head, eyelids, legs, digits Horse: perineal skin and underside of root of tail Feline: head Angora goat: dorsal ear, face, perineum	Dog and cats: single Horse: multiple Macules to nodules Usually dark brown or black	Epithelioid to spindle-shaped cells containing variable quantity of pigment Nests of these cells bordered by thin collagen septae Malignant are anaplastic and may be amelanotic	Canine: oral, mucocutaneous, subungual, often malignant; haired skin often benign Gray horses: usually progressive and multicentric Location, size, mitotic index and cell morphology help predict behavior	Melanin pigment in cytoplasm Common in horses that fade to gray

Fibroma Fibrosarcoma (malignant fibrous histiocytoma may be a variant with histiocytic and spindle-shaped cells)	Fibrosarcoma: 1 FeLV* and FeSV† are associated with development of multiple sarcomas in young cats 2 Vaccination in cats	Adult to aged All domestic animals Fibrosarcomas: common in cats, less common in dogs, rare other species	Head, legs, and sites of vaccination in cats	Circumscribed (fibroma) Firm to soft Resilient Gray-white	Interlacing bundles of fibroblasts and collagen Fibrosacrcoma may have multinucleated giant cells	Fibromas benign Fibrosarcomas are infiltrative and often recur, but metastasis is uncommon	Fibrosarcomas in cats have been caused by FeLV plus FeSV and by vaccination
Equine sarcoid	Bovine papillomavirus	Most common skin tumor of horses Horse, donkey, mule	Skin of legs, head, ventral trunk	Types: verrucous, fibroblastic, flat, or occult, mixed	Fibroblastic proliferation with pseudoepitheliomatous hyperplasia	Locally invasive Frequently recur Do not metastasize	Autotransplantable Rare spontaneous regression
Myxoma Myxosarcoma	Unknown	Rare in domestic animals Adult to aged	Any location, often limbs	Poorly defined and infiltrative Soft and mucoid Gelatinous	Fusiform and stellate cells within mucinous matrix	Infiltrative Recur frequently Myxosarcomas metastasize uncommonly	Some consider myxomas (sarcomas) to be a type of fibroma (sarcoma)
Hemangiopericytoma (cell of origin is controversial, probably perictye or possibly neural)	Unknown Some consider this to be a malignant peripheral nerve sheath tumor	Dogs Adult to aged More in females Cats, rare	Dermis and subcutis of extremities	Gray to pink Lobulated Firm and nodular or more gelatinous	Concentric laminations of spindle cells	Often recur Locally invasive Rarely metastasize	Concentric laminations of spindle cells around vessels
Nerve sheath tumors Neurofibroma Schwannoma	Unknown	Dogs; less others	Cutaneous tumors are uncommon; more on head of cats, legs of dogs, and eyelids of horses	Nodular Firm to gelatinous White-gray Associated with nerve	Bundles, whorls, and palisades of spindle cells	Dogs and cats: locally invasive; may recur	Cells arranged in palisades Associated with nerves
Lipoma Infiltrative lipoma Liposarcoma	Unknown	Lipoma: common in adult to aged dogs; less common in horse and cow; rare in cat, sheep, pig Infiltrative lipoma: adult dogs Liposarcoma: rare	Legs, thorax, abdomen	Lipoma: circumscribed, greasy, soft, white, slightly translucent; floats in formalin Infiltrative lipoma: poorly delineated soft enlargements of muscle or soft tissue Liposarcoma: firmer, nondiscrete, gray to white	Lipoma: mature fat cells Infiltrative lipoma: mature fat cells replacing normal muscle or collagen Liposarcoma: round to spindle cell tumor; cellular, vacuolated cytoplasm	Lipomas do not recur Infiltrative lipomas are locally invasive and recur but do not metastasize Liposarcomas are locally invasive, may recur, and rarely metastasize	Fatty tumor Float in formalin

*FeLV = feline leukemia virus.
†FeSV = feline sarcoma virus.

Continued

Table 11-3 Selected Cutaneous Neoplastic and Neoplastic-like Lesions of Domestic Animals—cont'd

Lesion	Cause	Species, Age, Breed, Sex	Location	Gross Pathology	Histopathology	Biologic Behavior	Unique Features
Hemangioma Hemangiosarcoma	Unknown Trauma or solar radiation for some types	Adult to aged More in dogs, Less in cats, horses, cattle, sheep, pigs Foals congenital hemangiomas	Hemangioma: dermis or subcutis Hemangiosarcoma: primary to skin or metastatic from visceral tumor Some, more in white, poorly haired dermis, especially of dogs	Red, brown to black Circumscribed (hemangioma) Soft Ooze blood on cut surface Dermal may bleed	Interconnecting blood-containing channels lined by endothelium Hemangiosarcoma may resemble fibrosarcoma or have benign appearance (especially if metastatic)	Hemangiomas do not recur Hemangiosarcomas in white cat eartip and eyelid recur Metastatic potential is high in canine hemangiosarcomas	Thrombosis frequent in hemangioma Coagulation disorder may be associated with these tumors, especially if tumors are large, malignant, or multifocal
Lymphangioma Lymphangiosarcoma	Some are believed to be congenital in young animals	Uncommon to rare	Lymphatics associated with skin	Poorly defined Cavernous or spongy Soft May dissect along fascial planes	Interconnecting channels lined by endothelium usually without erythrocytes May be difficult to distinguish benign and malignant types	May be difficult to remove because of dissection along fascia, so tumors tend to recur	
Leiomyoma Leiomyosarcoma	Unknown	Rare	Skin associated with arrector pili muscles or cutaneous blood vessels	Circumscribed Solitary Firm	Interlacing bundles of smooth muscle fibers tend to intersect at right angles; nuclei have blunt ends	Leiomyoma benign Leiomyosarcoma is locally invasive	

resemblance to a systemic granulomatous dermatosis of undetermined cause in human beings in which granulomas, comprised largely of epithelioid macrophages bordered by very few lymphocytes (sarcoidal granulomas), are a characteristic feature.

Diseases of the Nail Bed and Lupoid Onychodystrophy

Onychodystrophy refers to abnormal formation of the nail (claw), onychomadesis to sloughing of nails, and paronychia to inflammation of the skin of the nail fold. These conditions are rare. Onychodystrophy and paronychia of multiple nails on multiple feet have a variety of causes including infections (e.g., bacterial, fungal), immune-mediated disorders (e.g., pemphigus, lupus erythematosus), systemic disease (e.g., hyperadrenocorticism, disseminated intravascular coagulation), and disorders of unknown cause (e.g., lupoid onychodystrophy, idiopathic onychodystrophy). Diagnosis may require amputation of the third phalanx and the adjacent skin proximal to the nail fold for histopathologic evaluation. Lupoid onychodystrophy is probably the most common cause of onychomadesis that leads to onychodystrophy of multiple nails involving multiple feet in dogs. The condition affects many breeds of dogs of varying ages; the dogs are healthy otherwise. History includes sudden loss of nails, eventually involving all nails on all feet. There is partial regrowth of misshapen, friable nails that continue to slough. Paronychia is usually absent. Histologic lesions are more prominent on the dorsal aspect of the nail and nail bed skin; characteristics include interface lymphoplasmacytic inflammation with basal cell vacuolation and apoptosis and pigmentary incontinence. Secondary bacterial infection and osteomyelitis may develop.

Plasma Cell Pododermatitis

Feline plasma cell pododermatitis is an uncommon condition of undetermined pathogenesis. It is characterized clinically by exuberant soft tissue swelling of multiple footpads that may lead to collapse of the footpad and ulceration, hemorrhage, and lameness. Histologically, the skin of the footpad is heavily infiltrated by plasma cells with variable numbers of Russell body plasma cells, neutrophils, and lymphocytes. This condition is sometimes accompanied by plasmacytic stomatitis, hypergammaglobulinemia, immune-mediated glomerulonephritis, or renal amyloidosis. A recent study indicated 50% of cases are positive for feline leukemia virus.

Feline Ulcerative Dermatitis Syndrome

Feline ulcerative dermatitis syndrome is an uncommon syndrome of unknown cause that affects skin of the dorsal neck or interscapular regions. Self-trauma contributes but is not likely the only source of the lesion. The gross lesion consists of an ulcer with exudate that may mat hair. Microscopic lesions consist of an ulcer covered by fibrinonecrotic crust. The dermis subjacent to the ulcer contains components of necrotic epidermis or adnexa intermixed with degenerate neutrophils. Inflammation in adjacent and deeper dermis is variable, but often scant, and consists of a few neutrophils, eosinophils, and mixed mononuclear cells. In chronic cases, there is acanthosis of adjacent epidermis and a linear band of fibrosis beneath and parallel to the epidermis.

CUTANEOUS MANIFESTATIONS OF SYSTEMIC DISEASE

Laminitis

The term, "laminitis" refers to inflammation of the laminar structures of the hoof, but laminitis is a complex disease in which inflammation is only a part of the disease process. Laminitis may be seen in any hoofed animal, but is of greatest importance in horses and cattle. Laminitis occurs in three phases (developmental or preclinical, acute, and chronic). By definition, chronic laminitis (also called "founder") refers to the stage of laminitis associated with radiographic or physical evidence of rotational or vertical displacement of the third phalanx relative to the hoof wall. In severe laminitis, rotation may occur as early as 24 hours after the appearance of lameness. There are a variety of systemic causes of laminitis including, but not limited to, alimentary carbohydrate overload, toxemia, and sepsis. Repeated trauma to the foot may also cause laminitis. The pathogenesis of laminitis is complex, not completely understood, and controversial. There are two basic hypotheses, vascular and toxic-metabolic, that address mechanisms responsible for the systemic causes of laminitis. The vascular hypothesis argues that digital ischemia is the primary event. The toxic-metabolic hypothesis argues that there is direct damage to epithelial cells of the laminae or to the basement membrane, and that the vascular lesions are secondary. The principal clinical sign of laminitis is pain manifested as lameness, abnormal stance, or reluctance to move. Gross findings of the external foot in acute laminitis may be minimal. Swelling or edema of the coronary band may be seen; extravasation of serum through the skin above the coronary band is indicative of severe laminitis. Chronic lesions are highly variable, ranging from minimal gross changes to a totally gangrenous foot. Common gross lesions include circumferential hoof rings (ridges), altered foot shape, separation of the wall from the epidermis at the coronet, depression of coronary band, flattened sole, and, in some cases, penetration of the third phalanx through the sole. Diagnosis of laminitis is based principally on clinical, radiographic, and gross findings. Histopathology is used to facilitate understanding of the pathogenesis of laminitis. Regardless of whether the initial damage is ischemic or direct injury to the epithelium or basement membrane, the lesions of acute laminitis are degeneration and necrosis of epithelial cells of the laminae, separation of epithelial cells from the basement membrane, and loss of the basement membrane. If the epithelial and basement membrane damage is minor and patchy, regeneration of the damaged cells and basement membrane occurs preserving structural integrity of the epithelial laminae and hoof, and the animal does not enter into the chronic stage of laminitis. If the epithelial and basement membrane damage is more severe and confluent, the stability created by the interdigitating epithelial laminae attaching the hoof wall to the dermis and third phalanx is disrupted and the structural integrity of the foot is weakened. In addition, the epithelial necrosis causes release of inflammatory mediators such as cytokines, which result in congestion, edema, and an influx of a small to moderate number of neutrophils and mixed mononuclear cells. The edema adds to the soft tissue swelling and, in the confines of the rigid hoof wall, further compromises digital perfusion. If the tissue damage is subtotal, remaining epithelial cells regenerate. The hyperplasia and increased cornification of epithelial cells of the primary and secondary laminae cause broadening and fusion of the laminae, which reduces the surface area of the laminae and weakens the structural support of the hoof wall. The weakened structure of the epithelial laminae and basement membrane as a result of degeneration, necrosis, and subsequent epithelial hyperplasia, combined with the weight of the animal on the hoof and pulling force of the digital flexor tendon, contributes to displacement of the third phalanx, the hallmark of chronic laminitis, and to the altered shape of the foot in chronic laminitis.

Cutaneous Paraneoplastic Syndromes

Cutaneous paraneoplastic syndromes are rare dermatoses that occur in association with internal malignancies. Confirmation of a dermatosis as a paraneoplastic syndrome requires strict adherence to established clinical, histopathologic, and in some instances, immunologic criteria. Conditions meeting these criteria currently recognized in animals include paraneoplastic pemphigus (discussed in section on autoimmune diseases), cutaneous flushing associated with pheochromocytoma or mast cell tumor in the dog, and superficial necrolytic dermatopathy in the dog and cat, paraneoplastic pruritus with alopecia and bullous stomatitis in the horse, and paraneoplastic alopecia and exfoliative dermatosis in the cat. Dermatofibrosis in the dog and multisystemic eosinophilic epitheliotropic disease in the horse have also been associated with underlying neoplasia; however, they have not yet been proven to be true paraneoplastic syndromes. This list is exclusive of the endocrine dermatoses associated with functional tumors of endocrine organs. Many other syndromes are documented in man, and it is likely more will be documented in animals in the future. The refractory nature of these syndromes and their significance as a indicator of systemic disease underscores the importance of their recognition.

Paraneoplastic Alopecia Associated with Internal Malignancies in the Cat (Pancreatic Paraneoplastic Syndrome)

Rapidly progressive, ventrally distributed, symmetric alopecia has been reported as a marker of metastatic pancreatic or biliary carcinomas in older cats. Histologically, skin from the ventrum demonstrates marked follicular and adnexal atrophy and an absence of the stratum corneum that is thought to lead to the characteristic clinical appearance of "glistening alopecia."

Exfoliative Dermatitis and Thymoma in the Cat

A generalized exfoliative dermatitis has been documented as paraneoplastic syndrome of older cats with thymomas. The lesions begin as scaling and erythema of the head and ears and progress to generalized alopecia with scales, crusts, and ulcers. Histologically, the lesions are basal cell hydropic degeneration, lymphocyte exocytosis, lymphocyte clustering around apoptotic keratinocytes of the epidermis and outer follicular root sheath, which are suggestive of an immune system dysregulation. The lesions are compatible with erythema multiforme or a graft-versus-host–type reaction.

Nodular Dermatofibrosis and Renal Disease in the Dog

A syndrome of multiple cutaneous nodules composed of excessive dermal collagen coexistent with cystic renal disease has been described in German shepherd dogs, mixed-breed dogs, boxer and golden retriever. Renal lesions vary from multiple cysts with epithelial hyperplasia to cyst-adenomas, or cyst adenocarcinomas. Renal lesions are often bilateral and may not be detectable clinically for months or years after the appearance of dermal nodules. The condition in the German shepherd is thought to be inherited as an autosomal dominant trait. Whether the condition is a true paraneoplastic syndrome with the renal neoplasm-inducing dermal fibrosis or the simultaneous occurrence of two independent conditions with a common hereditary linkage is undetermined.

Superficial Necrolytic Dermatopathy (Diabetic Dermatopathy, Hepatocutaneous Syndrome, Necrolytic Migratory Erythema)

This disorder has been reported primarily in older dogs in association with deranged nutrient metabolism due to diabetes mellitus, hepatic dysfunction, or less commonly with glucagon-secreting pancreatic islet tumors. A single case of the condition in a cat with concurrent pancreatic endocrine carcinoma has been reported. Lesions of scaling, crusting, erythema, and alopecia develop on the face, distal extremities, and genitalia. Footpad lesions consist of crusting and fissuring or ulceration (Fig. 11-61). Microscopic lesions, when fully developed, are considered diagnostic and consist of a trilaminar thickening of the epidermis in which the outermost layer is parakeratotic, the intermediate epidermal layer is pale with reticular

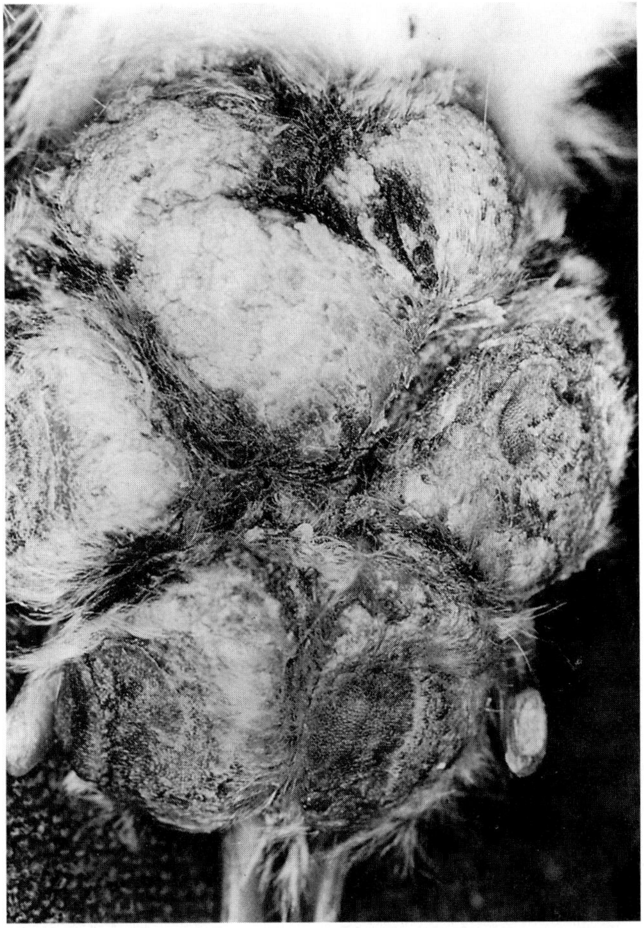

Figure 11-61 Skin, foot pad; dog. Superficial necrolytic dermatitis. Crusting and fissuring are present.

degeneration, and the innermost layer is hyperplastic (see Fig. 11-5). Dermatophytes, probably a secondary infection, have been identified in the footpads of some dogs with this syndrome.

CUTANEOUS NEOPLASIA

The skin is a common site of neoplastic growth in most animals; the neoplasms are of ectodermal, mesodermal, and melanocytic origin. Ectodermal neoplasms of the epidermis and adnexa are most often benign with the exception of the neoplasms of the apocrine sweat glands, apocrine glands of the anal sac, and neoplasms of the surface epithelium (squamous cell carcinomas).

Benign neoplasms do not metastasize or invade adjacent tissue. In general, benign neoplasms are circumscribed, grow by expansion, and are composed of well-differentiated cells that closely resemble the cells or tissue of origin. Malignant neoplasms are locally invasive and often metastasize. They are more often composed of anaplastic cells with a high mitotic index that no longer resemble the cells of origin. Anaplastic cells are pleomorphic (vary in cell size and shape) and have a large, vesicular nucleus with increased size and number of nucleoli. Malignant cells develop surface alterations such as altered antigenicity, decreased numbers or altered location of receptors for adjacent cells, and increased receptors for components of the extracellular matrix. Changes such as these allow malignant cells to detach from the primary site of tumor growth, move through tissues, and in some cases escape detection by the host's immune system. A specific example is the loss of E-cadherins (proteins responsible for epithelial cell to cell attachment) by some types of carcinomas. E-cadherins are partially responsible for the "contact inhibition" that leads to density control and inhibits uncontrolled proliferation of epithelial cells.

Neoplasms of the skin develop secondary to the same basic molecular changes, leading to the development of neoplasms of any tissue. The neoplastic transformation of a cell is the end result of a series of events causing damage to the cellular DNA. Most agents that are known to be carcinogenic target and damage DNA. Solar radiation, x-radiation, viral infections, and continued trauma are important contributors to neoplastic transformation of components of the skin. Continued trauma contributes to tumor development by increasing cell turnover, which in turn increases the chance of mutations. Not all factors contributing to the development of cutaneous neoplasms are known.

Four categories of genes encode for a large number of proteins responsible for regulation of cellular proliferation and differentiation. These categories are the tumor suppressor genes, the protooncogenes, genes that regulate apoptosis, and genes that regulate DNA repair. Damage to these genes results in deranged cellular proliferation by the abnormal expression or function of proteins such as growth factors, growth factor receptors, signal-transducing proteins, cell cycle regulators, and nuclear transcription factors. The majority of malignant neoplasms have evidence of damage (mutation) of multiple genes within these categories. Mutations are often collected by cells in a stepwise manner that imparts increasing degrees of malignant potential. These molecular changes are known to correlate with morphologic changes and the clinical behavior of some neoplasms. For example, it is known that squamous cell carcinomas often develop in a stepwise manner and progress through several recognizable stages: hyperplasia (excessive number of cells present; no cellular atypia or tissue disorganization) → dysplasia (cellular atypia and tissue disorganization present) → carcinoma in situ (marked cellular atypia and disorganization present, but no invasion of underlying basement membrane) → invasive squamous cell carcinoma (disruption of the basement membrane with dermal invasion by anaplastic carcinoma cells). The progression of the disease from mere hyperplasia to an invasive carcinoma represents a series of molecular events whereby the population of cells harbors an increasing number of damaged genes belonging to the four categories of genes listed. This series of changes takes place over long periods of time, often years, before a tumor reaches full malignant potential. The process may be halted in the early stages if the agents causing continued genetic damage can be removed (for example, exposure to UV radiation).

Most cutaneous neoplasms are primary, as the skin is an uncommon to rare site for metastasis; however, the skin can be the site of secondary tumor growth. Examples include mammary gland neoplasms that invade into adjacent skin, feline pulmonary bronchogenic carcinomas that metastasize to multiple digits of the feet, and canine visceral hemangiosarcomas that may metastasize to the skin. Table 11-3 gives an abbreviated listing of the salient features of cutaneous neoplasms.

GLOSSARY

Acantholysis loss of cohesion between keratinocytes due to the breakdown of intercellular bridges via immune destruction or due to neutrophilic enzymatic destruction

Acanthosis thickening of the spinous cell layer (stratum spinosum)

Acral distal parts of the extremities

Alopecia hair loss

Anagen phase of hair cycle in which hair synthesis takes place

Anaplasia lack of cellular differentiation and organization, a feature of neoplastic cells

Apoptosis programmed cell death

Atrophy reduction in size of a cell, tissue, organ, or part

Blister (vesicle or bulla) localized collection of fluid usually in or beneath epidermis

Bulla large blister (>0.5 cm)

Catagen transition phase of the hair cycle between growth and resting phases

Comedo (comedones) plug of keratin and dried sebum in a hair follicle

Cornification production of stratum corneum by terminal epidermal differentiation

Crust material formed by drying of exudate or secretion on the skin surface

Cytokines small molecular weight protein molecules (generally ≤ 30 kDa) that are mediators of inflammation and growth

Dematiaceous naturally pigmented black or brown mycelium or conidium

Dermatosis noninflammatory lesion of the skin

Dermatophytosis infection of the keratin of the epidermis, hair, or nails with fungi of the genera *Microsporum, Epidermophyton,* or *Trichophyton*

Dyskeratosis abnormal, premature, or imperfect keratinization

Dysplasia abnormal development

Effluvium shedding of hair

Epidermal collarette peripheral expanding ring of scaling

Epidermolysis separation of the epidermis from the dermis

Eruption rapid development of skin lesion associated with redness

Erosion loss of all or part of the thickness of the epidermis

Erythema redness of skin due to congestion of capillaries

Excoriation superficial loss of epithelium due to physical trauma (scratching)

Exfoliation shedding of layers or scales

Exudation escape of fluid, cells, or debris from blood vessels and its deposition in or on other tissues

Fissure cleft or groove

Folliculitis inflammation of a hair follicle

Furuncle circumscribed, painful nodule (accumulation of pus) in the dermis secondary to follicular rupture

Genodermatosis a genetically determined disorder of the skin

Glabrous smooth skin, hairless skin

Gynecomastia excessive development of mammary glands in the male

Hydropic degeneration intracellular edema of basal epidermal cells

Hyperhidrosis excessive sweating

Hyperkeratosis histologic term for thickening of stratum corneum (keratin layer)

Hyperplasia increase in the number of normal cells

Hypoplasia incomplete development

Hypotrichosis less hair than normal

Ichthyosis congenital skin disorder associated with marked hyperkeratosis

Impetigo bacterial dermatitis characterized by pustules

Indurated hardened

Interface mild dermal inflammation arranged in a layer close to and often obscuring the epidermal-dermal junction (interface), and with vacuolar and sometimes apoptotic basal cells. There is controversy regarding the meaning of the terms interface and lichenoid. Some use the terms interchangeably, and others define interface as much milder inflammation that is tightly associated with the epidermal dermal interface, often obscuring the interface, and associated with vacuolar and apoptotic basal cells.

Intertrigo dermatitis that develops due to friction between apposing skin surfaces (e.g., adjacent folds)

Keratinocytes the epidermal cells that synthesize keratin and comprise more than 90% of epidermal cells

Keratosis excessive formation of keratin in localized areas of epidermis

Langerhans' cells antigen-presenting cells of the skin

Lichenification thickening of skin with accentuation of skin creases

Lichenoid dense "bandlike" dermal inflammation parallel to the epidermis that may or may not obscure the epidermal dermal interface. There is controversy regarding the meaning of the terms lichenoid and interface. Some use the terms interchangeably, and others define lichenoid as a much denser band of subepidermal inflammation that does not necessarily obscure the epidermal dermal interface.

Macule flat, circumscribed lesion of altered skin color

Melanin dark, amorphous pigment consisting of dihydroxy indoxylic acid

Melanophage macrophage containing ingested melanin

Merkel cell a neuroendocrine cell found in the stratum basale

Mycelium a mass of hyphae

Myxedema nonpitting edema of the skin due to abnormal deposits of mucin in the dermis

Nevus circumscribed malformation of the skin assumed to be of congenital or inherited origin, and consisting of any component of the skin; most common are pigmented epidermal nevi and collagenous nevi

Onychodystrophy abnormal formation of the nail

Onychomadesis sloughing of nails

Panniculitis inflammation of subcutaneous adipose tissue

Papule small, circumscribed, solid elevation of skin

Parakeratosis retention of pyknotic nuclei in epidermal cells of the stratum corneum due to faulty or accelerated cornification

Paronychia inflammation of skin around the nails

Pemphigus cutaneous disease associated with blistering

Phaeohyphomycosis mycotic disease caused by pigmented fungi (dematiaceous) of a variety of genera and species that do not form sclerotic bodies or granules

Pigmentary incontinence melanin released from previously injured basal layer cells is phagocytized by dermal macrophages or remains free in the dermis

Plaque a flat-topped, solid elevation in the skin that occupies a relatively large surface area in comparison with its height

Pruritus itching
Pyoderma pyogenic (pus-producing) bacterial infection of the skin (e.g., luminal folliculitis)
Pustule small, circumscribed accumulation of pus within the epidermis
Scale a thin, platelike accumulation of keratin on surface of skin
Sebaceous pertaining to sebum
Seborrhea nonspecific term for clinical signs of scaling, crusting, and greasiness. Primary seborrhea is a more specific term applied to inherited cornification disorders.
Sebum secretion of sebaceous glands; thick semifluid substance composed of fat and epithelial debris
Spongiosis intercellular edema which, by widening of the intercellular space and stretching of the "intercellular bridges," creates a spongelike appearance to the epidermis
Telogen resting phase of the hair cycle
Ulcer loss of epidermis and at least superficial portion of dermis
Urticaria vascular reaction in dermis consisting of transient wheals (hives)
Vesicle small blister within the epidermis or at or below the dermal-epidermal interface (<0.5 cm)
Vibrissa (sinus hair) long, coarse hair located about the muzzle
Vitiligo acquired disorder characterized by circumscribed areas of depigmentation in the skin
Wheal smooth, circumscribed, slightly elevated area on skin caused by dermal edema
Yeast unicellular budding fungus

Suggested Readings

Campbell KL. Feline dermatology. Veterinary Clinics North America (Small Animal Practice). 1999; 29.

Fadok VA. Dermatology. Veterinary Clinics North America (Equine Practice) 1995;11.

Goldschmidt MH, Shofer FS. Skin tumors of the dog and cat. New York: Pergamon, 1992.

Gross TL, Ihrke PJ, Walder EJ. Veterinary dermatopathology: A macroscopic and microscopic evaluation of canine and feline skin disease. St. Louis: Mosby–Year Book, 1992.

Kunkle GA. Feline dermatology. Veterinary Clinics North America (Small Animal Practice) 1995;4.

Pascoe RRR, Knottenbelt DC. Manual of equine dermatology. Philadelphia: Saunders, 1999.

Ruoslahi E. Fundamental understandings: How cancer spreads. Sci American September 1996; 72-77.

Scott DW. Large animal dermatology. Philadelphia: Saunders, 1988.

Scott DW, Miller WH, Griffin CE. Muller & Kirk's Small Animal Dermatology. 6th ed. Philadelphia: Saunders, 2000.

Stannard AA, Pulley LT. Tumors of the skin and soft tissues. In: Moulton JE, ed. Tumors in domestic animals. 3rd ed. Berkeley: University of California Press, 1990:23-87.

Weinberg RA. Fundamental understandings: How cancer arises. Sci American September 1996; 61-70.

Yager JA, Scott DW. The skin and appendages. In: Jubb KVF, Kennedy PC, Palmer N, eds. Pathology of domestic animals. 4th ed. New York: Academic, 1993:531-738.

Yager JA, Wilcock BP. Color atlas and text of surgical pathology of the dog and cat. St. Louis: Mosby–Year Book, 1994.

CHAPTER 12

Reproductive System: Female

HELEN M. ACLAND

DEVELOPMENTAL ANOMALIES OF THE FEMALE SYSTEM

The sex of an individual can be defined at several different levels: genetic, chromosomal, gonadal, ductal, and phenotypic. Normal mammalian chromosomal sex is XX for female and XY for male. On the Y chromosome, a gene (sex-determining region Y, Sry) for the testis-determining factor has been identified. The differentiation of a gonad to a testis is dependent on this gene. In its absence, the indifferent embryonic gonad differentiates into an ovary, by default or under the influence of as yet unidentified factors. In the normal mammalian female, the Wolffian ducts regress in the absence of the Sry gene product and the cascade of events it stimulates. The Müllerian ducts persist.

Intersexes

Gonadal sex is based on the histologic components of the gonad. Ductal sex is based on whether the tissue elements are derived from the Müllerian (female) or the Wolffian (male) system. The appearance of the external genitalia is the criterion used for determination of phenotypic sex. The gender can be uncertain when the various components are of mixed male and female types.

Abnormalities of Phenotypic Sex

Pseudohermaphrodites have the chromosomes and gonads of one sex and the tubular organs modified toward those of the opposite sex. They are classified according to the gonadal tissue. Female pseudohermaphrodites are rare. The best known example is the masculinization of female fetuses by sex steroid hormones given to the dam during pregnancy or shortly before conception. Human female pseudohermaphrodites occur in the adrenogenital syndrome, caused by a defect in one of the enzymes responsible for cortisol production. Cortisol precursors accumulate because of excess adrenocorticotropic hormone (ACTH) production in response to low cortisol concentrations. These precursors are converted to androgen rather than to cortisol, and the androgens masculinize the fetal genitalia.

Segmental aplasia of the Müllerian-derived duct system can have a variety of forms. Segmental aplasia of the Müllerian duct system most often occurs in shorthorn cattle, in which it is associated with the recessive gene for white coat color. The simplest form is failure of the Müllerian duct to make a proper connection with the urogenital sinus, leaving a persistent hymen, the division between the two precursor tissues. A perforated hymen often persists and is of no clinical significance. However, if the hymen membrane is completely imperforate, the vagina, cervix, and uterus fill with normal secretions, become atonic, and are likely to become infected because of the potential microbial growth medium in the tract. In the more severe forms, one or more segments of the vagina, cervix, uterine body, and uterine horns are absent or rudimentary (Fig. 12-1). Generally, the ovaries, uterine tubes, and most anterior parts of the uterine horns are present and normal, except the horns can be distended by secretion.

Aplasia of a segment of the uterus can affect the ovaries. Prostaglandin can be synthesized and released from a uterine horn made blind by the absence of a segment, just as it would be produced by a normally connected uterine horn. In species such as the pig in which systemic transmission of prostaglandin $F_{2\alpha}$ from the endometrium to the corpus luteum is important, prostaglandins from the blind uterine horn can have a lytic effect on the corpora lutea of pregnancy in the contralateral ovary. In species such as the cow in which the local utero-ovarian pathway is important for luteolysis, the absence of a large segment of the uterus could result in $PGF_{2\alpha}$ insufficient for regression of the corpus luteum. Even a small segment of uterine aplasia can have the same effect, if the cranial segment becomes distended with fluid and does not synthesize prostaglandins. In the dog and cat, the uterus does not play a role in the regression of the corpus luteum.

Imperfect fusion of the paired Müllerian ducts is a common cause of anomalies. Normally, the two ducts unite first at the cloacal end to form the vagina and the process moves cephalad to form the cervix and the uterine fundus. A double uterine fundus, called uterus didelphys, and a double cervix are normal structures at an early stage of development. Malformations due to imperfect fusion are most common in and adjacent to the cervix. They range

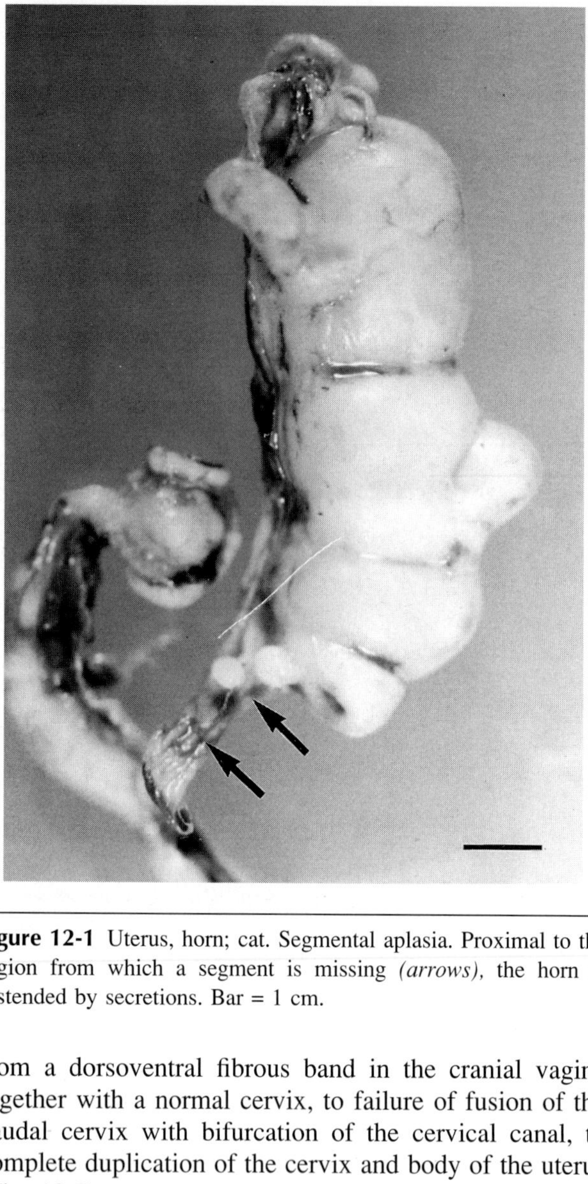

Figure 12-1 Uterus, horn; cat. Segmental aplasia. Proximal to the region from which a segment is missing *(arrows)*, the horn is distended by secretions. Bar = 1 cm.

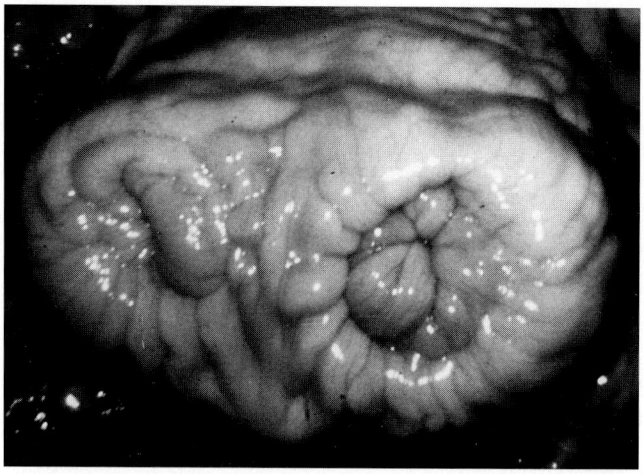

Figure 12-2 Cervix; cow. Double cervices, side by side, caused by failure of normal fusion of the paired Müllerian ducts. *Courtesy Dr. R. Zemjanis.*

from a dorsoventral fibrous band in the cranial vagina together with a normal cervix, to failure of fusion of the caudal cervix with bifurcation of the cervical canal, to complete duplication of the cervix and body of the uterus (Fig. 12-2).

Abnormalities of Gonadal Sex

Hermaphrodites have both ovarian and testicular tissue in their gonads. They are further classified into three types: "bilateral" or "unilateral," according to whether a combined organ, called an ovotestis, is present on one or both sides, and "lateral," with a testis on one side and an ovary on the other. Hermaphrodites have a genital tract that cannot be easily classified as male or female. True hermaphrodites are rare. In many cases, the mechanism for the development of hermaphrodites is unknown, but the mechanism for some are known. Examples include chimera formation and partial sex reversal produced by small amounts of testis-determining factor in an animal with XX chromosomes. Hermaphrodites occur in canine, porcine, and caprine XX sex reversals.

Animals in which the gonadal sex does not follow the chromosomal sex are termed "sex reversed." Examples are XX true hermaphrodites and XX males. In these animals, the testis-determining factor gene is present on an X chromosome or an autosome. Partial or complete sex reversals have been described in several species, including dogs (American cocker spaniel, Chinese pug, German shorthaired pointer, Kerry blue terrier, Norwegian elkhound) pigs, goats, horses, and a llama. From work in dogs, in which XX true hermaphrodites and XX males were found in the same family of cocker spaniels, it is likely that the two phenomena represent varying degrees of severity of the same defect. In cocker spaniel dogs, XX sex reversal is inherited as an autosomal recessive trait. Most are XX true hermaphrodites, and 10% are XX males. Some of the hermaphrodites have female appearance and are fertile. The testes of the XX males do not have germ cells. XX male dogs have penile malformations, including hypoplasia and abnormal curvature. In affected cocker spaniels, Müllerian duct derivatives persist, and the ductus deferens is embedded in the myometrium.

In sex-reversed goats, the gene with the Y effect is close to the gene for hornlessness ("polled"), a dominant gene. Heterozygotes are hornless and have normal genitalia; homozygous hornless goats are either XY normal males or XX hermaphrodites or pseudohermaphrodites with testes or ovotestes. The extreme variability in gonadal differentiation frequently seen among intersex goats could be explained by variability in the dose of the factor with the sex-determining effect. Sry cannot be identified in some intersex goats. The external appearance of these goats ranges from that of a normal male to that of a female with an enlarged clitoris.

Abnormalities of Chromosomal Sex

Animals with abnormal chromosomal sex generally have underdeveloped rather than ambiguous organs. Examples are XXY males (Klinefelter's syndrome), XO females (Turner's syndrome), and XXX females.

Animals that are chimeras or mosaics for the sex chromosomes do have ambiguous reproductive organs. Chimeras and mosaics have two or more cell types, each with a different chromosomal constitution. The cells of a chimera come from two different sources (such as from male and female members of a set of twins in the bovine freemartin), whereas the cells of a mosaic come from the same source. Several cases of canine chimeras have been described.

The most common chimera in domestic animals is the **freemartin** calf. Placental vascular anastomoses, which allow exchange of blood between fetuses, are a requirement for the occurrence of a freemartin. These anastomoses occur most often in the bovine species, and less frequently in other ruminants. The freemartin is the female of a set of male and female twins. The percentage of male cells in freemartins varies widely. Müllerian inhibitory substance from the male twin's testes causes the differentiation of fetal Sertoli cells and seminiferous cordlike structures in the female twin's ovaries. The ovaries are small, ranging from organs with reduced number of or no germ cells, to organs partially converted to testes, or to organs composed entirely of structures resembling seminiferous tubules. The Müllerian duct derivatives vary from almost normal to cordlike structures, but communication is never made with the vagina (Fig. 12-3). The vagina, vestibule, and vulva are hypoplastic. Seminal vesicles are always present; other Wolffian structures are present to varying degrees. Externally the animal appears female, but the vestibule and vagina are short, the vulva is hypoplastic, and the clitoris is enlarged. The male twin is minimally affected.

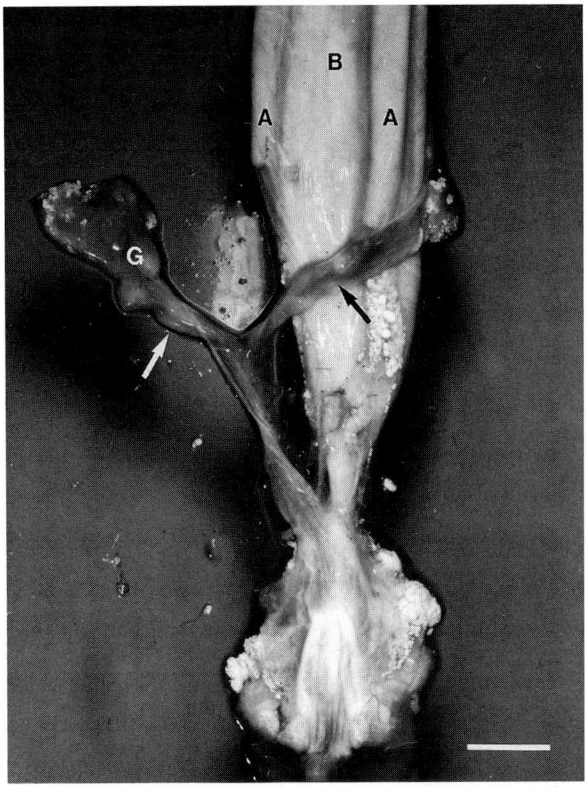

Figure 12-3 Urogenital tract; freemartin newborn calf. Compared with the normally sized urinary bladder *(B)* and umbilical arteries *(A)*, the genital tract is very small. Seminal vesicles are present but not visible in this case because of the surrounding fat. (*G*, gonad; uterine horns indicated by *arrows*). Bar = 2 cm.

VAGINA AND VULVA

Cysts in the vaginal wall of the cow arise from Gartner's ducts (Wolffian remnants) or Bartholin's glands. Causes of cyst formation include inflammation of the lining of the duct or gland, and hyperestrogenism, in which edema due to estrogen stimulation is prolonged. Gartner's ducts normally do not open into the vagina. When they become cystic, they form single or multiple cysts or a tortuous channel in the floor of the vagina somewhere between the cervix and near the urethral opening (Fig. 12-4). Bartholin's glands become cystic when edema, inflammation, or scar tissue obstructs their openings into the lateral wall of the vagina or vagina-vulva junction.

Tumefaction of the vulva is normal during estrus. Overly large or persistent swelling is abnormal. Abnormal tumefaction occurs in hyperestrogenism. An example is poisoning of pigs by the mycotoxin zearalenone found in moldy corn. Other effects of the mycotoxin are precocious mammary development, tenesmus leading to rectal prolapse, and the luteotrophic activities that induce anestrus or pseudopregnancy.

Ingestion of moldy corn by pig → mycotoxin zearalenone toxicity → hyperestrogenism → vulvar swelling, precocious mammary development, tenesmus leading to rectal prolapse, & luteotrophic activity leading to anestrus or pseudopregnancy.

Inflammation

The vagina and vulva are lined by stratified squamous epithelium that is fairly resistant to infection.

Postparturient vulvitis and vaginitis occur when these organs are lacerated during dystocia and become infected (Fig. 12-5). Trauma unrelated to parturition also can progress similarly. Inflammation of the cervix and posterior vagina following dystocia can have a more serious outcome because of the possible local spread of infection into and through the vaginal wall into the peritoneal cavity.

Granular vulvitis in cows has no established cause, but *Mycoplasma* and *Ureaplasma* spp. have been proposed. Granular vulvitis, associated with *Ureaplasma* infection, characteristically in the acute stage has a profuse purulent vulvular discharge and a hyperemic vulvular mucosa with 2-mm raised granules. The disease can become chronic and lesions resolve within 3 months. However, the acute signs can recur. In about 10% of affected cows, discrete, raised, white epithelial inclusion cysts, 2 to 5 mm in diameter, occur in rows or clusters on the dorsolateral wall of the vulva. Reduced fertility is likely due to persistence of the organisms in the uterus for up to 7 days following contamination of the uterus from the vulvular lesions at breeding.

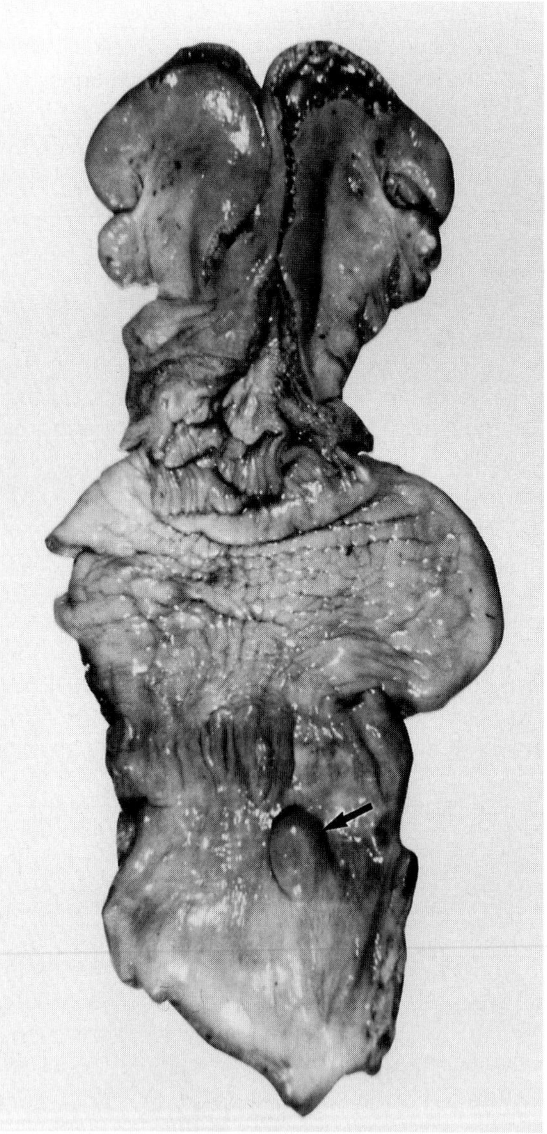

Figure 12-4 Genital tract; cow. Cystic Gartener's duct. A unilateral cystic duct *(arrow)* is present on the floor of the vagina. Gartener's ducts, which are Wolffian remnants, are normally not visible and become apparent only when hyperplastic, inflamed, or obstructed.

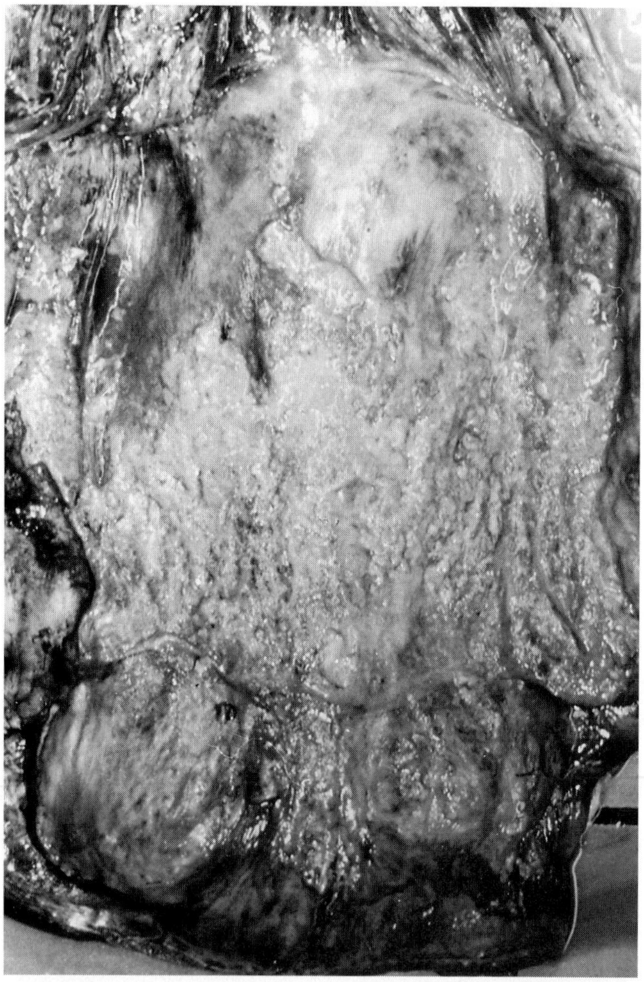

Figure 12-5 Vagina; mare. Acute vaginitis. The vaginal mucosa is thick, rough, and irregular because of severe, diffuse, acute, necrotizing vaginitis. Infection followed the trauma of dystocia and manual delivery of a foal.

Infectious pustular vulvovaginitis of cattle is caused by bovine herpesvirus 1, which is similar to the BHV-1 that is the cause of infectious bovine rhinotracheitis (IBR). The two diseases behave as separate entities, but their occurrence can overlap in a herd or in an individual. Vulvovaginitis is transmitted by coitus, artificial insemination, and possibly nose to vulva contact. The first evidence of the disease includes hyperemia and edema of the vagina and vulva; these lesions are followed by petechial hemorrhages and slight nodularity of the mucosal surfaces. A rapidly coalescing multifocal erosion and ulceration of the mucosa follows, beginning over the lymphoid nodules. Microscopically, changes can be detected in the epithelium, the lamina propria, and the lymphoid nodules. The epithelium with eosinophilic intranuclear inclusions undergoes ballooning degeneration followed by necrosis, neutrophil infiltration, and desquamation, but without a discrete stage of vesicle or pustule formation. The lamina propria is hyperemic, edematous, and infiltrated by inflammatory cells, mostly lymphocytes and plasma cells. The subepithelial lymphoid nodules are hyperplastic. Resolution of the disease is rapid, and the lesions that remain are slightly thickened epithelium and hyperplastic lymphoid nodules. Lesions are similar in the penis of affected bulls. Caprine herpesvirus 1 causes lesions in goats similar to those of bovine vulvovaginitis. In the equine species, equine

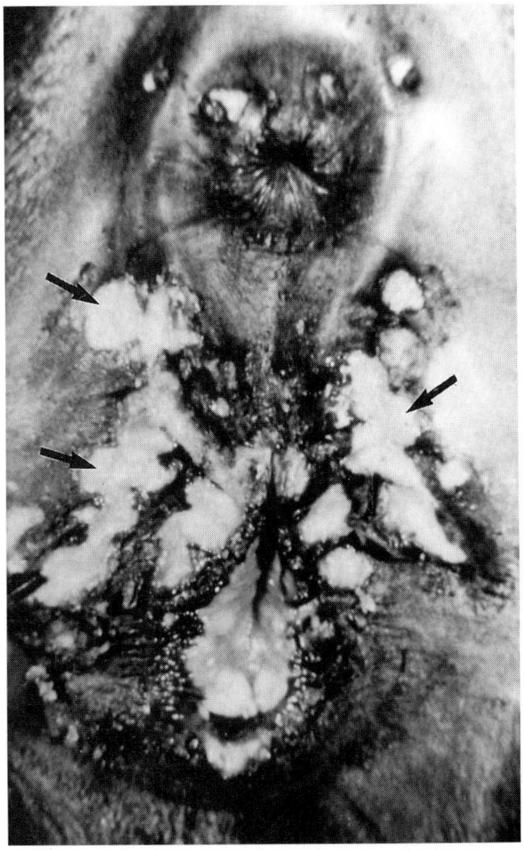

Figure 12-6 Vulva; mare. Coital exanthema. Note the multiple, circular ruptured vesicles *(arrows)*. *Courtesy Dr. L.J. Gleeson.*

herpesvirus 3 (as distinct from equine herpesvirus 1, responsible for respiratory disease, nervous disease, and abortion) is the cause of coital exanthema characterized by transient vesicles and erosions, morphologically similar to those observed in IBR, on the external genitalia of both mares and stallions (Fig. 12-6). Infectious bovine cervicovaginitis, or "epivag," occurs in Africa and is likely caused by bovine herpesvirus 4. It is transmitted only by coitus. Lesions of intense congestion and abundant purulent exudate develop first in the anterior vagina and rapidly spread to the uterus, uterine tubes, and ovarian bursae.

Dourine, caused by *Trypanosoma equiperdum,* is a venereal disease of equidae that is enzootic in Africa, Asia, southeastern Europe, and South America. *T. equiperdum* can penetrate the intact vaginal mucosa and multiply locally in the wall before becoming systemic. Trypanosomes can be found in male and female genital discharges and in blood of infected animals. Lesions are found in the skin and nervous system as well as in the genital tract. The virulence of the organism, resistance of the host, incubation period, persistence of the trypanosomes in the blood, length and severity of the clinical disease, and severity of the lesions vary tremendously. In the male and female external genital organs, the acute lesion is extensive edema. With time, the areas with edema become fibrotic. Lymphoid nodules of the genital tract are hyperplastic, and the overlying mucosa is ulcerated. Ulcers heal without repigmentation of the epithelium.

Neoplasms

Transmissible venereal tumor (TVT) of the dog is transmitted by coitus and by the transfer of intact neoplastic cells. A viral cause has been investigated. TVT cells have 59 chromosomes compared with the normal canine number of 78. Both sexes are affected. The neoplasm begins as a nodule beneath the genital mucosa and, when enlarged, breaks through the overlying mucosa. In the bitch, the lesion often begins in the dorsal wall of the vagina at the junction with the vestibule. It proliferates into the lumen of the vagina and can protrude through the vulva as an ulcerated, friable mass. Microscopically, the neoplastic cells are large, round or oval, uniform in size but with occasional large, bizarre nuclei. Cytoplasm is poorly defined and lightly staining. The number of cells in mitosis is increased. Spontaneous regression of the neoplasm is the rule, and neoplasms have multifocal necrosis, infiltration of lymphocytes, likely cell-mediated neoplastic cell lysis, and deposition of collagen. A few neoplasms have metastases in other sites, although in countries with stray dogs and dogs in poor health, neoplasms with metastases are relatively common. An explanation for the patchiness of the worldwide distribution of the disease has not been developed.

Squamous cell carcinoma of the vulva occurs in the mature cow, ewe, and the mare (Fig. 12-7). Solar radiation has been established as an etiologic factor. Ewes subjected to the Mules' operation (surgery to the perineum and inguinal areas intended to redirect the tip of the vulva to prevent urine wetting the wool) and to short tail docking have a greater exposure of the vulva and greater incidence of squamous cell carcinoma of the vulva. Correlation can be made of incidence with exposure to sunlight, and, at least in the cow, with the lack of pigmentation of the vulva. The squamous cell carcinoma originates on the hairless and less pigmented skin of the vulva and has the appearance and biologic behavior of squamous cell carcinomas in other sites. The neoplasm metastasizes late in the course of disease to the iliac lymph nodes.

CERVIX

Anomalies. Two entire or a single bifurcated cervix along with a divided vagina and two uteri can result from failure of proper fusion of the paired elements of the Müllerian system. In cows, some developmental abnormalities are restricted to the cervix. These include hypertrophy or hypoplasia of the whole structure, aplasia of one or more of the usual five rugae, tortuosity, and dilation or diverticulum formation of the cervical canal.

Cervicitis usually occurs as a minor lesion concurrently with more severe endometritis or vaginitis. This distribution is observed in specific infectious diseases, such as contagious equine metritis caused by *Taylorella equigenitalis,* and in nonspecific postparturient metritis, cervicitis, and vaginitis. As a single lesion, inflammation of the cervix can result from poorly performed traumatic artificial insemination. In cows with acute cervicitis, the caudal rugae are edematous and prolapse into the vagina. Inflammatory exudate covers the cervical mucosa and collects in the vagina. The cervical mucosa is relatively thin, and the underlying fibromuscular tissue is relatively impervious to infection; thus most cases of cervicitis resolve readily. Those infections that follow traumatic dystocia are likely to involve the muscle layer from the onset and have potential for production of severe lesions. These lesions include pericervical abscesses, local peritonitis with granulating tracts into the connective tissue of the pelvic canal, stenosis with adhesions across the lumen of the cervix in areas denuded of epithelium, or cysts filled with mucus in the lining.

Neoplastic disease of the cervix of domestic animals is rare.

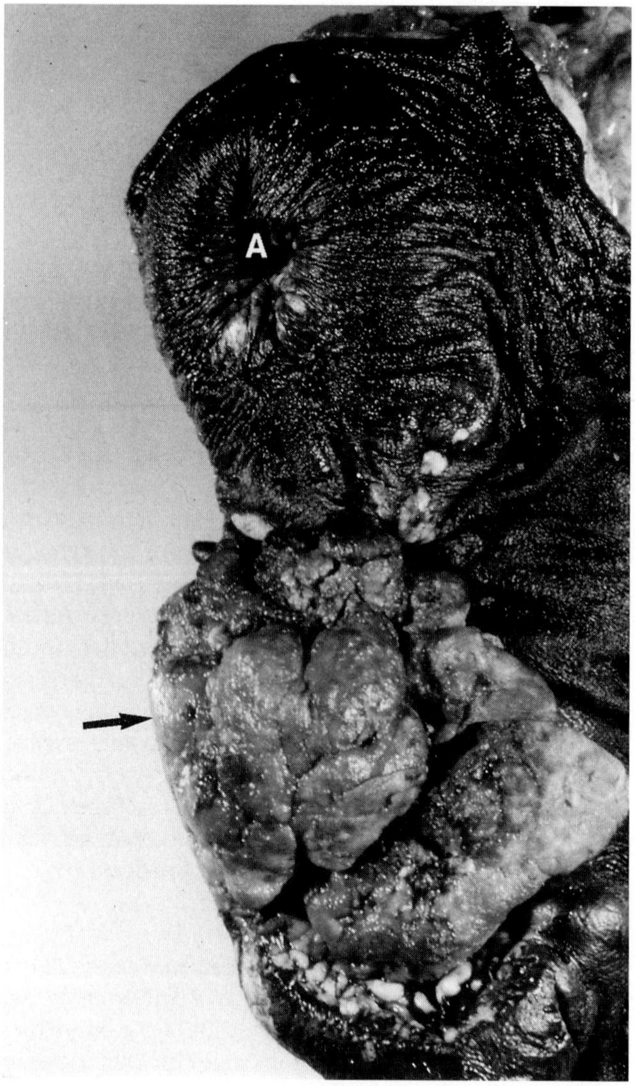

Figure 12-7 Vulva; mare. Squamous cell carcinoma. The opening of the vagina is filled by neoplastic tissue *(arrow).* (*A,* anus).

UTERUS

Noninflammatory Abnormalities

Torsion of the uterus occurs mostly in pregnant animals, mainly in the cow, and to a lesser extent in the bitch and queen (Fig. 12-8), and when the uterus is enlarged by pyometra (accumulation of pus in the uterine lumen) or mucometra (accumulation of mucus in the uterine lumen). The mesovarium is a fixed point in both the cow and the bitch, with the other fixed point influenced by the length of the horns and the presence and rigidity of the ligament between the horns. Rotation tends to occur about the cervix in the cow and the junction of the uterine horn and body in the bitch. The result of torsion is circulatory compromise; the veins, being thinner walled, are compressed and occluded before the arteries. The uterine wall and placenta become congested and edematous. The fetus dies and mummifies or putrefies if the cervix is open enough to allow the entrance of bacteria or fungi to colonize the fetus. The uterine wall is friable and prone to rupture. Rupture of the uterus is also likely in severe dystocia and during treatment of uterine diseases by infusion of drugs and fluids. Rupture can be incomplete, involving just the mucosa, or complete. The torsion and dystocia-related ruptures are likely to be in the caudal part of the uterus and are often fatal because of hemorrhage or infection. The rupture that follows overvigorous infusion of medications into the uterus occurs at the lesser curvature of a horn, dissects beneath the serosa and into the mesometrium, and results in perimetritis.

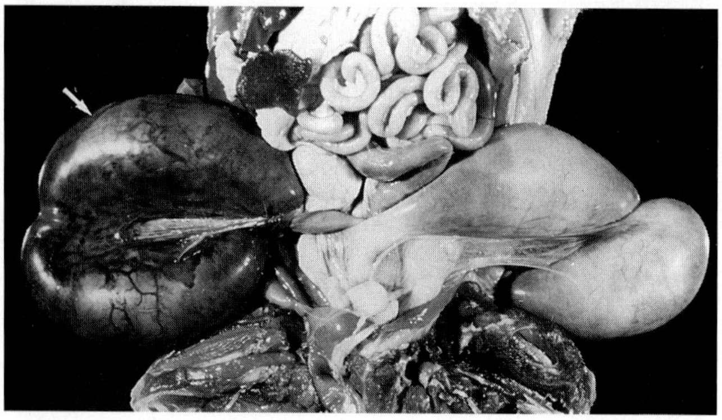

Figure 12-8 Uterus; pregnant cat. Torsion. The affected (right) horn *(arrow)* is purple-black, whereas the normal horn is pink.

Prolapse of the uterus is important in the ewe, cow, and sow after parturition. Factors that cause uterine inertia, such as prolonged dystocia, hypocalcemia, and ingestion of estrogenic plants, usually contribute to prolapse of the uterus. The anatomic structures that are prolapsed can be restricted to the previously pregnant horn, or also include all of the uterus, the bladder, and sometimes some small intestine. Vascular compromise, shock, trauma, and infection follow prolapse.

Subinvolution of placental sites is the longer than normal persistence and deeper than normal penetration of trophoblast-like cells in the uterus after parturition. In the normal placenta, trophoblasts are found in the endometrium and around the small blood vessels of the myometrium, but they rapidly degenerate in the postpartum period. In the bitch, subinvolution of placental sites is characterized clinically by a bloody vaginal discharge that lasts for weeks or months after delivery. Grossly, subinvoluted placental sites are about twice the size of normal sites for the same time after parturition. Also, multiple segmental thickenings of the walls of the uterine horns are identifiable from the serosal surface (Fig. 12-9) and are interspersed with normal areas. The luminal surface of each site is a raised, rough, ragged, gray to brown plaque.

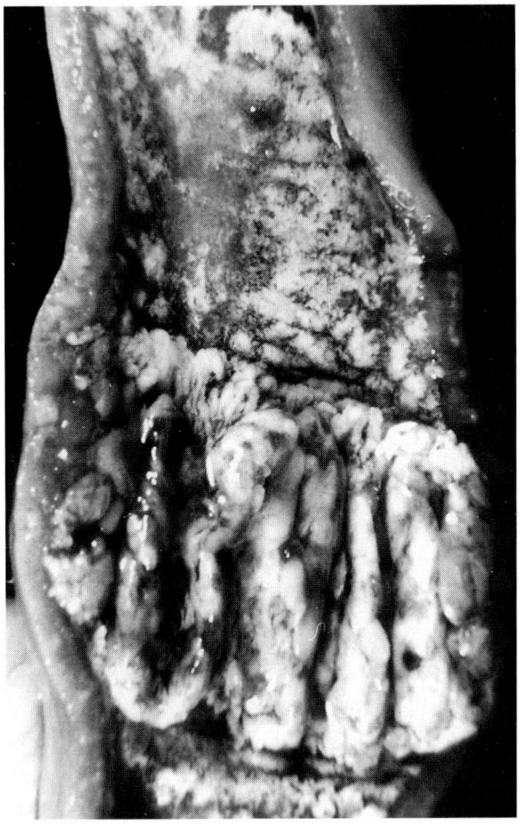

Figure 12-9 Uterus; bitch. Subinvolution of placental site. The placental site is a circumferential band that is more raised and rough surfaced than a normal placental site at the same time after parturition.

Microscopically, the superficial part of the plaque near the lumen is composed of cell debris, hematoma, thrombus, and regenerating endometrium. In the deeper part of the site, the changes are collagen deposition, hemorrhage, and distension, and decreased density of endometrial glands. Trophoblast-like cells are more numerous in subinvolution sites than in the normal placental sites and are abundant at the base of the deposited collagen; these cells invade the myometrium and penetrate the full thickness of the wall and perforate the uterus.

Endometrial atrophy is usually due to loss of ovarian function secondary to hypopituitarism as the endometrial atrophy of old age is not seen in domestic species. In the mare, diffuse endometrial atrophy occurs in anestrus and also occurs, but much less commonly, because of the ovarian inactivity of debility and chromosomal aberrations. Focal endometrial atrophy of unknown cause sometimes occurs in the mare. Atrophic endometrium is thin and flat. In the mare, the longitudinal folds are indistinct in atrophic areas, and in the cow, the caruncles are flattened. The uterus of the mare has been most studied microscopically because data from uterine biopsies are frequently used for the management of breeding. The endometrium of the uterus of the anestrous mare has cuboidal luminal and glandular epithelium, with short straight glands.

Endometrial hyperplasia is an important lesion in the ewe and bitch, occurs in the cow, cat, and sow, and is rare in the mare. In farm animals, it is caused by prolonged hyperestrogenism. Ingested clover is the most likely source of estrogen in the ewe. Cystic follicles, granulosa cell tumors, and estrogens from plants are causes of endometrial hyperplasia in the cow. The mycotoxin zearalenone obtained from moldy feed is a cause in the sow. In the bitch, endometrial hyperplasia occurs under the influence of progesterone, but with priming by estrogen from the ovaries. Some bitches can have a normal-appearing corpus luteum and experience pseudopregnancy. In the queen, which is an induced ovulator, strong association has been found between endometrial hyperplasia and actively secreting corpora lutea. However, because endometrial hyperplasia has been found in older queens, the lesion in the feline uterus is likely due to chronic stimulation of the endometrium by estrogen. These cats often have not been bred, and, thus, their follicles have not been induced to ovulate. Their blood estrogen concentrations change with follicular growth, but no corpora lutea are present, and progesterone concentrations remain low.

Simple endometrial hyperplasia can be overlooked or be recognizable grossly when mild and patchy or diffuse thickening involves the endometrium. When it progresses to the stage of cystic endometrial hyperplasia, the lesion is readily recognized at necropsy (Fig. 12-10). Endometrial cysts, about 1 cm in diameter in the ewe and up to 5 mm in diameter in the bitch, are filled with clear fluid. In the ewe, the cysts are both beside and beneath the caruncles (Fig. 12-11). Because of the local influence of progester-

Cystic endometrial hyperplasia

↑ estrogen
ewe: clover
cow: cystic follicles, GCT, plant estrogen
pig: zearalenone (moldy feed)

↑ progesterone
bitch: w/estrogen priming

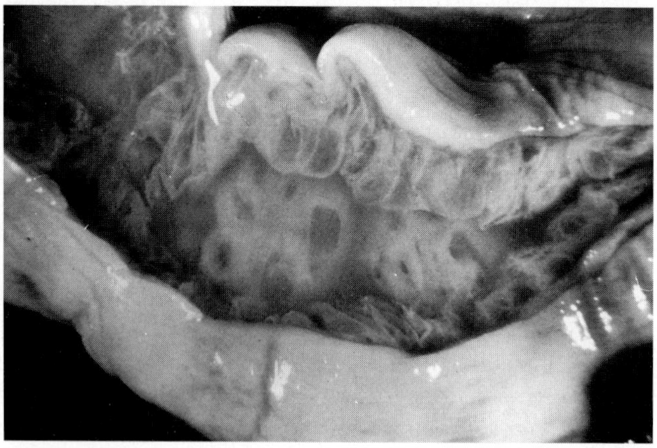

Figure 12-10 Uterus; bitch. Cystic endometrial hyperplasia. The endometrium is diffusely thickened by numerous cysts. Progesterone is the dominant hormone.

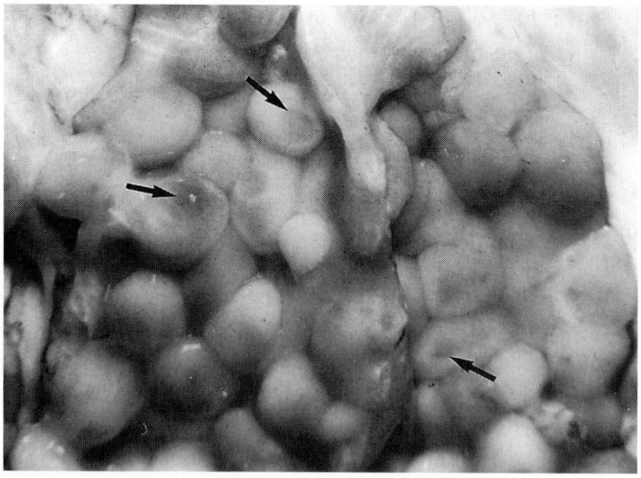

Figure 12-11 Uterine body; ewe. Cystic endometrial hyperplasia. Cystic glands *(arrows)* are beside, between, and beneath caruncles. Estrogen is the dominant hormone.

one in the bitch and queen, infection can be superimposed, resulting in cystic hyperplastic endometritis. Microscopically, the main component of endometrial hyperplasia is an increase in the size and number of glands with no change in the stroma except for edema. In the bitch and queen, the glandular epithelium is progestational in appearance, that is, the cells are columnar, hypertrophic, and hyperplastic, and have clear cytoplasm. As the glands become cystic, the pressure of retained secretion is increased, and the glands' epithelium becomes flattened. Bitches and queens are likely to develop endometritis and then pyometra and, in some cases, endometrial polyps, thought to arise from focal areas of endometrial hyperplasia. In all species, the cystic lesions are probably irreversible. In ewes, endometrial hyperplasia results in reduced fertility, dystocia, and uterine prolapse due to uterine hypotonicity. Glands of endometrial type can develop in the cervical mucosa. Even when nonpregnant, ewes have mammary gland enlargement. Endometrial hyperplasia is not precancerous in domestic animals, as it can be in women.

Mucometra is the accumulation of mucus in the uterine lumen. The cause is congenital or acquired obstruction of the outflow of mucus initially produced in normal amounts. However, mucometra can be due to the production of excessive amounts of mucus in cases of hyperestrogenism.

Adenomyosis and **endometriosis** are lesions of importance only in primates. However, adenomyosis at least is occasionally encountered in domestic animals, notably the queen, cow, and bitch, and is probably a result of prolonged estrogen stimulation. Adenomyosis is the presence of nests of endometrium within the myometrium, and the effect generally is negligible in domestic animals, which do not menstruate. Sometimes, the uterus undergoes diffuse, symmetric or focal, asymmetric enlargement. Microscopically, endometrial glands or stroma or both have extended from the basal endometrium beyond the junction between endometrium and myometrium. Endometriosis is the presence of endometrial glands or stroma in locations outside the uterus, such as the ovary, the mesometrium, the peritoneum, and peritoneal surgical scars. The mechanism for development of endometriosis is unknown; proposed mechanisms include metaplasia of celomic epithelium, transformation of tissue rests, regurgitation of endometrium through the infundibulum of the oviduct at the time of menstruation, implantation at the time of uterine surgery, and dissemination of endometrium by lymph or blood vessels. The abnormally placed endometrium can have menstrually shed debris and cause adhesions between organs.

Inflammation

Most uterine infections begin in the endometrium and are related to introduction of semen contaminated with bacteria or to metabolic disturbances that favor an environment for bacterial organisms in pregnancy, parturition, or postpartum involution. Resistance of the uterus to infection is influenced by humoral and cellular immune mechanisms, by the hormonal environment, and by physical factors.

Humoral and Cellular Immune Mechanisms

Following infection, changes include hyperemia and a rapid influx of edema fluid into the uterine wall and lumen. Recruitment of neutrophils from the blood occurs in response to chemotactic substances released by bacteria and to leukotriene B_4 from endometrium and leukocytes. Attracted neutrophils infiltrate the endometrium and enter the uterine lumen and contribute additional amounts of leukotriene B_4, providing additional chemotactic stimuli. Neutrophils release substances that are toxic to gametes and embryos. Complement activation, directly by bacteria by the alternate pathway or by specific antibody by the classical pathway, can eliminate bacteria either by lysis following attack on their membranes or by phagocytosis enhanced by opsonization. Leakage of serum into the uterine lumen from the inflamed endometrium contributes to the antibody content of the uterine fluid. Opsonization of bacteria by antibodies, especially IgG, promotes more efficient phagocytosis by neutrophils and macrophages.

The role of immunoglobulins in protecting the female genital tract of domestic animals has been most studied in the mare. IgG and IgA predominate in uterine secretions in the mare, but IgM has been detected. Immunoglobulins in the uterine lumen apparently are produced by cells in the endometrium rather than being derived from the blood. Local uterine immunity seems better developed in the mare than in other species. The influence of the estrous cycle on antibodies in the uterus is controversial, but much data suggest that concentrations of luminal immunoglobulins and immunoglobulin-containing cells in the endometrium are not influenced by the stage of the estrous cycle. Demonstration of greater concentrations of IgA and IgG in the uterine secretions of mares more susceptible to infection has led investigators to conclude that immunoglobulins play only a minor role in the defense of the uterus against infection.

Locally produced IgA is not directly bactericidal and neither acts as an opsonin nor as a macrophage activator. It can, however, interfere with attachment of bacteria to mucosal surfaces and can activate complement via the alternate pathway. Variations occur among species on the position in the tract where the concentration of IgA is greatest, but the sites correspond to the site of semen deposition (uterus in mares, vagina in cows).

Hormonal Influences

Infections of the uterus are more easily overcome at estrus than at other stages of the cycle. This increased response is due in part to better drainage through an open cervix under estrogen stimulation and to the increase in leukocytes in the uterine wall at estrus. In different studies, leukocytic phagocytosis has been unchanged or increased under the influence of estrogen, but it is generally accepted that neutrophil activity is reduced under the influence of progesterone. Generally, the uterus is more susceptible to infection during the progestational phase of the estrus cycle because progesterone reduces the migration of blood neutrophils and reduces phagocytosis and killing of bacteria by uterine neutrophils. The mechanism for effect of sex hormones on neutrophils is unknown, and receptors for sex hormones have not been demonstrated. The nonpregnant uterus is highly resistant to infection.

Prostaglandins are normally produced by components of the endometrium. Probably, the epithelium secretes the majority of PGF and the endometrial stroma secretes the majority of PGE. In most species (excluding the dog, cat, and primates), prostaglandins are responsible for lysis of the corpus luteum. In acute inflammation, prostaglandin production by the endometrium is increased, via the release of arachidonic acid from the phospholipids of cell membranes; under these circumstances, lysis of the corpus luteum occurs sooner. When chronic inflammation progresses to the stage of epithelial and mucosal surface loss, production of prostaglandins is decreased and the corpus luteum persists.

Conformation of the external genitalia is the physical factor that has received the most attention in relation to uterine infections. In the mare, a large proportion of the vulva is higher than the floor of the pelvic canal, and the vulva tends to become horizontal and to suck air and contaminants, including feces, into the vagina or even into the uterus. Urine can pool in the vagina of mares with defective function of the muscles of the vestibule and vulva. When contamination and pooling of urine occur, the vestibule and vagina become inflamed and the cervix and uterus either become inflamed at the onset from direct contact with environmental organisms or from local spread of the inflammation. An additional physical factor that is an aid to the female to resist infection is the drainage allowed by the hormonally controlled normal relaxation and opening of the cervix and contraction of the myometrium during estrus.

Organisms that cause inflammation of the uterus can enter through the vulva (ascending infection) or can arrive via the blood (hematogenous infection). Ascending infections are initiated at breeding and parturition, whereas hematogenous infections are most of the specific infections, such as *Brucella abortus* or bovine viral diarrhea virus infection in cows, that occur during pregnancy. A few specific organisms, such as *Streptococcus equi* in the mare, are ascending infections, but most ascending infections are due to a mixture of organisms. Organisms that cause placentitis, fetal infection, and abortion, in most cases, also spread and cause inflammation of the endometrial component of the placenta. In those species with a zonary (dog, cat) or cotyledonary (ruminant) rather than a diffuse placenta (horse, pig), endometritis extends beyond the bounds of the part of the endometrium making close contact with the fetal part of the placenta. Postpartum metritis occurs to some extent even after a normal pregnancy and parturition, but metritis is especially common and more severe following an abnormal parturition (Fig. 12-12). Lochia, the debris that is discharged from the uterus for a short time after parturition, is an excellent nutrient medium for bacterial growth.

Endometritis is inflammation limited to the endometrium. Almost all uterine infections begin as endometritis. Mild cases of acute endometritis are not detected grossly. In more severe cases of acute endometritis, the mucosa is swollen and has a rough surface, often with adherent

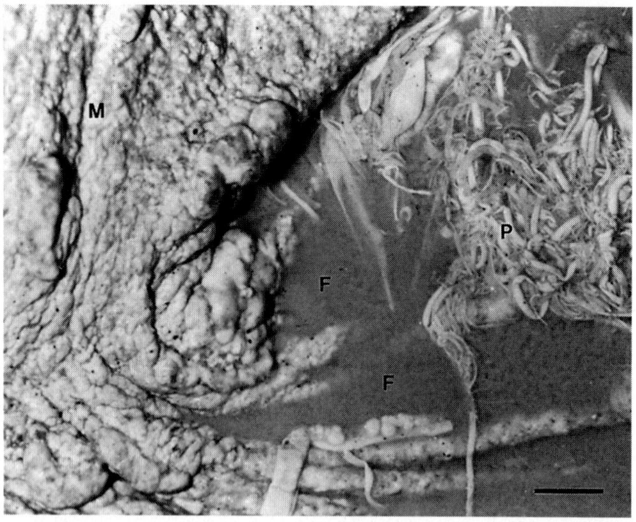

Figure 12-12 Uterus; cow. Severe, postcalving metritis. The mucosa *(M)* is coarsely nodular and is subacutely to chronically inflamed. Strings and shreds of disintegrating placenta *(P)* and brown fluid *(F)* are present in the lumen. Bar = 2 cm.

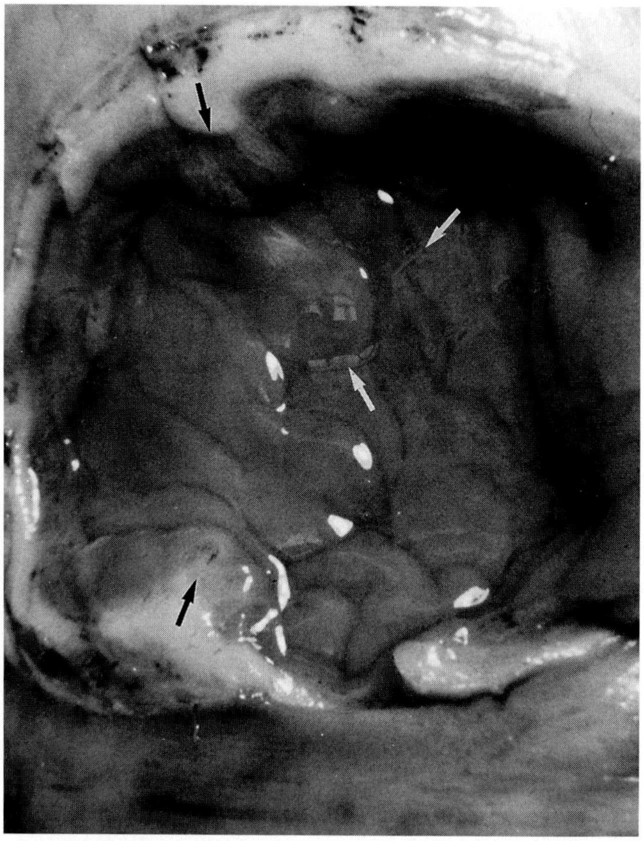

Figure 12-13 Uterus; mare. Contagious equine metritis. In the acute stage, the endometrial folds are swollen because of edema, best seen at the cut edge *(black arrows)*. The lumen contains increased amount of mucus and inflammatory debris *(white arrows)*.

shreds of fibrin and necrotic debris (Fig. 12-13). At microscopic examination a few to many neutrophils are found in the stroma and in the glands, with a range of surface changes from desquamation of a few surface epithelial cells to severe necrosis of the endometrium. Mild lesions resolve completely or incompletely with residual changes of cystic glands and periglandular fibrosis (Fig. 12-14). Severe acute endometritis often becomes chronic (Fig. 12-15) and the necrotic endometrium is replaced by granulation tissue devoid of glands and ultimately by fibrous tissue. Acute endometritis can stimulate the synthesis of prostaglandin $F_{2\alpha}$ in large animals that have had 4 or 5 days of progesterone priming causing premature regression of the corpus luteum and shortening of the estrous cycle. The loss of endometrium in chronic endometritis can result in reduced production of $PGF_{2\alpha}$, and this decrease in $PGF_{2\alpha}$, especially in the mare and the cow, results in a persistent corpus luteum.

In the mare, endometrial biopsy is used as a breeding management tool, because the severity of endometritis is correlated directly with the inability of the uterus to carry a fetus to term. To give a prognosis based on the features of the endometrium, focal and diffuse inflammatory cell infiltration of the stroma, contents of the glands, and frequency and severity of periglandular fibrosis are scored. Kenney used the score to place the endometrium of individual mares into a category that predicted high, reduced, or low likelihood of the animal completing pregnancy.

Persistent endometritis is a problem in mares. Affected animals are unable to resolve the acute endometritis that usually follows mating. This persistence is likely due to defects in both cellular and humoral response to infectious agents. Neutrophils, the principal phagocytic cells in the uterus, could be less able to migrate from the blood in susceptible compared with resistant mares. Also, uterine neutrophils in susceptible mares might be less competent at phagocytosis of bacteria. Uterine secretions appear deficient in promoting neutrophil bactericidal activity, unrelated to the generation of opsonizing complement components. The density of lymphocytes in the endometrium is increased in persistent endometritis and large lymphoid nodules are formed with an even greater preponderance of $CD4^+$ cells over $CD8^+$ cells than in the scattered lymphocytes in the normal endometrium.

Metritis is inflammation of all layers of the uterine wall. In the acute stage, the serosa is dull, finely granular, and has petechial hemorrhages and fine adhering strands of fibrin. Microscopically, the subserosal tissue and muscle layers are edematous and infiltrated by neutrophils. Endometritis, as described above, is present.

Pyometra occurs as a sequel to endometritis or metritis. It is an acute or chronic infection of the uterus with accumulation of pus in the lumen as the result of a closed cervix. The closure of the cervix is not always complete and some discharge occurs. In some instances, the obstruction of the cervix is mechanical, but most cases are

Cat & dog:
• Excess progesterone → cystic endometrial hyperplasia (± pseudopregnancy → secondary bacterial endometritis → pyometra

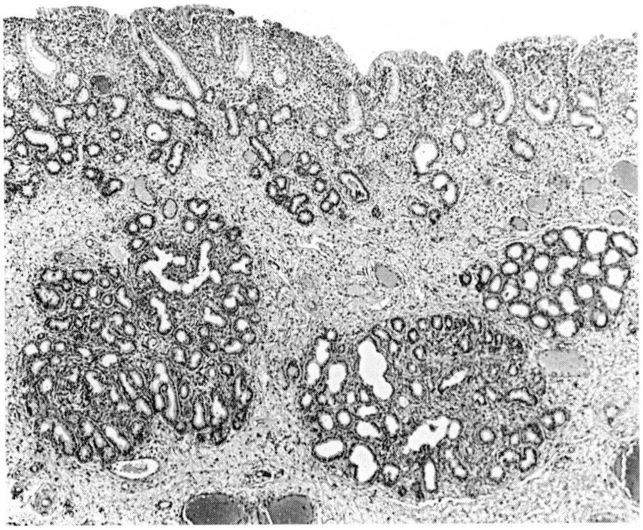

Figure 12-14 Endometrium; mare. Moderate endometrial fibrosis. The stratum compactum beneath the surface epithelium is diffusely hypercellular because of infiltrating lymphocytes and plasma cells. In the stratum spongiosum, three large nests of distended glands have collagen deposited between and around their coils. H & E stain.

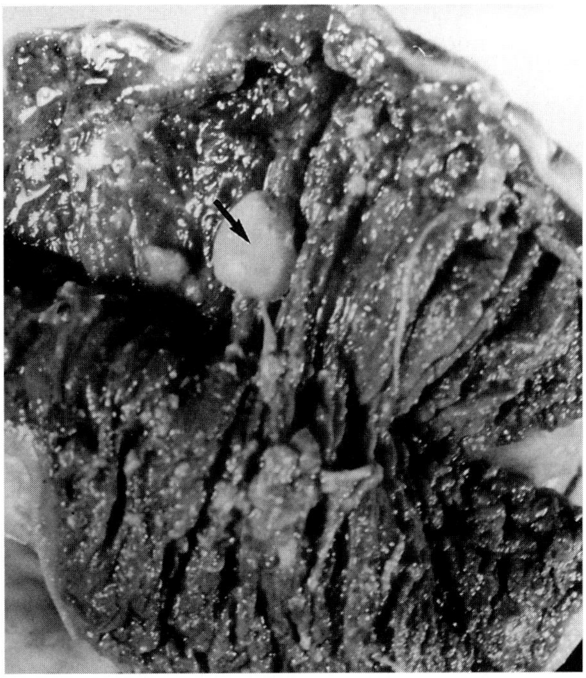

Figure 12-15 Uterus; sow. Chronic staphylococcal endometritis. The endometrium is thickened and granular. Remnants of a macerated fetus, notably the cranium *(arrow)*, are present.

caused by a functional obstruction of the cervix under the influence of progesterone produced by a retained corpus luteum. In the cow, the persistence of the corpus luteum is usually secondary to a pathologic process in the uterus. In the bitch and queen, most cases of pyometra are the result of bacterial infection secondary to endometrial hyperplasia, and most occur during pseudopregnancy. The color and consistency of the exudate vary with the infecting bacteria. Exudate is viscid and brown with *Escherichia coli* infection and creamy yellow with streptococcal infection. The uterus can be greatly distended (Fig. 12-16) but not necessarily uniformly. Grossly, necrotic, ulcerated, and hemorrhagic areas are present in the uterine mucosa, as well as dry, white, thickened, finely cystic areas. Microscopically, the dry white areas have changes of hyperplasia and squamous metaplasia of surface epithelium, a common occurrence in chronic inflammation of any mucous membrane, and the cystic areas are due to cystic endometrial hyperplasia. Lesions outside the genital tract, such as bone marrow depression, widespread extramedullary hematopoiesis, and immune complex glomerulopathy are common in the bitch.

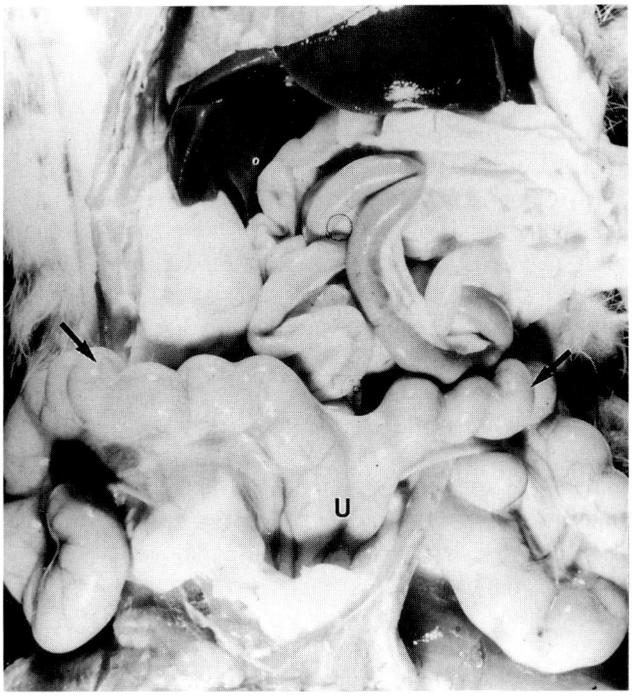

Figure 12-16 Uterus; cat. Pyometra. The pus filled uterine body *(U)* and horns *(arrows)* occupy a large proportion of the abdomen.

Neoplasms

Uterine neoplasms are not common in domestic animals. The primary ones that do occur with any significant frequency are carcinoma in the cow and leiomyoma in the bitch. Lymphosarcoma in the cow is the most often encountered metastatic neoplasm.

Leiomyomas in the bitch are multiple neoplasms, not only in the uterus, but also in the cervix and vagina, and are often associated with other abnormalities such as endometrial hyperplasia, follicular cysts, or mammary gland neoplasms. Estrogens likely have a role in provoking and maintaining these neoplasms in the bitch. In other species, however, these neoplasms are rare, tend to be single, and have no unusual hormonal background. The neoplasms are well demarcated but not encapsulated, are usually spherical, and vary greatly in size. Depending on size, they can be confined within the wall of the vagina, cervix, or uterus, or protrude into the lumen or project to the serosal surface or into the pelvic canal. Some luminal neoplasms, especially those in the vagina, are pedunculated, making them liable to trauma or torsion. They are usually firm, pink or white, and occasionally calcified or edematous. The color is related to the amount of fibrous tissue present along with the whorled smooth muscle cells; in the grossly white neoplasms, fibrous tissue is the predominant component.

Carcinoma of the endometrium is rare in domestic animals as a clinical problem, but it is well known as a lesion of the bovine uterus found at the time of meat inspection. In the cow, the early carcinoma is found most often in the depths of the endometrial glands of the horns and less often in the body of the uterus. As it increases in size, the neoplasm thickens the uterine wall without any distortion of the overlying endometrium. A scirrhous response, the deposition of large amounts of fibrous tissue, is a characteristic lesion and makes the neoplasm firm and causes localized constriction bands on the external surface. The neoplasms can be small and annular or involve a large area of the uterine wall (Fig. 12-17). Microscopically, the neoplasm is readily distinguished from normal endometrium by the increased size, pleomorphism, and disarray of the glandular epithelial cells and the accompanying scirrhous reaction. Metastases occur to the regional lymph nodes, lungs, and seed the serosal surfaces of the abdomen.

Lymphosarcoma in the cow in the enzootic form is caused by the bovine leukemia retrovirus and commonly affects a tetrad of organs, namely the heart, abomasum, lymph nodes, and uterus. In the uterus, as in other locations, infiltration of neoplastic cells can be focal, multifocal, or multifocally coalescing (Fig. 12-18). Affected areas are light yellow, slightly friable, sometimes centrally necrotic, and thicken or replace any or all layers of the uterine wall. It is not uncommon for the cervix and vagina to have lesions as well as the uterus. In such cows, the vaginal lesions are multiple, small, often hemorrhagic, but nonulcerated nodules. An extensively involved uterus can support pregnancy even to an advanced stage.

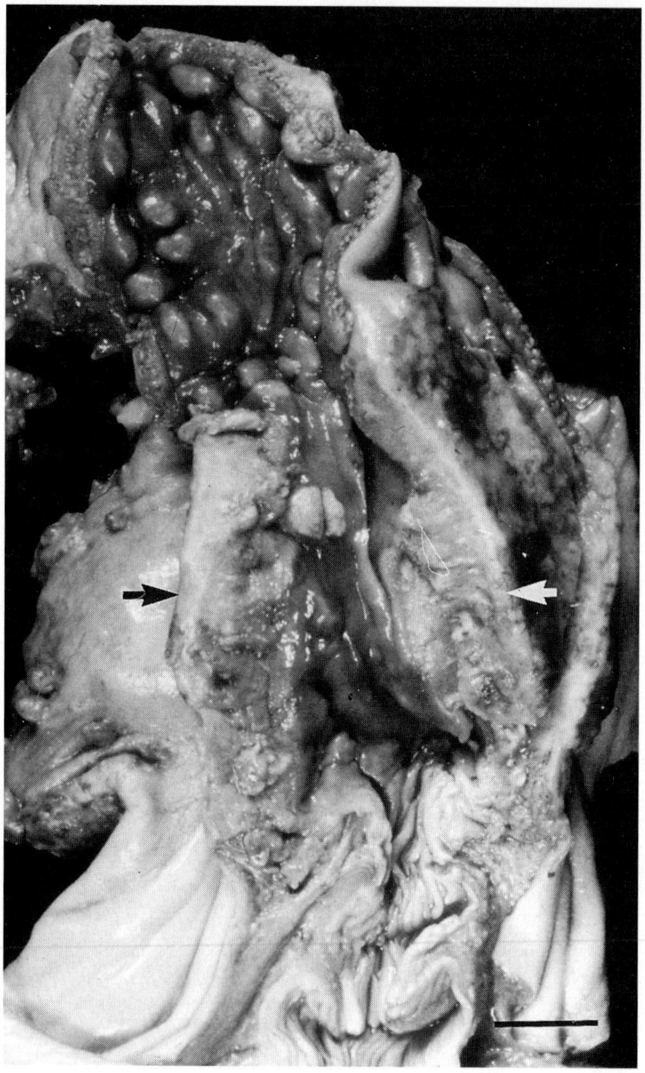

Figure 12-17 Genital tract; cow. Endometrial carcinoma. Cut surface shows the wall of the uterine body is thickened by the neoplasm and fibrous tissue *(arrows)*. Bar = 2 cm.

PLACENTA AND FETUS
Noninflammatory Diseases

Retention of fetal membranes for longer than normal after parturition is common, especially in the cow. In cows, membranes are considered retained if not expelled by 12 hours postpartum. The cause of the retention is uncertain, but infectious, nutritional, hormonal, circulatory, hereditary, and weather factors have been proposed. The membranes can act as a nutrient medium for growth of contaminant bacteria and for the development of severe endometritis from the transient mild postparturient endometritis. The endometritis can even cause systemic disease such as septicemia or disseminated intravascular coagulation. Normal shedding of the placenta involves separation of the maternal caruncles from the fetal cotyledons. The

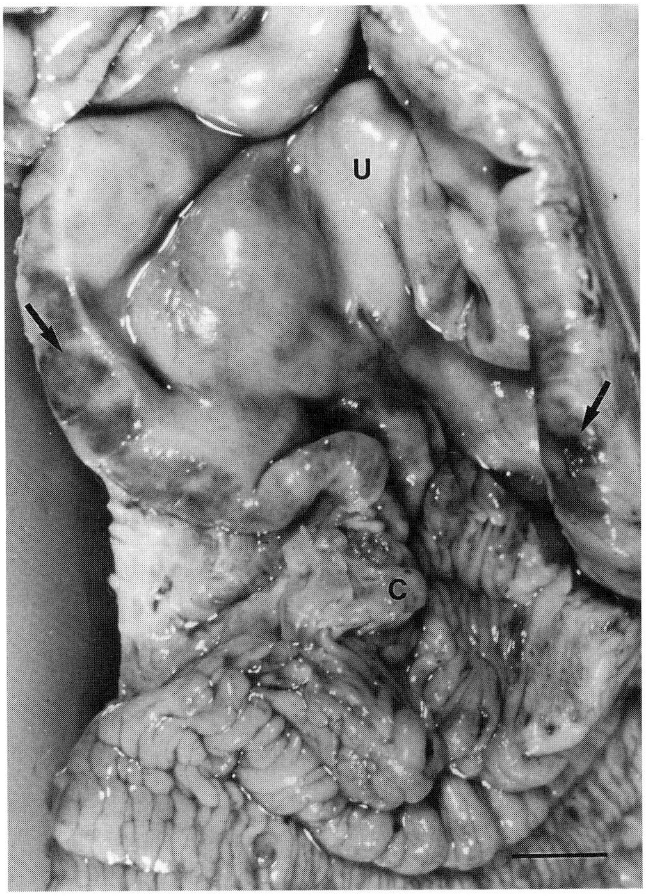

Figure 12-18 Cervix *(C)* and uterine body *(U)*; cow. Enzootic lymphosarcoma. The uterine wall is diffusely thickened by light yellow neoplastic tissue with streaks of hemorrhage, best seen on cut surface *(arrows)*. Bar = 2 cm.

caruncles become smaller as a result of the decreased blood supply that occurs in early uterine involution and because of degeneration of the tips of the caruncular septa. None of the morphologic changes define the cause of the retention of the placenta. No microscopic differences have been detected prepartum between placentomes (caruncles plus cotyledons) from cows that have shed their placentas normally and placentomes from cows that have retained the placenta. In normal cows, a marked decline in the number of binucleate giant cells occurs in the placentomes by 1 hour postpartum, but reduction to the same extent does not occur in cows that have retained their membranes. Possibly these giant cells are concerned with maintaining cell attachment at the fetomaternal placental interface, and their reduction aids in separation as necrosis of these cells releases enzymes that destroy the ligands at the interface and allows separation to occur.

Twinning in the mare is the most common noninfectious cause of abortion. Normally, chorionic villi develop where contact is made between the endometrium and the chorion. In other areas, such as the contact area between chorion and endocervix and the contact area between the placentas of twins, chorionic villi do not develop and the chorionic surface is smooth. Thus, the combined functional area of the chorions of both twins is only slightly larger than that for a normal nontwin foal. Twin fetuses often have growth retardation. Aborted twin equine fetuses often appear to have died at different times. Death is thought to be due to placental insufficiency. When the available space in the uterus is divided evenly, which is approximately 80% of cases, both twins usually die and are aborted in midgestation. In cases in which great disparity exists in the apportioning of space, the favored twin has a chance of survival, while the other dies and mummifies.

In the mare, **endometrial fibrosis,** often the result of a previous endometritis, reduces the area of the endometrium available for formation of a diffuse placenta. Chorionic villi do not develop where there is no endometrium with glands for the formation of interdigitations between fetal and maternal parts of the placenta. In large areas of endometrial fibrosis, the chorion does not develop microcotyledons and their villi. Clearly demarcated and smooth areas of chorionic surface mirror the affected areas of the endometrium. Severely affected mares become pregnant, but do not carry the fetus to term because the functional area of the placenta is too small.

Premature placental separation in the mare has been described in two forms. One form occurs around the time of parturition, causing the chorioallantois to appear at the vulva with the cervical star intact. While the caudal part of the chorioallantois is detached from the uterus, the cranial part remains in place, and there is tearing of the chorioallantois across its body. The other form occurs some time before parturition. Prematurely detached areas become brown and dehydrated. Another equine disease, albeit a rare one, in which fetal death and abortion occur as a result of placental insufficiency and fetal malnutrition is **uterine body pregnancy.** The fetus occupies the uterine body rather than the body and horns, and the placenta is underdeveloped in the horns.

Torsion of the umbilical cord is a cause of equine abortion. In torsion, the cord is long, excessively twisted, and the twists are difficult to undo. For a twisted cord to qualify as pathologic, lesions caused by compromise of the umbilical vessels must be present (Fig. 12-19). The cord is edematous and hemorrhagic, and congested, distended segments alternate with constricted twisted segments. Fibrin is often present on the surface of affected areas of the cord. Lesser degrees of torsion occur without seriously affecting the umbilical blood vessels and killing the fetus.

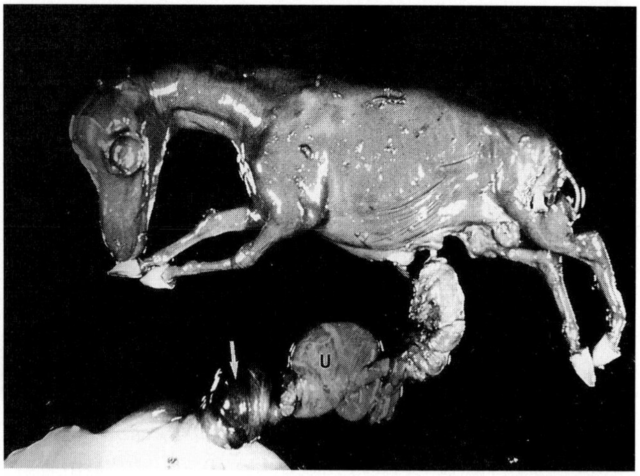

Figure 12-19 Fetus; horse. Umbilical cord torsion. Fetal death and mummification. Early mummification is most easily recognized by the paucity of orbital contents. The vessels of the cord are congested in the twisted area *(arrow)*, and the urachus *(U)* is ballooned on the fetal side of the twist.

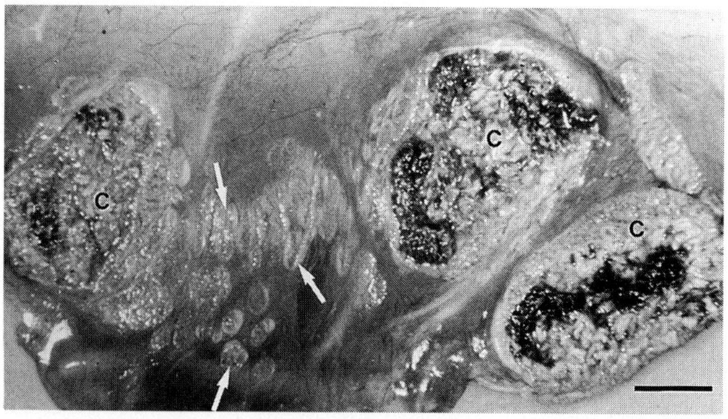

Figure 12-20 Chorioallantois; cow. Adventitial placentation. Very severe inflammation and necrosis of cotyledons. Small adventitial cotyledons *(arrows)* are in between the major cotyledons *(C)*. Bar = 2 cm.

The urachus is thinner and more pliable than the umbilical arteries or vein and is more easily constricted. Local distentions of the urachus can occur anywhere along its course in the cord from the umbilicus to the allantoic cavity.

Adventitial placentation in ruminants is the formation of additional areas of fetal and maternal placental contact as a response to inadequacy of the conventional placentomes. This inadequacy is most likely due to loss of caruncles as a result of endometritis (Fig. 12-20). Compensation can be achieved by enlargement of the existing functional maternal caruncles and the establishment of additional areas of contact by simple villous interdigitation. These adventitious areas form initially adjacent to the placentomes, but can expand to involve much of the surface.

Hydramnios and **hydrallantois** refer to the excessive accumulation of fluid in the amnionic and allantoic sacs, respectively. These lesions occur mostly in the cow, are rare, and usually do not occur together. Amnionic fluid is viscid, resembling fetal saliva from which it is formed. Accumulation of excessive amnionic fluid occurs in association with some fetal facial muscle and skeletal abnormalities. The implication is that serious nervous abnormalities impair the muscles responsible for the fetal drinking reflex. An association has been found between fetal adrenal insufficiency and hydramnios. Allantoic fluid is formed from fetal urine received through the urachus. In the cow, hydrallantois occurs in conjunction with adventitial placentation and in some twin pregnancies. Abortion or dystocia follow, with a dead and sometimes small anasarcous and ascitic fetus. The allantoic fluid composition changes from normal to that closely resembling maternal or fetal extracellular fluid. When these membranes are retained after delivery of a fetus, fluid sometimes continues to accumulate.

Embryonic and **fetal death** deprive the fetomaternal unit of whatever contribution the conceptus makes to the continuation of pregnancy. Parturition or abortion in most large animal species is brought about by synthesis and release of $PGF_{2\alpha}$ from the endometrium, causing in turn regression of the corpus luteum and decreased progesterone production. In large animals, the loss of very small embryos does not influence the time of return to estrus. If embryonic loss occurs later, the interval to the next estrus will be somewhat increased because the corpus luteum will have been programmed for prolongation of its life. The importance of the fetal component and the necessity of the presence of a corpus luteum for the entire pregnancy vary with species. For instance, the corpus luteum of the sow in needed throughout pregnancy, as progesterone production by the placenta is small, but in the mare, the corpus luteum regresses halfway through pregnancy and placental progesterone maintains pregnancy. Regardless of the source of hormones responsible for maintaining pregnancy in large animals, embryonic or fetal death are likely to permit the release of $PGF_{2\alpha}$ and expulsion of the embryo or fetus. The exact outcome is unpredictable and is influenced, among other things, by species, stage of gestation, and number of fetuses. In the bitch and queen, the life span of the corpus luteum is not very different between pregnant and nonpregnant animals. When embryonic or fetal death occurs in domestic carnivores, the demise of the corpus luteum is not a direct consequence and dead products of conception are retained until approximately the normal time of parturition.

Hydramnios
- Fluid in amnionic sac
- Fetal saliva
- Fetal facial muscle & skeletal abn.
- Fetal nervous abn. → impair fetal drinking reflex
- Fetal adrenal insufficiency

Hydrallantois
- Fluid in allantoic sac
- Fetal urine
- assoc. w/ adventitial placentation or twinning
- abortion/dystocia
- sm. anasarcous & ascitic fetus

The products of embryonic death have received relatively little study, because they are not available before decomposition has advanced, or they are resorbed, or they are passed per vaginum unnoticed. In animals as well as human beings, many of the embryos die because of chromosomal abnormalities.

Mummification is one of the possible outcomes of fetal death. Rather than being expelled soon after death, the fetus is retained and progressively dehydrates to become a firm, dry mass, colored brown or black by degraded hemoglobin, and consisting of leathery skin enclosing the harder parts of the fetus. The cause of death can be infectious or noninfectious, but requisites for mummification are that organisms that promote lysis of dead tissue be absent and that the cervix be closed to prevent the entry of putrefactive organisms. The situations in which mummification most commonly occurs are in twin pregnancy in the mare and in parvovirus infection in the sow. In twin pregnancy in the mare, the mummified fetus and the longer surviving fetus are aborted together before term. In parvovirus infection in the sow, mummified fetuses are retained and born at term along with live fetuses. In any species with a pregnancy with a single fetus, the mummified fetus can be expelled at any time or retained indefinitely.

Maceration of a dead fetus requires the presence of bacterial organisms in the uterus. These bacteria could be the ones that caused the fetal death in the first place, or putrefactive organisms that entered the uterus via the cervix after the death of the fetus. In addition to disintegration of the fetus, the uterus has lesions also. Endometritis or pyometra is present; the type of lesion depends on whether the cervix is open or closed. Endometritis and pyometra tend to become severe and chronic, with voluminous pus in the case of pyometra. Emphysema occurs with the invasion of the fetus by clostridial organisms, and maternal toxemia and death are likely. Fetal bones resist maceration, and if the uterus eventually regains some muscular tone, the bones can cause perforation.

Abortion in domestic animals is expulsion of the fetus before its development is sufficiently advanced to allow survival. An aborted fetus can be alive or dead at the time of abortion, but most are dead. **Stillbirth** is defined as the delivery of a dead fetus at a stage of development at which it should have been viable. Although these are useful terms, they do not provide pathogenetic or diagnostic information. Uterine infections cause a spectrum of effects from fetal mummification, abortion, or stillbirth to the birth of a live, but sick, fetus.

Fetal anomalies can take innumerable forms. Some of those that directly influence the reproductive process are mentioned here. First, certain anomalies cause prolonged gestation because a fetal organ does not make the necessary hormonal contribution to the birth process. One mechanism is aplasia or hypoplasia of the adrenal glands, and another mechanism is displacement, dysgenesis, or absence of the anterior pituitary gland. The classic example of a displaced gland causing prolonged gestation is in the fetal lamb when the dam had ingested the plant *Veratrum californicum* on the fourteenth day of gestation. Absence of the pituitary gland occurs, probably as an inherited disease, in Guernsey and Jersey cattle. Absence of the pituitary gland can occur alone or as part of anencephaly. Anencephaly is literally absence of the brain, but the term is used loosely to cover the far more common situation of absence of a forebrain, variable presence of a midbrain, and presence of brain stem. The neurohypophysis adenohypophysis are absent. The second large group of fetal anomalies interferes with the reproductive process by causing mechanical problems at parturition (dystocia). Examples are hydrocephalus, hydrops fetus, and arthrogryposis.

Inflammatory Diseases

Bacterial Causes

Bacterial species causing inflammation of the placenta and fetus are numerous. Almost any organism that causes septicemia can infect the uterus, but the following discussion concerns those organisms that target the placenta or fetus, or both. The route of invasion of the uterus and fetus for many animal species and many bacteria is hematogenous, after the organisms have entered the dam either through the digestive or genital tract. For some diseases, the method of spread can be either venereal or by ingestion. In the mare, most placental pathogens enter the pregnant uterus through the cervix.

Campylobacter fetus var. *venerealis* can be a long-term inhabitant of the exterior of the bovine penis and the preputial cavity. It is transmitted venereally and can survive for some time on the vaginal mucosa, but the cow must become pregnant for it to establish itself in the uterus. Embryonic or early fetal death is the most likely manifestation of campylobacteriosis and often the only clinical abnormalities are irregular estrus cycles or the return to estrus of an animal thought to be pregnant. Much less frequently abortion occurs at a later stage of pregnancy. Cows become resistant to subsequent infections by the bacteria. Gross and microscopic lesions in placentas are similar to those described in brucellosis (edema of the intercotyledonary chorioallantois and necrosis of cotyledons with microscopic inflammation of both), but are less severe and with fewer organisms in the desquamated chorionic epithelial cells. Fetal lesions are nonspecific.

Campylobacter fetus subsp. *fetus* and *Campylobacter jejuni* are primarily intestinal inhabitants and cause similar lesions in sheep. The organisms are transmitted by ingestion and abortions occur in outbreaks. Infection of the pregnant uterus results in late-term abortion or the birth

Fetal anomalies → prolonged gestation
- aplasia/hypoplasia of adrenals
- displacement/dysgenesis/absence of ant. pit.
↳ lamb: in utero Veratrum californicum on day 14 → displaced ant. pit.
↳ Guernsey/Jersey: absence of pituitary

of live, but sick lambs. Immunity is gained after the first infection. The placentitis is characterized by an edematous intercotyledonary chorioallantois and friable, yellow cotyledons. Grossly, about 25% of the fetuses have multiple yellow areas of hepatic necrosis from 10 to 20 mm in diameter with red, depressed centers. Microscopically, the chorioallantois is infiltrated by a mixture of cells, mostly neutrophils, but many cells are necrotic and cannot be identified. Inflammation is especially severe in the chorionic villi. *Campylobacter* organisms are abundant among the inflammatory cells. A diagnostically useful lesion in campylobacterial infection is the presence of large, dense emboli of bacteria in the capillaries of the chorionic villi. The fetal lesions are those of a severe multifocal necrotizing hepatitis with abundant organisms. *Flexispira rappini* causes similar lesions in the ovine placenta and fetus, but infections are sporadic.

Brucella abortus in cattle is ingested with feed contaminated by an infected aborted fetus or placenta. The initial lesion is a persistent nasopharyngeal lymphadenitis. Bacteria are released into the blood in waves causing bacteremia and bacteria colonize the spleen, lymph nodes, mammary glands, testes, accessory male glands and joint capsules, bursae, and tendon sheaths. *Brucella* organisms are removed from most organs, but a small nidus of infection usually persists in some organ. The pregnant uterus is particularly susceptible to infection and the uterine disease process becomes chronic, eventually resolving after abortion or parturition. Gross lesions in the placenta are edema of the intercotyledonary chorioallantois that is opaque with a leathery texture, light brown exudate on the chorionic surface, and various extents of necrosis of the cotyledons. A placenta with such lesions is grossly indistinguishable from the placenta of cases of mycotic abortion or the rare case of campylobacteriosis with a late-term abortion. The fetal lesions are nonspecific and consist of edema and fluid accumulation in body cavities; often more specific lesions include bronchopneumonia and pleuritis. Microscopic lesions include inflammation with edema and infiltration of mononuclear cells and a few neutrophils of both the intercotyledonary chorion and the chorionic villi. A striking feature is the presence of numerous coccobacilli within chorionic epithelial cells, many of which are desquamated and form the considerable debris between maternal and fetal tissues. In ruminants, *B. abortus* moves from the maternal circulation into the hematomas that occur at the tips of the maternal septa within the placentome. Organisms are then phagocytosed by the erythrophagocytic trophoblasts at the nearby base of the chorionic villi. Replication occurs in adjacent periplacentomal chorioallantoic trophoblasts (Fig. 12-21). Replication is followed by trophoblast necrosis and chorioallantoic ulceration and organisms enter the uterine lumen and chorionic villi to finally disseminate hematogenously to fetal viscera. *B. abortus* appears to be taken up by endocytosis by erythrophagocytic trophoblasts and replicates in the rough endoplasmic reticulum of the periplacentomal and interplacentomal trophoblasts, a unique mechanism of intracellular parasitism. Vasculitis occurs in both maternal and fetal tissues and the lesion could be a response to endotoxin released from the *Brucella* organisms. Most fetuses have pneumonia that ranges from minimal to severe. Microscopically, the pneumonia is either a chronic bronchopneumonia with an exudate of numerous mononuclear cells and some neutrophils or a fibrinous pneumonia. Microscopic granulomas that include multinucleate giant cells occur in various organs such as the liver, spleen, and lymph nodes.

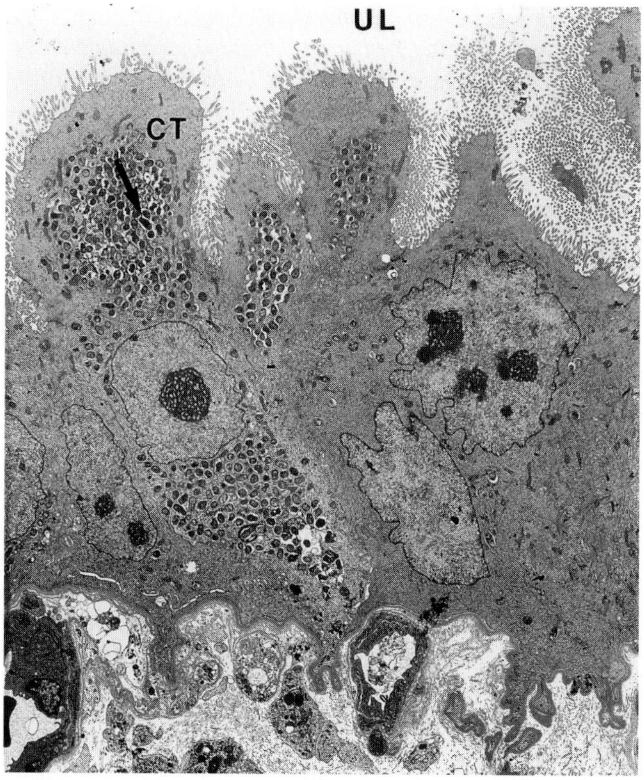

Figure 12-21 Transmission electron micrograph. Chorioallantois; goat. *Brucella abortus* infection. In the nonplacentomal chorioallantois, the trophoblasts contain numerous *B. abortus* in dilated cisternae of the rough endoplasmic reticulum *(arrow)* and perinuclear envelope. A trophoblast *(CT)* is in the process of desquamating into the uterine lumen *(U)*. Fetal capillaries and connective tissue are normal. *Courtesy Dr. T.D. Anderson.*

Brucella canis is acquired by the dog either by ingestion or venereally. Both sexes have lymphadenitis, especially of the nodes of the head and neck, and bacteremia. Epididymitis and testicular degeneration are the lesions in male dogs and females have placentitis and fetal endocarditis, pneumonia, and hepatitis. Microscopically, chorionic epithelial cells are packed with *Brucella* organisms. Other fetal lesions include renal hemorrhage,

Sheep:
- Campylobacter fetus subsp. fetus
- Campylobacter jejuni
- Flexispira rappini

↳ cotyledonary necrosis & intercotyledonary edema
↳ lg. dense (B) emboli in chorionic villi capillaries
↳ Fetus: MF necrotizing hepatitis → yellow foci w/ red depressed centers

subacute inflammation of the pelvic connective tissue, and lymphadenitis.

Brucella ovis in sheep is probably transmitted venereally from a ram with epididymitis shedding large numbers of organisms in the semen. Gross placental lesions are essentially similar to those produced by *B. abortus* in cattle. Fetal lesions at necropsy are nonspecific, i.e., edema and fluid accumulation in the body cavities. Calcified plaques on the hooves have been noted, but there is some doubt as to their specificity. Microscopically, as with *Brucella* sp. infections in other species, large numbers of coccobacilli are found in chorionic epithelial cells and are free in the chorionic mesenchyme. Vasculitis involves the larger chorionic vessels. Lesions in the fetus are pneumonia, lymphadenitis, interstitial nephritis, and pericholangitis. In younger fetuses, infiltrates of monocytes and macrophages are present, whereas older fetuses have well-formed nodules of lymphocytes and plasma cells. *Brucella melitensis* infectionin sheep and goats occurs mainly in Mediterranean countries. The infection has a septicemic phase but inflammation is localized to the mammary gland and pregnant uterus. Goats have more severe febrile disease and more severe mastitis than do sheep.

Brucella suis causes a disease in pigs that differs in several respects from brucellosis in ruminants. The lesions are more widespread and have a predilection for bones and joints. Necrosis with caseation occurs in many lesions. Pregnancy is not a prerequisite for endometritis in porcine brucellosis. Miliary granulomas in the endometrium are mixed with multiple hyperplastic lymphoid nodules. Endometrial glands become distended with mucous and leukocytes and the surface epithelium is partly desquamated and focally has squamous metaplasia. Between placentas of the pregnant uterus, the lumen has a mucopurulent exudate in which intracellular and free organisms are plentiful. The chorioallantoic membranes have nonspecific lesions of edema and congestion.

Coxiella burnettii, the cause of Q fever in human beings, is sometimes responsible for abortion or the birth of dead or weak lambs or kids. Abortion occurs in newly exposed animals and repeat infection with abortion is possible. Infection of goats is more common. Transmission of the organism is either by ingestion or by inhalation. The organism is shed in vaginal discharges at parturition and in the milk. In affected goats, the intercotyledonary chorioallantois is thick, leathery, yellow, and covered with a moderate amount of surface exudate. Gross fetal lesions are nonspecific. Microscopically, the placental lesions of acute inflammatory infiltration are most severe in the intercotyledonary areas. Hypertrophic chorionic epithelial cells are filled with *Coxiella* organisms. Fetal lesions, if present, consist of peribronchiolar, renal medullary, and hepatic portal lymphoid accumulations.

Enzootic abortion of ewes is caused by *Chlamydophila psittaci* and occurs in small outbreaks in Britain and the United States producing late-term abortion in ewes. Transmission is probably oral and ewes seem to be immune to reinfection after the first abortion. The placenta in affected ewes grossly is similar to the placenta in *Coxiella* infection and in ovine brucellosis. Microscopically, the chorioallantois is infiltrated by neutrophils. Cotyledons have more severe inflammation than the intercotyledonary areas. The organisms distend the chorionic cells, but are difficult to visualize without special stains, such as modified Ziehl-Neelsen or Gimenez stains. In the fetus, subacute inflammatory foci are present in several organs, especially the liver, lungs, and muscle.

Epizootic bovine abortion, also known as foothills abortion, occurs in California and adjacent states. For many years a chlamydial organism was considered the cause of the disease. However, it was discovered that normal bovine fetuses could harbor the same organism. Attention then was shifted to a *Borrelia*-like spirochete and later to an unidentified tick-transmitted virus. Abortion or the birth of weak calves occurs only in cows newly introduced into the territory of the tick *Ornithodorus coriaceus*. The fetal disease is chronic with marked microscopic lesions 50 days after tick exposure of the dam. The lesions are of sufficient specificity for a diagnosis after 100 days. Gross lesions include ascites, an enlarged nodular liver, and enlarged lymph nodes and spleen. Lymphoid follicles are hyperplastic and have large numbers of macrophages. The thymus is atrophic because of loss of cortical lymphocytes. The thymic parenchyma and interstitium are infiltrated by macrophages. Foci of acute necrosis are present in several organs, especially the lymph nodes and spleen. These foci frequently develop into pyogranulomas. Vasculitis, acute or subacute, occurs in several organs. Deposits of IgG and IgM are present in the vascular lesions.

Leptospirosis is another possible cause of abortion. Results of serologic studies indicate that a large percentage of cattle and pigs are infected, but most animals do not have clinical signs. Several different serovars are associated with abortion, especially *Leptospira interrogans* serovar *hardjo* in cattle and serovar *pomona* in swine. In adult animals, the organisms localize in the kidneys after the septicemic phase. Pregnant sows or cows abort weeks after the septicemic phase, usually in the last trimester. Placental lesions are usually limited to edema. Fetal lesions often are mild and obscured by autolysis. Some dead fetuses expelled near term without extensive autolysis have gross lesions of ascites and fibrinous peritonitis. Microscopic lesions include subacute interstitial nephritis and subacute necrotizing hepatitis. With or without morphologic changes in the fetal kidneys, leptospiral organisms can be demonstrated in tubular lumens by silver stains or by immunohistochemical techniques.

Listeriosis caused by *Listeria monocytogenes,* is a cause of sporadic abortions in cattle, sheep, and goats and

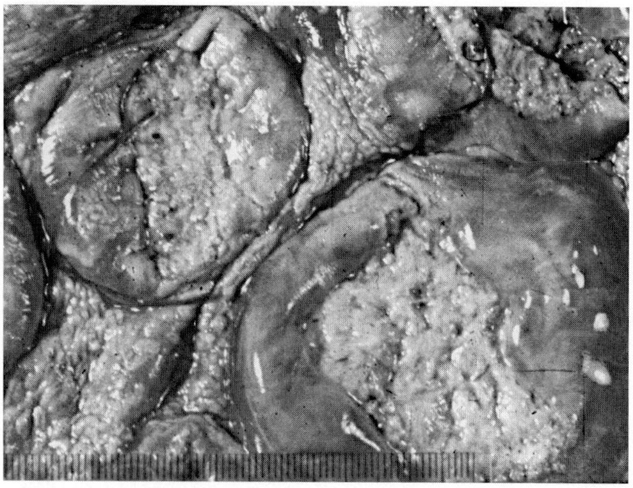

Figure 12-22 Chorioallantois; cow. Mycotic placentitis. The intercotyledonary tissue is thickened and in parts is either leathery or edematous. The cotyledons are enlarged and friable and have surface inflammatory exudate. Gradations = 1 mm.

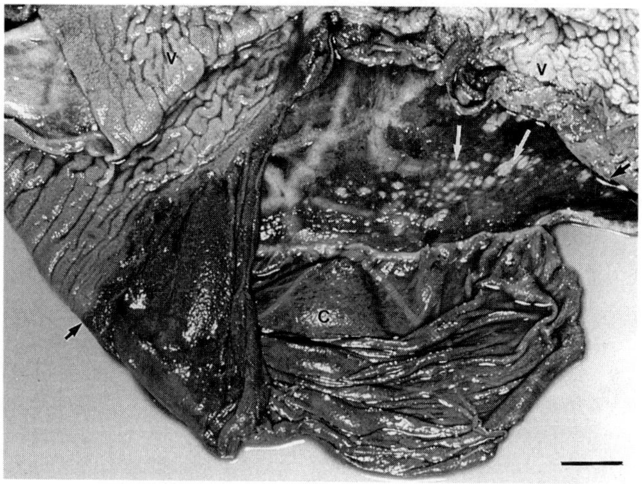

Figure 12-23 Placenta, cervical area; mare. Mycotic abortion. The allantochorion *(C)* opposite to the cervix is torn, dehydrated, and friable and is clearly demarcated *(black arrow)* from the viable *(V)* allantochorion. Note the fungal plaques *(white arrows)* on the allantoic surface. Bar = 1 cm.

of outbreaks of abortion in sheep. Although both nervous disease and reproductive disease occur in the same flock or herd, this is rare. Listerial abortions occur in the last trimester of pregnancy. Some aborting dams are septicemic and have endometritis. The placental lesions include severe diffuse necrotizing and suppurative inflammation of both the cotyledons and the intercotyledonary areas. Fetal lesions are an enlarged liver with numerous 1-mm yellow foci. Microscopically, severe inflammation involves the mesenchyme of the villi and the upper intercotyledonary chorion, with some of the cells neutrophils and others degenerated beyond recognition. Chorionic epithelial cells, especially in the areas between the villi, are filled with gram-positive listerial bacilli. The cells in areas of acute multifocal necrotizing hepatitis are also filled with organisms. Other fetal organs have similar microscopic lesions.

Organisms that cause bacteremia in adult animals are capable of causing lesions in the placenta and fetus. Thus, in cattle, bacteria such as *Salmonella* and *Pasteurella* spp and *Haemophilus somnus* are potential causes of placentitis, fetal inflammatory lesions, and abortion. In pigs, various *Streptococcus* spp. can cause similar lesions. Ureaplasmas can cause abortion in cattle. The placental lesions include focal or diffuse reddening of the amnion and chorioallantois, accompanied by thickening and yellow discoloration of the amnion. Fibrosis, edema, inflammation, and necrosis of the amnion occur together with focal inflammation and necrosis of the cotyledons and the intercotyledonary chorioallantois.

Various bacterial organisms can cause abortion in the mare. Hemolytic streptococci are the most frequently recovered from fetal organs, placentas, and uterine discharges. Other commonly encountered organisms are *E. coli* and *Pseudomonas, Klebsiella,* and *Staphylococcus* spp. Although some infections are hematogenous, the ascending route of infection, through the cervix, is the rule. Inflammation of the chorioallantois is most severe opposite the cervix and the area involved usually extends further ventrally than dorsally because of gravity spread. Affected parts of the placenta are edematous and brown and covered by small amounts of fibrinonecrotic exudate. Gross fetal lesions are enlarged liver and increased abdominal and thoracic fluid. Microscopically, the lesions are a moderately severe subacute inflammation of the stroma of the chorionic microcotyledons and desquamation of chorionic epithelium. Microscopic fetal lesions are rare, despite the ease with which bacteria can be recovered from many fetal organs. The prelude to abortion is either fetal death from septicemia or placental insufficiency.

Fungal Causes

Aspergillus and phycomycetes *(Absidia, Mortierella, Mucor, Rhizopus)* cause sporadic abortions in cows and mares. In cows, the organisms spread to the placenta hematogenously, as indicated by the fact that the placentomes are involved first and the random involvement of the placentomes. In the mare, as with bacterial placentitis, the fungi enter through the cervix because the lesions in the chorioallantois are most severe in or even confined to the cervical area. In the affected bovine placenta, the cotyledons become enlarged, brown, and friable and the intercotyledonary chorioallantois becomes leathery and covered with a brown exudate (Fig. 12-22). Thus, the gross appearance of the placenta is similar to the classic descriptions of the placenta in bovine brucellosis.

Table 12-1 Herpesviruses and Fetal Disease

Species	Virus	Disease in the Fetus	Disease in the Adult
Cattle	Infectious bovine rhinotracheitis virus (Bovine herpesvirus 1)	Abortion; fetus is usually autolysed when expelled; multifocal inflammation and necrosis in lung, liver, adrenal, with intranuclear inclusions	Neonatal gastrointestinal ulceration Rhinotracheitis Vulvovaginitis Pneumonia
Horses	Equine herpesvirus 1	Abortion; multifocal inflammation and necrosis in liver, lung, adrenal, lymphoid organs, with intranuclear inclusions	Rhinopneumonitis Encephalomyelitis
Pigs	Pseudorabies virus (Suid herpesvirus 1)	Abortion; affected and unaffected litter members; inclusion bodies in chorionic epithelium; multifocal inflammation and necrosis in liver, lung, adrenal, lymphoid organs; one of the causes of congenital tremor	Dermatitis in pigs (rare) Encephalitis in pigs and cattle
Goats	Caprine herpesvirus 1	Abortion; multifocal inflammation and necrosis in multiple organs	Vulvular erosions, ulcerative balanoposthitis Ulcerative enteritis, mesenteric lymphadenitis in kids
Dogs	Canine herpesvirus 1	Multifocal inflammation and necrosis in many organs; newborn pups most susceptible.	Balanitis, vaginitis, conjunctivitis

Affected areas of the equine chorioallantois are brown, initially thickened, and, later, shrunken and friable (Fig. 12-23). In both bovine and equine species, the amnion has thick, white or yellow, leathery areas. Small, white, raised plaques are present on the bovine fetal skin, and sometimes, on equine fetal skin. Microscopically, the lesions include inflammatory cell infiltration of allantoamnionic and chorionic mesenchyme and desquamation of chorionic epithelium. In the bovine species, the lesions of vasculitis and fungal vascular invasion involve the larger vessels at the base of the cotyledons. Lesions in the fetus are confined to the skin and include subacute dermatitis and hyperkeratosis. Fungal hyphae, septate in the case of *Aspergillus* and nonseptate in the case of the phycomycetes, are abundant in the lesions of the placenta and the skin of the fetus. Fungi can be recovered from the fetal stomach, presumably from swallowed amnionic fluid.

Viral Causes

Herpesviruses are well established as causes of outbreaks of abortion in cows, mares, and sows and described in goats and dogs (Table 12-1). Generally, the lesions in affected fetuses are lymphoid necrosis in spleen, thymus, and lymph nodes and multiple small foci of necrosis, mild acute inflammation, and intranuclear inclusion bodies in parenchymal cells in a wide range of organs, but especially the liver, lungs (Fig. 12-24), and adrenal glands. Often the fetal liver is enlarged, and the focal lesions are large enough to be visible as 1- to 2-mm white areas. Vascular lesions vary in severity, but even when slight the damage can cause pleural and peritoneal effusion and subcutaneous edema. Pulmonary lesions usually include hyperplasia, focal necrosis, and desquamation of bronchiolar epithelium. Fibrinous bronchiolitis, grossly visible, is present in some fetuses, especially equine. The placenta can be

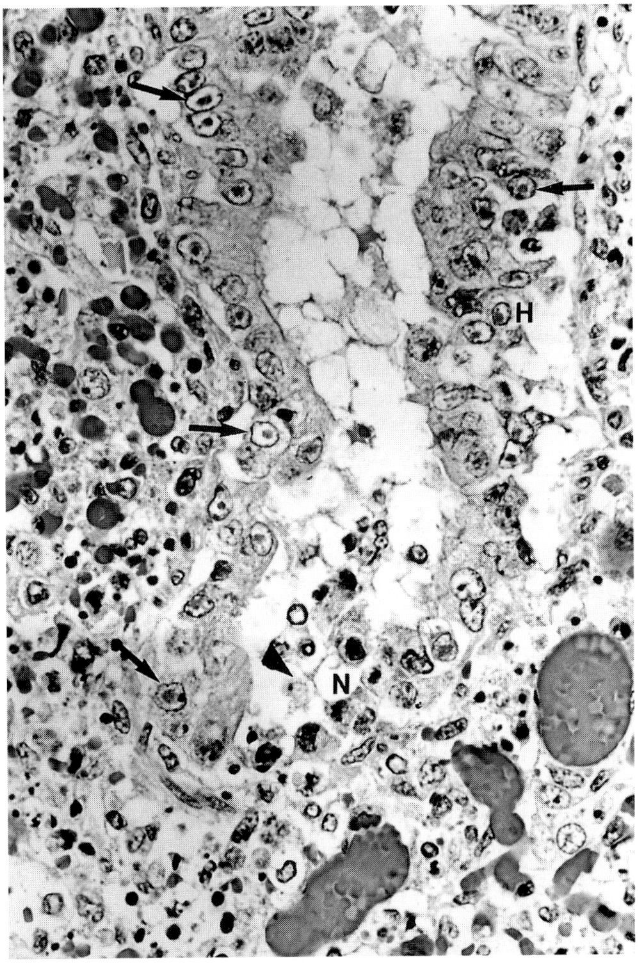

Figure 12-24 Fetal lung; foal. Equine herpesvirus abortion. Bronchiolar epithelium is hyperplastic, and some necrotic epithelial cells have desquamated into the lumen. Intranuclear inclusions are numerous *(arrows)*.

edematous, but only in the sow are inflammation and inclusion bodies readily observed in the chorion.

Equine herpesvirus 1 (EHV-1) could be the most economically significant abortigenic animal herpesvirus. Viral infection of maternal uterine endothelial cells has a major role in the pathogenesis of abortion. Damage to these endothelial cells results in thromboses accompanied by perivascular infiltration of lymphocytes, neutrophils, and monocytes and perivascular edema and subsequent infarction of the endometrium. The fluid that escapes through the damaged endometrium causes separation of the maternal and fetal layers of the placenta and this separation could allow virus from maternal leukocytes and lysed endothelial cells to enter the fetus. Fetal endothelial cells and the cells of a wide range of parenchymatous organs are targets for the virus.

In the cow, an affinity of herpesvirus for the endometrium has been demonstrated. After experimental intrauterine inoculation, infectious bovine rhinotracheitis virus (bovine herpesvirus 1) produces an acute necrotizing endometritis in the uterine body or caudal parts of the uterine horns of the cow. Microscopically, the lesions range from mild focal lymphocytic endometritis to severe diffuse necrotizing metritis.

Pestiviruses in cattle (bovine viral diarrhea [BVD] virus), sheep (border disease virus), and pigs (hog cholera virus) can cause fetal death or malformation, depending on viral strain, fetal age, and stage of development of the fetal immune system (Table 12-2). In the mare, equine viral arteritis virus causes abortion, but in the majority of cases no lesions are in the fetus. In this species, the mechanism is probably fetal anoxia due to compression of uterine blood vessels by virus-induced myometritis, although a few cases of arteritis in the chorion and myocardium of aborted fetuses have been described.

Porcine parvovirus is an important cause of embryonic and fetal loss and causes death and mummification of a proportion of affected litters. Pig fetuses infected before immunocompetence have widespread necrotizing lesions, together with inflammation and inclusion bodies, especially in the liver, lungs, kidneys, and cerebellum. Damage to the fetal circulatory system results in edema, hemorrhage, and the accumulation of serosanguinous fluid in body cavities.

Transplacental infection of pig fetuses with porcine reproductive and respiratory syndrome (PRRS) virus, an arterivirus, causes segmental or diffuse hemorrhage in the umbilical cords as a result of necrotizing arteritis. Few stillborn fetuses have specific microscopic lesions; lesions are more common in live littermates. Gross lesions include ascites, hydrothorax, and edema of perirenal tissue, splenic ligament, and mesentery. Microscopically, mild to moderate segmental arteritis occurs in the lungs, heart, and kidneys. Alveolar septa in the lungs are thickened by mononuclear cell accumulation and proliferation of type 2 pneumocytes. Aggregates of lymphocytes, plasma cells, and macrophages are about blood vessels in the heart, portal tracts, and cerebellar white matter. Various degrees of endometritis and myometritis also occur with lymphohistiocytic perivascular cuffs and edema.

Akabane virus and **Cache Valley virus** are bunyaviruses that cause fetal infection and abortion in sheep and other ruminants. The virus produces a range of lesions in the developing fetal central nervous system (CNS) including hydranencephaly, microencephaly, cerebellar hypoplasia, and loss of spinal cord ventral horn neurons. The loss of ventral horn neurons causes denervation muscle atrophy. The atrophy and myositis are responsible for arthrogryposis (fixation of limb joints) and skeletal deformities such as torticollis and scoliosis. Fetal lambs with hydranencephaly due to infection with bluetongue virus (an orbivirus) have viral antigen in immature neural cells in areas of necrosis in the subventricular zone of the cerebral hemispheres.

Protozoal Causes

Toxoplasma gondii is an important cause of abortion in ewes. The organism has a cat-sheep life cycle, with contamination of sheep feed by cat feces and the ingestion of sheep fetal membranes by cats. Gross lesions in the fetal

Table 12-2 Pestiviruses and Fetal Disease

Species	Virus	Disease in the Fetus	Disease in the Adult
Cattle	Bovine virus diarrhea virus	Abortion; cerebellar hypoplasia, microphthalmia, retinal dysplasia	BVD/mucosal disease; hemorrhagic thrombocytopenic disease in calves
Sheep	Border disease virus	Abortion; hypomyelination of CNS; decreased secondary hair follicles; skeletal immaturity	Depressed levels of thyroid hormones; immunodeficiency; specific immunotolerance for BDV, with persistent shedding
Pigs	Hog cholera virus	Abortion; one of the causes of congenital tremor; hypomyelinogenesis; cerebellar hypoplasia; head deformity; arthrogryposis	Hog cholera

BVD, Bovine virus diarrhea.

membranes include edema of the intercotyledonary chorioallantois and white 1- to 2-mm foci in the cotyledons (Fig. 12-25). Leukoencephalomalacia in the fetus is likely a nonspecific effect of fetal anoxia secondary to placentitis. Microscopically, the cotyledonary lesions are distinctive and consist of chorionic epithelial hypertrophy and hyperplasia with rare groups of toxoplasma organisms within chorionic epithelial cells. Other lesions are inflammation common to many intrauterine infections and foci of necrosis and desquamation.

Neospora caninum has become an increasingly frequently recognized cause of abortion in cows. Fetuses are of 3 to 9 months gestation and have no gross lesions. In the fetal brain, multiple foci of necrosis or proliferated microglial cells are often adjacent to capillaries with hyperplastic endothelium. Groups of *N. caninum* (Fig. 12-26) in or around these foci are either extracellular or occur in neural cells or endothelial cells. In the heart, the lesions include subacute multifocal epicarditis, myocarditis, endocarditis, and protozoal organisms either in myofibers or endothelial cells. Mononuclear portal hepatitis, multifocal hepatocellular necrosis, and fibrin thrombi in sinusoids are common. Foci of mononuclear inflammatory cells are present in additional organs, including the placenta.

Tritrichomonas foetus in cattle is another protozoal organism that can cause abortion. Mild placentitis, with no fetal lesion, is present. The standard method of diagnosis is the demonstration of protozoa in the contents of the fetal stomach. Endometritis can be severe, and pyometra is a possible sequela. Infiltration of the endometrium with mononuclear cells is moderate to severe. Lymphoid nodules and secondary follicles develop; these are likely sites of local production of IgA.

UTERINE TUBES

Most lesions of the uterine tubes are either incidental or secondary to lesions elsewhere in the reproductive tract. In dogs and cats, lesions of the uterine tubes are unlikely to affect reproductive performance. Lesions commonly encountered in dogs and cats are duct remnants in the mesosalpinx, more often Wolffian (simple tubular structures lined by low columnar to cuboidal cells) than Müllerian (lined by a folded mucosa similar to the uterine tube mucosa).

Congenital or acquired **hydrosalpinx,** distension of the uterine tubes by clear fluid, is caused by mechanical or functional obstruction of the lumen. The obstruction can be at either end of an uterine tube. The distention can be uniform or irregular; the wall is thin, and the tube increases in length and tortuosity. Multiloculated cysts are numerous in the mucosa. The congenital type result from segmental aplasia of the uterine tube as present in freemartins or more likely to segmental aplasia of the horn of the uterus. The acquired type is secondary to trauma or chronic inflammation; acute inflammation will cause pyosalpinx rather than hydrosalpinx. Trauma by manual interference with a corpus luteum in cows can cause an organizing hematoma about the uterine tube, resulting in obstruction by external pressure. This same manipulation can force inflammatory exudate from the uterus into the uterine tube, causing inflammation of tubular mucosa and obstruction of the lumen. Inflammatory exudate can be forced manually or under the pressure of therapeutic uterine infusion, not only into the uterine tube, but also into the ovarian bursa, where the ensuing

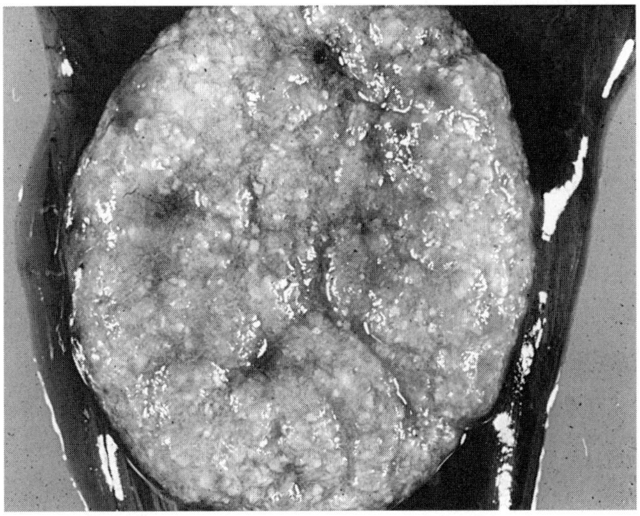

Figure 12-25 Placenta; ewe. Placentitis and abortion due to *Toxoplasma gondii* infection. The cotyledon has characteristic 1- to 2-mm white foci of inflammation, necrosis, and mineralization.

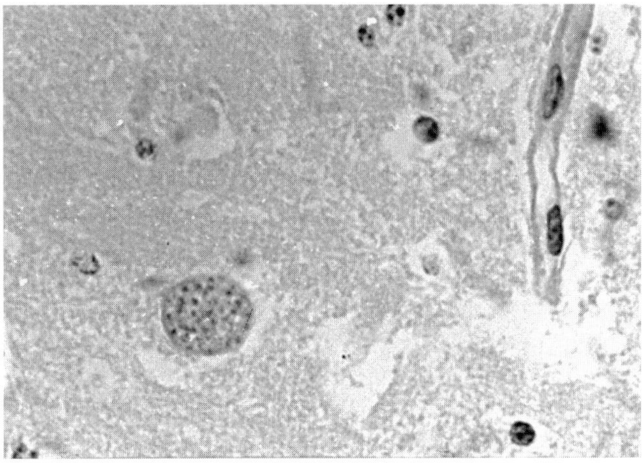

Figure 12-26 Brain; bovine fetus. A *Neospora caninum* tissue cyst with multiple organisms is in the brain. A small focus of subacute encephalitis was present in an adjacent field. *Courtesy Dr. P.L. Habecker.*

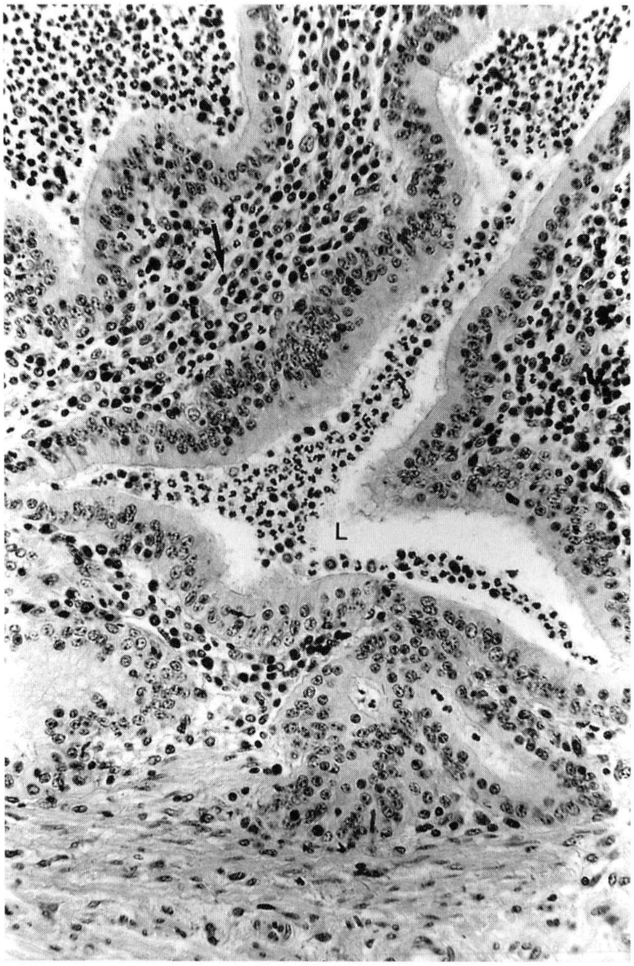

Figure 12-27 Uterine tube; mare. Subacute salpingitis, contagious equine metritis. The lamina propria of the folds of the uterine tube is hypercellular and is infiltrated by inflammatory cells, mainly mononuclear *(arrow)*, and the lumen *(L)* has an inflammatory exudate that includes many neutrophils. Hematoxylin-eosin (H & E) stain.

inflammation can result in fibrous bands that compress the uterine tube. Hydrosalpinx, or a bacteriologically sterile pyosalpinx, is one of the commonest causes of sterility in swine. It occurs almost exclusively in nulliparous animals and is almost always bilateral. The cause is unknown, but some evidence points to obstruction by embryonal rests of the Wolffian system.

Salpingitis results from spread of infection from the uterus to the uterine tubes and is usually bilateral. Generally, gross lesions are few, except perhaps for some hyperemia and thickening of the mucosa and small amounts of lumenal exudate. Probably, even very mild inflammation can reduce fertility. Microscopically, the inflammation ranges from mild to severe and from acute to chronic (Fig. 12-27). Early mild lesions are loss of cilia and desquamation of epithelial cells at the tips of the

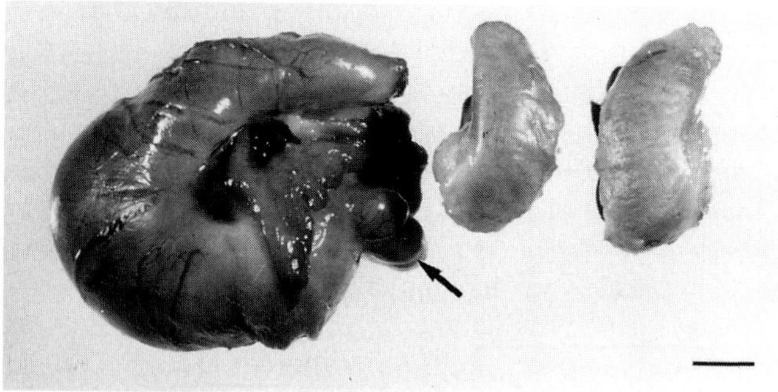

Figure 12-28 Ovaries; two mares. Hypoplastic ovaries on the right, and normal ovary on the left for comparison. Associated with the normal ovary are cysts *(arrow)* in the attached fimbriae of the uterine tube. Bar = 1 cm.

mucosal folds. When severe, salpingitis involves other parts of the mucosa and sometimes the muscle layer. Exudate is present in the lumen. With time, adhesions form between the denuded areas and adjacent mucosa becomes cystic, reepithelializes, or is replaced by granulation tissue.

Pyosalpinx has similar pathogenetic events as salpingitis. Grossly, pus accumulates in the lumen, filling irregularities created by inflammation, scarring, and obstruction. Microscopically, numerous neutrophils are present along with other inflammatory cells, both within the mucosa and in mucosal cysts. Much of the mucosa is lost; some of the epithelium undergoes squamous metaplasia.

OVARY

Developmental Anomalies

Occasionally, agenesis from unknown cause involves one or both ovaries. The reproductive tract can be absent as part of the defect. In cases of bilateral agenesis, the tubular genitalia remain infantile. Duplication of an ovary is a rare anomaly, arising by two different mechanisms: by originating separately or by splitting from an already developing ovary. The latter type, an accessory ovary, is located close to the normally located organ and is usually connected to it.

Hypoplasia of the ovaries occurs most commonly in cows and to a lesser extent in other species. It is usually bilateral but nonsymmetric. The affected ovaries are small (Fig. 12-28), lack follicles or surface scars from ovulation, but sometimes have cysts. Microscopically, cortical stroma and ova are absent or poorly developed. Because the embryonic development of the female system happens passively in the absence of testis-determining factor and is not under the direction of gonadal hormone, it follows that ovarian hypoplasia does not result in hypoplasia of the remainder of the female genital tract. The tract, however, will remain infantile after puberty. Other causes of an infantile reproductive tract are malnutrition or other forms of debility. Ovaries in these animals, however, have numerous primordial follicles and can respond to gonadotrophic hormones after the debilitating factor is removed.

Hypoplasia because of genetic and chromosomal abnormalities has been reported. Ovarian hypoplasia occurs in Swedish Highland cattle as an autosomal recessive trait with incomplete penetrance. The ovarian defect is either unilateral or bilateral. The number of primordial follicles and the proportion of graafian follicles are less then normal. Luteinization tends to occur without ovulation. Ovarian hypoplasia has been associated with cytogenetic anomalies such as XXX chromosomes in the mare and cow and XO chromosomes in the mare. The latter type is similar to the XO disease in human females, called Turner's syndrome, with such features as small stature, lack of uterine cyclic activity, and underdevelopment of the endometrium. The fetal gonad is normal, but the adult ovary has no follicles.

Vascular hamartomas of the ovary are incidental findings in the cow, sow, and mare (Fig. 12-29). They occur as a dark red mass on the surface of the ovary and are composed of connective tissue and vascular channels lined by mature endothelial cells.

Cysts in the mesovarium adjacent to the ovary, called paraovarian cysts, arise from either mesonephric or paramesonephric ducts. These cysts are common in the mare and can be several centimeters in diameter. Those from the paramesonephric duct have less smooth muscle in their wall and occur near the fimbriae of the oviduct. Cysts within the ovary are of three types, non-gonadal stromal, gonadal stromal, and neoplastic. The latter two are described later. The nongonadal stromal cysts are of two different types. One is the serous inclusion cyst, seen mostly in the bitch, and formed by a small area of surface epithelium lagging behind the remainder in growth and losing continuity with the surface. The other is formed by cystic rete tubules. These rete tubular cysts can reach follicular size in both the bitch and queen. Cystic rete ovarii is more common in the queen than previously thought. It expands into the ovarian stroma rather than into the mesovarium and is lined by ciliated columnar to flattened epithelium.

Acquired Ovarian Lesions

Oophoritis, inflammation of the ovary, is rare in domestic animals. Experimentally, infectious bovine rhinotracheitis virus (bovine herpesvirus 1) can induce necrotizing oophoritis in the postestrus cow, subsequent to viremia. The corpus luteum is hemorrhagic and thick cloudy fibrinous fluid fills some follicles. Microscopically, the lesions in the corpus luteum range from focal necrosis and infiltration of mononuclear cells to diffuse hemorrhage and

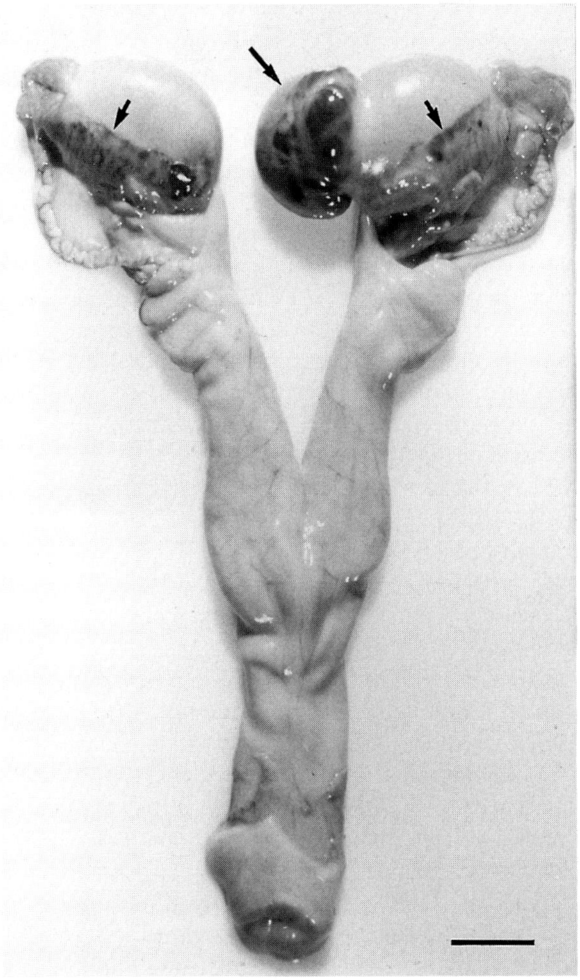

Figure 12-29 Ovary; fetal foal. Vascular hamartoma *(long arrow)*. The margin between germinal epithelium and well-vascularized attachment zone is clearly demarcated *(short arrows)*. Bar = 2 cm.

necrosis. Most affected ovaries also have necrotic follicles and diffuse mononuclear cell infiltrates in the stroma. BVD virus, a vertically and horizontally transmitted virus responsible for mild to fatal enteric disease and reproductive failure, can localize in bovine oocytes and cumulus cells and cause chronic oophoritis. Infection of ovarian oocytes with BVD virus is one of several possible routes of transmission of the virus from cow to fetus.

Ovarian bursal adhesions vary from thin bands to large sheets of fibrous tissue binding together the walls or crossing the cavity of the ovarian bursa, a peritoneal pouch formed around the ovary by the broad ligament and the mesosalpinx. The lesion is often bilateral in cows and could result from an ascending uterine infection that follows a retained placenta as a complication of pregnancy. Physical trauma from manipulations of the ovary is another possible cause. Bursal adhesions are common in beef heifers.

Lesions Related to Cyclic Changes

Hemorrhages into follicles are sometimes present in calves, and hemorrhages into cystic follicles happen occasionally in the bitch. Some hemorrhages, usually small and few, occur at the time of ovulation in all species. The mare is an exception because normally much blood is present in the cavity of the follicle, forming the corpus hemorrhagicum. In the mare and cow, a focal area of serositis is detectable at the point of ovulation. Progression through a fibrinous to a fibrous stage is rapid, and an "ovulation tag" is formed. The manual expression of a persistent corpus luteum in the cow sometimes is followed by severe hemorrhage. Organization of the blood clot can result in adhesions between the ovary and adjacent structures such as fimbriae of the oviduct or ovarian bursa.

Atretic follicles are those that become arrested at any stage of development and then regress. Atretic follicles are, in most cases, normal. In any estrus cycle, only one or a small number of follicles is destined to mature, while the others undergo atresia at various stages of maturation. A similar process occurs in seasonal anestrus and in all domestic species during pregnancy except for the mare. Follicular atresia is considered abnormal when it is a part of any disease process that interferes with the release of, or the pituitary response to, gonadotropin-releasing hormone. Development of the follicle can be arrested at any stage and after an undetermined amount of time, it degenerates. The ovum and zona pellucida undergo apoptosis first; then the granulosa cells become pyknotic, vacuolated, and desquamate. The follicle either persists as a cyst with a partial thin lining of granulosa cells, or is infiltrated by macrophages, theca cells, and fibrous connective tissue, eventually becoming a small scar.

Cystic graafian follicles are important in cows and sows. In dairy cows, the prolongation of the postpartum interval to first estrus is the main consequence of cystic follicles. Ovulation does not occur. Bovine cystic follicles are 2.5 cm or more in diameter and persist for 10 or more days without the formation of a corpus luteum (Fig. 12-30). They probably develop because of a deficiency of luteinizing hormone (LH), although the mechanism is not defined. An analysis of LH receptors, especially determining if a full complement is acquired, could contribute to the understanding of the pathogenesis of cystic follicles. Cystic follicles were common lesions in a large slaughterhouse survey of beef heifers. Cystic follicles were associated with use of melengestrol acetate, a compound resembling progesterone, that was used to inhibit estrus by suppressing LH release.

Evidence is available that postpartum uterine infection can cause cystic ovaries in dairy cows. Cystic ovaries have been linked with the recovery of *Escherichia coli* from the uterus and increased concentrations of serum prostaglandin $F_{2\alpha}$ metabolites and cortisol. Because of these findings, it has been proposed that bacterial endotoxins, or the prostaglandins produced because of damage caused by endotoxins, stimulate the adrenal cortical secretion of cortisol; cortisol excess suppresses the preovulatory release of LH, resulting in the development of cysts.

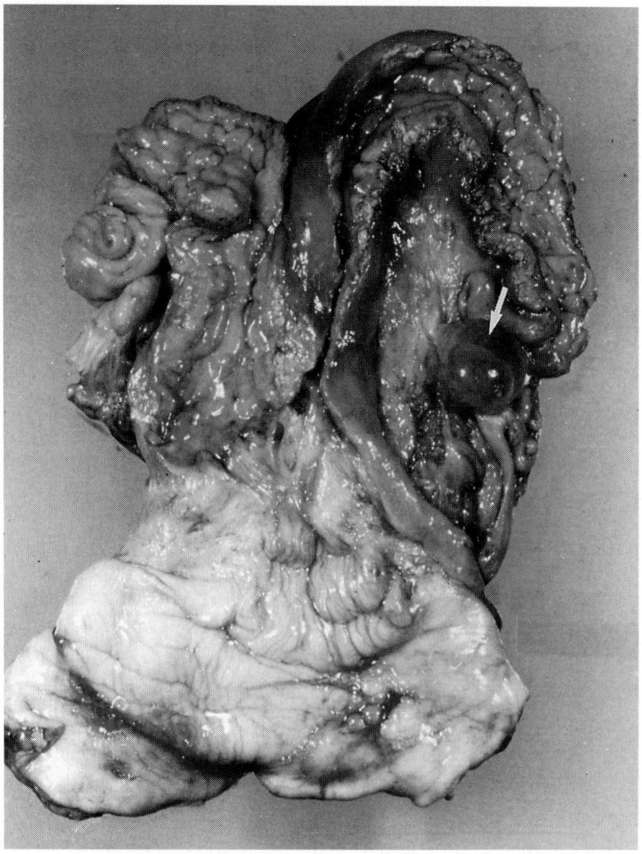

Figure 12-30 Genital tract; cow. Cystic ovary. A large, thin-walled follicular cyst *(arrow)* is present in the right ovary.

Follicular cysts in cows can be single or multiple, unilateral or bilateral, and usually thin walled. Microscopically, the granulosa cell layer is thicker than normal or is degenerating and eventually becomes a flattened single cell layer with no luteinization. The surrounding theca cell zone is thin and can become partially luteinized. Luteinization of the theca cell zone is more common when the granulosa cell zone is absent. It is possible that only the theca interna cells become luteinized. Follicular cysts can undergo spontaneous regression; however, cysts that develop after the first postpartum ovulation are likely to be replaced by other cystic follicles. Rather than persist as static structures, most cysts regress and are replaced by other cysts during subsequent follicular waves. The remainder of the reproductive system can have lesions of long-term estrogen stimulation.

Anovulatory luteinized cyst is likely caused by delayed or insufficient release of LH. It occurs in cows and sows more than in other species. Ovulation does not occur.

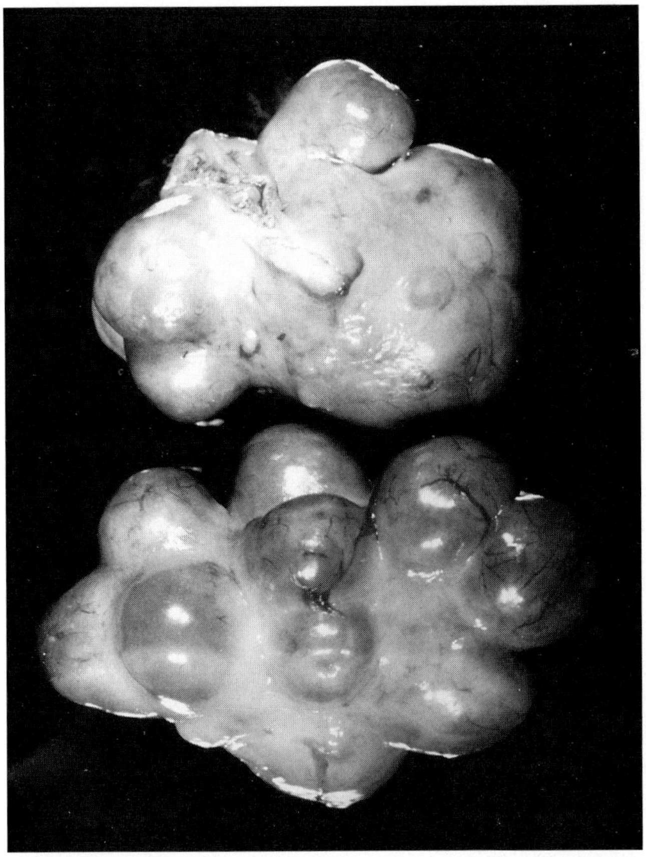

Figure 12-31 Ovaries; cow. Numerous corpora lutea instead of the normal one or two. The cow has been treated with drugs that caused superovulation.

The cystic cavity is lined by fibrous tissue, surrounded by an adjacent zone of luteinized theca cells. Cystic follicles and luteinized cysts can occur in the same ovary. The extent of luteinization that must occur in a cystic follicle to justify its designation as a luteal cyst has not been defined.

Cystic corpus luteum is of uncertain pathogenesis. In cows, it must be distinguished from anovulatory luteinized cyst and from the small central cyst that can occur normally in a corpus luteum. Ovulation occurs and a large irregular cyst develops, but without interference with the length of the estrous cycle. It has been suggested that in sows, at least, the cysts found in ovaries are different stages of the same aberration. The morphologic form, whether ovulated or unovulated follicle or a corpus luteum, is determined by the stage at which the physiologic process became abnormal.

Supernumerary follicles are induced in bovine ovaries by chorionic gonadotropin or follicle-stimulating hormone used in doses to cause superovulation in preparation for embryo transfer. In these cows, it is not unusual for more than a dozen well-developed follicles or corpora lutea of the same age to be present (Fig. 12-31).

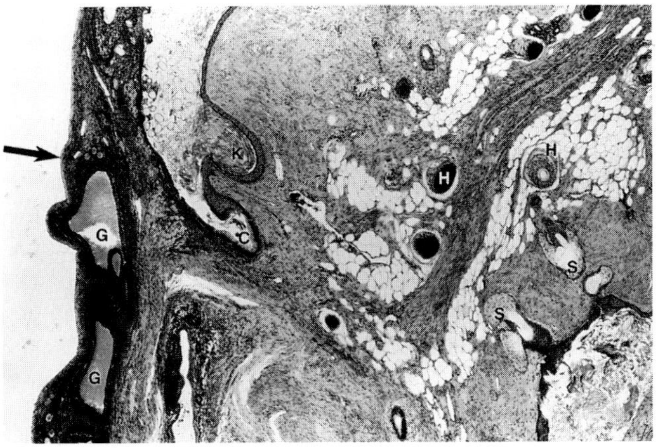

Figure 12-32 Ovary; monkey. Teratoma. Note normal ovarian structures such as primordial follicles *(arrow)*, and graafian follicles *(G)*. Among the nonovarian elements are hair follicles *(H)*, sebaceous glands *(S)*, and keratinizing squamous epithelium *(K)* merging with columnar epithelium *(C)*. *Courtesy Dr. T.G. Hodge.*

Neoplasms

Germ Cell Neoplasms

The ovum following fertilization differentiates to form embryonic and extraembryonic (placental or yolk sac) tissues. It would be expected that neoplasms arising from germ cells could differentiate along either embryonic or extraembryonic lines and could be benign or malignant or undifferentiated. In practice, in domestic animals, the great majority of neoplasms of germ cells are benign undifferentiated (dysgerminoma) or benign with somatic differentiation (teratoma).

Dysgerminoma is a rare neoplasm of bitches, sows, cows, and mares composed of cells resembling primitive germ cells. The neoplasm is usually a solid lobulated mass with areas of hemorrhage and necrosis. It is analogous to seminoma in the male. Mitotic rate is high, but metastases are rare.

Ovarian teratomas are rare, usually well differentiated, and benign. They arise from totipotential primordial germ cells and have disorganized elements of at least two of the three embryonic germ layers. Skin is often a significant component (Fig. 12-32). Malignant teratomas occur less often, except in the bitch.

Gonadal Stromal Neoplasms

Granulosa cell neoplasms are the most common ovarian neoplasms in large animals. They are unilateral, smooth surfaced, round, and can be 20 to 30 cm in diameter. They can be solid, cystic, or polycystic (Fig. 12-33). The cysts can vary from microscopic size to several centimeters in diameter. Often the fluid within the cysts is red-brown. Microscopically, the granulosa cells are not different from normal granulosa cells and often are arranged as they would be in normal graafian follicles, i.e., in single or multiple rows of round to columnar cells lining fluid-filled spaces. In less differentiated areas, the neoplastic cells are arranged in sheets (Fig. 12-34). Sometimes, especially in queens, Call-Exner bodies are present in the fluid. These bodies are rosettes of granulosa cells, some containing an eosinophilic body in the central space. The stroma can be sparse or plentiful; if the stroma predominates, the neoplasm is a thecoma. The cytoplasm of some thecoma cells contains lipid droplets. Areas of luteinization in granulosa–theca cell neoplasms are not uncommon, but luteomas, neoplasms with a uniform population of luteinized cells, are rare. Luteomas can probably develop from either granulosa or theca cells. Granulosa cell neoplasms are often malignant in the queen and sometimes in the bitch, but in the cow and mare, sex cord stromal neoplasms are usually benign. Many stromal neoplasms produce estrogens or androgens. The mare can have signs of anestrus, nymphomania, or stallionlike behavior; the bitch is likely to have prolonged estrus as well as cystic endometrial hyperplasia and pyometra, as lesions of progesterone stimulation.

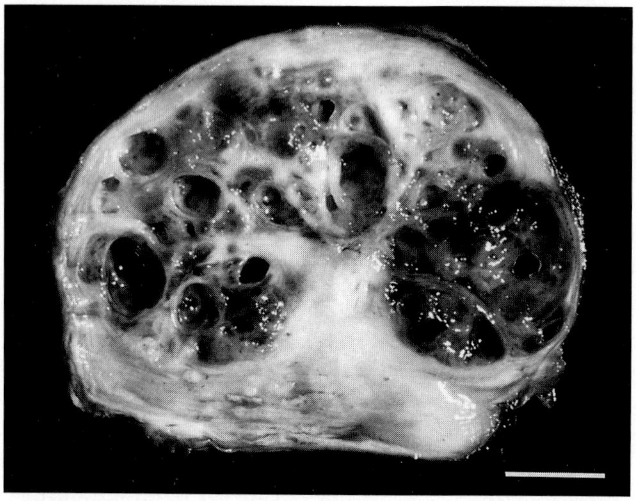

Figure 12-33 Ovary; mare. Granulosa cell tumor. The ovary is greatly enlarged by multiple fluid-filled cysts. The polycystic form is the most frequently encountered granulosa cell tumor. Bar = 1 cm. *Courtesy Dr. M.D. McGavin.*

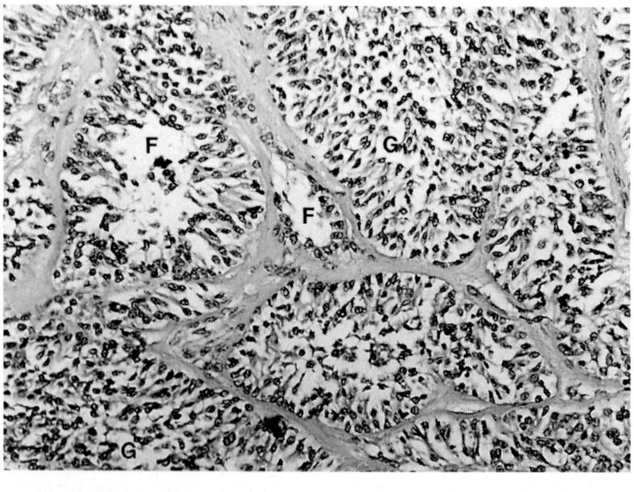

Figure 12-34 Ovary; mare. Granulosa cell tumor. Granulosa cells are in large groups *(G)* without a central cavity as well as in structures resembling normal follicles *(F)*. H & E stain.

Surface Neoplasms

The ovaries are covered by coelomic epithelium, the same layer of tissue that invaginates in early fetal life to form the lining of the reproductive tract. Neoplasms of the ovarian surface epithelium can thus resemble the several neoplasm types of the endometrium. In practice, the serous type is the only important one in animals. Serous papillary cystadenoma and cystadenocarcinoma occur commonly in the bitch (Fig. 12-35). They originate from the surface

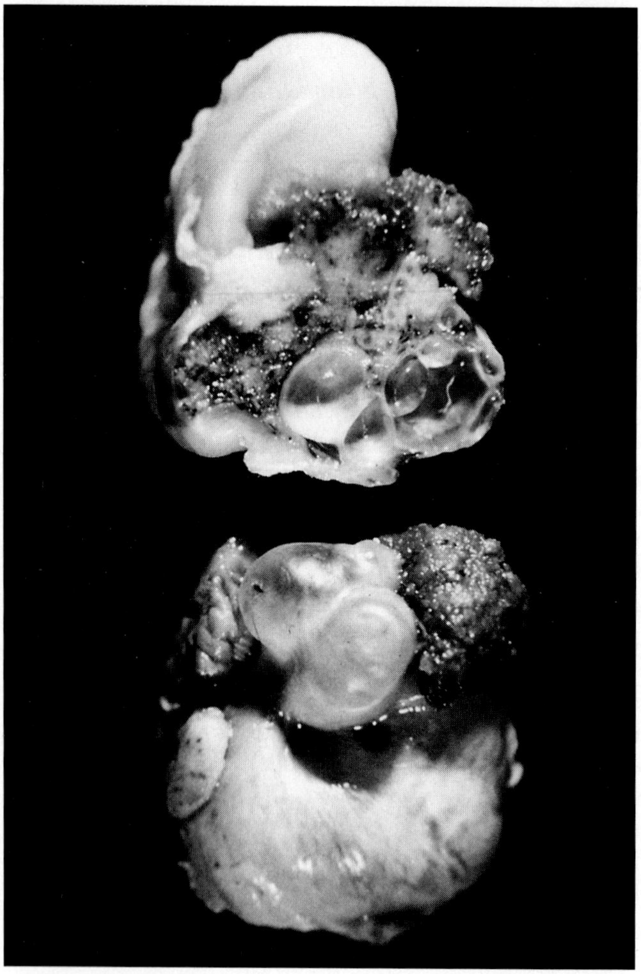

Figure 12-35 Ovaries; bitch. Bilateral papillary cystadenocarcinoma. Large cysts and finely cystic tissue project from the surface of the ovaries.

epithelium or from subsurface rests within the ovary or from the rete ovarii. The neoplasms are frequently bilateral, with a shaggy surface and up to 10 cm in diameter. Malignant forms spread over the peritoneal surface by both lateral extension and seeding. Ascites results either from obstruction of the diaphragmatic lymph vessels, which reabsorb peritoneal fluid, or from excess fluid secretion by the neoplasm.

MAMMARY GLAND

Inflammation

Inflammation of the mammary gland is called mastitis. Mastitis in domestic animals is almost solely due to infection by microorganisms. Because of increased vascular permeability, plasma components enter the milk, ionic balance is altered, and the products of inflammation enter the milk, altering its appearance. Alveolar epithelium that is damaged by inflammation or by pressure from adjacent inflammation secretes less milk. Thus, bovine mastitis is a cause of great economic loss. The following is a discussion of mastitis in the cow, with notes on the disease in other species.

Most of the organisms responsible for mastitis are bacteria. These bacteria can be divided into three groups. In one group are those organisms such as *Streptococcus agalactiae, Staphylococcus aureus,* and *Mycoplasma* species for which the mammary gland is the principal site of persistence or reservoir. Coliforms organisms are in the group that has the environment as reservoir. An overlap group has members such as *Streptococcus uberis* and *Streptococcus dysgalactiae* capable of persisting in either location. Cow-to-cow transmission is important for the mammary reservoir group, whereas contamination of the teat end is important for disease caused by the environmental group. The rates of new mammary gland infections in dairy cows caused by environmental pathogens are greatest during the first and the last 2 weeks of a 60-day nonlactating period. Coliform and streptococcal infections that are established during the nonlactating period with organisms from the environment are present at the time of parturition and cause clinical mastitis soon afterward.

Although hematogenous and percutaneous entries of infection into the mammary gland are possible, the usual route is via the opening of the ductus papillaris, the approximately 1-cm long keratinized, stratified squamous epithelium–lined duct between the exterior and the lactiferous sinus in the teat. Bacteria colonizing the lining of the ductus papillaris multiply and persist and later cause intramammary infections.

Non-Immune-Mediated Defense Mechanisms in the Mammary Gland of the Cow

The teat orifice and the ductus papillaris offer mechanical resistance to the entry of organisms. In cows, a long ductus possibly protects against mammary gland infection. The keratin of the ductus papillaris can be protective by having bactericidal fatty acids, by adsorbing bacteria and desquamating when coated with bacteria, and by desiccating. Infection and inflammation of the ductus papillaris are rare.

The mammary gland has some intrinsic defense mechanisms that are not immune mediated. Regular milking out of the mammary gland probably is a natural defense mechanism because of the flushing of organisms and products of inflammation from the gland. Lactoferrin, the major iron-binding protein of saliva and milk, is a nonspecific natural protective factor in milk. Mammary gland epithelial cells produce the bulk of lactoferrin in milk. Lactoferrin concentration is increased in acute mastitis and in the involuting gland. The binding of iron withholds an essential nutrient from pathogenic bacteria and thus has a bacteriostatic effect. The lactoperoxidase-thiocyanate-H_2O_2 system temporarily inhibits some streptococci and coliforms and *Staphylococcus aureus.* Lactoperoxidase is synthesized by mammary gland epithelium, thiocyanate is derived from certain green feeds, and H_2O_2 is produced by streptococci or comes from an exogenous source. Hypothiocyanite produced by the system damages the inner bacterial membrane killing the bacteria. Lysozyme, synthesized locally or from blood, destroys bacteria by lysis of cell wall peptidoglycan. Of minor importance is complement activated by the alternate pathway in response to the presence of bacterial endotoxin.

Immune-Mediated Defense Mechanisms in the Mammary Gland

The mechanisms can be divided into cellular and humoral types.

Cellular Immune Defense Mechanisms

After the epithelial lining, the first elements of the ductus papillaris that bacteria encounter in the cellular defense system are the cells of the lamina propria of the ductus papillaris and the rosette of Furstenberg. The rosette is a circle of cells at the base of the lactiferous sinus in the teat, immediately proximal to the junction between stratified squamous epithelium lining the ductus papillaris and the one or two layers of cuboidal or columnar cells lining the lactiferous sinus in the teat. The rosette area can be regarded as where the mammary gland proper begins. The lamina propria of the ductus papillaris and Furstenberg's rosette have greater numbers of immunoglobulin-bearing leukocytes than parenchymal mammary gland tissue in both uninfected and infected quarters. The number of leukocytes is greater for Furstenberg's rosette in infected compared with uninfected quarters. In one study, the cells of Furstenberg's rosette were neutrophils and macrophages and not plasma cells. Thus, the antibody detected was considered cytophilic or endocytosed, already used or unavailable for defense against bacteria. In another study, the subepithelial cells in the lamina propria near Furstenberg's rosette were predominantly plasma cells, and the principal antibody produced was IgG_1.

In the mammary gland, macrophages are the resident detector cells against invading bacteria. Macrophages can be found in the alveoli and the interstitium, as well as in the lamina propria of the lactiferous sinus and interlobular and intralobular lactiferous ducts. Macrophages are the most numerous cells in normal milk. In a lactating cow, apparently at least 500,000 phagocytes per milliliter of milk are needed for defense of the mammary gland against invading bacteria. In an uninfected bovine mammary gland, 50,000 to 200,000 neutrophils and macrophages are found per milliliter in milk, with the macrophages predominating.

Upon stimulation by the presence of microorganisms, macrophages in any tissue produce interleukin 1, which causes increased membrane phospholipase activity, releasing arachidonic acid, a substrate for the synthesis of prostaglandins and leukotrienes. Milk macrophages secrete less interleukin 1 than blood macrophages, a property common to macrophages from healthy or inflamed quarters of the mammary gland. Leukotriene B_4 produced by typical macrophages in any tissue is a powerful attractant of neutrophils. Whether leukotriene B_4 is produced by macrophages in milk has not been determined with certainty.

Neutrophils are the principal effector cells in eliminating bacteria from the mammary gland. The primary method by which neutrophils kill bacteria is by phagocytosis after opsonization by antibody from blood, with or without complement from blood. A method of minor importance is lysis by antibody plus complement.

Recruitment of neutrophils from the blood to an infection site is one of the first steps in an inflammatory response. Recruitment can be rapid, so that neutrophils are the dominant cells as early as 2 hours after infection. Cell counts in milk can average 700,000/ml in subclinically infected quarters, and millions of neutrophils per milliliter are common in clinical infections (Fig. 12-36).

The numbers of inflammatory cells (mostly neutrophils) in milk cycle up and down every several days in experimental staphylococcal mastitis, with a corresponding inverse cycling of the number of viable bacteria. When cell counts are at a peak, bactericidal activity per cell is most efficient, by as much as 10,000-fold, and phagocytosis is optimal. The frequency and periodicity of the cycle, as well as the amplitude of the cell and bacterial counts, are independent for each infected quarter. The likely source of reinfection of the mammary gland is those neutrophils that are inefficient at killing intracellular bacteria at the time of low cell count. As these cells undergo necrosis and lysis, their previously protected intracellular viable bacteria are released to multiply, and the inverse cycling of neutrophils and bacterial numbers continues.

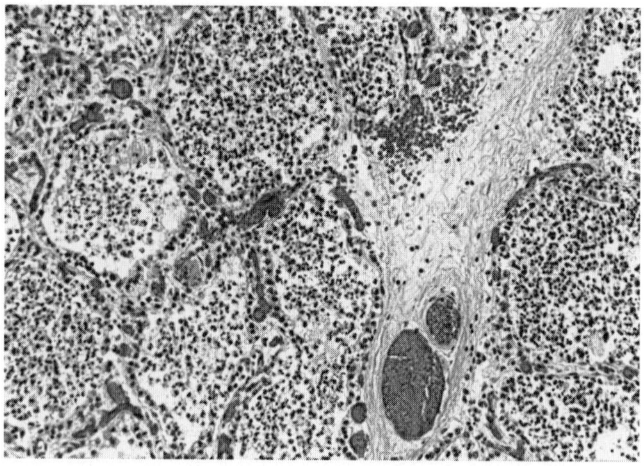

Figure 12-36 Mammary gland; cow. Severe, acute mastitis. Neutrophils are present in the alveoli, congestion and hemorrhage in the intralobular interstitial tissue, and edema in the interlobular septum.

Although neutrophils recruited from the blood are so important in fighting infection in the mammary gland, they do not kill bacteria as well in milk as they do in blood. Milk seems to be a poor medium for the functioning of neutrophils. Some possible reasons include the absence of glucose in milk for the glycolytic metabolism of neutrophils, decreased amounts of glycogen in milk neutrophils, deficiency of opsonins and complement in milk, coating of the surface of neutrophils with casein, loss of neutrophil pseudopodia caused by phagocytosis of fat, and decrease of hydrolytic enzymes within neutrophils after phagocytosis of casein and fat.

In the first week after parturition, when neutrophils are likely most needed to deal with mammary gland infections, bovine blood neutrophils already are defective before they pass into the mammary gland. They have significantly impaired chemokinesis and decreased superoxide anion production, antibody-dependent cell-mediated cytotoxicity, and phagocytosis of bacteria. The causes are probably some combination of the effects of stress, energy, and protein demands of early lactation, and the hormonal fluxes of this stage of the reproductive cycle. In the parturient period, the concentration of glucocorticoids is increased. This means that leukocyte function is less effective, because expression of L-selectin and CD18 on neutrophils are downregulated by glucocorticoids. This downregulates adhesion between blood neutrophils and vascular endothelium and transendothelial migration of neutrophils.

The amount of tumor necrosis factor (TNF) in mammary gland secretions increases toward the end of gestation. The increase is in concert with the increase in the number of macrophages, the source of TNF. Bovine neutrophils do not seem to respond to TNF in the same way as do neutrophils of other species. (Cattle treated with

TNF have neutrophils that are decreased in numbers in blood, have decreased migration, and decreased synthesis of reactive oxygen species.) The large amount of TNF could contribute to the poor performance of bovine mammary gland neutrophils in the postparturient period, leading to establishment of bacteria in the gland.

Interleukin 1 from mammary gland macrophages stimulates the immune system by activating T and B lymphocytes. Only a few B lymphocytes are present in the mammary gland and milk. T lymphocytes in normal mammary gland tissue and milk have a large proportion of $\alpha\beta CD8^+$ cells. The $CD4^+/CD8^+$ ratio is <1, reversed from the ratio in blood. The mammary gland can thus be regarded as having selective lymphocyte trafficking, favoring $CD8^+$ cells, which have either cytotoxic or suppressor function. $CD4^+$ (T helper) T lymphocytes, which activate B lymphocytes, T lymphocytes, and macrophages, are underrepresented in normal mammary gland tissues and milk. $CD8^+$ T lymphocytes are found in lactiferous duct and alveolar epithelium, while the lesser numbers of $CD4^+$ lymphocytes and B cells are in clusters in the connective tissues. In early lactation, the $CD8^+$ lymphocytes in milk function more as suppressor cells (express interleukin 4) than cytotoxic cells (express interferon-γ), but the situation is reversed in mid and late lactation. Suppressor T cells control, modulate, or suppress the immune response, and cytotoxic T cells can act as scavengers, removing damaged mammary cells. In response to bacterial infection, an influx of $CD4^+$ T cells occurs in milk, and these cells eventually outnumber $CD8^+$ T lymphocytes. $\gamma\delta$T lymphocytes preferentially migrate to epithelial surfaces and can destroy altered epithelial cells. $\gamma\delta$ T cells are present in greater numbers in mammary gland secretions and parenchyma when compared with blood. The percentage of $\gamma\delta$ T lymphocytes of mammary parenchymal lymphocytes decreases in the postpartum period, a time of increased susceptibility of the mammary gland to disease, suggesting that $\gamma\delta$ T lymphocytes can be important in defense against infection.

Humoral Immune Defense Mechanisms

Antibody concentration in normal bovine milk is small, about 1 mg/ml. Most IgG is serum derived; IgG_1 is selectively transferred into mammary gland secretion and is the major immunoglobulin class in milk obtained from healthy mammary glands. IgG_2 is both serum derived and locally produced by resident plasma cells. IgA and IgM are synthesized locally in the mammary gland. Local production is caused by stimulation of subepithelial lymphocytes. Particulate antigens, such as bacteria, stimulate an antibody response in the mammary gland of the cow, whereas soluble antigens do not. In colostrum and in milk from inflamed mammary glands, antibody concentration approaches 50 mg/ml. Early in inflammation, IgG_1 and IgG_2 opsonize bacteria to enhance phagocytosis by macrophages, but later the importance of IgG_2 as an opsonin increases as neutrophils enter the gland. Neutrophils can transport IgG_2 to the mammary gland as they move to the site of inflammation. IgM also functions as an opsonin. IgA does not opsonize, but could prevent bacterial adherence to epithelium, inhibit bacterial multiplication, neutralize leukocyte-inhibiting bacterial toxins, and agglutinate bacteria.

Specific Pathogens in Mastitis

Streptococcus agalactiae was the most important pathogen of the bovine mammary gland in the era before adequate mammary gland hygiene and efficient antibacterial drugs. Resistance of cows to mastitis caused by this organism is subject to great individual variation; in general, resistance decreases with age. The mammary gland is the only organ affected by this organism. *S. agalactiae* does not persist long in the environment. Once a cow is infected, however, the organism persists in the lactiferous sinus, with periodic waves of multiplication, increase in virulence, and tissue invasion. The initial response to invasion of *S. agalactiae* is interstitial edema and influx of neutrophils into the interstitium and alveoli. The alveolar epithelium undergoes either brief hyperplasia or vacuolation, and then is desquamated. Macrophages quickly become a component of the cell population of infected alveoli, and fibrosis rapidly obliterates the lumen of these alveoli. Edema, cellular infiltration, and fibrosis are lesions found in infected and adjacent alveoli, so that pressure is increased within the lobule and within adjacent lobules. The increased pressure causes stagnation of milk flow, thereby initiating premature involution of a portion of the gland. After the acute phase, periductal fibrosis occurs and granulation tissue replaces part of the normal cuboidal to columnar epithelium of smaller ducts. Fibrous polyps can completely obstruct milk flow. Restoration of ductal epithelium can occur after the granulation tissue has matured and contracted. The lobar ducts and sinuses, with their normally two-layered columnar epithelium, are similarly but less severely affected, often going through a phase of squamous metaplasia of the epithelium.

The gross appearance of a mammary gland with mastitis caused by *S. agalactiae* depends on the stage of the disease; different stages are to be expected in different areas of a gland. Usually more than one quarter is involved. In the acute stage, hyperemia involves the mucosa of the sinuses. Milk quality is altered and strands or clumps of debris are present in the milk, or the milk is transformed into pus. The areas of parenchymal edema and cellular infiltration are gray and turgid. Groups of alveoli in which the secretion is retained because of obstruction of the duct by granulation tissue resemble small abscesses. Involuting parenchyma and fibrotic parenchyma appear similar to one another and can be difficult to differentiate grossly. Duct and sinus mucosae become granular and thickened because of underlying projecting areas of granulation tissue and surrounding fibrosis.

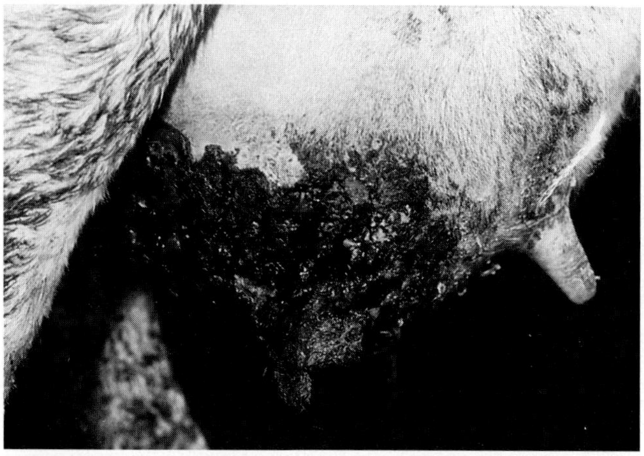

Figure 12-37 Mammary gland; cow. Gangrenous mastitis. Acute staphylococcal or coliform mastitis has resulted in necrosis of the right hind quarter of the gland. Eventually, it will slough. *Courtesy Dr. M.D. McGavin.*

Isolates of *Staphylococcus aureus* obtained from the bovine mammary gland range from nonpathogenic to highly pathogenic. Hemolysis and production of coagulase in microbiologic culture are useful guides to evaluating the virulence of the isolates. Products released by staphylococci during their growth and the ability of the organisms to adhere to epithelial surfaces are important virulence factors. The severest form of staphylococcal mastitis is the gangrenous form (Fig. 12-37), usually seen shortly after parturition, and involving a variable proportion of the udder. Severe acute inflammation, with classical heat, redness, swelling, and pain, progresses to necrosis with its coldness of the affected area, blue-black color, fluid exudation, and crepitation.

Microscopically, during the first 48 hours after infection with toxigenic *S. aureus,* the infected tissue has severe interstitial edema that increases interalveolar stromal area and reduces alveolar luminal area. Progressive swelling, vacuolar degeneration, and focal erosion and ulceration occur throughout the duct system and are most prominent near the junction of stratified squamous epithelium and columnar epithelium in the area of the rosette of Furstenberg. The organism attaches to epithelial cells, causing focal damage, and later can be seen on, within, and below ductal and alveolar epithelium. Inflammatory cellular response is rapid, with neutrophils initially in the subepithelial tissues of the distal parts of the duct system, then within the epithelium, and, later, in the interstitial and epithelial tissue of alveoli.

Staphylococcal mastitis in the less acute form follows a course similar to that of the streptococcal mastitis. Initially, damage occurs to the epithelium of the lactiferous sinus and larger lactiferous ducts. Organisms extend along the ducts rapidly and produce acute inflammation in groups of adjacent terminal alveoli. In chronically infected quarters, macrophages are the principal inflammatory cell type in epithelial lining, lumens, and, especially, in the glandular interstitium. Lymphocytes also increase in number, but some investigators have reported a lack of increase in plasma cells. These observations suggest that mammary gland lymphocytes could become hyporesponsive to antigenic stimulation in quarters chronically infected with *S. aureus*. Some data indicate that mammary gland lymphocyte function is compromised; blastogenesis is depressed in lymphocytes recovered from quarters infected with *S. aureus*. Studies have documented that plasma cells are prevalent in the stroma of mammary glands with chronic *S. aureus* mastitis; more cells produce IgA than IgG antibodies, and IgA-containing cells increase in number as the disease progresses. The extent of regeneration is uncertain; it is unclear whether damaged alveoli redevelop secretory tissue or remaining healthy tissue undergoes compensatory hypertrophy, or both processes occur.

Staphylococcus aureus has a greater propensity than *Streptococcus agalactiae* for invading the interstitial tissue between alveoli. The initial inflammatory reaction is necrotizing; abscess formation can follow. Abscesses, scattered and often coalescing, vary in size from those that are microscopic to those grossly visible. Sometimes the staphylococcal organisms are surrounded by rosettes of immunoglobulin-containing club-shaped material. (The obsolete term botryomycosis was applied to such lesions.) An equally important and parallel set of events occurring in the lobules not invaded by bacteria is the obstruction of milk flow by granulation tissue and pressure from surrounding fibrosis, resulting in involution of those uninvaded lobules. Multiple, small, soft cream to pink nodules, some containing pus, are separated by bands of fibrous tissue. Disease caused by less pathogenic strains of staphylococci, such as nonhemolytic coagulase-negative strains, progresses less dramatically, not necessarily with obvious abscess formation. However, the same components of granulation tissue and fibrosis are present, causing obstruction and pressure, which in turn cause atrophy of adjacent lobules.

Coliform mastitis is caused after organisms from the environment contaminate the opening of the papillary duct at the distal end of the teat and ascend the duct. The most common organisms are *Escherichia coli, Enterobacter aerogenes,* and *Klebsiella pneumoniae*. The coliform organisms probably exert their damaging effect via endotoxin acting on the vasculature. In the acute form of the disease, the lesions are hyperemia, hemorrhages, and edema of the affected areas centered around the lactiferous ducts (Fig. 12-38). The secretion in the lactiferous sinus is cloudy and blood stained and has clumps of fibrin. Microscopically, interlobular septa are edematous and fibrin thrombi are in lymph vessels. Epithelium of ducts

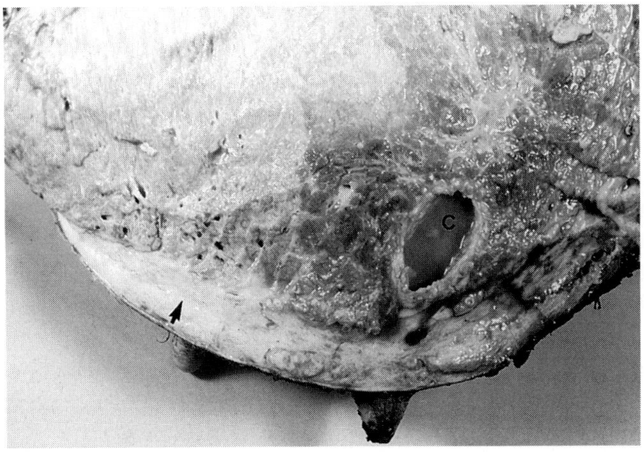

Figure 12-38 Mammary gland; cow. Severe, acute coliform mastitis. Watery milk, flecked with fibrin, is in the lactiferous sinus *(C)*. Note the subcutaneous edema *(arrow)*. *Courtesy Dr. M.D. McGavin.*

and alveoli is necrotic and very few inflammatory cells are present in the alveoli. Coliform organisms are numerous in the alveoli. Large numbers of organisms are phagocytosed by the secretory epithelium. The severity of the disease in postparturient cows is attributed to a delay in the influx of neutrophils. The cow's response to endotoxin is influenced by the stage of the reproductive cycle. The nonlactating mammary gland is much less sensitive to the effects of endotoxin than the lactating gland.

If the cow survives endotoxemia, the necrotic mammary tissue, which can be a large portion of a quarter, becomes separated from the viable tissue and eventually sloughs. Cows in early lactation with less severe coliform mastitis often develop chronic mastitis that has alterations of hyperplasia, disorganization, and filiform processes of the epithelial lining of the papillary duct and lactiferous sinus.

Actinomyces pyogenes causes a mastitis in lactating, nonlactating, and even immature bovine mammary glands that is characterized by abscesses in the tissue about the large and small lactiferous ducts. Abscesses range from those microscopic in size to those grossly visible. Fistulas from the abscesses can form at the base of the teat. Fibrosis of the abscess walls can result in loss of small affected ducts and involution and fibrosis of the parenchyma they drain. The wall of large abscesses is thickened by granulation tissue.

Mycoplasma mastitis in cows occurs in herds in which the conventional forms of bacterial mastitis have been eliminated. Several mycoplasmas are capable of causing bovine mastitis, but *Mycoplasma bovis* is by far the most prevalent. The disease caused by *M. bovis* tends to involve the whole gland, with a pronounced purulent exudate in the early stages. Affected quarters initially are enlarged, firm, light brown, and have a nodular parenchyma. Abscesses can be up to 10 cm in diameter. Exudation of neutrophils into the lobular interstitium and alveoli is intense in the early stages. The exudate changes with chronicity to include mononuclear cells. Early vacuolation and degeneration of alveolar epithelium is followed by hyperplasia of alveolar and ductular epithelium, and, then, by metaplasia to a relatively undifferentiated multilayered epithelial lining. Focal erosions of duct epithelium are filled in by granulation tissue. Aggregates of lymphocytes occur in the lobular interstitium and around ducts. Interstitial fibrosis and lobular atrophy are found in the late stages.

Granulomatous mastitis occurs naturally, with bovine tuberculosis as the prime example, a disease now rare in the United States. Iatrogenic granulomatous mastitis is produced by the introduction through the teat of the cow of therapeutic products contaminated with bacteria or fungi that can cause granulomatous inflammation.

Tuberculous mastitis, whether in the form with multiple nodules less than 1 cm in diameter (miliary tuberculosis), the form with larger nodules (organ tuberculosis), or the form with large irregular caseous areas (caseous tuberculosis), involves the lactiferous ducts. In the cow, *Mycobacterium bovis* probably arrives at the mammary gland hematogenously from organs with previously established tubercles. In most cases, it appears that the first lesions are in the interalveolar or interlobular connective tissue with later spread to the ducts, although progression in the opposite direction, with primary involvement of ducts and secondary involvement of alveoli, is evident in those few animals with minimal glandular involvement. Most cases are of the organ type, but a few are of the miliary type, which occurs with the massive release of organisms into a relatively naive organ, or of the caseous type, which occurs when the immune response of the organ to the bacteria is especially suppressed. Microscopically, the miliary type consists of classical tubercles, with central caseation surrounded by a zone of epithelioid macrophages and multinucleate giant cells, bounded by lymphocytes and fibrous tissue. In the more common organ type, the same cellular elements are present but are not organized into tubercles.

The algal organism *Prototheca zopfii* can cause outbreaks of granulomatous mastitis in cattle. Affected animals are discovered in screening of milk samples or at slaughter. *Prototheca* spp. organisms have been found commonly in dairy environments in North and South America and in Europe, particularly in wet areas contaminated with manure. Lesions occur in the mammary glands and the supramammary lymph nodes. In the early lesions, algae are within macrophages in mammary gland alveoli, but not in neutrophils, mammary epithelial cells, or myoepithelial cells. In older lesions, inflammation is mostly interstitial. The algae lack chlorophyll and are unstained with hematoxylin and eosin, but stain with Gomori methenamine silver or periodic acid–Schiff stains. The protothecal organisms occur as single cells with a large nucleus, or endosporulating forms with daughter cells, or as empty, collapsed and crescent shaped structures.

Iatrogenic granulomatous mastitis in the cow occurs when drugs for mastitis treatment are introduced through the teat and are contaminated with *Nocardia asteroides, Cryptococcus neoformans, Mycobacterium* sp. other than *M. bovis,* or *Candida* sp. Nocardiosis can also be a spontaneous mammary gland disease, from organisms normally resident in the soil. Features of the disease are systemic illness and the presence of discharging sinuses from the mammary gland through the skin. An udder affected with cryptococcal mastitis has the same yellow gelatinous material that is typical of cryptococcal lesions elsewhere.

Nonbovine Mastitis

Ovine progressive pneumonia virus can cause mastitis in sheep. Clinical signs and gross lesions often are absent, but microscopic lesions include a diffuse interstitial accumulation of lymphocytes and focal degeneration of ductal epithelium in the mammary gland. In more severe cases, lesions include periductal lymphoid nodules with germinal centers and hyperplasia, vacuolation, and focal necrosis of overlying epithelium. The mammary gland is a highly susceptible target organ of this nononcogenic lentivirus and spread of the virus is facilitated through the milk. Caprine arthritis–encephalitis virus, a closely related lentivirus found in goats, has been associated with diffuse and nodular infiltrates of lymphocytes and a few macrophages around ducts in the mammary gland. The virus can be recovered from the mammary gland of goats that have antibody to the virus. In this disease, too, the mammary gland is an important target organ from an epidemiologic standpoint, allowing transmission of the virus through the colostrum from doe to kid.

Mycoplasma agalactiae causes mastitis in sheep and goats, especially goats, in Mediterranean countries and in the United States. In the systemic disease, localization of inflammation occurs in the joints and eyes as well as the mammary gland. Edema of the interstitium is the first mammary gland lesion. The glands are firm, swollen, and have thick yellow secretions. Systemically, microthrombi and occasional foci of necrosis occur in the liver and pulmonary alveoli are filled with proteinaceous fluid. If the animal survives, interstitial fibrosis and glandular atrophy ensue in the mammary gland.

Pasteurella haemolytica causes mastitis in lactating sheep and sometimes also causes rhinitis and pneumonia in their lambs. Usually only one of the two sides of the mammary gland is affected. The acute phase is characterized by swelling of the gland and by a watery secretion instead of milk. The affected gland has a blue discoloration due to necrosis. If the disease is not fatal, abscess formation is followed by sloughing of the affected side of the gland.

It is likely that coliform mastitis plays a part in the important clinical syndrome of mastitis-metritis-agalactia in sows. Some mastitis is present in at least one gland in more than 50% of affected sows, although metritis might not be a significant component. The lesions in the mammary gland have not received much descriptive attention, but it is likely that they are similar to those of acute coliform mastitis in the cow. The pathogenesis of the agalactia could be the suppression of prolactin production by the lipopolysaccharide of bacterial endotoxin acting on cells of the adenohypophysis or hypothalamus.

Mastitis is not common in dogs and cats. When it does occur, it is likely to be a sequela to minor lesions of the nipples, or to be superimposed on mammary hyperplasia or neoplasia. The organisms most responsible are streptococci and staphylococci, which in the acute phase tend to cause suppurative or necrotizing inflammation, respectively.

References

Al-Bassam MA, Thomson RG, O'Donnel L. Involution abnormalities in the postpartum uterus of the bitch. Vet Pathol 1981;18:208-218.

Al-Dahash SYA, David JSE. Histological examination of ovaries and uteri from cows with cystic ovaries. Vet Rec 1977; 101:342-347.

Allen GP, Bryans JT. Molecular epizootiology, pathogenesis, and prophylaxis of equine herpesvirus-1 infections. Prog Vet Microbiol Immunol 1986; 2:78-144.

Anderson JC. Progressive pathology of staphylococcal mastitis with a note on control, immunization and therapy. Vet Rec 1982; 110: 372-376.

Anderson ML, BonDurant RH, Corbeil RR, Corbeil LB. Immune and inflammatory responses to reproductive tract infection with *Tritrichomonas foetus* in immunized and control heifers. J Parasitol 1996; 82:594-600.

Anderson TD, Cheville NF, Meador VP. Pathogenesis of placentitis in the goat inoculated with *Brucella abortus*. 11. Ultrastructural studies. Vet Pathol 1986; 23:227-239.

Anderson TD, Meador VP, Cheville NF. Pathogenesis of placentitis in the goat inoculated with *Brucella abortus*. 1. Gross and histologic lesions. Vet Pathol 1986; 23:219-226.

Barlow RM, Patterson DSP. Border disease of sheep: a virus-induced teratogenic disorder. Berlin: Hamburg: Parey, 1982.

Barr BC, Anderson ML, Blanchard PC, Daft BM, Kinde H, Conrad PA. Bovine fetal encephalitis and myocarditis associated with protozoal infections. Vet Pathol 1990; 27:354-361.

Bosu WTK, Peter AT. Evidence for the role of intrauterine infections in the pathogenesis of cystic ovaries in postpartum dairy cows. Theriogenology 1987; 28:725-736.

Carmichael LE, Kenney RM. Canine abortion caused by *Brucella canis*. JAVMA 1968; 152:605-616.

Coignoul FL, Cheville NF. Pathology of maternal genital tract, placenta, and fetus in equine viral arteritis. Vet Pathol 1984; 21:333-340.

Collins RA, Parsons KR, Bland AP. Antibody-containing cells and specialised epithelial cells in the bovine teat. Res Vet Sci 1986; 41:50-55.

Cullor JS, Tyler JW, Smith BP. Disorders of the Mammary Gland. In: Smith BP, ed. Large Animal Internal Medicine. St. Louis: Mosby, 1990: 1047-1067.

Cutlip RC, Lehmkuhl HD, Brogden KA, Bolin SR. Mastitis associated with ovine progressive pneumonia. Am J Vet Res 1985; 46:326-328.

Daley MJ, Oldham ER, Williams TJ, Coyle PA. Quantitative and qualitative properties of host polymorphonuclear cells during experimentally induced *Staphylococcus aureus* mastitis in cows. Am J Vet Res 1991; 52:474-479.

Deyoe BL. Brucellosis. In: Leman AD, et al, eds. Diseases of Swine. 6th ed. Ames: Iowa State University Press, 1986: 599-607.

Edington N, Smyth B, Griffiths L. The role of endothelial cell infection in the endometruim, placenta and foetus of equid herpesvirus 1 (EHV-1) abortions. J Comp Pathol 1991; 104:379-387.

Edwards JF, Livingston CW, Chung SI, Collisson EC. Ovine arthrogryposis and central nervous system malformations associated with in utero Cache Valley virus infection: Spontaneous disease. Vet Pathol 1989; 26:33-39.

Ellis WA. Leptosporosis. In: Leman AD, Straw BE, Mangeling WL, et al, eds. Diseases of Swine. 7th ed. Ames: Iowa State University Press, 1992:529-536.

Fray MD, Prentice H, Clarke MC, Charleston B. Immunohistochemical evidence for the localization of bovine viral diarrhea virus, a single-stranded RNA virus, in ovarian oocytes in the cow. Vet Pathol 1998; 35:253-259.

Frost AJ, Brooker BE. Hyperacute *Escherischia coli* mastitis of cattle in the immediate post-partum period. Aust Vet J 1986; 63:327-331.

Garverick HA. Ovarian follicular cysts in dairy cows. J Dairy Sci 1997; 80:995-1004.

Gelberg HB, McEntee K. Pathology of the canine and feline uterine tube. Vet Pathol 1986; 23:770-775.

Gelberg HB, McEntee K, Heath EH. Feline cystic rete ovarii. Vet Pathol 1984; 21:304-307.

Grooms DL, Brock KV, Ward LA. Detection of bovine viral virus in the ovaries of cattle acutely infected with bovine viral diarrhea virus. J Vet Diagn Invest 1998; 10:125-129.

Gudding R, Mc Donald JS, Cheville NF. Pathogenesis of *Staphylococcus aureus* mastitis: Bacteriologic, histologic, and ultrastructural pathologic findings. Am J Vet Res 1984; 45:2525-2531.

Hanson LE, Tripathy DN. Leptospirosis. In: Leman AD, et al, eds. Diseases of Swine. 6th ed. Ames: Iowa State University Press, 1986: 591-599.

Hartley WG, Kater J. The pathology of toxoplasma infection in the pregnant ewe. Res Vet Sci 1963; 4:326-332.

Herenda D. An abattoir survey of reproductive organ abnormalities in beef heifers. Can Vet J 1987; 28:33-37.

Hill AW, Frost AJ. Progressive pathology of severe *Escherichia coli* mastitis in dairy cows. Res Vet Sci 1984; 37:179-187.

Hunter RH. Aetiology of intersexuality in female (XX) pigs, with novel molecular interpretations. Mol Reprod Dev 1996;45:392-402.

Jasper DE. The role of *Mycoplasma* in bovine mastitis. J Am Vet Med Assoc 1982; 181:158-162.

Jeffcott LB, Whitwell KE. Twinning as a cause of foetal and neonatal loss in the thoroughbred mare. J Comp Pathol 1973; 83:91-106.

Kehrli ME, Nonnecke BJ, Roth JA. Alterations in bovine lymphocyte function during the periparturient period. Am J Vet Res 1989a; 50:215-220.

Kehrli ME, Nonnecke BJ, Roth JA. Alterations in bovine neutrophil function during the periparturient period. Am J Vet Res 1989b; 50:207-214.

Kennedy PC, Casaro AP, Kimsey PB, Bon Durant RH, Bushnell RB, Mitchell GM. Epizootic bovine abortion: Histogenesis of the fetal lesion. Am J Vet Res 1983; 44:1040-1048.

Kennedy PC, Richards WPC. The pathology of abortion caused by the virus of infectious bovine rhinotracheitis. Pathol Vet 1964; 1:7-17.

Kennedy-Stoskopf S, Narayan O, Strandberg JD. The mammary gland as a target organ for infection with caprine arthritis-encephalitis virus. J Comp Pathol 1985; 95:609-617.

Kenney RM. Cyclic and pathologic changes of the mare endometrium as detected by biopsy, with a note on early embryonic death. J Am Vet Med Assoc 1978; 172:241-262.

Kesler DJ, Garverick HA. Ovarian cysts in dairy cattle: A review. J Anim Sci 1982; 55:1147-1159.

Lager KM, Halbur PG. Gross and microscopic lesions in porcine fetuses infected with porcine reproductive and respiratory syndrome virus. J Vet Diagn Invest 1996; 8:257-282.

Lascelles AK. The immune system of the ruminant mammary gland and its role in the control of mastitis. J Dairy Sci 1979; 62:154-160.

Lawler DF, Evans RH, Reimers TJ, Colby ED, Monti KL. Histopathologic features, environmental factors, and serum estrogen, progesterone, and prolactin values associated with ovarian phase and inflammatory uterine disease in cats. Am J Vet Res 1991; 52:1747-1753.

Lenghaus C, Forman AJ, Hale CJ. Experimental infection of 35, 50 and 60 day old pig foetuses with porcine parvovirus. Aust Vet J 1978; 54:418-422.

MacLachlan NJ. Ovarian disorders in domestic animals. Environ Health Perspect 1987; 73:27-33.

Mahaffey LW, Adam NM. Abortions associated with mycotic lesions of the placenta in mares. J Am Vet Med Assoc 1964; 144:24-32.

Mattila T, Frost AJ. Induction by endotoxin of the inflammatory response in the lactating and dry bovine mammary gland. Res Vet Sci 1989; 46:238-240.

MacMillan AP. Brucellosis. In: Leman AD, Straw BE, Mangeling WL, et al, eds. Diseases of Swine. 7th ed. Ames: Iowa State University Press, 1992:446-453.

McEntee K, Nielsen SV. Tumors of the female genital tract. Bull WHO 1976; 53:217-226.

Meyers-Wallen VN, Patterson DF. Disorders of sexual development in the dog. In: Morrow DA, ed. Current Therapy in Theriogenology. 2nd ed. Philadelphia: WB Saunders, 1986: 567-574.

Miller JM. Bovine leukemia virus. In: Howard JL, ed. Current Veterinary Therapy: Food Animal Practice 2. Philadelphia: WB Saunders, 1986: 506-508.

Miller JM, Van Der Maaten MJ. Reproductive tract lesions in heifers after intrauterine inoculation with infectious bovine rhinotracheitis virus. Am J Vet Res 1984; 45:790-794.

Nickerson SC. Immune mechanisms of the bovine udder: An overview. J Am Vet Med Assoc 1985; 187:41-45.

Nickerson SC, Heald CW. Cells in local reaction to experimental *Staphylococcus aureus* infection in bovine mammary gland. J Dairy Sci 1982; 65:105-116.

Nickerson SC, Heald CW. Histopathologic response of the bovine mammary gland to experimentally induced *Staphylococcus aureus* infection. Am J Vet Res 1981; 42:1351-1355.

Nielsen SW, Misdorp W, McEntee K. Tumors of the ovary. Bull WHO 1976; 53:203-215.

Nonnecke BJ, Harp JA. Effect of chronic staphylococcal mastitis on mitogenic responses of bovine lymphocytes. J Dairy Sci 1985; 68:3323-3328.

Osburn BI. The relation of fetal age to the character of lesions in fetal lambs infected with *Brucella ovis*. Pathol Vet 1968; 5:395-406.

Osebold JW, Osburn BI, Spezialetti R, Bushnell RB, Stott JL. Histopathologic changes in bovine fetuses after repeated reintroduction of a spirochete-like agent into pregnant heifers: Association with epizootic bovine abortion. Am J Vet Res 1987; 48:627-633.

Palmer NC, Kierstead M, Key DW, Williams JC, Peacock MG, Vellend H. Placentitis and abortion in goats and sheep in Ontario caused by *Coxiella burnetti*. Can Vet J 1983; 24:60-61.

Park YH, Fox LK, Hamilton MJ, Davis WC. Bovine mononuclear subpopulations in peripheral blood and mammary gland secretions during lactation. J Dairy Sci 1992; 75:998-1006.

Pattison IH. The progressive pathology of bacterial mastitis. Vet Rec 1958; 70:114-117.

Politis I, Mc Bride BW, Burton JH, Zhao X, Turner JD. Secretion of interleukin-1 by bovine milk macrophages. Am J Vet Res 1991; 52:858-862.

Potter K, Hancock DH, Gallina AM. Clinical and pathologic features of endometrial hyperplasia, pyometra and endometritis in cats: 79 cases (1980-1985). J Am Vet Med Assoc 1991; 198:1427-1431.

Rooney JR. Autopsy of the horse. Baltimore: Williams & Wilkins, 1970:120-134.

Ruhnke HL, Palmer NC, Doig PA, Miller RB. Bovine abortion and neonatal death associated with *Ureaplasma diversum*. Theriogenology 1984; 21:295-301.

Sandholm M, Vasenius H, Kivisto A-K. Pathogenesis of canine pyometra. J Am Vet Med Assoc 1975; 167:1006-1010.

Shalev A, Short RV, Hamerton JL. Immunogenetics of sex determination in the polled goat. Cytogenet Cell Genet 1980; 28:195-202.

Smith BB. Pathogenesis and therapeutic management of lactation failure in periparturient sows. Comp Cont Educ 1985; 7:S523-533.

Smith KL, Schanbacher FL. Lactoferrin as a factor of resistance to infection of the bovine mammary gland. J Am Vet Med Assoc 1977; 170:1224-1227.

Smith KL, Todhunter DA, Schoenberger PS. Environmental pathogens and intramammary infection during the dry period. J Dairy Sci 1985; 68:402-417.

Sordillo LM, Doymaz MZ, Oliver SP. Distribution of immunoglobulin-bearing leukocytes in bovine mammary tissue infected chronically with *Staphylococcus aureus*. J Vet Med B 1990; 37:473-476.

Sordillo LM, Doymaz MZ, Oliver SP. Morphological study of chronic *Staphylococcus aureus* mastitis in the lactating bovine mammary gland. Res Vet Sci 1989; 47:247-252.

Sordillo LM, Redmond MJ, Campos M, Warren L, Babiuk LA. Cytokine activity in bovine mammary secretions during the periparturient period. Can J Vet Res 1991; 55:2298-301.

Sordillo LM, Shafer-Weaver K, DeRosa D. Immunobiology of the mammary gland. J Dairy Sci 1997; 80:1851-1865.

Taylor BC, Keefe RG, Dellinger JD, Nakamura Y, Cullor JS, Stott JL. T cell populations and cytokine expression in mild derived from normal and bacteria-infected bovine mammary glands. Cell Immunol 1997; 182:68-76.

Vaiman D, Koutita O, Oustry A, Elaen JM, Manfredi E, Fellous M, Cribiu EP. Genetic mapping of the autosomal region involved in XX sex-reversal and horn development in goats. Mamm Genome 1996; 7:133-137.

Van Der Maaten MJ, Miller JM. Ovarian lesions in heifers exposed to infectious bovine rhinotracheitis virus by non-genital routes on the day after breeding. Vet Microbiol 1985; 10:155-163.

Varner DD, Blanchard TL. An update on uterine defense mechanisms in the mare. J Equine Vet Sci 1990; 10:169-175.

Vermooten MI. Canine transmissible venereal tumor (TVT): A review. J South Afr Vet Assoc 1987; 58:147-150.

Vigier B, Tran D, Legeai L, Bezard J, Josso N. Origin of anti-Müllerian hormone in bovine freemartin fetuses. J Reprod Fertil 1984; 70:473-479.

Watson ED. Uterine defence mechanisms in mares resistant and susceptible to persistent endometritis: A review. Equine Vet J 1988; 20:397-400.

Watson ED, Thomson SR. Lymphocyte subsets in the endometrium of genitally normal mares and mares susceptible to endometritis. Equine Vet J 1996; 28:106-110.

Whitwell KE. Investigations into fetal and neonatal losses in the horse. Symposium on equine reproduction. Vet Clin North Am 1980; 2:213-331.

Williams WF, Margolis MJ, Manspeaker J, Douglass LW, Davidson JP. Peripartum changes in the bovine placenta related to fetal membrane retention. Theriogenology 1987; 28:213-223.

Zimmerman J, Yoon K-J, Stevenson G, Dee SA. PRRS Compendium. Des Moines, Iowa: National Pork Producers Council, 1998: 46-47.

CHAPTER 13

Reproductive System: Male

Helen M. Acland

NORMAL MALE REPRODUCTIVE SYSTEM

For a normal placental mammalian male reproductive system to develop, it is necessary for **the gene for the testis-determining factor (Sry)** to be present. This gene is located on the Y chromosome that is acquired at fertilization. The expression of Sry occurs briefly, in the somatic cells of the indifferent gonads (or genital ridges). Because expression ceases shortly before Sertoli cells can be recognized, it is proposed that the functional gene product (SRY) influences other genes, such as Sox9, that ensure the differentiation and maintenance of Sertoli cells. Sox9 is expressed on the genital ridges of both sexes, and is upregulated in XY individuals and downregulated in XX individuals just before gonad differentiation. Sertoli cells signal the other supporting cell precursor lines to differentiate along the male pathway. Without the presence of SRY, the supporting cell precursor lineage differentiates instead into ovarian granulosa or follicle cells.

Early in sex differentiation, the embryo has a double set of ducts. The Müllerian or paramesonephric ducts are female precursors, arising by invagination of the celomic cavity; the **Wolffian ducts** are male precursors, arising from the duct of the primitive kidney, the mesonephros. After germ cells migrate from the yolk sac and the testes develop in genital ridge tissue, the testes produce two hormones. **Sertoli cells** secrete the polypeptide hormone **Müllerian-inhibiting substance (MIS)** during embryonic development and at lower concentrations postnatally. MIS causes regression of the ipsilateral Müllerian duct, indirectly through action on mesenchymal tissue. Sertoli cells stimulate differentiation of **Leydig cells** from the testicular interstitial cells. Leydig cells secrete the steroid hormone **testosterone,** which causes persistence and differentiation of the Wolffian ducts. Testosterone is likely transported down the Wolffian ducts rather than moving by simple diffusion. A third hormone, **dihydrotestosterone,** which is a metabolite of testosterone, is required for formation of the prostate gland, the closing of the urethral folds, and the formation of the penis and scrotum. The enzyme **steroid 5α-reductase** is produced by cells in the urogenital sinus, genital tubercle, and genital swellings, respectively, and reduces testosterone to dihydrotestosterone. Functional androgen receptors on target tissues are needed for androgen-dependent differentiation and growth. Species differences exist in whether the production of testosterone by Leydig cells is under the control of gonadotropin produced by the fetal pituitary gland or the placenta. Fetal Leydig cells are replaced by postnatal Leydig cells, which are relatively quiescent until puberty. The production of testosterone is regulated by luteinizing hormone (LH), which is under the control of LH-releasing hormone (LHRH) from the hypothalamus. Also under the control of LHRH is follicle-stimulating hormone (FSH), produced by the anterior pituitary gland. FSH regulates the activity of Sertoli cells, and can thus influence MIS production. Sertoli cells stimulated by FSH produce a glycoprotein, androgen-binding protein, which fosters high testosterone concentration around the germ cells for the progression of spermatogenesis.

DEVELOPMENTAL ABNORMALITIES OF THE MALE SYSTEM: INTERSEXES

In normal individuals, the process of sexual differentiation runs to completion and there is concordance between genetic, chromosomal, gonadal, and phenotypic sex.

Abnormalities of Phenotypic Sex

Individuals that are clearly male or female with respect to their chromosomes (XY or XX) and gonads (testes or ovaries) but whose reproductive tract's phenotypic appearance is ambiguous are termed pseudohermaphrodites (Fig. 13-1). They are male pseudohermaphrodites or female pseudohermaphrodites according to the gonad present. (Individuals with both male and female gonadal tissue are termed hermaphrodites.) The differentiation of the tract can be slightly or greatly abnormal. In many cases, the mechanism for the abnormal differentiation is unknown. Ample scope exists for deficiencies in enzymes, hormones, or receptors to cause imperfect differentiation of the tract to match the gonads.

Three **male pseudohermaphrodite** syndromes in which the pathogenesis is understood are persistent Müllerian duct syndrome, androgen insensitivity, and steroid 5α-reductase deficiency.

Persistent Müllerian duct syndrome (PMDS) is a rare disorder of MIS production or function. MIS can be

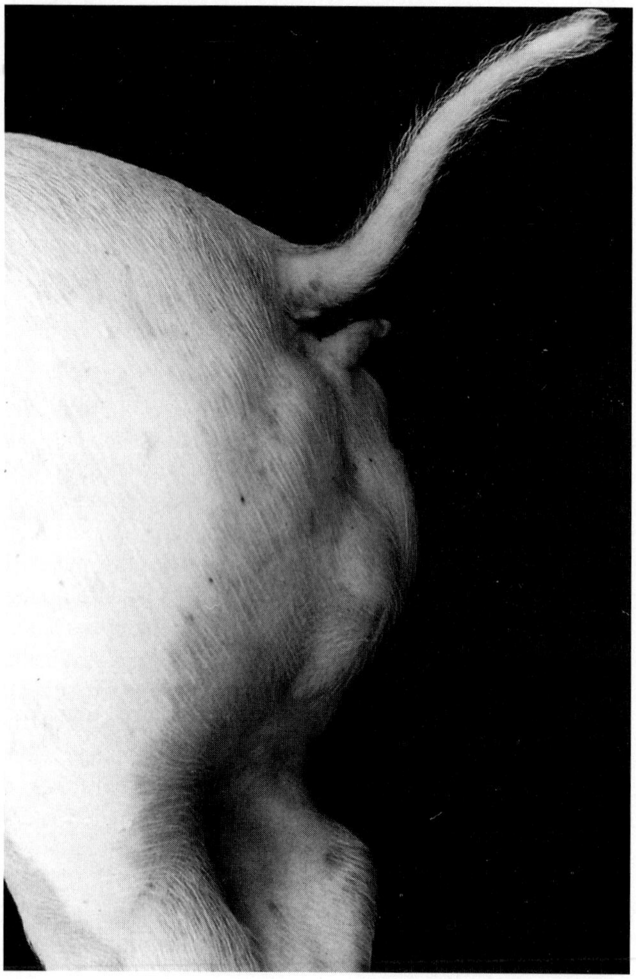

Figure 13-1 External genitalia; pig. Pseudohermaphroditism. The external appearance is ambiguous, as the penis is short, is clitoris-like in length, but has a terminal urethral opening. Testes are in the scrotal sacs.

absent or present in affected humans beings, with the syndrome being due to either a mutation in the MIS gene or the MIS gene receptor, respectively. In animals, the syndrome is described in miniature schnauzer dogs, with an autosomal recessive mode of inheritance, and in a goat, with unknown mode of inheritance. Affected dogs have XY (or XXY) chromosomes, and externally are normal males with the common exception of unilateral or bilateral cryptorchidism. The testes, however, are attached to the cranial ends of uterine horns. When a testis has descended into the scrotum, the uterine horn passes through the inguinal ring. Ductus deferens can be found microscopically within the myometrium. Cranial vagina and prostate gland are often present. MIS is present in the testes of normal male dogs up to 143 days of age. MIS is present in the testes of young affected dogs also and is bioactive. A mutation in the structural gene for the MIS receptor results in MIS resistance in PMDS-affected dogs. Dogs with unilateral or bilateral scrotal testes can be fertile. Sertoli cell tumor and pyometra are diseases to which PMDS-affected dogs are subject. Testicular abnormalities in PMDS, such as reduced spermatogenesis and tubular sclerosis, could be attributable to cryptorchidism. Cryptorchidism could be due to interference with the MIS-controlled first phase of the function of the gubernaculum, the phase in which the testis migrates to the inguinal area.

Deficiency of 5α-reductase type 2, inherited as an autosomal recessive trait in humans beings, has not yet been documented in animals, but in all likelihood exists. The enzyme converts testosterone to dihydrotestosterone, which is required for the masculinization of the urogenital sinus, tubercle, and genital swellings. Without dihydrotestosterone, these structures passively become caudal vagina, vestibule, clitoris, and vulva. Internally, Wolffian structures (ductus deferens, epididymis) develop. The testes are likely to be cryptorchid.

Androgen receptor defects. Androgen receptor disorders are becoming increasingly recognized as causes of male pseudohermaphroditism. Most cases are due to a mutation in the androgen receptor gene, which is located on the X chromosome and thus in a single copy. Hundreds of mutations have been identified, and the effects range from complete androgen insensitivity with female external genitalia (testicular feminization) to mild male pseudohermaphroditism. Affected individuals are chromosomally male and have testes. The testes produce testosterone, but the stimulation of the Wolffian system is not normal because of defective androgen receptors. The normal androgen receptor has a hormone-binding and a DNA-binding domain; once activated by androgen, the domain changes shape and is able to bind to specific DNA sequences and regulate the transcription of other specific genes, leading to normal male differentiation. In human beings with androgen insensitivity, the gene is rarely deleted, but numerous point mutations in the receptor gene have been identified, mostly in the hormone-binding and DNA-binding domains. Whether the result is partial or complete androgen insensitivity depends on the location of the mutation and the change in function of the receptor. Dihydrotestosterone binds to the androgen receptor with greater affinity than testosterone does, and the receptor, when it acts as a transcriptional factor, might interact with different genes than the testosterone-bound receptor. In domestic animals, complete androgen insensitivity has been described in the equine, bovine, and feline species. The testes are often cryptorchid and are in the inguinal area. The first phase of testicular migration, which is under the control of MIS, is normal. The inguinoscrotal second phase, which is under the control of androgens, does not occur. MIS produced by

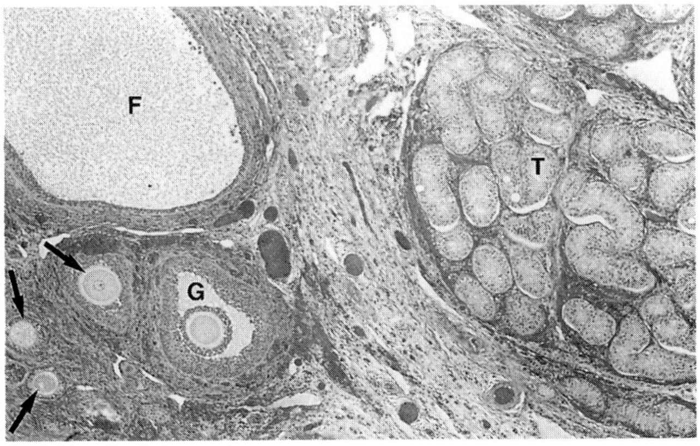

Figure 13-2 Gonad; dog. In this ovotestis, seminiferous tubules *(T)* are adjacent to a cluster of follicles. Two or more layers of nuclei of granulosa cells surround the oocyte in growing follicles *(arrows)*. The antrum of a small Graafian follicle can be seen *(G)*, as well as the cavity of a large follicle *(F)*. H & E stain. *Courtesy of Dr. M.H. Goldschmidt.*

the testes causes regression of the Müllerian ducts. External genitalia are female in complete androgen insensitivity, with a cranial blind end to the vagina, and neither Müllerian nor Wolffian ductal system is present.

Embryonal and fetal testicular regression syndromes are described in men. Five overlapping subtypes are related to absence of, or cessation of, testicular function at a particular stage of development. These are genotypic males in which the testes might have never developed, or could have developed but regressed in early, mid, or late gestation. The forms of the duct system and external genitalia depend on the timing of regression of the testes. With absence of testes, the phenotype is female. With very early regression of the testes, after some secretion of MIS but before much secretion of testosterone, neither male nor female duct system is present and the external genitalia are female. With a little later regression, Wolffian duct derivatives and ambiguous external genitalia are present. Later still, the external genitalia are male, and the penis is small. With regression in late fetal life, the external genitalia are normal male.

Abnormalities of Gonadal Sex

Hermaphrodites have abnormal gonads, and the gonads possess both testicular and ovarian tissues. There can be separate testis and ovary, or one or both gonads can be mixed. The mixed organ is termed an ovotestis (Fig. 13-2). Most ovotestes have an end-to-end arrangement of ovarian and testicular tissues, with clear demarcation between the two. Each type of gonadal tissue is well developed and easily recognizable. Bilateral hermaphrodites have an ovotestis on each side, unilateral hermaphrodites have an ovotestis on one side, and lateral hermaphrodites have a testis on one side and an ovary on the other. The genital tract in hermaphrodites is ambiguous. Hermaphrodites occur in canine, porcine, and caprine XX sex reversals and bovine freemartin XX/XY chimeras. In many other cases, the basic mechanism for the production of hermaphrodites is unknown.

Sex reversal is the term used when the gonad is not the type corresponding to the XX or XY chromosomal makeup of the individual. XX males have been identified in several species. They are discussed under the female system. XY females are rare, but they have been identified in mice, horses, and human beings and have a deletion or mutation of the testis-determining region of the Y chromosome. XY females have hypergonadotropic hypogonadism with no secondary sexual characteristics. The gonad is a streak of ovarian stroma.

Abnormalities of Chromosomal Sex

Sex chromosomes can be abnormal in structure or number. Two examples of abnormal structure of the Y chromosome are deletion of the short arm and isochromosome formation (duplication of one arm and loss of the other). Affected individuals have female phenotype and extremely hypoplastic gonads. A few cattle have been identified with an isochromosome Y. With duplication of one of the sex chromosomes in an individual with an Y chromosome (XYY or XXY), the external genitalia are male in character. Klinefelter's syndrome (XXY) is discussed under testicular hypoplasia. Chimeras such as XX/XY are phenotypically sexually ambiguous.

TESTIS

Developmental Abnormalities

Descent of the testes into the scrotum is facilitated by the **gubernaculum,** a cord of mesenchymal tissue that attaches the developing testis and epididymis to the forming scrotal pouch. MIS controls the swelling reaction of the gubernaculum, which is responsible for movement of the testis to the inguinal area. The second phase of descent, the movement of the testis from the inguinal to the scrotal area, is androgen dependent. Part of the mechanism of descent is the slower growth rate of the gubernaculum than surrounding pelvic structures. Also, the gubernaculum develops an enlargement just distal to the external inguinal ring, which allows for traction to be exerted. The pulling is passive, as no contractile tissue is present in the gubernaculum. The interplay between intraabdominal pressure, the patency of the processus vaginalis, and the androgen-dependent regression of the gubernaculum results in descent of the testes.

Cryptorchidism is incomplete descent of the testis. In most mammalian species, the testis normally has descended into the scrotum by the time of birth. Cryptorchidism is more often unilateral than bilateral. The undescended testis can be anywhere along its path from caudal to the kidney to the scrotum, including just inside the inguinal ring and just outside the inguinal ring but not in the scrotal sac. Epididymal differentiation is coordinated with testicular descent and, consequently, epididymal differentiation is slowed in some cases of cryptorchidism.

Cryptorchidism is the most common disorder of sexual development in the dog, occurring in as many as 13% of male dogs. It is likely to have a genetic basis, and a reasonable working hypothesis is a sex-limited autosomal recessive mode of inheritance. It has been suggested that one gene might control internal testicular descent and placement of the epididymis and ductus deferens and another gene might control external testicular descent.

In the horse, left unilateral cryptorchidism predominates over right. This predominance can be explained by the relatively slower rate of descent of the left epididymis and testis and the fact that the internal inguinal ring consistently closes at about the time of birth. In some studies in the horse, the left and right testicular retention are almost equal in occurrence and the left retained testis is more likely to be abdominal than inguinal in location. Three breeds (Percheron, American saddle horse, and American quarterhorse), ponies, and crossbred horses were significantly overrepresented in a large hospital-based study of cryptorchidism.

The gubernaculum could cause cryptorchidism by its failure to develop, improper position, excessive growth, or failure to regress. Some other possible predisposing or contributing factors for cryptorchidism include testicular hypoplasia, estrogen exposure in pregnancy, breech labor compromising blood supply to the testes, and late closing of the umbilicus, delaying the ability to increase abdominal pressure.

Degeneration occurs in the cryptorchid testis after puberty. The testis is small and fibrotic and has alterations of interstitial collagen deposition, hyaline thickening of the tubular basement membranes, and atrophy of germinal epithelium so that only a few spermatogonia remain along with the normal complement of Sertoli cells (Fig. 13-3). Spermatogenesis is dependent on the relatively cool scrotal temperature. Apoptosis (programmed cell death) of germ cells in the higher temperature environment of the abdomen is probably mediated by the regulatory protein p53. Leydig cells appear relatively more numerous than in descended testes.

Cryptorchid testes are much more prone to neoplasia than scrotally placed ones, and the tendency is increased with the extent to which the testis is retained in the abdomen. In the dog, Sertoli cell tumors are more likely to occur in the testes present in the abdomen, while seminomas tend to develop more commonly in inguinally placed testes. In men, undescended testes are prone to develop germ cell neoplasms (seminomas and teratomas). The contralateral testis is also at increased risk for developing a neoplasm, even if the testis is located in the scrotum. A retained testis enlarged by a neoplasm is prone to torsion.

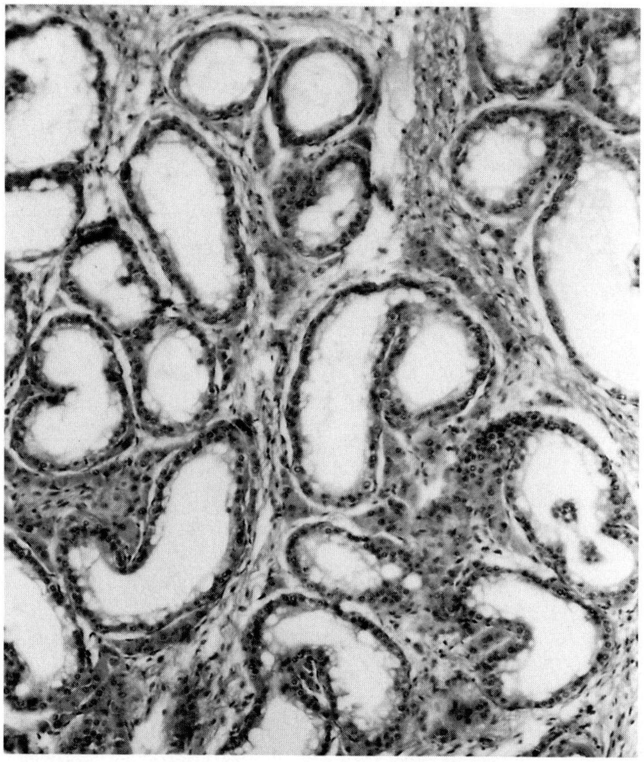

Figure 13-3 Testis; horse. Cryptorchidism. Tubules are lined by Sertoli cells and a few spermatogonia. Note the numerous interstitial cells and moderate interstitial fibrosis. H & E stain.

Intersex individuals (both hermaphrodites and pseudohermaphrodites) commonly have cryptorchid testes. The greater the ratio of testicular to ovarian tissue, the more likely an ovotestis will have descended into the scrotum. A pure testis most often lies in the scrotum, and an ovary is in its normal position. The ovary or ovarian portion of an ovotestis is histologically normal, but the seminiferous tubules of a testis or ovotestis are abnormal because of a combination of cryptorchidism and the effects of estrogen produced by the ovarian tissue. Except for a few cases of scrotal testes, the tubules of testis or ovotestis are lined by Sertoli cells with only rare spermatogonia.

Hypoplasia of the testes is difficult to distinguish from testicular degeneration by using morphologic features. Either testicular hypoplasia or degeneration can occur alone, with no apparent contributing or influencing factors; either can also be associated with, secondary to, or as part of some other lesion. Testicular hypoplasia has been causally related to cryptorchidism, intersex development, poor general nutrition, zinc deficiency, specific genes in the Swedish red and white breed of cattle, and endocrine and cytogenetic abnormalities. Endocrine disturbances causing testicular hypoplasia are those related to reduced

Cryptorchid testis in dog:
↳ intra-abdominal → Sertoli cell tumor
↳ inguinal → seminoma

production of either luteinizing hormone by the pituitary gland, which in turn influences testosterone production by the Leydig cells, or follicle-stimulating hormone by the pituitary gland, which stimulates the nurturing function of the Sertoli cells.

A wide range of cytogenetic abnormalities, from translocations and mosaics to nondisjunctions causing polysomies of sex chromosomes, result in testicular hypoplasia. The best known example of polysomy is the XXY karyotype of **Klinefelter's syndrome,** seen in several cats, bulls, dogs, a boar, and a horse. In cats, the syndrome is recognized in male cats with the tricolor, tortoiseshell, or calico coat types. These cats can be XXY, XX/XXY, or more complex chimeras or mosaics with two or more X chromosomes and one or more Y chromosomes. The gene for black and the gene for orange are carried one per X chromosome, and so a normal male cat should not have hair of both colors. In adult men with Klinefelter's syndrome, some degree of eunuchoidism is observed, and about half of the affected men have gynecomastia (enlargement of the breasts). Before puberty, the testicular tubules have only Sertoli cells. At puberty, the tubules undergo an irregular progressive sclerosis and become collagenous cords without the elastic fibers that are found in sclerotic but previously normal tubules. Leydig cells are hyperplastic and clumped.

Hypoplasia of the testes often is not apparent until after puberty. Unilateral hypoplasia is more common than bilateral hypoplasia, but this difference in prevalence could be a reflection of the relative ease of recognizing a size abnormality when the normal is available for ready comparison. Unilateral hypoplasia is difficult to explain because most of the causes seem to act systemically and, therefore, should produce a bilateral effect. The size range of a hypoplastic testis generally is from one quarter normal to near-normal. Consistency of a hypoplastic testis is near to normal.

The severity of the hypoplasia can be graded histologically by the proportion of hypoplastic tubules scattered through the organ. Hypoplastic tubules have a small diameter, are lined by Sertoli cells and a few stem cells and spermatogonia, have a thickened basement membrane, and are surrounded by collagen. Leydig cells appear proportionally more numerous. In severe testicular hypoplasia, most or all of the tubules are abnormal; the tubules have a small diameter, and a uniform microscopic appearance with only infrequent vacuolation of Sertoli cells and without a thickened basement membrane. In moderate hypoplasia, fewer tubules are small, those of normal size have some differentiation of the seminiferous epithelium, and a few tubules reach an advanced stage of development. In most tubules, however, when the stage of spermatocyte formation is reached, the spermatocytes undergo degeneration, leaving tubules lined by Sertoli cells with vacuolated cytoplasm. The lumen of such tubules can have cellular debris and multinucleate cells that are formed when dividing cells fail to separate. When hypoplasia is mild, only a few small tubules are lined mostly by Sertoli cells; while most of the tubules are active, many producing spermatozoa, multinucleate giant cells can be present in the tubular lumens of some of these testes. Mild hypoplasia is difficult to distinguish from testicular degeneration. The number of hypoplastic tubules would not be expected to increase with age, as hypoplastic tubules do not arise after puberty.

Degeneration

Testicular degeneration (testicular "atrophy") is a relatively common lesion. Mild testicular degeneration can be detected only microscopically, but when it is severe and chronic, the testis is small and firm. The causes are many, and in a particular individual the specific cause is often unknown. Degeneration can be unilateral or bilateral, depending on whether the cause is local or systemic. In young growing males, the distinction between testicular degeneration and hypoplasia is often difficult to make using morphologic features. Both lesions are often present together because hypoplastic testes are prone to degeneration. Inflammation also can be superimposed on degeneration when the cause is obstruction, leading to back pressure, rupture of seminiferous tubules, and spermatic granuloma formation. Recovery of a testis with degeneration back to a normal testis is possible if the injurious agent is eliminated and damage is not too severe.

Specific causes of testicular degeneration are numerous, and accumulating data indicate that many agents act via apoptosis of germ cells. Fever or local heat from inflammation of the scrotal skin can injure the testis. Obstruction of flow of spermatozoa causes testicular degeneration. Obstruction can be due to developmental anomalies such as segmental aplasia of mesonephric duct derivatives, local injury or inflammation of the epididymis, or vascular impairment from age-related mineralization of the spermatic cord or testicular vessels. More dramatic vascular events such as torsion or severe crushing of the spermatic cord can cause obstruction. Systemic injurious factors include nutritional deficiency, hormonal aberrations, toxins, and irradiation. Vitamin A and zinc are specific nutritional deficiencies; general malnutrition also causes testicular degeneration. Interference with gonadotropin-releasing hormones, or luteinizing hormone and its control of androgen production by Leydig cells, or follicle-stimulating hormone and its effect on the production of androgen-binding protein by Sertoli cells can have a deleterious effect on the seminiferous epithelium. Such interference could happen, for instance, when a neoplasm of the pituitary gland causes local compression of the pituitary gland, the hypothalamus, or both. Estrogen produced by Sertoli cell tumors induces testicular degeneration. Some therapeutic drugs, such as amphoteracin B, gentamicin, and chemotherapeutic compounds, cause testicular degeneration.

Of the many toxins capable of causing testicular degeneration, most damage the spermatogonia and dividing primary spermatocytes, but some damage later stages, spermatocytes and spermatids, or injure Sertoli cells. Degeneration of seminiferous epithelium can occur secondary to severe injury of Sertoli cells.

A testis undergoing degeneration initially is swollen and softer than normal, but as the degeneration progresses, the testis becomes smaller. The cut surface of the normal testis and the acutely degenerated testis bulges slightly. After the acute phase, the testis becomes firmer and has small flecks or large areas of calcification. Degeneration due to obstruction of efferent ducts occurs in the dorsal part of the testis. If the degeneration is due to ischemia after a vascular accident in the spermatic cord, small islands of parenchyma can survive the infarction because of diffusion of oxygen from vessels of the epididymis and tunica albuginea. Degeneration can occur locally around a lesion such as a neoplasm that expands and causes compression.

Microscopically, testicular degeneration has similar features to testicular hypoplasia; small seminiferous tubules have a thickened basement membrane, decreased numbers of seminiferous epithelial cells, vacuolated Sertoli cells, intratubular giant cells, and interstitial fibrosis (Figs. 13-4 and 13-5). The severity of the vacuolation of the Sertoli cells is likely to be more severe in the testis undergoing degeneration than in testicular hypoplasia because of the degeneration of Sertoli cells and the loss of germinal cells. A key lesion in the differentiation of testicular degeneration from testicular hypoplasia is the redundant basement membrane found in testicular degeneration because affected tubules had at some stage reached full size and, then, subsequently collapsed. Because the basement membranes are thickened, they can be seen without special staining. At the end stage of testicular degeneration, Sertoli cells are the only lining cells remaining, but with time, these also disappear, leaving only the basement membranes. Calcification can involve intratubular cellular debris, tubular basement membranes, or the interstitium.

Inflammation

Spermatozoa are sequestered within the seminiferous tubules and isolated from the general circulation by Sertoli cells. More mature stages of spermatogenesis thus can be protected from immune cells and antibody or from toxins. The **Sertoli cell barrier** (blood-testis barrier) has two permanent compartments: a basal compartment bounded by peritubular myoid cells and Sertoli cells below their tight junctions with associated spermatogonia and preleptotene spermatocytes and an adluminal compartment beyond the tight junctions between Sertoli cells, with the later stages of spermatogenesis. A temporary intermediate compartment is formed by the successive formation and breakdown of tight junctions as spermatocytes move from the basal to the adluminal compartment. Cell surface antigens undergo many changes during spermatogenesis, and mature sperm cells have a set of surface antigens not present at the time in fetal life when immune self-

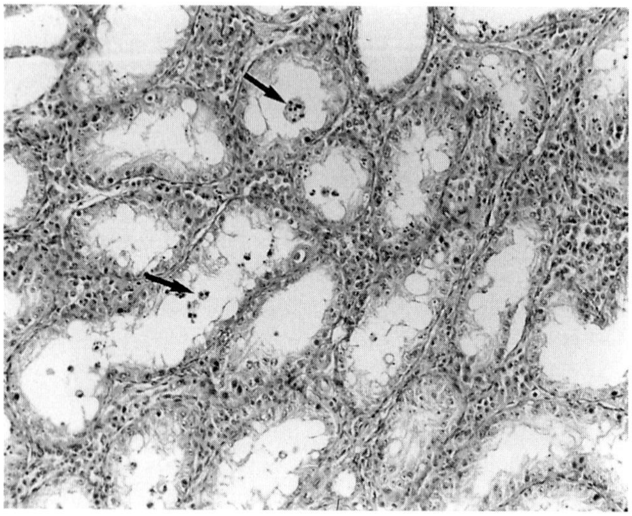

Figure 13-4 Testis; horse. Testicular degeneration. Much of the seminiferous epithelium lining the tubules has disappeared and the remaining Sertoli cells are vacuolated (fenestrated). Intratubular multinucleate giant cells have formed *(arrows)*. H & E stain.

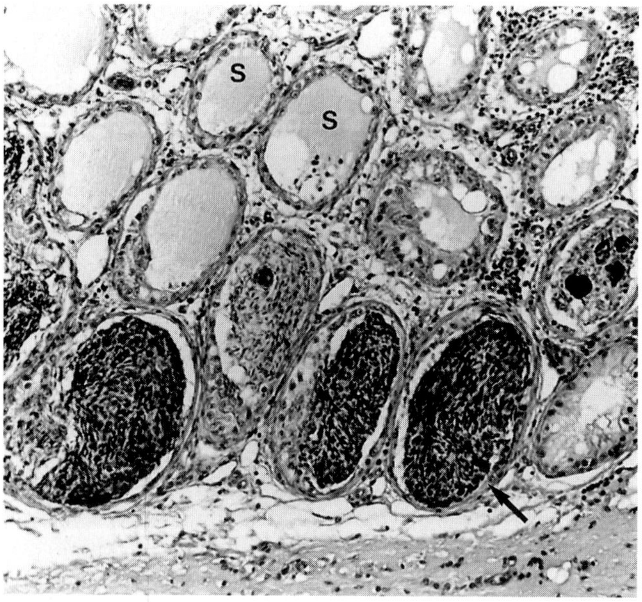

Figure 13-5 Testis; ram. Testicular degeneration. Obstruction of seminiferous tubules has caused impaction of sperm *(arrow)*. Most tubules *(S)* are lined by Sertoli cells and have only remnants of seminiferous tubular epithelium. Tubular atrophy is mild. H & E stain.

recognition takes place. Yet, spermatozoa in normal locations are not recognized as foreign by the immune system of the male animal. Sequestration of mature spermatozoa from the immune system is the mechanism most widely believed responsible, as lymphocytes have not been identified in the testicular interstitium. The absence of T lymphocytes has been proposed as a mechanism that lessens the possibility of immune stimulation by sperm cells in the testis. Another theory is that minute amounts of soluble spermatozoan antigen pass into the host via the numerous tight junctions of the Sertoli cells, and this soluble antigen activates suppressor lymphocytes involved in downregulating cytotoxic immune responses.

The formation of antispermatozoan antibodies in human males has been found associated with major disruption of the blood-testis barrier. Antibodies against spermatozoa can form after testicular damage caused by trauma, neoplasms, and infections. Disruption of the ductus deferens following obstruction or surgical vasectomy allows immune cells and antibody to gain access to spermatozoa. Antibody attached to the cell surface can interfere with spermatozoan function. Antispermatozoan antibodies have been identified in the seminal fluid or the serum of stallions that had low sperm cell viability following trauma to the testis.

If **autoimmune** orchitis occurs in domestic animals, it seems likely from data obtained in experimental studies that the rete testis or efferent ducts are the starting sites for the process. When the disruption of the blood-testis barrier is so severe that spermatozoa are outside their normal containment within the testis, epididymis, ductus deferens, and urethra, a foreign body granulomatous reaction occurs.

Nonspecific orchitis, a mild, multifocal, subacute intertubular inflammation of unknown cause, is relatively common in bulls and stallions. There are no gross lesions. Microscopically, lymphocytic foci are present between tubules and around vessels. Other forms of orchitis that produce grossly apparent lesions are much less common.

Intratubular orchitis probably arises by an infection ascending from the urethra, urinary bladder, ductus deferens, and epididymis. It starts as inflammation in the seminiferous tubules, which then spills over into the interstitium. Intratubular orchitis appears grossly as poorly defined up to 1 cm yellow foci that become firm and white as the lesions become chronic. Initially, the affected tubules have acute inflammatory debris. The lining of the tubules is lost, but the tubular outlines are present for some time. Spermatic granulomas can form any time spermatozoa make contact with extratubular tissue. In the center of these granulomas, spermatozoa can be seen free and within macrophages. Macrophages and lymphocytes infiltrate around the core of spermatozoa and macrophages and, with time, collagen is deposited at the edge of the lesion.

Necrotizing orchitis, the most severe form of orchitis, can begin as an intratubular disease or can arise hematogenously. In some cases, the affected areas are so severely inflamed and the necrosis is so extensive that the original structures have formed a caseous mass. Gray-brown, initially soft and later firm, necrotic debris replaces an irregular, but large, portion of the testis. In a few extremely severe cases, a fistula develops through the scrotum.

Granulomatous orchitis includes the formation of multiple, possibly coalescing, inflammatory nodules displacing and replacing parenchyma. Inflammation of the tunica vaginalis or the epididymis can be secondary to intratubular, necrotizing, or granulomatous orchitis. Orchitis in bulls caused by *Brucella abortus* is probably the most important example of granulomatous orchitis in domestic animals. It is a hematogenous intratubular orchitis that becomes necrotizing. Initially, swelling of the testis occurs to the limit permitted by the tunica albuginea. Fibrinous exudate distends the cavity of the tunica vaginalis. Foci of necrosis of the parenchyma expand and can coalesce so that much of the testis is involved, becoming either liquefied or caseous and gritty. The surrounding tunics and any surviving parenchyma become densely fibrous. Eventually, the testes become small and suspended in abundant fluid or semifluid exudate. Microscopically, bacteria are clustered in the cytoplasm or in cytoplasmic vacuoles of macrophages in the areas of necrotizing pyogranulomatous inflammation.

Brucella canis causes inflammation of the testis, epididymis, and prostate gland in dogs. The bacteria multiply in the cytoplasm of macrophages and epithelial cells in these organs. The heads of agglutinated spermatozoa in the epididymal duct and semen are coated with IgA antibody, considered an anti-spermatozoan autoantibody locally produced. Serum agglutinating antibody is also detectable.

Organisms that commonly cause orchitis in domestic animals are listed in Table 13-1.

Table 13-1 Common Causes of Infectious Orchitis in Domestic Animals

Bull	**Ram**
Actinomyces pyogenes	*Brucella ovis*
Bluetongue virus	*Chlamydia psittaci*
Brucella abortus	*Corynebacterium ovis*
Lumpy skin disease virus	Sheeppox virus
Mycobacterium tuberculosis	
Nocardia asteroides	**Boar**
	Brucella suis
Buck	*Pseudomonas pseudomallei*
Brucella melitensis	Rubulavirus
Dog	**Stallion**
Brucella canis	Equine infectious anemia virus
Canine distemper virus	Equine viral arteritis virus
Escherichia coli	*Salmonella abortus equi*
Proteus vulgaris	*Strongylus edentatus*
Pseudomonas pseudomallei	

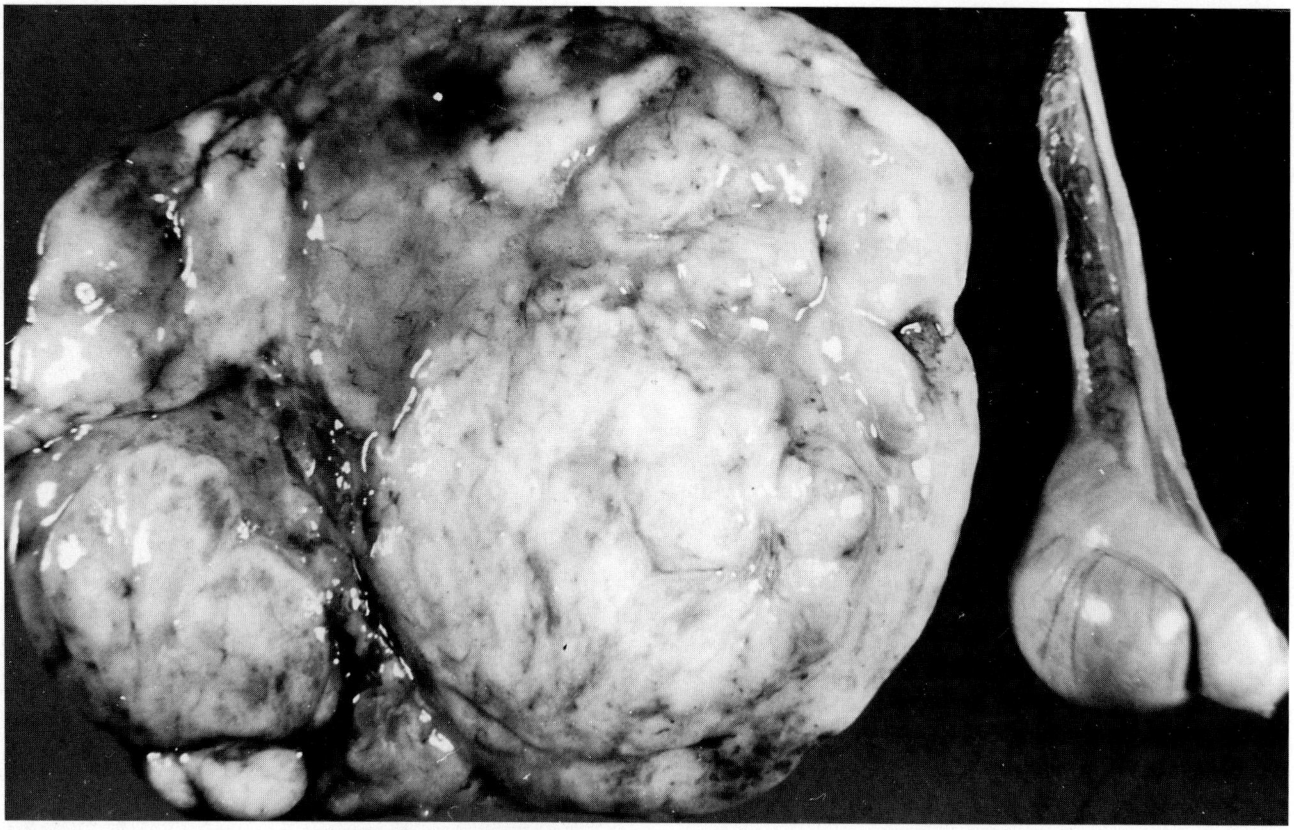

Figure 13-6 Testis; dog. Seminoma. The neoplasm bulges from the cut surface, is discrete, and is divided by a few fibrous trabeculae. Normal testis is included for comparison.

Neoplasms

Testicular neoplasms are common in older dogs, occur in older bulls, and are rare in other species. They can arise from germ cells or from gonadal stroma (Sertoli cells or Leydig cells). Occasionally, neoplasms of testicular mesenchymal structures or metastatic neoplasms are found. The three common primary testicular neoplasms, which are seminoma, Leydig cell adenoma, and Sertoli cell tumor, can occur singly or in combination.

Germ cell neoplasms are seminoma, teratoma, and other less common types.

Seminomas are the second most common canine testicular neoplasm and the most common testicular neoplasm in the aged stallion. These neoplasms have been observed in other species, but are rare. They are more prevalent in cryptorchid testes than in descended testes. Arising from primitive seminiferous tubules, they do not produce hormones. Multicentric origin within the testis and local invasiveness are characteristic. The neoplasm is white or pink-gray, firm, bulging when cut, and has fine fibrous trabeculae (Fig. 13-6). Seminomas microscopically have an intratubular or diffuse arrangement of large, polyhedral, discretely demarcated cells with a large nucleus, variable nuclear size, and very little cytoplasm. Giant cells, with either a single nucleus or multiple nuclei, are sometimes present (Fig. 13-7). Lymphoid nodules are often present in seminomas. These neoplasms are seldom malignant. Pain from pressure created by the enlarging neoplastic mass can be the presenting sign.

Teratomas arise from totipotential primordial germ cells. They are uncommon, but are best known in the horse, especially in the cryptorchid testis of the young horse. The neoplasms can be large, cystic or polycystic and can contain recognizable hair, mucus, bone, or even teeth. Histologically, at least derivatives of two of the three embryonic germ layers (ectoderm, mesoderm, and endoderm) are present. Most teratomas have well-differentiated organoid structures and are benign.

Neoplasms of germ cell origin other than seminoma and teratoma are rare in animals. Embryonal carcinoma is the stem cell type for nonseminoma germ cell neoplasms. Derivatives of embryonal carcinoma can be of one histologic type or more than one histologic type, and can differentiate in placental or embryonic directions. Teratoma is an example of the latter.

Gonadal stromal neoplasms are Leydig cell adenoma, Sertoli cell tumor, and some other less common types.

Leydig cell tumors (interstitial cell tumor) are the most common testicular neoplasms of the dog and bull. They are relatively rare in the stallion, in which most cases are in

Testicular neoplasms

Dog
1. Leydig cell tumor
2. Seminoma
3. Sertoli cell tumor

Horse
1. Seminoma

Bull
1. Leydig cell tumor

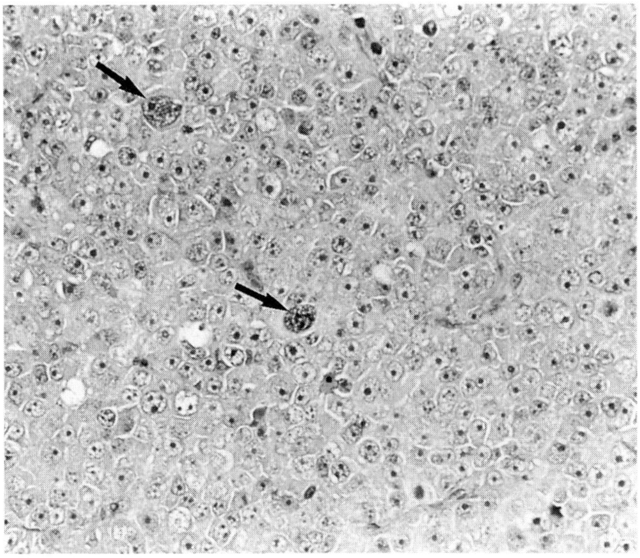

Figure 13-7 Testis; dog. Seminoma. The neoplastic cells are large, polyhedral, discrete and their nuclei vary in size. A few giant cells *(arrows)* are present. H & E stain.

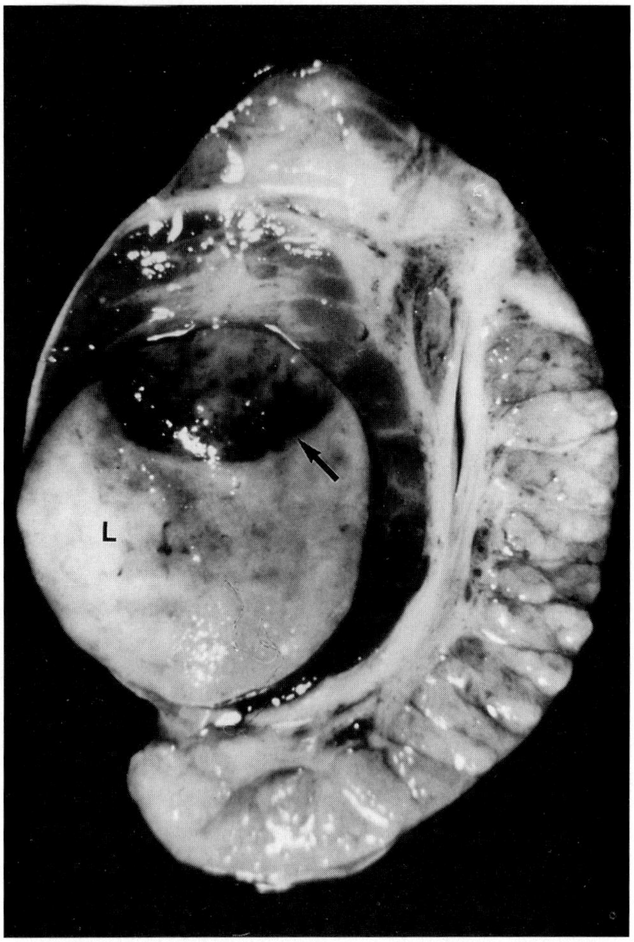

Figure 13-8 Testis; dog. Interstitial cell (Leydig cell) adenoma *(L)*. The neoplasm is distinctly demarcated and has an area of hemorrhage *(arrow)*.

undescended testes. They are readily identifiable grossly by their tan to orange color. The neoplasm is spherical and well demarcated (Fig. 13-8). These neoplasms are almost always benign. In fact, the distinction between nodular hyperplasia of Leydig cells and Leydig cell adenoma is problematic. Whether the neoplasm produces hormones or not is unsettled. Microscopically, the cells of the bovine neoplasms vary little, but in the dog, the cells can be large, round, polyhedral, or spindle shaped. The cells have abundant cytoplasm that is often finely vacuolated and often has brown pigment. The cells are arranged in solid sheets or divided into small groups by fine fibrovascular trabeculae (Fig. 13-9). Although hemorrhage, necrosis, and cyst formation are common, Leydig cell adenomas are noninvasive and finely encapsulated.

Sertoli cell tumor is the third most common testicular neoplasm of the dog. It is rare in other species, but occurs in stallions and shorthorn bulls. In the dog, more than 50% of Sertoli cell tumors are located in undescended testes. The neoplasm is firm, white, lobulated by fibrous bands, and can cause enlargement of the affected testis (Fig. 13-10). The neoplasm can invade the spermatic cord and occasionally metastasize to the local internal iliac lymph node. Metastases beyond the local lymph node have been reported, but are rare. The neoplastic Sertoli cells either resemble normal Sertoli cells, or are more pleomorphic. They can have an intratubular or a diffuse arrangement. The abundant fibrous connective tissue in Sertoli cell tumors distinguishes them from the other two common types of testicular neoplasm. Neoplastic cells tend to palisade along the fibrous stroma (Fig. 13-11).

In addition to the effects of pressure and local invasion, the other important consequence of the presence of Sertoli cell tumors is that about a third of them produce estrogen, which can have a feminizing effect, causing gynecomastia (enlargement of the mammary glands). A possibly life-threatening effect of estrogen secretion is myelotoxicity, resulting in nonregenerative anemia, granulocytopenia, and thrombocytopenia. Other effects of estrogen are induction of hypothyroidism and alopecia, hyperplasia, or squamous metaplasia of the acini of the prostate gland, and adenomyosis of the epididymis. The amount of hormone produced is generally proportional to the size of the neoplasm.

Mixed germ cell–stromal neoplasms have been described in old dogs. The neoplasm-bearing testis is large and often cryptorchid. The testis is partially or completely replaced by a firm, gray-white to tan, single multilobed mass. Intimate intermingling of germ cells and Sertoli cells occurs in tubular structures of various sizes. The germ cell component extends into the surrounding tissue. Staining for neuron-specific enolase identifies Sertoli cells, and focal or perinuclear staining for vimentin helps to identify germ cells.

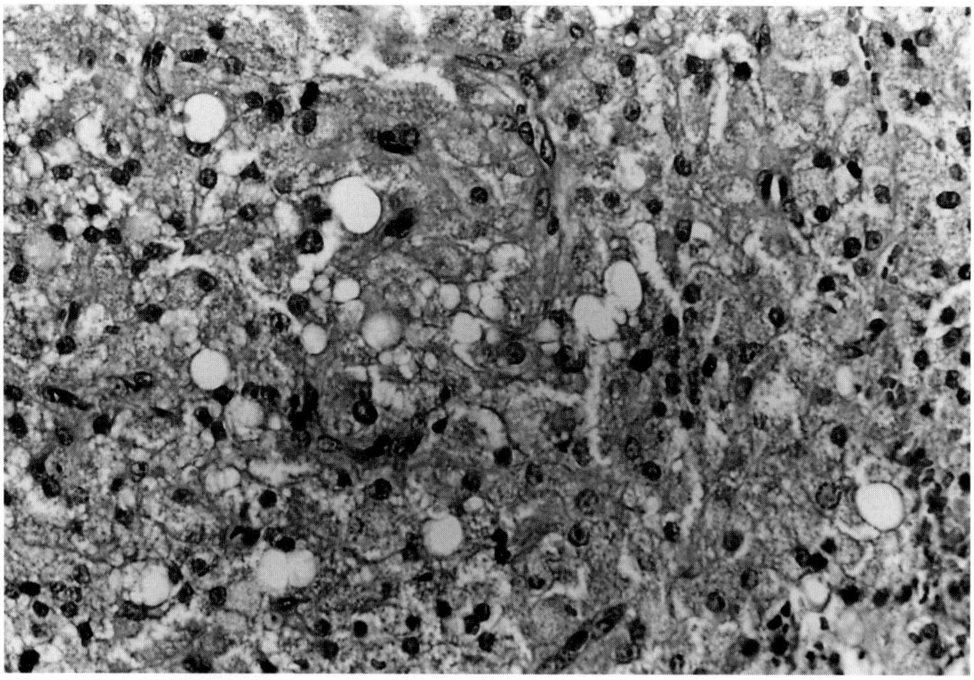

Figure 13-9 Testis; dog. Interstitial cell (Leydig cell) adenoma. Neoplastic cells are in a sheet and their cytoplasm is finely vacuolated, a characteristic of Leydig cells. H & E stain.

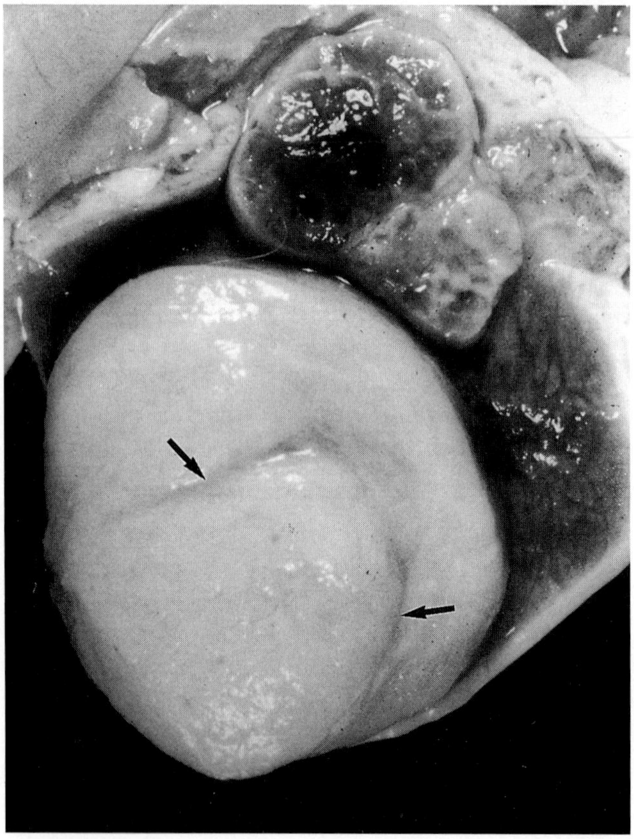

Figure 13-10 Testis; dog. Sertoli cell tumor. Numerous white bands of fibrous tissue *(arrows)* dissect through the neoplasm.

SCROTUM

The scrotum is an outpouching of the perineum, composed of skin, tunica dartos, and scrotal fascia. It is fused with the parietal layer of the tunica vaginalis. The skin has a thin dermis, few hairs, and many sweat glands.

Developmental Anomalies. The fusion of the paired primordia of scrotal skin depends on hormones produced by cells of the gonad after it has differentiated into a testis. Disturbances in the formative stages can lead to various defects in the scrotum, such as failure of fusion, cleft formation, or bifurcation of the scrotum. Defects can be local, confined to the scrotum and penis, or part of a wider range of defects in an intersex animal.

Dermatitis of the scrotal skin is common. Often it is nonspecific, the result of trauma, frostbite, or exposure to environmental irritants such as cement dust. Some pathogens have the scrotum as a predilection site. These include *Dermatophilus congolensis* and *Besnoitia besnoiti* in the bull, and *Chorioptes ovis* in the ram (Fig. 13-12). The heat generated in scrotal dermatitis can interfere with the thermoregulatory function of the scrotum, leading to testicular degeneration.

Neoplasms of any of the types that occur in the skin can occur in the scrotum, but are much less common in the scrotal skin. Neoplasms occasionally encountered are mast cell tumors, melanomas, and hemangiomas in the dog and papillomas in the boar. Vascular abnormalities, which could be hemangiomas, occur on the scrotum of the dog. The scrotal veins of bulls sometimes become varicose.

Scrotal dermatitis
- Ram → Chorioptes ovis
- Bull → Dermatophilus congolensis
  → Besnoitia besnoiti

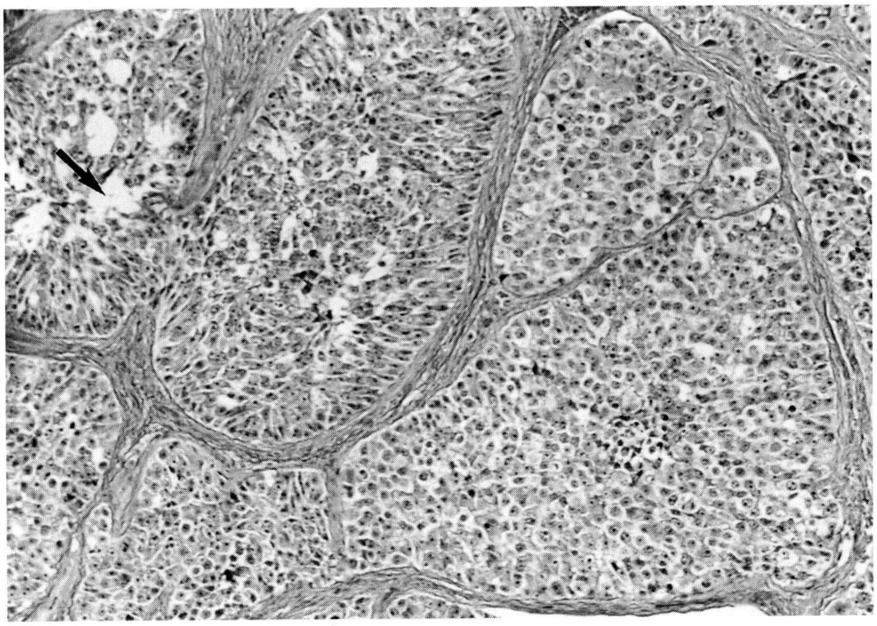

Figure 13-11 Testis; dog. Sertoli cell tumor. Neoplastic Sertoli cells palisade along fibrous trabeculae and form solid tubules or tubules with a central space *(arrow)* or lumen. H & E stain.

TUNICA VAGINALIS

The tunica vaginalis is the extension of the peritoneum that lines the scrotal sac as the parietal layer and covers the testis, epididymis, and spermatic cord as the visceral layer. The cavity between the two layers is continuous with the peritoneal cavity. The tunics and the cavity thus are subject to all the inflammatory and neoplastic diseases of the peritoneum and peritoneal cavity. Neoplastic lesions are uncommon; mesothelioma is the most frequently encountered.

Inflammation of the tunica vaginalis as part of a systemic disease will have the characteristics of that disease. Inflammation of the tunica vaginalis without initial inflammation of the abdominal peritoneum can have a noninfectious, i.e., traumatic, or infectious cause. The latter is likely to be an extension from an orchitis or epididymitis. Especially well-known causes are *Brucella ovis* and *Actinobacillus seminis* in rams, and trypanosomes in bulls, rams, and male goats. In general, traumatic inflammation of the tunica vaginalis is mild and focal, and inflammation with an infectious cause is severe and diffuse. Adhesions between the parietal and visceral tunica vaginalis, fibrinous at first and later fibrous, are common.

SPERMATIC CORD

Varicocele is the local dilatation of the spermatic vein in the pampiniform plexus. In the ram, associated lowered fertility has been proposed, with poor spermatozoan motility, immature spermatozoa in the semen, and testicular degeneration. The dilatation in the venous plexus is located near the inguinal ring and does not involve the

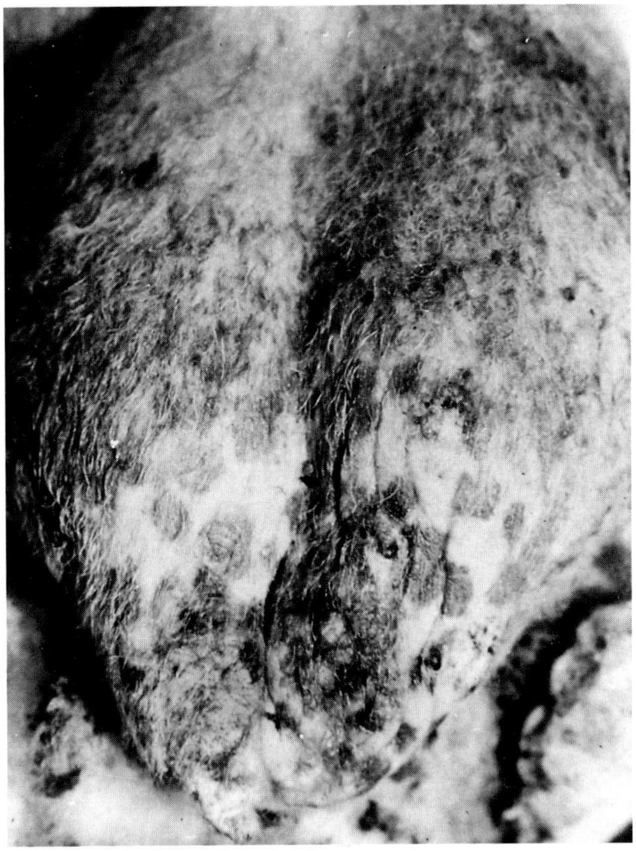

Figure 13-12 Scrotum; ram. Dermatitis. The multiple coalescing areas of hyperkeratosis and inflammation are caused by *Chorioptes ovis* mites.

complex distal part. About half the cases are bilateral, and the unilateral cases are evenly divided between the left and right side. Thrombosis of affected vessels is common. Varicoceles can cause enlargement of the scrotum, even to the extent that the scrotum touches the ground.

Torsion of the spermatic cord can occur when the testis is undescended. Torsion causes vascular occlusion, which can involve just the spermatic vein or both the vein and artery, and results in necrosis (infarction) of the testis.

Inflammation of the spermatic cord occurs after the contamination of a castration wound. Sometimes the lesion is acute and necrotizing, but more often it is chronic and a scirrhous cord is encountered. Great enlargement of the distal part of the cord is due to exuberant granulation tissue in which numerous small pockets of pus are scattered. Staphylococci are the organisms frequently recovered from the pus in the horse. The term "botryomycosis" has been used for these staphylococcal pyogranulomas. Radiating club-shaped eosinophilic deposits (Splendore-Hoeppli material) are present around the central clusters of bacteria.

MESONEPHRIC DUCT DERIVATIVES: EPIDIDYMIS, DUCTUS DEFERENS, AMPULLA, SEMINAL VESICLE

The mesonephric duct forms the epididymis, ductus deferens, ampulla, and seminal vesicle on each side. The seminal vesicle is an outpouching of the ductus deferens. The ducti deferentia open in common or along side each other into the prostatic urethra. The prostatic utricle or uterus masculinus is a Müllerian duct remnant located centrally between the two ducti deferentia. Cats and dogs lack seminal vesicles.

Developmental Abnormalities

Improper Linkage of Derivatives of Mesonephric Tubules and Duct

The testis is derived from gonadal cords that form between the gonadal ridge on the medial side of the mesonephros and remnants of mesonephric tubules. The rete testis and efferent ducts are derived from mesonephric tubules. Within the mesonephros, many mesonephric tubules enter the single mesonephric duct. It is from the within-mesonephros part of the duct that the epididymis is derived. The ductus deferens, ampulla, and seminal vesicle are derived from the more posterior part of the mesonephric duct, outside the mesonephros. In the developed testis, about 20 efferent ducts are found, but the number varies with species. Efferent ducts normally link in the head of the epididymis. Blind efferent ducts result when the connection to the epididymis is not made properly. The blind efferent ducts can be resorbed or can persist, and enlarge to form cysts or rupture. In the bull, stallion, and dog, blind-ending efferent ducts can be present in sufficient numbers to cause enough spermiostasis to reduce fertility. Spermatozoa outside normal containment are treated as foreign bodies and incite an inflammatory response.

Unconnected with the lumen of the epididymal tubule or efferent ducts, remnants of tubules of the mesonephros can form **cysts** adjacent to the head of the epididymis (paradidymis externus) or within the head of the epididymis (paradidymis internus). Cysts, both connected and unconnected with the ductular system, are lined by ciliated columnar epithelium. They are clinically significant if they become large enough to cause stasis of spermatozoa in adjacent structures, or if they rupture and liberate spermatozoa into the surrounding tissue. Of no clinical significance is the remnant of the Müllerian duct, called the appendix testis, located on the anterior or anteroventral surface (depending on the species orientation of the testes) of the testis near the head of the epididymis. Sometimes this small nodule of tissue can appear cystic.

Segmental Aplasia of Mesonephric Duct Derivatives

Segmental aplasia of the epididymis, ductus deferens, ampulla, or seminal vesicle can involve any of the structures, but most commonly involves the epididymis alone, and less commonly the epididymis and other structures. Segmental aplasia is reported mainly in the bull and most commonly involves the body and tail of the epididymis and is unilateral. Spermatozoa become impacted because of obstruction; local dilation or rupture of the structure occurs secondarily, allowing escape of spermatozoa and formation of spermatic granulomas.

Spermatocele is a local distension of the epididymis, containing accumulated spermatozoa. It can follow congenital or acquired (such as by vasectomy performed to manage "teaser" males) occlusion or obstruction of the lumen and often is followed by escape of spermatozoa into the connective tissue outside the duct when degeneration causes rupture of the wall. Spermatic granulomas can form in the connective tissues about the rupture site.

Immotile cilia syndrome, a rare disease identified in human beings, dogs, pigs, mice, and rats, is caused by one or more of several defects in the axoneme of cilia throughout the body and of the flagellum of spermatozoa. An autosomal recessive mode of inheritance is proposed. In dogs, heterogeneity of ultrastructural abnormalities of microtubule doublets and their dynein arms or central microtubules is reported. The effect on the reproductive system is immotile or hypomotile spermatozoa due to flagellar lesions or to oligospermia (a subnormal concentration of spermatozoa) or azoospermia (no spermatozoa), presumably due to defective cilia in the epididymis and ductus deferens. Because of defective cilia in the nasal mucosa, bronchial and bronchiolar mucosa, and ependyma, commonly associated lesions are rhinitis, bronchopneumonia, bronchiectasis, and hydrocephalus. Also associated is situs inversus (reversal of the normal left and right orientation of organs), but the pathogenesis is unclear. Female infertility is related to defective function of cilia of the uterine tube.

Inflammation

Because the epididymis is only a single coiled tubule, any lesion along its length has potential for causing obstruction of spermatozoan flow. **Epididymitis** can be focal, multifocal, or diffuse, unilateral, or bilateral. It is most frequently encountered in unilateral, chronic, focal, or multifocal form and thus can be recognized by comparing the size and shape of the abnormal organ with the normal one. In acute inflammation, the epididymis is soft and swollen; in chronic inflammation, it is firm and enlarged because of the deposition of fibrous tissue and likely to be nodular because of distension of segments of the duct and the presence of spermatic granulomas and abscesses. Obstruction of the outflow of spermatozoa is one of the causes of testicular degeneration. The testis on gross appearance is atrophic. Focal fibrinous or fibrous adhesions occur between the visceral tunica vaginalis over the epididymis and the parietal tunica vaginalis lining the scrotal sac. If an abscess ruptures into the cavity of the tunica vaginalis, diffuse inflammation of the tunics can result, followed by adhesions across the cavity. In some cases, fistulas discharge through the scrotum.

Noninfectious causes of epididymitis include trauma, influx of urine along the ductus deferens, rupture of impacted blind-ending efferent ductules, as well as any lesion in which spermatozoa escape from the lumen of the epididymis. Spermatozoa that have escaped from the lumen of the epididymis incite a foreign body response (Fig. 13-13). Congenital and acquired obstructions account for most of the cases of escape of spermatozoa from the epididymal tubule. A less common mechanism involves adenomyosis. In adenomyosis, the epithelium of the epididymis invades the muscular layer, creating extensions of the lumen in which spermatozoa can become entrapped. If these outpouchings rupture, spermatozoa escape into the lamina propria. Adenomyosis of the epididymis is often associated with presence of Sertoli cell tumors of the testis and is probably a response to estrogen secretion by the neoplasm.

Microscopically, in epididymitis the lumen has a mixture of inflammatory cells, in which neutrophils are present and macrophages are prominent, together with desquamated epithelial cells, intact and fragmented spermatozoa, and spermatozoa within multinucleate giant cells. If the wall of the tubule is breached, inflammation spreads to the interstitium, and macrophages become more numerous in the inflammatory exudate and collagen is deposited. Hypertrophy of the smooth muscle layer of the wall of the epididymis occurs, together with hyperplasia of the luminal epithelium of the epididymis. The epithelial cells proliferate irregularly, so that thick areas of epithelium appear to enclose thin areas, leading to "intraepithelial lumen" formation. Squamous metaplasia of the epithelium is another possible outcome in chronic epididymitis.

Infectious epididymitis is more likely to result from the entry of organisms from the urinary tract rather than from hematogenous spread. *Brucella ovis, Actinobacillus seminis,* or *Histophilus ovis* infections in rams produce epithelial hyperplasia and intraepithelial lumen formation as lesions of the early infection and later lesions of spermatic granuloma and abscesses. Abscesses are more likely to be in the tail of the epididymis and can be palpated. Testicular atrophy occurs secondarily. In *Brucella abortus* infection in bulls, epididymitis is accompanied by orchitis. Epididymitis occurs in mature dogs as a nonspecific infection (Fig. 13-14) or as part of a specific disease such as canine distemper. Intranuclear and intracytoplasmic inclusions can be found in the epithelial cells of the epididymis in canine distemper. *Brucella canis* infection causes epididymitis, followed by testicular degeneration and atrophy. The lesions are often unilateral

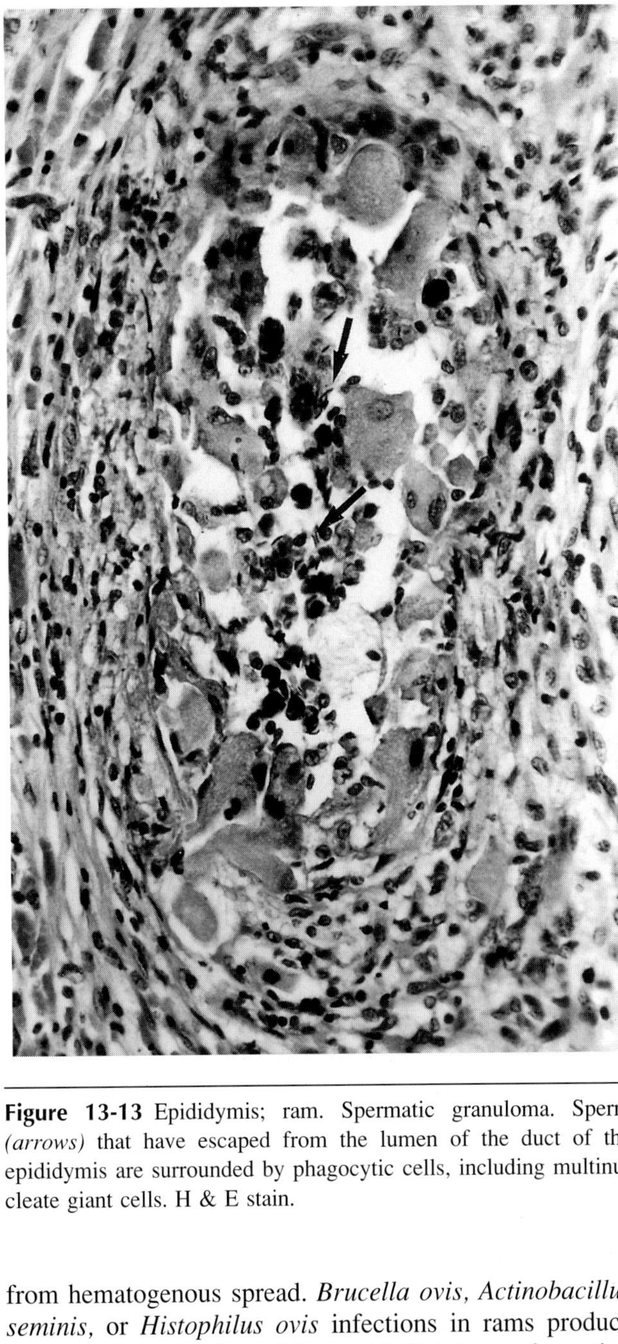

Figure 13-13 Epididymis; ram. Spermatic granuloma. Sperm *(arrows)* that have escaped from the lumen of the duct of the epididymis are surrounded by phagocytic cells, including multinucleate giant cells. H & E stain.

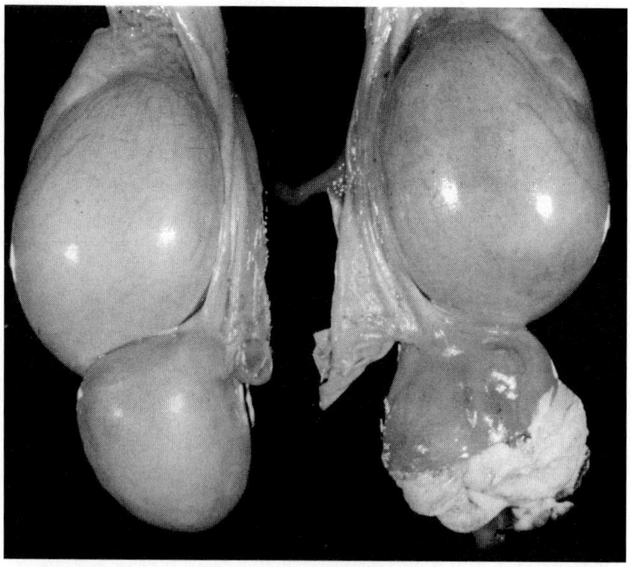

Figure 13-14 Epididymis; ram. The tail of both epididymides are enlarged by inflammation caused by bacterial infection. One epididymal tail has ruptured and pus is visible.

and occur together with scrotal hyperemia, dermatitis, and prostatitis. The epididymis can become greatly enlarged, especially the tail, as a result of interstitial lymphocytic infiltration and fibrosis.

Seminal vesiculitis is a significant problem in the bull because fertility is reduced after the seminal vesicles contribute pus to the semen, and inflamed seminal vesicles are the most common source of inflammatory cells in bovine semen. The cause is most likely infectious; various organisms including viruses, protozoa, *Chlamydia, Ureaplasma, Mycoplasma, Brucella abortus,* and other bacteria having been investigated over the years. The pathogenesis is uncertain, but hypotheses include ascending infection, descending infection, hematogenous spread, congenital malformation preventing excretion of fluid and spermatozoa, and reflux of spermatozoa or urine into the glands.

The common form of seminal vesiculitis is a chronic interstitial inflammation. In some cases, the glands are enlarged, firm, and have loss of lobulation. Collagen is deposited between the acini. Lymphocytes, plasma cells, macrophages, and a few neutrophils and eosinophils are present in the interstitium. The lumens have neutrophils, desquamated epithelial cells, and debris. Metaplasia of glandular epithelium to a stratified squamous type is common. In some bulls, much disorganization and denuding involve the epithelium of inflamed seminal vesicles.

The seminal vesicles in bulls can be among the organs involved in *Brucella abortus* and *Mycobacterium bovis* infections. In other species, seminal vesiculitis can be part of the range of lesions caused by *Pseudomonas pseudomallei* and *Brucella abortus* in the boar and by *Brucella melitensis* and *Actinobacillus seminis* in the ram.

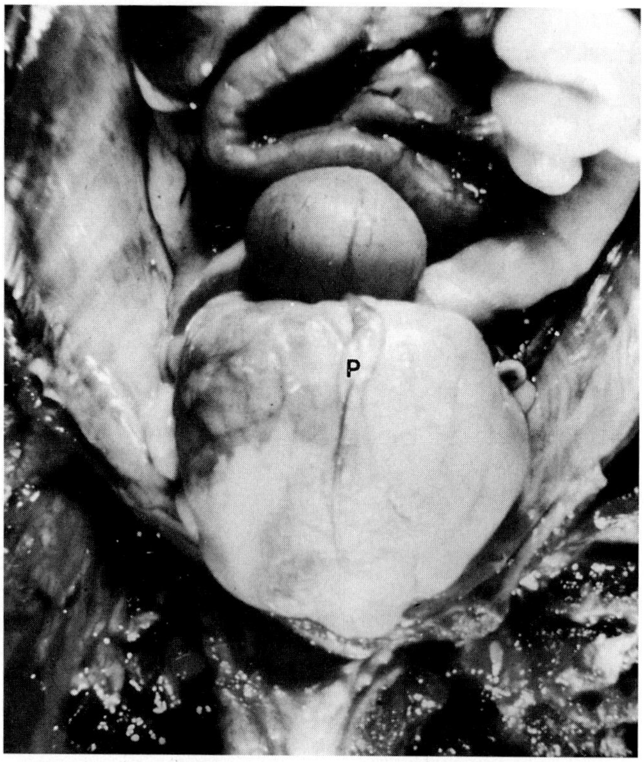

Figure 13-15 Prostate gland; dog. The prostate *(P)* is greatly enlarged. The prostate gland normally is smaller than the urinary bladder, even when the latter is empty.

PROSTATE GLAND

The prostate gland and the bulbourethral gland are derived from the urogenital sinus. Most domestic animals have both glands. The dog and cat, however, have only the prostate gland. The central part of the prostate gland is of Müllerian origin. Both estrogens and androgens have trophic action on the prostate gland.

Prostatitis can be clinically significant if toxemia accompanies the infection or if the gland becomes large enough to cause urinary obstruction. In the dog, prostatitis can be found in old animals, often together with hyperplasia, or in young animals without hyperplasia. Although increased concentrations of zinc in prostatic fluid are associated with antimicrobial properties in men and dogs, resistance to infection and resolution of infection are not correlated with zinc concentrations in prostatic tissue in the dog. Men with bacterial prostatitis have lowered prostatic zinc concentration. Prostatitis can usefully be divided into acute, chronic, abscess formation, and specific *(Brucella canis)* forms. Organisms such as *Escherichia coli, Proteus vulgaris,* and others invade from the urethra. The affected organ can be diffusely or focally involved, swollen, congested, and edematous (Fig. 13-15). The early microscopic lesion is catarrhal inflammation of the acini, expanding later to involve the interstitium, with abscess formation. The abscesses can persist or be replaced by fibrous tissue. Prostatitis is part of the spectrum of lesions caused by *Brucella canis* in the dog, and the prostate can be the site of persistence of the organism. A subacute interstitial inflammation causes enlargement and fibrosis of some lobules. Dogs have a common, clinically insignificant, chronic prostatitis of unknown cause.

Hyperplasia and metaplasia of the prostate. Enlargement of the prostate is relatively common in old dogs, and the dog is the only domestic animal species that spontaneously develops prostatic hyperplasia with age. Clinical consequences of prostatic hypertrophy are obstruction and infection of the urinary tract and development of hydronephrosis. Partial obstruction of the rectum causes constipation. Enlargement of the prostate is hormone related, but the precise cause is unknown. Hypertrophy of the gland does not occur in castrated dogs, and removal of androgens by castration of affected dogs is therapeutic. Administration of estrogens causes enlargement of the gland. Acinar hyperplasia possibly is caused by androgen excess, and fibromuscular hyperplasia is caused by estrogen excess, but the contribution of these two elements to the enlargement of the gland can overlap considerably. Enlargement of the gland need not be uniform. A large single cyst or multiple small cysts are common.

Microscopically, hyperplasia of the interlobular and, to a lesser extent, the intralobular fibromuscular stroma occurs, together with hyperplasia of the acinar epithelium, often with the formation of papillae. Some acini are distended with fluid and have a flattened epithelium. The presence of dilated cystic acini with attenuated epithelium is the basis for classifying prostatic hyperplasia as benign complex rather than benign glandular. In a study of the age-related changes in laboratory beagles, complex **benign prostatic hyperplasia** was found in all dogs over 6 years of age. Increases in size and weight of the prostate are primarily attributable to increases in interstitial tissues and to inflammation that is located primarily in the interstitial tissues. Increase in the glandular component is due to cystic dilation, not to the volume of glandular epithelium.

Estrogen-induced hypertrophy of the canine prostate gland, most often due to the presence of Sertoli cell tumor, has the added feature of squamous metaplasia of acinar epithelium, ducts, prostatic urethra, and uterus masculinus. Flattened keratinized epithelial cells are desquamated into the acini, and neutrophils and other inflammatory cells are present. Squamous metaplasia of the prostate gland in dogs is not preneoplastic. Castrated male sheep grazing clover pasture with a large estrogen content have hypertrophy, squamous metaplasia, and cyst formation in the accessory sex glands, especially the bulbourethral glands.

Adenocarcinoma of the prostate gland in the dog is the only prostatic neoplasm of any importance in domestic animals, and it is uncommon. The cause, possibly related to abnormal hormonal environment, has not been well defined. Prostatic hyperplasia appears not to precede prostatic carcinoma, although the two lesions can be found together. Some of the clinical signs of prostatic carcinoma are similar to those of prostatic hyperplasia, because of the enlargement of the organ. But, in addition, adenocarcinoma and its metastases cause cachexia and locomotory abnormalities through pressure and invasion of nearby structures, especially bones. Grossly, the neoplasm is responsible for increased firmness, nonsymmetric enlargement, partial or complete loss of the median raphe, and cystic cavities in the prostate gland. Some of these alterations can be detected by rectal palpation. The outgrowing neoplasm can rupture the capsule, and often the prostate gland becomes attached to the floor of the pelvis.

Microscopically, areas of hyperplasia of epithelial cells and fibroplasia are present. Differentiating between hyperplasia and neoplasia can sometimes be a problem; in hyperplasia, orientation of epithelial cells against a basement membrane is regular, with little fibrosis and no invasion. Prostatic intraepithelial neoplasia, described as a precursor of human prostatic cancer, has been recognized in the dog. The features are disruption of basal cell layer, increased mitotic index, and increased density of small blood vessels. Microscopically, prostatic adenocarcinomas can form acini, or undifferentiated sarcoma-like sheets, or single cells can invade the connective tissue. In men, it is recognized that the inner mass of the gland is subject to estrogen stimulation and the outer mass to androgen stimulation; hyperplasia most often occurs in the inner mass and neoplasia in the outer mass. In dogs, no specific regions of the prostate have been associated with the development of hyperplasia or neoplasia.

PENIS AND PREPUCE

Developmental Abnormalities

The penis is subject to many abnormalities of size and form, such as congenital absence, hypoplasia, duplication, directional deviations, and, in ruminants, absence of the sigmoid flexure and abnormal locations of the insertions of the retractor muscles. None of these lesions is common.

Hypoplasia of the penis and prepuce can be the result of early castration. In intersex states, hypoplasia of these structures is part of a spectrum of abnormalities.

Persistent frenulum is a minor anatomic abnormality rather than a serious defect, but it can have an important deleterious effect in limiting the extent to which the penis can be protruded from the sheath (Fig. 13-16) and in causing the erect penis to be curved instead of straight. Persistent frenulum is of importance in bulls. Judging by the frequent occurrence of large flaps and tags of tissue on the ventral raphe of the penis, transitory persistence of the frenulum is quite common. The raphes of the penis and prepuce are remnants of the frenulum, a thin membrane ventral to the penis that normally ruptures at puberty, probably as the result of a simple mechanical cause. Persistent segments of frenulum are well vascularized, usually occur at the distal end of the penis, and can connect the penis to the prepuce or the penis to itself.

Hypospadias and epispadias are malformations of the urethral canal that create abnormal openings of the urethra on the ventral surface of the penis (hypospadias) or on the dorsal surface (epispadias). Hypospadias can be regarded as a mild form of pseudohermaphroditism, with minimal gender ambiguity, as there is failure of proper closure of the urethral fold. In hypospadias, the urinary opening is ventral and proximal to its usual location, anywhere from the glans to the penile shaft, penoscrotal junction, or the perineum. Either hypospadias or epispadias can occur in individuals with other malformations incompatible with survival, or they occur alone. Their importance is in the potential for causing urinary obstruction and in interference with normal insemination.

Phimosis and paraphimosis are terms that in men refer, respectively, to inability to retract the prepuce over the penis because of too small a preputial opening, and to inability to replace the prepuce over the penis because of penile swelling. True congenital phimosis does not occur in animals because of the larger preputial cavity and opening. Inflammatory phimosis in animals occurs when inflammation causes swelling of the penis or prepuce so that the penis cannot be extruded from the prepuce.

Inflammation

Inflammation of the glans penis is called **balanitis;** inflammation of the prepuce is called **posthitis.** Nonspecific inflammation of the penis and prepuce **(balanoposthitis)** occurs in a number of situations. A large and diverse microbial flora normally inhabits the preputial cavity and can be a source of infection causing inflammation secondary to trauma, such as bite wounds in dogs and boars. Traumatic lesions occur in bulls of breeds such as Brahmin that have a pendulous sheath easily torn by sticks or other sharp objects. Because temporary protrusion of the penis from the sheath is common in these and other bulls, the everted preputial mucosa is subject to injury. In males with phimosis, the initial problem is greatly exacerbated by urination into and retention of urine in the preputial cavity, creating an environment for the overgrowth of bacterial organisms. Repeated protrusion of the penis into the normal preputial diverticulum of the boar, because of malformation or masturbation, likewise will predispose this diverticulum to local infection. Depending on the cause, balanoposthitis takes several forms: mild to severe, focal to diffuse, acute to chronic, possibly ulcerative, necrotizing, diphtheritic, catarrhal, or suppurative. Lymphoid nodules are located in the preputial lamina propria of the bull and could be important in cell-mediated immunity in the preputial cavity.

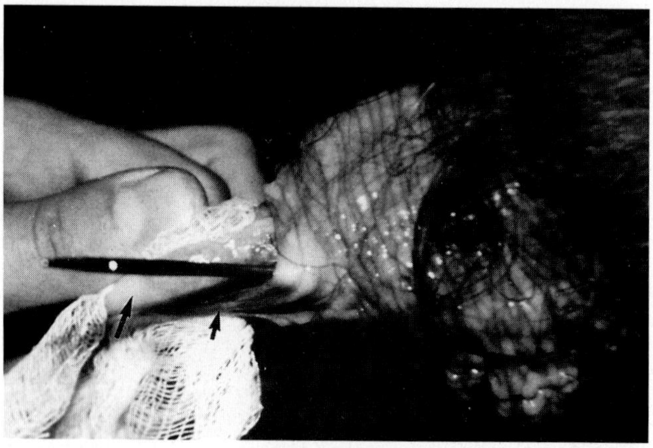

Figure 13-16 Penis; bull. Persistent frenulum. The persistent frenulum *(short arrow)* is ventral, between the penis *(long arrow)* and the prepuce, and permits only limited protrusion of the penis. A probe has been inserted between the penis and frenulum. *Courtesy Dr. E.A. Usenik.*

Herpesviruses can cause balanoposthitis in several species. Bovine herpesvirus 1 causes a balanoposthitis in the bull, progressing over the course of a few days from hyperemia and swelling to pustules and then 1- to 2-mm ulcers, especially of the glans penis. In the pustule stage, intranuclear inclusion bodies are present briefly in epithelial cells of the penis and prepuce. Ulcerative balanoposthitis with acidophilic intranuclear inclusions has been observed in goats and is considered due to caprine herpesvirus infection. Equine herpesvirus 3 is the cause of equine coital exanthema, a disease of stallions and mares with a similarly short clinical course, but with larger (15 mm) pustules with a predilection for the body rather than the glans of the penis. Canine herpesvirus causes inflammation at the base of the penis and the reflection of the prepuce, but does not cause the formation of pustules or ulcers. Resolution of these lesions in the affected species is rapid, leaving only hyperplastic mucosal lymphoid nodules and small areas of depigmented mucosa. Bovine herpesvirus 1, suid herpesvirus 1 (pseudorabies virus) in pigs, caprine herpesvirus 1, and canine herpesvirus can persist in a latent state, capable of becoming reactivated by stress or treatment with corticosteroids.

Ovine ulcerative posthitis is caused by urease-producing *Corynebacterium renale.* When the urine has a high concentration of urea, it produces ulceration of the prepuce near the orifice. A high-protein diet predisposes to the disease. Lack of testosterone is also involved because the disease occurs mainly in wethers. If the preputial orifice becomes blocked by swelling, the disease becomes much more severe, spreading beyond the initial small ulcer on the hairless skin of the prepuce to diffusely involve the mucosa, with ulceration of the glans penis and loss of the urethral process.

Other organisms are capable of causing balanoposthitis. These include *Strongyloides papillosus* in the bull and the larvae of *Habronema* spp. in the horse. In equine habronemiasis, the gross lesion has the same elevated nodular bleeding surface as granulation tissue or a sarcoid. Microscopically, however, the lesions are distinct tracks of larval migration filled with debris and surrounded by fibrovascular tissue rich in eosinophils. The well-known bovine venereally transmitted diseases of **vibriosis** and **trichomoniasis** cause no lesions or minimal nonspecific lesions of the male external genitalia.

Neoplasms

The penis and prepuce can be involved in metastatic or multicentric neoplasms such as mast cell tumor, melanoma, and lymphosarcoma. The following are the most important primary neoplasms of the penis and prepuce.

Transmissible venereal tumor of the dog is a neoplasm of histiocytic immunophenotype cells. The primary neoplasm is usually on the external genitalia, but extragenital primaries do occur, as well as metastatic neoplasms. In the male dog, the neoplasm is found on the penis, more often on the proximal parts, and not often on the prepuce (Fig. 13-17). The neoplasm can be single or multiple, a few millimeters to 10 cm in diameter, with an inflamed, ulcerated, cauliflower-like surface. Microscopically, the neoplasm is the same as it is in the bitch, composed of sheets of neoplasm cells and minimal stroma. The neoplastic cells are large, uniform, with a large nucleus and nucleolus, indistinct cell outline, and numerous mitotic figures. Regression and recovery are the rule, with the expression of major histocompatibility complex class II antigen by the neoplastic cells and the infiltration of inflammatory cells, including increased numbers of T lymphocytes during the regression of the neoplasm. The neoplasm is thought to arise from a specific genetic alteration of dog histiocytes, followed by the transmission of abnormal cells from dog to dog. The neoplasms are very similar around the world, based on data obtained from immunologic, cytogenetic, and nucleotide sequence studies.

Squamous cell carcinoma of the penis is of importance in the horse and to a lesser extent in the dog. In the horse, both stallions and geldings have neoplasms, and the common site is the glans penis. Rather than producing a proliferative mass, the neoplasm in this location in invasive, necrotic, and ulcerating (Fig. 13-18). Microscopically, the neoplasm is well differentiated, with well-developed keratin pearls. Metastases to the inguinal and iliac lymph nodes usually can be found. The sheath

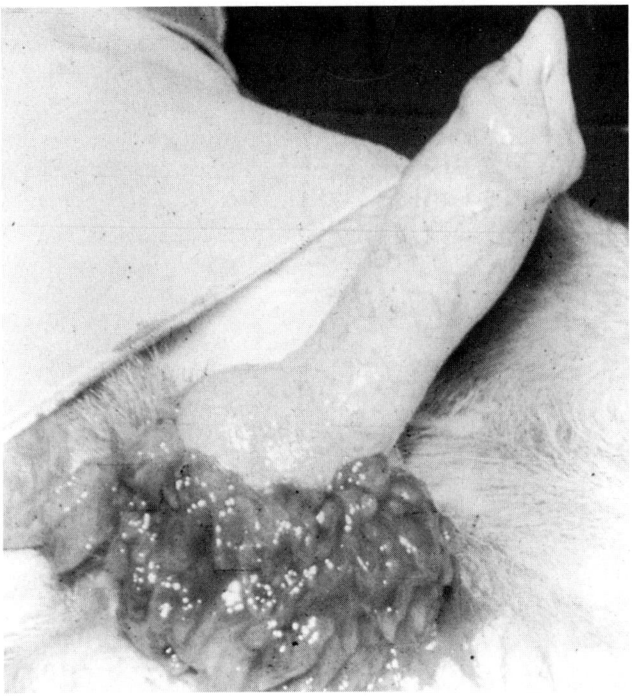

Figure 13-17 Penis; dog. Transmissible venereal tumor. Soft, neoplastic masses have formed in a cluster on the mucosa over the proximal end of the shaft of the penis. *Courtesy Dr. M.H. Goldschmidt.*

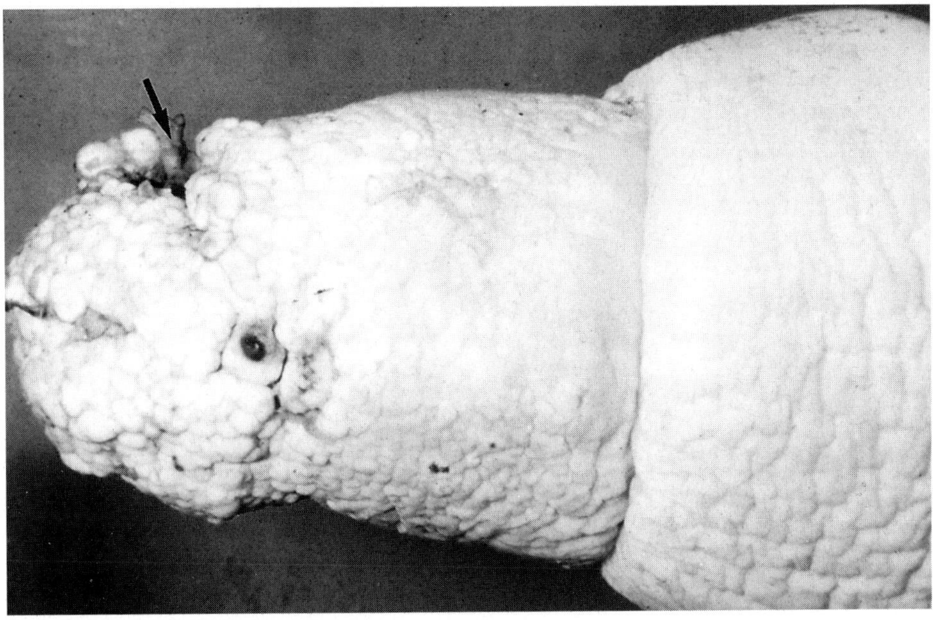

Figure 13-18 Penis; horse. Squamous cell carcinoma. The carcinoma has invaded and has caused necrosis and subsequent ulcerations of the glans penis *(arrow).*

becomes edematous because of lymph vessel obstruction, and the preputial cavity becomes distended by retained smegma, inflammatory debris, and urine.

Papilloma (or fibropapilloma) occurs on the glans penis of young bulls. The age of the affected animals and the occasional observation of inclusion bodies suggest a viral cause. The single or multiple warty growths have a significant fibrous core and a papilliferous epithelial covering. The proportions of epithelial and fibrous tissue vary greatly from case to case. Surface ulceration is often extensive following spontaneous necrosis or trauma. Larger neoplasms can interfere with breeding or cause phimosis or paraphimosis. Other untoward possible sequels are preputial hairs entangling the prolapsed penis and causing strangulation and compression of the phimotic penis resulting in rupture of the urethra.

Acknowledgments

Photographs or material for photographs were kindly contributed by D. M. Gillette (Figure 13-1), M. H. Goldschmidt (Figure 13-19), L. J. Lowenstine (Figure 13-12), R. G. Thomson (Figure 13-5), and E. A. Usenik (Figure 13-17). In addition, photographs from the files of the Laboratory of Pathology and the Laboratory of Large Animal Pathology, University of Pennsylvania, were taken by A. L. Hattel (Figure 13-8), K. L. Hawkins (Figure 13-17), C. C. Morse (Figure 13-15), and K. L. Woods (Figure 13-16).

References

Aquilina JW, McKinney L, Pacelli A, Richman LK, Waters DJ, Thompson I, Burghardt WF Jr, Bostwick DG. High grade prostatic intraepithelial neoplasia in military working dogs with and without prostate cancer. Prostate 1998; 36:189-193.

Barsanti JA, Finco DR. Canine prostatic diseases. Vet Clin North Am Small Anim Pract 1986; 16:587-599.

Brown TR, Migeon CJ. Androgen receptors in normal and abnormal male sexual differentiation. Adv Exp Med Biol 1986; 196: 227-255.

Clarnette TD, Sugita Y, Hutson JM. Congenital anomalies in human and animal models reveal the mechanisms and hormones governing testicular descent. Br J Urol 1997; 79:99-112.

Cohen D. The mechanism of transmission of the transmissible venereal tumour of the dog. Transplantation 1974; 17:8-11.

Cowan LA, Barsanti JA, Brown J, Jain A. Effects of bacterial infection and castration on prostatic tissue zinc concentration in dogs. Am J Vet Res 1991; 52:1262-1264.

da Silva SM, Hacker A, Harley V, Goodfellow P, Swain A, Lovell-Badge R. Sox9 expression during gonadal development implies a conserved role for the gene in testis differentiation in mammals and birds. Nat Genet 1996; 14:62-68.

Edwards DF, Kennedy JR, Patton CS, Toal RL, Daniel GB, Lothrop CD. Familial immotile-cilia syndrome in English springer spaniel dogs. Am J Med Genet 1989; 33:290-298.

Ezzi A, Ladds PW, Hoffmann D, Foster RA, Briggs GD. Pathology of varicocele in the ram. Aust Vet J 1988; 65:11-15.

Gelberg HB, McEntee K. Equine testicular interstitial cell tumors. Vet Pathol 1987; 24:231-234.

Haas GG, Beer AE. Immunologic influences on reproductive biology: Sperm gametogenesis and maturation in the male and female genital tracts. Fertil Steril 1986; 46:753-766.

Humphrey JD, Ladds PW. Pathology of the bovine testis and epididymis. Vet Bull 1975; 45:787-795.

Jones TC. Sex chromosome anomaly, Klinefelter's syndrome. In Jones TC, Hackel DB, Migaki G, Pendleton M, eds. Animal Models of Human Disease. Washington, DC: Registry of Comparative Pathology, 1972: model no. 5.

Kahrs RF. Effects of infectious bovine rhinotracheitis on reproduction. In: Morrow DW, ed. Current Therapy in Theriogenology. 2nd ed. Philadelphia: WB Saunders, 1986:250-254.

Koopman P, Munsterberg A, Capel B, Vivian N, Lovell-Badge R. Expression of a candidate sex-determining gene during mouse testis differentiation. Nature 1990; 348:450-452.

Leav I, Ling GV. Adenocarcinoma of the canine prostate. Cancer 1968; 22:1329-1345.

Lowseth LA, Gerlach RF, Gillett NA, Muggenburg BA. Age-related changes in the prostate and testes of the beagle dog. Vet Pathol 1990; 27:347-353.

Madrid M, Ott RS, Rao Veeramachaneni DN, Parrett DF, Vanderwert W, Willms CL. Scrotal circumference, seminal characteristics, and testicular lesions of yearling Angus bulls. Am J Vet Res 1988; 49:579-585.

Marshall LS, Oehlert ML, Haskins ME, Seldon JR, Patterson DF. Persistent Müllerian duct syndrome in miniature schnauzers. J Am Vet Med Assoc 1982; 181:798-801.

McEntee K. Pathology of the testis of the bull and stallion. Proc Soc Theriogenol 1979; 80-91.

Meyers-Wallen VN, Donahoe PK, Ueno T, Manganaro TF, Patterson DF. Müllerian inhibiting substance is present in testes of dogs with persistent Müllerian duct syndrome. Biol Reprod 1989; 41:881-888.

Meyers-Wallen VN, Patterson DF. Disorders of sexual development in the dog. In: Morrow DW, ed. Current Therapy in Theriogenology. 2nd ed. Philadelphia: WB Saunders, 1986:567-573.

Meyers-Wallen VN, Patterson DF. Sexual differentiation and inherited disorders of sexual development in the dog. J Reprod Fertil 1989; Suppl 39:57-64.

Meyers-Wallen VN, Wilson JD, Griffin JE, Fisher S, Moorhead PH, Goldschmidt MH, Haskins ME, Patterson DF. Testicular feminization in a cat. J Am Vet Med Assoc 1989; 195:631-634.

Mozos E, Mendez A, Gomez-Villamandos JC, Martin de las Mulas J, Perez J. Immunohistochemical characterization of canine transmissible venereal tumor. Vet Pathol 1996; 33:257-263.

Nielsen SW, Lein DH. VI. Tumors of the testis. Bull WHO 1974; 50:71-78.

Paitnaik AK, Mostofi FK. A clinicopathologic, histologic, and immunohistochemical study of mixed germ cell-stromal tumors in the testis of 16 dogs. Vet Pathol 1993; 30:287-295.

Papa FO, Alvarenga MA, Lopes MD, Campos Filho EP. Infertility of autoimmune origin in a stallion. Equine Vet J 1990; 22:145-146.

Post K, Kilborn SH. Canine Sertoli cell tumor: A medical records search and literature review. Can Vet J 1987; 28:427-431.

Postorino NC. Tumors of the male reproductive tract. In: Withrow SJ, MacEwen EG, eds. Clinical Veterinary Oncology. Philadelphia: JB Lippincott, 1989:305-311.

Reif JR, Brody RS. The relationship between cryptorchidism and canine testicular neoplasia. J Am Vet Med Assoc 1969; 155:2005-2010.

Romagnoli SE. Canine cryptorchidism. Vet Clin North Am Small Anim Pract 1991; 21:533-545.

Rutgers JL, Scully RE. Pathology of the testis in intersex syndromes. Semin Diagn Pathol 1987; 4:275-292.

Wiener JS, Teague JL, Roth DR, Gonzales ET, Lamb DJ. Molecular biology and function of the androgen receptor in genital development. J Urol 1997; 157:1377-1386.

Weiner JS, Marcelli M, Lamb DJ. Molecular determinants of sexual differentiation. World J Urol 1996; 14:278-294.

Zhang J, Ricketts SW, Tanner SJ. Antisperm antibodies in the semen of a stallion following testicular trauma. Equine Vet J 1990; 22:138-141.

CHAPTER 14

The Eye and Ear

James A. Render
William W. Carlton

COMPONENTS OF THE EYE

The components of the eye include the globe (eyeball), optic nerve, and accessory structures, including the eyelids, lacrimal apparatus, orbital fascia, and extraocular muscles. The globe detects light, which is converted into an electrical signal (phototransduction). This signal is transmitted to the brain via the optic nerve, allowing vision to occur. The eyelids and the lacrimal apparatus protect the rostral components of the globe, and the extraocular muscles allow the globe to move. The orbit is a fossa that contains fascia and separates the globe from the cranial cavity.

The globe is composed of three concentric tunics—fibrous, vascular, and nervous—that surround an anterior space containing transparent media: aqueous humor, the lens, and the vitreous body. The rostral aspect of the outer fibrous tunic is composed of the transparent cornea and the remainder of the tunic is composed of the opaque sclera. Epithelium covering the cornea is continuous with the epithelium of the conjunctiva that covers the rostral aspect of the sclera. The middle, vascular, and pigmented tunic (uvea) is composed of the iris, ciliary body, and choroid. The inner nervous tunic (retina) lines the portion of the globe caudal to the lens. The lens is suspended in the interior of the globe by zonular fibers extending from the processes of the ciliary body.

The intraocular space rostral to the lens houses the aqueous humor, and the intraocular space (vitreous cavity) caudal to the lens contains the vitreous body. Aqueous humor is continuously produced by ciliary processes throughout life. This fluid moves from the space between the iris and the lens (posterior chamber), through the central hole in the iris (pupil), and into the space between the cornea and iris (anterior chamber). From here it flows into the angle formed by the iris and the cornea, through filtration spaces, and, eventually, into the scleral vasculature.

The retina is composed of two layers. The outer layer is composed of a row of neuroepithelial cells that are pigmented, except where they cover the tapetum lucidum, a specialized, light-reflective part of the choroid in certain species. This outer layer of neuroepithelium is the retinal pigment epithelium (RPE). The other inner portion of the retina is the neurosensory retina. The potential intraretinal space between these two retinal layers is referred to as the subretinal space.

The neurosensory retina is transparent to allow light to stimulate photoreceptors located in the outer portion of this layer. The neurosensory retina is composed of nine histologically identifiable layers. The outer and inner segments of photoreceptors form a layer (of rods and cones) that is adjacent to the RPE. The layer of rods and cones is separated from the layer of photoreceptor cell nuclei (outer nuclear layer) by the outer limiting membrane. This membrane consists of cellular junctions between processes of Müller cells and the inner segments of photoreceptor cells. Müller cells are retinal glial cells. Terminals of photoreceptors synapse with dendrites of neurons (horizontal and bipolar cells) in the outer plexiform layer. The cell bodies of these neurons and the cell bodies of Müller cells are located in the inner nuclear layer. Neurons with nuclei in the inner nuclear layer synapse with ganglion cells in the inner plexiform layer. The cell bodies of ganglion cells are located in the ganglion cell layer, and axons of ganglion cells form the nerve fiber layer. The nerve fiber layer is separated from the vitreous body by the inner limiting membrane, a basement membrane of Müller cells. Axons in the nerve fiber layer converge at the optic disc to form the optic nerve. In the dog, the main retinal vessels are located in the nerve fiber and ganglion cell layers, but in cattle, sheep, and pigs, retinal vessels can protrude into the vitreous cavity.

Certain terms are used to describe the location of normal ocular structures or ocular lesions. The central points of the anterior and posterior curvatures of the globe, or lens, are referred to as the anterior pole and posterior pole, respectively. An imaginary line drawn around the globe, or lens, midway between the anterior and posterior poles is the equator. The plane passing through these poles is the meridional plane, and planes parallel to this plane are sagittal planes. Structures near the center of the globe are inner and structures farther away from the center are outer. Structures that are rostral are referred to as anterior, and structures that are caudal are referred to as posterior.

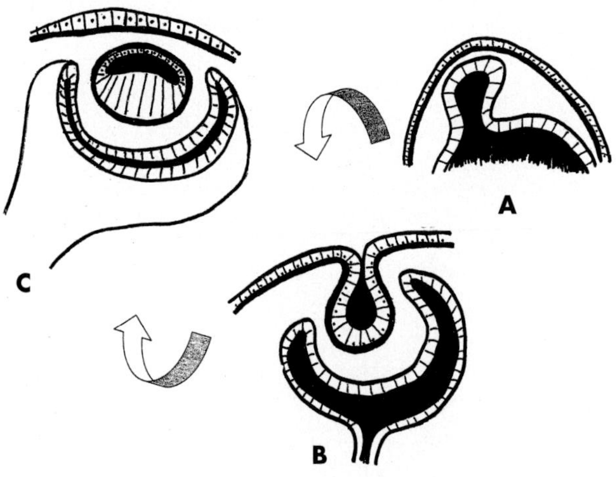

Figure 14-1 Eye. Embryologic development. **A,** Optic vesicle lined by neuroectoderm evaginates from the developing forebrain. **B,** Surface ectoderm is induced to invaginate to form the lens vesicle, while the optic vesicle becomes the optic cup. **C,** Epithelial cells along the posterior of the optic vesicle elongate to fill the space and form the nucleus of the lens, leaving lens epithelium only beneath the anterior part of the basement membrane that surrounds the lens, the lens capsule.

OCULAR EMBRYOLOGY

The globe develops from several embryonic tissues including neural crest cells (ocular mesenchyme), neuroectoderm (retina and neuroepithelium of the iris and ciliary body), surface ectoderm (epithelial structures and the lens), and mesoderm (extraocular muscles and vascular endothelium). Paired evaginations of neuroectoderm from the developing forebrain form optic vesicles, which are connected to the forebrain by optic stalks (Fig. 14-1). Optic vesicles induce the surface ectoderm to invaginate and form the lens vesicles. Lens vesicles are lined by epithelium and are completely surrounded by a basal lamina, which becomes the lenticular capsule. The lenticular epithelial cells along the posterior capsule elongate, fill in the space of the lens vesicle, and form the embryonic nucleus of the lens. Lenticular epithelial cells along the anterior lens capsule undergo mitosis, migrate to the equator of the lens, move inward, elongate, and form the outer layer of the lens (lens cortex). This process continues throughout life.

The formation of the lens vesicle causes the optic vesicle to invaginate and form the optic cup. The optic cup has a ventral linear fissure (choroidal or optic fissure) that closes as the globe matures. The neuroepithelial cells at the rostral margin of the optic cup form two layers of iridal epithelium, which are continuous with two layers of ciliary epithelium. Both layers of iridal epithelium are pigmented, but only the outer ciliary epithelial layer is pigmented. The outer ciliary epithelium is continuous with the retinal pigment epithelium, and the inner ciliary epithelium is continuous with the neurosensory retina at the ora ciliaris retinae (ora serrata in primates).

After formation of the optic cup, changes occur in the ocular mesenchyme of the anterior portion of the globe (anterior segment). Portions of the cornea (stroma and endothelium), the iridal stroma, the posterior chamber, anterior chamber, and structures of iridocorneal angle are formed. A portion of this mesenchyme forms a vascular bridge across the future pupil (pupillary membrane). In the posterior segment, development of the choroid and sclera is influenced by the retinal pigment epithelium. The developing avascular lens is surrounded by a vascular plexus of capillaries (tunica vasculosa lentis) that receives blood from the hyaloid vascular system. The vessels of the hyaloid system extend through the optic fissure and are surrounded by mesenchymal cells forming the primary vitreous. The primary vitreous and the tunica vasculosa lentis eventually regress as the globe matures. The tertiary vitreous, composed of collagen fibers, forms between the equator of the lenticular capsule and the basal lamina of the nonpigmented ciliary epithelium. The tertiary vitreous eventually differentiates into zonular fibers (zonules).

ANOMALIES OF THE GLOBE

Anophthalmia, Congenital Cystic Globe, and Microphthalmia

Disruption of the normal evagination of the optic vesicle can result in complete absence of the globe (anophthalmia or anophthalmos), a congenital cystic globe lacking intraocular structures, or a congenitally small globe (microphthalmia or microphthalmos). Anophthalmia is rare. It occurs when the optic vesicle either fails to develop or undergoes atrophy at an earlier point in embryologic development. Most reports of "clinical anophthalmia" are really severe microphthalmia because rudiments of recognizable intraocular structures, such as pigmented uvea and neuroepithelium, are found in orbital tissue.

If the neuroepithelium of the optic vesicle fails to interact with surface ectoderm, no induction of the lens vesicle occurs. Without the formation of a lens vesicle, developmental interactions fail to occur. The result is a congenital cystic globe.

Microphthalmia occurs sporadically in domestic and wild animals, including dogs, horses, swine, cattle, and white-tailed deer. This anomaly has been reported in calves as the result of in utero infections by bovine virus diarrhea virus and has been linked to a maternal vitamin A deficiency in piglets. The lesion can be unilateral or bilateral, and the size of the globe and the extent of associated ocular malformations can vary (Figs. 14-2 and 14-3). Associated ocular lesions include anterior segment dysgenesis, cataract, persistent primary vitreous, retinal dysplasia, retinal detachment, intraocular cartilage, and intraocular glandular tissue. A concurrent failure in the fusion of the optic fissure can result in an area devoid of tissue (coloboma) or a small globe with cysts located posterior to the globe (retrobulbar cysts). Microphthalmia

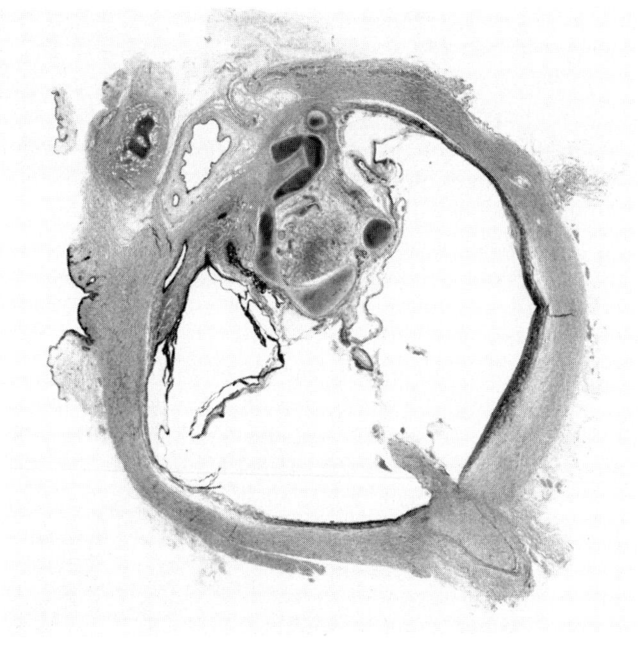

Figure 14-2 Globe; equine. Microphthalmia. Multiple intraocular anomalies including anterior segment dysplasia, intraocular cartilage, and retinal nonattachment. H & E stain.

must be differentiated from phthisis bulbi, the small, distorted, "end-stage" globe that occurs as a sequela to severe intraocular trauma or inflammation.

Cyclopia and Synophthalmia

A defect in the development of the brain before evagination of the optic vesicles can result in improper separation of the developing globes. Cyclopia is a rare developmental anomaly characterized by the presence of a single medial globe within a single median orbit. Most lesions of "clinical cyclopia" are really two globes merged together (synophthalmia or synophthalmus). Synophthalmia is a rare anomaly characterized by incomplete separation, or early fusion, of paired globes. The ocular lesion can be accompanied by other malformations including malformed pinnas, anomalies of the brain, a median proboscis, cranioschisis, and palatoschisis.

Cyclopian lesions can occur following the ingestion of *Veratrum californicum*. The feeding of fresh or dried plant to ewes on gestational day 14 results in the birth of lambs with the lesions. Lesions similar to those in lambs were produced in the offspring of goats and cows fed *V. californicum*. The teratogenic compounds in *V. californicum* are steroidal alkaloids (e.g., cyclopamine).

Anterior Segment Dysplasia

Anomalies of the structures of the anterior segment (cornea, iris, and ciliary body) can be caused by abnormal development of mesenchyme or defective development associated with the optic cup. Anomalies of the anterior segment are numerous and variable in severity. Failure in

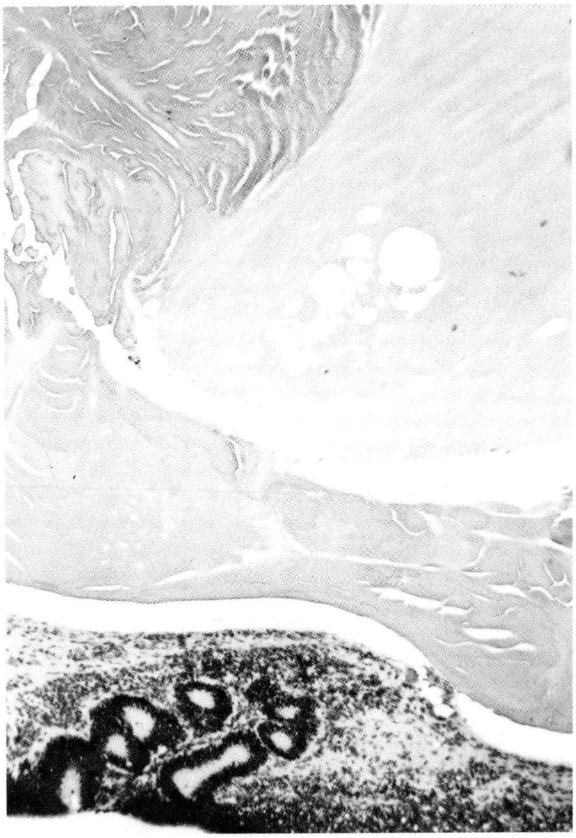

Figure 14-3 Globe; canine. Microphthalmia. Multiple ocular anomalies include retinal detachment, retinal dysplasia, and cataract with retina focally adhered to lens. H & E stain.

complete regression of mesenchyme to form the anterior chamber results in strands of tissue extending from the iris to the inner cornea, causing a focal corneal opacity **(adherent leukoma).** Severe anterior segment dysplasia can be a feature of microphthalmia. Lesions consist of cysts lined by multiple layers of squamous epithelium and connective tissue containing ectopic cartilage and lacrimal gland epithelium in the region of the anterior segment.

Coloboma

Coloboma is the term used for the absence of ocular tissue that normally should be present. Although colobomas occur in many locations, typical coloboma refers to the absence of ocular tissue resulting from a failure of fusion of the edges of the optic fissure. Normally, the optic fissure begins to close near the equator and proceeds rostrally and caudally. Coloboma of the iris and ciliary body occur if there is a failure in closure of the anterior aspect of the optic fissure. Coloboma of the iris rarely alters ocular function but can produce variations in pupillary shape.

Failure of the posterior aspect of the optic fissure to close completely results in a notchlike defect in the area of the optic disc. This defect can be associated with posterior thinning and outpouching of the sclera **(sclera ectasia)** and

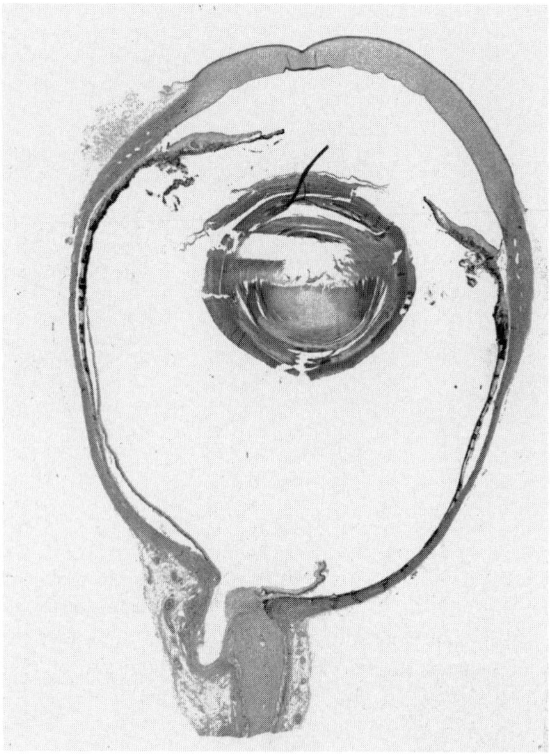

Figure 14-4 Globe; canine. Collie eye anomaly. Coloboma of the optic nerve with scleral ectasia. H & E stain.

can cause large, multilocular cysts to form caudal to the globe **(retrobulbar cysts).** Thin, disorganized (dysplastic) neuroepithelium can line the defect. Faulty induction by the retinal pigment epithelium is considered a cause of coloboma in this location.

Collie Eye Anomaly

Collie eye anomaly is a common disease of both smooth and rough collie dogs and is inherited as an autosomal trait. The main lesion **(choroidal hypoplasia)** is a relatively common lesion in dogs. The hypoplastic choroid will be poorly pigmented and thin. Other lesions include posterior coloboma, scleral ectasia, retinal dysplasia, retinal folds, retinal detachment, and vitreous hemorrhage (Fig. 14-4). Ocular lesions are bilateral, although the severity of the lesions can vary between globes.

LESIONS OF THE CORNEA

The cornea is the transparent portion of the fibrous tunic that refracts light entering the globe. The outer cornea consists of a layer of nonkeratinized stratified squamous epithelium that is protected and nourished by an overlying precorneal tear film. Basal epithelial cells are firmly attached to a basal lamina by hemidesmosomes, which secure the epithelial layer to the underlying corneal stroma. The rostral aspect of the corneal stroma is referred to as the anterior limiting membrane. In most domesticated animals, this is a poorly differentiated, thin, cell-free zone. In primates and birds, this is a prominent structure composed of condensed collagen fibers known as Bowman's membrane. Ninety percent of the entire corneal thickness is composed of stroma. This layer consists of collagenous lamellae arranged in parallel sheets interspersed with flat fibroblasts (keratocytes). No blood vessels are present.

The posterior boundary of the corneal stroma is covered by a homogeneous, acellular basement membrane (Descemet's membrane). The layer is covered by a single layer of mesenchymal cells (corneal endothelium). The corneal endothelium and the corneal epithelium contain a physiologic pump involving Na^+, K^+-ATPase that maintains a certain state of corneal dehydration or deturgescence needed for corneal transparency.

Corneal lesions can occur when the eyelids fail to prevent an injury, the outer surface of the cornea fails to stay moist, or intraocular disease is present. Corneal injuries, such as abrasions or ulcers, have a loss of epithelium. Deeper corneal wounds, such as a **laceration** or **penetration,** can cause bacteria, fungi, or foreign bodies to become embedded in the corneal stroma. Projectile injuries cause **perforation** of the entire cornea or globe.

Because the corneal epithelium contains numerous naked nerve endings, the cornea is sensitive to pain. Even mild irritation can result in marked clinical signs. Clinical signs of corneal disease include keeping the eyelids tight together **(blepharospasm),** excessive lacrimation with overflow of tears **(epiphora),** avoidance of light **(photophobia),** withdrawal of the globe into the orbit **(endophthalmos)** that causes protrusion of the nictitating membrane, conjunctival congestion or hyperemia, conjunctival edema **(chemosis),** and a small pupil **(miosis).** Corneal lesions often include inflammation **(keratitis)** that is manifested by edema and vascularization of the corneal stroma.

Anomalies of the Cornea

Anomalies of the cornea include abnormalities of size, shape, or transparency. **Microcornea** is a cornea proportionally smaller than the expected size, and **macrocornea** (megalocornea) is a congenitally larger than expected cornea. Macrocornea needs to be differentiated from corneal enlargement secondary to an enlarged globe (buphthalmos) that can occur at birth. Congenital corneal opacities include dermoid and stromal deposits and can occur along with anomalies of the anterior chamber.

Corneal Dermoid

Corneal dermoid is a congenital choristoma characterized as skin in the cornea, conjunctiva, or both locations. The lesion has been described in several animal species, but is probably most common in cattle (e.g., polled Hereford cattle). Corneal dermoids are either unilateral or bilateral

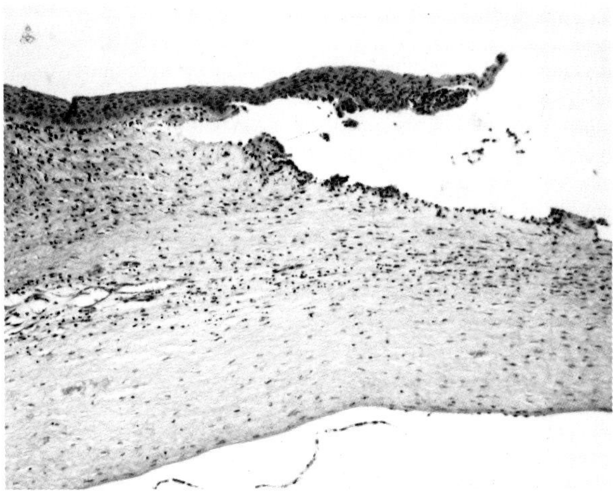

Figure 14-5 Globe, cornea; bovine. Ulcerative keratitis. Portion of cornea is missing, the corneal epithelium is elevated (artifact), and the corneal stroma has vessels and cellular infiltrates. H & E stain.

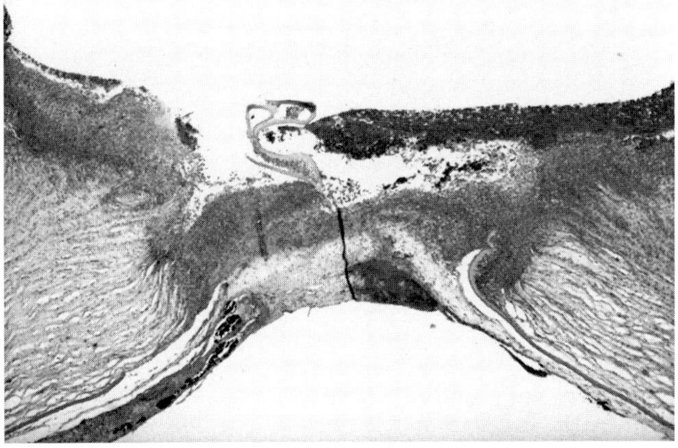

Figure 14-6 Globe, cornea and iris; canine. Ruptured descemetocele and keratitis. Central cornea is missing, and the space is filled with an inflammatory exudate containing a wrinkled, exteriorized, ruptured Descemet's membrane. The iris is adhered to the cornea and extends into the space (iris prolapse). The corneal stroma is edematous, and a severe keratitis surrounds the site of rupture. H & E stain.

and are often located in the temporal region in dogs. Dermoids are visible when the eyelids are open, but because of irritation, the lesion is often associated with a mucopurulent discharge and blepharospasm. Microscopically, the lesion consists of pigmented or nonpigmented keratinized squamous epithelium that overlies dermal tissue with hair follicles, sweat glands, and sebaceous glands.

Corneal Ulceration

Corneal ulcers can be classified by their depth of involvement, progressive behavior, or cause (Fig. 14-5). Superficial corneal ulcers, or erosions, can be further classified as uncomplicated or refractory. Most uncomplicated corneal ulcers heal within 2 to 6 days. Refractory corneal ulcers heal slowly and tend to recur. Deep corneal ulcers extend deeper into the stroma and can be progressive or nonprogressive. Progressive corneal ulcers can extend deeply down to Descemet's membrane. When this occurs, Descemet's membrane often bulges outward forming a **descemetocele.** Rupture of a descemetocele results in corneal perforation, loss of aqueous humor, loss of intraocular pressure **(hypotony),** and collapse of the globe (Fig. 14-6). The iris adheres to the corneal endothelium **(anterior synechia)** or extends into the corneal lesion **(iris prolapse).**

Corneal ulcers can be caused by abrasions, chemical burns, and infections. Few infectious agents are capable of causing primary corneal lesions, but those that can include herpesviruses and the bacterium, *Moraxella (Branhamella) bovis*. Many bacterial and mycotic microorganisms cause keratitis as secondary infections, especially in animals whose immune systems have been suppressed by use of corticosteroids.

Feline herpesvirus type I (FHV-1) is a common cause of upper respiratory tract disease, conjunctivitis, and keratitis in the cat. Conjunctivitis consists of hyperemia, blepharospasm, chemosis, and ocular discharge. Corneal lesions include dendritic ulcers, which are pathognomonic for the disease. Other corneal lesions associated with an infection by FHV-1 include neonatal ophthalmia, corneal sequestrum, and eosinophilic keratitis.

Infectious bovine keratoconjunctivitis (bovine pinkeye) is caused by *M. bovis*. This disease has worldwide distribution and is a possible cause of economic loss because of blindness. Infections occur primarily during the summer months. Predisposing factors include dust, sunlight, and various insects, such as flies. The central corneal lesions are often unilateral, but can be bilateral. Clinical signs include epiphora, blepharospasm, photophobia, and conjunctival hyperemia and chemosis. The cornea of affected cattle develops superficial axial defects that progress into abscesses, which can rupture, leaving an ulcer. The corneal ulcers can either heal within 3 weeks leaving a scar, or progress to keratoconjunctivitis with or without secondary iridocyclitis and hypopyon.

Feline Corneal Sequestrum

Feline corneal sequestrum is either a unilateral or bilateral, central, black corneal lesion (Fig. 14-7). Although the lesion is well characterized, the cause is still unknown. Because it occurs at a high incidence in cats with shallow orbits (e.g., Persian or Himalayan), it can have a hereditary basis, even though other breeds (e.g., domestic shorthair) can have the lesion. Other factors, such as FHV-1 infection, could be involved. The lesion is a superficial, circular,

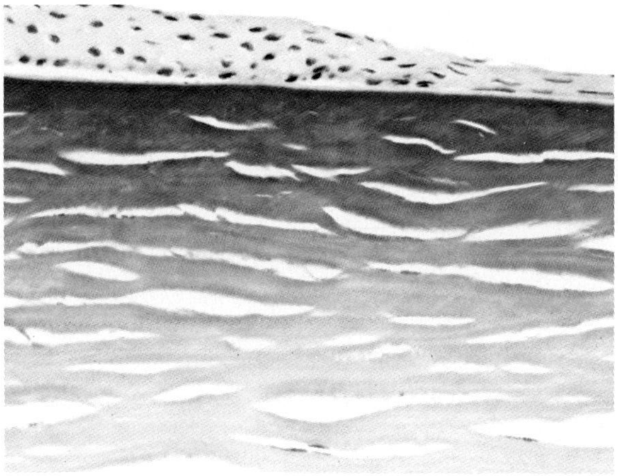

Figure 14-7 Globe, cornea; feline. Feline sequestrum. Corneal epithelial cells have migrated to cover the ulcer. The sequestrum of pigmented necrotic tissue is acellular and avascular. H & E stain.

black focus in the center of the cornea. Microscopically, the discrete, tan to black, ulcerated lesion is devoid of keratocytes and other cells. Inflammatory cells, especially neutrophils, can be present at the borders of the lesion, and the corneal epithelium can extend partially under the lesion. A similar lesion has been reported in the horse.

Refractory Corneal Ulcer

Refractory corneal ulcer (recurrent erosion syndrome or indolent ulcer) occurs in the dog and horse. This lesion is characterized by focal erosion or ulceration of the central cornea, which is covered by nonadherent corneal epithelium and bordered by hyperplastic corneal epithelium. The epithelium has swirls of squamous epithelium (squamous eddies), and the basement membrane can be absent, thinned, or thickened. The corneal stroma beneath the basement membrane can have a hypereosinophilic, acellular zone. The cause of this zone is unknown, but it is proposed that the corneal stroma is somehow defective and prevents the attachment of the epithelium by hemidesmosomes. The lesion is treated by a method that fosters attachment of the epithelium to underlying stroma.

A common treatment for refractory corneal ulcer is grid keratotomy. This surgical procedure involves removal of the nonadherent epithelium and making superficial incisions into the exposed corneal stroma in a grid pattern. The purpose is for epithelial cells to adhere to a bed of new collagenous connective tissue formed by activated stromal fibroblasts. Microscopically, granulation tissue fills in the surgical incisions, which will, hopefully, result in attachment of the corneal epithelium.

Keratitis

Inflammation of the cornea (keratitis) is similar to inflammation elsewhere in the body and can be divided into acute keratitis and chronic keratitis (Fig. 14-8). Acute keratitis is a response to corneal injury, bacterial infection, or mycotic infection. Neutrophils gain access to the cornea from conjunctival blood vessels, limbal blood vessels, and the tear film. Neutrophils appear within the corneal stroma within 5 hours after corneal injury and are important sources of fibroblastic and angioblastic growth factors. An addition to neutrophils, acute keratitis is also characterized by stromal edema and stromal vascularization. Corneal vascularization is either superficial or deep, depending on the cause. Chronic keratitis is characterized by the accumulation of lymphocytes, plasma cells, stromal fibroblasts, and melanin-containing cells. Melanin can be in melanocytes or in basal epithelial cells, fibroblasts, or macrophages. The presence of melanin in the cornea is referred to as **corneal pigmentation, corneal melanosis,** or **pigmentary keratitis.**

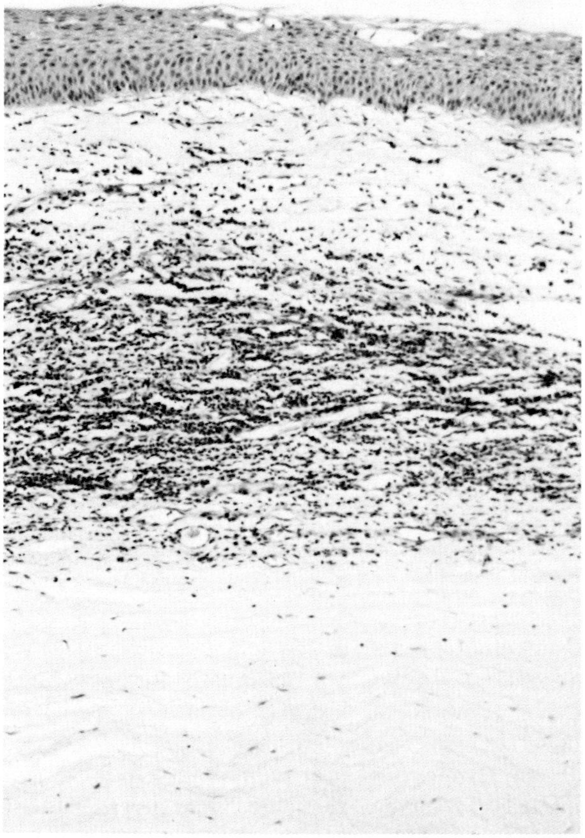

Figure 14-8 Globe, cornea; equine. Keratitis. Dense cellular infiltrates along with vessels are present in the edematous corneal stroma beneath a focally vacuolated corneal epithelium. H & E stain.

Keratitis can be superficial or deep. Superficial keratitis can be the result of corneal ulceration (ulcerative keratitis), secondary to drying of the corneal epithelium and conjunctiva from a paucity of the precorneal tear film (keratoconjunctivitis sicca) and a lesion of an immune-mediated disease (degenerative pannus or chronic super-

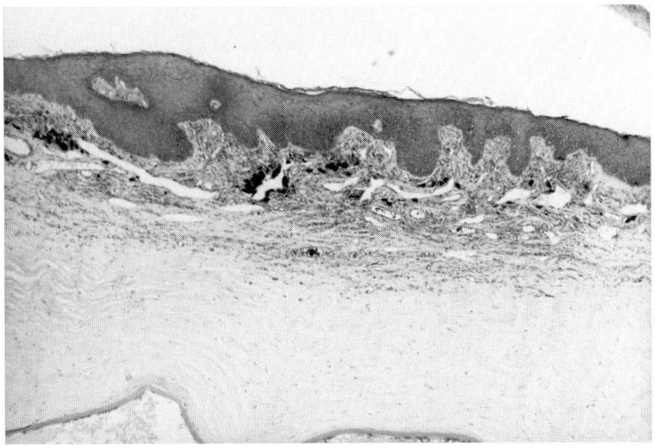

Figure 14-9 Globe, cornea; canine. Chronic keratitis. Epidermalization of corneal epithelium, superficial vascularization, and infiltration of inflammatory cells, with accumulation of melanocytes. H & E stain.

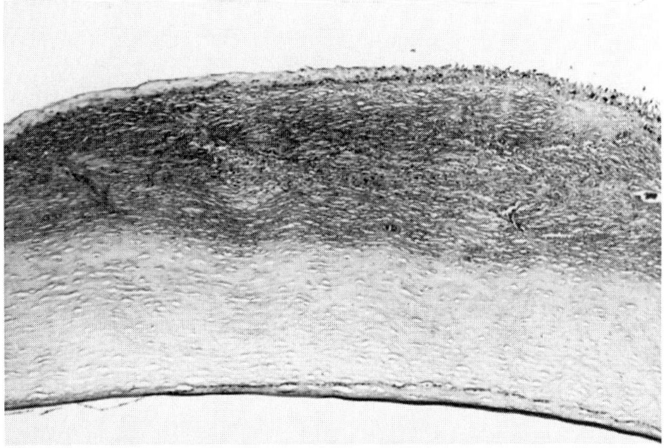

Figure 14-10 Globe, cornea; canine. Chronic superficial keratitis (degenerative pannus). H & E stain.

ficial keratitis). Deep keratitis is inflammation of the deep corneal stroma that can be caused by mycotic or bacterial infections or intraocular inflammation.

Keratoconjunctivitis Sicca

This disease (dry eye, xerophthalmia), common in the dog but rare in other domestic animals, is a chronic disease of the cornea and conjunctiva due to inadequate tear production. Keratoconjunctivitis sicca can be primary, secondary, or of unknown cause. The primary type results from congenital lack of lacrimal secretion or in response to spontaneous senile atrophy of the lacrimal glands (inadequate production of aqueous layer). Secondary keratoconjunctivitis sicca follows destruction of the lacrimal glands. Causes include canine distemper, trauma to the lacrimal glands or their nerve supply, occlusion of the lacrimal ducts as the result of chronic bacterial conjunctivitis, toxicity by certain drugs, and an immune-mediated inflammation.

The clinical signs vary greatly, depending on the severity of the reduced tear production. Reduction in serous tear production results in decreased lubrication of the cornea and conjunctiva; these tissues become painful, resulting in blepharospasm and endophthalmos. With decreased tear production, flushing of the surface of the cornea by tears is inadequate and a mucous residue accumulates, adheres to the conjunctiva, and accumulates on the central cornea. The corneal epithelium keratinizes, becomes thickened, and forms rete pegs similar to skin **(epidermalization)** (Fig. 14-9). As the disease progresses, the cornea becomes opaque, ulcerated, vascularized, and, possibly, pigmented. Similar corneal lesions occur if the globe is displaced anteriorly **(exophthalmos)** by retrocorneal, space-occupying lesions, especially if the eyelids do not cover the cornea **(lagophthalmos).**

Chronic Superficial Keratitis

Chronic superficial keratitis (Uberreiter's syndrome, degenerative pannus) is a progressive, bilateral inflammatory disease beginning at the temporal or inferior temporal limbus of the dog, especially the German shepherd breed. The lesion consists of corneal epithelial cells proliferating over a membrane of vascularized and pigmented granulation tissue that extends into the peripheral cornea (Fig. 14-10). Lymphocytes, plasma cells, and mast cells accompany the infiltrating fibrovascular tissue, which extends across the cornea. The cause is unknown but appears to be an immune-mediated disease with cell-mediated immunity to corneal antigens that is exacerbated by prolonged exposure to ultraviolet light.

Mycotic Keratitis

Mycotic keratitis **(keratomycosis)** occurs most often in the horse and rarely in other domesticated animals. Fungi of the genera *Aspergillus, Penicillium, Fusarium,* and *Cylindrocarpon* are reported causes of keratitis in the horse, but other fungi, such as *Candida albicans,* have been reported to cause keratitis in several species. Fungi such as *Aspergillus* sp. gain access to the corneal stroma during trauma, but have an affinity for Descemet's membrane, resulting in a deep stromal abscess (Fig. 14-11). Fungal hyphae are present along Descemet's membrane and are often surrounded by neutrophils. Lysis of Descemet's membrane is possible, but fungi are rarely found in the anterior chamber.

Bacterial Keratitis

The precorneal tear film of animals contains numerous bacteria. Some bacteria are nonpathogenic and others are opportunistic organisms that colonize the corneal stroma after gaining access following trauma. Examples of

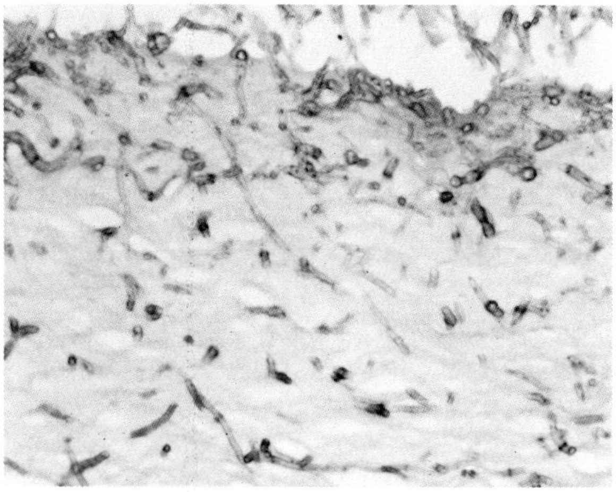

Figure 14-11 Globe, cornea; avian. Aspergillosis. Fungal hyphae are extending into the corneal stroma. H & E stain.

opportunistic bacteria isolated from neutrophilic keratitis include *Staphylococcus, Streptococcus, Bacillus,* and *Klebsiella* spp., and *Escherichia coli,* to mention a few. Other bacteria, such as *Moraxella bovis,* are considered primary pathogens. Bacteria, such as *Pseudomonas aeruginosa,* adhere, invade, and cause extensive destruction of the corneal stroma because of proteases, exotoxins that attract neutrophils. The liberation of collagenases result in collagenolysis, causing the corneal stroma to become clinically opaque and soft ("melting"). This type of keratitis is usually followed by corneal ulceration and is common in the horse.

Eosinophilic Keratitis

Eosinophilic keratitis is a unique type of keratitis that occurs in cats and horses. In cats, the lesion is referred to as proliferative keratoconjunctivitis. The typical lesion is a white to pink, irregular, raised, vascularized mass arising from the limbus. Microscopically, the lesion consists of plasma cells and lymphocytes with a variable number of eosinophils, macrophages, and mast cells. The cause is unknown, but feline herpesvirus-1 could be involved in the pathogenesis.

In horses, eosinophilic keratitis is manifested as a raised, white, subepithelial plaque covering a corneal ulcer. Accompanying clinical signs include blepharospasm, chemosis, and conjunctivitis. Microscopically, the plaques consist of coalescing foci of eosinophils, areas of collagenolysis and other inflammatory cells including mast cells, lymphocytes, plasma cells, and, possibly, neutrophils. The cause is unknown, but an allergic response, immune-mediated response, or inflammatory response to parasites are possibilities.

Corneal Edema

Corneal edema is a lesion caused by an uptake of fluid into the corneal stroma from the precorneal tear film, stromal

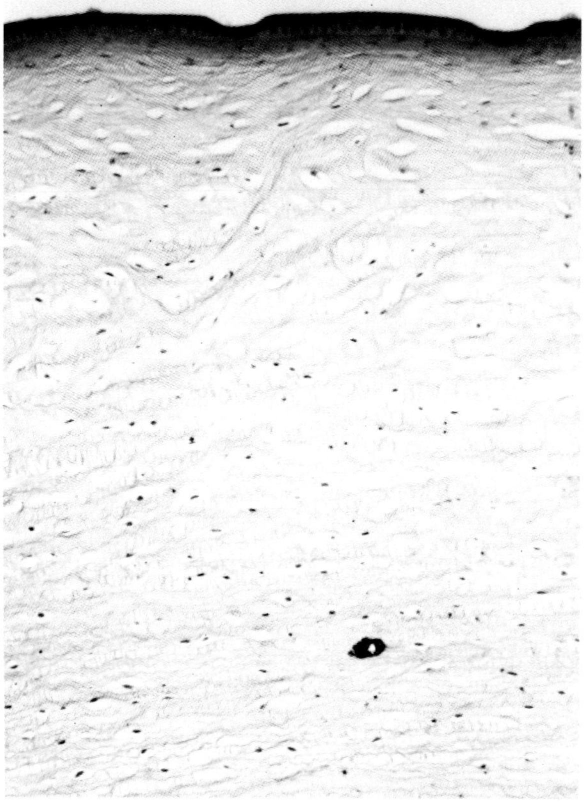

Figure 14-12 Globe, cornea; canine. Canine viral hepatitis. The pale-staining corneal stroma is thickened by edema. H & E stain.

blood vessels, or aqueous humor. The fluid disrupts the densely packed, parallel arrangement of lamellae of collagen needed for transparency. Clinically, corneal edema causes blue-gray opacification of the cornea. Microscopically, individual collagen fibers are separated, resulting in a thicker and paler-staining corneal stroma. This is in contrast to the fusiform unstained spaces in the corneal stroma, which are artifacts of fixation. Corneal edema can be secondary to corneal ulceration, keratitis, or endothelial dysfunction. Corneal edema resulting from superficial corneal injuries is usually restricted to the superficial corneal stroma immediately adjacent to the lesion. In contrast, corneal edema due to endothelial dysfunction is diffuse and tends to involve the deeper corneal stroma. Causes of endothelial dysfunction can include endothelial dystrophy that occurs in certain breeds of dog (e.g., Boston terrier, Chihuahua and dachshund), adherence of the iris to the corneal endothelium (anterior synechia), adherence of an anteriorly displaced lens to the corneal endothelium (anterior lens luxation), inflammation involving the corneal endothelium (e.g., infectious canine hepatitis, malignant catarrhal fever), aggregates of inflammatory cells adhered to the corneal endothelium (**keratic precipitates**), intraocular surgery, certain toxicants, and glaucoma (Fig. 14-12).

Corneal Response to Injury

The response of the cornea to injury depends on the extent of the lesion. Disruption of the continuity of the corneal epithelium, such as an abrasion, superficial ulcer, or laceration, is healed by a process of sliding and mitosis of adjacent corneal epithelial cells. This could be in response to epidermal growth factor. After approximately 1 hour, polygonal epithelial cells slide and flatten to cover the defect. If the defect is large, bulbar conjunctival epithelium at the limbus participates. Most small corneal defects are covered by epithelium between 48 and 72 hours after the injury.

Keratocytes within the corneal stroma are transformed into fibroblasts and vessels are formed from limbal angioblasts. Cytokines involved in this response include fibroblast growth factor and transforming growth factor-β. Recruitment begins within 24 hours after corneal stromal injury; the maximum rate of corneal migration by limbal blood vessels is 1 mm/d. Corneal vessels are not clinically noticeable for 2 to 5 days. Superficial vascularization is a response to superficial corneal disease, and deep stromal vascularization is a response to deep corneal stromal or intraocular disease.

Fibroblasts, transformed from keratocytes, often accompany migrating corneal vessels and form corneal granulation tissue. This new highly cellular corneal tissue is eventually remodeled to ensure the cellularity and organization of normal corneal stroma. Failure in this healing process results in a scar that appears as a corneal opacity of variable density. A **nebula** is a slight, diffuse, hazy superficial cornea opacity. A **macula** is a well-circumscribed, moderately dense corneal scar, and a **leukoma** is a white, dense corneal scar. If the iris adheres to the posterior surface of the cornea (anterior synechia), the scar is an **adherent leukoma.**

Healing of corneal perforation or other breaks in Descemet's membrane can involve fibroplasia. Fibroblasts within the defect spread along the inner surface of Descemet's membrane, forming a fibrous **retrocorneal membrane.** This membrane can result from proliferation of keratocytes or possibly from metaplasia of corneal endothelial cells.

Corneal Pigmentation

Black pigmentation of the cornea **(corneal melanosis)** is commonly associated with chronic inflammation of the cornea **(pigmentary keratitis).** Melanocytes migrate with blood vessels from the limbus, but as the vascularization resolves, the melanocytes remain. Corneal pigmentation also can occur when melanin is present in the cytoplasm of infiltrating macrophages or deposited within the cytoplasm of basal epithelial cells. Melanin also can be within the cytoplasm of stromal fibroblasts or possibly corneal endothelial cells. Corneal melanosis is a common lesion associated with chronic buphthalmos and chronic superficial keratitis.

In some cases, corneal pigmentation is not due to limbal melanocytes. Corneal pigmentation can be due to uveal pigment or possibly tear film. Black corneal lesions involving the iris include the adherence of the iris to the cornea **(anterior synechia),** incorporation of the iris into the corneal stroma **(anterior staphyloma),** and prolapse and incarceration of the iris through a site of corneal perforation **(iris prolapse).** Central black corneal lesions can be areas of corneal sequestration in cats.

Corneal Deposits

Deposits of calcium or lipid can occur in the cornea. Corneal deposits can be secondary to penetrating wounds or from topical applications or blood or can be the result of defective corneal metabolism. Microscopically, calcium appears as granular, basophilic deposits, often along basement membranes. Lipid, which is usually cholesterol, is removed during tissue processing, leaving fusiform, unstained spaces (cholesterol clefts).

Calcium is deposited adjacent to the basement membrane of the corneal epithelium. This results in a clinical gray-white, granular superficial corneal opacity. The distribution of the deposition is often oriented in a central horizontal zone within the area of the palpebral fissure **(band keratopathy),** and the overlying corneal epithelium can be nonadherent. The cause can be associated with localized keratitis (dystrophic calcification) or systemic hypercalcemia (metastatic calcification). Band keratopathy is reported in the dog and horse.

Certain strains of mice and rats have spontaneous subepithelial deposition of calcium within the cornea. In some mice, the deposits can be observed as early as 3 weeks of age. In rats, the deposits often occur between 7 and 26 weeks of age. Although the cause is unknown, genetic factors and environmental influences, such as exposure to excessive ammonia in cage bedding, are possible contributing factors.

Corneal lipidosis (lipid keratopathy) occurs either because of a metabolic defect within the corneal stroma (dystrophy), secondary to altered vascular permeability, or secondary to systemic hyperlipidemia (degeneration). Lipid corneal dystrophy is characterized by deposits rich in cholesterol. Clinically, the deposits are white to yellow and are oval. Lipid corneal degeneration can occur in dogs with hypothyroidism (arcus lipoides corneae) and in rabbits fed cholesterol-rich feed. Clinically, arc-shaped deposits occur adjacent to the limbic vasculature. Lipid also can accumulate from vascular leakage and can be present as cholesterol clefts within granulomatous inflammation **(xanthomatous keratitis)** (Fig. 14-13).

LESIONS OF THE CONJUNCTIVA

The conjunctiva (palpebral conjunctiva) is a mucous membrane that covers the posterior surface of the eyelids and both surfaces of the nictitating membrane. Bulbar conjunctiva is the conjunctiva that covers the episclera and

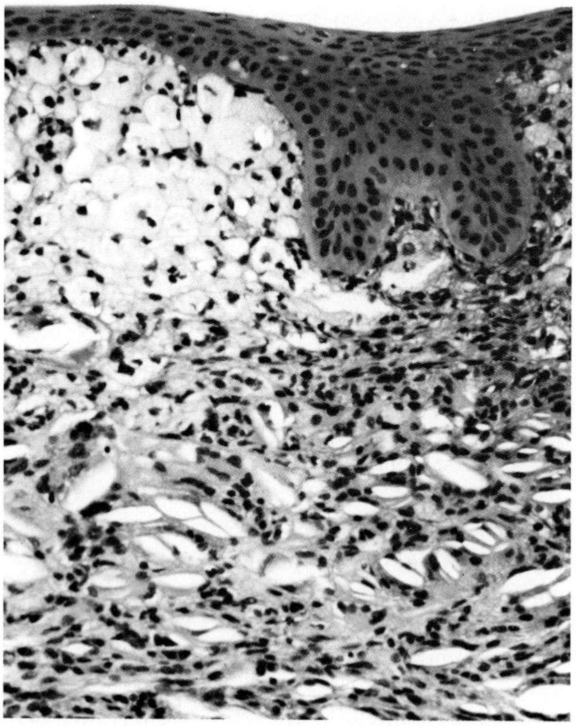

Figure 14-13 Globe, cornea; canine. Lipid keratopathy. Granulomatous keratitis has lesions of cholesterol clefts and large foamy macrophages with epidermalization of corneal epithelium. H & E stain.

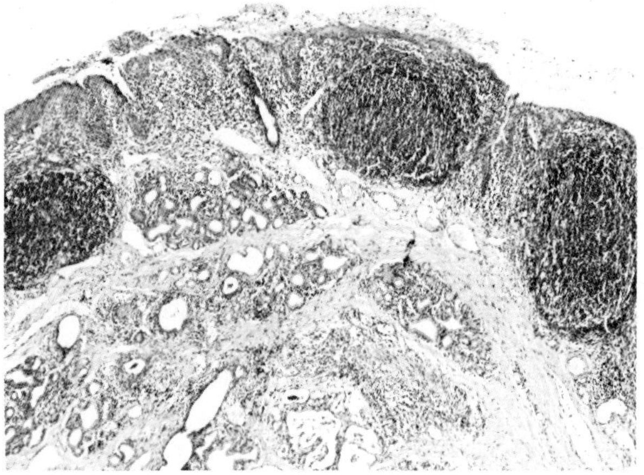

Figure 14-14 Eyelid, conjunctiva; canine. Follicular conjunctivitis. The lymphoid tissue is hyperplastic with follicle formation. H & E stain.

underlying anterior sclera of the globe. Palpebral conjunctiva becomes bulbar conjunctiva at the fornix. The epithelium of the bulbar conjunctiva abruptly becomes corneal epithelium at the limbus. Conjunctival goblet cells are plentiful in the fornix and produce the mucus portion of the precorneal tear film. Conjunctival-associated lymphoid tissue (CALT) is present beneath the conjunctival epithelium of the bulbar surface of the nictitating membrane and has immunologic functions.

Anomalies of the Conjunctiva

Congenital anomalies of the conjunctiva are rare, but include dermoid and pseudopterygium. **Dermoid** is a choristoma. Tissue resembling skin is present in the conjunctiva instead of normal conjunctival epithelium. **Pseudopterygium** is a fold of normal-appearing conjunctiva that extends over an unremarkable cornea. The lesion is rare, but reported in Dutch belted rabbits.

Conjunctivitis

The principal abnormality of the conjunctiva is inflammation **(conjunctivitis).** Acute conjunctivitis is often characterized by congestion of vessels, edema **(chemosis),** and possibly an overflow of tears **(epiphora).** An ocular discharge can be serous, mucoid, or mucopurulent. Chronic conjunctivitis is characterized by an increased number of goblet cells, epithelial cell hyperplasia, squamous metaplasia with keratinization, and subepithelial accumulation of lymphocytes and plasma cells. Lymphocytes can form subepithelial aggregates **(follicular conjunctivitis),** especially along the bulbar surface of the nictitating membrane, and give the conjunctiva a cobblestone appearance (Fig. 14-14). Conjunctivitis can be associated with inflammation in other locations. For example, conjunctivitis is often a manifestation of an upper respiratory tract disease and occurs with concurrent inflammation of the cornea **(keratoconjunctivitis).** Possible sequelae, especially of neonatal conjunctivitis, are adhesion between the upper and lower eyelids **(ankyloblepharon)** and adhesion of the palpebral conjunctiva to the cornea or bulbar conjunctiva **(symblepharon).**

Causes of conjunctivitis are numerous. Conjunctival blood vessels become engorged with blood and fluid accumulates within the loose connective tissue quickly after trauma, exposure to mechanical irritants, allergens, toxins, or pathogenic microbes. Conjunctival congestion ("red eye") is a common and nonspecific clinical sign of conjunctivitis. Causes include drying of the conjunctiva from an inadequate covering of tears. This occurs secondary to an outward deviation of the margin of the eyelid (ectropion), an inability to blink (lagophthalmos), or an inadequate quantity of tears (keratoconjunctivitis sicca). Other causes of conjunctival congestion, or underlying episcleral congestion, include corneal irritation from abnormal eyelids or cilia, other corneal disease, anterior uveitis, glaucoma, or orbital disease. Infectious conjunctivitis occurs in all species and is more common in cats and cattle than other domesticated animals. Viruses, mycobacteria, chlamydiae, other bacteria, fungi, and parasites are all potential causes of conjunctivitis. Conjunctival infections caused by more than one infectious agent are possible. For example, neonatal conjunctivitis, an acute inflammatory diseases of neonatal kittens characterized by copious mucopurulent ocular discharge, is caused by several infectious agents including feline herpesvirus-1, bacteria, and chlamydial organisms.

Viral Conjunctivitis

Conjunctivitis can be a manifestation of a viral disease. Transient intracytoplasmic viral inclusions can be present in the conjunctiva of dogs or other susceptible animals (raccoons) with canine distemper. Cats with feline immunodeficiency viral infection can have mild conjunctivitis. Conjunctivitis can be a manifestation of equine viral arteritis, equine adenovirus infection, and an infection by herpesvirus-1 in cattle (infectious bovine rhinotracheitis).

In addition to keratitis and tracheobronchitis, conjunctivitis is a lesion of an infection by feline herpesvirus-1 in neonatal and adolescent cats. Cats develop latent viral infections and have periodic recrudescent of clinical disease later in life. The infection is characterized by conjunctival congestion and serous ocular discharge, which can be mucoid or mucopurulent. Microscopic lesions include epithelial necrosis, neutrophil infiltration, dendritic ulceration of the cornea, and transient intranuclear inclusions within conjunctival and corneal epithelial cells.

Bacterial Conjunctivitis

Bacterial conjunctivitis is a common disease in many animal species. Although numerous bacteria, and other microbes are isolated from the conjunctiva of animals, many are nonpathogenic or only cause mild, transient disease. For example, *Moraxella (Branhamella) ovis* is isolated from the conjunctiva of healthy sheep and from sheep with conjunctivitis. Pathogenic bacteria include *Pasteurella multocida* in rabbits and *Staphylococcus* sp. and other gram-positive bacteria in dogs. These bacteria cause mucopurulent conjunctivitis. In poultry, conjunctivitis with ocular discharge and associated blepharitis can be clinical signs of fowl cholera, a disease caused by *P. multocida.* Similar clinical signs can be caused by *Bordetella avium* in young turkeys and *Haemophilus paragallinarum,* the cause of infectious coryza in chickens. Other bacteria causing conjunctivitis in birds include *Staphylococcus aureus, Streptococcus* sp., *Erysipelothrix rhusiopathiae,* and *Pseudomonas aeruginosa.*

Chlamydial Conjunctivitis

Infections by *Chlamydophila (Chlamydia) psittaci* occur in birds and other animals, especially cats, sheep, goats, and swine and can be manifested as conjunctivitis. In birds, the conjunctiva can be infiltrated with heterophils, macrophages, lymphocytes, and plasma cells. In cats, acute lesions are characterized by conjunctival congestion, chemosis, serous ocular discharge, and infiltration of the conjunctiva with neutrophils. Intracytoplasmic inclusions can be present, and lymphocytic nodules (follicular conjunctivitis) develop as the infection becomes chronic. In sheep and goats, the infection is known as infectious keratoconjunctivitis, but polyarthritis also can occur. The characteristic lesion is follicular conjunctivitis. Similar lesions can be caused by *M. ovis.*

Mycoplasmal Conjunctivitis

Different species of *Mycoplasma* have been reported to cause conjunctivitis in birds, cats *(M. felis),* sheep *(M. conjunctivae* and *M. agalactiae),* goats *(M. mycoides* subsp. *mycoides),* and cattle *(M. bovis, M. laidlawii,* and *M. bovirhinis).* A similar infectious agent, *Ureaplasma* sp., has been associated with conjunctivitis in cattle. Poultry and house finches can develop conjunctival congestion and chemosis and an ocular discharge as clinical signs of an infection with *Mycoplasma gallisepticum.* Microscopic findings include epithelial hyperplasia and proliferation of conjunctival-associated lymphocytes. Microcolonies of mycoplasmal organisms adhere to the surface of the conjunctival epithelium. Concurrent keratitis (keratoconjunctivitis) and uveitis can occur, as well as concurrent secondary bacterial conjunctival infections. Similar lesions (acute conjunctival congestion, chemosis, epiphora, and neutrophilic infiltration progressing to follicular conjunctivitis) are present in cats and food animals with conjunctival mycoplasmal infections. Intracytoplasmic coccobacillary and ring-shaped bodies can be observed cytologically in epithelial cells.

Parasitic Conjunctivitis

Parasitic conjunctivitis occurs in many different mammalian and avian species. The cause can be coincidental invasion by a migrating nematode larvae (e.g., *Oestrus ovis* in sheep) or because the conjunctival sac is the normal location for an adult parasite. Mammals, especially cattle and horses living in the western United States and Canada, can have *Thelazia* sp. within the conjunctival sac and nasolacrimal ducts. Some species of this small, slender, white nematode have been reported in dogs and cats. Although the role of *Thelazia* sp. in causing ocular disease is uncertain, the parasites are generally reported as nonpathogenic or mildly pathogenic, resulting in mild lymphoplasmacytic conjunctivitis. Mild to severe ocular lesions have been reported in wild and domestic birds infested with the nematode *Oxyspirura* sp. or the trematode *Philophthalmus gralli.*

Allergic Conjunctivitis

Allergic conjunctivitis occurs frequently in the dog, especially as a component of a type I hypersensitivity reaction to pollen, dust, or bacterial toxins. Clinical signs include conjunctival congestion, chemosis, pruritus, and serous ocular discharge. Microscopic findings include lymphocytes, plasma cells, and a few eosinophils within the conjunctiva.

Lipogranulomatous Conjunctivitis

Lipogranulomatous conjunctivitis occurs in cats and is characterized by the deposition of lipid within the connective tissue of the conjunctiva. Associated with this deposition is granulomatous inflammation and goblet cell hyperplasia. The source of the lipid can be the Meibomian gland, adipose sites in the connective tissue, or possibly lipid from a subconjunctival injection. When an aggregate of lipid-laden foamy macrophages occurs in the palpebral conjunctiva, the lesion is termed **xanthoma,** or **xanthelasma.**

Ligneous Conjunctivitis

Ligneous conjunctivitis is a unique inflammatory lesion seen in dogs, especially in Doberman pinschers. It is characterized by an eosinophilic pseudomembrane and subconjunctival exudate composed of fibrin and amorphous material intermixed with lymphocytes and plasma cells. The lesion must be distinguished from amyloidosis, which occurs as amorphous eosinophilic, hyaline deposits; amyloidosis rarely occurs within subconjunctival connective tissue.

Conjunctival Neoplasms

Except for squamous cell carcinoma in cattle, horses, and cats, neoplasms of the conjunctiva are uncommon. Conjunctival neoplasms are not common in the dog, but include squamous epithelial neoplasms (papilloma and squamous cell carcinoma), mast cell tumor, and vascular neoplasms (hemangioma, hemangiosarcoma and angiokeratoma). Conjunctival lymphosarcoma can also occur, but is often an extension of an orbital or intraocular lesion.

Squamous epithelial neoplasms of the conjunctiva include primary neoplasms (squamous cell papilloma, carcinoma in situ, and squamous cell carcinoma) and metastatic ones (e.g., canine transmissible venereal tumor). Squamous cell papilloma is more common in cattle than other animals and appears as a soft or hard, pedunculated or sessile, gray, red, or black mass. Microscopically, it consists of a stalk of fibrous connective tissue covered by well-differentiated stratified squamous epithelium.

Squamous cell carcinoma of the conjunctiva is a pink or white, variable size, irregular mass that is often ulcerated. It is common in the horse and reported in dogs and cats. The greatest incidence of squamous cell carcinoma is in cattle lacking circumocular and periocular pigmentation and living in geographic areas that have prolonged exposure to sunlight, especially ultraviolet radiation. The neoplasm arises from the conjunctiva of the nictitating membrane and lower eyelid, but many of the lesions are at the limbus, and some involve the cornea (Fig. 14-15). Lesions have a tendency to expand along the edge of the eyelids at the palpebral fissure. Lesions can begin as an area of epithelial dysplasia but develop into carcinoma and, eventually, invasive carcinoma. Untreated squamous cell carcinoma gradually enlarges and infiltrates into adjacent tissues. Invasion into lymph vessels also occurs with the formation of emboli of neoplastic cells. Metastasis to regional lymph nodes and other sites occurs late in the disease. Genetic and viral factors have been suggested in the pathogenesis of the lesion, but prolonged exposure to solar ultraviolet radiation appears to be a major cause.

Conjunctival vascular neoplasms include hemangioma, hemangiosarcoma, and angiokeratoma. Hemangiomatous lesions occur in the bulbar conjunctiva of dogs, usually at the lateral limbus. Grossly, they appear as a smooth, red or black nodule. Small lesions are focal clusters of vessels or well-circumscribed blood-filled spaces (hematocysts). Large lesions are composed of variably sized spaces filled with blood and lined by well-differentiated flat endothelial cells (hemangioma). Large lesions are composed of poorly differentiated cells

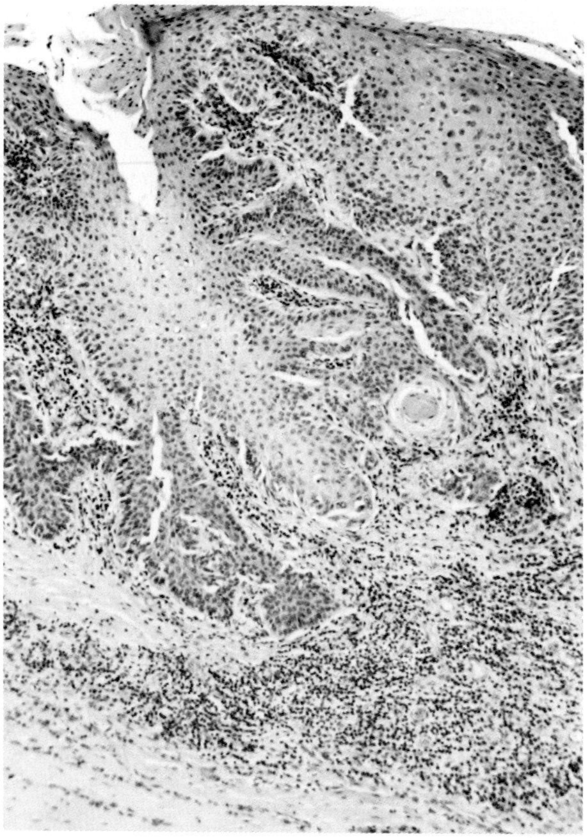

Figure 14-15 Globe, cornea; bovine. Squamous cell carcinoma. Infiltrating cords of neoplastic squamous cells are accompanied by an inflammatory cell infiltrate in the corneal stroma. H & E stain.

arranged in a sheet with poorly defined vascular spaces. Cellular anisokaryosis, pleomorphism, and mitotic activity are present (hemangiosarcoma). Angiokeratoma is a discrete, superficial focus of large, dilated, and engorged vascular spaces adjacent to an overlying hyperplastic epithelium. Complete surgical excision of these neoplasms appears to be curative.

Transmissible venereal tumor (TVT) is a disease that is endemic in areas with large populations of stray dogs. The lesions of TVT occur on the exernal genitalia of both sexes and on the head and seldom metastasize. Intraocular metastasis can occur in addition to direct spread to palpebral conjunctiva. Grossly, the lesion consists of numerous, red nodules, 2 to 6 mm in diameter. The lesion consists of a uniform population of discrete, round to polygonal cells with either abundant clear cytoplasm or moderate with fine granular eosinophilia.

LESIONS OF THE SCLERA AND EPISCLERA

Both the sclera and cornea form the outer, supportive, fibrous tunic of the globe. The sclera is composed of interwoven bundles of collagen. To help maintain the normal shape of the globe, cartilage and bone are present within the sclera of birds and some reptiles. The sclera contains passageways (emissaria) for vessels and nerves and for the optic nerve (lamina cribrosa). The uvea can extend along the vessels in the scleral emissaria; therefore, inflammatory cells can be present around vessels during uveitis without scleritis, and neoplastic uveal cells can surround scleral vessels without neoplastic infiltration into these vessels.

The junction between the transparent cornea and the opaque sclera is the limbus. At the limbus the corneal epithelium abruptly changes into bulbar conjunctiva. The bulbar conjunctiva covers the underlying episclera, which covers the rostral aspect of the sclera. The episclera is a layer of well-vascularized connective tissue.

Scleral Thinning, Scleral Ectasia, and Staphyloma

The shape of the sclera can be diffusely or focally altered. Diffuse scleral thinning occurs as the globe becomes enlarged (buphthalmos) from persistent increased intraocular pressure (glaucoma). Focal thinning and outward bulging of the sclera (scleral ectasia) can be related to coloboma or can be the result of an acquired lesion in which the thinned sclera is lined by uvea (staphyloma). Clinically, staphyloma is a localized black lesion in the sclera and needs to be differentiated from outward extension of intraocular melanoma or limbal melanoma.

Scleritis

Inflammation of the sclera (scleritis) is usually secondary and the result of an extension of inflammation from the uvea (uveitis), episclera (episcleritis), conjunctiva (conjunctivitis), or orbit (orbital cellulitis). When inflammation involving the uvea and other intraocular structures (endophthalmitis) extends outward to include the sclera, the condition is referred to as panophthalmitis. Primary scleritis is rare, but does occur in the dog.

Primary scleritis in the dog is granulomatous and classified as either nonnecrotizing or necrotizing. The cause is unknown, but considered to be immune mediated. Nonnecrotizing granulomatous scleritis is characterized by infiltration of lymphocytes, plasma cells, and epithelioid macrophages into the sclera with possible associated lymphoplasmacytic uveitis. Necrotizing granulomatous scleritis is a rare lesion in dogs and characterized by collagenolysis surrounded by palisading granulomatous inflammation with giant cells (Fig. 14-16).

Episcleritis

Lesions of the episclera occur most often in the dog and include inflammation (episcleritis) and limbal melanoma. Episcleritis can be divided into primary episcleritis and secondary episcleritis. Primary episcleritis is either simple nodular episcleritis, an infrequent and possibly self-limiting lesion, or nodular granulomatous episcleral keratoconjunctivitis, which has been diagnosed as nodular fasciitis, fibrous histiocytoma, or proliferative keratoconjunctivitis. This lesion is a firm, nodular, pink solitary mass that is composed of a mixture of histiocytes (macrophages), lymphocytes, and a variable number of plasma cells, neutrophils, and fibroblasts. The lesion usually occurs at the limbus with extension into the cornea and can be bilateral, especially in the collie and Shetland

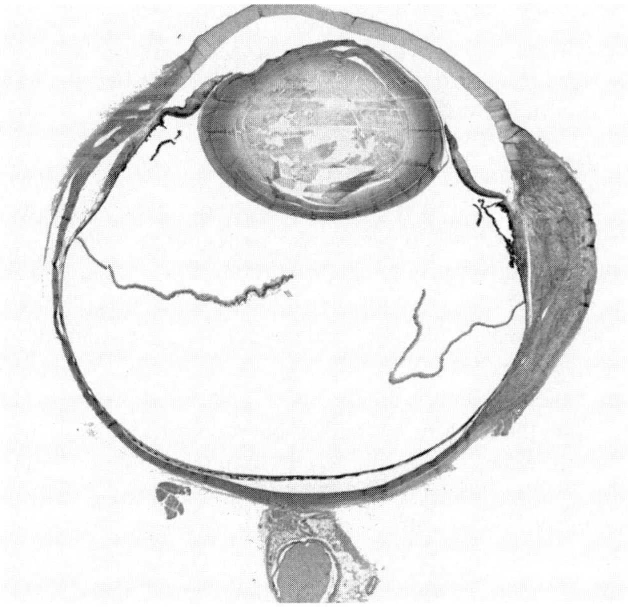

Figure 14-16 Globe; canine. Necrotizing granulomatous scleritis. Focal inflammation of the sclera *(right)* around an area of scleral collagenolysis. H & E stain.

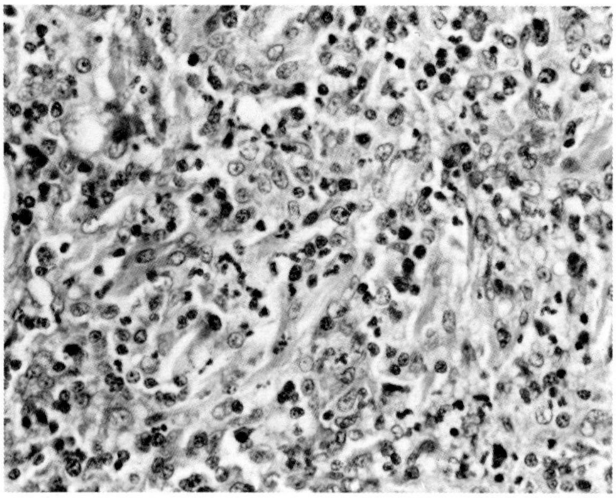

Figure 14-17 Eyelid; canine. Nodular granulomatous blepharitis. Mass is composed of fibroblasts, histiocytes, lymphocytes, and plasma cells. H & E stain.

sheepdog. A similar lesion can be present in the conjunctiva of the eyelid and nictitating membrane or within the orbital connective tissue (Fig. 14-17). The cause is unknown, but appears to be immune mediated.

Limbal Melanoma

Limbal melanoma (epibulbar melanoma) is a fairly common lesion in the dog, especially in certain breeds (e.g., German shepherd) and occasionally has been reported in cats (Fig. 14-18). The morphologic appearance is similar to melanocytoma of the canine anterior uvea. Limbal melanoma is composed of many plump cells and some spindle cells. All cells have an abundance of intracytoplasmic melanin. The neoplasm is benign, but because it will extend inward, the removal of the globe is often required.

LESIONS OF THE UVEA

The uvea is the pigmented vascular tunic of the globe that provides nutrients to intraocular structures. It consists of the iris, ciliary body, and choroid. The iris and ciliary body are termed the anterior uvea, and the choroid is the posterior uvea. The ciliary body and choroid are adjacent to the inner aspect of the sclera. The iris is anterior to the lens and extends from the anterior portion of the ciliary body to separate the anterior chamber from the posterior chamber. The iris serves as a diaphragm to limit the amount of light to the retina. The edge of the pupil is called the pupillary margin (pupillary ruff). The base of the iris (root of the iris) is internal to the peripheral cornea and the anterior sclera. The pectinate ligament extends from the root of the iris to the peripheral edge of Descemet's membrane.

The anterior surface of the iris, which can be viewed clinically, can be divided into the pupillary zone and the ciliary zone. The pupillary zone is located between the pupillary margin and the collarette. The ciliary zone is

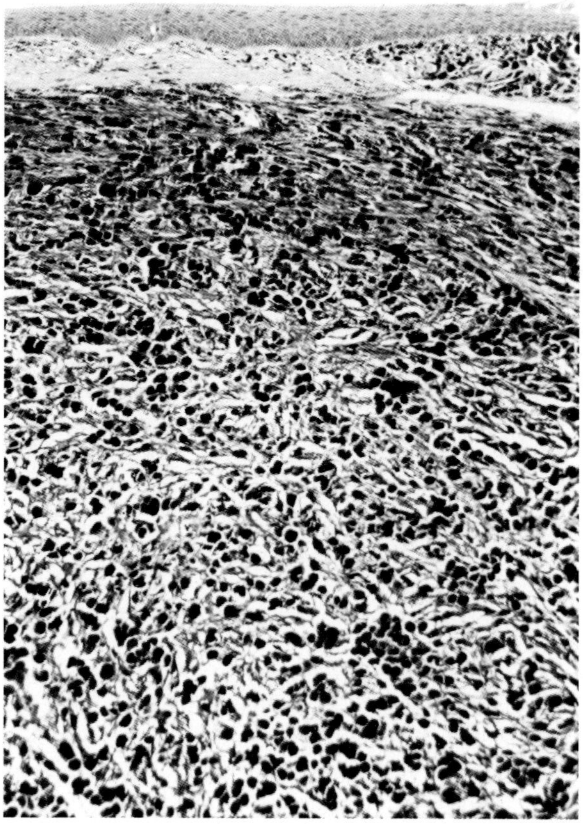

Figure 14-18 Globe, bulbar conjunctiva and episclera; canine. Limbal (epibulbar) melanoma. Neoplasm composed of pigment-filled spindle and round cells. H & E stain.

located between the collarette and the root of the iris. The anterior border of the iris is devoid of epithelium, but the posterior surface is covered by two layers of iridal epithelium. The iridal epithelium is continuous with the two layers of ciliary epithelium. Herbivores have black nodules along the dorsal margin of the pupil (granula iridica, corpora nigra). These masses are composed of iridal epithelial cells and are normal structures.

The stroma of the iris contains blood vessels, muscles, and nerves. Iridal muscles are composed of smooth muscle fibers in mammals and striated muscle fibers in birds. The sphincter muscle surrounds the pupil, and contraction causes the pupil to be small. Microscopically, the sphincter is located near the pupillary margin. The dilator muscle is located in the iridal epithelium. Contraction of this muscle causes the pupil to become large. These muscles are controlled by the autonomic nervous system.

The ciliary body is located between the iris and the choroid. This component of the anterior uvea is divided into an anterior pars plicata and the posterior pars plana. The ciliary body is responsible for continuous formation of aqueous humor and for changing the shape of the lens. The ciliary body is covered by two layers of ciliary epithelium. The inner ciliary epithelium is nonpigmented and is continuous with the inner pigmented iridal epithelium and the sensory retina. The outer pigmented ciliary epithelium is continuous with the outer iridal epithelium and the retinal pigment epithelium. The pars plicata is composed of ciliary processes. Zonular fibers extend from the basement membrane of the inner ciliary epithelium and attach to the lens capsule.

The ciliary body has a muscle located mainly in the outer aspect of the pars plicata. The size of the muscle varies among species. For example, the muscle is well developed in primates and poorly developed in rodents. The myofibers are striated in mammals but nonstriated in birds. When the ciliary muscle contracts, tension on the zonular fibers and the lens capsule is decreased, thus causing the lens to have a more spherical shape suitable for near vision. Relaxation of the ciliary muscle increases tension on the zonular fibers and the lens capsule, thus causing the lens to have a flattened shape suitable for distance vision.

The choroid is continuous with the stroma of the pars plana and forms the layer of vessels and melanocytes sandwiched between the retina and the sclera. The innermost layer is the choriocapillaris. The basal lamina of the capillaries in this layer combine with collagen, and the basal lamina of the retinal pigment epithelium form Bruch's membrane. Some animals have specialized, reactive tissue beneath Bruch's membrane in the superior half of the ocular fundus (tapetum lucidum). The tapetum lucidum is absent in some species (e.g., rodent, rabbit, pig, primate, bird, reptile) and varies in its histologic appearance. In dogs and cats, the tapetal cells have an epithelial appearance with intracytoplasmic reflecting rods (tapetum cellulosum). In ungulates, the layer is composed of regularly arranged collagenous fibers (tapetum fibrosum). The entire retina overlying the tapetum lucidium is transparent because the retinal pigment epithelium is nonpigmented. Therefore, light is reflected back through the retina, thus allowing for maximal stimulation by available light, especially at night.

Blood-eye Barrier

The blood-eye barrier is actually two barriers, which restrict the amount of ocular antigens that reach the general circulation. There are two components for each barrier, each relying on tight junctions. The barriers are the blood-aqueous barrier and the blood-retina barrier. The blood-aqueous barrier is composed of an endothelial portion involving iridal vessels and the epithelial component involving the nonpigmented epithelium of the ciliary body. The two components of the blood-retina barrier are the endothelium of the retinal capillaries and the retinal pigment epithelium. Breakdown of the endothelial blood-aqueous barrier results in protein and cells accumulating in the anterior chamber. Breakdown of the epithelial blood-aqueous barrier results in an inflammatory exudate overlying the ciliary processes. Breakdown of the epithelial blood-retina barrier results in serous or exudative retinal detachment as the subretinal space is expanded. Breakdown of the endothelial blood-retina barrier results in edema of the retina.

Iridal Hypopigmentation

The color of the iris is determined mainly by the amount of stroma pigmentation. The variation in the number or distribution of melanocytes within the iris causes the variation in the color of the iris. The lack of the expected color within a part or all of the iris of the same animal, or between the irises of an animal and other animals of the same breed is called **heterochromia iridis,** or **irides,** respectively. This cause of hypopigmentation of the iris can be unilateral or bilateral and has been described in many domestic animal species. The lesion can be congenital and associated with white coat color and deafness, idiopathic, or due to atrophy following trauma or inflammation. The microscopic changes include pigment abnormalities, hypoplasia of the iridal stroma, reduction in iridal pigment, and clumping, irregular distribution, or partial absence of pigment in the iridal stroma or possibly other portions of the uvea.

Pale irides, hypopigmentation of the fundus, and photophobia are ocular manifestations of **Chédiak-Higashi syndrome,** an autosomal recessive disorder of cats, cattle, mink, and mice. Systemic manifestations include cutaneous hypopigmentation, increased susceptibility to infections, and abnormal coagulation. Microscopically, melanocytes and neutrophils contain giant cytoplasmic granules, and tapetal cells can be decreased in number and disorganized. The ocular hypopigmentation has been associated with fusion of premelanosomes with lysosomes. Remaining melanosomes are irregular.

Iridociliary Cysts

Congenital iridociliary cysts are variably sized, spherical, unilateral or bilateral, single or multiple hollow masses that develop along the posterior border of the iris, especially near the pupillary margin and within the ciliary epithelium, especially along the pars plicata. The cysts are lined by attenuated cuboidal epithelium and originate when fluid accumulates within the potential space between the epithelial layers derived from the neuroectoderm of the anterior border of the optic cup. Iridociliary cysts are usually darkly pigmented, but can be nonpigmented and progressively enlarge. Some become dislodged and float in the anterior chamber and are possible causes of glaucoma. The cyst is common in retriever breeds of dog and might be clinically apparent only after the dog is several years old.

Aniridia and Iridal Hypoplasia

An arrest in the differentiation of the layers of the anterior optic cup can cause malformation of the iris. The iris can be partially (**iridal hypoplasia**) or totally (**aniridia**) absent because of a failure of induction of the anterior segment

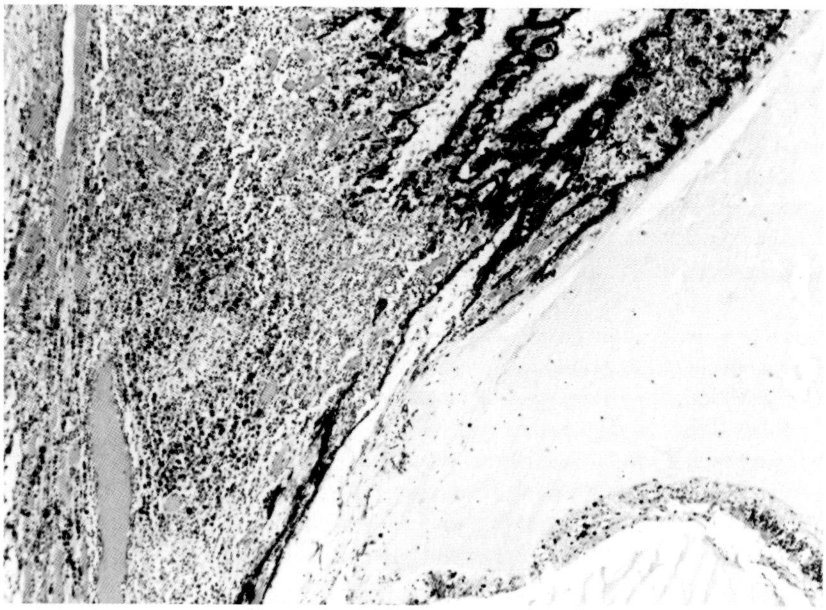

Figure 14-19 Globe, ciliary body, vitreous body and retina; canine. Lymphoplasmacytic cyclitis, plasmoid vitreous, and retinal detachment. Proteinaceous exudate fills the subretinal space beneath the detached retina with peripheral atrophy. H & E stain.

mesenchyme. Aniridia and iridal hypoplasia are rare and can be associated with other anomalies, including microphthalmia, corneal opacities, glaucoma, and cataract.

Persistent Pupillary Membrane

Mesenchyme in the region of the developing iris contains vessels that normally undergo atrophy in the dog by 6 months of age. Failure to undergo atrophy results in persistent pupillary membrane that is common in certain breeds of dog (e.g., basenji dog). The lesion consists of thin, threadlike vascular strands covered by a thin adventitial stroma that extends from the region of the iris collarette or minor anterior circle of the iris to the cornea. The strands can insert on the iris, extend into the anterior chamber, and possibly bridge the iris.

Choroidal Hypoplasia

Faulty differentiation of the retinal pigment epithelium results in a failure in the normal induction of the choroid. Choroidal hypoplasia is manifested as a thin choroid and a thin or absent tapetum lucidum. This is a relatively common lesion in collie dogs and is associated with genes for color dilution. Choroidal hypoplasia is a lesion of ocular dysgenesis and the collie eye anomaly.

Ocular Trauma

Injuries to the globe follow blunt trauma (contusion) or perforation. Contusion can result in tears or stromal necrosis of the iris with intraocular hemorrhage. Separation of the root of the iris from the ciliary body **(iridodialysis)** causes marked hemorrhage, especially into anterior chamber **(hyphema).** Blood can be present in all chambers of the globe **(hemophthalmos),** and hemosiderin from previous intraocular hemorrhage can be present **(hemosiderosis bulbi).** With excessive hemorrhage, iridal adhesions form and result in glaucoma. Contusion of the ciliary body results in hemorrhage and separation of the ciliary body from the sclera **(cyclodialysis),** or rupture of zonular fibers and dislocation of the lens. Contusion of the choroid causes choroidal hemorrhage and possibly hemorrhagic retinal detachment. If injuries are the result of perforation, aqueous humor is lost with collapse of the anterior chamber and intraocular pressure is markedly decreased **(hypotony).** Iris prolapse, lens prolapse, or incarceration of the iris into the wound **(iridencleisis)** are possible lesions resulting from perforation.

Ocular Inflammation

Maintenance of intraocular structures in a normal state is essential for the maintenance of vision. Although pathologic processes, especially inflammation, involving the globe are similar to those in other parts of the body, the potential for serious consequences, such as the eye becoming nonfunctional (blind), are much greater.

Because the uvea is the vascular layer of the globe, ocular inflammation **(ophthalmitis)** usually involves this layer **(uveitis).** Inflammation can involve one or more of the components of the uvea, for example the iris **(iritis),** ciliary body **(cyclitis),** iris and ciliary body **(iridocyclitis** or **anterior uveitis),** choroid **(choroiditis),** or entire uvea **(panuveitis)** (Fig. 14-19). When structures interior to the sclera are inflamed, including the uvea, the condition is endophthalmitis. When inflammation involves all tunics of the globe, the lesion is panophthalmitis (Fig. 14-20).

In the eye, as well as other parts of the body, inflammation occurs in stages. The first stage is acute and characterized by hyperemia and increased vascular permeability. Fluid and protein move from vessels into the

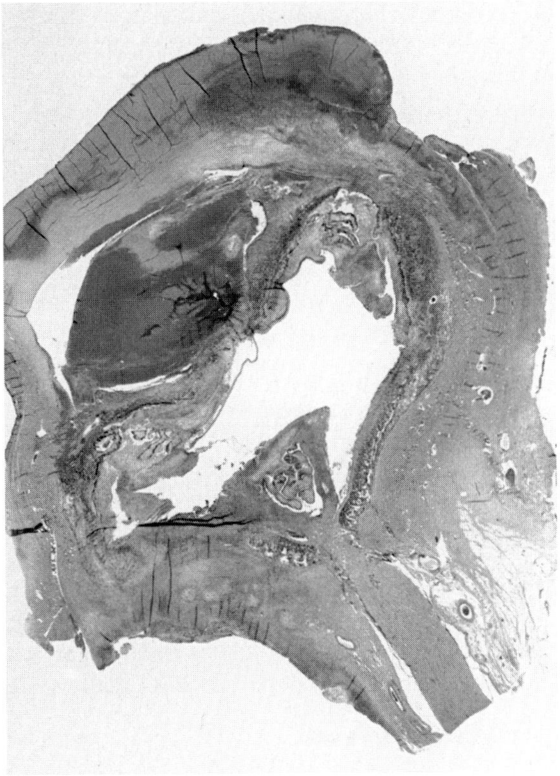

Figure 14-20 Globe; canine. Panophthalmitis, orbital cellulitis, and early phthisis bulbi. Keratitis, exudate in anterior chamber, panuveitis, no distinct lens, hyalitis, retinal scleritis, detachment and retinitis, and orbital cellulitis are other lesions. The globe is distorted and shrunken, early stage of phthisis bulbi. H & E stain.

surrounding tissue. Hemorrhages also can occur. This stage is followed by a cellular stage that involves chemotaxis and movement of inflammatory cells from vessels into intraocular tissues and spaces. The final stage involves resolution and repair.

Even though ocular inflammation is dynamic and ever changing, the characteristics of the inflammatory response are often indicative of certain diseases. Increased vascular permeability, especially in the iris, results in secondary lesions. Along the anterior surface of the iris, there is no barrier to fluid movement. Fluid, protein, blood, and cells can move easily into the anterior chamber. Vascular leakage of protein into the anterior chamber can be observed clinically **(aqueous flare).** Blood can occur in the anterior chamber **(hyphema)** or in several intraocular chambers **(hemophthalmos).** Neutrophils also can accumulate in the anterior chamber **(hyphema).**

Increased vascular permeability in the ciliary processes results in swelling of these structures from edema. Fluid is held in the ciliary stroma by the epithelial component of the anterior blood-eye barrier (tight junctions between the ciliary epithelial cells). If the inflammation becomes severe, this barrier can be breeched.

The type of exudate and the pattern of inflammation are helpful in determining the cause of ocular disease. Focal to multifocal granulomatous inflammation is a lesion indicating the possible presence of certain intraocular parasites, fungi, or bacteria. The parasites can be migrating larvae of roundworms, for example, larvae of the raccoon roundworm, *Baylisascaris procyonis* and the canine roundworm, *Toxocara canis.* Discrete granulomas can be found in the vitreous body, retina, or choroid. These lesions consist of macrophages, multinucleated giant cells, and possibly eosinophils, lymphocytes, and plasma cells. Multifocal coalescing pyogranulomas are typical ocular manifestation of coccidioidomycosis. Higher bacteria, such as *Mycobacteria* sp., incite granulomatous inflammation when present in the globe. Multinucleated giant cells can be present, depending on the mycobacterial and animal species.

Ocular Vasculitis

Vasculitis is usually associated with a systemic bacterial infection (septicemia) or a systemic viral infection. Necrosis of vascular walls with accumulation of fibrin and fibrin thrombosis are common findings of bacterial infections that result in septicemia (e.g., *Hemophilus somnus* in cattle, *Salmonella* sp. in several species, and coliforms in calves). Bacterial vasculitis can also occur secondary to contaminated penetrating intraocular wounds. Viral diseases with ocular vasculitis include malignant catarrhal fever in cattle and feline infectious peritonitis.

Neutrophilic Inflammation

Neutrophils can be present within ocular tissues or ocular chambers and can occur concurrently with the exudation of fibrin and tissue necrosis. Causes of neutrophilic inflammation include the presence of intraocular bacteria, septicemia, or an immune-mediated response. Bacteria can gain access to the interior of the globe through penetrating or perforating wounds, corneal ulcers, or via the vascular system. The extent and severity vary depending on the route of exposure, size of the inoculum, virulence of the infectious organism, and host response.

Neutrophils are prominent inflammatory cells in type III hypersensitivity reactions. Complement fixation and neutrophil chemotaxis are involved in the pathogenesis of certain viral diseases, such as canine infectious hepatitis. This mechanism is the cause of the destruction of corneal endothelial cells that results in the diffuse corneal edema typical of the disease. Neutrophils are a part of the suppurative uveitis secondary to septicemia and pyogranulomatous uveitis caused by intraocular infection by systemic fungi (e.g., *Blastomyces dermatitidis), Prototheca* sp., or higher bacteria (e.g., *Nocardia* sp.). Neutrophils are the major inflammatory cells involved in the response to a ruptured lens capsule.

Acute uveitis is often an anterior uveitis. Neutrophilic anterior uveitis is characterized by numerous neutrophils and fibrin within the anterior chamber **(hypopyon).** Neutrophils can adhere to corneal endothelium. The exudate often extends into the iridocorneal angle and ciliary cleft. Iridal vessels, and possibly ciliary vessels, are dilated and congested and, in some cases, fibrin thrombi can be present in uveal vessels. The ciliary stroma can be edematous. Neutrophilic anterior uveitis is often a feature of an immune-mediated response (e.g., lens-induced uveitis and infectious canine hepatitis).

Acute uveitis can involve the choroid. Neutrophilic choroiditis often involves the retina and is better characterized as chorioretinitis. Causes of chorioretinitis include infections by bacteria, such as *Haemophilus somnus* and *Salmonella* sp. These bacteria cause necrosis of uveal and retinal vessels, resulting in hemorrhage. Intraocular inflammation characterized by numerous neutrophils and a variable number of macrophages within the choroid, retina, and vitreous body are typical of certain systemic mycotic infections and algal infections. Examples include blastomycosis and protothecosis, respectively. The vitreous body liquefies and a suppurative to pyogranulomatous exudate accumulates within the subretinal space, causing retinal detachment.

Lymphocytic-Plasmacytic Uveitis

Lymphocytic-plasmacytic (lymphoplasmacytic) anterior uveitis is a common, chronic lesion that is characterized by numerous lymphocytes and plasma cells in the stroma of the iris and the ciliary body. Lymphocytes can accumulate as nodules in the anterior uvea, especially in cats. In cats, the lymphocytic nodules can involve the ciliary cleft and are often associated with secondary glaucoma. The cause of lymphoplasmacytic anterior uveitis is often unknown (idiopathic), but can be the result of intraocular or systemic viral or protozoal infections, intraocular parasitic infections, ocular trauma, cataract, or intraocular neoplasia. For example, lymphoplasmacytic anterior uveitis occurs in dogs that have immature forms of *Dirofilaria immitis* in their aqueous humor and cats that test serologically positive for *Toxoplasma gondii.*

Granulomatous Inflammation

Granulomatous uveitis is characterized by the presence of epithelioid macrophages. The macrophages can be accompanied by multinucleated giant cells, neutrophils, lymphocytes, and plasma cells. The pattern and extent of inflammation can be variable, but are often associated with the inciting antigen. Macrophages can surround an area of necrosis, form an inflammatory nodule, or form a diffuse sheet of inflammatory cells throughout the entire uvea (granulomatous panuveitis). Aggregates of macrophages can adhere to the corneal endothelium (keratic precipitates) secondary to granulomatous anterior uveitis (e.g., feline infectious peritonitis). Macrophages are often intermixed with neutrophils, especially when the uveitis is a manifestation of an ocular disease (e.g., nocardiosis, blastomycosis, protothecosis), or is intermixed with lymphocytes and plasma cells, especially if the uveitis is an ocular manifestation of an immune-mediated disorder. Diffuse granulomatous panuveitis is caused by antigens or organisms that are located in the cytoplasm of macrophages. Examples of diseases with this pattern of uveal inflammation include Volt-Koyanagi-Harada-like syndrome (dog) and ocular histoplasmosis (cat).

Feline Infectious Peritonitis

Ocular lesions of the feline coronaviral disease, feline infection peritonitis, include perivascular aggregates of lymphocytes and plasma cells and pyogranulomatous vasculitis, especially of anterior scleral vessels (Fig. 14-21). A similar mixture of neutrophils, macrophages, lymphocytes, and plasma cells occurs as an infiltrate in the ciliary body, choroid, retina, and optic meninges. Aggregates of macrophages can be found as small aggregates on the corneal endothelium **(keratic precipitates).**

Malignant Catarrhal Fever

Malignant catarrhal fever is a disease affecting many cloven-hoofed animals. The cause involves an infection by a herpesvirus and an immunologic reaction characterized as type IV hypersensitivity. The disease is manifested as acute vasculitis. Lymphocytes and lymphoblasts are present in the uvea, especially uveal vessels, and in vessels of the conjunctiva and retina. Similar inflammatory cells are present in the corneal endothelium, resulting in diffuse, bilateral corneal edema.

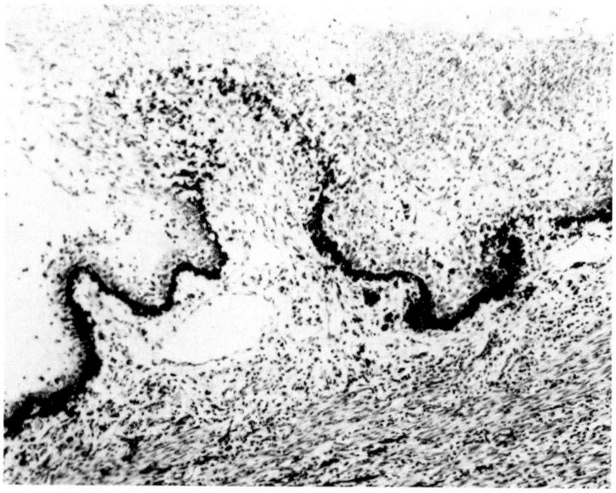

Figure 14-21 Globe, ciliary body; feline. Feline infectious peritonitis. Uveal necrosis includes ciliary epithelium and is accompanied by exudate in posterior chamber about ciliary process. H & E stain.

Vogt-Koyanagi-Harada-like Syndrome

Uveodermatologic, or Vogt-Koganagi-Harada-like (VKH-like), syndrome occurs in dogs (e.g., Akita) and is similar to VKH syndrome in human beings. The cause is unknown, but antimelanin autoimmunity appears to be involved in the pathogenesis. Clinical signs consist of bilateral panuveitis with chorioretinitis, depigmentation of the skin (vitiligo), loss of pigmentation of the hair (poliosis), and neurologic signs. The target of the inflammation appears to be uveal, retinal, and epidermal melanin-containing cells. Ocular lesions consist of diffuse dispersal and phagocytosis of melanin throughout the entire uvea. Effacement of the retinal pigment epithelium is a common finding, and retinal detachment can occur. The granulomatous inflammation is intermixed with lymphocytes and plasma cells, and secondary lesions such as cataract, synechiae, and glaucoma can occur.

Lens-Induced Uveitis

Lenticular proteins, such as soluble α-crystallin and insoluble albuminoid, are antigenic. Normally, some lenticular proteins escape from the lens and induce immunologic tolerance. With cataract formation, the amount of soluble lenticular protein leaking through an intact lens capsule can overwhelm the immunologic tolerance and cause uveitis. The severity of the uveitis depends on the amount of lenticular antigen, persistence of lenticular antigen, or both. Lens-induced uveitis is divided into two types: phacolytic uveitis and phacoclastic uveitis.

Phacolytic uveitis occurs in dogs and other species and is characterized as a mild anterior uveal lymphoplasmacytic uveitis. Although this type of ocular inflammation is nonspecific, the presence of cataract and an absence of other causes of uveitis, such as systemic disease, are helpful in making the diagnosis. The lesion can be granulomatous in old dogs with rapidly progressive or long-standing cataracts.

Phacoclastic uveitis occurs in response to the release of large amounts of lenticular protein (Fig. 14-22). The inflammatory reaction is concentrated around the lens and is most severe at the point of rupture of the lens capsule. The lesion is characterized by numerous neutrophils that dissect between lenticular fibers **(neutrophilic phakitis)** along with liquefaction of the lens cortex. Neutrophils intermixed with lymphocytes and plasma cells form a zone of perilenticular inflammation. This inflammation can include fibroplasia from the anterior uvea and fibrous metaplasia from the lenticular epithelium. This can lead to the formation of posterior synechiae. Granulomatous inflammation is not the typical response in the dog, but is more typical of the response in the rabbit. Although the cause of the lenticular capsule rupture is not always known, intraocular bacterial infection can be a contributing factor in the dog, and an intraocular infection by *Encephalitozoon cuniculi* can be a contributing factor in the rabbit.

Histoplasmosis

Histoplasmosis occurs in North and South America and is endemic in the Ohio, Missouri, and Mississippi River valleys. The disease, caused by *Histoplasma capsulatum,* is characterized by involvement of the gastrointestinal tract, liver, and lungs. Ocular involvement is infrequent. Ocular lesions consist of a diffuse granulomatous uveitis that can be panuveitis, but is often chorioretinitis (Fig. 14-23). The optic nerve can be involved. The organisms are round yeasts with a diameter of 2 to 4 μm. The central dense body is surrounded by a thin-nonstaining halo.

Blastomycosis

Ocular lesions of blastomycosis are most commonly observed in dogs and consist of pyogranulomatous chorioretinitis and hyalitis with exudative retinal detachment. The disease is caused by *Blastomyces dermatitidis,* and yeast forms are variable in number but associated with neutrophils in the vitreous body and subretinal space (Fig. 14-24). The organisms are spherical, thick walled, and approximately 8 to 20 μm in diameter (Fig. 14-25). Reproduction is by budding. Although inflammatory lesions can involve the anterior segment of the globe, the principal and severe lesions involve the posterior segment.

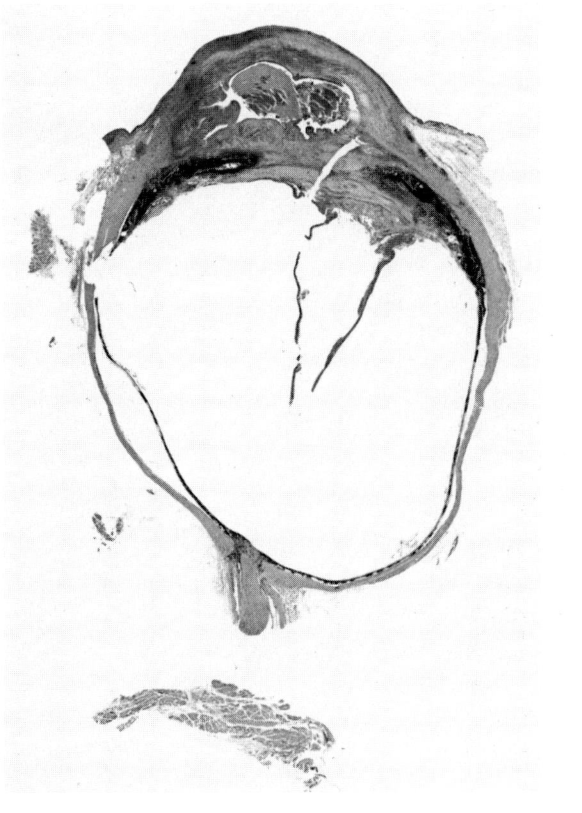

Figure 14-22 Globe; canine. Phacoclastic uveitis. Cataract, rupture of the lens capsule, severe perilenticular anterior uveitis, keratitis, and retinal detachment are present. H & E stain.

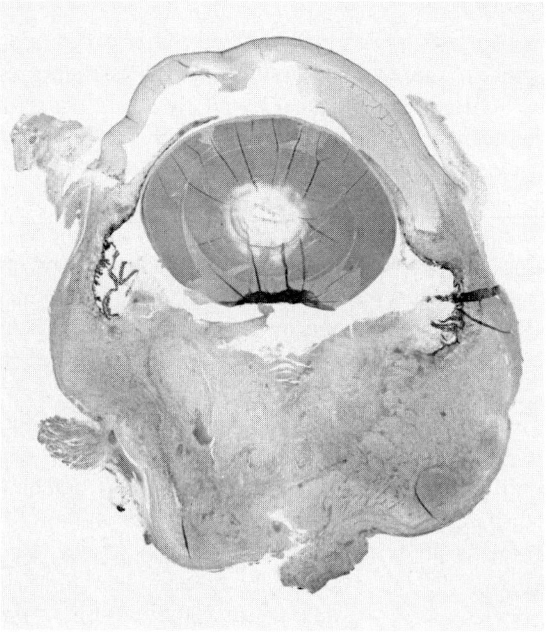

Figure 14-23 Globe; canine. Histoplasmosis. Granulomatous panuveitis that extends outward (scleritis and retrobulbar orbital cellulitis) and inward (retinitis and hyalitis). H & E stain.

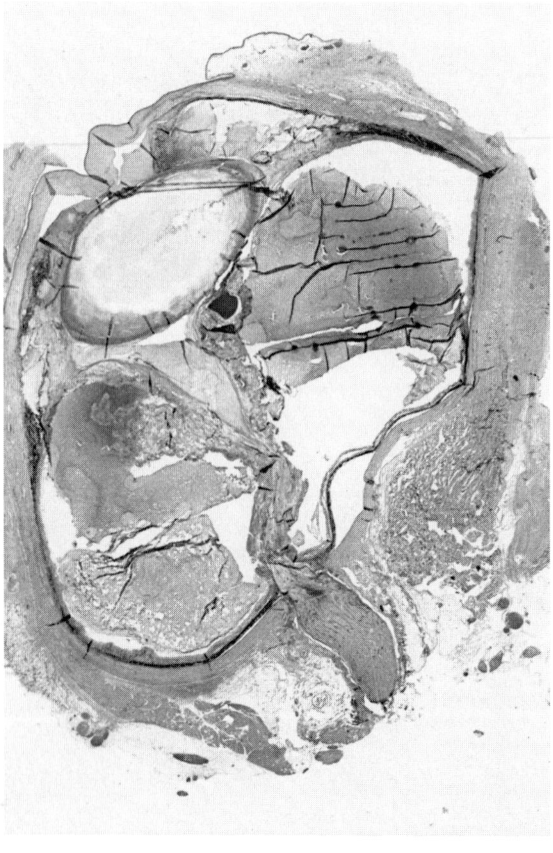

Figure 14-24 Globe; canine. Blastomycosis. Pyogranulomatous hyalitis, exudative retinal detachment, and anterior uveitis are illustrated. H & E stain.

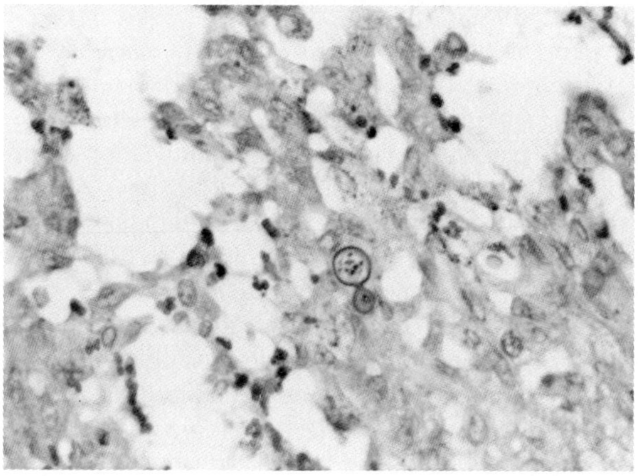

Figure 14-25 Globe; canine. Blastomycosis. Budding blastospore of *Blastomyces dermatitidis* is in granulomatous exudate. H & E stain.

Cryptococcosis

The lack of inflammation and the location of the lesions are unique features of ocular cryptococcosis, a fungal disease caused by *Cryptococcus neoformans*. Focal or multifocal lesions involve the choroid and overlying retina, but also involve the optic meninges (Fig. 14-26). Lesions are composed of numerous spherical to ovoid, sometimes folded, thin-walled yeasts, each 5 to 10 μm in diameter with a thick mucinous capsule and minimal inflammatory cells. The organisms are often found as focal or multifocal subretinal aggregates in the optic meninges. Occasionally, the lesions are extensive with numerous macrophages and fewer organisms. The organisms most likely gain access to the globe hematogenously and become trapped in the choriocapillaris.

Coccidioidomycosis

Ocular infection with the fungus *Coccidioides immitis* has been rarely reported, although disseminated infection in dogs is common in endemic areas. The ocular lesions of pyogranulomatous endophthalmitis involve the cornea, ciliary body, iris, choroid, and retina (Fig. 14-27). The lesions are nodular granulomas that have large (up to 60 μm in diameter), thick-walled spherules and sporangia containing sporangiospores (Fig. 14-28). In some areas, especially about spherules, the inflammatory cellular reaction is mainly neutrophilic. Much exudate can be present in the anterior and posterior chambers and in the vitreous cavity. Exudate accumulating in the choroid causes detachment of the retina. Extensive involvement of tissues of the iridocorneal angle results in glaucoma.

Protothecosis

Ocular protothecosis is characterized by marked inflammation and numerous organisms within the choroid, retina, and subretinal space (Fig. 14-29). Different species of

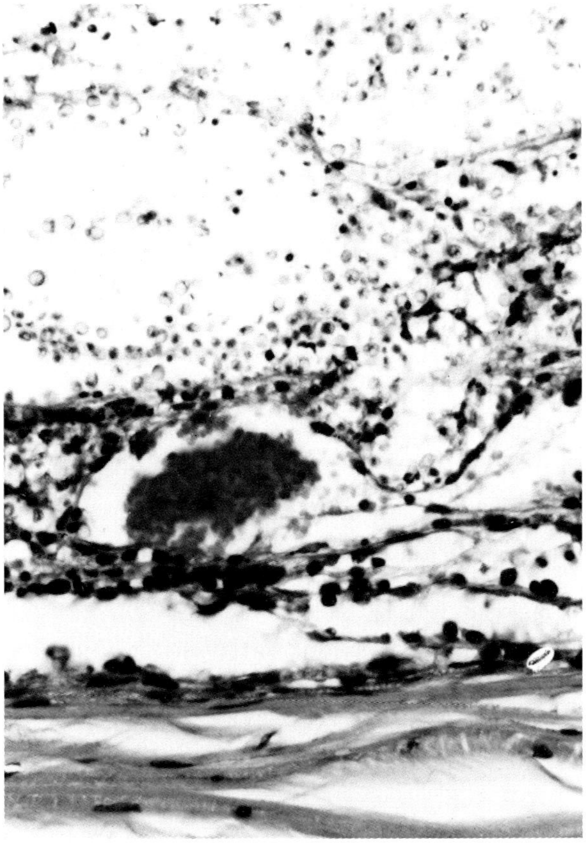

Figure 14-26 Globe, choroid; canine. Cryptococcosis. Yeast forms of *Cryptococcus neoformans* are in the choroid, with little associated inflammatory reaction. H & E stain.

Prototheca have been the cause, but most often *P. zopfii* have been identiifed. The ovoid or angular organisms are approximately 8 to 20 μm in diameter and have refractile walls. Each organism has a central nucleus with granular cytoplasm or multiple daughter cells that form from multiple asexual fission (morula). The inflammatory response is characterized by numerous neutrophils intermixed with macrophages and mainly involves the posterior segment of the globe.

Equine Recurrent Uveitis

Equine recurrent uveitis (periodic ophthalmia) is a common ocular disease of horses manifested by recurring periods of acute uveitis that are separated by quiescent periods of variable duration. The acute stage of the disease consists of neutrophilic anterior uveitis and hypopyon with infiltration of lymphocytes into the stroma of the iris and ciliary body. Similar inflammatory cells can be present in the vitreous body, which can contain an increased amount of protein (plasmoid vitreous). After repeated episodes of uveitis, perivascular cuffs of lymphocytes can be present in the optic papilla. Degenerative changes can occur in the retina and optic nerve, but the hallmark lesion is a hyalinized membrane covering the inner aspect of the

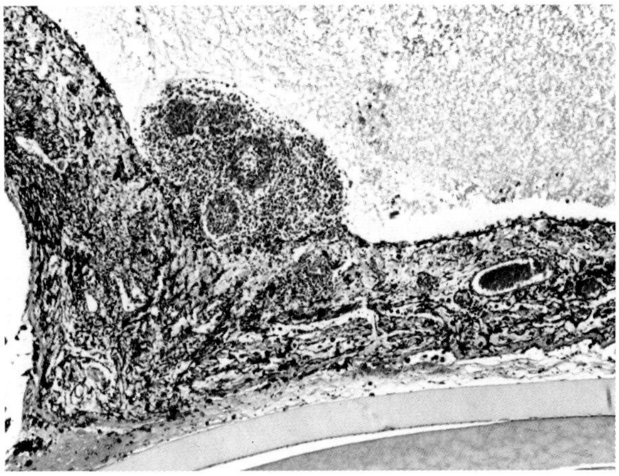

Figure 14-27 Globe, iris; canine. Coccidioidomycosis. Granulomatous iritis, posterior synechiae, nodules on the anterior surface of the iris, and proteinaceous exudate in the anterior chamber are illustrated. H & E stain.

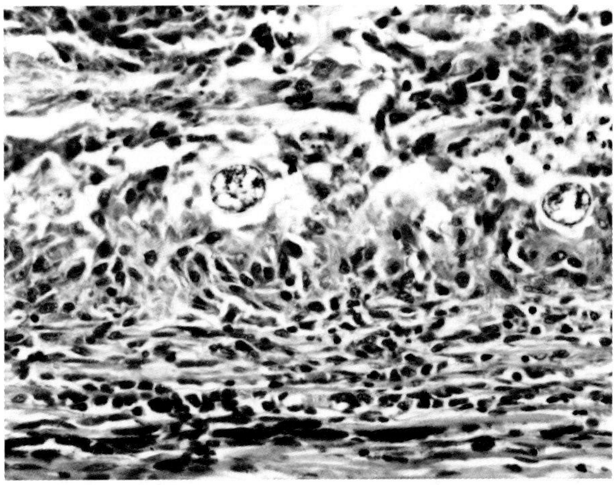

Figure 14-28 Globe, choroid; canine. Coccidioidomycosis. Granulomatous choroiditis has spherules of *Coccidioides immitis*. H & E stain.

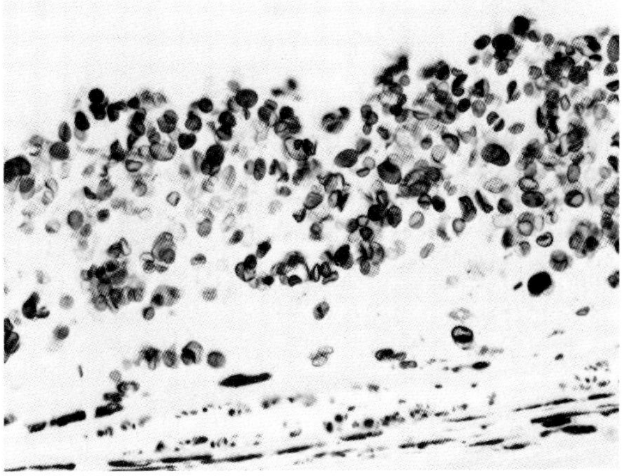

Figure 14-29 Globe, choroid; canine. Protothecosis. *Prototheca zopfii* organisms are in the choroidal exudate. Gomori's methenamine silver (GMS) stain.

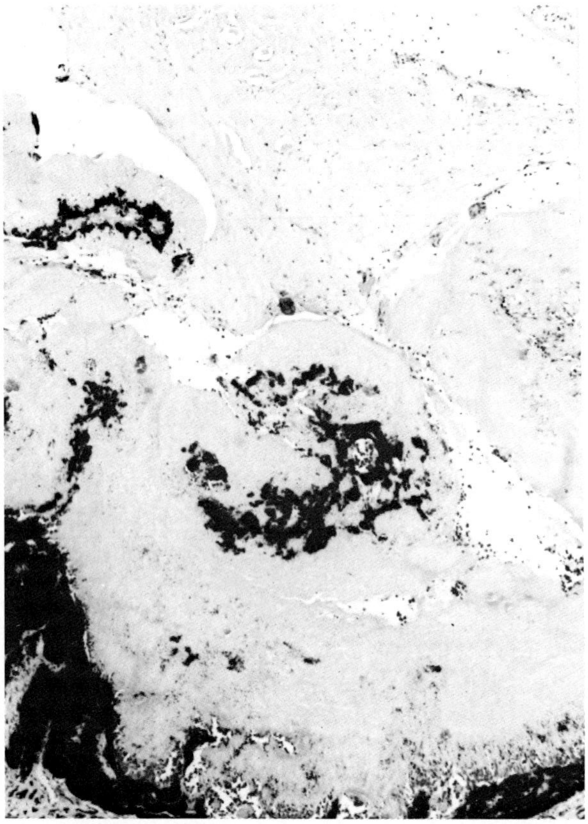

Figure 14-30 Globe, ciliary processes; equine. Equine recurrent uveitis. A hyalinized membrane that will stain positive for amyloid covers the ciliary processes. H & E stain.

ciliary epithelium (Fig. 14-30). The membrane stains positive for amyloid. Crystalline proteinaceous inclusions develop in the cytoplasm of the inner ciliary epithelium; secondary lesions include cataract, corneal vascularization, retinal detachment, loss of photoreceptors, gliosis, and hypertrophy and hyperplasia of the retinal pigment epithelium. With the loss of the posterior epithelial blood-eye barrier, there is localized accumulation of circulating immune complexes and a subsequent type III hypersensitivity reaction. Antigens reported to be involved in the disease include those of several serovars of *Leptospira interrogans serovar pomona* and dead microfilaria of *Onchocerca cervicalis*.

Toxoplasmosis

Ocular manifestations of toxoplasmosis has been described in many animal species, but especially in the cat. The cause is an obligate intracellular protozoal parasite, *Toxoplasma gondii*. In human beings, the principal ocular lesion is necrotizing retinochoroiditis, but in cats ocular lesions includes multifocal granulomatous or lymphoplasmacytic chorioretinitis and lymphoplasmacytic anterior uveitis. The role of *T. gondii* in causing anterior uveitis is controversial, since organisms have not been identified in the globes by microscopic examination. An association between exposure to *T. gondii* and anterior uveitis seems likely, and an aberrant ocular immune response could occur in cats exposed to *T. gondii*.

Sequelae of Uveitis

Sequelae of intraocular inflammation include adhesions and fibrovascular membranes. The presence of fibrin in the anterior and posterior chambers can cause adherence of the iris to the anterior lens capsule **(posterior synechia).** If this adhesion completely surrounds the pupil, the flow of aqueous humor from the posterior chamber into the anterior chamber will be blocked. The accumulation of aqueous humor in the posterior chamber causes the iris to bow anteriorly **(iris bombé).** This narrows the iridocorneal angle, possibly to the point of forming an adhesion between the iris and the peripheral cornea **(peripheral anterior synechia).** Closure of the iridocorneal angle, along with compression of the ciliary cleft, results in **secondary glaucoma.**

The accumulation of fibrin on the surface of intraocular structures can serve as a scaffold for the formation of fibrovascular membranes. Angiogenic and fibroblastic growth factors are released under conditions such as intraocular neoplasia, intraocular inflammation, and retinal detachment. These mediators diffuse through the ocular media to stimulate angiogenesis within the uvea, especially the iris. Cytokines that are thought to be involved include basic fibroblastic growth factor (bFGF), epidermal growth factor (EGF), transforming growth factor-β (TGF-β), platelet-derived growth factor (PDGF), and vascular endothelial growth factor (VEGF). Membranes that extend from the iris near the pupillary border can cause outward **(ectropion uveae)** or inward **(entropion uveae)** deviation of this border. One type of membrane, **preiridal fibrovascular membrane,** forms along the anterior surface of the iris. This membrane can extend across the iridocorneal angle and along the peripheral cornea, causing peripheral anterior synechia and **secondary glaucoma.** Newly formed vessels within these membrane are fragile and a cause of **hyphema.** Similar fibrovascular membranes can extend along the posterior surface of the iris and along the surface of the anterior lens capsule **(iris membrane).** Membranes can originate from the ciliary body and extend along the surface of the posterior lens capsule **(cyclitic membrane).**

Lesions can occur in other ocular structures concurrently with uveitis or as a result of uveitis. The corneal endothelium can be destroyed by the inflammatory process that results in secondary corneal edema. Other lesions, including vascularization of the corneal stroma, keratitis, cataract, vitreous syneresis, hyalitis, retinitis, and retinal detachment, also can occur. Atrophy of the ciliary processes can result in reduced production of aqueous humor and reduced aqueous to cataract and decreased intraocular pressure **(hypotony).** The entire globe can undergo shrinkage and distortion to become an "end-stage globe" **(phthisis bulbi),** and osseous metaplasia can occur in the posterior segment.

Uveal Neoplasia

Intraocular neoplasms often involve the uvea and either arise from a component of the uvea (primary intraocular neoplasm) or are the result of metastasis to the uveal vasculature (secondary intraocular neoplasm). Primary intraocular neoplasms arise from uveal melanocytes, the neuroepithelium, or smooth muscle. In general, most intraocular neoplasms in the dog are benign. Enucleation is necessary in some cases, but the prognosis is good as metastasis is rare. In contrast, many of the intraocular neoplasms in cats are malignant and the likelihood of metastasis is much greater. Less is known about uveal neoplasms in other animal species.

Anterior Uveal Melanoma

The most common primary intraocular neoplasm in animals is melanoma; the anterior uvea is the most common site of involvement. This is in contrast to human beings, in whom the choroid is the most common site for development. Intraocular melanoma occurs most commonly in the dog and cat, although it occurs rarely in other species (e.g., horse and rat). In the dog and cat, anterior uveal melanoma is usually unilateral, although bilateral anterior uveal melanoma has been reported.

In the dog, anterior uveal melanoma is usually benign and has been referred to as **melanocytoma** (Fig. 14-31). Typically, these neoplasms are composed of numerous large, spherical cells, intermixed with a variable number of fusiform cells. The cells are arranged in sheets that form a mass that effaces the intraocular architecture. Secondary lesions, such as retinal detachment, glaucoma, and cataract, are common sequelae. Neoplastic cells extend along vessels into the scleral emissaria. The majority of canine anterior uveal melanomas have very few mitotic figures and no tendency for metastasis.

Malignant anterior uveal melanoma is an invasive neoplasm that has features of malignancy, such as an increased mitotic activity (2 or more mitotic figures per 10 high-power fields), cellular atypia, and anaplasia. Malignant anterior uveal melanoma metastasizes to multiple sites, including the lungs, liver, and the other globe. Dogs with this lesion have a decreased life span.

Feline intraocular melanoma almost always involves the iris, although atypical primary ocular melanoma, resembling canine melanocytoma, occurs in the ciliary body and choroid. Clinically, the lesion begins as focal or multifocal, asymmetric hyperpigmentation of the iris. These areas gradually coalesce and become **diffuse iris melanoma.** This lesion generally occurs in older cats and represents a proliferation of melanocytes throughout the iridal stroma. The melanocytes are polygonal to fusiform and can vary in their amount of intracytoplasmic melanin. As a result, **feline anterior uveal melanoma** can vary from amelanotic to heavily pigmented. Feline anterior uveal melanoma is considered benign unless the ciliary body is involved. Extension into the ciliary body usually involves extension into the ciliary cleft and secondary glaucoma. Extension into scleral vessels and metastasis is also possible. Distant metastasis to the lungs, liver, and other organs can occur months to years after the initial diagnosis. When anterior uveal melanoma extends into scleral vessels, the cats have a decreased survival rate. Cats with extensive ocular involvement have the lowest survival rate.

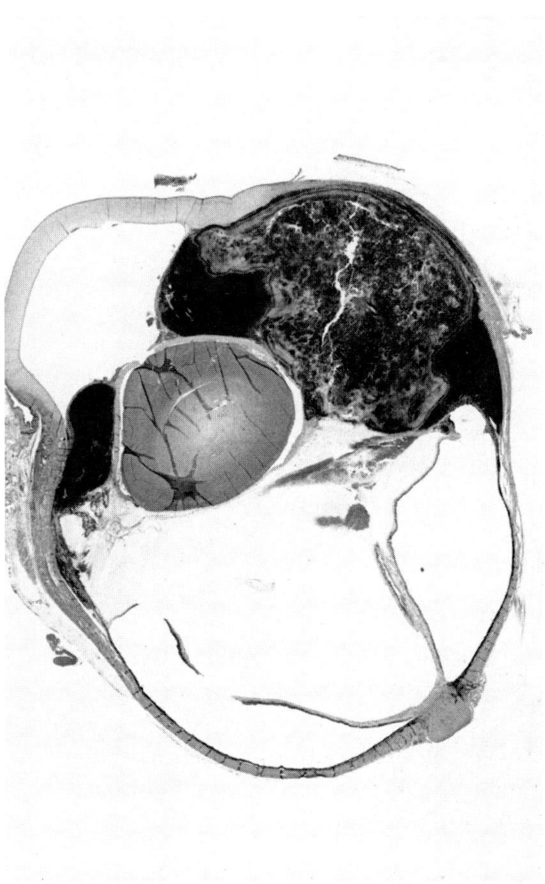

Figure 14-31 Globe; canine. Benign anterior uveal melanoma. Melanocytoma effaces the anterior uvea with diffuse posterior synechiae and retina detachment. H & E stain.

In animals, **choroidal melanoma** is less common than anterior uveal melanoma and occurs most often in the dog. Canine choroidal melanoma has morphologic features and biologic behavior similar to that of benign anterior uveal melanoma. Their biologic behavior of lesions is benign, but they can extend into the optic meninges and the optic nerve. Secondary retinal detachment is a common concurrent ocular lesion.

Intraocular melanoma occurs in other species but is less common than those in dogs and cats. In the horse the melanoma involves the anterior uvea and is composed of large plump cells with an abundance of intracytoplasmic melanin. The neoplasm grows within the globe, resulting in effacement of involved ocular structures.

Ocular Melanocytosis

Ocular melanocytosis is a tumorlike proliferation of plump melanocytes within the stroma of the iris and ciliary body (Fig. 14-32). These melanocytes extend into the sclera and peripheral cornea. The accumulation of melanocytes effaces the ciliary cleft, resulting in secondary glaucoma, and extension into the choroid causes secondary retinal detachment. This lesion is sporadic and unilateral in the dog, but occurs more commonly as an asymmetric, bilateral lesion in the cairn terrier. This indicates a possible genetic predisposition.

Iridociliary Epithelial Tumors

Neoplasms arising from the anterior uveal neuroepithelium are the second most common type of primary intraocular neoplasms. Most occur in the dog, and fewer occur in the cat. Both iridociliary adenoma and iridociliary carcinoma occur, but iridociliary adenoma is more common. **Iridociliary adenoma** occurs as a well-demarcated, solid, space-occupying mass located posterior to the iris and extending from the ciliary body (Fig. 14-33). This neoplasm is white, but lesions in the dog can contain melanin pigment. Microscopically, the neoplasm is composed of cuboidal cells with round to ovoid nuclei and a moderate amount of cytoplasm (Fig. 14-34). The cells palisade along a basement membrane forming a solid, papillary or microcystic, noninvasive mass. Some pig-

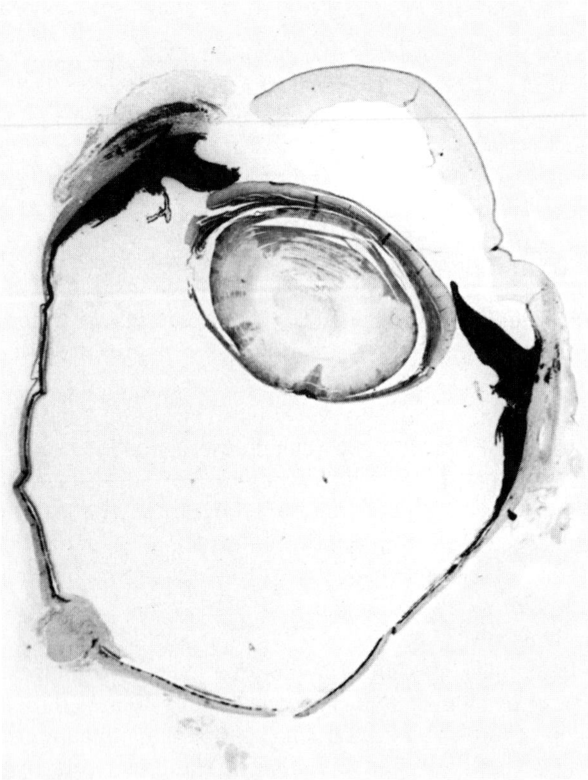

Figure 14-32 Globe; canine. Melanocytosis. Diffuse thickening of the anterior uvea by melanocytes that have extended through the sclera into the episclera. The ciliary cleft is filled with melanocytic cells, leading to secondary glaucoma. H & E stain.

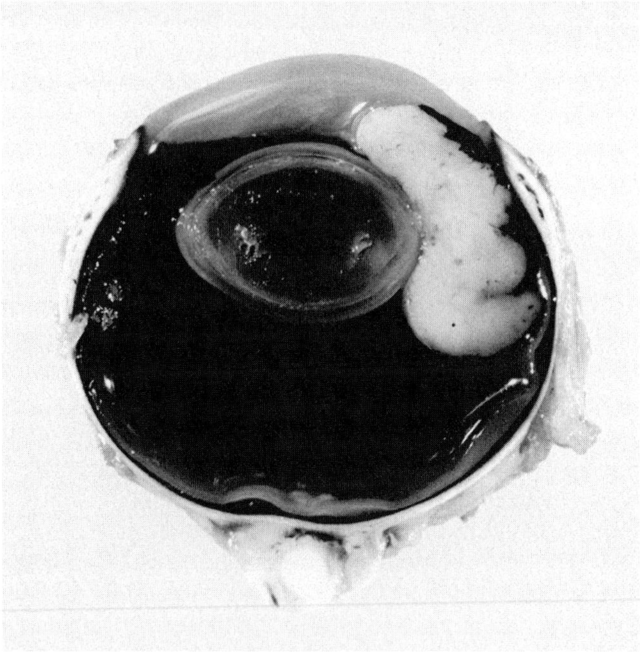

Figure 14-33 Globe; canine. Iridociliary adenoma *(right)*. White, well-demarcated adenoma extending from the posterior iris and ciliary body.

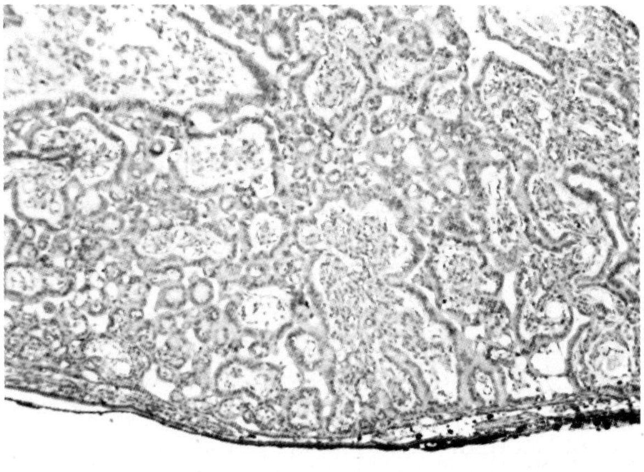

Figure 14-34 Globe, anterior uvea; canine. Iridociliary adenoma. Neoplasm composed of glandular and papillary formations of closely packed cuboidal epithelium. H & E stain.

mented epithelial cells and clusters of swollen epithelial cells with clear cytoplasm can be present. **Iridociliary adenocarcinoma** has morphologic features similar to iridociliary adenoma, but is invasive, especially into the sclera. This neoplasm has cellular features of anaplasia and can be distinguished from metastatic adenocarcinoma because of the presence of basement membranes. Although the potential for metastasis exists, the actual occurrence is rare. Concurrent lesions in the dog include preiridal fibrovascular membrane and asteroid hyalosis.

Medulloepithelioma and Teratoid Medulloepithelioma

Medulloepithelioma is a rare neoplasm arising from neuroepithelium. It arises from the anterior uvea, especially in young dogs and horses, and from the retina and optic disc in young horses. These neoplasms are composed of densely packed neuroblastic cells with indistinct cytoplastic borders. These cells are arranged in sheets and can form pseudorosettes around congested blood vessels (Fig. 14-35). Rosettes and areas of necrosis can be present, and the continuity between neoplastic cells and iridociliary epithelium or retina can be observed. Teratoid medulloepitheliomas have morphologic features similar to those of medulloepitheliomas, but also have tissues resembling neuropil, cartilage, or other tissues. These are usually benign neoplasms.

Feline Primary Ocular Sarcoma

Sarcomas have been observed in the globes of cats months to years after trauma to the globe. These posttraumatic ocular sarcomas are almost always associated with rupture of the lens capsule. The affected globes can be normal, bulging, or shrunken and irregular in shape (Fig. 14-36). Microscopically, the sarcoma can efface the entire globe and extend into the optic nerve and orbital contents. The histologic features of the sarcomas are variable and include fibrosarcoma, anaplastic sarcoma, round cell sarcoma, giant cell sarcoma, and osteosarcoma (Fig. 14-37). The origin of the sarcoma appears to be lenticular epithelium, although pigmented neuroepithelium could also be the origin. In addition to local infiltration, distant metastasis is common; therefore, posttraumatic ocular sarcoma is considered a life-threatening neoplasm in cats.

Primary Mesenchymal Ocular Neoplasms

Primary mesenchymal neoplasms of the globe are rare and few cases have been reported. These include hemangioma, hemangiosarcoma, leiomyoma, leiomyosarcoma, and fibrosarcoma. Neoplasms of smooth muscle need to be differentiated from amelanotic spindle cell melanoma, especially in the rat.

Metastatic Intraocular Neoplasms

Metastatic intraocular neoplasms are of epithelial, mesenchymal, or melanocytic origin. Most are the result of hematogenous spread, although extension from orbital or adnexal neoplasia is possible. Although ocular metastasis is possible whenever disseminated neoplasia is observed at necropsy, reports are limited, possibly because globes are

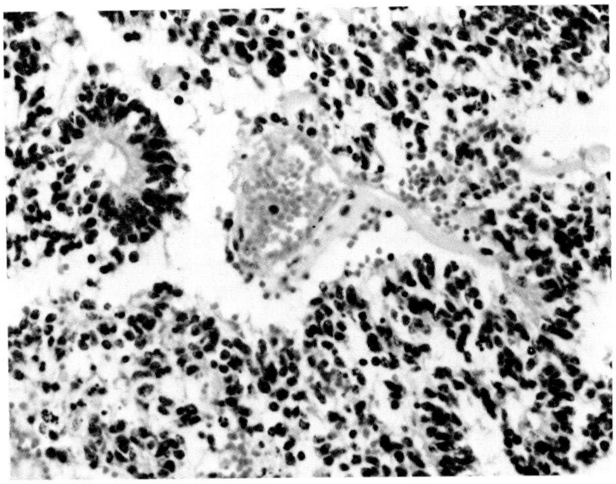

Figure 14-35 Globe, anterior uvea; canine. Medulloepithelioma. Neoplasm composed of bands of undifferentiated epithelial cells with some ill-defined rosettes. H & E stain.

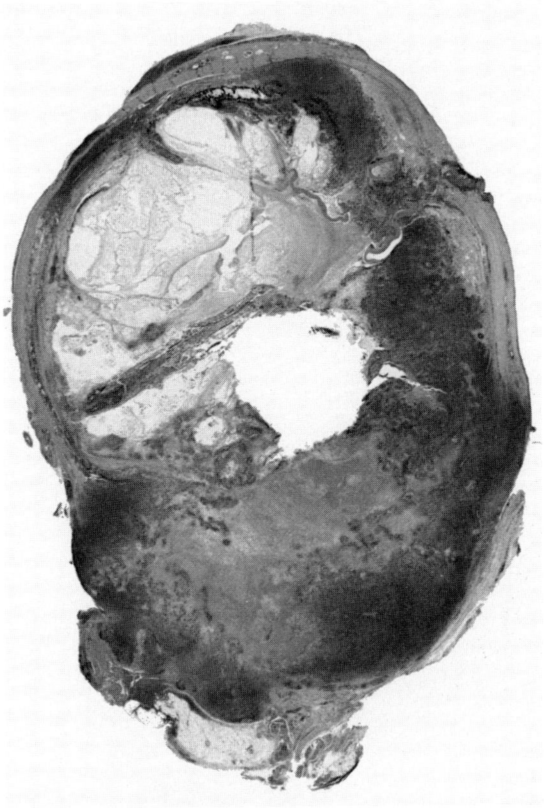

Figure 14-36 Globe; feline. Trauma-associated sarcoma. The architecture of the entire globe is effaced by a sarcoma with areas of necrosis. A metal shot was present in the central space. H & E stain.

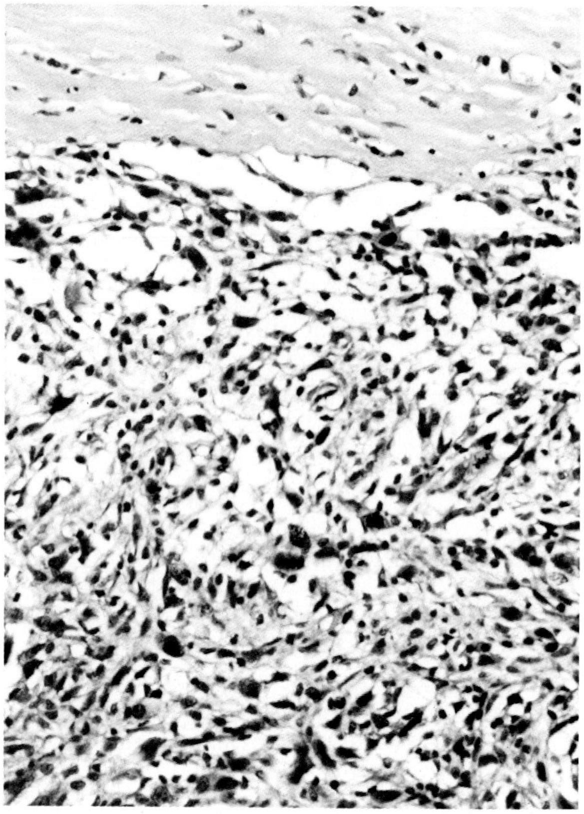

Figure 14-37 Globe, anterior uvea; feline. Trauma-associated sarcoma. Neoplasm is composed of anaplastic, mesenchymal, spindle-shaped cells that filled the anterior chamber and invaded the cornea. H & E stain.

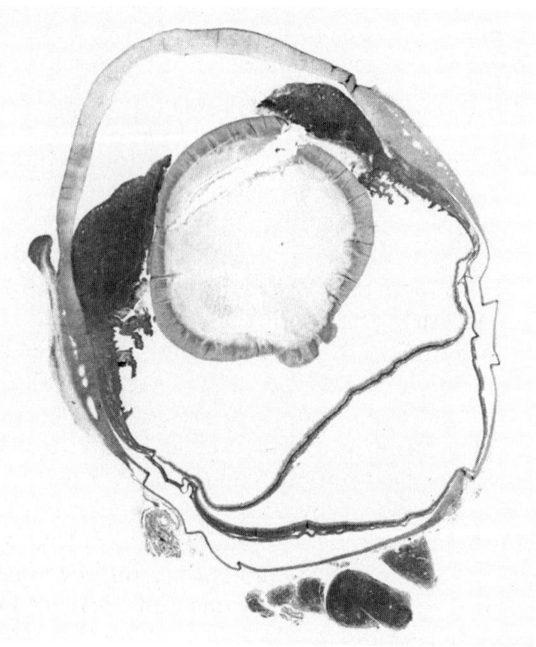

Figure 14-38 Globe; feline. Ocular lymphosarcoma. Diffuse thickening of the iris and ciliary body by an accumulation of neoplastic lymphocytes. H & E stain.

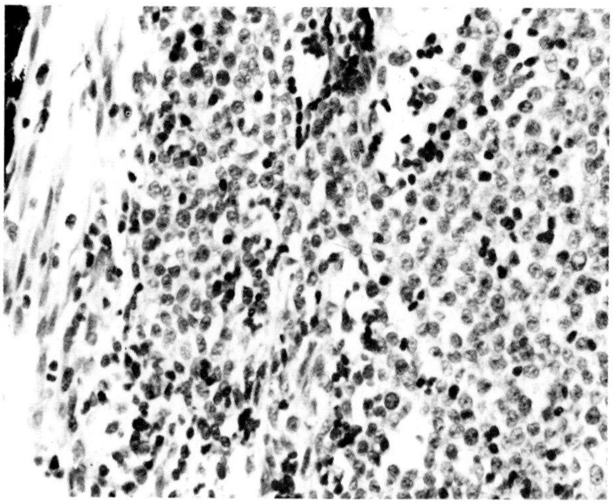

Figure 14-39 Globe, iris; canine. Lymphosarcoma. Nodule composed of sheets of lymphoid cells. H & E stain.

not often examined. Reports of metastasis to the globe include mammary carcinoma, pulmonary carcinoma, hemangiosarcoma, oral malignant melanoma, osteosarcoma, among others. Metastatic lesions often involve the ciliary body. Metastatic epithelial neoplasms can cover the iris and ciliary body and extend onto the corneal endothelium. Neoplastic epithelial cells of either glandular or squamous origin can fill vessels of the choroid and optic nerve in cats with primary pulmonary carcinoma (metastatic angioinvasive pulmonary carcinoma).

Although on rare occasions lymphosarcoma can be primary intraocular disease, **ocular lymphosarcoma** is usually secondary and is the most common intraocular metastatic neoplasm, especially in the dog and cat. Clinically, neoplastic cells infiltrating the iridal stroma cause a color change of the iris and a distorted pupil **(dyscoria),** similar to the ocular manifestations of Marek's disease in chickens. It occurs as solid, white to tan nodules in the iris and often is bilateral and involves the ciliary body (Fig. 14-38). Neoplastic lymphocytes have scant cytoplasm, although some neoplasms have a mixed population of cells, with some having an epithelioid appearance (Fig. 14-39). The initial site of involvement is most often the iris and ciliary body. The trabecular meshwork often is effaced, resulting in secondary glaucoma.

LESIONS OF THE LENS

The lens is a transparent, avascular, biconvex structure, which refracts light rays and focuses them on the retina. The center of the anterior curvature of the lens is the anterior pole, and the center of the posterior curvature is the posterior pole. The anterior portion of the lens is bathed by aqueous humor, and the posterior portion of the lens is located within a shallow depression in the vitreous body. The anterior and posterior curvatures of the lens merge at the equator. The lens has a highly ordered, cellular structure that allows for transparency. It is surrounded by a basement membrane (lens capsule), and zonular fibers are attached to the lenticular capsule at the equator.

Beneath the anterior lenticular capsule is a monolayer of cuboidal epithelial cells. These cells cause thickening of the anterior lenticular capsule. Lenticular epithelial cells immediately anterior to the equator of the lens proliferate to form new epithelial cells. These epithelial cells elongate and extend beneath the lenticular epithelium and the posterior lenticular capsule. These long, prismatic lenticular fibers are tightly packed and form a cortex of the lens. Since the formation of new lenticular fibers is a continuous process, older lenticular fibers are gradually moved inward toward the center (nucleus) of the lens. With time, this compression of lenticular fibers gradually causes hardening of the nucleus **(nuclear sclerosis).** Clinically, a lens with nuclear sclerosis has a white-blue appearance when viewed with diffuse illumination because of the scattering of light rays.

Energy is derived from anaerobic glycolysis, especially in the lenticular epithelium. The major end products of glycolysis in the lens are lactic acid and energy. Energy is in the form of adenosine triphosphate, which is mainly used for active transport of cations. Water passively moves with the cations. Approximately 65% of the lens is water, and most of the remainder of the lens is composed of protein (soluble crystallins and insoluble albuminoid).

Anomalies of the Lens

Congenital anomalies of the lens usually occur because of alterations in the formation of the lens vesicle. Abnormal development of the lens often results in the formation of other intraocular defects. The complete absence of a lens **(aphakia)** is rare, but can occur through failure of the optic vesicle to induce surface ectoderm. An abnormally small lens **(microphakia)** is often also abnormally spherical **(spherophakia)** and can even be located in an abnormal location **(ectopia lentis).** The normal contour of the lens can be altered by absence of a portion of the lens **(lenticular coloboma).** This lesion can occur with uveal coloboma. Other abnormalities of the lenticular shape include coning of the lens **(lenticonus).** Posterior lenticonus is a lesion that occurs with persistent perilenticular vessels and persistent primary vitreous, especially in certain breeds of dog (e.g., Doberman pinscher). Other anomalies, including congenital opacification of the lens (congenital cataract), can occur with other ocular anomalies. Congenital cataract can be the result of an in utero viral infection (e.g., bovine diarrhea viral infection) or caused by teratogenic compounds, nutrient deficiencies (e.g., vitamin E deficiency), or genetic abnormalities.

Persistent Tunica Vasculosa Lentis

The embryonic lens is surrounded by a vascular network (tunica vasculosa lentis) that communicates with the hyaloid vascular system. This vascular network should regress, but can persist, especially along the axial posterior surface of the lens as a focal posterior subcapsular opacity **(Mittendorf's dot).** When the vessels are present with fibrous connective tissue, or possibly metaplastic cartilage, the lesion is referred to as persistent hyperplastic tunica vasculosa lentis.

Cataract

A cataract is a permanent opacity of the lens that results from increased hydration due to alterations in nutrition, metabolism, or osmotic balance of the lens. Cataracts can be inherited or acquired. Acquired cataracts occur in systemic metabolic diseases, nutritional deficiencies, exposure to radiation, the effects of toxins, aging, glaucoma, uveal inflammation, retinal disease, lens luxation, trauma, and electric shock. In diabetes mellitus, excessive amounts of glucose in the aqueous humor enter the lens and are metabolized via the sorbitol pathway. This results in the production of polyalcohol, which creates an osmotic gradient, causing water to accumulate within the lens. Excessive fluid disrupts the lenticular fiber membranes. Some animals fed excessive galactose develop similar cataracts and lesions. Radiation, which increases membrane permeability, causes an imbalance in cations and water. Other cataracts are associated with dietary deficiencies such as tryptophan, phenylalanine, valine, histidine, or arginine. Intraocular diseases, such as uveitis, glaucoma, and retinal degeneration, can cause cataract by disruption of lenticular nutrition or formation of harmful metabolites. In fish, cataract can be the result of infestation by nematode larvae (*Diphostomun* sp.).

Morphologic changes of cataract are often similar, regardless of cause, and involve the lenticular epithelium and fibers. The lenticular epithelium can flatten and form a multilayered plaque along the lenticular capsule. The cells of the plaque have the histologic appearance of fibroblasts; therefore, the process is referred to as **fibrous metaplasia** (Fig. 14-40). Lenticular epithelial cells can migrate to an abnormal locations, especially along the posterior capsule **(posterior subcapsular epithelial cell migration)** and can swell to form **bladder cells** (Figs. 14-41 and 14-42).

Cataract usually involves alterations of lenticular fibers. As proteins aggregate in the cytoplasm of lenticular fibers, the fibers stain more intensely. Cell membranes of lenticular fibers undergo lysis, resulting in release of proteinaceous contents **(liquefaction).** An extracellular spherical globule **(morgagnian globule)** develops, and proteinaceous fluid accumulates between lenticular fibers as clefts, vacuoles, and lakes (Fig. 14-43). Necrotic debris within the lens can undergo **mineralization,** and with time the volume decreases, causing the lenticular capsule to become wrinkled.

Cataracts can be classified by age of the animal at the time of appearance, stage of maturation, and location within the lens. Cataracts can be present at birth **(congenital).** These are usually bilateral and can coexist

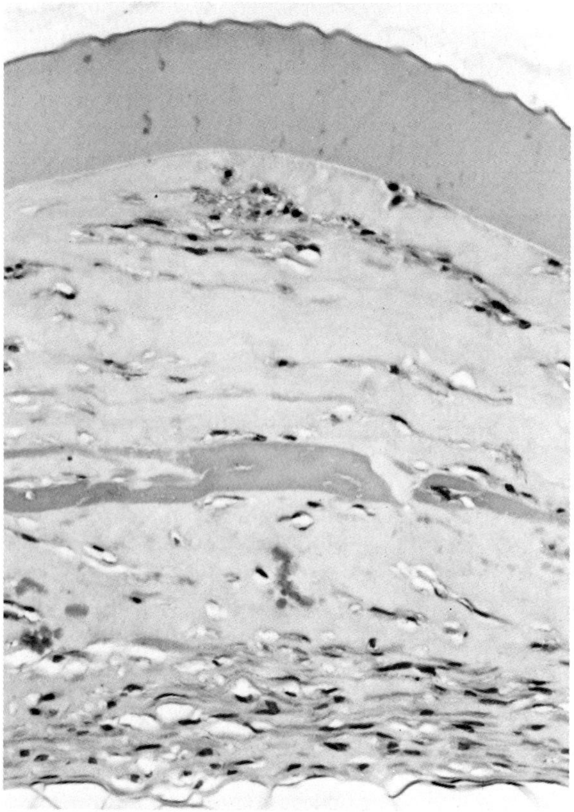

Figure 14-40 Globe, lens; equine. Cataract. Lenticular epithelium is hyperpalstic and metaplastic, resembling fibrocytes. H & E stain.

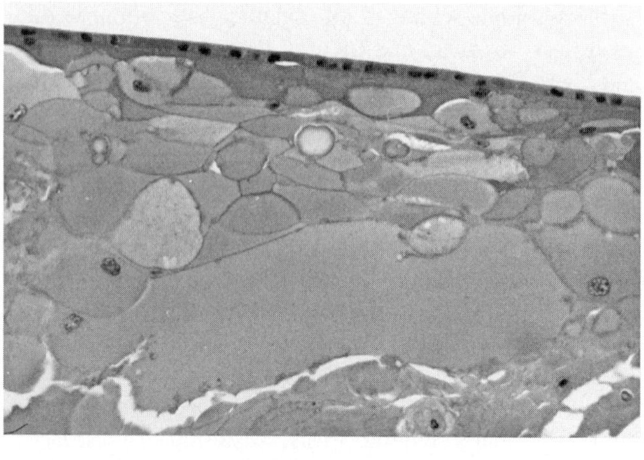

Figure 14-41 Globe, lens; canine. Cataract. Thick anterior lens capsule (aging change), bladder cells, and liquefaction of lenticular cortex are present. H & E stain.

with other ocular anomalies (e.g., persistent pupillary membrane and microphthalmia), or be a solitary lesion. Cataracts can develop in young animals (**juvenile**) or in old animals (**senile**). An **incipient cataract** involves only a small portion of the lens. An **immature cataract** involves

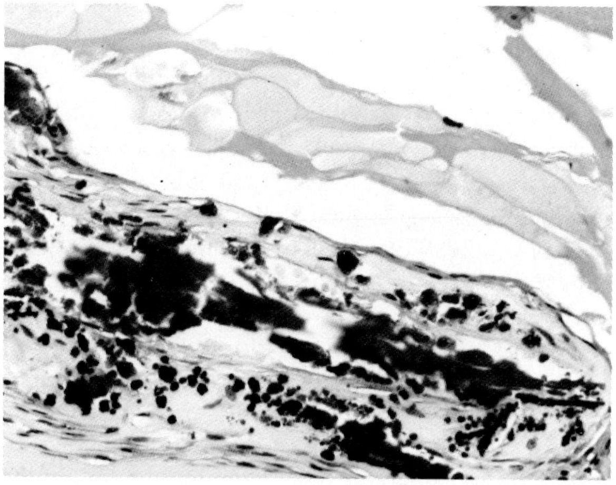

Figure 14-42 Globe, lens; canine. Lenticular epithelium has proliferated along posterior lenticular capsule; some necrotic lenticular fibers are calcified, and some hyperplastic lenticular cells are swollen, finely granular, and have well-defined cellular membranes (bladder cells). H & E stain.

more of the lens than the incipient cataract, and clinically, a tapetal reflection is still visible. A **mature cataract** is a diffuse opacity of the lens, which clinically obscures the tapetal reflex. Cataract can involve the imbibition of water, which causes the lens to swell **(intumescence),** or cortical lenticular fibers can undergo liquefactive necrosis. Loss of cortex results in a wrinkled lenticular capsule **(hypermature cataract)** or ventral displacement of the lenticular nucleus **(morgagnian cataract).** A cataract can involve any part of the lens. Opacities can involve in the capsule **(capsular),** or the **cortex** beneath the capsule **(subcapsular),** the **equator,** or the region of the **anterior or posterior poles.** The anterior lenticular capsule becomes thicker as a part of the aging process.

Rupture of the Lens Capsule

Rupture of the anterior lenticular capsule can occur as the result of a penetrating wound to the globe, and rupture of the posterior lenticular capsule can occur concurrently with interocular infections. In rabbits, rupture of the lenticular capsule occurs in infections by the protozoan, *Encephalitozoon cuniculi;* in dogs lenticular capsular rupture occurs with interocular bacterial infections. Although the type of inflammatory response varies among species, neutrophils are usually found dissecting between lenticular fibers and necrotic lenticular debris outside of the lens. Although the lens is avascular, this neutrophilic response is referred to as **phakitis.** Fibrous metaplasia of lenticular epithelium also occurs with rupture of the lenticular capsule. This fibroblastic response can result in the formation of fibrous membranes. In cats, primary intraocular sarcomas often develop after traumatic rupture of the lens capsule. One possible origin of the sarcomas is

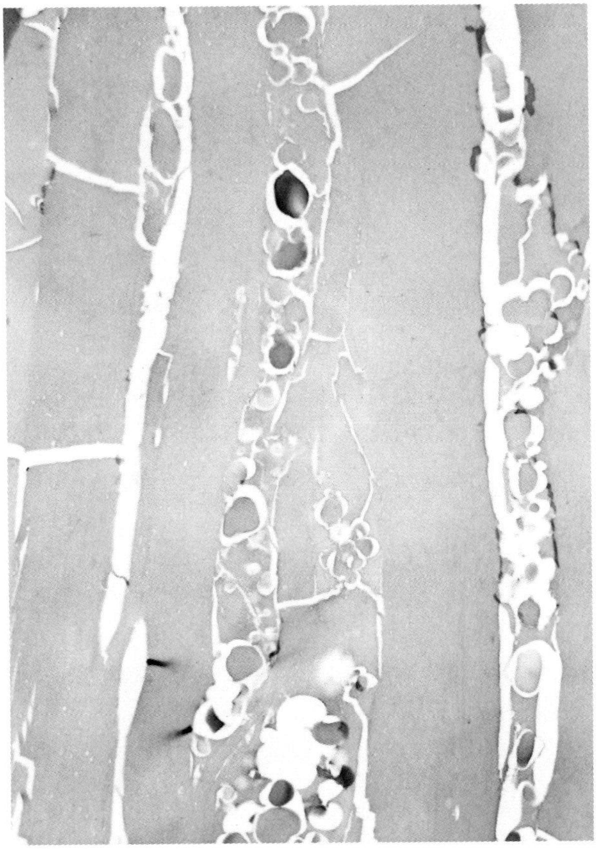

Figure 14-43 Globe, lens; canine. Cataract. Morgagnian globule formation (irregular, variably sized masses) from necrotic lenticular fibers. H & E stain.

the lenticular epithelium that has undergone malignant transformation after fibrous metaplasia.

Lens Dislocation

Displacement of the lens from its normal location in the patellar fossa of the vitreous body can be partial **(subluxation)** or complete **(luxation)** and can be characterized as primary or secondary. The displacement is usually ventral, which allows for the clinical visualization of the dorsal margin of the lens. This ventral displacement of the lens creates an arch-shaped space dorsal to the lens **(aphakic crescent).** Displacement of the lens is secondary to pathologic alterations in zonular fibers. Primary lens luxation is considered to be hereditary and can occur at birth **(ectopia lentis).** The cause is poorly formed or weak zonular fibers. Primary lens luxation occurs in certain breeds of dogs (e.g., terriers). Secondary lens luxation occurs after ocular trauma, or because of stretching from buphthalmos that results in tearing of zonular fibers. Chronic inflammation can cause zonulolysis, and all these lesions can result in lens displacement.

Lesions accompanying lens dislocation are dependent on the direction of the lens displacement. Subluxation and anterior luxation can occlude the outflow of aqueous humor and cause glaucoma. Movement of the lens into the anterior chamber can cause contact with the corneal endothelium and, thus, secondary corneal edema. A concurrent iritis can accompany anterior lens luxation. Posterior luxation of the lens creates fewer lesions, but is often associated with liquefaction (syneresis) of the vitreous body.

LESIONS OF THE VITREOUS BODY

The vitreous body (vitreous) is a transparent, avascular hydrogel filling the vitreous chamber. The vitreous consists of a fine network of collagen fibrils with hyaluronic acid and water filling the interfibrillar spaces. The anterior surface is concave (patellar fossa), and collagen fibrils from the vitreous attach to the posterior lens capsule, forming the hyaloideocapsular ligament. The center of the vitreous is the nucleus, and the peripheral portion of the vitreous, next to the retina, is the cortex. Collagen fibrils from the cortex join the inner limiting membrane of the retina. The vitreous helps to keep the lens and the retina in their proper locations. The base of the vitreous is located near the ora ciliaris retinae. Changes in the consistency of the vitreous can affect the positioning of these structures.

The vitreous normally contains few cells. A few histiocytes (hyalocytes) can be found in the cortex near the vitreous base, and some fibrocytes and glial cells are found near the ciliary body and optic disc. The hyaluronic acid can serve as a barrier, which prevents diffusion of cells into the vitreous, and thus maintains transparency. When the hyaluronic acid concentration decreases as the result of some disease process or the aging process, this barrier is disrupted.

The vitreous body of mammals develops in three stages. A primitive vascular structure is first formed (primary vitreous), then a nonvascular mass of vitreous develops (secondary vitreous), and, later during embryonic growth, the tertiary vitreous develops as the zonular fibers. Development of the primary vitreous ceases and, in time, the hyaloid vessels atrophy. The avascular secondary vitreous continues to be formed by retinal Müller cells and, possibly, by hyalocytes.

Persistent Primary Vitreous

The hyaloid artery and its branches enter the developing globe through the optic fissure and ramify over the posterior lenticular capsule to form the posterior aspect of the perilenticular vascular tunic. These vessels normally atrophy before complete development of the globe, but sometimes persist and appear as a fine thread of fibrous and glial elements extending from the region of the optic disc. In rodents the vestigial hyaloid artery can persist and be patent to 3 months after birth, resulting in vitreous hemorrhage. A glial remnant of the hyaloid system can be present in the region of the optic disc (**Bergmeister's papilla**). These remnants are common in cattle and not associated with clinical disease.

Persistent Hyperplastic Primary Vitreous

Persistent hyperplastic primary vitreous (PHPV) is an uncommon lesion in domestic animals except for certain breeds of dogs, especially the Doberman pinscher. It consists of a fibrovascular membrane along the posterior surface of the lens and hyaloid vessels. Pathologic features of PHPV include posterior lenticonus, posterior polar subcapsular cataract, and retrolental pigment deposition. Microscopically, the retrolental fibrous plaques can extend to the equator of the lens and consist of fibrous connective tissue with cartilage and bone (Fig. 14-44). In some cases, the fibrous tissue has collections of lenticular cells.

Vitreous Syneresis and Detachment

The aging process and certain pathologic processes, such as inflammation, can result in the denaturation of hyaluronic acid and the lysis of collagen fibrils within the vitreous. The vitreous body undergoes liquefaction (syneresis), which can cause separation of the posterior vitreous from the retina (vitreous detachment). This has an adverse effect on the metabolism of the sensory retina and can cause separation of the sensory retina from the retinal pigment epithelium (retinal detachment).

Hyalitis

Even though the vitreous is devoid of blood vessels, the presence of an inflammatory exudate within the vitreous is referred to as hyalitis. Hyalitis often is an extension of inflammation of the retina alone or concurrently with the choroid. Breakdown of the posterior blood-eye (blood-retina) barrier occurs with retinitis and chorioretinitis, and proteinaceous fluid leaks into the vitreous causing opacification (**plasmoid vitreous**). The type of inflammatory cell infiltrate is dependent on the cause. For example, suppurative or pyogranulomatous hyalitis commonly occurs with ocular blastomycosis and ocular protothecosis. Hyalitis can be diffuse or focal, as with ocular migration of the raccoon roundworm, *Baylisascaris procyonis*. Regardless of the distribution, hyalitis often causes liquefaction of the vitreous, which can lead to vitreous detachment and retinal detachment.

In addition to an extension of ocular inflammation, hyalitis can be caused by penetrating or perforating wounds. Foreign bodies and contaminating microbial organisms can be deposited within the vitreous. This can stimulate localized neutrophilic inflammation (**vitreous abscess**). The vitreous can prolapse into wounds of the anterior uvea and adhesions can form between the iris and the prolapsed vitreous. Fibrovascular membranes can form from inflammatory mediators. Adhesions or contraction of these membranes can result in rhegmatogenous retinal detachment from traction on the retina.

Asteroid Hyalosis

Asteroid hyalosis consists of numerous, minute (0.01 to 0.10 mm), spherical opacities suspended throughout the vitreous by attachment to the collagenous framework (Fig. 14-45). Although the cause is unknown, asteroid hyalosis commonly occurs with primary epithelial neoplasms of the ciliary body. Microscopically, the amorphous particles stain weakly basophilic with a routine stain (hematoxylin-eosin) and positive for lipid and acid mucopolysaccharides. The particles appear crystalline (birefringent) under polarized light.

Blood within the vitreous can come from hemorrhage of vessels in the anterior uvea or from vessels of the retina and choroid. Causes include leakage from a patent hyaloid vessel in young animals (e.g., common in young rats),

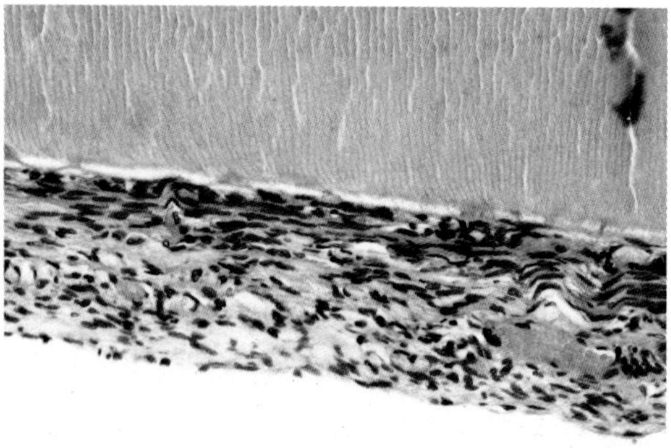

Figure 14-44 Globe, lens; canine. Persistent hyperplastic primary vitreous. A fibrovascular membrane extends along the posterior surface of the lens. H & E stain.

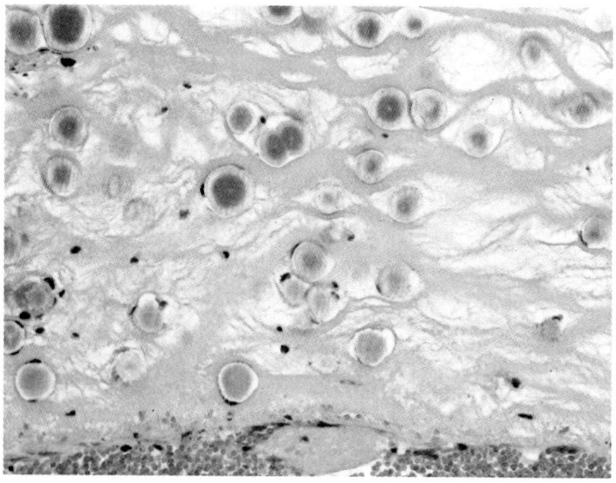

Figure 14-45 Globe, vitreous; canine. Asteroid hyalosis. Spherical crystalline bodies (calcium-lipid) in liquefied vitreous. H & E stain.

vasculitis associated with ocular inflammation, trauma, or leakage from newly formed fibrovascular membranes. With time, extensive hemorrhage can result in the deposition of cholesterol (synchysis scintillans) or hemosiderin (hemosiderosis) within the vitreous.

Synchysis Scintillans

Synchysis scintillans (cholesterosis bulbi) is a rare lesion that consists of numerous cholesterol particles within a liquefied vitreous. Because the particles are not attached to the collagenous framework of the vitreous, they settle inferiorly when the globe is immobile. Microscopically, they appear as nonstaining clefts, since the cholesterol crystals are removed during processing. The cause of synchysis scintillans can be the incomplete resolution of previous vitreous hemorrhage.

LESIONS OF THE RETINA

Usually, the term retina is used to refer to the entire retina, including the RPE, and the neurosensory retina. The neurosensory retina is also referred to as the neural retina or sensory retina.

Retinal Dysplasia

Retinal dysplasia is the faulty differentiation of the retina, especially photoreceptor cells, and proliferation of one or more of its constituent elements. Morphologic alterations occur before the retina reaches maturity. It is characterized by rosettes composed of a variable number of neuronal retinal cells, often with accompanying retinal folds (Fig. 14-46). Microscopically, retinal dysplasia can consist of rosettes with primitive, undifferentiated neuronal cells surrounding a lumen, or retinal folds. Spontaneous retinal dysplasia occurs in several breeds of dog including certain types of terriers and spaniels. It can be associated with a singular ocular defect or with multiple ocular anomalies, such as microphthalmia and posterior coloboma. Retinal dysplasia is often the result of an inherited defect, but can occur secondary to in utero viral infections, vitamin A deficiency, x-ray irradiation, certain drugs, and intrauterine trauma. Retinal dysplasia can be unilateral or bilateral and characterized as focal, multifocal, geographic, or complete with detachment. An in utero infection causes necrosis followed by astrocytosis and distortion of the retina. Examples of in utero infectious disease, which can be manifested by postinflammatory retinal dysplasia, include bovine virus diarrhea in calves and bluetongue in lambs. Lambs born of ewes given bluetongue virus vaccine during the first half of gestation can have the ocular lesions as well as lesions in the brain. Initially, inflammation of the retina (retinitis) with perivascular cuffing of lymphocytes and focal necrosis eventually leads to the formation of a glial scar.

Retinal Degeneration

Retinal degeneration is a broad term that includes degenerative changes in the retina, such as the loss of photoreceptors and other retinal neurons, and the formation of spaces within the retina. When retinal neurons are lost, the thickness of the neurosensory retina is decreased **(retinal atrophy).** Retinal atrophy is characterized by the layers of the retina that are lost. **Inner retinal atrophy** refers to loss of ganglion cells and their axons, and possibly loss of neurons, which have nuclei in the inner nuclear layer. Inner retinal atrophy is usually caused by glaucoma, but occlusion of retinal vessels or retrograde atrophy from disease involving the optic tract or optic nerve are possible causes. **Outer retinal atrophy** results from loss of photoreceptors. Because normal photoreceptors appear to be required for maintenance of other retinal neurons, outer retinal atrophy often progresses to panretinal atrophy (Fig. 14-47).

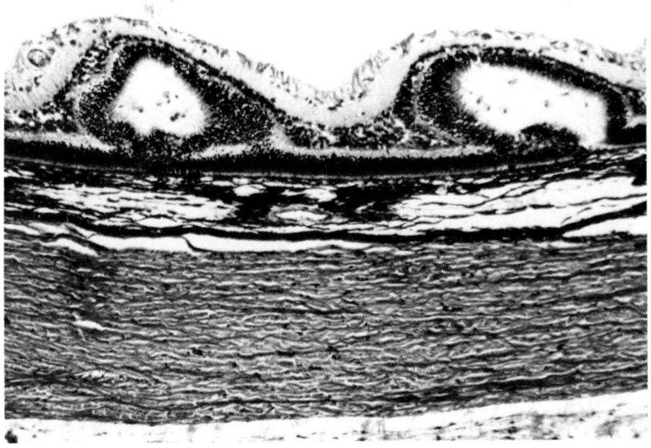

Figure 14-46 Globe, retina; bovine. Retinal dysplasia. Rosettes present in retina have central, irregular to oval cavity. H & E stain.

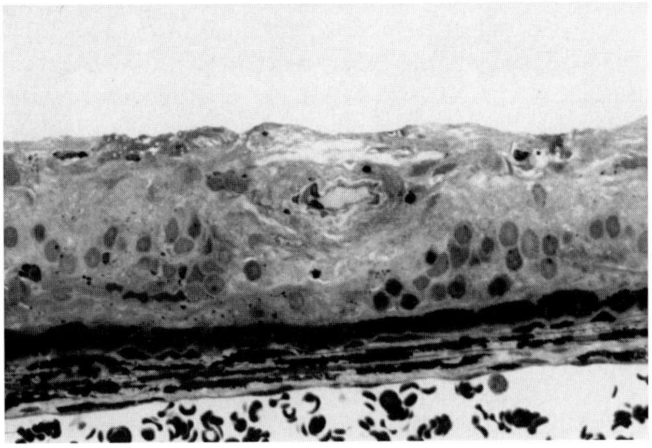

Figure 14-47 Globe, retina; canine. Severe retinal atrophy. Marked loss of cells in all retinal layers. H & E stain.

With time, retinal degeneration leads to thinning or atrophy of the neurosensory retina. A thin neurosensory retina allows more light to be reflected off the tapetum lucidum and results in tapetal hyperreflectivity seen at ophthalmic examination. As retinal atrophy progresses, retinal vessels become smaller. Regardless of the cause, degeneration of photoreceptors results in similar retinal alterations. Initially, photoreceptor outer segments are shortened, fragmented, and distorted. Lamellae, outer segments, and eventually whole photoreceptor cells are lost. Nuclei of degenerating photoreceptor cells migrate past the outer limiting membrane and into the layer of the rods and cones. Inner segments swell and nuclei become pyknotic. Eventually photoreceptors are lost, decreasing the number of nuclei in the outer nuclear layer. Posterior cortical cataract occurs as a result of retinal degeneration.

Retinal degeneration can be classified according to the cause. Causes include heredity, aging, nutritional deficiency, toxicity, excessive exposure to light, high oxygen tension, and exposure to radiation.

Developmental Retinal Degeneration

Developmental degeneration of photoreceptor cells occurs as an inherited lesion in the dog, cat, rodent, and chicken. Dysplasia of photoreceptor cells is a disorder in which photoreceptor cells never mature normally. The onset of dysfunction occurs at a young age. Types of **retinal dysplasia** in the dog include rod-cone dysplasia in the Norwegian elkhound, cone dysplasia in the Alaskan malamute, and photoreceptor cell dysplasia of rodents. Other types of inherited degeneration of photoreceptor cells occurs in middle-aged dogs. These disorders, referred to as **progressive retinal atrophy (PRA),** occurs in certain breeds (e.g., miniature poodle and cocker spaniel). Most types are inherited as simple autosomal conditions, but the ocular phenotype is similar. Often there is initial loss of function of rod photoreceptor cells (i.e., night blindness), but eventually function of cone photoreceptors is lost and blindness is complete. Similar conditions occur in cats and rodents. Diseases under the heading of PRA can be divided into two types: generalized PRA and central PRA (CPRA). The term CPRA has been replaced by the designation retinal pigment epithelial dystrophy (RPED).

Some inherited retinal disorders in animals are similar to human retinal diseases. For example, some retinal disorders in animals are similar to the human disease, retinitis pigmentosa. One canine disease, rod-cone dysplasia type 3 (rcd 3), occurs in Cardigan Welsh corgis. Affected dogs are blind by 3 years of age. The cause is a mutation in the gene encoding the alpha subunit of cyclic guanosine monophosphate (cGMP) phosphodiesterase. A similar disorder occurs in the Irish setter. Dogs affected with this disease have a mutation in the beta subunit of the cGMP phosphodiesterase gene. This condition is designated as rod-cone dysplasia type 1 (rcd 1) and is similar to the defect in a certain strain of mouse (rd mouse). Rod-cone dysplasia type 2 (rcd 2) occurs in the collie dog and is the result of a mutation of a different gene.

Retinal pigment epithelial dysplasia is a disorder that develops early in life and is the result of a defect in the retinal pigment epithelium. Lipofuscin accumulates within the cytoplasm of retinal pigment epithelial cells and alters their function. The disease occurs in the collie dog, spaniels, retrievers, and the Royal College of Surgeons (RCS) rat. The retinal pigment epithelial cells become hypertrophied and form multicellular nests. Secondary degenerative changes occur within photoreceptor cells.

Retinal degeneration can be characterized by distribution (e.g., focal multifocal or diffuse), or by etiology. Some causes of outer retinal degeneration are unknown, but other causes include aging, toxins, nutritional deficiencies, excessive light, exposure to radiation, and exposure to excessive amounts of oxygen. Retinal degeneration can occur as a result of vascular lesions of diabetes mellitus or as a sequela to retinal inflammation.

Sudden Acquired Retinal Degeneration

Sudden acquired retinal degeneration syndrome (SARDS) is a disease in dogs that results in acute blindness from degeneration of photoreceptor cells. Blindness occurs over a period of days to weeks. The disease often develops in dogs around a mean age of 9 years with a greater tendency of occurrence in neutered females and dachshunds. The ocular fundus has a normal or near-normal appearance and the electroretinographic response is extinguished. Affected dogs can have polydipsia, polyuria, polyphagia, and weight gain. The cause is unknown, and therapy fails to stop the progression of the disease.

Senile Retinal Degeneration

Senile retinal degeneration is characterized by gradually expanding **cystoid degeneration of the peripheral retina** and retinal breaks. The microcystoid spaces are mainly in the outer retinal layers and are caused by intraretinal edema. Retinal breaks can be complete without retinal detachment and includes holes, ruptured peripheral retinal cysts, holes associated with vitreous strands, and breaks associated with choroidal coloboma. The retina can have large patches of retinal atrophy associated with holes. The holes can spread and coalesce, leading to **retinoschisis.**

Nutritional Retinopathy

Vitamin A, vitamin E, and taurine are important nutrients for the maintenance of photoreceptors. Vitamin A (retinol) is stored in the retinal pigment epithelium and combines with opsin to form rhodopsin, a visual pigment. A systemic vitamin A deficiency is characterized by night blindness in several species. Additional ocular lesions associated with a vitamin A deficiency include corneal hyperkeratosis and a decrease in the number of conjunctival goblet cells.

Vitamin E is an antioxidant that maintains the stability of cell membranes by preventing lipid peroxidation. Puppies fed a feed deficient in vitamin E developed retinal changes consisting of tapetal hyperreflectivity and attenuation of retinal vessels. Microscopically, photoreceptors are lost and an accumulation of autofluorescent pigment is within the cytoplasm of cells of the RPE.

Taurine is a sulfur-containing amino acid essential to cats. Unlike other animals, cats have a limited ability to synthesize it from cystine. In addition to the heart, taurine is found in high tissue concentration in the retina, especially the photoreceptors. It is now accepted that deficiency of taurine results in the condition known as nutritional feline degeneration and feline central retinal degeneration. Lesions begin as focal degeneration of photoreceptors in the "area centralis." This has an ophthalmoscopic appearance of an ellipsoidal, hyperreflective lesion that progressively enlarges. Microscopically, degeneration and loss of photoreceptors are present, and the changes begin with vesiculation and disorientation of cone outer segment discs. With time, rod photoreceptors can be affected.

Many drugs, compounds, and some poisonous plants are associated with adverse effects on the retina. Some, such as ethambutol and hydroxypyridinethione, target the cells of the tapetum lucidium causing swelling, disorientation, and possibly necrosis. These changes cause serous retinal detachment. Drugs, such as azalide, causes swelling of cells in the tapetum lucidium, but also the accumulation of lysosomal bodies within retinal ganglion cells. In sheep, ingestion of locoweed *(Astragalus mollissimus)* causes vacuolation of retinal ganglion cells, bipolar cells, ciliary epithelial cells, and lacrimal gland acinar cells. Ingestion of bracken fern *(Pteridium aquilinum)* by sheep results in bright blindness, a disease characterized by degeneration of rod and cone photoreceptors.

Light-Induced Retinopathy

Photoreceptors are sensitive to an excessive amount of fluorescent and incandescent light, especially the photoreceptors of albino rats (Fig. 14-48). This effect appears to be enhanced by increased ambient temperature, lack of ocular pigmentation, mydriasis, increased age of the animal, and sex (e.g., higher incidence in female rats). Several types of lasers are also capable of producing retinal damage.

The extent of damage to the retina is modified by many variables, such as wavelength of light. The wavelengths most efficient in producing retinal damage are those most efficient in bleaching rhodopsin. The rate of degeneration is also directly related to such variables as the intensity of the illumination, duration of exposure, increased body temperature, and increased age of the animal.

Continuous light produces early effects in the outer segments of the photoreceptor cells. Microscopically, photoreceptors undergo typical degenerative changes beginning with the outer segments and progressing to loss of photoreceptor cells resulting in atrophy of the outer retina.

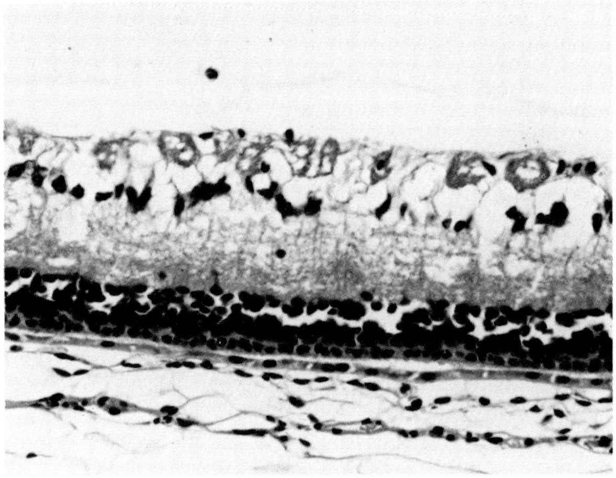

Figure 14-48 Globe, retina; murine. Light-induced retinopathy. Atrophy involves the outer retinal layers (loss of layer of rods and cones and much of outer nuclear layer) in a rat exposed to continuous light for several weeks. H & E stain.

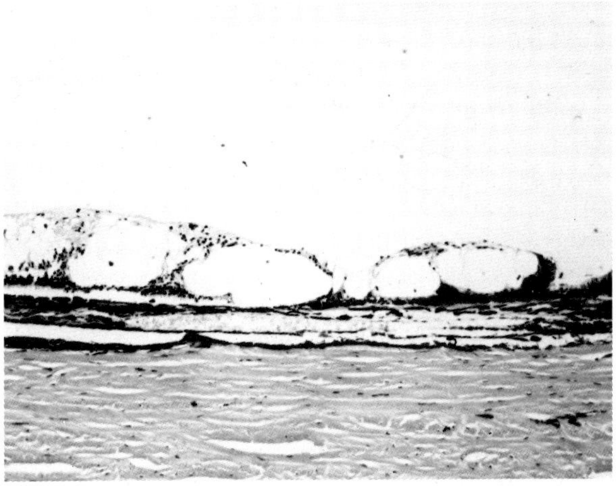

Figure 14-49 Globe, retina; canine. Cystoid degeneration of peripheral retina consists of multiple variably sized cysts with replacement of retina. H & E stain.

Peripheral Cystoid Retinal Degeneration

Peripheral cystoid retinal degeneration is a common intraocular lesion that begins in young animals, but increases in size with age. It consists of a variable number of small cysts, which begin within the middle layers of the retina (Fig. 14-49). With time, the cysts extend to the inner limiting membrane and into the external layers of the retina. Microscopically, the spaces often are empty. Coalescence of numerous microcysts results in retinoschisis.

Retinal Cysts and Retinoschisis

A focal space within the neurosensory retina is referred to as a retinal cyst, even though the space is not lined by epithelial cells. Microscopically, retinal cysts are often in the middle and inner retinal layers and free of contents (content is usually lost during processing). The contents are usually fluid from retinal vessels. Retinoschisis is an intraretinal space that has a smaller internal-external thickness than width.

Retinal Detachment

The neurosensory retina is attached to the optic disc and abruptly becomes the inner ciliary epithelium at the ora ciliaris retinae. The RPE stops at the optic disc and abruptly becomes the pigmented ciliary epithelium at the ora ciliaris retinae. Retinal detachment (RD) is the separation of the neurosensory retina from the RPE. This expands the potential space (subretinal space) between the two portions of the retina.

There are four types of retinal detachment—congenital, tractional, exudative, and rhegmatogenous. Congenital RD is most likely nonattachment of the neurosensory retina. This lesion is often observed with microphthalmia. The cause is believed to be improper induction of the choroid and sclera by the RPE. This causes an imbalance between the size of the neurosensory retina and the size of the choroid and sclera combined. The result is focal linear areas of nonattachment of the neurosensory retina **(retinal folds)** or diffuse nonattachment of the neurosensory retina (retinal detachment).

Tractional RD can occur with vitreous syneresis. The neurosensory retina that is attached to the vitreous is pulled away as the vitreous shrinks. Exudative RD occurs if fluid or an inflammatory exudate accumulates within the subretinal space (Fig. 14-50). Rhegmatogenous RD occurs when the peripheral neurosensory retina tears away from the ora ciliaris retinae. Microscopically, the edges of the neurosensory retina around the tear are rounded. A lesion associated with retinal tears is proliferative vitreoretinopathy. This is a membrane that forms from glial cells and other retinal cells that proliferate on the inner limiting membrane.

Complete retinal detachment is recognized as a ballooning anterior displacement of the neurosensory retina. The neurosensory retina forms a posteriorly directed "funnel" that is attached at the ora ciliaris retinae and the optic disc. Separation of the neurosensory retina from the RPE disrupts an intimate and essential association between the photoreceptor cells and the RPE. Retinal detachment also results in displacement of the photoreceptor cells from their source of nutrients, the choriocapillaris. This results in changes in the photoreceptor cells. The outer segments of photoreceptor cells undergo degenerative changes and gradually shorten. If retinal detachment persists, photoreceptor cells eventually become necrotic and are lost. The RPE undergoes a reactive change. Microscopically, the retinal pigment epithelial cells become individualized and slightly elongated, resulting in a distinctive "cobblestone" or "tombstone" appearance (Fig. 14-51). If retinal detachment persists, hyperplasia of the RPE and retinal cysts can occur.

Artifactual retinal detachment is common. As the period between surgical enucleation and death of the animal and fixation increases, the possibility of artifactual retinal detachment also increases. The neurosensory retina can be easily detached from the RPE if an enucleated globe is handled roughly or incised before fixation. After fixation, artifactual retinal detachment can occur when the globe is trimmed. Microscopically, lesions, such as photoreceptor atrophy, hypertrophy of the RPE, protein, or cells within the subretinal space are not present in cases of artifactual retinal detachment.

Retinitis

Inflammation of the retina **(retinitis)** is often characterized by perivascular cuffing of retinal vessels by lymphocytes that is seen concurrently with a similar vascular lesion in

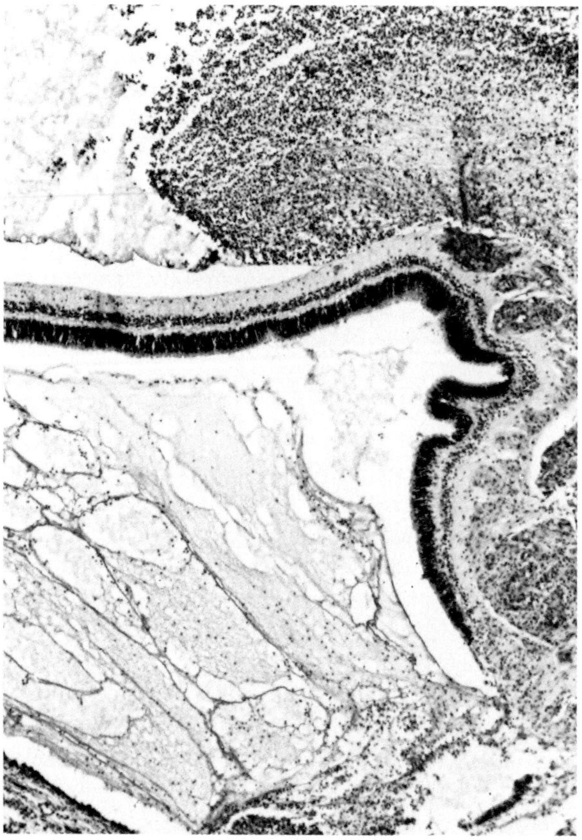

Figure 14-50 Globe, equine. Suppurative endophthalmitis. The lesions include papillitis, perivascular retinitis, and hyalitis with exudate extending into the vitreous, retinal detachment, and a subretinal exudate. H & E stain.

the iris and ciliary body (anterior uveitis). Retinitis occurs with idiopathic lymphoplasmacytic anterior uveitis in cats and is seen with ocular toxoplasmosis and viral diseases, such as malignant catarrhal fever in cattle (Fig. 14-52), feline infectious peritonitis, and canine distemper.

Inflammation of the retina also occurs concurrently with inflammation of the choroid **(chorioretinitis).** This inflammation results in detachment of the neurosensory retina by accumulation of an exudate in the subretinal space. Chorioretinitis with retinal detachment occurs in thromboembolic meningoencephalitis in cattle (Fig. 14-53), mycobacterial infections in cats and horses, systemic mycoses (e.g., blastomycosis), protothecosis, and the ocular migration of certain ascarids. Cryptococcal organisms tend to accumulate in the subretinal space, but the associated inflammation is often minimal. Ocular lesions of canine distemper involve the retina and optic nerve, but eosinophilic intranuclear and intracytoplasmic inclusions occur in other cells of the eye including ciliary, conjunctival, and corneal epithelium. Lesions include necrosis and loss of retinal cells and lymphocytic perivascular cuffing. Other viral diseases and toxoplasmosis can produce similar retinal lesions (e.g., pseudorabies in pigs).

Retinal Neoplasia

In animals, retinal neoplasia is rare. Retinal neoplasms include medulloepithelioma, and secondary neoplasia

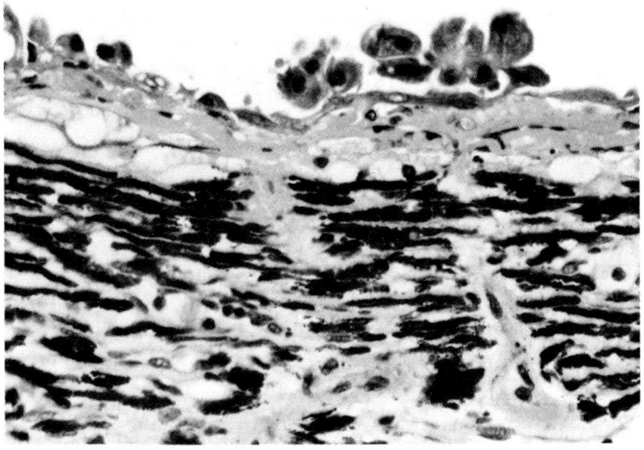

Figure 14-51 Globe, choroid and retinal pigment epithelium; canine. Retinal detachment. Hypertrophy and hyperplasia of retinal pigment epithelium occur when the retina is detached. H & E stain.

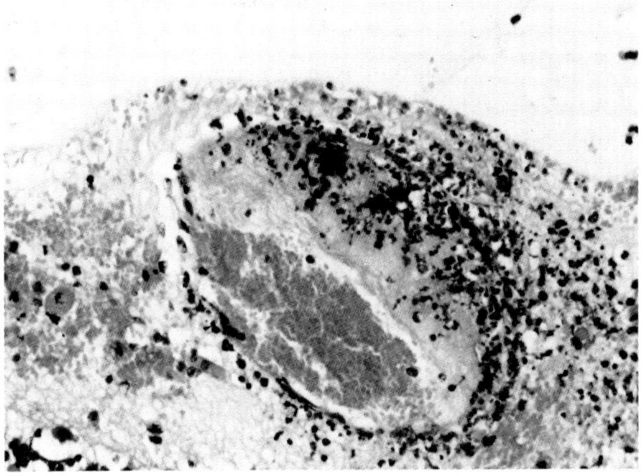

Figure 14-52 Globe, retina; bovine. Malignant catarrhal fever. Retinitis characterized by mononuclear cells within the walls and forming cuffs about retinal vessels. H & E stain. *Courtesy Dr. H.E. Whiteley.*

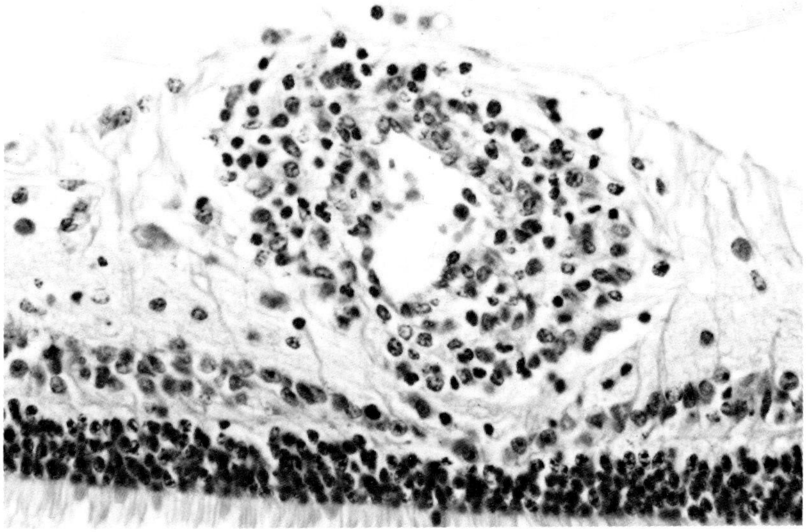

Figure 14-53 Globe, retina; bovine. Thromboembolic meningoencephalitis. *Haemophilus somnus* infection results in vasculitis, thrombosis, and retinal hemorrhage and necrosis. H & E stain.

from hematogenous metastatic spread or extension from neoplasia in another part of the eye. Medulloepithelioma arises from neuroepithelium, as well as retinoblastoma, but most retinal neoplasms in animals fail to meet the characteristics of human retinoblastoma.

LESIONS OF THE OPTIC NERVE

Axons of retinal ganglion cells converge at the optic disc (optic papilla, optic nerve head), traverse the lamina cribrosa, and form the optic nerve. The optic nerve is a white fiber tract of the central nervous system extending from the globe to the optic chiasma. Axons of the optic nerve continue beyond the optic chiasma to form the optic tracts. The optic nerve consists of ocular, orbital, and intracranial portions. The orbital and intracranial portions are covered by the optic meninges that are continuous with the meninges of the brain. The optic disc, optic nerve, and lamina cribrosa vary in morphologic appearance among species. The optic disc has a depression (physiologic cup) in the dog and rabbit. In most species, the axons of the ocular optic nerve are unmyelinated and become myelinated in the region of the lamina cribrosa. In the dog and the rabbit, myelinated fibers occur within the optic disc. Primates have a function central retinal artery and vein, but in other species, vessels enter the nerve through the sclera. The lamina cribrosa is dense and prominent in the horse, cow, and dog, but almost nonexistent in the rabbit and rodents.

In cross section (H & E stain), the axis cylinders of the nerve fibers appear as small, faintly stained eosinophilic dots surrounded by clear halos—the myelin sheath. The normal nerve is rather pale with a microscopic spongiform appearance. Glial cells are inconspicuous, and the nerve appears hypocellular.

Anomalies of the Optic Nerve

Aplasia of the optic nerve is rare in animals. The optic nerves are thin, fragile strands that extend from the globe to the brain with no recognizable chiasma. Retinal ganglion cells and their axons in the optic nerve, optic chiasma, and optic tracts are absent.

Hypoplasia of the optic nerve is rare. It can result from failure of development of the ganglion cell layer and absence of a corresponding number of optic nerve fibers. The extent of the reduction in size of the nerve varies from a severe form, in which only a thin fragment remains, to a mild form, in which the reduction in size is slight. The optic chiasms and optic tracts have a similar amount of reduced size.

Coloboma of the optic nerve is a focal absence of the optic disc and ocular optic nerve, which results in cavitation of these structures. The anomaly can produce outward retrobulbar ectasia of the sclera and is often accompanied by dysplasia of the adjacent retina. The colobomatous cavities are lined by thinned retina and choroid. Coloboma of the optic nerve can occur alone, but is often associated with microphthalmia, especially in the dog, in which it is part of the collie eye anomaly syndrome. Coloboma of the optic disc has also been described in cattle and cats.

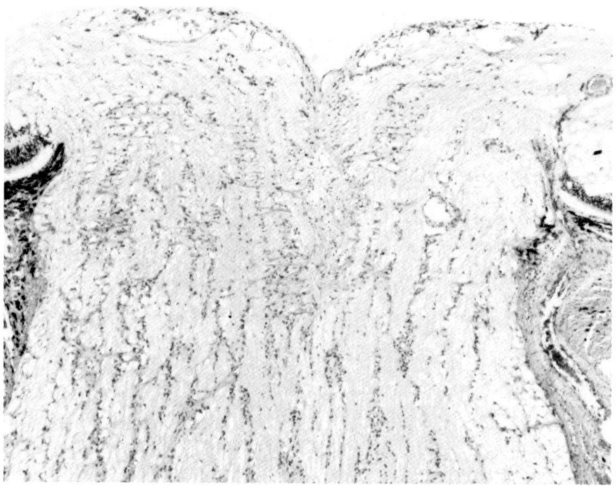

Figure 14-54 Globe, optic nerve; canine. Papilledema. Optic nerve head is pale staining, swollen, and protrudes into vitreous (rafoxanide toxicity). H & E stain. *Courtesy Dr. R. Brown.*

Papilledema

Swelling of the optic disc because of edema is termed papilledema (Fig. 14-54). The cause is an increase in the pressure posterior to the lamina cribrosa so that the flow of the tissue fluid is outward (from the optic nerve into the globe). This is the result of space-occupying intracranial lesions, increased venous pressure, meningitis, and orbital neoplasms. Microscopically, the vessels of the optic disc can be congested, and the optic disc is swollen and pale staining. The optic disc bulges into the vitreous cavity and can cause buckling of the retina. Chronic papilledema causes degenerative changes resulting in optic atrophy and astrogliosis.

Inflammation of the Optic Nerve

Inflammation can involve any portion of the optic nerve. Inflammation of the optic disc is **optic papillitis,** which can occur alone or as part of inflammation of the optic nerve, retina, or globe. It is characterized by cellular infiltrates, edema, and astrogliosis. Inflammation of the optic nerve **(optic neuritis)** usually occurs along with lesions in the globe or brain and can be subdivided into **optic meningitis** (perineuritis; leptomeningitis of the optic nerve), periaxial optic neuritis (extension of meningeal inflammation along the pial septa into the parenchyma of the optic nerve), axial neuritis (selective involvement of the inner portions of the optic nerve), and transverse neuritis (severe and extensive inflammation of the optic nerve).

When inflammation of the optic nerve occurs, it is often a manifestation of a systemic disease or an extension of a

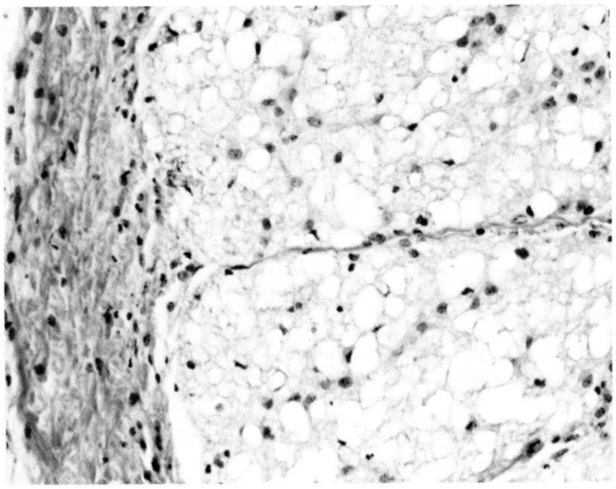

Figure 14-55 Globe, optic nerve; bovine. Male fern optic neuropathy. Spongy degeneration (edema, demyelination, vacuolation) involves the peripheral portion of the optic nerve. H & E stain. *Courtesy Dr. D.R. Lucas.*

localized lesion. Optic neuritis occurs with certain infectious diseases, such as encephalitozoonosis in rabbits, toxoplasmosis in several species, and canine distemper, and produces lesions similar to those within the brain. Granulomatous optic neuritis occurs with some cases of granulomatous optic meningitis and also occurs in cases of feline infectious peritonitis. Optic meningitis with minimal inflammation but with numerous organisms occurs in cats with ocular cryptococcosis. Usually concurrent accumulations of yeast cells occurs within the subretinal space. Optic meningitis also can be an extension of cerebral leptomeningitis, especially when leptomeningitis is caused by bacteria. Optic meningitis also can be a direct extension of localized inflammation from the sinuses, orbital space, or globe.

Degeneration of the Optic Nerve

Because the optic nerve is a part of the central nervous system, the nerve fibers have no Schwann cells and little or no capacity for regeneration. Glial, meningeal, and connective tissue components of the optic nerve respond to injury by proliferation. Optic nerve degeneration can be ascending when lesions affect retinal ganglion cells (Wallerian degeneration) and can vary in severity. The result is optic atrophy with reduction in the diameter of the optic nerve because of a loss of axons. Microscopically, the optic nerve becomes less spongy, more compact, and more eosinophilic because of wallerian degeneration, loss of axons, an increased number of glial cells, and an increased amount of connective tissue. Similar changes also occur as an aging change, especially in the dog, and include decreased diameter of axons, increased thickness of pial septa, and astrogliosis.

Degenerative optic neuropathy can occur as the result of optic neuritis, vascular disease near the globe, retinal degeneration, prolonged papilledema, glaucoma, or certain toxicologic diseases, such as rafoxanide and male fern toxicoses. Rafoxanide is a halogenated salicylanilide with fasciolicidal activity that causes increased cerebrospinal fluid pressure in the dog and sheep. The increased pressure causes papilledema and status spongiosus of the corpus callosum, fornix, periventricular areas of the brain, and optic nerves. Male fern *(Dryopteris [Aspidinum] felix-mas; Dryopteris austriaca)* is a plant that contains a complex mixture of phloroglucin derivatives (Fig. 14-55). Calves ingesting the rhizomes of male fern develop acute peripapillary hemorrhage and papilledema. In the chronic stage, the optic disc is depressed and light gray and contains degenerative changes.

Optic neuropathy occurs in calves from dams fed a vitamin A–deficient feed. These calves are blind because of constriction of the orbital optic nerve that increases the cerebrospinal fluid pressure. This results in papilledema. The blindness in calves can vary in severity from a reversible night blindness to the irreversible blindness of retinal degeneration and optic nerve atrophy (Fig. 14-56). Calves deficient in vitamin A have bones with an increased thickness and reduced density.

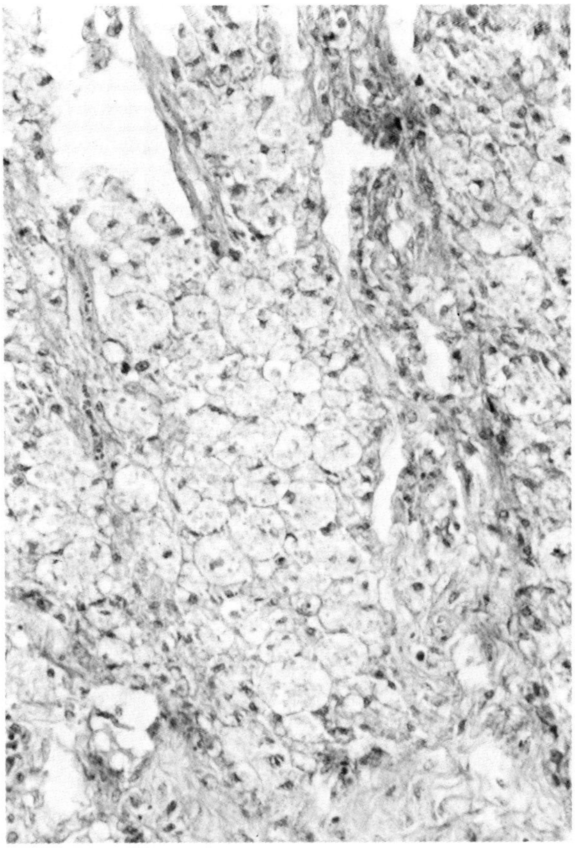

Figure 14-56 Globe, optic nerve, bovine. Vitamin A deficiency. Necrosis of optic nerve is accompanied by replacement with large foamy macrophages ("gitter cells"). H & E stain. *Courtesy Dr. S. Nielsen.*

Proliferative Optic Neuropathy

Proliferative optic neuropathy is a white or white-gray, round or oval, elevated mass partially covering the optic disc. The lesion is usually unilateral, and visual disturbances are not detected. The thinly encapsulated mass is composed of large, plump, round to ovoid cells with small, dense, eccentrically placed nuclei and palely eosinophilic, foamy to vacuolated cytoplasm (Fig. 14-57).

Neoplasms of the Optic Nerve

Neoplasms of the optic nerve are rare. The most common neoplasm is optic meningioma in the dog (Fig. 14-58).

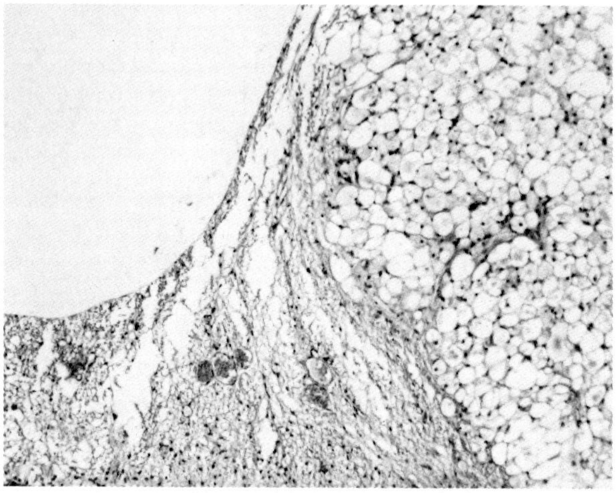

Figure 14-57 Globe, optic disc; equine. Proliferative optic neuropathy. Circumscribed lesion is composed of sheet of large cells with vacuolated cytoplasm. H & E stain.

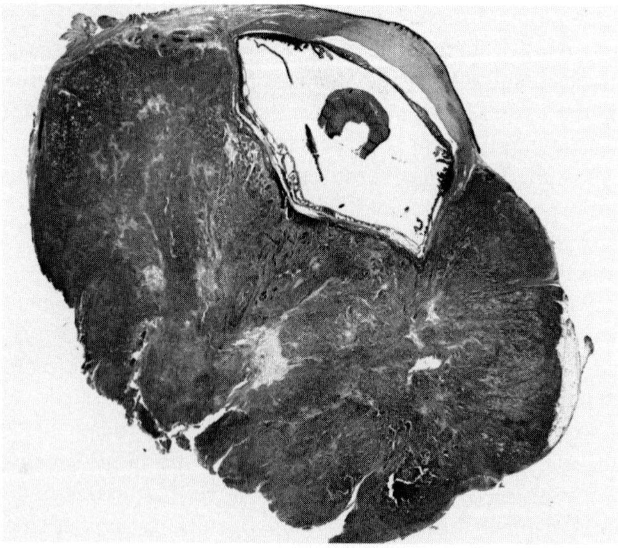

Figure 14-58 Globe; canine. Optic meningioma. Retrobulbar meningioma surrounds the optic nerve, filling the space within the orbit, and results in exophthalmos and exposure keratitis. H & E stain.

This neoplasm is glossy white and surrounds the retrobulbar optic nerve. Microscopically, the neoplasm consists of whorls of meningoepithelial cells, scattered lamellated mineralized foci (psammoma bodies), or foci of metaplastic bone or cartilage. These neoplasms can enlarge, fill the orbit, cause exophthalmos, and extend along the optic nerve.

Other neoplasms of the optic nerve include medulloepithelioma, especially in the horse, and rarely, astrocytoma.

Metastatic neoplasms of the optic nerve or optic meninges are rare. Metastatic carcinoma, including squamous cell carcinoma, occurs in cats.

GLAUCOMA

Aqueous humor is the transparent fluid that is similar to an ultrafiltrate of plasma. It is continuously formed by the ciliary processes through a combined process of active secretion, ultrafiltration, and simple diffusion. From the posterior chamber, aqueous humor flows through the pupil and into the anterior chamber. Aqueous humor then flows into the iridocorneal angle and through the openings in the pectinate ligament that extends between the peripheral edge of Descemet's membrane and the root of the iris. Aqueous humor then flows through the filtration spaces between the uveal trabecular meshwork in the ciliary cleft and eventually through the corneoscleral meshwork and into the scleral vascular structures (angular aqueous plexus). The rate of aqueous humor formation varies among species, but the rate of formation equals the outflow so that intraocular pressure (IOP) is maintained at a relatively constant level. In addition to the abovementioned conventional outflow, there are nonconventional routes that are used to a variable degree by various species. Obstruction to net outflow increases the IOP.

Glaucoma is considered a group of related diseases. The common feature of these diseases is sustained increase in IOP and the resultant changes produced in various ocular structures. The main change is progressive loss of retinal ganglion cells and their axons. Elevated IOP is considered the primary recognized cause of glaucoma, although abnormalities in microcirculation or extracellular matrix of the optic disc and the presence of excitotoxic amino acids could be contributing factors. Because the elevated IOP is almost always caused by changes that reduce aqueous outflow, types of glaucoma can be classified by the type of obstruction. This classification scheme includes congenital glaucoma, primary glaucoma, and secondary glaucoma.

Congenital Glaucoma

Congenital glaucoma is rare and occurs shortly after birth. The elevated IOP results from abnormal development of the anterior segment. The cause is usually unknown, although some cases of congenital glaucoma in animals are the result of intraocular inflammation from an intrauterine bacterial infection.

Primary Glaucoma

Primary glaucoma is considered an inherited, bilateral disease, although both globes do not always have lesions of equal severity. This type of glaucoma has been described in several breeds of dog (eg., basset hound) and is commonly associated with goniodysgenesis. **Goniodysgenesis** is a term used to imply abnormal development of the pectinate ligament, trabecular meshwork, ciliary cleft, or some combination (Fig. 14-59). Microscopically, the pectinate ligament can be shortened, thickened, or nonexistent. The root of the iris can be positioned immediately adjacent to the corneoscleral junction. The peripheral edge of Descemet's membrane can have multiple abnormalities including thickening, fibriation, and elongated projections extending into the ciliary cleft. The ciliary cleft is partially or totally collapsed.

Secondary Glaucoma

Most cases of glaucoma in animals are of the secondary type and unilateral and are due to complications of traumatic, inflammatory, degenerative, or neoplastic disease. Obstruction of aqueous outflow can occur at the pupil, iridocorneal angle, ciliary cleft, or trabecular meshwork. Anterior displacement of the vitreous and obstruction of aqueous flow from the posterior chamber can occur following subluxation or anterior luxation of the lens.

A dislocated lens can cause pupillary blockage and closure of the iridocorneal angle. Extreme pupillary block occurs when the lens is dislocated into the anterior chamber with the iris pressed against the posterior surface of the lens. It is not always possible in the late stages of glaucoma to distinguish primary from secondary lens luxation.

Secondary closure of the iridocorneal angle can be caused by pupillary block, which obstructs the flow of aqueous between the posterior and anterior chambers. Annular adhesions, because of organization of inflammatory exudate, develop between the lens and the pupillary part of the iris in certain cases of iritis and, if complete, the pressure increase in the posterior chamber pushes the iris forward, producing **iris bombé** (Fig. 14-60). If iris bombé is chronic, collapse of the ciliary cleft occurs and peripheral anterior synechiae form at the site of contact between the iris and peripheral cornea. Adhesions form because of iridal swelling and exudates in the iridocorneal angle. As the IOP increases, the root of the iris is displaced forward to further decrease the width of the iridocorneal angle.

Preiridal fibrovascular membrane causes secondary glaucoma by extending over the pectinate ligament. Vasogenic factors released by a hypoxic retina, neoplastic cells, or inflammatory cells stimulate endothelial cells to extend along the anterior surface of the iris. These

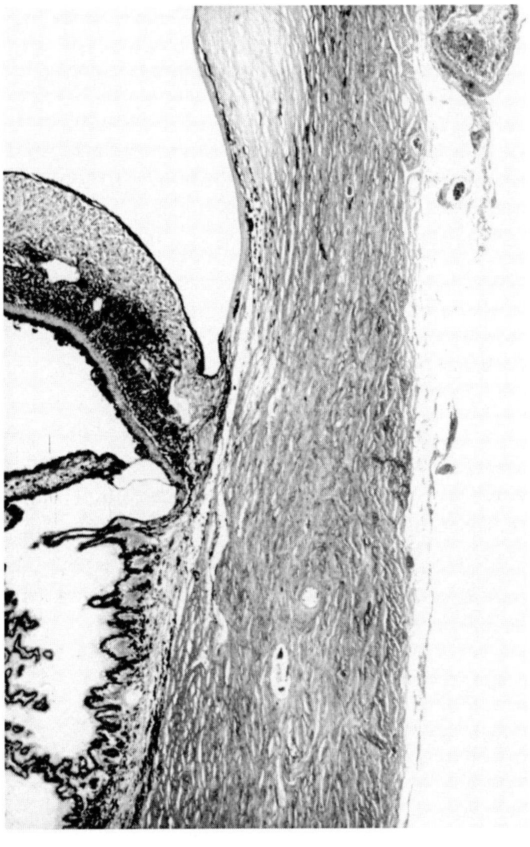

Figure 14-59 Globe; canine. Primary glaucoma. Goniodysgenesis with collapse of the ciliary cleft. H & E stain.

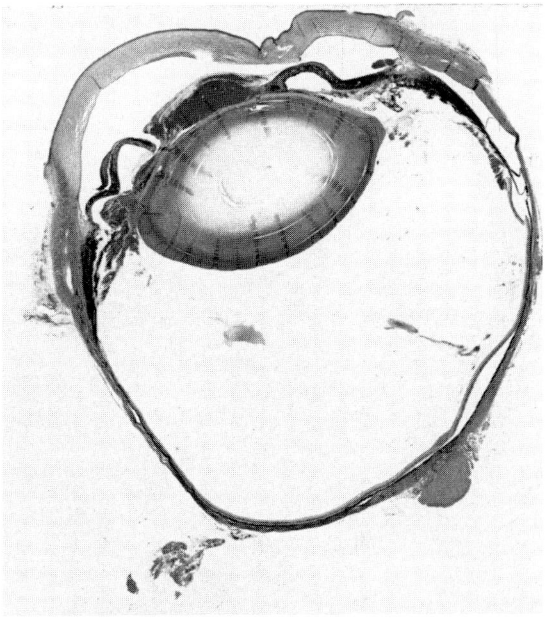

Figure 14-60 Globe; canine. Iris bombé. Diffuse peripupillary posterior synechiae with blood in anterior and posterior chambers. H & E stain.

endothelial cells give rise to a fibrovascular membrane, which becomes more fibrous with time. The membrane contracts as it matures, causing the pupillary margin of the iris to fold inward **(entropion uveae)** or fold outward **(ectropion uveae).** The membrane's vessels are fragile and bleed into the anterior chamber **(hyphema).**

Glaucoma often develops in globes with a neoplasm of the anterior segment. Intraocular neoplasms produce peripheral anterior synechiae by displacing the iris forward against the trabecular meshwork or cause the formation of a preiridal fibrovascular membrane (e.g., ciliary adenoma). Intraocular neoplasms of the iris and ciliary body, whether primary or metastatic, can invade and obstruct the iridocorneal angle, ciliary cleft, or trabecular meshwork.

Ocular Effects of Glaucoma

Regardless of cause, persistent elevated **IOP** causes changes in intraocular structures. The globe enlarges (buphthalmos, buphthalmia), and the sclera and uvea are stretched outward by the pressure. The root of the iris is displaced in an outward and posterior direction, which causes collapse of the ciliary cleft and trabecular meshwork. **Uveal atrophy** occurs with time. The iridal stroma becomes thin and there is gradual atrophy of the ciliary body (Fig. 14-61). With buphthalmos, tension on zonular fiber increases and leads to tearing and eventually to **subluxation or luxation of the lens.** Increased IOP changes the composition and rate of aqueous humor formation; these changes can be contributing factors in the formation of cataract associated with glaucoma. As the IOP increases, the metabolism of the corneal endothelial cells decreases and edema of the corneal stroma develops. **Corneal edema** causes the corneal stroma to be thicker. This change, combined with buphthalmos, results in failure of the eyelids to cover the cornea **(lagophthalmos).** This lack of coverage causes evaporation of the precorneal tear film, corneal vascularization, migration of melanocytes into the cornea, keratitis, and, possibly, corneal ulceration. As glaucoma persists, gradual loss of corneal endothelial cells occurs and focal, linear breaks develop in Descemet's membrane **(Haab's striae).**

Changes occur in the vitreous, retina, and optic nerve associated with glaucoma. The vitreous undergoes liquefaction (vitreous syneresis). As the globe enlarges, the sclera stretches and the scleral lamina cribrosa is pushed posteriorly. Because the retina cannot stretch, the sensory retina becomes detached and axons of retinal ganglion cells undergo wallerian degeneration (Fig. 14-62). The optic disc develops a posterior cup and loculated cavities containing proteinaceous material can occur (Schnabel's cavernous atrophy).

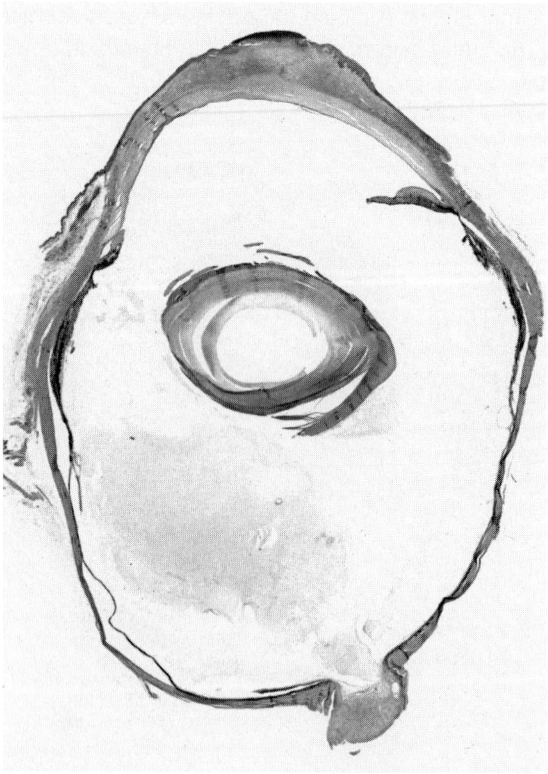

Figure 14-61 Globe; canine. Glaucoma. Exposure keratitis, ciliary body atrophy, lens luxation, and cupping of the optic disc are present. H & E stain.

OCULAR MANIFESTATIONS OF STORAGE DISEASES

Inborn errors of metabolism are rare in animals and result from a deficiency in a specific enzyme that causes the enzyme substrate to accumulate in many different cells of the globe, optic nerve, and other tissues. The substrate is usually a complex lipid, glycoprotein, or polysaccharide. The defect is usually inherited as a recessive trait. These animal diseases can serve as animal models of human disease.

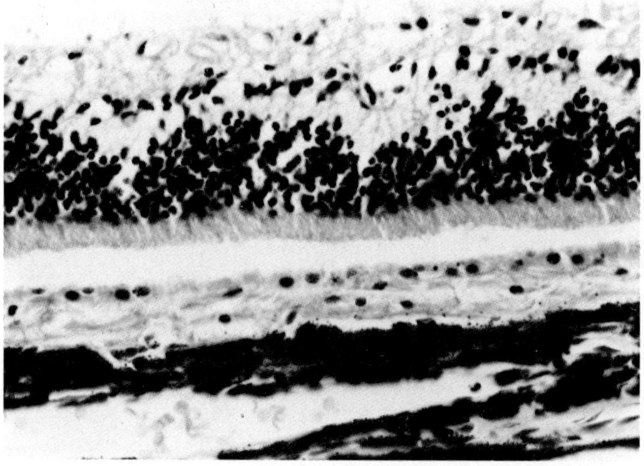

Figure 14-62 Globe, retina; canine. Secondary glaucoma. The inner layers of the retina are atrophied with only a single row of nuclei remaining of inner nuclear layer. Outer nuclear layer and layer of rods and cones appear unaffected. H & E stain.

Gangliosidosis

Gangliosidosis is caused by a deficiency of lysosomal hydrolase, ß-galactosidase, and is characterized by an accumulation of GM_1 ganglioside in the cerebral cortex and the eye of the dog, cat, and cattle. Retinal ganglion cells are enlarged and swollen and have granular cytoplasm caused by the presence of membranous inclusions (Fig. 14-63). Affected cats have unique, faint corneal opacity associated with intracellular vacuoles within keratocytes and corneal endothelial cells.

Mannosidosis

Mannosidosis is a recessively inherited disease caused by a deficiency of mannosidase, resulting in lysosomal storage of mannose-rich glycoproteins, glycopeptides, and oligosaccharides. Ocular lesions have been described in animals with deficiencies of the α and β forms of mannosidase. Aberdeen Angus and Murray Grey cattle affected with α-mannosidosis have vacuolated retinal cells. Nubian goats affected with α-mannosidosis have small palpebral fissures, a paucity of myelin in the optic nerves, and the presence of numerous, nonstaining, spherical, intracytoplasmic vacuoles in retinal ganglion cells, ciliary epithelium, retinal pigment epithelium, keratocytes, corneal endothelial cells, other retinal cells, and other mesenchymal cells. Similar lesions, except for vacuolation of the retinal pigment epithelium, have been observed in affected Salers cattle.

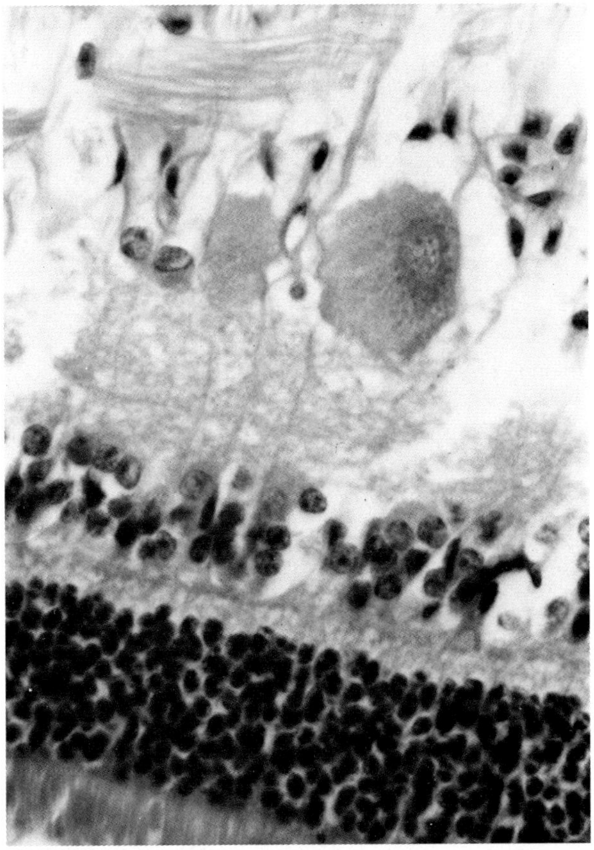

Figure 14-63 Globe, retina; bovine. GM_1 gangliosidosis. Retinal ganglion cells are enlarged, swollen, and have granular cytoplasm. H & E stain. *Courtesy Dr. B. Sheahan.*

Mucopolysaccharidoses

Mucopolysaccharidoses (MPS) are a group of diseases characterized by defective glycosaminoglycan catabolism. Ocular lesions have been described in cats and dogs with MPS I. Affected animals have diffuse corneal opacities as the result of the accumulation of mucopolysaccharide due to an α-L-iduronidase deficiency. Cats affected with MPS I have intracytoplasmic vacuoles in connective tissue cells of the cornea, conjunctiva, sclera, choroid, iris, ciliary body, in the epithelium of the iris and ciliary body; and in the retinal pigment epithelium. Cats with MPS IV have similar lesions. Vacuolated cells and retinal degeneration is reported in dogs affected by MPS VII, a deficiency of β-glucoronidase.

Fucosidosis

Fucosidosis is a recessively inherited disease in the English springer spaniel in Australia and England. It is caused by a deficiency of α-L-fucosidase, which results in an accumulation of a fucose substrate within cells, including retinal ganglion cells. Clinically, affected dogs have visual impairment, although no ophthalmoscopic lesions have been observed.

Ceroid Lipofuscinoses

Ceroid lipofuscinoses are a group of metabolic diseases characterized by the accumulation of an autofluorescent lipopigment (ceroid) in neurons, including those of the retina. The disease occurs in cattle, sheep, dogs, and cats. Affected English setters are blind at approximately 1 year of age and have cellular inclusions within retinal ganglion cells, other retinal neuronal cells, and retinal pigment epithelial cells.

LESIONS OF THE EYELIDS

Eyelids have an outer layer composed of skin and an inner layer composed of palpebral conjunctiva. Between these layers is dense fibrous connective tissue referred to as the tarsal plate. The meibomian sebaceous glands secrete the major component of the outer layer of the preocular tear film and are located within the tarsal plate at the junction of the epidermis of the skin and the palpebral conjunctiva at the margin of the palpebral fissure. Within the tarsal plate is the orbicularis oculi muscle that encircles the space between the eyelids, called the palpebral fissure. This muscle closes the fissure. Cilia (eyelashes) are found along the margin of the eyelids near the opening of the meibomian glands within the superior eyelids of domesticated animals, except for cats, which do not have cilia. The glands of Zeiss are sebaceous, and the glands of Moll are modified sweat glands located within the conjunctiva. They contribute serous fluid to the precorneal tear film.

Most animals, except fish and snakes, have superior and inferior eyelids. Snakes have a transparent spectacle that covers the cornea. The spectacle is separated from the cornea by a space and is periodically shed with the skin (ecdysis). Faulty shedding of the skin (dysecdysis), which is often the result of improper hydration during this period, can result in retention of the spectacles. **Retained spectacles** are a cause of blindness.

Anomalies of the Eyelids

Abnormalities of the eyelids can be congenital or acquired. Congenital anomalies include an absence of an eyelid **(agenesis),** adhesion of the margins of the eyelid to each other **(ankyloblepharon),** inversion of the margin of the eyelid **(entropion),** eversion of the margin of the eyelid **(ectropion),** micropalpebral fissure, and macropalpebral fissure. Abnormalities can involve cilia and include cilia arising from an opening of the meibomian gland **(distichiasis),** cilia misdirected toward the cornea **(trichiasis),** and cilia that erupt through the palpebral conjunctiva **(ectopic cilia).** An inability to open the palebral fissure completely **(blepharophimosis)** and an inability to blink **(lagophthalmos)** can be congenital lesions or lesions resulting from inflammation or neoplasia.

Blepharitis

Inflammation of the eyelid (blepharitis) can be focal or diffuse and can be a manifestation of a systemic or cutaneous disease. Blepharitis is often characterized by hyperemia, edema, blepharospasm (keeping the palpebral fissure closed), and excessive lacrimation. Alopecia, ulceration, and scabs occur because of secondary self-trauma. In dogs, blepharitis can be a lesion of an allergic or pemphigoid disease. Purulent blepharitis in puppies can be a manifestation of juvenile pyoderma, and in adult dogs bacterial blepharitis can be caused by *Streptococcus* or *Staphylococcus* sp. Mycotic blepharitis is uncommon, but can be caused by dermatophytes. Hyperemia, alopecia, and pruritus of the eyelids are lesions of demodectic and sarcoptic mange. Other causes of blepharitis include viral infections (e.g., avian pox) and trauma. Multifocal pyogranulomatous blepharitis, referred to as marginal blepharitis, can be a distinct lesion in the dog of unknown cause.

Hordeolum

Purulent inflammation of glandular tissue within the eyelid is referred to as hordeolum. External hordeolum (stye) refers to inflammation of the glands of Zeiss or Moll. Internal hordeolum is purulent inflammation of the meibomian gland. Affected eyelids are swollen and abscesses form in the follicles of cilia. The cause is often a staphylococcal infection.

Chalazion

Chalazion refers to chronic granulomatous inflammation of meibomian glands or glands of Zeiss (Fig. 14-64). The release of sebaceous secretion into the adjacent connective tissue initiates this response, which is characterized by macrophages and multinucleated giant cells. Chalazion is a common lesion of dogs and often develops adjacent to neoplasms of the meibomian glands.

Neoplasms of Eyelids

Neoplasms of eyelids are common in the dog but occur less commonly in other domesticated animals. The most common ones are benign meibomian gland neoplasms, neoplasms of skin, and neoplasms of the palpebral conjunctiva. Almost all neoplasms arising from meibomian glands are either adenoma or epithelioma (Fig. 14-65). **Meibomian gland adenoma** is composed of well-differentiated sebaceous epithelial cells arranged in lobules (Fig. 14-66). Hyperkeratotic papillary projections often extend from the margin of the eyelid. **Meibomian gland epithelioma** is similar to meibomian gland adenoma except it is composed of poorly differentiated basal cells arranged in sheets with areas of differentiation toward keratinizing squamous epithelium and sebaceous

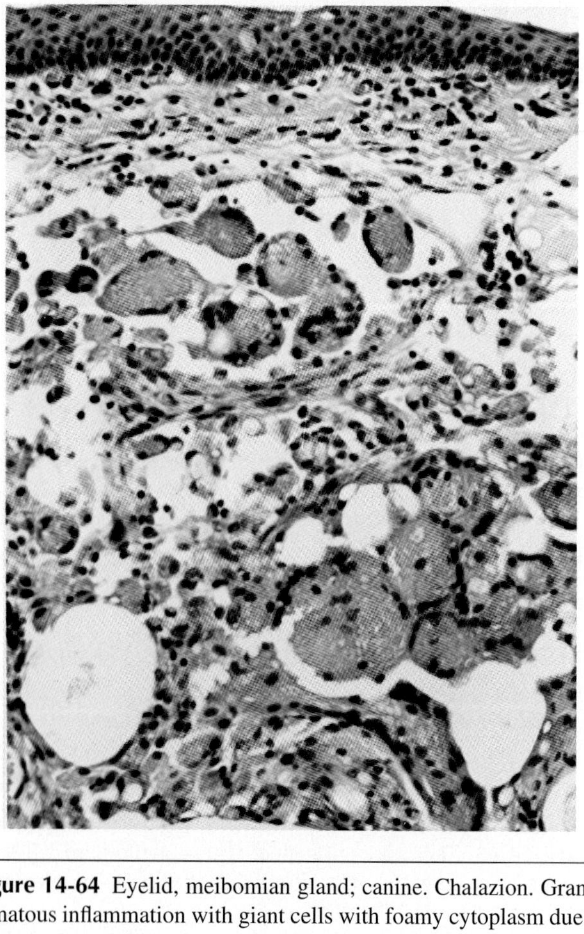

Figure 14-64 Eyelid, meibomian gland; canine. Chalazion. Granulomatous inflammation with giant cells with foamy cytoplasm due to sebum released from necrotic meibomian glands. H & E stain.

epithelium. When melanin is dispersed throughout the epithelioma, it is grossly black. Meibomian gland neoplasms in the dog form masses that cause corneal irritation, but have a benign biologic behavior.

Melanoma can arise from either the skin or the palpebral conjunctiva of the eyelid. Melanoma of the skin of the eyelids is similar to melanoma of the skin in other locations. It is composed of plump, discrete, round to polygonal to fusiform cells. All cells have an abundance of intracytoplasmic melanin pigment. Mitotic figures are observed rarely. Melanoma of the skin of the eyelid is almost always benign, but melanomas of the conjunctiva are sometimes malignant. Benign conjunctival melanoma is a heavily pigmented neoplasm with little stromal invasion. Malignant conjunctival melanoma is infiltrative and has anaplastic cells, mitotic figures, and less pigmentation. Local recurrence and distant metastasis occur in some cases.

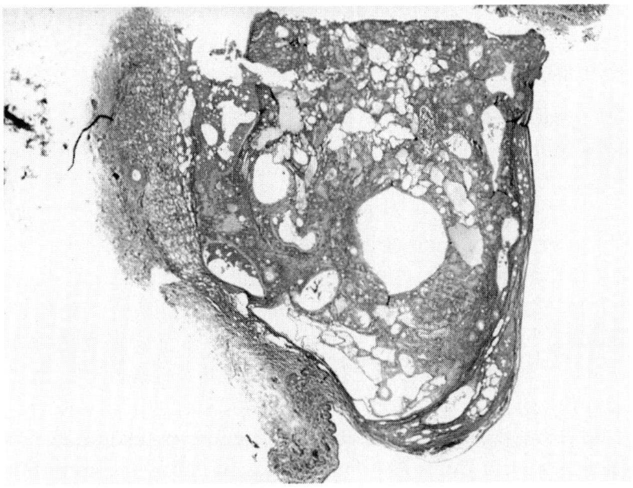

Figure 14-65 Eyelid; canine. Sebaceous (meibomian) adenoma and chalazion. Well-demarcated mass in the location of the meibomian gland is surrounded by granulomatous inflammation and lipid accumulation. H & E stain.

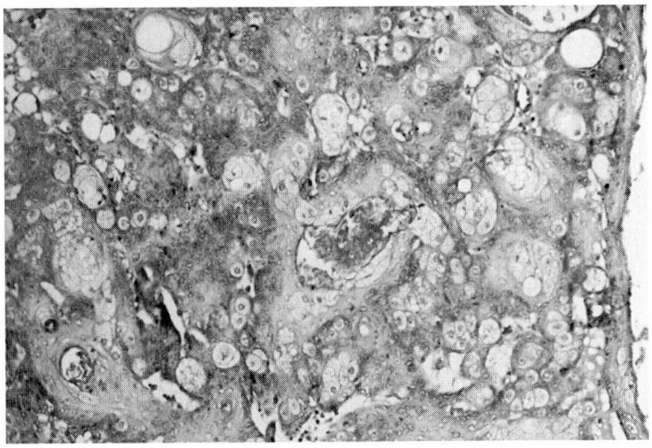

Figure 14-66 Eyelid; canine. Sebaceous (meibomian) adenoma. Adenoma with sebaceous differentiation. H & E stain.

Any neoplasm that can occur in the skin generally can arise in the skin of the eyelids. The morphologic features and biologic behavior of those of the eyelids are the same as those arising in the skin elsewhere. Neoplasms of the eyelids that occur more frequently include mast cell tumor, fibrosarcoma, lymphosarcoma, canine histiocytoma, equine sarcoid, and neoplasms of the epidermis, hair follicle, and sweat glands. Neoplasms of the palpebral conjunctiva also occur.

LESIONS OF THE NICTITATING MEMBRANE

In mammals, the nictitating membrane (membrana nictitans, third eyelid) is a flat triangular structure covered by conjunctiva. It extends over the cornea in the conjunctival sac from the medial canthus when the globe is recessed in the orbit. The shape is maintained by a T-shaped plate of cartilage surrounded by fibrous connective tissue. The anterior (palpebral) surface and the posterior (bulbar) surface are covered by squamous epithelium. Lymphocytes are present beneath the conjunctiva. The rostral leading edge is unattached and the caudal attached end of the nictitating membrane is surrounded by a lacrimal gland (gland of the nictitating membrane). In birds, the nictitating membrane is often transparent and protects the cornea during flight or diving.

Anomalies of the Nictitating Membrane

Abnormalities of the nictitating membrane include congenital or inherited anomalies, inflammation, and neoplasia. The nictitating membrane can be encircling in certain breeds of dogs (e.g., American cocker spaniel) and the cartilage can curl inward (inversion) or outward (eversion). Prolapse of the gland of the nictitating membrane ("cherry eye") is a common disorder thought to be due to weak connective tissue anchoring the gland (Fig. 14-67).

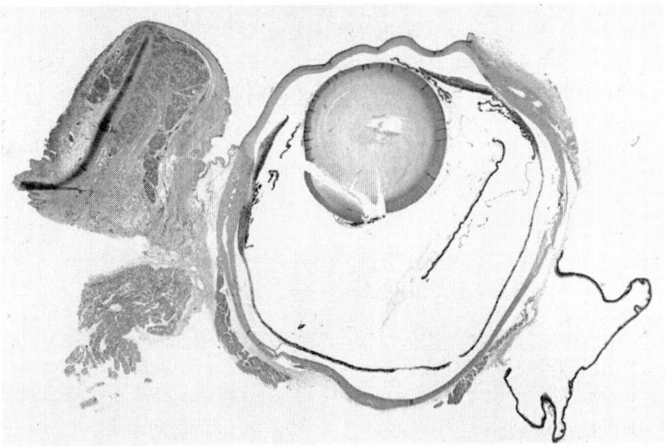

Figure 14-67 Globe and nictitating membrane; canine. Prolapse of the gland of the nictitating membrane. H & E stain.

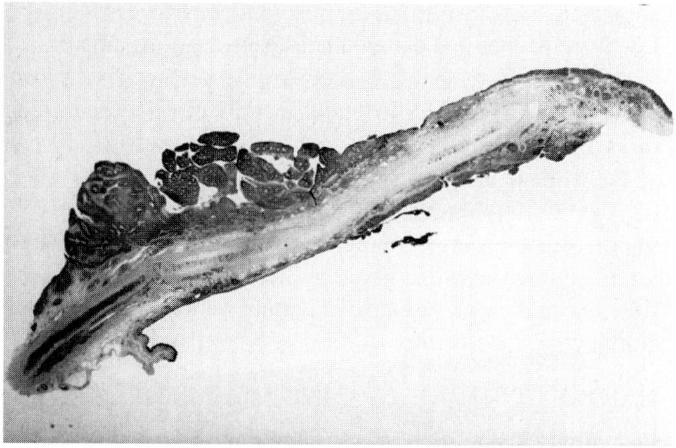

Figure 14-68 Nictitating membrane; canine. Squamous cell carcinoma. Proliferative mass extends from the surface of the palpebral surface of the nictitating membrane. H & E stain.

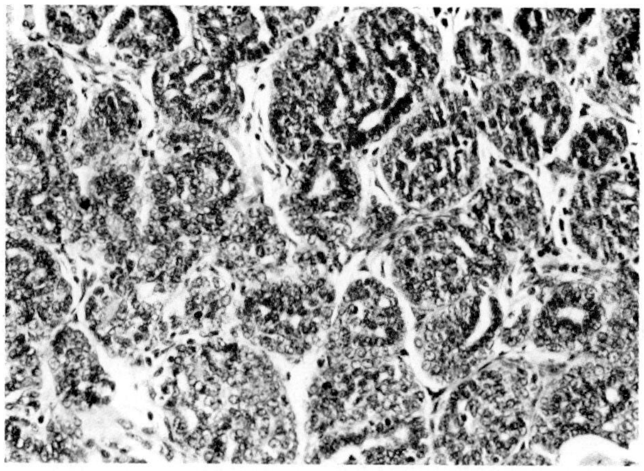

Figure 14-69 Nictitating membrane, lacrimal gland; canine. Adenocarcinoma. Neoplastic epithelial cells are in nests of closely packed cuboidal cells, forming tubular profiles. H & E stain.

The prolapsed gland of the nictitating membrane appears as a red (congested) mass at the medial canthus.

Protrusion of the Nictitating Membrane

Protrusion of the nictitating membrane occurs when the globe becomes recessed into the orbit (anophthalmus). This occurs because of loss of retrobulbar fat (e.g., emaciation), dehydration, contraction of the retrobulbar muscle (e.g., associated with corneal pain), and abnormally small globe (microphthalmia or phthisis bulbi), or as a clinical sign of systemic disease (e.g., tetanus, rabies, or cannabis intoxication).

Inflammation of the Nictitating Membrane

Inflammation of the nictitating membrane can be due to chronic irritation or have an unknown cause. Lymphoid follicles can develop beneath the bulbar surface as the result of chronic irritation **(follicular conjunctivitis).** These follicles are observed grossly as numerous, small, white nodules. In some cases, plasma cells instead of lymphocytes form aggregates within the connective tissue of the nictitating membrane and macrophages and epithelioid cells are intermixed with lymphocytes and plasma cells. This latter type of inflammation is periodically observed and the cause is unknown.

Neoplasms of the Nictitating Membrane

Neoplasms of the nictitating membrane are uncommon in the dog. Neoplasms include those of the conjunctiva (e.g., squamous cell carcinoma) (Fig. 14-68), papilloma, melanoma, vascular neoplasms and mast cell tumors, lymphosarcoma, and neoplasms of the gland of the nictitating membrane. Adenocarcinoma of the gland of the nictitating membrane is locally invasive and slow to metastasize in the dog (Fig. 14-69). It is rare in the cat, but appears to be very infiltrative and sometimes metastasizes to local lymph nodes.

LESIONS OF THE ORBIT

The orbit is the osseous fossa that separates the eye from the cranial cavity. Blood vessels, peripheral nerves, and the optic nerve extend through foramina in the orbital bone. In addition to the globe and the optic nerve, the orbital contents include orbital fascia, orbital adipose tissue, extraocular muscles, the lacrimal gland, and the gland of the third eyelid. Orbital fascia includes periorbita, Tenon's capsule, and fascial sheaths of the extraocular muscles. The periorbita is a fibrous membrane that lines the orbit and covers the globe and the extraocular muscles. Tenon's capsule is condensed connective tissue on the outer aspect of the sclera that extends from near the limbus and becomes continuous with the fascia surrounding the extraocular muscles. Orbital structures vary among species. The orbit of some species (e.g., dog) contains a zygomatic salivary gland, and the orbit of rats and mice contain a porphyrin-secreting lacrimal gland, the Harderian gland.

Orbital diseases occur in many species, but especially dogs. Orbital lesions such as atrophy of orbital fat secondary to cachexia can be confined only to the orbit or can develop as an extension of a disease involving the oral cavity, tooth roots, nasal cavity, or paranasal sinuses. Loss of orbital mass causes the globe to sink into the orbit (endophthalmos), but since most lesions of the orbit occupy retrobulbar space, the globe is deviated from the normal visual axes (strabismus), or protrudes anteriorly (i.e., exophthalmos). Exophthalmos can be severe enough that there is an inability to close the eyelids (lagophthalmos). If prolonged, exophthalmos can cause drying of the cornea (exposure keratitis).

Orbital lesions include retrobulbar dermoid cyst, vascular anomalies, orbital inflammation, salivary retention cysts and mucoceles, myositis, trauma, and retrobulbar neoplasms. **Dermoid cysts** have a wall of keratinized squamous epithelium. Vascular anomalies occur in animals, but are rare. Orbital **varix** is an enlarged and tortuous vessel, which form as a congenital anomaly or as the result of trauma. Orbital inflammation **(orbital cellulitis)** is often suppurative and often bacterial in origin. If inflammation is localized, a **retrobulbar abscess** can form. The cause can be infected teeth, spread of infection from the paranasal sinuses or the globe, penetrating foreign bodies, fungi, or parasites. Leakage of saliva from the zygomatic salivary gland or its ducts can also cause orbital cellulitis. If salivary outflow is obstructed, **salivary retention cyst** or **salivary mucocele** form. Inflammation can also extend to the lacrimal gland **(dacryoadenitis),** especially the Harderian gland in rats. Orbital trauma can cause orbital hematoma or orbital emphysema, and these can displace the globe anteriorly (proptosis).

Because no lateral bony orbital wall is present in dogs, swelling of the masticatory muscles or the extraocular muscles with inflammation can laterally displace the globe. **Canine masticatory eosinophilic myositis** and **canine extraocular polymyositis** are both thought to be immune-mediated myopathies. Extraocular polymyositis results in swelling of the superior and inferior recti and oblique muscles but not the retractor bulbi muscle. Grossly, affected muscles are enlarged and pale. Microscopic lesions include myofiber necrosis and infiltration by lymphocytes, plasma cells, histiocytes, and a few eosinophils.

Orbital neoplasms can develop from any orbital tissue. Dogs develop optic meningioma, a neoplasm that develops from optic meninges. The neoplasm surrounds the optic nerve and fills the orbit, resulting in remodeling of the orbital bone. Microscopically, meningiomas are characterized by sheets, nests, and whorls of meningoepithelial cells, possibly with mineralized lamellated concretions (psammoma bodies). Areas of osseous and cartilagenous metaplasia are often scattered throughout the neoplasm. Intraocular extension occurs, but intracranial extension is rare.

Other retrobulbar neoplasms include extra-adrenal paraganglioma in the horse, neurofibrosarcoma in the dog, and metastatic neoplasms. Orbital neurofibrosarcoma is an uncommon, firm, white, infiltrative malignant neoplasm. Microscopically, it is composed of fusiform cells arranged in interwoven cords containing whorls of cells and mitotic figures.

LESIONS OF THE LACRIMAL APPARATUS

Tears are needed to maintain an optical uniform corneal surface, to remove debris from the corneal surface and conjunctival sac, to provide nutrients to the outer cornea, and for antimicrobial activity. The precorneal tear film is composed of three layers. The outer lipid layer is produced by sebaceous glands of the eyelids, especially the meibomian glands. The outer lipid layer helps to provide smooth movement of the eyelids while reducing evaporation from the underlying aqueous layer. The middle aqueous layer is composed mainly of secretion from the lacrimal glands, but a contribution is also made by the gland of the nictitating membrane. The aqueous layer provides oxygen and nutrition to the superficial cornea. The inner mucinous layer is composed of mucin from the conjunctival goblet cells. The mucinous layer absorbs the tears to the surface of the cornea. As the precorneal tear film is produced, it is continuously spread over the surface of the cornea. Tears collect in the medial cul-de-sac and flow through puncta into canaliculi that drain into the lacrimal sac. Finally, tears flow from the lacrimal sac into the nasal lacrimal duct to the nose.

Lesions of Lacrimal Gland

Lesions involving the lacrimal gland are infrequent and include congenital hypoplasia, neoplasia, and degeneration secondary to inflammation (dacryoadenitis), drug toxicity (e.g., sulfadiazine), facial nerve damage (e.g., iatrogenic during blastotomy), or trauma. Neoplasms of the lacrimal gland are rare, can be adenoma or adenocarcinoma, and are located in the dorsal lateral aspect of the orbit. Dacryoadenitis can be secondary to systemic diseases (e.g., canine distemper), autoimmune disease, or inflammation of orbital contents (orbital cellulitis). A deficiency in the volume of tears causes the cornea and conjunctiva to become dry (keratoconjunctivitis sicca), a common ocular disorder, especially in the dog.

Lesions of Harderian Gland

In addition to lacrimal glands, the tears of rodents are formed, in part, by the secretion of a large, retrobulbar gland, the Harderian gland. The secretion from this gland contains porphyrins that cause the tears of rodents to be red. This is noticed when excessive red tears are formed **(chromodacryorrhea)** in rats with disease. Lesions of the Harderian gland include inflammation that is common in rats and neoplasms that occur in mice and hamsters (Harderian gland adenoma) and rarely in rats. In rats, inflammation of the salivary gland and lacrimal glands (sialodacryoadenitis) is a common lesion caused by a coronaviral infection. This highly contagious, nonfatal infection spreads rapidly among susceptible rats, especially suckling and weaning rat pups, but causes few deaths. As the Harderian gland becomes swollen from the inflammation, the globe is extruded rostrally (exophthalmos). This causes drying of the cornea (exposure keratopathy). At the same time, "red tears" are increased (chromodacryorrhea). Lesions of the Harderian gland include necrosis of acinar epithelium, infiltration with neutrophils, lymphocytes, and macrophages, and squamous metaplasia of ductular epithelium.

Lesions of Lacrimal Drainage System

Congenital anomalies and acquired lesions can involve any of the structures of the lacrimal apparatus. The puncti and canaliculi can be absent **(atresia),** small **(hypoplasia),** or **misplaced.** Obstruction of this drainage results in an overflow of the tears onto the adjacent skin **(epiphora).** Congenital required cystic dilations of the lacrimal sac **(dacryops)** or canaliculi **(canaliculops)** can occur. Acquired lesions include lacerations from trauma, inflammation of the lacrimal sac **(dacryocystitis),** and neoplasia. Ocular parasites, such as *Thelazia* sp. in cattle and horses, can cause chronic irritation of the nasal lacrimal duct. Primary neoplasms of the nasal lacrimal duct are rare, but obstruction occurs from neoplasms of adjacent structures.

Lesions of Gland of Nictitating Membrane

Inflammation, glandular atrophy, and neoplasms of the gland of the nictitating membrane are uncommon. Neoplasms are either adenomas or adenocarcinomas. Some are complex neoplasms and have epithelial and myoepithelial components. **Adenocarcinoma of the gland of the nictitating membrane** can be locally invasive. Metastasis to lymph nodes and possibly other locations is uncommon, but more likely to occur in cats than in dogs.

PREPARATION OF OCULAR TISSUES FOR HISTOLOGIC EXAMINATION

The structures of the globe, especially the retina, undergo postmortem autolysis rapidly after enucleation or death of the animal. Thus, enucleation must be done quickly; the globe should be handled gently and placed in a fixative as soon as possible. The most commonly used fixative is neutral buffered 10% formalin (NBF), but this fixative does not penetrate rapidly enough to fix intraocular structures when the globe is submerged. To achieve maximum fixation, the globe should be slowly injected with a small amount (0.3 to 0.5 ml for canine globe) of 10% NBF into the vitreous cavity. The globe should be cleaned of all extraocular tissue. A 25- to 27-gauge needle attached to a syringe should be inserted into the vitreous cavity at a point posterior to the lens along the long posterior ciliary artery. Injection of the 10% NBF is done slowly and continued until the globe is firm. After injection, the globe should be submerged in 10% NBF at a 10:1 to 20:1 fixative:globe ratio.

Other ocular tissues collected for histologic study include eviscerated intraocular contents and corneal samples from a keratectomy. The contents of eviscerated globes should be examined microscopically for evidence of neoplasia. Biopsies of ulcerated cornea, especially from horses, should be stained with a combination of hematoxylin and eosin and Gomori's methenamine silver to demonstrate fungal hyphae.

COMPONENTS OF THE EAR

The ear is a sensory organ composed of the external ear, middle ear, and the inner ear. Any portion of the ear can be involved in disease. To understand lesions of the ear, one must have an appreciation of the embryology, gross and microscopic anatomy, function, and terminology of the ear. The ear has two functions: the sense of hearing and the sense of balance. The external ear captures sound waves and funnels them to the tympanic membrane, which vibrates and moves the ossicles in the middle ear. One of the ossicles is attached to the oval window, and movement of the oval window causes movement of perilymph within the inner ear, which causes movement of the basilar membrane and of the specialized cilia of sensory hair cells.

LESIONS OF THE EXTERNAL EAR

The external ear is composed of the auricle (pinna) and the external auditory meatus, which ends medially at the tympanic membrane. All of these structures can be examined easily grossly. The pinna is composed of a flat sheet of elastic cartilage covered by skin. The anterior (concave) surface contains numerous sebaceous glands and hairs that become less frequent toward the external auditory meatus. The external auditory meatus is supported laterally by cartilage and medially by bone and is lined by epidermis containing some hair follicles, numerous sebaceous glands, and numerous modified, apocrine sweat glands (i.e., ceruminous glands). Rodents do not have ceruminous glands but have lobulated sebaceous glands (i.e., Zymbal's glands) ventral to the base of the external ear.

Congenital Anomalies of the Ear

At birth, the pinna can be normal, abnormally large **(macrotia),** or abnormally small **(microtia).** Absence of the pinna **(anotia)** can be an inherited defect in sheep and can occur with other deformities in the dog. Extra pinnae **(polyotia)** can result from a recessive mutation in the cat. An abnormally shaped pinna is a characteristic lesion of Nubian goats affected with β-mannosidosis. Multiple, hard, spherical intracartilaginous pseudocysts can occur in the auricular cartilage of dogs. Deafness can result from the absence of the external auditory meatus **(atresia)** or failure of the meatal plug to be shed **(persistent meatal plug).** In the dog, the meatal plug is shed between 14 to 17 days after birth.

Auricular Chondritis

Auricular chondritis is a disorder of unknown etiology that occurs in several strains of laboratory rats. The disorder is characterized by focal necrosis of auricular cartilage that is eventually replaced by numerous mononuclear inflammatory cells. Eventually, the inflammatory tissue is replaced by disorganized cartilagenous tissue that causes a thickened, malformed nodular pinna. An immunologic reaction to type II collagen has been proposed as a possible factor in the pathogenesis.

Auricular Necrosis

Necrosis of the tip of the pinna occurs with frostbite in pigs and cattle, ergot poisoning in cattle, septicemia in pigs, or trauma. Trauma results from scratching, rubbing, or head shaking. These are clinical signs associated with inflammation of the external ear (otitis externa). Trauma also causes fissures to develop along the distal edge of the canine pinna.

Auricular Hematoma

An auricular hematoma can result from an intrachondral fracture of the pinnal cartilage. This fluctuant, blood-filled swelling commonly occurs on the concave surface of the canine pinna near the apex. With time, the blood is replaced by granulation tissue. Contraction of this granulation tissue can distort the pinna. Auricular hematoma is the result of violent head shaking and scratching, although an immune-mediated reaction also has been suggested as a contributing factor.

Auricular Lesions of Dermatologic Diseases

The external ear is sometimes involved in either generalized or regional dermatologic diseases. Regional diseases include idiopathic auricular alopecia in Siamese cats, feline solar dermatitis, marginal seborrhea, and equine aural plaques, to mention a few. **Feline solar dermatitis** is a chronic actinic disorder of the margin of the pinna characterized by erythema, acanthosis, scaling, epithelial necrosis, ulceration, and superficial perivascular dermatitis with basophilic degeneration of superficial dermal collagen. The disease progresses through epithelial hyperplasia, dysplasia, and carcinoma in situ to invasive squamous cell carcinoma.

Marginal seborrhea is characterized by numerous, small, greasy nodules of orthokeratotic and parakeratotic hyperkeratosis of the pinnae of dogs. In severe cases, the lesions become inflamed, necrotic, ulcerated, and result in auricular deformity.

Equine aural plaques are solitary or multiple, raised, flat-surfaced, nonpigmented, scaly to crusty lesions of the inner aspects of the pinna caused by infection with a papilloma virus. The lesions consist of epithelial hyperplasia and hypertrophy. The enlarged cells have clear cytoplasm and keratohyaline-like granules in the stratum spinosum and granulosum.

Otitis Externa

Inflammation of the external ear (otitis externa) is common in the dog and involves many factors and causes. Certain predisposing factors that increase the risk of developing otitis externa include hair in the external auditory meatus, a pendulous concave pinna, excessive moisture in the external auditory meatus, and inappropriate treatment of otitis media. Primary causes of otitis externa include foreign bodies, such as awns of certain grasses (e.g., foxtail grass in the western United States), parasites, fungi, bacteria, hypersensitivity, metabolic disorders, and chronic inflammation.

Parasitic Otitis Externa

A variety of parasites, including ticks (e.g., *Amblyomma* sp., *Boophilus* sp., *Dermacentor nitens, Haemaphysalis leporis-palustris, Otobius megnini,* and *Rhipicephalus* sp.), skin mites (e.g., *Demodex canis, Demodex cati, Notoedres cati, Ixodes cati,* and *Sarcoptes scabiei),* and ear mites (e.g., *Otodectes cynotis, Psoroptes cuniculi,* and *Rallietia auris*) infect the external ear, resulting in disease (otoacariasis). The ear mite, *Otodectes cynotis,* is a common cause of otitis externa in young cats, whereas the incidence of ear mites as a cause of otitis externa in dogs is much less. Otitis externa developing from parasitic infections has an allergic basis. For example, feline otoacariasis can involve Arthus-type hypersensitivity. Other external auditory lesions associated with parasites are irritation from biting insects (e.g., sandflies) or the formation of auricular granulomatous nodules (e.g., leishmaniasis).

Otomycosis

Mycotic infections of the external ear (otomycosis) are caused by fungi of the genera *Microsporum, Candida, Trichophyton, Aspergillus,* and *Peyronella* (i.e., *Sporothrix*). A fungus frequently cultured from the external ears of dogs and cats, with or without otitis externa, is *Malassezia pachydermatis* (Fig. 14-70). Although the importance of this yeast infection is controversial, it was found pathogenic to the tissues of the canine external auditory meatus.

Bacterial Otitis Externa

Bacterial infections are usually secondary causes of otitis externa and have been reported in dogs, cats, pigs, and ruminants. In the dog, gram-positive cocci, but not gram-negative bacteria, have been cultured from the external auditory meatus. Bacteria reported to cause otitis externa in dogs and cats include *Staphylococcus intermedius, S. aureus,* β-hemolytic *Streptococcus* sp., *Proteus* sp., *Pseudomonas* sp., *Escherichia coli,* and *Klebsiella* sp. Granulomatous auricular dermatitis that thickens and distorts the pinnae of food animals is caused by *Actinomyces (Arcanobacterium) bovis.*

Another cause of otitis externa is hypersensitivity (e.g., atophy, food allergy, and contact allergic dermatitis). An allergic reaction causes erythema, edema, and mild accumulation of cerumen. Atophy is a frequent cause of canine otitis externa and is limited to the pinna or vertical external auditory meatus. Food allergy is a common allergic cause of otitis externa, especially in certain breeds of dog (e.g., cocker spaniel, Labrador retriever), and contact allergic dermatitis results from certain topical medications.

Otitis externa also has been associated with metabolic and epithelial disorders. Certain endocrinopathies, including hypothyroidism, male-feminizing syndrome, Sertoli cell tumor, and certain ovarian disorders, cause chronic ceruminous otitis externa.

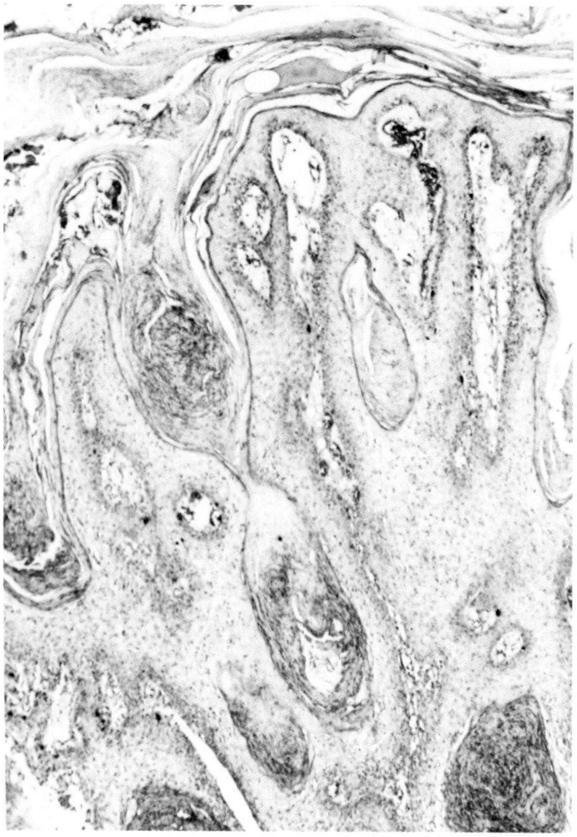

Figure 14-70 External ear, pinna; canine. Otitis externa. Epidermal hyperplasia and hyperkeratosis due to infection with *Malassezia pachydermatitis.* H & E stain.

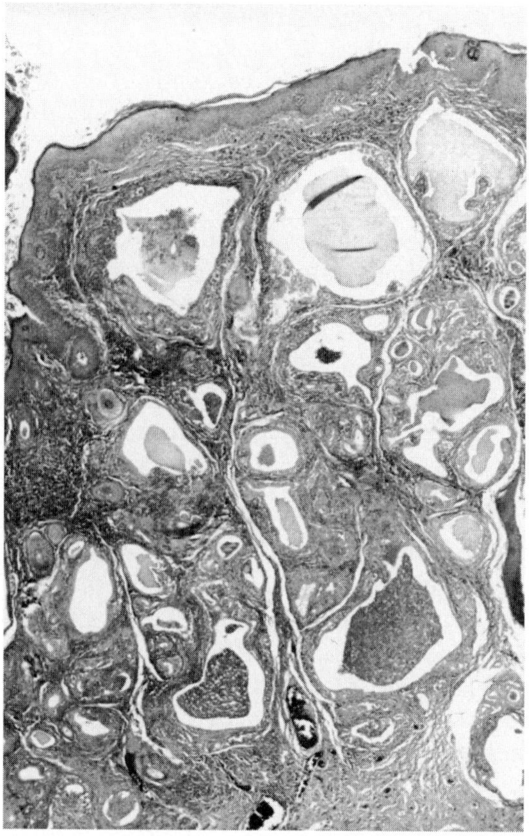

Figure 14-71 External ear; canine. Chronic otitis externa. Marked thickening of the wall of the external meatus with lymphoplasmacytic inflammation, interstitial fibrosis, and dilatation and proliferation of ceruminous glands. H & E stain.

Perpetuating factors that prevent resolution of otitis externa and contribute to the chronic nature of the disease include obstructive lesions (e.g., polyps, neoplasms), excessive ceruminous secretion secondary infections, reactions to topical medication, and trauma, which is worse when foreign bodies (e.g., hair, dirt) are introduced. Pathologic responses associated with chronic otitis externa include epidermal hyperkeratosis, acanthosis, dermal fibrosis, edema, inflammation of apocrine glands (hidradenitis), and apocrine gland hyperplasia (Fig. 14-71). The inflammation is characterized by the presence of lymphocytes, plasma cells, macrophages, and neutrophils. With time, fibrosis, and, possibly, calcification occurs, leading to stenosis of the external auditory meatus. Contributing factors include a thickened meatal wall with obstruction of the meatal lumen by a coagulum of exfoliated debris, tenacious brown cerumen, exfoliated keratocytes, dried serum, and leukocytes. Mites or other parasites, bacteria, or fungi can be present in the debris. The inflammation of the external auditory meatus can cause the formation of inflammatory polyps and rupture of the tympanic membrane with secondary inflammation of the middle ear (otitis media). Otitis media can be difficult to treat, resulting in eventual surgical removal of the external ear (ablation of the external ear canal). If the middle ear is involved, the surgical procedure can involve opening the tympanic bulla (bulla osteotomy).

Neoplasms of the External Ear

Neoplasms of the skin of the external ear are uncommon, but originate from the pinna or from ceruminous glands. Although any neoplasm of the skin can arise from auricular skin, an important one because of its invasive behavior is **squamous cell carcinoma.** This neoplasm occurs commonly in the pinnae of white cats exposed to sunlight for prolonged periods. Precancerous lesions consist of ulcers along the margin of the pinnae (feline solar or actinic dermatitis) that progress to epithelial hyperplasia and dysplasia, carcinoma in situ, and eventually invasive squamous cell carcinoma. The progression of the lesion can take years, and metastasis occurs late in the course of the disease. Other neoplasms of the pinna include canine histiocytoma, basal cell carcinoma, mast cell tumor, sebaceous adenoma and adenocarcinoma, trichoepithelioma, apocrine adenocarcinoma, fibroma, fibrosarcoma, papilloma, chondroma, chondrosarcoma, and rhabdomyoma. In horses auricular equine sarcoid can develop. In laboratory rats, neoplasms of the Zymbal's gland develop at the ventral base of the external ear. Microscopically, these neoplasms are sebaceous adenoma or adenocarcinoma, or squamous cell carcinoma.

Adenoma and Adenocarcinoma

Ceruminous gland neoplasms occur in older dogs and cats, especially those with chronic otitis externa. The neoplasms appear as nodular or pedunculated masses, usually less than 2 cm in diameter, that protrude into the external auditory meatus. The majority of the neoplasms in dogs are benign, whereas more of the ceruminous gland neoplasms in cats are malignant. Microscopically, adenomas are composed of cuboidal epithelium arranged in well-differentiated tubules and acini containing eosinophilic to golden brown pigment. Adenocarcinoma is invasive, and therefore has the potential of spreading to regional lymph nodes.

LESIONS OF THE MIDDLE EAR

The middle ear is separated from the external ear by the translucent tympanic membrane that is composed of three layers. The outer layer is composed of squamous epithelium of the external auditory meatus. The middle layer is connective tissue, and the inner layer is composed of mucosa from the middle ear.

The middle ear develops from a lateral extension of the first pharyngeal pouch, which connects with the first pharyngeal cleft to form the tubotympanic recess. This widens to become a cavity within the temporal bone and communicates with the nasopharynx via the **auditory** (eustachian) **tube.** In the horse, a portion of the auditory tube develops into a diverticulum, the **guttural pouch.** The middle ear is lined in part by squamous and in part by cuboidal epithelium. The cuboidal epithelium is ciliated or nonciliated and has goblet cells. This mucosa resembles modified respiratory mucosa. Defense mechanisms of the middle ear include a mucociliary system and a cellular defense system. The manubrium of the malleus, one of the three tympanic ossicles, is attached to the tympanic membrane. The **malleus** articulates with the **incus,** which articulates with the **stapes.** The footplate of the stapes is attached to the membrane of the **vestibular (oval) window** of the cochlea. Collectively, the ossicles communicate and amplify sound-induced vibrations of the tympanic membrane to perilymph of the inner ear. Lesions of the middle ear are often inflammatory, and treatment can involve surgical opening of the tympanic bulla (i.e., bulla osteotomy).

Gross examination of the middle ear includes examination of the tympanic cavity, including its contents and delineating structures. The **tympanic cavity** is normally filled with air. The boundaries include the **tympanic membrane** (laterally), the **petrous temporal bone** (dorsally), and the thin and smooth-walled osseous diverticulum, the **tympanic bulla** (ventrally). The **auditory ossicles** form a bridge from the tympanic membrane to the oval (vestibular) window of the cochlear promontory. The cochlear promontory is an osseous prominence extending from the dorsomedial wall of the tympanic cavity. The promontory is covered by postganglionic sympathetic nerve fibers from the cranial cervical ganglion. In the cat, the tympanic cavity is divided into two compartments, the dorsolateral compartment and the larger ventromedial compartment. The tympanic bullae of cattle and swine contain numerous interconnecting osseous septa separating the cavity into many air spaces.

The middle ear also includes the auditory tube. In horses, each auditory tube has a large diverticulum, the guttural pouch. The guttural pouch can be examined by viewing the caudal aspect of the head at necropsy. The guttural pouch is lined by a thin mucous membrane containing pseudostratified ciliated epithelium. The underlying connective tissue contains numerous lymphatic nodules, especially in young horses. The internal carotid artery is located in a fold along the caudal border.

Otitis Media

Inflammation of the middle ear (otitis media) is the principal lesion involving the middle ear. Otitis media can occur as an extension of otitis externa across the tympanic membrane. This is a common occurrence in the dog. Other cases of otitis media are rarely from hematogenous spread, or by spread via the auditory tube from the pharynx. This latter route is common in pigs, cats, ruminants, rats, and rabbits and occurs with a concurrent pneumonia. Otitis media is often due to a bacterial infection. Many different bacterial and mycoplasmal species have been isolated from the middle ear of animals with otitis media. Some of the more common isolates include *Arcanobacterium pyogenes* (ruminants, swine), *Mycoplasma bovis* (calves), *Mycoplasma hyorhinis* (swine), *Mycoplasma pulmonis* (rats, mice), *Pasteurella multocida* (cats, cattle, rabbits, swine), *Pseudomonas aeruginosa* (dogs, swine), *Staphylococcus* sp. (dogs), and *Streptococcus* sp. (dogs, pigs). Otitis media can also be caused by *Candida* sp., *Aspergillus* sp., and *Malassezia pachydermatis.* Regardless of the cause, the tympanic cavity fills with exudate. The inflammation can spread into the adjacent bone, causing osteomyelitis and osteolysis of osseous septa in calves and pigs. Otitis media in the horse can extend through the surrounding bone and involve the stylohyoid bone, resulting in fusion of the temporohyoid joint. Fusion of the joint predisposes to fractures of the petrous temporal bone. These fractures can cause vestibulocochlear and facial nerve dysfunction.

Lesions of the auditory tube, **eustachitis,** are inflammation of the auditory tube, including the guttural pouch in horses. Eustachitis can precede otitis media in cattle and swine; therefore, causes include *Pasteurella multocida* (swine), *Arcanobacterium pyogenes* (swine, cattle), *Myco-*

plasma hyorhinis (swine), and *Mycoplasma bovis* (calves). Inflammation of the guttural pouch can be caused by *Streptococcus* sp. and *Aspergillus* sp., and the inflammation can extend into the wall of the adjacent internal carotid artery. The resulting arteritis weakens the wall, resulting in rupture. Hemorrhage from the carotid artery into the guttural pouch can be severe and result in death.

Other lesions of the guttural pouch include empyema and tympany. **Empyema** is the accumulation of suppurative exudate within the guttural pouch and is usually caused by an upper respiratory tract infection. **Tympany** is the entrapment of air within the guttural pouch and occurs more commonly in young horses.

Nasopharyngeal Polyp

Nasopharyngeal polyps arise in cats from the mucosa of the tympanic cavity, often the dorsolateral compartment, and can be unilateral or bilateral. The polypoid mass can fill the tympanic cavity, extend through the auditory tube, and protrude into the nasopharynx (Fig. 14-72). Polyps present in the nasopharynx can be ulcerated and superficially infiltrated by neutrophils. The polyps also can rupture through the tympanic membrane and into the external auditory meatus. The polyps are composed of well-vascularized, fibrous, or myxomatous connective tissue, diffusely infiltrated by lymphocytes and covered by squamous epithelium or nonciliated or ciliated columnar epithelium. The polyps can contain mucous glands and lymphoid nodules.

Aural Cholesteatoma

Aural cholesteatoma is a nodule that resembles an epidermal inclusion cyst and is located in the cavity of the middle ear. Occasionally, the mass protrudes into the external auditory meatus. The lesion is composed of white, pastelike, keratinized debris. Cholesteatomas arise spontaneously but often are associated with chronic otitis externa or chronic otitis media. The cavity of the middle ear has inflammatory debris, cholesterol clefts, and blood. The pathogenesis involves hyperplasia of squamous epithelium within a confined space (e.g., stenotic external auditory meatus). In human beings, cholesteatoma occurs as the result of congenital displacement of squamous epithelium within the middle ear (i.e., congenital aural cholesteatoma), squamous metaplasia of tympanic mucosa, or as the result of migration of squamous epithelium through a ruptured tympanic membrane. Aural cholesteatoma has been reported in gerbils, rabbits, guinea pigs, dogs, and cats.

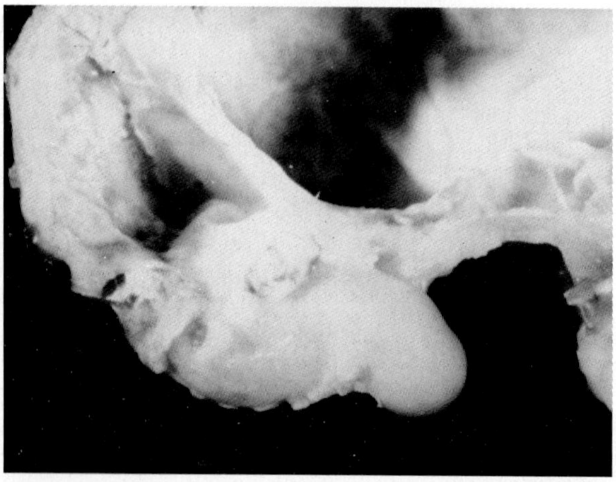

Figure 14-72 Ear, middle ear; feline. Nasopharyngeal polyp. The polyp is located within the opened tympanic bulla, auditory tube, and nasopharynx.

Neoplasms of the Middle Ear

Neoplasms are found rarely in the middle and inner ears of domestic animals. Neoplasms have been reported in older animals and include squamous cell carcinoma of the middle and inner ears of domestic cats and adenoma of the middle ear of dogs. Vestibular dysfunction in the cat has been caused by infiltrative squamous cell carcinoma extending to the inner ear from a primary location in the middle ear. Adenomas can arise from the wall of the tympanic cavity but are rare. They are solid or papillary and composed of cuboidal epithelial cells arranged in small tubules. An invasive, malignant neoplasm can arise from the jugulotympanic paraganglion in the dog, and metastatic neoplasms such as lymphosarcoma occur but are rare.

LESIONS OF THE INNER EAR

The inner ear (labyrinth) consists of membranous channels (membranous labyrinth) that line cavities within the petrous temporal bone (osseous labyrinth). Portions of the membranous labyrinth are separated from the osseous labyrinth by a fluid (perilymph). The osseous labyrinth is divided into three parts—the cochlea, semicircular canals, and the vestibule. The membranous cochlear duct lies within the cochlea, and the membranous semicircular canals lie within the osseous semicircular canals. The vestibule contains the endolymphatic duct, the utricle, and the saccule of the membranous labyrinth.

The sensory organ of hearing is the organ of Corti, a portion of the cochlear duct. It is supported by the basilar membrane and consists of external hair cells, internal hair cells, and supportive cells. The hair cells are stimulated by movement of the stereocilia, which extend into the overlying gelatinous tectorial membrane. Hair cells then stimulate the nerve endings of bipolar neurons that have their cell bodies in the spiral ganglion (cochlear ganglion) in the central osseous core of the cochlea, modiolus. Axons of these neurons constitute the auditory portion of the eighth cranial nerve.

The sensory end organs of the vestibular system include the macula within the utricle and saccule and the cristae ampullares within the ampulla of the semicircular canals. The macula contains a gelatinous mass with calcareous bodies (i.e., otoliths or otoconia) that are affected by gravity during accelerated motion. The cristae ampullares contain a gelatinous mass (i.e., cupula) that moves during shifts in the position of the head. On stimulation, impulses are transmitted through the bipolar neurons with cell bodies located in the vestibular ganglion (Scarpa's ganglion) of the vestibular nerve.

Deafness

The loss of hearing, or deafness, can be from a lesion involving the external or middle ears (e.g., otitis externa or otitis media, respectively) and is referred to as conductive deafness. Deafness also can be the result of a neurologic abnormality. If the cause of the deafness involves the brain or auditory pathway, the condition is referred to as central deafness; if the cause is a lesion involving the cochlea, the condition is referred to as peripheral deafness. Causes of peripheral deafness are hereditary, toxic, acoustic, inflammatory, neoplastic, and senile. Inherited dysplasia of the cochlear duct has been reported in several species including cats, Dalmations and other breeds of dog, Hedlund mink, Japanese dancing (shaker) mice, and waltzing guinea pigs. Deafness can be associated with a white haircoat, especially in cats and mink (Fig. 14-73). The cause is a deficiency of pigmented cells in the stria vascularis, resulting in secondary collapse of the organ of Corti. Numerous compounds are ototoxic, including aminoglycoside antibiotics, loop diuretics, salicylates, and other analgesics. Loss of sensory hair cells occurs in older animals. Cochlear findings are similar, irregardless of the specific cause. Lesions include a loss of inner and outer hair cells, a loss of supporting cells in the organ of Corti, vacuolation of hair cells, collapse of Reissner's membrane, distortion of the tectorial membrane, and generalized atrophy of the organ of Corti. Abnormalities in the organ of Corti that result in deafness can be detected clinically by determining the patter of auditory-evoked brain stem responses (AEBR).

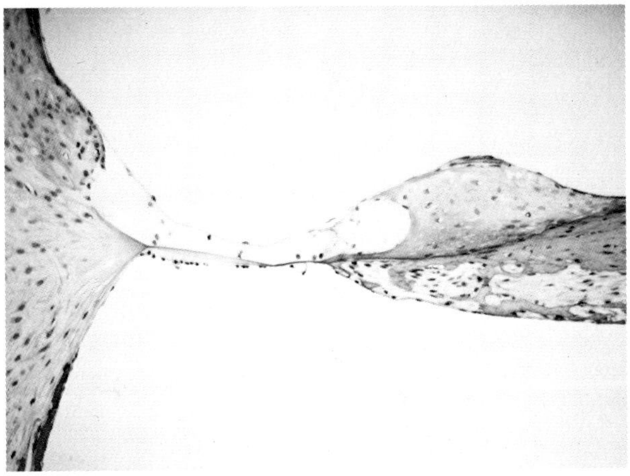

Figure 14-73 Ear, inner ear, cochlear duct; canine. Dysplasia of organ of Corti. The organ of Corti and tectorial membrane are underdeveloped, and there is collapse of Reissner's membrane. H & E stain. *Courtesy Dr. D.J. Zappia.*

The inner ear and middle ear can be abnormal in certain storage diseases, such as β-mannosidosis. This storage disease has been observed in Nubian goat kids and Salers calves. Affected goats have a tympanic cavity narrowed by numerous coalescing mucosal folds. Epithelial and connective tissue cells contain intracytoplasmic vacuoles, as well as hair cells. Affected Salers cattle have similar vacuolated cells.

Inflammation of the inner ear (**otitis interna** or **labyrinthitis**) is uncommon, but can cause effacement of the cochlear duct. The inflammation can spread to cause vestibular labyrinthitis, vestibulocochlear neuritis, or temporal osteomyelitis. Infections can be caused by viruses, bacteria, fungi, or algae. Infectious agents that cause otitis media or meningitis are potential causes of otitis interna.

Vestibular Dysfunction

In addition to vestibular labyrinthitis, vestibular dysfunction occurs with or without identifiable vestibular lesions. Idiopathic vestibular syndrome is an example of a common disorder in dogs, cats, and horses characterized by clinical signs of vestibular dysfunction. The cause is often unknown. Clinical signs include acute onset of head tilt, nystagmus, ataxia, and occasionally, facial paralysis. Animals recover spontaneously or after treatment with antibiotics.

Vestibular lesions can be the result of nutritional disorders. Congenital vestibular disorders have been reported in dogs and cats and have been associated with the "screwneck syndrome" in pastel mink. This syndrome is characterized by a reduction in the number or by the absence of otoliths and can be prevented by a dietary supplement of manganese. Vitamin A deficiency in guinea pigs results in progressive metaplastic changes in the macular epithelium and loss of hair cells.

References

The Eye or Ear: General Review

Gelatt KN, ed. Veterinary Ophthalmology. 3rd ed. Baltimore: Lippincott Williams & Wilkins, 1999.

Hockwin O, Green K, Rubin LF, eds. Manual of Oculotoxicity Testing of Drugs. New York: Gustav Fischer Verlag, 1992.

Jones TC, Hunt RD, King NW. Organ of special sense. In: Jones TC, Hunt RD, King NW, eds. Veterinary Pathology, 6th ed. Baltimore: Williams & Wilkins, 1996:1299-1329.

Jones TC, Mohr U, Hunt RD, eds. Eye and Ear, Monographs on Pathology of Laboratory Animals, International Life Science Institute. New York: Springer-Verlag, 1991.

McKeever PJ, Torres SMF. Ear disease and its management. Vet Clin North Am Small Anim Pract 1997; 27:1523-1536.

Prince JH, Diesem CD, Eglitis L, Ruskell GL. Anatomy and Histology of the Eye and Orbit in Domestic Animals. Springfield, Ill.: Charles C Thomas, 1960:13.

Sanders LZ, Rubin LF. Ophthalmic Pathology of Animals. Basel: Karger, 1975:158-176.

Wilcock BP. The eye and ear. In: Jubb KVF, Kennedy PC, Palmer N, eds. Pathology of Domestic Animals. Vol 1, 4th ed. New York: Academic, 1993:441-530.

Ocular Embryology and Anomalies

American College of Veterinary Ophthalmologists. Ocular Disorders Proven or Suspected to Be Hereditary in Dogs. CERF (ACVO Book). West Lafayette, Ind.: Purdue University, 1992.

Boevé MH, Stades FC, van der Linde-Sipman JS, Vrensen GFJM. Persistent hyperplastic tunica vasculosa lentis and primary vitreous (PHTVL/PHPV) in the dog: A comparative review. Prog Vet Comp Ophthalmol 1992; 2:163-172.

Brown TT, Bistner SL, DeLahunta A, Scott FW, McEntee K. Pathogenetic studies of infection of the bovine fetus with bovine viral diarrhea virus. II. Ocular lesions. Vet Pathol 1975; 12:394-404.

Cook CS. Microphthalmia and anophthalmia, mouse and rat. In: Jones TC, Mohr U, Hunt RD, eds. Monographs on Pathology of Laboratory Animals, Eye and Ear. Heidelberg: Springer-Verlag, 1991:125-132.

Leipold HW, Huston K. Congenital syndrome of anophthalmia microphthalmia with associated defects in cattle. Pathol Vet 1968; 5:407-418.

Martin CL, Stiler J, Willis M. Feline colobomatous syndrome. Vet Comp Ophthalmol 1997; 7:39-43.

Peiffer RL, Fischer CA. Microphthalmia, retinal dysplasia, and anterior segment dysgenesis in a litter of Doberman pinschers. J Am Vet Med Assoc 1993; 183:857-878.

Peters M. Dipsosopia with triophthalmia in a newborn kitten. Kleintierpraxis 1998; 43:609-615.

Roberts SR. Color dilution and hereditary defects in collie dogs. Am J Ophthalmol 1967; 63:1762-1775.

Roberts SR, Bistner SI. Persistent pupillary membrane in Basenji dogs. J Am Vet Med Assoc 1968; 153:533-542.

Rubin LF, Nelson EJ, Sharp CA. Collie eye anomaly in Australian shepherd dog. Prog Vet Comp Ophthalmol 1991; 1:109-118.

Van der Linde-Sipman JS, Stades FC, de Wolff-Rouenduall D. Persistent hyperplastic tunica vasculosa lentis and persistent hyperplastic primary vitreous in the Doberman pinscher: Pathological aspects. J Am Anim Hosp Assoc 1983; 19:791-802.

Eyelids, Sclera, Episclera, and Orbit

Carpenter JL, Schmidt GM, Moore FM, Albert DM, Abrams KL, Elner VM. Canine bilateral extraocular polymyositis. Vet Pathol 1989; 26:510-512.

Deykin AR, Guandalini A, Ratto A. A retrospective histopathologic study of primary episcleral and scleral inflammatory disease in dogs. Vet Comp Ophthalmol 1997; 7:245-248.

Gilger BC, McLaughlin SA, Whitely RD, Wright J. Orbital neoplasms in cats: 21 cases (1974-1990). J Am Vet Med Assoc 1992; 201:1083-1091.

Goodhead AD, Venter IJ, Nesbit JW. Retrobulbar extra-adrenal paraganglioma in a horse and its surgical removal by orbitotomy. Vet Comp Ophthalmol 1997; 7:96-100.

Jones JC, Smith MM, Sponenberg DP, Smith EM. Orbital multibular tumor of bone in a basset hound. Vet Comp Ophthalmol 1997; 7:111-116.

Kern TJ. Orbital neoplasia in 23 dogs. J Am Vet Med Assoc 1985; 186:489-491.

Ratto A, Peiffer JR. RL, Peruccio C, Rossi L. Zygomatic salivary gland adenocarcinoma in a dog. Prog Vet Comp Ophthalmol 1991; 1:59 62.

Schmidt GM, Betts CW. Zygomatic salivary mucoceles in the dog. J Am Vet Med Assoc 1978; 171:940-942.

Schmidt GM, Krehbiel JD, Coley SC, Leid RW. Equine ocular onchocerciasis: Histopathologic study. Am J Vet Res 1982; 43:1371-1375.

Walde J, Hittmair K, Henninger W, Czedik-Eysenberg T. Retrobulbar dermoid cyst in a Dachshund. Vet Comp Ophthalmol 1997; 7:239-244.

Cornea, Conjunctiva, Lacrimal Apparatus, and Nictitating Membrane

Aguirre GD, Carmichael L, Bistner S. Corneal endothelium in viral induced anterior uveitis. Utrastructural changes following canine adenovirus type-1 infection. Arch Ophthalmol 1975; 93:219-224.

Aguirre GD, Laties A. Pigment epithelial dystrophy in the dog. Exp Eye Res 1976; 23:247-256.

Boscos CM, Ververidis HN, Tondis DK, Stamou AI, Samartzi FC. Ocular involvement of transmissible venereal tumor in a dog. Vet Ophthalmol 1998; 1:167-170.

Brightman AH. Keratoconjunctivitis sicca. J Am Vet Med Assoc 1980; 176:710-711.

Collins BK, Collier LL, Miller LA, Canton LL. Biologic behavior and histologic characteristics of canine conjunctival melanoma. Prog Vet Comp Ophthalmol 1993; 3:135-140.

Cook CS, Rosenkrantz W, Peiffer RL, MacMillan, A. Malignant melanoma of the conjunctiva in a cat. J Am Vet Med Assoc 1985; 186:505-506.

Elad D, Yeruham I, Bernstein M. Moraxella ovis in cases of infectious bovine keratoconjunctivitis (IBK) in Israel. J Vet Med 1998; 35:431-434.

Gelatt KN, Peiffer RL, Stevens J. Chronic ulcerative keratitis and sequestrum in the domestic cat. J Am Anim Hosp Assoc 1973; 9:204-213.

Gelatt KN, Samuelson DA. Recurrent corneal erosions and epithelial dystrophy in the boxer dog. J Am Anim Hosp Assoc 1982; 18:453-460.

Grahn B, Wolfer J, Keller C, Wilcock B. Equine keratomycosis: Clinical and laboratory findings in 23 cases. Prog Vet Comp Ophthalmol 1993; 3:2-8.

Hamor RE, Ramsey DT, Wiedmeyer CE, Gerding Jr. PA, Knight B, Whileley HE. Melanoma of the conjunctiva and cornea in a horse. Vet Comp Ophthalmol 1997; 7:52-55.

Hendrix DVH, Chmielewski NJ, Smith PJ, Brooks DE, Gelatt KN, Whittaker C. Keratomycosis in four horses caused by *Cylindrocarpon destructans*. Vet Comp Ophthalmol 1996; 6:252-257.

Hendrix DVH, Ward DA, Ouglick MA. Disseminated candidiasis in a neonatal foal with keratomycosis as the initial sign. Vet Comp Ophthalmol 1997; 7:10-13.

Keil SM, Olevero DK, McKeever PJ, Moore FM. Bilateral nodular eosinophilic granulomatous inflammation of the nictitating membrane of a cat. Vet Comp Ophthalmol 1997; 7:258-262.

Kerlin RL, Dubielzig RR. Lipogranulomatous conjunctivitis in cats. Vet Comp Ophthalmol 1997; 7:177-179.

Komaromy AM, Ramsey DT, Render JA, Clark P. Primary adenocarcinoma of the gland of the nictitating membrane in a cat. J Am Anim Hosp Assoc 1997; 33:333-336.

Martin CL. Canine epibulbar melanomas and their management. J Am Anim Hosp Assoc 1981; 17:83-90.

Martin CL. Conjunctivitis: Differential diagnosis and treatment. Vet Clin North Am 1973; 3:367-383.

Martin CL, Dice PF. Corneal endothelial dystrophy in the dog. J Am Anim Hosp Assoc 1982; 18:327-336.

Monlux AW, Anderson WA, Davis CL. The diagnosis of squamous cell carcinoma of the eye (cancer eye) in cattle. Am J Vet Res 1957; 18:5-33.

Morgan RV, Abrams KL, Kern TJ. Feline eosinophilic keratitis: A retrospective study of 54 cases (1989-1994). Vet Comp Ophthalmol 6:131-134.

Mughannam AJ, Hacker DV, Spangler WL. Conjunctival vascular tumors in six dogs. Vet Comp Ophthalmol 1997; 7:56-59.

Nasisse MP, Weigler BJ. The diagnosis of ocular feline herpesvirus infection. Vet Comp Ophthalmol 1997; 7:44-51.

Prasse KW, Winston SM. Cytology and histopathology of feline eosinophilic keratitis. Vet Comp Ophthalmol 6:74-81.

Ramsey DT, Ketring KL, Glaze MB, Knight B, Render JA. Ligneous conjunctivitis in four Doberman pinschers. J Am Anim Hosp Assoc 1996; 32:1-9.

Read RA, Dunn KA, Smith KC, Barnett KC. A histological study of nictitans glands from dogs with tear overflow of unknown cause. Vet Comp Ophthalmol 1996; 6:195-204.

Slatter DH, Lavach JD, Severin GA, Young S. Ubereiter's syndrome (chronic superficial keratitis) in dogs in the Rocky Mountain area: A study of 463 cases. J Small Anim Pract 1977; 18:757-772.

Wilcock BP, Peiffer RL. Adenocarcinoma of the gland of the third eyelid in seven dogs. J Am Vet Med Assoc 1988; 193:1549-1550.

Lens

Gelatt KN, Das ND. Animal models for inherited cataracts: A review. Curr Eye Res 1984; 3:765-778.

Gerardi JG, Colitz CMH, Dubielzig RR, Davidson MG. Immunohistochemical analysis of lens-epithelial-derived membranes following cataract extraction in the dog. Vet Ophthalmol 1999; 2:163-168.

Stiles J. Cataracts in a kitten with nutritional secondary hyperparathyroidism. Prog Vet Comp Ophthalmol 1991; 1:296-298.

Stiles J, Didier E, Ritchie B, Greenacre C, Willis M, Martin C. *Encephalitozoon cuniculi* in the lens of a rabbit with phagoclastic uveitis: Confirmation and treatment. Vet Comp Ophthalmol 1997; 7:233-238.

Taylor VL, Peiffer RL, Costello MJ. Ultrastructural analysis of normal and diabetic cataractous canine lenses. Vet Comp Ophthalmol 1997; 7:117-125.

Vitreous Body, Retina, and Optic Nerve

Adcock JL, Hibter CP. Vascular and neuroophthalmic pathology of elaeophorosis in elk. Pathol Vet 1969; 6:185-213.

Aguirre G. Hereditary retinal diseases in small animals. Vet Clin North Am 1973; 3:515-528.

Andrews SE, Abrams KL, Brooks DE, Kubilis PS. Clinical features of steroid responsive retinal detachments in twenty-two dogs. Vet Comp Ophthalmol 1997; 7:82-87.

Carlton WW, Feeney DA, Zimmerman JL. Disseminated cryptococcosis with ocular involvement in a dog. J Am Anim Hosp Assoc 1976; 12:53-59.

Chader GJ. Animal mutants of hereditary retinal degeneration. General considerations and studies on defects in cyclic nucleotide metabolism. Prog Vet Comp Ophthalmol 1991; 1:109-126.

Hayes KC, Nielsen SW, Eaton HD. Pathogenesis of the optic nerve lesion in vitamin A–deficient calves. Arch Ophthalmol 1968; 80:777-781.

Hogan RN, Albert DM. Does retinoblastoma occur in animals? Prog Vet Comp Ophthalmol 1991; 1:73-82.

Jubb KV, Saunders LZ, Coates HV. The intraocular lesions of canine distemper. J Comp Pathol 1957: 61:21-29.

Lanum J. The damaging effects of light on the retina. Empirical findings, theoretical and practical implications (review). Surv Ophthalmol 1978; 22:221-249.

Patz A, Maumenee AK. Studies on diabetic retinopathy. 1. Retinopathy in a dog with spontaneous diabetes mellitus. Am J Ophthalmol 1962; 54:532-541.

Rubin LF, Saunders LZ. Intraocular larva migrans in dogs. Pathol Vet 1965; 2:566-573.

Schmidt SY, Berson EL, Hayes KC. Retinal degeneration in cats fed casein. 1. Taurine deficiency. Invest Ophthalmol 1976; 15:47-52.

Smith RIE, Sutton RH, Jolly RD, Smith KR. A retinal degeneration associated with ceroid-lipofuscinosis in adult miniature Schnauzers. Vet Comp Ophthalmol 1996; 6:187-191.

Syed NA, Nork MN, Poulsen GL, Riis RC, George C, Albert DM. Retinoblastoma in a dog. Arch Ophthalmol 1997; 115:758-763.

Van der Lugt JJ, Oliver J, Jordaan P. Status spongiosis, optic neuropathy, and retinal degeneration in *Helichrysum argyrospaerum* poisoning in sheep and a goat. Vet Pathol 1996; 33:495-502.

Vestre WA, Turner TA, Carlton WW. Proliferative optic neuropathy in a horse. J Am Vet Med Assoc 1982; 181:490-491.

Watson WA, Terlecki S, Patterson DSP, Sweasey D, Herbert CN, Done JT. Experimentally produced progressive retinal degeneration (bright blindness) in sheep. Br Vet J 1972; 128:457-469.

Uvea and Ocular Inflammation

Bussanich MN, Rootman J, Dolman CL. Granulomatous panuveitis and dermal depigmentation in dogs. J Am Anim Hosp Assoc 1982; 18:131-138.

Carlton WW. A case of blastomycosis in a dog with pulmonary, cutaneous and ocular lesions. J Am Anim Hosp Assoc 1974: 10:586-590.

Carlton WW, Austin L. Ocular protothecosis in a dog. Pathol Vet 1973; 10:074-280.

Collier LL, Prieur DJ, King EJ. Ocular melanin pigmentation anomalies in cats, cattle, mink and mice with Chediak-Higashi syndrome: Histologic observations. Curr Eye Res 1984; 3:1241-1251.

Davidson MG, English RV. Feline ocular toxoplasmosis. Vet Ophthalmol 1998; 1:71-80.

Dubielzig RR, Render JA, Morreale RJ. Distinctive morphologic features of the ciliary body in equine recurrent uveitis. Vet Comp Ophthalmol 1997; 7:163-167.

Dukes TW. The ocular lesions in thromboembolic meningoencephalitis (TEME) of cattle. Can Vet J 1971; 2:180-182.

English RV. Regulation of intraocular immune responses. Prog Vet Comp Ophthalmol 1992; 2:41-49.

Halliwell RE, Brim TA, Hines MJ, Wolf D, White FH. Studies on equine recurrent uveitis. II: The role of infection with *Leptospiru interrogans* serovar *pomona*. Curr Eye Res 1985; 4:1033-1040.

Hendrix DV, Nassise MP, Cowen P, Davidson MG. Clinical signs, concurrent diseases, and risk factors associated with retinal detachment in dogs. Prog Vet Comp Ophthalmol 1993; 3:87-91.

Herrera HD, Duchene AG. Uveodermatological syndrome (Vogt-Koyanagi-Harada–like syndrome) with generalized depigmentation in a Dachshund. Vet Ophthalmol 1998; 1:47-51.

Millichamp NJ, Dziezyc J. Mediators of ocular inflammation. Prog Vet Comp Ophthalmol 1991; 1:41-58.

Murray JA, Blakemore WF, Barnett KC. Ocular lesions in cats with GM1-gangliosidosis with visceral involvement. J Small Anim Pract 1977; 18:1-10.

Peiffer RL, Belkin PV. Ocular manifestations of disseminated histoplasmosis in a cat. J Fel Pract 1979; 9:24-29.

Peiffer RL, Wilcock BP. Histopathologic study of uveitis in cats: 137 cases (1978-1990). J Am Vet Med Assoc 1991; 198:135-138.

Percy DH. Feline histoplasmosis with ocular involvement. Vet Pathol 1981; 18:163-169.

Romeike A, Brugmann M, Drommer W. Immunohistochemical studies in equine recurrent uveitis. Vet Pathol 1998; 35:515-526.

Rosenthal JJ, Herdgerd T, Peiffer RL. Ocular and systemic cryptococcosis in a cat. J Am Anim Hosp Assoc 1981; 17:307-310.

Rubin LF, Sanders LZ. Intraocular larval migrans in dogs. Pathol Vet 1965; 2:566-572.

Schultze AE, Ring RD, Morgan RV, Patton CS. Clinical, cytologic and histopathologic manifestations of protothecosis in two dogs. Vet Ophthalmol 1998; 1:239-243.

Shively JN, Whiteman C. Ocular lesions in disseminated coccidioidomycosis. Pathol Vet 1970; 7:1-6.

Silverstein AM. Immunogenic uveitis. Trans Ophthalmol Soc UK 1974; 94:496-517.

Spiess BM, Bollinger JO, Ouseetti F, Haessig M, Lackner PA, Ruehli MG. Multiple ciliary body cysts and secondary glaucoma in the Great Dane: A report of nine cases. Vet Ophthalmol 1998; 1:41-45.

Syed NA, Nork TM, Poulsen GL, Riis RC, George C, Albert DM. Retinoblastoma in a dog. Arch Ophthalmol 1997; 115:758-763.

Trevino GS. Canine blastomycosis with ocular involvement. Pathol Vet 1966; 3:652-658.

Van der Woerdt A, Nasisse MP, Davidson MG. Sudden acquired retinal degeneration in the dog: Clinical and laboratory findings in 36 cases. Prog Vet Comp Ophthalmol 1991; 2:11-18.

Whiteley HE, Young S, Liggitt HD, DeMartini JC. Ocular lesions of bovine malignant catarrhal fever. Vet Pathol 1985; 22:219-225.

Wilcock BP, Peiffer RL. The pathology of lens induced uveitis in dogs. Vet Pathol 1987; 24:549-553.

Intraocular Neoplasia

Bjerkas E, Arnesen K, Peiffer Jr. RL. Diffuse amelanotic iris melanoma. Vet Comp Ophthalmol 1977; 7:190-191.

Brooks DE, Patton CS. An ocular ganglioneuroblastoma in a dog. Prog Vet Comp Ophthalmol 1991; 1:299-302.

Cassotis NJ, Dubielzig RR, Gilger BC, Davidson MG. Angioinvasive pulmonary carcinoma with posterior segment metastasis in four cats. Vet Ophthalmol 1999; 2:125-131.

Collinson PN, Peiffer Jr RL. Clinical presentation, morphology and behavior of primary choroidal melanomas in eight dogs. Prog Vet Comp Ophthalmol 1993; 3:158-164.

Corcoran KP, Peiffer RL, Koch DA. Histopathologic features of feline ocular lymphosarcoma in 49 cats. (1978-1992). Vet Comp Ophthalmol 1995; 5:35-41.

Davidson HJ, Blanchard GL, Wheeler CA, Render JA. Anterior uveal melanoma with secondary keratitis and glaucoma in a horse. J Am Vet Med Assoc 1991; 199:1049-1050.

Dubielzig RR. Ocular sarcoma following trauma in three cats. J Am Vet Med Assoc 1984; 184:578-581.

Dubielzig RR, Aquirre GD, Gross SL, Diters RW. Choroidal melanomas in dogs. Vet Pathol 1985; 22:582-587.

Dubielzig RR, Hawkins KL, Toy KA, Rosebury WS, Mazur M, Jasper TG. Morphologic features of feline ocular sarcomas in 10 cats: Light microscopy, ultrastructure, and immunohistochemistry. Prog Vet Comp Ophthalmol 1994; 4:7-12.

Dubielzig RR, Steinberg H, Garvin H, Deehr AJ, Fischer B. Iridociliary epithelial tumors in 100 dogs and 17 cats: A morphologic study. Vet Ophthalmol 1998; 1:223-231.

Duncan DE, Peiffer RL. Morphology and behavior of anterior uveal melanomas in cats. Prog Vet Comp Ophthalmol 1991; 12:25-32.

Duncan DE, Peiffer RL. Morphology and prognostic indicators of anterior uveal melanomas in cats. Prog Vet Comp Ophthalmol 1991; 1:25-32.

Eagle RC, Font RL, Swerezek TW. Malignant medulloepithelioma of the optic nerve in a horse. Vet Pathol 1978; 15:488-494.

Fulton LM, Bromberg NM, Goldschmidt MH. Soft tissue fibrosarcoma with intraocular metastasis in a cat. Prog Vet Comp Ophthalmol 1991; 1:129-132.

Giuliano EA, Chappell R, Fischer B, Dubielzig RR. A matched observational study of canine survival with primary intraocular melanocytic neoplasia. Vet Ophthalmol 1999; 2:185-190.

Harris BP, Dubielzig RR. Atypical primary ocular melanoma in cats. Vet Ophthalmol 1999; 2:121-124.

Kalishman JB, Chappell R, Flood LA, Dubielzig RR. A matched observational study of survival in cats with enucleation due to diffuse iris melanoma. Vet Ophthalmol 1998; 1:25-29.

Krohne SG, Henderson NM, Richardson RC, Vestre WA. Prevalence of ocular involvement in dogs with multicentric lymphoma. Prospective evaluation of 94 cases. Vet Comp Ophthalmol 1994; 4:127-135.

Langloss JM, Zimmerman LE, Krehbiel JD. Malignant intraocular teratoid medulloepithelioma in three dogs. Vet Pathol 1976; 13:343-352.

Mohr U, ed. International Classification of Rodent Tumors, part I—the rat, 7. Central Nervous System; Heart, Eye; Mesothelium. Lyon, France: World Health Organization, International Agency for Research on Cancer, 1994.

Nell B, Suchy A. 'D-shaped' and 'reverse-D-shaped' pupil in a cat with lymphosarcoma. Vet Ophthalmol 1998; 1:53-56.

Peiffer RL. Ciliary body epithelial tumors in the dog and cat: A report of 13 cases. J Small Clin Pract 1983; 24:347-370.

Render JA, Ramsey DT, Ramsey CC. Contralateral uveal metastasis of malignant anterior uveal melanoma in a dog. Vet Comp Ophthalmol 1997; 7:263-266.

Ryan AM, Diters RW. Clinical and pathologic features of canine ocular melanomas. J Am Vet Med Assoc 1984; 184:60-67.

Saunders LZ, Barron CN. Intraocular tumors in animals. IV. Lymphosarcoma. Br Vet J 1964; 126:25-35.

Wilcock BP, Peiffer RL. Morphology and behavior of primary ocular melanomas in 91 dogs. Vet Pathol 1986; 23:418-424.

Glaucoma

Deehr AJ, Dubielzig RR. A histopathological study of iridociliary cysts and glaucoma in Golden Retrievers. Vet Ophthalmol 1998; 1:153-158.

Halenda RM, Grahn GH, Sorden SD, Collier LL. Congenital equine glaucoma: Clinical and light microscopic findings in two cases. Vet Comp Ophthalmol 1997; 7:105-109.

Martin CL, Wyman M. Primary glaucoma in the dog. Vet Clin North Am 1978; 8:257-286.

Peiffer RL, Wilcock BP, Yin H. Pathogenesis and significance of pre-iridal fibrovascular membranes in domestic animals. Vet Pathol 1990; 27:41-45.

Samuelson DA. A reevaluation of the comparative anatomy of the eutherian iridocorneal angle and associated ciliary body musculature. Vet Comp Ophthalmol 1996; 6:153-173.

Smith RIE, Peiffer Jr. RL, Wilcock BP. Some aspects of the pathology of canine glaucoma. Prog Vet Comp Ophthalmol 1993; 3:16-28.

Wilcock BP, Peiffer RL, Davidson M. The causes of glaucoma in cats. Vet Pathol 1990; 27:35-40.

Storage Diseases

Aguirre G, Stramm L, Haskins M, Jezyk P. Animal models of metabolic eye disease. In: Goldberg MF, ed. Genetic and Metabolic Eye Disease. Boston: Little, Brown, 1986:139-167.

Haskins ME, Desnick RJ, DiFerrante N, Jezyk P, Patterson DF. Beta-glucoronidase deficiency in a dog: A model of human mucopolysaccharidosis. VII. Pediatr Res 1984; 18:980-984.

Jolly RD, Palmer DN, Studdert VP, Sutton RH, Kelly WR, Koppung N, Dahme G, Hartley WJ, Patterson JS, Riis RC. Canine ceroid-lipofuscinoses: A review and classification. J Small Anim Pract 1994; 35:299-306.

Keller CB, Lamarre J. Inherited lysosomal storage disease in an English Springer Spaniel. J Am Vet Med Assoc 1992; 200:194-195.

Render JA, Lovell KL, Jones MZ, Wheeler CA. Ocular pathology of caprine beta-mannosidosis. Vet Pathol 1989; 26:444-446.

Shull RM, Munger RJ, Spellacy E, Hall CW, Constantopoulos G, Neufeld E. Canine alpha-L-iduronidase deficiency: A model of mucopolysaccharidosis. I. Am J Pathol 1982; 109:244-248.

External Ear

Chiu T. Auricular chondriits. In: Jones TC, Mohr U, Hunt RD, eds. Monographs on Pathology of Laboratory Animals, Eye and Ear. Berlin: Springer-Verlag, 1991;149-155.

Chiu T, Lee KP. Auricular chondropathy in aging rats. Vet Pathol 1984; 21:500-504.

Griffin CE, Song MD. Management of otitis externa. Advances in Veterinary Dermatology. Vol 3. Proceedings of the Third World Congress of Veterinary Dermatology, Edinburgh, Schotland, Sept. 11-14, 1996. Oxford, United Kingdom: Butterworth-Heinemann Ltd, 1998:369-375.

Kirpensteijn F. Aural neoplasms. Semin Vet Med Surg (Small Anim) 1993; 8:13-17.

Legendre A, Krahwinkel DJ. Feline ear tumors. J Am Anim Hosp Assoc 1981; 17:1035-1037.

McKeever PJ, Torres S. Otitis externa, part 1: The ear and predisposing factors to otitis exerna. Companion Anim Pract 1988; 2:7-14.

Mansfield PD, Boosinger TR, Attleberger MH. Infectivity of *Malassezia pachydermatis* in the exteral ear canal of dogs. J Am Anim Hosp Assoc 1990; 26:97-100.

Marino DJ, MacDonald JM, Matthiesen DT, Patnaik DT, et al. Results of surgery and long-term follow-ups in dogs with ceruminous gland adenocarcinoma. J Am Anim Hosp Assoc 1993; 29:560-563.

Moisan PG, Watson GL. Ceruminous gland tumors in dogs and cats: A review of 124 cases. J Am Anim Hosp Assoc 1996; 32:448-452.

Powell MG, Weisbroth SH, Roth D, et al. Reaginic hypersensitivity in *Otodectes cynotis* infestation of cats and mode of feeding. Am J Vet Res 1980; 41:877-882.

Rogers KS. Tumors of the ear canal. Vet Clin North Am Small Animal Pract 1988; 18:859-868.

Rosser EJ. Diagnosis of food allergy in dogs. J Am Vet Med Assoc 1993; 203:259-262.

Scott DW. Observations on canine atopy. J Am Anim Hosp Assoc 1981; 17:91-100.

Shell LG. Otitis media and otitis interna. Etiology, diagnosis; and medical management. Vet Clin North Am Small Anim Pract 1988; 18:885-889.

Smeak DD, Dettoff WD. Total ear canal ablation: Clinical results in the dog and cat. Vet Surg 1986; 15:161-170.

Vail DM, Withrow SJ. Tumors of the skin and subcutaneous tissues. In: Withrow SJ, MacEwen EG, eds. Small Animal Clinical Oncology. Philadelphia: W.B. Saunders, 1996:185-186.

Willemse A, van den Brom WE. Investigations of the symptomatology and the significance of immediate skin test reactivity in canine atopic dermatitis. Res Vet Sci 1983; 34:261-265.

Middle Ear

Bacmeister C. Dyspnea in a cat with otitis. Feline Pract 1991; 19:508.

Bentz BG, Ross MW. Otitis media/interna in horses. Compend Contin Educ Pract Vet 1997; 19:524-534.

Cooley AJ, Fox LE, Duncan ID, England DM. Malignant jugulotympanic paraganglioma in a dog. J Comp Pathol 1990; 102:375-383.

Cox CL, Payne-Johnson CE. Aural cholesterol granuloma in a dog. J Small Anim Pract 1995; 36:25-28.

Evans HE. The middle ear. In: Evans HE, ed. Miller's Anatomy of the Dog. 3rd ed. Philadelphia: WB Saunders, 1993:994-999.

Fingland RB, Gratzek A, Vohries MW, Kirpensteijn J. Nasopharyngeal polypin in a dog. J Am Anim Hosp Assoc 1993; 29:311-314.

Hottendorf GH. Cholesteatoma, aural, gerbil. In: Jones TC, Mohr U, Hunt RD, eds. Eye, Ear, Monographs on Pathology of Laboratory Animals. Berlin: Springer-Verlag, 1991:156-158.

Kapatkin AS, Matthiesen DT, Noone KE, Church EM, Seavelli TG, Patnaik AK. Results of surgery and long-term follow-up in 31 cats with nasopharyngeal polyps. J Am Anim Hosp Assoc 1990; 26: 387-392.

Lim DJ. Functional morphology of the mucosa of the middle ear and eustachian tube. Ann Otol Rhinol Laryngol 1976; 85(Suppl 25, Pt 2):245-249.

Little CJL. Inflammatory middle ear disease of the dog. The pathology of otitis media. Vet Rec 1999; 128:293.

Little CJL. Inflammatory middle ear disease of the dog: the Clinical and pathological features of cholesteatoma, a complication of otitis media. Vet Rec 1991; 128:319-322.

Little CJL, Pearson GR, Lane JG. Neoplasia involving the middle ear cavity of dogs. Vet Rec 1989; 124:54-57.

Neer TM, Howard PE. Otitis media. Comp Cont Educ 1982; 4:4-10.

Parker NR, Binnington AG. Nasopharyngeal polyps in cats: Three case reports and a review of the literature. J Am Anim Hosp Assoc 1985; 21:473-478.

Rose WR. Otitis media. Vet Med Small Anim Clin 1976; 71:1443.

Simpson D. Atresia of the external acoustic meatus in a dog. Aust Vet J 1997; 75:18-20.

Walz PH, Mullaney TP, Render JA, Walker RD, Baker JC. Otitis media in pre-weaned Holstein dairy calves in Michigan due to *Mycoplasma bovis*. J Vet Diagn Invest 1997; 9:250-254.

Inner Ear

Branis M, Burda H. Inner ear structures in the deaf and normally hearing dalmation dog. J Comp Pathol 1985; 95:295-299.

Burke EE, Moise NS, deLahunta A, Erb HN. Review of idiopathic feline vestibular syndrome in 75 cats. J Am Vet Med Assoc 1985; 187:941-943.

Delack JB. Hereditary deafness in the white cat. Compend Cont Educ Pract Vet 1984; 6:609-619.

Knowles K, Blauch B, Leipold H, Cash W, Hewett J. Reduction of spiral ganglion neurons in the aging canine with hearing loss. J Vet Med 1989; 36:188-199.

Powers HT, Watrous BJ, de Lahunta A. Facial and vestibulocochlear nerve disease in six horses. J Am Vet Med Assoc 1983; 183:1076-1080.

Saunders LZ. The histopathology of hereditary congenital deafness in white mink. Pathol Vet 1965; 2:256-263.

Schunk KL, Averill DR. Peripheral vestibular syndrome in the dog: A review of 83 cases. J Am Vet Med Assoc 1983; 182:1354-1357.

Strain GM. Congenital deafness in dogs and cats. Compend Contin Educ Pract Vet 1991; 13:245-254.

Index

E

I

S